TENDON AND NERVE SURGERY IN THE HAND

A Third Decade

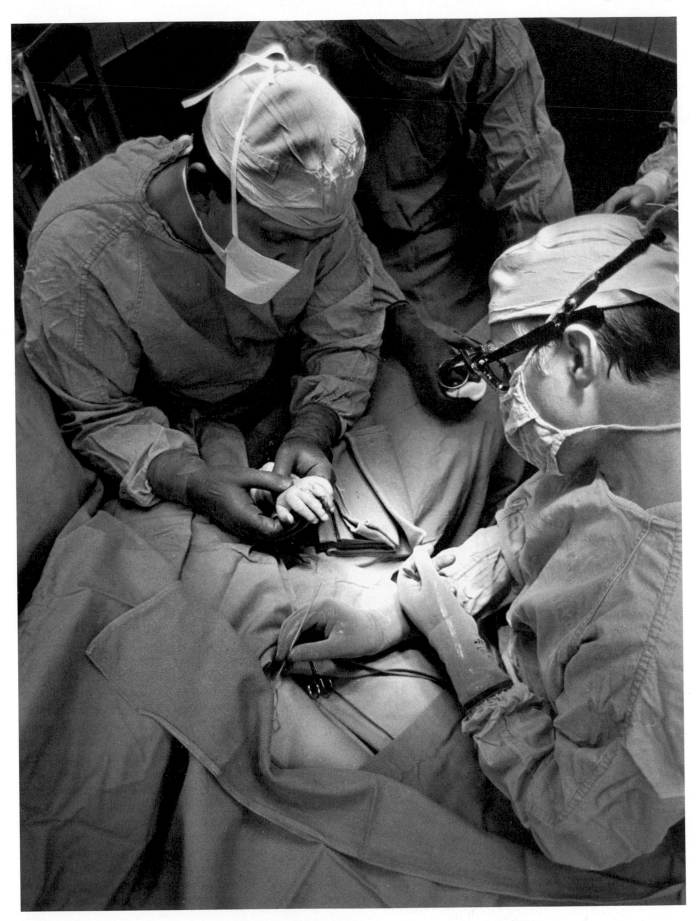

Dr. William Littler at the Roosevelt Hospital in New York City, circa 1970.

TENDON AND NERVE SURGERY IN THE HAND

A Third Decade

James M. Hunter, M.D.

Distinguished Professor of Orthopaedic Surgery
Former Director, Division of Hand Surgery
Jefferson Medical College of Thomas Jefferson University
Philadelphia, Pennsylvania

Lawrence H. Schneider, M.D.

Clinical Professor
Department of Orthopaedic Surgery
Director, Division of Hand Surgery
Jefferson Medical College of the Thomas Jefferson University
The Philadelphia Hand Center, P.C.
Philadelphia, Pennsylvania

Evelyn J. Mackin, P.T.

Executive Director
Hand Rehabilitation Foundation
Former Director of Hand Therapy
The Philadelphia Hand Center, P.C.
Philadelphia, Pennsylvania

with 804 illustrations including 10 in color

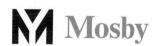

St. Louis Baltimore Boston Carlsbad Chicago Naples New York Philadelphia Portland
London Madrid Mexico City Singapore Sydney Tokyo Toronto Wiesbaden

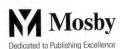

Mosby
Dedicated to Publishing Excellence

A Times Mirror
Company

Vice President and Publisher: Anne S. Patterson
Senior Managing Editor: Kathryn H. Falk
Developmental Editor: Carolyn M. Kruse
Project Manager: Linda Clarke
Production Editor: Jennifer Harper
Production: Graphic World Publishing Services
Designer: Carolyn O'Brien
Manufacturing Manager: William A. Winneberger, Jr.

Printed in the United States of America
Composition by Graphic World, Inc.
Printing/binding by Maple-Vail Book Manufacturing Group

Mosby–Year Book, Inc.
11830 Westline Industrial Drive
St. Louis, Missouri 63146

Library of Congress Cataloging-in-Publication Data

Tendon and nerve surgery in the hand : a third decade / [edited by]
    James M. Hunter, Lawrence H. Schneider, Evelyn J. Mackin.
        p.   cm.
        Proceedings of a conference held in 1994 in Philadelphia, Pa.
        Includes bibliographical references and index.
        ISBN 0-8151-4740-6
        1. Hand–Wounds and injuries–Surgery–Congresses.   2. Tendons–
    Surgery–Congresses.   3. Nerves, Peripheral–Surgery–Congresses.
    4. Hand–Innervation–Congresses.   I. Hunter, James M. (James
    Megargee), 1924- .   II. Schneider, Lawrence H.   III. Mackin,
    Evelyn.
        [DNLM: 1. Hand Injuries–surgery–congresses.   2. Hand–surgery–
    congresses.   3. Tendon Injuries–surgery–congresses.
    4. Peripheral Nerves–surgery–congresses.   WE 830 T2903 1996]
    RD559.T444   1997
    617.5′75059–dc20
    DNLM/DLC
    for Library of Congress   96-36163
                                                                       CIP

97 98 99 00 01 / 9 8 7 6 5 4 3 2 1

CONTRIBUTORS

Sven-Olof Abrahamsson, M.D., Ph.D.
University of Lund
Department of Hand Surgery
University Hospital in Malmo
Malmo Allmanna Sjukhus
Malmo, Sweden
Chapter 35

Yves Allieu, M.D.
Chef de Service, Centre Hospitalier Universitaire
    de Montpellier
Chirurgie Orthopedique et Traumatologique II
Chirurgie de la main et du membre Superier
Montpellier, France
Chapters 49, 63

Peter C. Amadio, M.D.
Professor, Department of Orthopaedic Surgery
Mayo Clinic and Mayo Foundation
Rochester, Minnesota
Chapters 20, 31

Kai-Nan An, Ph.D.
John and Posy Krehbiel Professor of Orthopedics
Professor of Bioengineering
Orthopedic Biomechanics Laboratory
Mayo Clinic and Mayo Foundation
Rochester, Minnesota
Chapter 31

Wayne Bauerle, M.D.
The Philadelphia Hand Center, P.C.
Philadelphia, Pennsylvania
Chapter 37

John M. Bednar, M.D.
Assistant Professor of Orthopaedic Surgery
Jefferson Medical College of Thomas Jefferson University
The Philadelphia Hand Center, P.C.
Philadelphia, Pennsylvania
Chapter 38

Judith A. Bell-Krotoski, O.T.R., C.H.T., F.A.O.T.A.
CAPTAIN, United States Public Health Service
Chief, Hand and Occupational Therapy Department
Clinical Research Therapist
Rehabilitation Research Department
Gillis W. Long Hansen's Disease Center
Carville, Louisiana
Chapter 7

Vilmos Biró, M.D.
Debreceni Orvostudományi Egyetem
Traumatológiai Tanszék
Debrecen, Hungary
Chapter 54

F. William Bora, Jr., M.D.
Chief of Hand Surgery
Professor of Orthopaedic Surgery
Hospital of the University of Pennsylvania
Penn Hand Specialists
Philadelphia, Pennsylvania
Chapter 6

Joseph H. Boyes, M.D.†
Emeritus Clinical Professor of Surgery
University of Southern California
Los Angeles, California
Chapter 47

Paul W. Brand, M.D.
Clinical Professor, Emeritus
Department of Orthopaedics
University of Washington
Seattle, Washington
Chapters 9, 48

Paul W. Brown, M.D.
Clinical Professor of Orthopaedics and Rehabilitation
Clinical Professor of Plastic and Reconstructive Surgery
Yale University School of Medicine
Colonel (Retired), Medical Corps
United States Army
New Haven, Connecticut
Chapter 26

Giorgio A. Brunelli, M.D.
Professor and Chairman
Department of Orthopaedics
Brescia University Medical School
Brescia, Italy
Chapter 27

Giorgio R. Brunelli, M.D.
Director, Department of Clinical Orthopaedics
Facolta' di Medicina e Chirurgia
Brescia University Medical School
Brescia, Italy
Chapter 27

†Deceased.

v

Frank D. Burke, M.D., M.B., B.S., F.R.C.S.
Consultant Hand Surgeon
The Pulvertaft Hand Centre
The Derbyshire Royal Infirmary NHS Trust
London Road
Derby, United Kingdom
Chapter 18

Patricia M. Byron, M.A., O.T.R./L., C.H.T.
Director of Hand Therapy
The Philadelphia Hand Center, P.C.
Philadelphia, Pennsylvania
Chapters 16, 57

Giuseppe Caserta, M.D.
Istituto di Clinica Ortopedica
Modena, Italy
Chapter 53

M. Chammas, M.D.
Division of Orthopedic and Hand Surgery
Lapeyronie University Hospital
Montpellier, France
Chapter 49

J.H. Coert, M.D.
Department of Surgery and Traumatology
University Hospital, Leiden School of Medicine
Leiden, The Netherlands
Chapter 31

Judy C. Colditz, O.T.R./L., C.H.T., F.A.O.T.A.
Clinical Director
Hand and Orthopaedic Rehabilitation Associates
Raleigh, North Carolina
Chapter 25

William P. Cooney, M.D.
Division of Hand Surgery
Department of Orthopedic Surgery
Mayo Clinic
Rochester, Minnesota
Chapters 31, 32

Randall W. Culp, M.D.
Associate Professor of Orthopaedic Hand and Microsurgery
Jefferson Medical College of Thomas Jefferson University
The Philadelphia Hand Center, P.C.
Philadelphia, Pennsylvania
Chapters 39, 61

Joe Dias, M.D., F.R.C.S.E.
Consultant Orthopaedic and Hand Surgeon
Glenfield Hospital
Leicester, United Kingdom
Chapter 18

James R. Doyle, M.D.
Professor Emeritus
Department of Surgery
Division of Orthopaedics
John A. Burns School of Medicine
University of Hawaii
Honolulu, Hawaii
Adjunct Professor, Orthopaedic Surgery
University of California Medical School
San Diego, California
Chapter 30

Ronald Drozdenko, Ph.D.
Vice President, Research and Development
NeuroCommunication Research Laboratories, Inc.
Western Connecticut University
Danbury, Connecticut
Chapter 8

Marco Esposito, M.D.
Istituto di Clinica Ortopedica
Modena, Italy
Chapter 53

Roslyn B. Evans, B.S., O.T.R./L., C.H.T.
Director
Indian River Hand Rehabilitation
Vero Beach, Florida
Chapter 43

Elaine Ewing Fess, M.S., O.T.R., F.A.O.T.A., C.H.T.
Private Practice, Hand Research
Zionsville, Indiana
Chapter 12

Frank Fleming, M.D.
Plastic and Reconstructive Surgery
Seattle, Washington
Chapter 60

Guy Foucher, M.D.
Head of SOS Main
Strasbourgh, France
Chapter 52

Gary K. Frykman, M.D.
Clinical Professor
Department of Orthopaedic Surgery
Loma Linda University School of Medicine
Chief, Hand Surgery
Jerry L. Pettis Memorial Veterans Administration Medical
    Center
Loma Linda, California
Chapter 4

Richard H. Gelberman, M.D.
Professor and Chairman of Orthopaedic Surgery
Washington University
St. Louis, Missouri
Chapter 46

Eric R. George, M.D.
Hand Surgical Associates
Metairie, Louisiana
Chapter 22

Karan Gettle, M.B.A., O.T.R., C.H.T.
The Hand Rehabilitation Center of Indiana
Indianapolis, Indiana
Chapter 42

Carl Göran-Hagert, M.D., Ph.D.
Associate Professor
Chief Hand Surgeon, Hand Surgery Unit
Department of Orthopaedics
University Hospital
Lund, Sweden
Chapter 66

Richard M. Gray, M.D.
Matthews Orthopaedic Clinic
Tampa, Florida
Chapter 21

Maureen A. Hardy, P.T., M.S., C.H.T.
Hand Management Center
St. Dominic Hospital
Jackson, Mississippi
Chapter 23

James M. Hunter, M.D.
Distinguished Professor of Orthopaedic Surgery
Jefferson Medical College of Thomas Jefferson University
President, The Philadelphia Hand Center, P.C.
Department of Orthopaedics
Thomas Jefferson University Hospital
Philadelphia, Pennsylvania
Chapters 21, 33, 55, 57

François Iselin, M.D.
Chirurgien de l'hopital de Nanterre
Centre de Chirurgie de la Main Paris-Ouest
Paris, France
Chapter 62

Michael E. Jabaley, M.D.
Clinical Professor of Surgery (Plastic)
Clinical Professor of Orthopaedic Surgery
University of Mississippi
Jackson, Mississippi
Chapters 3, 11

Scott H. Jaeger, M.D.
National Medical Director
HealthSouth Rehabilitation Corporation
Birmingham, Alabama
Chapter 57

Michael E. Joyce, M.D.
Assistant Clinical Professor of Orthopaedic Surgery
University of Connecticut School of Medicine
Willimantic, Connecticut
Chapter 34

László Józsa, M.D.
Országos Traumatológiai Intézet
Budapest, Hungary
Chapter 54

Emanuel B. Kaplan, M.D., F.A.C.S.†
Former Associate Professor of Anatomy
College of Physicians
Columbia University
Former Chief of Hand Surgery
Hospital for Joint Diseases
Chapter 29

Mary C. Kasch, O.T.R., C.V.E., C.H.T., F.A.O.T.A.
Clinical Director
Hand Rehabilitation Center of Sacramento
Sacramento, California
Chapter 19

Michael W. Keith, M.D.
Professor of Orthopaedic and Biomedical Engineering
Case Western Reserve University
Cleveland Veterans Affairs Medical Center
MetroHealth Medical Center
Cleveland, Ohio
Chapter 28

Harold E. Kleinert, M.D.
Clinical Professor of Surgery
University of Louisville School of Medicine
Louisville, Kentucky
Clinical Professor of Surgery
Indiana University/Purdue University School of Medicine
Indianapolis, Indiana
Chapter 36

Raymond J. Kobus, M.D.
Hand and Microsurgery Associates
Clinical Instructor in Orthopaedics
The Ohio State University Hospitals
Riverside Methodist Hospital
Columbus, Ohio
Chapter 57

Sung Tack Kwon, M.D.
Department of Plastic Surgery
Seoul National University Hospital
Chongno-Gu, Seoul
Korea
Chapter 50

Antonio Landi, M.D.
Facolta' di Medicina e Chirurgia
Istituto di Clinica Ortopedica
Modena, Italy
Chapter 53

†Deceased.

J. William Littler, M.D.
Professor Emeritus of Clinical Surgery
Columbia University
Past Director, Hand Surgical Service
Roosevelt Hospital
New York, New York

Jueren Lou, M.D.
Department of Orthopaedic Surgery
Washington University School of Medicine
St. Louis, Missouri
Chapter 34

Göran Lundborg
Professor, Lund University
Department of Hand Surgery
Malmo University Hospital
Malmo, Sweden
Chapters 1, 17

Eveyln J. Mackin, P.T.
Executive Director
Hand Rehabilitation Foundation
Former Director of Hand Therapy
The Philadelphia Hand Center, P.C.
Philadelphia, Pennsylvania
Chapter 57

Glenn A. Mackin, M.D.
Assistant Professor
Department of Neurology
Director of Electromyography
University of Colorado Health Sciences Center
Denver, Colorado
Chapter 5

Paul R. Manske, M.D.
Department of Orthopaedic Surgery
Washington University School of Medicine
St. Louis, Missouri
Chapter 34

Stanley D. Marczyk, M.D.
The Philadelphia Hand Center, P.C.
Philadelphia, Pennsylvania
Chapter 37

Takeshi Matsui, M.D., Ph.D.
Matsui Orthopaedic Clinic
Shima-cho Mie Prefect
Japan
Chapter 33

Esther J. May, BAppSc(OT), Ph.D.
School of Occupational Therapy
University of South Australia
Adelaide, South Australia
Australia
Chapter 41

Fergal M. McGoldrick, M.Ch., F.R.C.S. Orth, F.R.C.S.I.
Blackrock Clinic
Dublin, Ireland
Chapter 36

Hanno Millesi, M.D.
Professor Emeritus
Medical Director
Vienna Private Hospital
Chairman, Ludwig Boltzmann Institute for Experimental
    Plastic Surgery
Vienna, Austria
Chapters 14, 24

A. Lee Osterman, M.D.
Professor, Orthopaedics/Hand Surgery
Thomas Jefferson Medical School
The Philadelphia Hand Center, P.C.
Philadelphia, Pennsylvania
Chapter 64

G. Padjardi, M.D.
University of Milan
Milan, Italy
Chapter 52

N. Paksima, D.O.
The Philadelphia Hand Center, P.C.
Philadelphia, Pennsylvania
Chapter 64

Nicholas H. Papas, M.D.
Clinical Instructor in Plastic Surgery
Northeastern Ohio Universities College of Medicine
Akron, Ohio
Fellow, Christine M. Kleinert Institute for Hand and
    MicroSurgery
Louisville, Kentucky
Chapter 36

Karen Stewart Pettengill, M.D., O.T., C.H.T.
Clinical Coordinator, Hand Therapy
NoraCare Outpatient Rehabilitation
Springfield, Massachusetts
Chapter 40

Jean Pillet, M.D.
Director
Pillet Hand Prostheses, France
Paris, France
Chapter 65

James S. Raphael, M.D.
Clinical Instructor
Thomas Jefferson University Hospital
The Philadelphia Hand Center, P.C.
Philadelphia, Pennsylvania
Chapter 37

Richard L. Read, P.T., E.C.S.
Electrophysiologic Clinical Specialist
The Philadelphia Hand Center, P.C.
Philadelphia, Pennsylvania
Chapter 21

Erik A. Rosenthal, M.D.
Hand and Upper Extremity Surgery
Pavilion Hand Surgeons, Inc.
Director Hand Surgery Service
Baystate Medical Center
Springfield, Massachusetts
Clinical Professor, Department of Orthopaedic Surgery
Tufts University School of Medicine
Boston, Massachusetts
Chapter 59

Jean-Claude Rouzaud, P.T.
Centre Hospitalier Universitaire de Montpellier
Chirurgie Orthopedique et Traumatologique II
Chirurgie de la Main et du Membre Superier
Chapter 63

Antal Salamon, M.D.
Professor
Vas Megyei Markusovszky Kórház
Baleseti Sebészeti Osztály
Szombathely, Hungary
Chapter 54

Roger E. Salisbury, M.D.
Hand Rehabilitation Foundation
Philadelphia, Pennsylvania
Chapter 55

Antonio Saracino, M.D.
Istituto di Clinica Ortopedica
Modena, Italy
Chapter 53

Steven C. Schmidt, M.D.
Hand Fellow, Department of Orthopaedic Surgery
Hospital of the University of Pennsylvania
Philadelphia, Pennsylvania
Chapter 6

Lawrence H. Schneider, M.D.
Clinical Professor
Department of Orthopaedic Surgery
Director, Division of Hand Surgery
Jefferson Medical College of Thomas Jefferson University
The Philadelphia Hand Center, P.C.
Philadelphia, Pennsylvania
Chapters 45, 50, 56

John Gray Seiler, III, M.D.
Associate Professor of Orthopaedic Surgery
Director of Orthopaedic Surgery Education
Emory University School of Medicine
Atlanta, Georgia
Chapter 46

Krister L. Silfverskiöld, M.D., Ph.D., F.R.A.C.S.
Blackwood, S.A.
Australia
Chapter 41

Kevin L. Smith, M.D., M.Sc.
Clinical Associate Professor
Department of Plastic Surgery
University of North Carolina—Chapel Hill
Charlotte Plastic Surgery Center
Charlotte, North Carolina
Chapter 2

James W. Strickland, M.D.
Clinical Professor
Department of Orthopaedic Surgery
Indiana University School of Medicine
Chairman, Department of Hand Surgery
St. Vincent Hospitals, Indianapolis
Staff Surgeon
The Indiana Hand Center
Indianapolis, Indiana
Chapters 42, 51

Sir Sydney Sunderland, M.D.†
Professor Emeritus
Department of Anatomy
University of Melbourne
Melbourne, Australia
Chapter 10

Alfred B. Swanson, M.D.
Professor of Surgery, Michigan State University
East Lansing, Michigan
Director of Orthopaedic Surgery Residency Training Program
   of the Grand Rapids Hospitals
Director of Hand Surgery Fellowship and Orthopaedic Re-
   search
Blodgett Memorial Medical Center
Grand Rapids, Michigan
Chapter 66

Genevieve de Groot Swanson, M.D.
Assistant Clinical Professor of Surgery
Michigan State University
East Lansing, Michigan
Coordinator of Orthopaedic Research Department
Blodgett Medical Center
Grand Rapids, Michigan
Chapter 66

Tatsuya Tajima, M.D.
Professor Emeritus, Niigata University
Chairman of the Board of Directors
Niigata Hand Surgery Foundation, Inc.
Niigata-Shi, Japan
Chapter 39

†Deceased.

John S. Taras, M.D.
Assistant Clinical Professor of Orthopaedic Surgery
Division of Hand Surgery
Jefferson Medical College of Thomas Jefferson University
The Philadelphia Hand Center, P.C.
Philadelphia, Pennsylvania
Chapter 37

David E. Thompson, Ph.D.
Professor and Chairman
Department of Mechanical Engineering
The University of New Mexico
Albuquerque, New Mexico
Chapter 43

Károly Trombitás, M.D.
Pécsi Orvostudományi Egyetem
Központi Elektronmikroszkópos Laboratórium
Pécs, Hungary
Chapter 54

Raoul Tubiana, Professor
Clinique Jouvenet
Chirurgie de l'Appereil Locomoteur
Institut de la Main
Paris, France
Chapters 44, 58

Shigeharu Uchiyama, M.D., Ph.D.
Vice-Director, Orthopedic Surgery
Suwa Red Cross Hospital
Suwa, Japan
Chapter 31

László Vámhidy, M.D.
Pécsi Orvostudományi Egyetem
Traumatológiai Klinika
Pécs, Hungary
Chapter 54

Janet Waylett-Rendall, O.T.R., C.H.T.
Director of Clinical Development
Rehabilitation Technology Works
San Bernardino, California
Chapter 13

Howard Webster, M.D.
Plastic Surgery Department
Monash Medical Centre
Melbourne, Australia
Chapter 18

Curt Weinstein, M.A.
President, Connecticut Bioinstruments, Inc.
Danbury, Connecticut
Chapter 8

Sir Sidney Weinstein, Kt. M., O.S.J., Ph.D.
Chief Executive Officer
NeuroCommunication Research Laboratories, Inc.
Danbury, Connecticut
Chapter 8

E.F. Shaw Wilgis, M.D.
Chief of Hand Surgery
Director of the Raymond Curtis Hand Center
Union Memorial Hospital
Baltimore, Maryland
Chapter 15

Robert Lee Wilson, M.D.
Lecturer in Surgery, University of Arizona
Tucson, Arizona
Hand Surgery Consultant
Maricopa Medical Center
Phoenix, Arizona
Chapters 22, 60

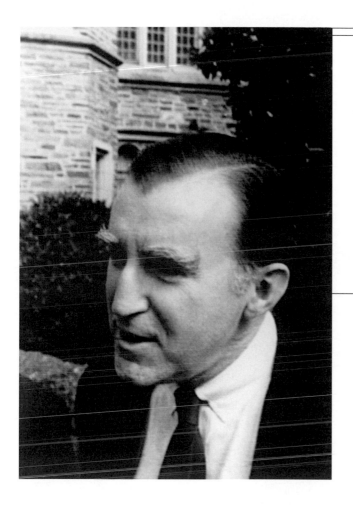

We dedicate this book to Dr. J. William Littler, Professor Emeritus of Clinical Surgery, Columbia University, College of Physicians and Surgeons, retired founder of the Hand Surgery Center at Roosevelt Hospital, New York City . . . master of hand surgery, enthusiastic teacher, and good friend. We thank him for his unparalleled contribution to hand surgery and the inspiration he has been to all who have followed in his footsteps.

FOREWORD

The splendid and cordial meetings organized by the team of the Philadelphia Hand Center have allowed many surgeons and physiotherapists to follow the evolution of tendon and nerve surgery in the Upper Extremity during the last decades. Exchanges between experts in physiology, kinesiology, and surgery have been extremely precious and fruitful. They have been a source of information and teaching for a number of surgeons and therapists all over the world.

One may say that the first decade has provided us with scientific information that had important implications for tendon and nerve surgery. The second decade has seen the development of new techniques of repair and of rehabilitation. The third decade allows the diffusion of these techniques. This does not mean that the cycle of progress is now closed. Many problems remain to be solved in tendon and nerve surgery, for example, in tendon surgery, early postoperative active motion or artificial tendons.

In nerve surgery, results are yet far from satisfactory. Moberg used to say that the term "nerve repair" is not semantically precise, "nerve surgery" seemed to him more appropriate. Although improving the orientation and coaptation of nerve ends is necessary, it may not be sufficient. Basic scientists and surgeons are trying to improve other factors that may influence the quality of functional recovery following nerve surgery.

We are always happy during these meetings to see again our hosts: James Hunter, Lawrence Schneider, Evelyn Mackin, as well as our colleagues from the first decade: Paul Brand, Paul Brown, Harold Kleinert, William Littler, Hanno Millesi, Alfred Swanson, Tatsuja Tajima, and many others, as well as younger bright surgeons from the second decade.

Unfortunately, some of our dearest friends, who were also pioneers in these fields have left us: Guy Pulvertaft, Erik Moberg, Joseph Boyes, Algimantas Narakas.

It is a particular pleasure for me to know that the editors of this book have dedicated it to William Littler, because Bill is one of my oldest and closest friends and he is a great surgeon whom I admire.

There are now many good technicians in hand surgery, but only a few have, when operating, the qualities of preci-

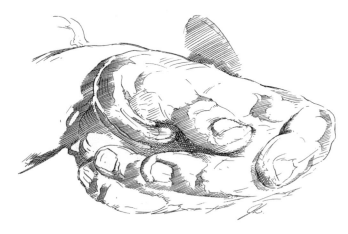

One of Dr. Littler's favorite pen sketches (made circa 1961) of Michelangelo's left (resting) hand of the sculpture, "il Giorno," in the Medici Chapel, Florence, Italy. (From Converse JM: *Reconstructive plastic surgery: principles in correction, reconstruction and transplantation,* vol iv, Philadelphia, 1964, WB Saunders.)

sion, of elegance, and of ingenuity that give you this rare sensation of perfection. Bill is not only a marvelous surgeon and a master who taught hand surgery to numerous pupils. He is also an artist, who feels equally at his ease with a pencil or with a scalpel. What is even more exceptional is that he is above all a creator. His sound knowledge of physiology has allowed him to conceive a considerable number of new procedures. To give examples, in extensor tendon surgery, he laid down the principles that govern the surgical treatment of chronic boutonnière deformity (i.e., the component parts of the extensor mechanism to the proximal interphalangeal and distal interphalangeal joints should be separated), and he described with Richard Eaton an original operation. He has conceived for the treatment of swan-neck deformity the lateral band tenodesis technique and the spiral oblique retinacular ligament reconstruction, and also the distal intrinsic release and the extensor tendon release. He has described a number of new procedures in other fields of hand surgery. I personally think that Littler's contribution has been one of the most important for the development of hand surgery, in particular in the topics dealt with in this beautiful book.

Raoul Tubiana

PREFACE

Each decade is a witness to new techniques and concepts for the management of tendon and nerve injuries. Each decade builds on the others. The purpose of this book is to review the current state-of-the-art in reparative nerve and tendon surgery with an appreciation of the contribution of those in previous decades.

On March 11-13, 1964, Lee Ramsay Straub, Herbert Conway, and James W. Smith organized an international symposium focused on tendon surgery in the hand. In his keynote address, Joseph H. Boyes reviewed the past and summarized the problems that still remained for the hand surgeon. R. Guy Pulvertaft concluded the meeting with his view of tendon surgery of the future. The symposium took place at Rockefeller Center in New York City. It was the first symposium to bring together the masters of hand surgery since the founding of the American Society for Surgery of the Hand (ASSH) in 1946.

Following in the footsteps of the 1964 meeting was the 1974 Another Decade of Tendon Surgery symposium, then came the 1984 The Hand: Another Decade of Tendon Surgery, and in 1994 The Hand: Another Decade of Tendon and Nerve Surgery symposia, which took place in Philadelphia. The organizers of the symposia—James M. Hunter, Lawrence H. Schneider, and Evelyn J. Mackin—have continued this worthy endeavor through the third decade and shared the privilege of preparing the publications that followed.

The addition of peripheral nerve surgery and its postoperative management in the 1994 symposium has been a natural outgrowth of the original purpose of the 1964 symposium to refine the final aspects of returning function to the injured hand.

Each symposium has touched the past and future through the papers of those who have worked so diligently to bring the specialty of hand surgery to the state of progress that it enjoys today.

The Philadelphia meetings on Surgery and Rehabilitation of the Hand held during the ensuing years now number twenty-one. These educational ventures beginning in the footsteps of the 1974 tendon symposium have in no small way helped to encourage the development of the American Society of Hand Therapists (ASHT). It is with great pride that we consider this accomplishment.

In looking back to 1964, it is apparent that the first tendon symposium was a milestone in many ways. It created a network among a group of hand surgeons in the United States and Europe who would, in the future, speak and write on the subject of hand tendon surgery and rehabilitation in such a profound way that it would develop into a new direction for the surgeons of the future to follow.

In 1964 secondary tendon grafting was the preferred method for the treatment of flexor tendon injury in zone 2. Investigations into tendon healing and nutrition were discussed. The possibility of staged tendon reconstruction using an artificial tendon was presented. Speakers at this meeting were soon to develop many of the advances in hand surgery: Joseph H. Boyes, Robert E. Carroll, Herbert Conway, Martin A. Entin, J. Edward Flynn, William H. Frackelton, James M. Hunter, Allan E. Inglis, Emanuel B. Kaplan, J. William Littler, Erik Moberg, Erle E. Peacock, R. Guy Pulvertaft, Daniel C. Riordan, James W. Smith, Lee Ramsay Straub, Alfred B. Swanson, and Raoul Tubiana. The idea of new sheath and fluid formation around the gliding artificial tendon was based on the celloidin tube concept described by Leo Mayer, a dean of American orthopaedic surgery, who was in the audience and came to the stage to support the concept for future tendon reconstruction.

One decade later in 1974 the American Academy of Orthopaedic Surgeons sponsored the second tendon symposium in Philadelphia, out of which came the monograph *Symposium on Tendon Surgery in the Hand,* 1975, C.V. Mosby. At the 1974 symposium, Claude Verdan entered his plea for the trained team "to repair initially the tendons within the digital sheath." James R. Doyle introduced his research study concerning the proper reconstruction of the flexor pulley system. Howard S. Caplan's studies opened the door to future work by a succession of Japanese research fellows on the vincula and the intrinsic vascularity of the flexor tendons. François Iselin showed us how to preserve and to bank free tendon grafts. The European surgeons' strengths were brought closer together at the 1974 meeting and, importantly, the physical and occupational therapy concept of preoperative and postoperative care for hand surgery were woven into the theme of the meeting.

The 1984 symposium, The Hand: Another Decade of Tendon Surgery, brought together major research papers dealing with tendon nutrition, repair, and reconstruction. This meeting resulted in a scholarly publication *Tendon Surgery in the Hand,* put together by the current editors and published in 1987 by C.V. Mosby. The book with 111 authors, has a permanent place in many hand surgery and therapy libraries. Postoperative tendon gliding techniques were emphasized. Jacques Michon suggested a place for the passive tendon implant in certain acute tendon injuries. Harold Kleinert's work represented a further impetus for the early direct repair of the flexor tendon in zone 2.

At this meeting Robert E. Carroll asked us to look back through the history of tendon repair and be mindful of its progress. R. Guy Pulvertaft, in his address, "A Look to the Future," noted the beginning of hand therapy in Great Britain. He stated, "I have been fortunate throughout my professional life in having strong support with physical therapists and occupational therapists. Their skill and enthusiasm make up one of the most significant features of hand care as we enter this new decade."

The 1997 book includes 66 papers presented at the 1994 Tendon and Nerve Surgery in the Hand: A Third Decade symposium and begins with an eloquent introductory presentation by Göran Lundborg, "The Hand and the Brain." We have reprinted two historic teaching papers, dealing with reconstructive flexor tendon surgery that set the standards for flexor tendon reconstruction before the revolution of microsurgery and the Kleinert primary tendon repair changed our teaching and training programs: the 1960 paper from the *Journal of Bone and Joint Surgery,* "Flexor Tendon Grafts in Finger and Thumb," by Joseph H. Boyes and the July 1971 *Journal of Bone and Joint Surgery* publication, "Flexor Tendon Reconstruction in Severely Damaged Hands," using a gliding Dacron-silicone tendon prosthesis by James M. Hunter and Roger E. Salisbury.

The stature of this book has been enhanced by the superb drawings of J. William Littler, which include selections from his monograph, *A Surgical Diary: Viet Nam 1969.* All should read this beautiful monograph in its entirety; it contains Dr. Littler's skilled surgical techniques and special philosophy. The diary is a look back at World War II when Major William Littler developed this method of preparing the hand for reconstructive surgery while Sterling Bunnell looked over his shoulder. Careful personal planning for re-construction was a hallmark of Dr. Littler's remarkable surgical skill.

We are indebted to Alfred Swanson who never missed the opportunity to turn back to a colleague an honor that he deserves. Dr. Littler had served in Dr. Swanson's government-sponsored Vietnam program. After the program was finished, Dr. Swanson brought Major Littler's ledger to the United States. From the ledger's lined paper, Mosby reproduced Dr. Littler's sketches of the treatment of Vietnam hand injuries.

Our sincere appreciation goes to our dear friend Mrs. Dorothy B. Kaufmann whose contributions to the hand-disabled patients and the specialty of hand therapy and hand surgery for two decades has earned her the respect and love of the Hand Rehabilitation Foundation and also the American Society of Hand Therapists (ASHT) who awarded her honorary membership in the ASHT in 1996.

Special thanks to Barbara G. Sielaff for her infinite patience in typing and retyping much of the material, diligent attention to detail, and yeoman efforts in coordinating this endeavor with the publisher.

We continue to enjoy a close working relationship with Kathy Falk, Senior Managing Editor, whose editorial assistance, guidance, and skills through the years have made her a valuable member of our team.

Our special thanks to our good friend Raoul Tubiana who has written the foreword to this book and whose enthusiasm, vision, surgical skills, and wide clinical experience have contributed to the great advances in hand surgery.

The editors are very proud to present this stellar group of national and international contributing authors to *Tendon and Nerve Surgery in the Hand: A Third Decade* and warmly thank them. Despite commitments and busy schedules their great efforts and enthusiasm have created a text in keeping with the original purpose of the 1964 symposium. We look forward to hosting the turn-of-the-century symposium on Tendon and Nerve Surgery and Rehabilitation of the Hand in the year 2004 . . . another decade.

James M. Hunter, M.D.
Lawrence H. Schneider, M.D.
Evelyn J. Mackin, P.T.

CONTENTS

COLOR PLATE CONTENTS

(Color plates follow page 74 of the text.)

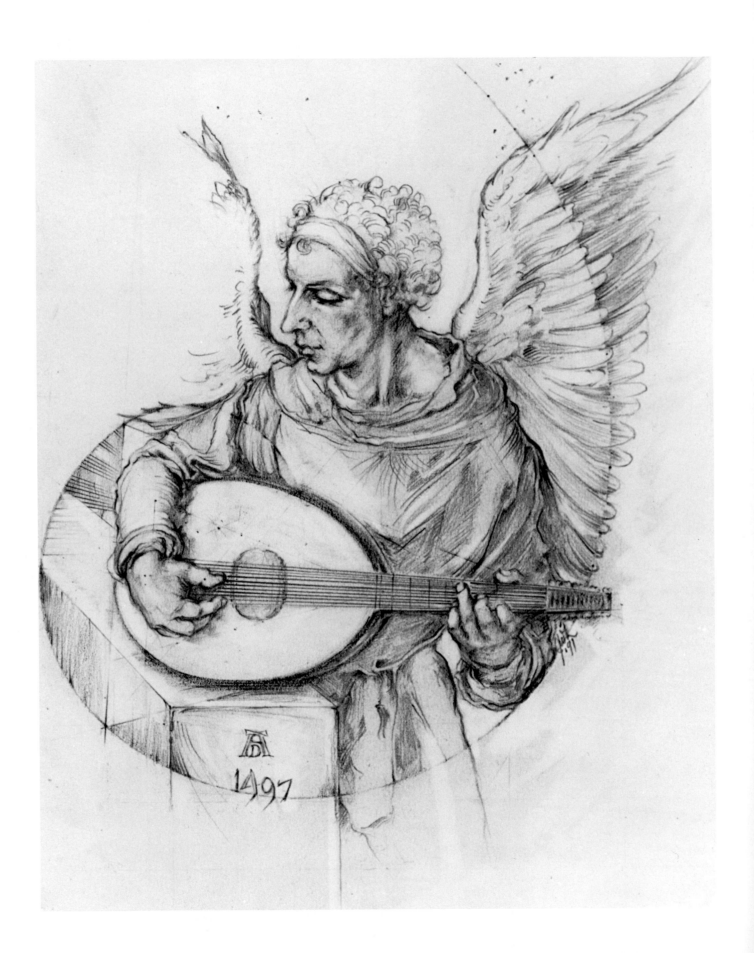

Part I

INTRODUCTION

Geometrical study of A. Durer's "Winged Lute Player." (From *J Hand Ther* 1992; 5(2) Hanley & Belfus [cover drawing].)

Chapter 1

THE HAND AND THE BRAIN

Göran Lundborg

The human hand can be described in various ways. The anatomist knows it as an extremely complicated anatomic structure with a remarkable capacity to perform precise movements because of a combined action of muscles, tendons, and joints. Hand surgeons and hand therapists describe the hand as a sense organ or an extension of the brain to the environment, being well aware of the specific sensory functions of the hand and the strong link between the hand and the psyche. This should be our perspective when we discuss hand injuries, and especially nerve injuries in the upper extremity: the hand, the brain, and the mind—the body and the soul together.

The face and the hand are the only structures of the body that are exposed to the environment. Both of them express thoughts and feelings. The expression of the face and the posture of the hands often have similarities, a phenomenon that has been well expressed in paintings by several great artists. Our ancestors also were aware of the importance of the hand and its function as a communication organ and perhaps also an organ essential for survival (Fig. 1-1).

THE HAND—A SENSE ORGAN

During evolution the human hand and brain developed into a unique, functionally combined unit making possible three-dimensional recognition of delicate structures and very small items (Fig. 1-2). The stereoscopic vision as well as the special three-dimensional sensibility called stereognosis or tactile gnosis[9,10] have developed parallel with an enormous expansion of the human brain cortex. The specific sensibility of the hand requires a large number of nerve cells in the brain. Together with the lips, the hands occupy more than half of the sensory cortex. With our fingertips we can detect the finest details of small structures, the quality and character

Acknowledgment: Peripheral nerve research in our laboratory is sponsored by the Swedish Medical Research Council, project 5188.

of plants and flowers, as well as the tiniest irregularity of a surface. The hand makes it possible to identify the shape of keys, small tools, and many other items (Fig. 1-2).

The ability to recognize and understand shape is dependent on the existence of permanent projections of each receptor site of the fingertip into one specific corresponding spot in the brain, and that these connecting nervous pathways, being wired during intrauterine life, remain intact. The newborn child watches, tastes, and touches structures in the immediate surroundings, and in this way a sensory education is carried out—a programming of the brain computer. The result is a capacity of the brain to understand and interpret the pattern of afferent impulses, which is initiated by touching certain structures. Erik Moberg and others have emphasized the ability of the fingertips to actually "see" small structures. In this respect the hand can even replace vision.

COMFORT AND CONSOLATION

The strong link between the hand and the brain is indicated by the importance of the hand for comfort, consolation, and satisfaction. As early as intrauterine life, the embryo has discovered that sucking the thumb provides comfort. It is wonderful to be covered and enclosed by hands. Hands symbolize safety and nearness; they create a link between generations. Friendship is the touch of hands. Sensitive, caring hands are necessary for social and family life. Hands express love.

HANDS IN COMMUNICATION

Hands are important for communication in social life. The hands express what the mind wants to say. At the terminal stage of a disease the touch of hands can sometimes be the only possible communication. We use hands to give instructions and to send signals. We clap our hands as a sign of appreciation. Applause is like fingerprints—extremely characteristic for each individual.

HANDS AND FEELINGS

Hands express enjoyment, happiness, and satisfaction. Together with facial expressions, they signal anxiety, despair, or deep sorrow. They indicate relaxation, comfort,

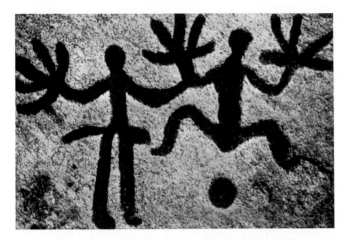

Fig. 1-1. Rock carving from the west coast of Sweden showing enlarged hands, one of them shared between two individuals (possibly a sign of communication). This rock carving is also the logo of the Scandinavian Society for Surgery of the Hand.

and satisfaction as well as intense concentration. They are the mirror of the mind. Their shape, position, and movements often say a great deal about the person.

ART AND MUSIC

Drawings and prints are memories from our ancient ancestors. Hand paintings by Australian aborigines date back to more than 8000 years BC. In Swedish rock carvings hands are often enlarged and are sometimes shared by two individuals, perhaps as a sign of the importance of communication (see Fig. 1-1).

In art such as Michelangelo's *Creation of Man* in the Sistine Chapel or in Rodin's God's hands modelling man hands illustrate creativity. In music the great conductors can, by using their hands, inspire and draw out the best performance of a full symphony orchestra. Piano players seem to have their brains in their fingertips. Playing the trumpet requires a combined action and coordination of the parts of the body dominating the sensory cortex—the hands and the lips (Fig. 1-3).

BRAIN PLASTICITY

In the brain the hand is represented in areas 3b and 1 in the somatosensory cortex.[5,6] Within this area the fingers are projected in well-defined bands. Until recently most neuroscientists believed that the brain was hardwired from shortly

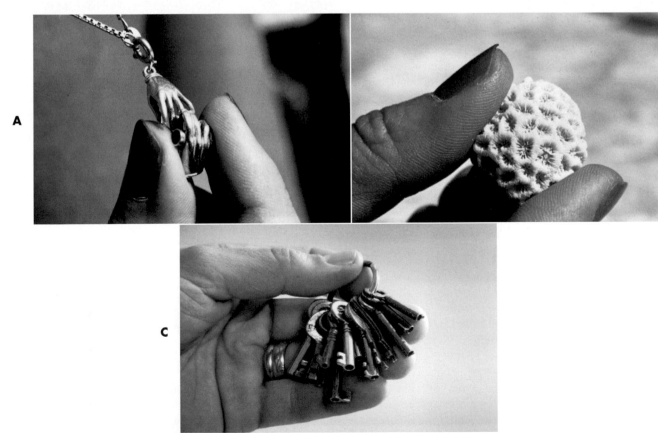

Fig. 1-2. With the fingertips it is possible to identify the structure, form, and texture of small items.

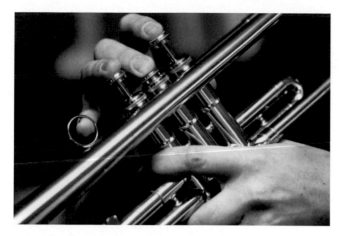

Fig. 1-3. Playing the trumpet requires interaction and coordination of the body parts dominating the sensory cortex: the hands and the lips.

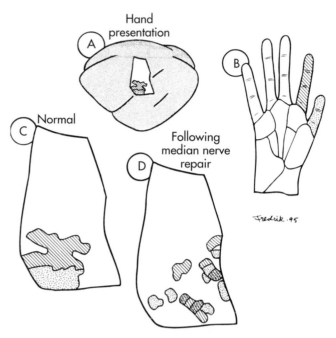

Fig. 1-4. Functional organization of the thumb and index finger in the somatosensory cortex normally (**A, B,** and **C**) and following median nerve transection, repair and regeneration in the owl monkey (**D**). Following nerve repair and regeneration there is a major topographic reorganization in the somatosensory cortex with the digit representations in small discontinuous patches instead of the previous bands. Based on information obtained from Wall, 1986.

after birth with old pathways firmly and immutably formed, and that the original projection of specific hand areas could not be changed. However, recent experiments and clinical experience indicate that this is not true. The brain is now regarded as a network that is continuously remodelling itself so that it can operate more efficiently when the demand is put on a particular body part.[3] There are several experiments illustrating this fact. In specific experiments monkeys were trained to use specifically the second, third, and fourth fingers for specific manipulative tasks over a period of 3 months.[5] During this period the monkeys rotated a disk for 1 hour a day using only the index, middle, and ring fingers. After 3 months of this activity the cortical area representing these three fingers in the brain had increased substantially, indicating a capacity of the brain to undergo rapid reorganizational changes.

Analogous phenomena have been observed in the adult human brain also. By the use of positron emission tomography (PET), a remarkable functional plasticity has been demonstrated in the cerebral cortex of blind people reading braille,[11] the projection of the reading finger increasing substantially in sensory as well as motor cortex. Following stroke, a remarkable capacity for such functional reorganization in the human brain also has been observed.[1,15] Thus, even the adult human brain can undergo dramatic functional reorganizational changes when there are new demands on hand function. Dramatic reorganizational changes are seen even more after peripheral nerve injuries.

It has been demonstrated in primate experiments that following transection and repair of the median nerve there is a considerable functional reorganization in the somatosensory cortex as a result of incorrect axonal reinnervation of targets.[13,14] Transection of the median nerve results in partial denervation of the hand, but also parts of the sensory cortex are denervated because of sudden absence of sensory input. There is a "black hole" in the brain corresponding to the median nerve territory. This area becomes occupied by

substitute tactile inputs from adjacent hand locations, still innervated by other nerves. With time, regenerating axons frequently do make peripheral connections with wrong peripheral receptor sites. This leads to a new phase—functional reorganization of the somatosensory cortex with major topographic changes, the individual fingers now being represented in several dispersed discontinuous patches rather than the previous well-defined bands (Fig. 1-4). Neurones with reinnervated cutaneous fields become abnormal in terms of numbers, location, and sizes of the skin areas to which they respond. Separate recording sites in the sensory cortex also may be abnormally located, and each of them may be associated with multiple cutaneous receptor fields.

REPROGRAMMING OF THE BRAIN COMPUTER

The functional cortical reorganization following nerve repair and regeneration implies that the hand "speaks a new language to the brain," it is no longer possible to interpret tactile stimuli to understand shapes, textures, and forms. Reprogramming is required to make it possible to regain functional hand sensibility.[8] To initiate and maintain such a relearning process, several types of reeducational programs have been suggested.[2,4,16] The concept is to combine visual and tactile stimuli to induce such a reprogramming process (Fig. 1-5). We are essentially dealing with a learning process analogous to learning a new language. In molecular terms

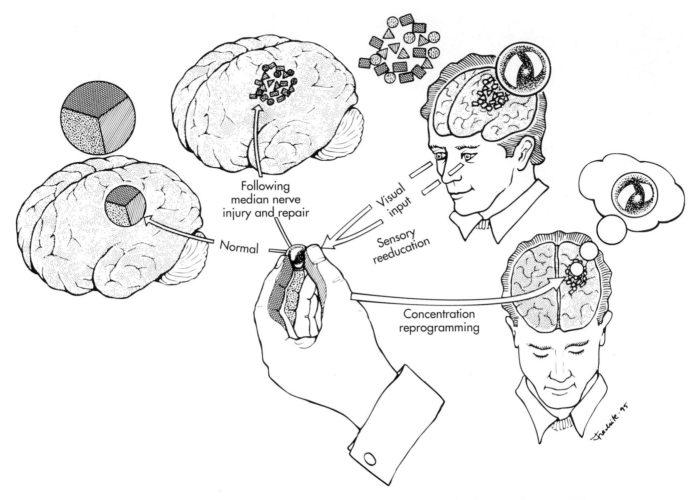

Fig. 1-5. Principles for sensory reeducation. Following the functional reorganization of the somatosensory cortex, resulting from a median nerve injury, the hand "speaks a new language to the brain." By relearning (sensory reeducational program) the mind can create a "visualization" of the structure the hand is touching in spite of the cortical remapping.

such a learning process may involve phenomena such as long-term potentiating (LTP) of existing synapses, formation of new synaptic connections, and probably even expression of new proteins in the brain cells caused by direct influence of the genes and their control of protein production in the cells.[3,7]

RECOVERY OF FUNCTIONAL SENSIBILITY AS RELATED TO SPECIFIC CENTRAL NERVOUS FUNCTIONS

It is well-known that there is an inverse relation between age and recovery of functional sensibility of the hand, superior results from nerve repair generally being achieved in children as compared with adults. Children are also able to learn a foreign language extremely rapidly as compared with adults. Following nerve injury the hand speaks a new language to the brain and there are reasons to believe that the capacity to learn such a new language may vary not only

between the young and adults but also between adult individuals. A possible hypothesis may be that variations in recovery of functional sensibility among adults after nerve injury and repair may correlate with variations in verbal learning capacity. In a recent study[8,12] it was found that age and peripheral nerve status (perception of cutaneous touch/ pressure thresholds by the use of Semmes-Weinstein monofilaments) explained 64% of the variance in outcome of functional sensibility tests, while verbal learning capacity explained a further 17%. Visuospatial capacity, reflected in the capacity to place colored cubes and triangles to form defined colored patterns (block design test)[12] explained 13% of the variance of the outcome of functional sensibility tests. Even this fact makes sense, since reorganization of the "finger bands" in somatosensory cortex into dispersed patches following nerve repair and regeneration requires specific abilities to make the mind adapt to changes in the original projectional pattern.

THE PAST AND THE FUTURE

From what has been said it is obvious that peripheral nerve injuries lead not only to severe functional impairment in the hand as a result of sensory and motor deficits but also to considerable reorganizational changes in the mind. Nerve injuries are especially crucial in this respect. Increasing knowledge of the dynamic properties of the brain may lead to modifications in future strategies for treatment of nerve injuries. Should we address primarily the peripheral structures or the brain?

Sometimes it is useful to put things in an evolutionary perspective. What have we lost and what have we gained during the evolutionary process? We have certainly not gained anything with respect to peripheral regeneration potential; instead we have lost such potential that was present in lower animal species. However, we have gained much by evolution in "brain capacity." It seems therefore logical that we should address the capacity and plasticity of the brain rather than only peripheral regeneration processes to achieve better results from nerve repair. Although microsurgery has contributed much to improve the results of nerve repair in many situations, the surgical techniques cannot be refined further. In addition, it seems that repair of human median and ulnar nerves by microsurgical techniques do not give more superior clinical results than intentionally leaving a short gap between the nerve ends inside a closed compartment (GL 1995). Thus, there are reasons to assume that the key to success when repairing nerves in the hand and forearm may be in the brain rather than in the peripheral nerve itself.

REFERENCES

1. Chollet F, DiPiero V, Wise RJS, et al: The functional anatomy of motor recovery after stroke in humans: a study with positron emission tomography, *Ann Neurol* 1991; 29:63.
2. Dellon AL: *Sensibility and re-education of sensation in the hand,* Baltimore, 1981, Williams & Wilkins.
3. Fischbach GD: Mind and brain, *Sci Am* 1992; 267:24 (editorial).
4. Imai H, Tajima T, Natsumi Y: Successful reeducation of functional sensibility after median nerve repair at the wrist, *J Hand Surg* 1991; 16A:60.
5. Jenkins WM, Merzenich NM, Ochs MT, et al: Functional reorganization of primary somatosensory cortex in adult owl monkeys after behaviorally controlled tactile stimulation, *J Neurophysiol* 1990; 63:82.
6. Jenkins WM, Merzenich NM, Recanzona G: Neocortical representational dynamics in adult primates: implications for neurophysiology, *Neuropsychologia* 1990; 28:573.
7. Kandel ER, Hawkins RD: The biological bases of learning and individuality, *Sci Am* 1992; 267:53.
8. Lundborg G, Rosén B, Dahlin J, Holmberg J: Functional sensibility of the hand following nerve repair correlates with visuospatial logic congnitive capacity, *Lancet* 1993; 342:1300.
9. Moberg E: Objective methods for determining the functional value of sensibility in the hand, *J Bone Joint Surg* 1958; 40B:454.
10. Moberg E: Criticism and study of methods for examining sensibility in the hand, *Neurology* 1962; 12:8.
11. Pasqual-Leone A, Torres F: Plasticity of the sensorimotor cortex representation of the reading finger in braille readers, *Brain* 1993; 116:39.
12. Rosén B, Lundborg G, Dahlin LB, et al: Nerve repair: correlation of restitution of functional sensibility with specific cognitive capacities, *J Hand Surg* 1994; 19B:452.
13. Wall JT, Kaas JH: Long-term cortical consequences of reinnervation errors after nerve regeneration in monkeys, *Brain Res* 1986; 372:400.
14. Wall JT, Kaas JH, Sur M, et al: Functional reorganization in somatosensory cortical areas 3b and 1 of adult monkeys after median nerve repair: possible relationships to sensory recovery in humans, *J Neurosci* 1986; 6:218.
15. Weiller C, Chollet F, Friston K, et al: Functional reorganization of the brain in recovery from striatocapsular infarction in man, *Ann Neurol* 1992; 31:463.
16. Wynn-Parry CB, Salter M: Sensory re-education after median nerve lesions, *Hand* 1976; 8:250.

DUCHENNE:
Physiology of Motion
Translated by
EMANUEL B. KAPLAN

To my
eternal friend
Dr. Hunter

E. Kaplan
4-11-77

Part II

NERVE ANATOMY

Professor Emanuel Kaplan turns the pages of his translation of Duchenne's *Physiology of Motion.*

Chapter 2

ANATOMY OF
THE PERIPHERAL NERVE

Kevin L. Smith

NEURAL MICROANATOMY

The peripheral nervous system serves as an interface between the central nervous system (CNS) and the environment and is designed to receive and relay information. It is a complex composite structure of cell bodies (neurons) and their cytoplasmic extensions, supportive connective tissue, cellular elements, and associated end organs.

The nerve cell bodies (or soma) are located in the spinal cord or in the outlying spinal ganglia and connect with the periphery via the nerve axon (Fig. 2-1). Axons are elongated cylindric processes of the nerve cells that facilitate communication between the neuron and the end organ by the initiation and propagation of electrical currents generated across their cell membranes. By this mechanism, information is transmitted quickly to and from the neuron. Information can be transmitted within the axon by axoplasmic transport as well, but it is a slow process. The nerve cell body contains the nucleus of the cell and its metabolic machinery and is the vital center for the control of the metabolic functions of the axon. The rate of impulse propagation (membrane depolarization and repolarization) is governed by the axon caliber and the configuration of the insulating myelin around each axon produced by the Schwann cell.

The CNS is joined to the peripheral nervous system through the dorsal and the ventral roots of the spinal cord (Fig. 2-2). Groups of motor axons leave the anterior spinal cord, join together to form the ventral root, and terminate at the motor end plate. The dorsal root is made up of fibers that emanate from the cell bodies that lie within the ganglia and terminate at the sensory end organs. Nerve fibers, either efferent (outgoing) or afferent (incoming), travel in bundles termed fascicles, bound by supportive connective tissues. Bundles of fascicles join together to form the peripheral nerves.

The connective tissue that supports and protects the nerve fiber bundles is arranged in three distinct layers: the endoneurium, the perineurium, and the epineurium (Fig. 2-3). These tissues support and protect the axons, and within these layers lies the nutritive vascular supply for the nerve.

The nerve fibers within each fascicle are densely packed within a mucopolysaccharide ground substance with longitudinally oriented collagen fibrils and smaller reticulin fibers—the endoneurium. The fibroblast is its principle cellular component and is responsible for the collagen synthesis. The endoneurium contains capillaries and lymphatics and is separated from each axon and Schwann cell complex by a basal lamina. Occasionally, mast cells and macrophages are found within the endoneurial layer.

The next layer is the perineurium. It is the organized connective tissue condensation around the individual nerve fascicles. The perineurium is composed of inner layers of lamellated squamous-like cells and collagen and is arranged in longitudinal, circumferential, and oblique bundles. Between each of the lamellae of cells there are longitudinal bundles of collagen, elastic fibrils, and occasional fibroblasts.

The perineurium is a very specialized structure with metabolic activity driving active transport of substances to and from the fascicles. This structure acts as the "blood-nerve" barrier that facilitates the regulation of the internal milieu of the fascicles and serves the protective function of excluding toxic macromolecules such as antigens and viruses. The perineurium is contiguous with the pia arachnoid mater at the

11

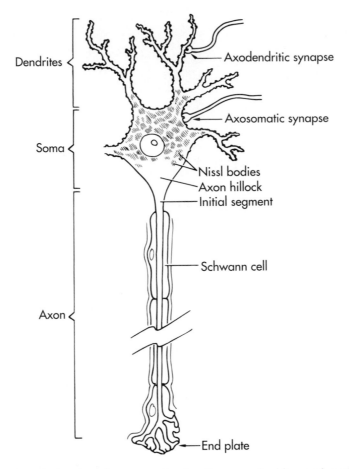

Fig. 2-1. Schematic drawing of a neuron showing the soma, dendrites, and myelinated axon with basal lamina. (From Terzis JK, Smith KL: *The peripheral nerve structure, function, and reconstruction,* New York, 1990, Raven.)

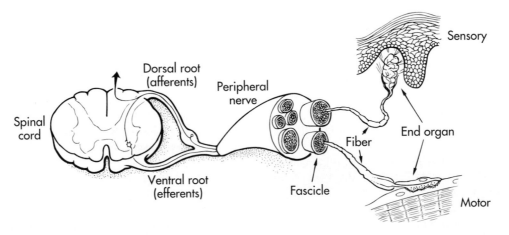

Fig. 2-2. The architecture of the peripheral nerve with central and peripheral connections. (From Terzis JK, Smith KL: *The peripheral nerve structure, function, and reconstruction,* New York, 1990, Raven.)

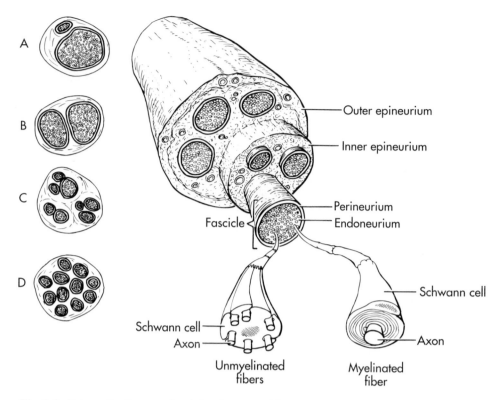

A

B

C

D

Outer epineurium

Inner epineurium

Perineurium

Fascicle ⟨

Endoneurium

Schwann cell

Schwann cell

Axon

Axon

Unmyelinated
fibers

Myelinated
fiber

Fig. 2-3. Schematic diagram of peripheral nerve architecture. The connective tissue elements consist of the endoneurium, the perineurium, and the inner and outer epineurium. Individual fascicles contain a heterogeneous mix of myelinated and unmyelinated fibers, but some fascicles demonstrate a preponderance of one type. Basic patterns of intraneural structure are demonstrated. A peripheral nerve is considered monofascicular if it holds one large fascicle *(A)* or oligofascicular for a few large fascicles *(B)*. Polyfascicular nerves consist of many fascicles, which may be grouped *(C),* or there may be no identifiable group patterns *(D).* (From Millesi H, Terzis JK: Problems of terminology in peripheral nerve surgery: committee report of the International Society of Reconstructive Microsurgery, *Microsurgery* 1983; 4:51-56.)

spinal angle. The perineurium furnishes the strong "skeletal" support for the enclosed neural tissue and is primarily responsible for the tensile strength of the peripheral nerve. This layer also maintains positive intraneural pressure that is necessary for the maintenance of endoneurial fluid pressure. As there are no lymphatics that cross the perineurial layer, perineurial pressure is necessary to counteract osmotic forces and to promote centrifugal flow toward the open distal end of the perineurium where excess endoneurial fluid can gain access to epineurial lymphatic drainage.

The outermost supportive ensheathment of the peripheral nerve is the epineurium. This is the loose outer sheath that comprises the perifascicular and interfascicular connective tissue around and between the nerve fascicles. The epineurium is a vascular structure that carries the nutrient blood vessels that supply the capillary plexus of the nerve. It also carries the lymphatics. The collagen fibrils of the epineurium are oriented parallel to the fascicles or in a shallow spiral. The epineurium is noted to be thicker in areas where the nerves cross joints, presumably as a protective function.

The outer layers of the epineurium are continuous with the mesoneurium—the suspensory mesentery of the peripheral nerve, which arises from the areolar connective tissue of the underlying fascia. The nerve lies loosely in its bed except where it is tethered by its branches or by entering blood vessels. During postural changes, the nerve glides within its bed. The mesoneurium is sufficiently "slack" to allow this gliding action without tethering.

There are four basic patterns of intraneural architecture that can be recognized (see Fig. 2-3). A peripheral nerve is considered monofascicular if it holds one large fascicle or oligofascicular if it contains a few large fascicles. Polyfascicular nerves consist of many fascicles that may be grouped or the fascicles may be found in random, nongrouped patterns.

Clinically, the peripheral nerve presents a confusing array of fascicular branchings and interconnections. Cross-sectional comparisons between the debrided ends of transected nerves rarely reveal fascicular matching. During nerve repair and reconstruction, the surgeon is often faced with two nerve ends that do not exactly match and the

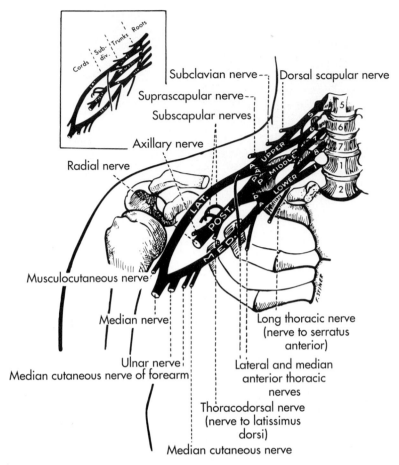

Fig. 2-4. Anatomy of brachial plexus. (From Hunter JM, Mackin EJ, Callahan AD, eds: *Rehabilitation of the hand: surgery and therapy,* ed 4, St Louis, 1995, Mosby.)

surgeon must make a decision about how to most appropriately coapt the fascicles.

Internal neuroanatomic studies have now shown that neural architecture is predictable. Despite considerable variability in fascicular patterns, there is a high degree of efferent and afferent segregation with fascicles of essentially pure motor or sensory axons. Axons are not chaotically or randomly oriented within fascicular bundles as once thought. It is now known that axonal location remains relatively constant within nerve quadrants.

Nerves are more heterogeneous proximally, and segments of extensive interfascicular interconnection do occur but not to the extent long thought to prohibit intraneural dissection, microcoaptation, or nerve grafting. Depending on the level of nerve, proximal to distal, a reduction in complexity can be expected when moving toward the periphery. In general, the nerves are not a jumble of interconnected and randomly arranged axons but have relatively homogeneous groups of fascicles that exist over appreciable lengths. Elaborate topographic maps have been created, which allow accurate group fascicular identification and proximal to distal match-up for reconstruction.

NEURAL GROSS ANATOMY

Fortunately for the diagnostician, the anatomy of the peripheral nerve is well documented and is remarkably consistent. Knowledge of this anatomy is essential for the diagnosis and treatment of the patient with a peripheral nerve lesion. It allows for precise determinations of the site of nerve lesions, and coupled with the history of the patient's injury a reasonable estimation of the patient's prognosis for recovery can be made.

Peripheral nerves course in predictable locations from their points of origin to their respective end organs, and they course in relatively protected positions. But as the nerves cross joints or leave or enter fascial compartments, they traverse specialized areas, which can present a potential danger to the enclosed nerve. There are some positions where the nerves are especially vulnerable because of their superficial location.

BRACHIAL PLEXUS ANATOMY

The nerves that supply the arm, forearm, and hand take their origin from the brachial plexus, which is formed by the merger of the ventral rami of the lower four cervical nerve roots (C5, C6, C7, C8) and part of the first thoracic nerve root (T1) (Fig. 2-4).

The five roots become three trunks (upper, middle, and lower), then the three trunks divide into anterior and posterior divisions at the level of the clavicle. The three posterior divisions unite to form the posterior cord (C5, C6, C7, C8, T1). The anterior divisions of the upper and middle trunks form the lateral cord (C5, C6, C7), and the anterior division of the lower trunk continues as the medial cord (C8, T1)—all named to correspond to their relationship with the axillary artery.

There are five major terminal branches of the brachial plexus. Most of the branches of the brachial plexus originate from the cords but do not contain fibers from all of the roots that are contained in that cord. The medial cord continues as the ulnar nerve after giving a branch to the median nerve. The branch to the median nerve contributes the innervation to the median innervated intrinsics of the hand.

The lateral cord of the plexus continues as the musculocutaneous nerve after contributing a branch to the median nerve. The posterior cord continues as the radial nerve after giving a terminal branch—the axillary nerve.

The roots have two clinically important branches—the long thoracic and dorsal scapular nerves (C5, C6, C7, and C5, C6, respectively). These nerve branches are important in the physical examination and diagnosis following a brachial plexus injury. If the muscles they innervate are functioning (the latissimus dorsi, serratus anterior, levator scapulae, and rhomboid muscles), the inference can be drawn that the nerve roots are intact. If these muscles are not functioning, it is highly probable that the injury has occurred very proximally and is at the root level.

At the trunk level, there is only one significant branch—the suprascapular nerve, which comes off the upper trunk. All of the remaining branches come off at the cord level or are the terminal extensions of the cords.

The brachial plexus is susceptible to compression at the trunk level as it exits between the scalene muscles and over the first rib, and it is subject to crush and laceration as it exits the axilla.

AXILLARY NERVE

The axillary nerve is the lateral terminal branch of the posterior cord of the brachial plexus and marks the point where the posterior cord continues as the radial nerve (Fig. 2-5). It joins the posterior circumflex artery as it travels around the surgical neck of the humerus, and together they form the neurovascular pedicle to the deltoid muscle and the teres minor. The nerve is susceptible to injury or compression in the axilla as it lies adjacent to the humerus.

RADIAL NERVE

The radial nerve is the continuation of the posterior cord of the brachial plexus and is made up of fibers from the C6, C7, C8, and T1 roots (see Fig. 2-5). It originates behind the

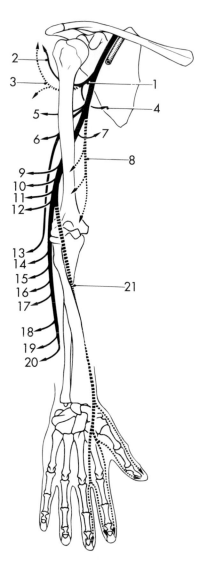

Fig. 2-5. The radial and axillary nerves; muscles supplied and cutaneous distribution. The forearm is pronated. *1*, Axillary nerve; *2*, Deltoid; *3*, Cutaneous branch to shoulder; *4*, Teres minor; *5*, Triceps (long); *6*, Triceps (lateral); *7*, Triceps (medial); *8*, Medial cutaneous branch; *9*, Brachioradialis; *10*, Extensor carpi radialis longus; *11*, Extensor carpi radialis brevis; *12*, Supinator; *13*, Anconeus; *14*, Extensor digitorum communis; *15*, Extensor digitorum to fifth digit; *16*, Extensor carpi ulnaris; *17*, Abductor pollicis longus; *18*, Extensor pollicis brevis; *19*, Extensor pollicis longus; *20*, Extensor indicis proprius; *21*, Anterior sensory branch. The sensory branches are shown as dotted lines. (From Tubiana, Thomme, Mackin: *Examination of the hand and upper limb,* Philadelphia, 1984, Saunders.)

axillary artery and then winds around the posterior aspect of the humerus in the spiral groove. Here the nerve is not in direct contact with the bone, but it is relatively immobile as it passes through the posterior intermuscular septum. The radial nerve's lack of mobility makes it especially susceptible to injury when there is a mid-shaft humeral fracture. The nerve then continues toward the forearm within the lateral bicipital groove and pierces the lateral intermuscular

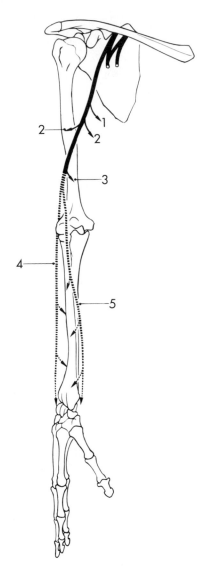

Fig. 2-6. The musculocutaneous nerve; muscles supplied and cutaneous distribution. *1,* Coracobrachial branch; *2,* Biceps brachii; *3,* Anterior brachial branch; *4,* Posterior branch (sensory); *5,* Anterior branch (sensory). The sensory branches are shown as dotted lines. (From Tubiana, Thomme, Mackin: *Examination of the hand and upper limb,* Philadelphia, 1984, Saunders.)

septum at the junction of the middle and distal thirds of the humerus where it continues between the brachialis and the brachioradialis muscles.

The radial nerve innervates the triceps muscle and provides a sensory branch to the medial aspect of the arm. Then it provides innervation to the brachioradialis, the extensor carpi radialis longus, the extensor carpi radialis brevis, and the supinator. At the level of the elbow, it branches into two terminal segments. One is motor to the extensor carpi ulnaris and to all of the extensors of the fingers (the extensor digitorum communis, the extensor digiti quinti, the abductor pollicis longus, the extensor pollicis brevis, the extensor

pollicis longus, and the extensor indicis proprius), and the other is sensory to the radial half of the dorsum of the hand.

As the radial nerve passes into the forearm below the supinator, it can be compressed by the most proximal edge of this muscle—the arcade of Frohse.

MUSCULOCUTANEOUS NERVE

Arising from the lateral cord of the brachial plexus and made up of contributions from C5, C6, and C7, the musculocutaneous nerve (Fig. 2-6) innervates the coracobrachialis, both heads of the biceps, and a portion of the brachialis. It then pierces the deep fascia distal to the elbow and provides cutaneous innervation as the lateral cutaneous nerve of the forearm.

MEDIAN NERVE

The median nerve is comprised of fibers originating in all of the roots of the brachial plexus (C5, C6, C7, C8, and T1) (Fig. 2-7). It travels through the anteromedial compartment of the arm with the brachial artery without branching. The nerve enters the forearm beneath the lacertus fibrosus (bicipital fascia), and it gives off sensory branches to the elbow. It then gives off motor branches to the pronator teres and passes between the superficial and deep heads of this muscle. Then, splitting into two branches, it innervates the major portion of the muscles of the hand and the wrist. The superficial branch passes through the origin of the flexor superficialis and lies deep to this muscle and its tendons. It gives off branches to the flexor digitorum superficialis (FDS) and the flexor carpi radialis. It then becomes superficial (palmar) in the distal forearm and becomes the most palmar structure within the carpal canal. After passing through the pronator teres muscle and dividing, the deep branch of the median nerve, the anterior interosseous nerve, courses along the anterior interosseous membrane and gives motor branches to the flexor digitorum profundus (FDP) to the index and long fingers and to the pronator quadratus. The final branch of the median nerve in the forearm is the palmar cutaneous nerve.

As the median nerve emerges from the carpal canal, it divides into its terminal branches to the radial thenar muscles, the radial two lumbrical muscles, and the skin of the radial three and one-half digits.

The median nerve passes through several specialized anatomic zones where it is susceptible to compression. Proximally, compression can occur as the nerve passes through the humeral origin of the pronator teres at the ligament of Struthers. At the elbow, the nerve can be compressed by a fibrous extension of the deep muscular fascia of the forearm, the lacertus fibrosus, and just distal to this, at the fibrous bridge between the heads of the FDS. Distally, compression can occur within the carpal canal. Throughout its course the median nerve is relatively well protected except where it is superficial in the distal forearm.

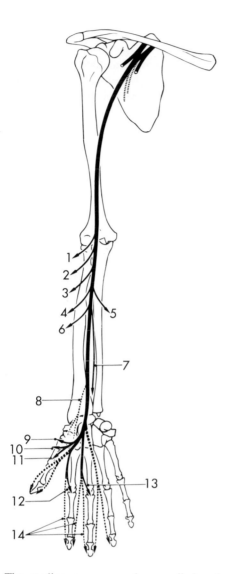

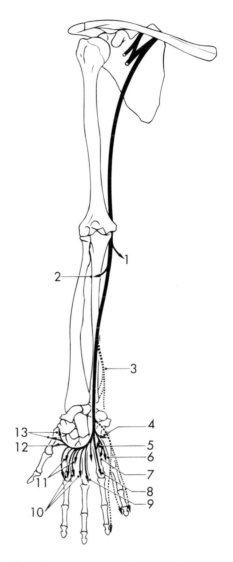

Fig. 2-7. The median nerve; muscles supplied and cutaneous distribution. *1*, Pronator teres; *2*, Palmaris longus; *3*, Palmaris brevis; *4*, Flexor digitorum superficialis; *5*, Flexor digitorum profundus to second and third digits; *6*, Flexor pollicis longus; *7*, Pronator quadratus; *8*, Palmar cutaneous branch; *9*, Abductor pollicis brevis; *10*, Superficial branch to flexor pollicis brevis; *11*, Opponens pollicis; *12*, First lumbrical; *13*, Second lumbrical; *14*, Digital nerves (sensory). The sensory branches are shown as dotted lines. (From Tubiana, Thomme, Mackin: *Examination of the hand and upper limb*, Philadelphia, 1984, Saunders.)

Fig. 2-8. The ulnar nerve; muscles supplied and cutaneous distribution. *1*, Branch to flexor carpi ulnaris; *2*, Branch to flexor digitorum profundus supplying fourth and fifth digits; *3*, Dorsal cutaneous branch; *4*, Palmar cutaneous branch; *5*, Branch to abductor digiti minimi; *6*, Branch to opponens digiti minimi; *7*, Branch to flexor digiti minimi; *8*, Fourth lumbrical branch; *9*, Third lumbrical branch; *10*, Branch to palmar interosseous muscles; *11*, Branch to dorsal interosseous muscles; *12*, Deep branch to flexor pollicis brevis; *13*, Branch to adductor pollicis. The sensory branches are shown as dotted lines. (From Tubiana, Thomme, Mackin: *Examination of the hand and upper limb*, Philadelphia, 1984, Saunders.)

ULNAR NERVE

The ulnar nerve arises from the medial cord of the brachial plexus and is made up of fibers from the C7, C8, and T1 roots (Fig. 2-8). It goes through the medial intermuscular septum and passes between the medial epicondyle of the humerus and the olecranon, the cubital tunnel. The nerve then enters the forearm between the humeral and ulnar origins of the flexor carpi ulnaris and proceeds through the anteromedial compartment of the forearm under the flexor carpi ulnaris (FCU). There, it supplies innervation to the

FCU and to the two ulnar heads of the FDP. In the distal forearm, it gives rise to the dorsal cutaneous branch, which supplies the dorsal ulnar aspect of the hand.

The ulnar nerve then passes into the hand through Guyon's canal, where it goes on to terminate in a deep branch that supplies all of the intrinsic muscles (except the radial two lumbricals), the adductor pollicis, and to the deep head of the flexor pollicis brevis, and a superficial branch that supplies the sensibility to the ulnar one and one-half digits.

The ulnar nerve can be compressed at several points along its course. In the lower third of the arm, the ulnar nerve enters the posterior compartment where it can be compressed as it passes through an osseofibrous foramen bound by the medial intermuscular septum, by a fibrous expansion of the coracobrachialis, and by the medial head of the triceps. Distal to this, there is an inconsistent insertion of the triceps that forms the arcade of Struthers, which can serve to compress the nerve. At the elbow, the nerve passes through the cubital tunnel, delineated by the medial epicondyle and the olecranon. The nerve enters the forearm between the humeral and ulnar heads of the FCU under a fibrous arcade that can serve to entrap the nerve. The ulnar nerve then passes into the hand through Guyon's canal, formed by the flexor retinaculum, the hook of the hamate, and an expansion of the FCU—another fixed volume compartment that can lead to compression neuropathy.

SUMMARY

Knowledge of the patterns of innervation and the gross and microscopic anatomy of the peripheral nervous system allows the surgeon and the therapist to accurately diagnose and treat patients with peripheral nerve injuries. As more is learned about the details of the anatomy of this system, treatments can be expected to become more predictable and the results of surgery and therapy will continue to improve.

SUGGESTED READING

Mackinnon SE, Dellon AL: *Surgery of the peripheral nerve,* New York, 1988, Thieme Medical Publishers.

Spinner M: *Kaplan's functional and surgical anatomy of the hand,* ed 3, Philadelphia, 1984, JB Lippincott.

Terzis JT, Smith KL: *The peripheral nerve—structure, function and reconstruction,* New York, 1990, Raven Press.

Tubiana R: *Examination of the hand and upper limb,* Philadelphia, 1984, Saunders.

Chapter 3

INTERNAL ANATOMY OF
THE PERIPHERAL NERVE

Michael E. Jabaley

Chapter 2 provides an excellent overall depiction of the nervous system and offers a springboard into the specific internal nature of peripheral nerves. In this chapter the vantage point will be that of the surgeon, but it should be read with the previous chapter in mind. It is written from a more clinical perspective and describes in detail the arrangement of specific nerve components and their importance in the clinical treatment of everyday problems, whether they result from trauma or compression.

The importance of internal anatomy in clinical nerve surgery is presently at its zenith and may become less important in the future (though this is by no means assured). As more is learned about trophic factors that control the nature and routes of regeneration, it is possible that sprouting axons in repaired nerves may be guided by something other than the mechanical efforts of surgeons. For the present, however, the goals of nerve repair can be simply stated: a tension-free juncture between viable nerve ends, held by as few sutures as possible; accurate alignment of fascicles, lying in a healthy, well-vascularized bed; and repair as soon as feasibly possible after injury since this leaves the least amount of time for scarring and degeneration.

The timing of repair always depends on a number of factors, including the nature of the wound, other injured structures, and most important, an assessment of the viability of the nerve ends, so one cannot be dogmatic on this point.

HISTORIC PERSPECTIVE

Early 20th-century anatomists were particularly interested in internal topography, and a number of studies were published which described the fascicular arrangement of various nerves.[12] Studies were of two types: (1) those that considered that "plexuses" of fascicles existed and that there was a constant interchange of nerve fibers between them and (2) those that presumed that there were few interconnections between fascicles and that they pursued more or less separate but parallel paths. There was less debate about the functional significance of plexuses, probably because this seemed of little practical importance at that time.

At the end of World War II, Sir Sydney Sunderland published his study on the internal topography of the radial, median, and ulnar nerves.[9] He examined and explained all of the previous studies that had been published on the subject, commented on their validity, and outlined the controversy. He then presented his detailed studies and effectively ended the debate. It remained for surgeons 25 years later to begin detailed examination of Sunderland's work and consideration of its clinical significance. In the 1980s, publications by many clinicians—Jabaley, Wallace, and Heckler,[5] Williams,[13] Chow et al.,[2] Watchmaker et al.[11]—all confirmed the surgical anatomy of peripheral nerves.

In his 1945 publication, Sunderland made serial sections and histologic examinations of each of the major forearm nerves, working in a distal to proximal direction and using the radial styloid as a reference point (Fig. 3-1). He noted the point of entry in millimeters of each branch from this landmark and followed it as it proceeded proximally until the branch ultimately merged with other fascicles and was no longer identifiable. With these studies, Sunderland documented the constantly changing pattern as fascicles joined or separated from one another, changed their locations, and generally resembled a plexus or network of fascicles. He stressed the plexus aspect of his examinations as typical of many nerves, but he also appreciated that the fibers

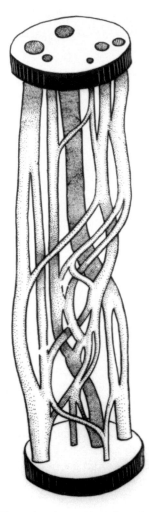

Fig. 3-1. Three-dimensional reconstruction of a 3-cm segment of the human musculocutaneous nerve. In this drawing Sunderland illustrates the "repeatedly uniting and dividing" of fascicles as they engage in plexus formation. (Reproduced with permission from Churchill Livingstone and the late Sir Sydney Sunderland.)

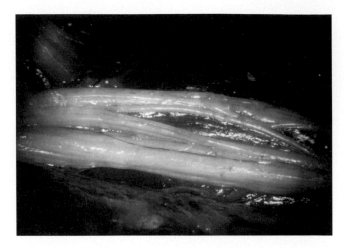

Fig. 3-2. Microscopic view of a partially dissected peripheral nerve. In contrast to the artist's drawing of the interconnections, this photograph shows clearly that individual fascicles may travel for several centimeters with few, if any, interconnections. When such uniting occurs, it can be easily seen.

eventually forming each branch proceeded for relatively long distances in an identifiable pattern and that their locations were more or less predictable as one moved proximally in the nerve. He also noted that plexus simplification occurred in the more distal portions of a nerve.

With the advent of microsurgery and interfascicular nerve grafting,[7] surgeons began to dissect and suture within nerves. Internal topography (or surgical anatomy) assumed a more practical significance. The clinical observations of surgeons working within the major forearm nerves suggested that fascicles could be separated for considerable distances (Fig. 3-2) and could be joined individually or in bundles by nerve grafts or direct suture, concepts at variance with the classic Sunderland illustrations (see Fig. 3-1). These observations prompted a relook at the subject of internal topography, this time by surgical investigators. They concluded that careful dissection was not only possible but that it permitted identification and separation of fascicles, thereby making

reconnection easier, more precise, and (hopefully) more effective.[2,5,11,13] It also allowed for internal neurolysis of chronically compressed nerves in a fashion that had not been previously possible.[3]

In examining the major nerves of the upper extremity, it appeared that the three-dimensional reconstruction of the musculocutaneous nerve that had been published by Sunderland was accurate for that nerve but was by no means typical of all peripheral nerves (as some had assumed). It is now believed that as one proceeds distally in a nerve trunk, fascicles tend to travel in parallel but separate pathways, gradually separating off groups of fibers that mingle with others to form specific branches. These fibers gradually segregate themselves into specific quadrants and move distally in an orderly fashion for some distance with few if any connections to their ultimate branch points. Because the majority of clinical injuries and symptomatic compressions (e.g., carpal tunnel syndrome) occur in the distal portions of extremities, this fact can be used by surgeons to facilitate repair or aid in decompression.

The explanation for the differences observed by Sunderland between the musculocutaneous and other more peripheral nerves seems quite simple: The musculocutaneous nerve, which branches from the lateral cord of the brachial plexus, initially arises from three or four cervical segments. It is a relatively short nerve, containing both motor and sensory fibers, innervating the biceps and brachialis muscles, and sending articular branches to the elbow before continuing distally as the lateral antebrachial cutaneous nerve. Fibers for these separate functions must segregate themselves in a relatively short distance to form these specific branches. This progressive segregation of fibers requires the sorting and intermingling of plexuses, which Sunderland correctly observed.

It has now been over 50 years since publication of Sunderland's study on internal topography. In addition to his concepts, the cross-sectional maps of the upper extremity nerves have been reproduced many times and serve as guides to investigators studying this area and surgeons operating within it. Sunderland's and other such studies comprise the major tome of peripheral nerve surgery, *Nerves and Nerve Injuries.*[10] The publication went through two editions in Sunderland's lifetime and, in this day of multiauthored textbooks, stands as a monument to the efforts of a single man.

PRACTICAL ANATOMY

What we call a *peripheral nerve* is, in fact, the long extension of cells that lie in the spinal cord, either in the dorsal root ganglia (sensory nerves) or in the anterior horn (motor nerves). These fibers may be long (up to several feet) and reach from the cell bodies to either sensory receptors or motor end plates of muscle. It is the meandering of these individual fibers as they arrange themselves in fascicles and prepare to exit through specific branches that accounts for the plexus formation described in the previous section.

An example of the functional consequences of this arrangement can be seen in the sensory nervous system. Specialized sensory receptors lie at the ends of these fibers in the dermis of the skin, the interface between the internal environment of the body and the outside world. It is here that the transduction of external stimuli into nerve impulses occurs. Volleys of impulses are generated at these distal levels and proceed proximally, first along branches, then in fascicles and finally to several segments of the spinal cord, where they continue centrally along specific tracts to the brain. It is in the brain that these sensory impulses, measurable as action potentials, eventually are elevated to the conscious level. Surgical repair and regeneration are limited to the afferent and efferent fibers of nerve cells. The remainder of the system is beyond the reach of surgeons.

A peripheral nerve is comprised of two parts: those portions that conduct the aforementioned impulses and those parts that perform a structural or supportive role. The conducting portions (axons and their Schwann cells) are derivatives of ectoderm, while all of the nonconducting portions arise from mesoderm. Mesodermal tissue, including epineurium and perineurium, serves several functions; it is supportive, structural, and nutritional, and it contains the circulation of the nerve. It is also the source of scarring when a nerve is injured.

It is important to keep in mind that mesodermal structures contain fibroblasts and the other cells necessary for collagen formation and wound healing. When injured, this portion of a nerve goes through the familiar sequence of inflammation, fibroplasia, and scar formation. The nerve fibers (ectodermal elements), on the other hand, restore themselves by regenerating along the Schwann cell tubes until they reach their termination. This intensely active metabolic process begins

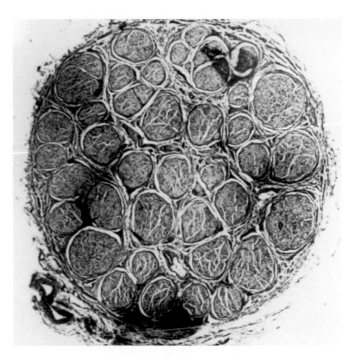

Fig. 3-3. A transverse section of a human median nerve, mid-forearm level. Individual fascicles, bound by perineurium, are of varying size. Some occur separately, surrounded by internal epineurium (2-4 o'clock). Others are in bundles of two or more fascicles (11-12 o'clock). All are encompassed by external epineurium, the investing layer of the nerve. A blood vessel in epineurium can be seen at 7 o'clock.

in the nerve cell body (which may be some distance from the injury) where axoplasmic flow and elongation of axons are stimulated. Restoration of function requires that regenerating fibers find their way into appropriate distal segments and that they reach appropriate end organs.

Individual fascicles or bundles of fascicles can be seen when examining the cut end of a peripheral nerve with the naked eye or low power magnification (Fig. 3-3). Some bundles may contain two to four fascicles, each encircled by a clearly defined perineurium. Perineurium is a strong, well-organized, relatively tight, laminated structure whose fibers run in different directions, much like the plies of an automobile tire.[1] It is the skeletal structure that separates the internal environment of the nerve from the external milieu. Perineurium also serves as a differential barrier, and the concentration of ions within the perineurium is quite different from the outside. There is a positive pressure inside perineurium, and surgeons are familiar with the resultant bulge of axoplasm that occurs when a fascicle is transected.

Within the perineurium are the nerve fibers themselves as well as their Schwann sheaths, both lying within the endoneurium. Fibers may be either myelinated or unmyelinated, but both require a strictly controlled chemical environment to function properly. One of the roles of perineurium is the maintenance of this environment, and conduction is severely impaired when it is injured.

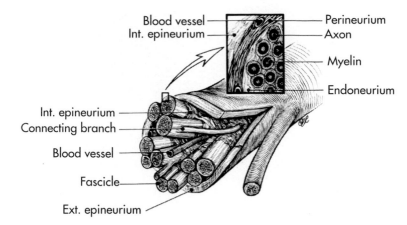

Fig. 3-4. Artist's rendition of a partially dissected nerve. Individual and groups of fascicles are shown within the partially opened epineurium. The insert is a magnified drawing of a portion of a single fascicle. The perineurium surrounds the contents. The conducting mechanism of the nerve consists of both myelinated and unmyelinated axons, lying within endoneurium. (Illustration by Elizabeth Roselius, 1991. Reprinted with permission from Gelberman RH: *Operative nerve repair and reconstruction,* Philadelphia, 1991, JB Lippincott.)

Surrounding the entire nerve is the epineurium, a more loosely organized adventitia-like structure that blends subtly into surrounding tissue (Fig. 3-4). Epineurium can be described as either external or internal epineurium, depending on its location. Internal epineurium lies between the fascicles, well within the nerve, while the external epineurium encircles the nerve and blends loosely with the surrounding adventitia. It is important to recognize the presence of both internal and external epineurium because it is the material which holds sutures in either an external epineurial (whole nerve suture) or in a group fascicular repair (see Fig. 11-1). The two are a continuum, and location determines their name.

CONTEMPORARY VIEW

In 1945, when Sunderland documented the fascicular arrangement of the major nerves of both the upper and lower extremities, he concluded that the longest section of any nerve with an unchanging internal pattern was 1.5 cm.[9] He observed, however, that fibers traveled for greater distances with little or no change in their overall position. In other words, they remained in the same quadrant of the nerve for much longer distances.

Beginning in the late 1970s, investigations were undertaken to ascertain what the practical significance of this information might be.[5] The serial section technique of Sunderland was repeated, noting carefully the entry point of each nerve and following it as far proximally as possible. These data were complimented with dissections of fresh cadaver extremities, in which the entry point of branches into a main trunk were noted and surgical separation carried out for as far as possible without transecting any interconnecting fibers. These interconnections were readily identifiable, so the end points were easily measured. In this way, the *dissection distances* (the distance within a nerve that a

branch can be traced before reaching the first interconnection) for each branch of all the major nerves between the hand and elbow were measured (Fig. 3-5). These data generally agreed with the previously published figures of both Sunderland and Seddon and are available for use in clinical nerve surgery.[8,10]

It is important to appreciate that dissection distances for any given branch vary from patient to patient and that they may even be different in the two extremities of the same patient. Nevertheless, they serve as guides which can be helpful to the surgeon in dealing with transected nerves. Since 1980, these data have been corroborated by other investigators using the same and similar techniques, so there seems to be little doubt about their validity.[2,11,13] A summary of the observations on each of the major forearm nerves follows.

INTERNAL TOPOGRAPHY OF SPECIFIC UPPER EXTREMITY NERVES
Radial nerve

Of the three major upper extremity nerves, the radial nerve terminates one joint more proximal, a point of clinical importance both in clinical handling and prognosis. Just below the elbow, the radial nerve separates into the posterior interosseous nerve (PIN) and the superficial radial nerve (SRN). The PIN is largely a motor nerve to the extensors of the wrist, fingers, and thumb, but it also contains sensory fibers to the wrist joint. The SRN is a pure sensory nerve to the thenar web and dorsal surfaces of the thumb, index, and long fingers.

Beginning below the elbow level, the terminal radial nerve can be separated proximally into its two major branches for a distance of 70 to 90 mm, approximately to the junction of the middle and distal thirds of the upper arm. Both of these nerves occupy predictable locations in the

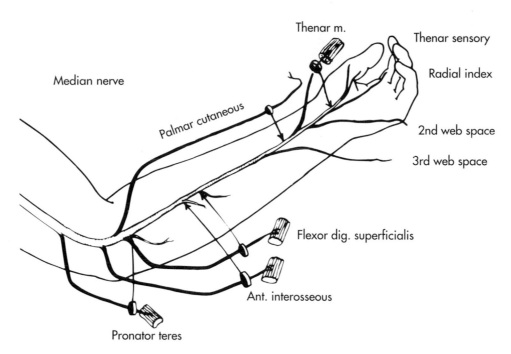

Fig. 3-5. Median nerve dissection distances. Some of the branches of the median nerve are illustrated in their dissected state. The ring and arrow on four branches show the original point of exit from the main trunk of the nerve. The branch is shown as a solid line, and the distance over which it can be separated without damaging connecting branches (the dissection distance) is shown. Interconnections with other fascicles occur where the branch joins the main trunk of the median nerve. (From Jabaley ME, Wallace WH, Heckler FR: Internal topography of major nerves of the forearm and hand: a current view, *J Hand Surg* 1980; 5:1-18.)

radial nerve trunk, making their separation relatively simple and their identification straightforward. If a transection occurs about the elbow, they can be correctly aligned and separately joined, either by direct suture or interfascicular nerve graft.

Interconnections between fascicles and separation becomes more difficult farther in the radial nerve in the upper arm, but the quadrantic relationship continues in a predictable fashion even further proximally. Sunderland noted that there are relatively few fascicles in the radial nerve in the upper arm, observing as few as one to three at the mid-humeral level. This may partly explain the much better prognosis for radial nerve injuries at this level compared to median and ulnar nerve transections.

Median nerve

A brief description of the median nerve is given from distal to proximal, emphasizing the dissection distances in areas of clinical importance (see Fig. 3-5). The sensory branches from the thumb, index, long, and ring fingers all fuse and are joined by the thenar motor branch at the level of the transverse carpal ligament. In most cases, the motor branch enters on the radial side of the nerve and occupies a radiopalmar position. As one proceeds proximally, motor fibers are gradually dispersed among other fascicles. The dissection distance for the motor branch of the median nerve averaged 84 mm in our cases, but they can sometimes be

shorter. The common digital nerves can be separated from each other for 40 to 90 mm although their fibers remain identifiable somewhat more proximal. Thus, fiber matching in the distal median nerve can be achieved for several centimeters. Beyond these distances, one must rely on alternative techniques to make the best possible union between groups of fascicles. This can be done by isolating fascicles as far as possible, noting their position relative to the whole nerve, and comparing to the cross-sectional maps of Sunderland.

As one proceeds more proximally in the median nerve, the next branch encountered is the palmar cutaneous branch. It may arise as one or two separate branches, usually containing one fascicle each. This branch commonly arises on the radial side, 20 to 30 mm proximal to the radial styloid, and remains quite discrete and well-localized along the radial border of the nerve for about 60 to 120 mm before the fibers merge into other fascicles of the median nerve. The palmar cutaneous branch can be easily separated from the median nerve in injuries at this level. It can (and should) be separately repaired because sensation to the proximal palm and thenar eminence can usually be restored. When specific branches of a terminal nerve can be identified for separate repair, the likelihood of functional recovery is measurably increased, other factors being equal.

No other branches exit from the median nerve in the mid forearm and the next area of fascicular activity is in the proximal one-third, just distal to the elbow. At this level, the anterior interosseus nerve exits the main trunk as do the branches to the other forearm flexor muscles. The pronator teres, flexor digitorum superficialis, and profundus branches are usually identifiable and can be followed for 45 to 140 mm within the nerve. The anterior interosseus nerve, remains a separate and identifiable structure within the median nerve proper for a distance of 50 to 150 mm. These branches can be separately joined in tidy wounds about the elbow.

Ulnar nerve

Like its functional role, the topographic anatomy of the ulnar nerve is quite different and distinct from that of the median nerve. In some ways it resembles the radial nerve or the sciatic nerve in the leg. Like the radial nerve, there is a clear separation between the motor and the sensory components in the palm and wrist. The sensory portion is comprised of the ulnar digital nerve of the small finger and the common digital nerve to the fourth web space. When these two join (as the terminal sensory portion), they remain separable for a distance of 25 to 30 mm within the main ulnar sensory trunk. In Guyon's canal they merge with the deep motor branch, containing fibers from most of the intrinsic muscles in the hand. This motor portion crosses dorsal to the sensory component and occupies a dorsi-ulnar position in the trunk of the ulnar nerve proper. The motor and sensory portions are bound within a common external epineurium, but they remain clearly separable for approximately 80 to 90 mm (as the motor and sensory portions of the radial nerve in the upper arm do).

As the terminal portions of the ulnar nerve proceed proximally, they are joined by the dorsal cutaneous branch (a "branch" that is actually separated from the rest of the ulnar nerve in the forearm). The ulnar nerve and dorsal cutaneous nerve travel in the same epineurium, but many dissections have shown them to be anatomically separate and identifiable for 170 to 200 mm from their point of union. The anatomic character of the dorsal cutaneous nerve is similar (though not its functional makeup) to the tibial and peroneal nerves in the leg. They travel the length of the posterior thigh in a common sheath as the terminal portion of the sciatic nerve, but there are no interconnections.

Because of the profound functional differences, it is wise to separate the dorsal cutaneous nerve from the ulnar nerve proper in the forearm and repair them separately. Likewise, the dorsal cutaneous nerve can be used as a donor for nerve grafting if it is irreparably injured and cannot be repaired.

The next area of branching activity in the ulnar nerve is at the elbow level, where motor branches to the flexor carpi ulnaris and half the flexor digitorum profundus muscles arise. These usually separate individually although a common trunk is sometimes seen. The motor branches can be separated from the main trunk for 75 to 90 mm, well above the elbow joint. With this information, surgeons who transfer the ulnar nerve to a more anterior position can safely do so

without fear of injuring these branches. In sharp transections at this level, repairs of motor branches can be successful (if they can be found) because of the short distances to the target muscles. When they can be identified (e.g., in acute cases), motor branches should be sutured separately.

DISCUSSION

In the past 50 years, little new information has come forth about internal topography, but its surgical importance and study have received great impetus from the technologic advances that have occurred. The subject has moved from the realm of anatomic interest only to one of clinical significance. The recent studies by hand surgeons have now confirmed the data originally promulgated by Sunderland and Seddon,[8,10] and its use in everyday nerve surgery is on solid ground. Based on these interpretations, the following points may be valuable to those undertaking nerve repair or decompression.

In virtually all clinical settings in the extremities, nerve branches can be expected to remain separable and identifiable for variable but significant distances proximal to their exit point, and their fibers occupy the same general location within the whole nerve for even greater distances as they proceed proximally. Knowledge of these dissection distances and quadrantic locations serves as the basis for internal dissection and allows for more accurate alignment in repair, either by direct suture or by nerve grafting.

In internal neurolysis at either the wrist or elbow, an appreciation of internal makeup makes the procedure easier and safer. It is now clear that there are instances where the external epineurium itself may be scarred and may be the constricting structure of its encased fascicles.[3] In such cases, it can be incised and the underlying bundles can be separated, so long as perineurium is not violated. When neurolysis is done, surgeons should recognize that scar formation is stimulated and that ultimate success and clinical improvement depend on other factors, including postoperative therapy, gliding exercises, and the circulation of the bed in which the nerve lies.

Dissection within a nerve is made easier by the knowledge of what those dissection distances might be for the branch in question. For example, the secondary repair of a median nerve transection at the wrist often begins with identification of the motor branch in the carpal canal. That branch might be separated off from the other branches in the distal segment for separate repair. In the proximal stump, the motor branch may no longer be separable but may still be identifiable by its location within the nerve trunk. Experience with awake stimulation has shown that this location can be confirmed in the compliant patient.[4] Thus, the surgeon has several guides for fiber localization: direct dissection of individual branches, electrical recordings of nerve action potentials, and direct electrical stimulation in awake patients, as well as the cross-sectional maps of Sunderland[10] and others. Each time functionally identifiable components are identified and joined after these maneuvers, the likelihood of a correct anatomic connection of the remaining nerve is increased.

It should be pointed out once again that the practical importance of a knowledge of internal topography is in rejoining transected ends by suture or interfascicular grafts. These techniques remain the standard of care for the present time, but the reader should be aware that this situation may not always pertain and that trophic factors may lessen or relieve the surgeon of some obligation to make unions in the future. Topographic identification and manual connection are not the ideal repair, but for the present, they are the best options available. Should trophic control and sutureless repair ever become a reality, the surgeon may have a biologic ally in obtaining correct fascicular lineups.[6] These thoughts are expanded in Chapter 11.

REFERENCES

1. Bunge MB, Wood PM, Tynan LB, et al: Perineurium originates from fibroblasts: demonstration in vitro with a retroviral marker, *Science* 1989; 243:229-231.
2. Chow JA, Van Beek AL, Meyer DL, Johnson MC: Surgical significance of the motor fascicular group of the ulnar nerve in the forearm, *J Hand Surg* 1985; 10A:867-872.
3. Curtis RM, Eversmann WW: Internal neurolysis as an adjunct to the treatment of carpal tunnel syndrome, *J Bone Joint Surg* 1973; 55A:733.
4. Jabaley ME: Electrical stimulation in the awake patient, *Bull Hosp Joint Dis* 1984; 44:248.
5. Jabaley ME, Wallace WH, Heckler FR: Internal topography of major nerves of the forearm and hand: a current view, *J Hand Surg* 1980; 5:1-18.
6. Lundborg G: *Nerve injury and repair,* Edinburgh, 1988, Churchill Livingstone.
7. Millesi H, Meissl G, Berger A: The interfascicular nerve-grafting of the median and ulnar nerves, *J Bone Joint Surg* 1972; 54A:727-750.
8. Seddon HJ: *Surgical disorders of the peripheral nerves,* Baltimore, 1972, Williams & Wilkins.
9. Sunderland S: The internal topography of the radial, median, and ulnar nerves, *Brain* 1945; 68:243-298.
10. Sunderland S: *Nerves and nerve injuries,* ed 2, Edinburgh, 1978, Churchill Livingstone.
11. Watchmaker GP, Gumucio CA, Crandall RE, et al: Fascicular topography of the median nerve: a computer-based study to identify branching patterns, *J Hand Surg* 1991; 16A:53-59.
12. Watchmaker GP, Jabaley ME: Topographic anatomy of peripheral nerves. In Omer GE, Spinner M, Van Beek AL, eds: *Management of peripheral nerve problems,* ed 2, Boston, Saunders (in press).
13. Williams HB: Peripheral nerve injuries in children. In Kernahan D, Thompson HG, Bauer B, eds: *Pediatric plastic surgery,* St Louis, 1982, Mosby.

Chapter 4

NERVE REGENERATION AFTER INJURY

Newer approaches to improving nerve regeneration

Gary K. Frykman

It has only been since the World War II era that peripheral nerves have been widely repaired. The classic studies of following large populations of nerve injuries performed by Seddon in England,[34] Sunderland in Australia,[39] and Woodhall and Beebe[46] in the United States have provided the basis for understanding the expected results from repair of peripheral nerve injuries by standard suture techniques from simple sharp injuries to complex war wounds. The results of these classic nerve repairs have frequently given less than ideal results.[34,39,46] Complete recovery following peripheral nerve suture is rare, except in children. Many so-called improved techniques of nerve repair have been tried over the past five decades. Improvements in results often have been only incremental. The expected improvement by better technical repairs using the operating microscope have shown at best modest improvement over conventional repairs.[7,13,25]

This chapter presents some of the newer approaches that are currently being used in the repair of peripheral nerve injuries. Technical improvements will be covered first and other techniques such as using biochemical manipulation of the nerve regeneration environment, using various tubules, stimulating nerve regeneration electrically, and combining some techniques studied experimentally and clinically will be examined.

NERVE REGENERATION REQUIREMENTS

Successful peripheral nerve regeneration has the following four requirements[16]:

1. The central cell body or neuron has to survive. Certain very proximal nerve injuries, such as nerve root and brachial plexus injuries, will kill the anterior horn cells and the dorsal root ganglion cells.
2. Axonal sprouting occurs from the proximal nerve, and the axons must grow into an environment that is conducive to nerve regeneration. The best naturally occurring environment for axonal growth is the distal nerve stump.
3. Appropriate distal connection of the regenerating axon has to occur (e.g., the motor axon, as it grows peripherally, has to connect to a motor end plate, or the distal growth of the axon will be wasted). Likewise, sensory axons can connect to only sensory end organs to give useful regeneration. Inappropriate distal connection is a reason mixed nerves do not regenerate as completely as pure sensory or motor nerves.
4. The appropriate central nervous system (CNS) understanding and integration of the peripheral nerve signal has to occur (e.g., the CNS, when axon regeneration is mixed up, has to be able to adapt to or learn what the new pattern of afferent signals mean). The brain must process the signals and send the appropriate messages back to the peripheral nervous system that will result in useful function.

SPECIFICITY

How specific is peripheral axonal growth following injury? Studies in the 1940s failed to show that there really

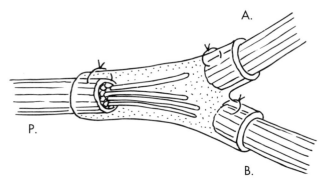

Fig. 4-1. Silicone Y chamber model. *P* is the proximal nerve. The *A* and *B* limbs are for distal tissues or nerves. More axons are growing toward *B* than *A*. (From Frykman GK: The quest for better recovery from peripheral nerve injury: current status of nerve regeneration research, *J Hand Ther* 1993; 6[2]:83-88; with permission.)

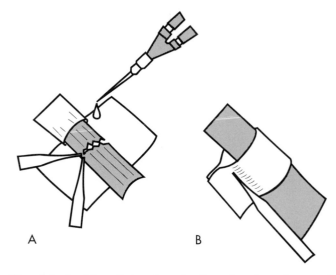

Fig. 4-2. Applying fibrin glue. **A.** Dropping the mixture of thrombin and fibrinogen onto the nerve junction site. **B.** A wrap is used to keep the low viscosity drops about the nerve junction until the fibrin clot forms.

was much specificity of nerve growth. For example, Weiss and Taylor,[42] were able only to find that the proximal nerve stump does prefer a distal nerve stump for a regenerating environment as opposed to tendon, bone, or other tissue. This tissue specificity has been identified, but they were unable to show any other specificity such as topographic or end organ specificity. Recent studies have supported other specificities. One experimental model to study specificities uses a Y chamber and puts the proximal end of a divided nerve into the proximal limb of the Y chamber and puts different nerves distally (Fig. 4-1). If the peroneal nerve of a rat is divided, and the distal peroneal nerve is placed in one end of the Y chamber and the tibial nerve is placed in the other limb, regenerating axons are allowed to "choose" which distal stump limb to grow toward. Seckel et al.[32] showed that the peroneal nerve axons tend to grow more toward the peroneal nerve. This study indicates there is some topographic specificity. There is evidence for at least some end organ specificity (e.g., the motor axon proximally tends to grow toward a motor nerve distally in preference to a sensory nerve distally[5,6]). So there is perhaps better specificity than previously thought. The mechanisms for specificities are not well understood. Since the specificity studies have been done in experimental animals, there is considerable uncertainty on how much specificity carries over to humans.

IMPROVING NERVE REGENERATION
Central approaches

The CNS adapts to the afferent signals from the injured nerve and sends the signals that go back. How the CNS changes is still not well understood. This process of CNS change is termed central plasticity (i.e., the brain is able to learn and adapt). Studies by Merzenich and Jenkins[26] have shown definite remodeling in the somatosensory cortex of the brain by different peripheral nerve manipulations, such as stimulating a certain area of the body peripherally, will make the cortical representation of that sensory area in the

brain actually grow larger. Conversely, if a finger is cut off or a nerve is cut and not allowed to regenerate, that area represented in the sematosensory cortex will decrease in size perhaps in response to less signals coming from the injured nerve. The brain seems to be adapting and changing, indicating somewhat of a competitive or fluid environment in the brain that accounts for central plasticity. Certainly central plasticity is much greater in infants and children than it is in adults. This is probably a major reason children experience better nerve regeneration than adults. It probably has very little to do with how well the peripheral nerve axons regenerate. Central plasticity is advantageous in applying a sensory reeducation program.[9,25]

Peripheral approaches

Approaches can be classified as technical, electrical, biochemical, or some combination.

Technical methods. It has been found that if a typical epineurial repair of the outer epineurial layer of a divided nerve is performed, it is like sewing together two tubes full of wet noodles. Instead of end-to-end apposition of the fascicles, they tend to be rather haphazardly distributed.[13] For instance, the cross-section of a peripheral nerve repair site reveals that the side of a proximal fascicle may be aligned with the end of a distal fascicle and vice versa. Nerves *do* regenerate in spite of this jumbled condition at a nerve repair site. Because of fascicular disorder at the epineurial suture site and the availability of the operating microscope, it seemed logical to do repairs of the individual fascicles or groups of fascicles to obtain better fascicular alignment and apposition.[43] Fascicle repairs have been done for a number of years, and there is some improvement, but the improvement has been modest at best. Repairing the

Silicone chamber

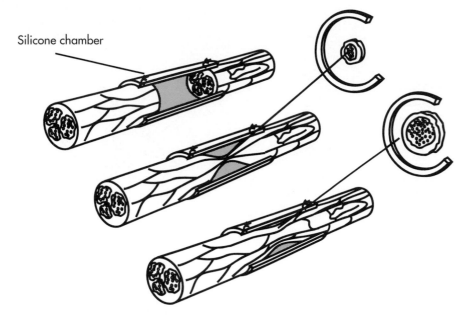

Fig. 4-3. Silicone chamber. A time sequence of a tube of silicone with the proximal and distal nerve stumps inserted with a gap provides an environment that attracts growth of axons across it. If not too great a distance, the gap will fill with axons.

groups of fascicles is most commonly done.[43] Individual fascicle repair is more difficult and tedious, and very few peripheral nerve surgeons do individual fascicle repairs. Tupper[40] has performed a sizable series of these repairs of median and ulnar nerves, and he has demonstrated they are somewhat better. However, he is still not enthusiastic about doing individual fascicular repair on a large multifasciculated nerve like a median nerve at the wrist, which has anywhere from about 40 to 100 fascicles.[40] There is a risk that putting in one to two sutures per fascicle may cause more scarring at the suture site. The present-day operating microscopes are very adequate for maximum magnification for fascicular repairs.

Nerve glue. There is considerable interest in gluing nerves together. The attempts to glue nerves together with fibrin clot began in the 1940s.[47] At present some surgeons are using a combination of fibrinogen and thrombin. If fibrinogen and thrombin contained in two different syringes are injected through a single needle, the drop that is produced will polymerize quickly into a fibrin clot—the natural glue of the vascular system. In Europe surgeons have been using fibrin glue for a number of years and found that it is faster than suturing nerves together.[12] Narakas[27] has published that it is about three times faster than suturing. In Narakas' published series, they obtained about 15% to 20% improved results over suturing nerve grafts. It is not commercially available in the United States yet because of fear of blood-borne disease transmission such as acquired immunodeficiency syndrome (AIDS) and hepatitis.[12,27] Patients can provide their own fibrin glue by donating their own unit of blood, and the blood bank prepares cryoprecipitate, which

is mostly fibrinogen. This can be placed in one syringe while another syringe holds commercially available thrombin. The contents of both syringes are injected through a single needle, and in a few seconds a fibrin clot will be obtained (Fig. 4-2). Another advantage of using fibrin is that fibrin is a neurotrophic factor that attracts axonal growth.[45]

Lasers. Lasers are a new technology in search of applications. Almquist and others have studied lasers and used many different types of lasers.[1,15,29] Using small fibrin strips and a laser beam, a nerve can be welded together. Another way is to weld the epineurium by using the laser directly on the site of apposition. At least a couple of epineurial sutures still have to be placed to properly orient the nerve. It is an attractive idea to weld the epineurium together, and the axons will grow across. One technical danger is that too deep a coagulation of the nerve may damage axons. It is doubtful that lasers will improve nerve regeneration, but with technical improvements it may be faster than the conventional suture.

Tubes. Lundborg,[22,23] among others, has had an interest in using tubes since he found that in a silicone tube into which the cut ends of a nerve are inserted with a small gap between the ends, the axons will grow across the gap. Analysis of the fluid between the nerve ends shows fibrin and other neurotrophic factors. With time the gap will fill up as the axons readily grow across a gap up to 1 cm (Fig. 4-3). In fact, Lundborg found that regeneration was even better than suturing in some instances. An interesting aspect of regeneration in a larger nerve treated this way is that the axons that grow across the gap will separate into individual fascicles across a gap like this. He is currently doing a prospective clinical series in Sweden comparing silicone tubes with suturing median and ulnar nerves at the wrist. Preliminary results show little difference in the results.[21] One concern with silicone and other nonabsorbable tubes is the possibility of long-term tolerance of the body to foreign material. There is an additional concern for compression of the nerve from the tube and the need for surgical removal. Many different materials have been tried over the years, including naturally occurring tubes such as collagen.[24,38] An attractive idea is to experimentally use a bioresorbable tube made out of suture materials such as polyglycolic acid and polylactate.[4,41] They have low reactivity to the body and are readily absorbed because they are not needed after regeneration has occurred. Absorbable nonreactive off-the-shelf tubes for nerve repair remain an attractive goal.

Muscle grafts. Muscle grafts as a substitute for nerve grafts have been studied mostly in England.[17] Why use a muscle for nerve graft? Muscle fibers are tubular structures that are rich in laminin and fibronectin, which both attract axonal growth and thus stimulate axons to grow along a muscle fiber. A published series of digital nerves in humans, using muscle grafts, shows that the results are better than those for direct nerve repair.[31] One advantage of using a muscle as a graft is that the deficit is negligible after harvesting a small section of muscle. In contrast, harvesting a sensory nerve as a graft will leave a variable sensory deficit.

Altering the environment. How can we alter the environment of nerve regeneration? There are many neurotrophic factors, hormones, neurite promoting factors, and other factors that are now becoming well known. These can be studied by looking in a silicone chamber at the various factors, analyzing them, and perhaps putting them back in the environment of the nerve ends[8,23] (Fig. 4-4). Nerve

growth factor, the best characterized one, has been known for many years.[20] It stimulates sensory and sympathetic neurite outgrowth.[14,30] It does not have any effect on motor nerves. Many other factors have been found,[8,18] including motor nerve growth factor[37] and ciliary neurotrophic factor.[35] Hormones also affect nerve regeneration.[3,33] Their mode of action is outside their classic endocrinologic function. Laminin and fibronectin are also neurite promoting factors.[19,33] Matrix factors such as fibrin are very strong attractants to axonal growth.[44]

Electrical fields. Electrical field stimulation is still being studied. There have been many studies done, using both direct currents[2] and electromagnetic fields[28,36] with several different signals, but there is nothing available of practical value yet. Perhaps in the future the type of signal that will enhance nerve regeneration will be elucidated.

Combination. deMedinaceli has proposed using cell surgery.[11] His technique uses a very sharp glass knife to cut the nerve, which is locally frozen under a physiologic solution. He found that the rat's nerves regenerated better.[11] There is at least one series of human nerve repairs that shows that nerves repaired by cell surgery have better regeneration.[10]

New bioresorbable tubes may become a technical advance. There are other avenues mentioned in the electrical or biochemical area or a combination procedure (e.g., cell surgery) that give cause for some optimism that nerve regeneration will be improved using one or more of these new techniques in the future.

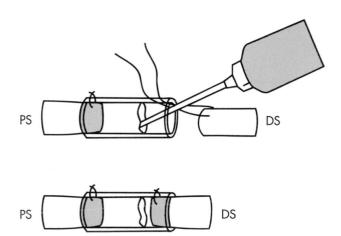

Fig. 4-4. Silicone tube can be used to collect and analyze the fluid between the nerve ends and as a model to alter the concentration of various neurotrophic factors to study the effects on nerve regeneration. (*PS,* Proximal stump of nerve; *DS,* distal stump of nerve.)

REFERENCES

1. Almquist EE: Nerve repair by laser, *Orthop Clin North Am* 1988; 19:201-208.
2. Beveridge JA, Politis MJ: Use of exogenous electric current in the treatment of delayed lesions in peripheral nerves, *Plast Reconstr Surg* 1988; 82(4):573-577.
3. Bijlsma WA, Jennekens FGI, Schotman P, Gispen WH: Neurotrophic factors and regeneration in the peripheral nervous system, *Psychoneuroendocrinology* 1984; 9(3):199-215 (review).
4. Bora FW Jr, Bednar JM, Osterman AL, et al: Prosthetic nerve grafts: a resorbable tube as an alternative to autogenous nerve grafting, *J Hand Surg* 1987; 12A:685-692.
5. Brushart TM: Preferential reinnervation of motor nerves by regenerating motor axons, *J Neurosci* 1988; 8(3):1026-1031.
6. Brushart TM, Seiler WA IV: Selective reinnervation of distal motor stumps by peripheral motor axons, *Exp Neurol* 1987; 97:289-300.
7. Cabaud HE, Rodkey WG, McCarroll HR, et al: Epineurial and perineurial fascicular nerve repairs: a critical comparison, *J Hand Surg* 1976; 1:131-137.
8. Cordeiro PG, Seckel BR, Lipton SA, et al: Acidic fibroblast growth factor enhances peripheral nerve regeneration in vivo, *Plast Reconstr Surg* 1989; 83(6):1013-1019.
9. Dellon AL: *Evaluation of sensibility and reeducation of sensation in the hand,* Baltimore, 1981, Williams & Wilkins.
10. deMedinaceli L, Merle M: Applying "cell surgery" to nerve repair: a preliminary report on the first ten human cases, *J Hand Surg* 1991; 16B(5):499-503.
11. deMedinaceli L, Wyatt RJ, Freed WJ: Peripheral nerve reconnection: mechanical, thermal, and ionic conditions that promote the return of function, *Exp Neurol* 1983; 81:469-487.

12. Diao E, Peimer CA: Sutureless methods of nerve repair. In Gelberman RH, ed: *Operative nerve repair and reconstruction,* New York, 1991, JB Lippincott.

13. Edshage S: Peripheral nerve suture: a technique for improved intraneural topography evaluation of some materials, *Acta Chir Scand* 1964; (suppl 331):75.

14. Fernandez, E, Pallini R, Mercanti D: Effects of topically administered nerve growth factor on axonal regeneration in peripheral nerve autografts implanted in the spinal cord of rats, *Neurosurgery* 1990; 26:37-42.

15. Fischer DW, Beggs JL, Kuishalo DL Jr, Shetter AG: Comparative study of micro-epineurial anastomosis with the use of CO_2 laser and suture technique in rat sciatic nerves, part 1, *Neurosurgery* 1985; 17:300-308.

16. Frykman GK: The quest for better recovery from peripheral nerve injury: current status of nerve regeneration research, *J Hand Ther* 1993; 6(2):83.

17. Glasby MA, Gschmeissner SE, Huang C, DeSouza BA: Degenerated muscle grafts used for peripheral nerve repair in primates, *J Hand Surg* 1986; 11B:347-351.

18. Hansson HA, Dahlin LB, Danielsen N, et al: Evidence indicating trophic importance of IGF-1 in regenerating peripheral nerves, *Acta Physiol Scand* 1986; 126:609-614.

19. Lander AD: Molecules that make axons grow, *Mol Neurobiol* 1987; 1:213-245.

20. Levi-Montalcini R: The nerve growth factor: thirty-five years later. *EMBO J* 1987; 6(5):1145-1154.

21. Lundborg G, Rosen B, Dahlin L, Holmberg J: *Tubular vs. conventional repair of median and ulnar nerves in the human forearm.* Read at Am Soc for Surgery of the Hand. Annual Meeting, San Francisco, Sept. 14, 1995.

22. Lundborg G, Dahlin LB, Danielsen N, et al: Nerve regeneration across an extended gap: a neurobiological view of nerve repair and the possible involvement of neuronotrophic factors, *J Hand Surg* 1982; 67:580-587.

23. Lundborg G, Dahlin LB, Danielsen N, et al: Nerve regeneration in silicone chambers: influence of gap length and of distal stump components, *Exp Neurol* 1982; 76:361-375.

24. Mackinnon SE, Dellon AL: A study of nerve regeneration across synthetic (Maxon) and biologic (collagen) nerve conduits for nerve gaps up to 5 cm in the primate, *J Reconstr Microsurg* 1990; 6:117-121.

25. Mackinnon SE, Dellon AL: *Surgery of the peripheral nerve,* New York, 1988, Thieme.

26. Merzenich MM, Jenkins WM: Reorganization of cortical representations of the hand following alterations of skin inputs induced by nerve injury, skin island transfers and experience, *J Hand Ther* 1993; 6(2):89.

27. Narakas A: The use of fibrin glue in repair of peripheral nerves, *Orthop Clin North Am* 1988; 19:187-199.

28. Orgel MG, O'Brien WJ, Murray HM: Pulsing electromagnetic field therapy in nerve regeneration: an experimental study in the cat, *Plast Reconstr Surg* 1984; 73:173-182.

29. Osedo M: An experimental study on nerve repair using carbon dioxide laser, *J Jpn Orthop Assoc* 1988; 62:653-663.

30. Owen DJ, Logan A, Robinson PP: A role for nerve growth factor in collateral reinnervation from sensory nerves in the guinea pig, *Brain Res* 1989; 476:248-255.

31. Pereira JH, Bowden REM, Gattuso JM, Norris RW: Comparison of results of repair of digital nerves by denatured muscle grafts and end-to-end sutures, *J Hand Surg* 1991; 16B:519-523.

32. Seckel BR, Ryan SE, Gagne RG, et al: Target-specific nerve regeneration through a nerve guide in the rat, *Plast Reconstr Surg* 1986; 78:793-798.

33. Seckel BR: Enhancement of peripheral nerve regeneration, *Muscle Nerve* 1990; 13:785-800.

34. Seddon HJ, ed: *Peripheral nerve injuries.* Medical Research Council Special Report Series, No. 282, London, 1954, Her Majesty's Stationery Office.

35. Sendtner M, Kreutzberg GW, Thoenen H: Ciliary neurotrophic factor presents the degeneration of motor neurons after axotomy, *Nature* 1990; 345:440-441.

36. Sisken BF: Effects of electromagnetic field on nerve regeneration. In Marino AA, ed: *Modern bioelectricity,* New York, 1988, Marcel Dekker.

37. Slack JR, Hopkins WG, Pockett S: Evidence for a motor nerve growth factor, *Muscle Nerve* 1983; 6:243-252.

38. Suematsu N: Tubulation for peripheral nerve gap: its history and possibility, *Microsurgery* 1989; 10:71-74.

39. Sunderland S: *Nerves and nerve injuries,* ed 2, New York, 1978, Churchill Livingstone.

40. Tupper JW, Crick JC, Matteck LR: Fascicular repairs: a comparative study of epineurial and fascicular (perineurial) techniques, *Orthop Clin North Am* 1988; 19:57-69.

41. Urban MA, Bora FW Jr: Nerve grafting through resorbable tubes. In Gelberman RH, ed: *Operative nerve repair and reconstruction,* Philadelphia, 1991, JB Lippincott.

42. Weiss P, Taylor AC: Further experimental evidence against "neurotropism" in nerve regeneration, *J Exp Zool* 1944; 95:233-257.

43. Wilgis EFS: Techniques of epineurial and group fascicular repair. In Gelberman RH, ed: *Operative nerve repair and reconstruction,* Philadelphia, 1991, JB Lippincott.

44. Williams LR, Danielsen N, Muller H, Varon S: Influence of the acellular fibrin matrix on nerve regeneration success within the silicone chamber model. In Gordon T, Stein RB, Smith PA, eds: *Neurology and neurobiology: the current status of peripheral nerve regeneration,* New York, 1988, Alan R. Liss.

45. Williams LR, Varon S: Modification of fibrin matrix formation in situ enhances nerve regeneration in silicone chambers, *J Comp Neurol* 1985; 231:209-220.

46. Woodhall B, Beebe GW, eds: *Nerve regeneration—a follow-up study of 3656 World War II injuries,* VA Monograph, Washington, DC, 1956, U.S. Government Printing Office.

47. Young JZ, Medawar PB: Fibrin suture of peripheral nerves, *Lancet* 1940; 2:126-128.

Chapter 5

ELECTROPHYSIOLOGIC TESTING OF INJURED AND REGENERATING NERVES

Glenn A. Mackin

PERIPHERAL NERVOUS SYSTEM ELECTROPHYSIOLOGY

Electrophysiologic studies are problem-oriented consultations that should consistently provide clinically useful insight into peripheral nervous system (PNS) structure and function. Their purpose is to extend the diagnostic sensitivity and specificity of even the most meticulous neurologic examination. Electrophysiologic studies are most useful when the presence, severity, and character of a neuropathy (e.g., compressive, traumatic, toxic-metabolic) or other neuromuscular disorder is uncertain. Properly performed by a physician, they are literally indispensable for directing diagnostic and therapeutic initiatives along the most efficient, cost-effective pathways.

Electrophysiologic studies refer to a *group* of diagnostic tests of PNS structure and function. *Electromyographic (EMG) study,* as used customarily and as ordered on lab requisition forms, is synonymous with electrophysiologic studies in this chapter. The specific components of a particular patient's study should depend on the individual's clinical problem as independently considered by an experienced electrophysiologist. Optimal studies should be tailored to the specific clinical problem and should never be limited to inflexible, cookbook protocols. Almost invariably, however, most studies consist of some selected sensory and motor nerve conduction studies (NCS) and some selected EMG. Depending on the clinical problem, additional components might be relevant or decisive, such as long latency responses (e.g., F-waves and H-reflexes), repetitive stimulation, quantitative EMG, and various new techniques

of motor unit number estimation (MUNE). Nevertheless, NCS and EMG form the core of most electrophysiologic studies. Because NCS and EMG provide *inextricably complementary data,* each is *rarely* indicated separately. Consultation requests specifying "NCS only" or "EMG only" are almost inherently self-defeating. The electrophysiologist's bottom line interpretation should follow as a logical proof from, and be as specific as justified by, all available meticulously recorded data.[31]

Conceptually, the PNS includes four discrete systems of nerve fibers and their supporting neurons (i.e., motor, large sensory, small sensory, and autonomic), Schwann cells, myelin sheaths, specialized or simple sensory fiber endings, neuromuscular junctions (NMJ), muscle membranes, and muscle fibers. Conventional electrophysiology tests clinically pertinent electrical properties of each system with the exception of sensory roots and small sensory and autonomic fibers. Fortunately, the testable properties are sufficient to characterize most PNS lesions.[50] Complementary sensibility tests of small unmyelinated axons (c-fibers), thinly myelinated sensory axons, and free nerve endings include thermal threshold tests.[48] Autonomic tests include the sympathetic skin response, cardiac R-R interval variation,[42] quantitative sudomotor axon reflex test (QSART),[33] among many others.[30] Intraneural-electrode microneurography is a powerful investigational method for directly studying electrical discharge patterns in small sensory and autonomic axons.[19]

Conventionally testable large sensory and motor nerve fibers may be evaluated as far proximally as their neuronal cell bodies. For PNS sensory axons, these are located in the dorsal root ganglia (DRG), which are relatively well protected in intervertebral foramina outside the central nervous system (CNS). For PNS motor axons, anterior horn cells (AHC) are located in the spinal cord within the CNS proper. These anatomic relationships explain why all but the most severe injuries to sensory roots spare the DRGs and thus pass undetected by conventional NCS and EMG, despite causing dermatomal numbness, tingling, and pain. By contrast, EMG is exquisitely sensitive to mild (often asymptomatic and incidental), acute, and chronic motor root injury, provided that the study is performed at the appropriate time. Before studying a patient with symptoms of purely small fiber dysfunction, including pain and burning dysesthesias but no objective neurologic signs, it is helpful for the electrophysiologist to state the reason for the test (i.e., to test for structural nerve injury, not to verify pain) to the patient.

SCOPE OF CHAPTER

This chapter is limited to the electrophysiologic evaluation of injured and regenerating nerves. Other applications of conventional PNS electrophysiology that are not covered include disorders of AHCs and NMJs, polyneuropathies, and myopathies. Electrophysiologic studies are best regarded as dynamic tests of living nerve (and muscle) tissues, which are biologically and functionally inseparable from nerve cell bodies that provide trophic support. This biologic dimension explains the predictable temporal progression of electrophysiologic findings after nerve injury—from demyelination and axon degeneration to remyelination and regeneration.

Electrophysiologic studies have definite strengths and limitations that referring physicians should understand but keep in perspective. They provide detailed information about localization, acuteness, severity, and prognosis of nerve injury, parameters that are directly relevant to PNS symptoms, particularly negative ones such as numbness and weakness. Compared with high-quality magnetic resonance imaging (MRI) scan results suggesting possible impingement of the nerve or root (possibly incidental in themselves), electrophysiologic data are closer to symptoms than imaged proximity of bone to nerve. When invasive treatment is being considered, purely clinical diagnoses are best reserved for clearcut syndromes after unrevealing electrophysiologic and appropriate sensibility testing. For example, although NCS and EMG may be normal occasionally with some suspected nerve entrapments being considered for surgery, more commonly they demonstrate mild, chronic, asymptomatic, truly incidental abnormalities that are better managed conservatively.

Omitting electrophysiology—an increasing temptation under managed care—sets the stage for avoidable misadventures like carpal tunnel releases, ulnar transpositions, and sympathectomies done without knowledge of concurrent or alternative diagnoses such as polyneuropathies, radiculopathies (e.g., "double crush" syndrome),[47] and even motor

neuron diseases. A case in point is the clinical diagnosis of reflex sympathetic dystrophy (RSD), best reserved for a strictly diagnosed pain syndrome without an identifiable underlying, possibly surgically remediable, nerve lesion.[22,46] Though electrophysiologic tests are blind to small sensory fibers, they remain integral to the assessment of neuropathic pain because of their exquisite sensitivity to associated structurally significant large fiber injuries. Other common examples include ubiquitous published uncontrolled studies claiming great efficacy for certain operative procedures supported only by subjective diagnostic criteria and sometimes radiographs but no preoperative and postoperative electrophysiologic or sensibility data. In the PNS diagnostic algorithm, electrophysiologic testing ranks second only to a careful history and examination.

QUALIFICATIONS FOR ELECTROPHYSIOLOGISTS

Electrophysiologic consultants should be physicians with appropriate fellowship training plus board certification. The United States now has two certifying boards, Special Qualifications in Neurophysiology offered by the American Board of Psychiatry and Neurology (ABPN) and the American Board of Electrodiagnostic Medicine (AAEM).[2] Quality fellowships require 1 to 2 years of formal, supervised postresidency training, including extensive hands-on experience evaluating a wide variety of nerve injuries and neuromuscular disorders.

Electrophysiologic consultants should have the time, interest, experience with neuromuscular diseases and EMG problem solving, and personal flexibility to tailor each study to account for more than just the referral question on the consult form. They should also account for unexpected neurologic signs and symptoms revealed during their brief focusing examinations before studies and unexpected results that occasionally arise during studies. Depending on the neurologic acumen of referring physicians, referral questions range from exceedingly precise to vague, misleading, and absent. Because of the risks involved, electrophysiologists should have the skill and personal commitment to respond to imprecise and errant questions with definite and intelligible answers. When symptoms, signs, and electrophysiologic findings disagree, that fact should be stated candidly. When the electrophysiologic study strongly indicates the need to consider a specific follow-up radiologic test, biopsy type, or biopsy site, that guidance should be provided as appropriate. Referring physicians should choose their electrophysiologists carefully, mindful that third party payers increasingly decline to authorize second opinions, even by better qualified and more thorough electrophysiologists.

PRINCIPLES OF NERVE CONDUCTION STUDIES[6,23]

After nerve injury, principal objectives of electrophysiologic tests are to determine whether there is axonal

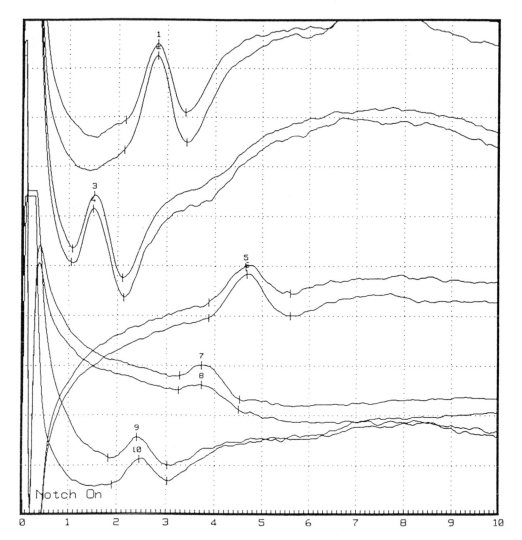

Fig. 5-1. Sensory nerve conduction studies (very mild CTS). This 46-year-old left-handed female symphony violinist with progressive right hand numbness with use was referred to exclude thoracic outlet syndrome. Stimulus artifact is at left, followed by distal latency (horizontal axis), then triphasic sensory nerve action potentials (SNAPs). From top to bottom, pairs of SNAPs are right median stimulating palm recording wrist (traces 1 and 2), ulnar palm to wrist (3 and 4), median wrist to elbow (5 and 6), median wrist to thumb (7 and 8), and radial wrist to thumb (9 and 10). Distal latencies to pairs 1 and 2 are twice those to 3 and 4 over identical distances. Latencies 7 and 8 are 50% longer than 9 and 10. Median sensory conduction across wrist calculated from 1 and 2 is 37.2 m/sec versus forearm (5 and 6) of 74.4 m/sec, proving focal slowing across carpal tunnel. Sensory amplitudes, motor nerve conduction studies and electromyography of selected right C5-T1 muscles are all normal. (For all traces, gain is 20 µV between horizontal divisions; temporal sweep is 1 msec between vertical divisions.)

continuity and whether the principal injury is *axon loss* or *demyelination*. The size, speed, and shape of NCS responses help identify the most likely principal nerve injury, whether caused by compression, stretch, or other mechanisms.

Conventional NCS are performed by electrically stimulating named nerves percutaneously at standard anatomic sites, inducing depolarization and propagation of the evoked impulse along large myelinated sensory and motor axons. Sensory nerve action potentials (SNAPs) represent the

summated conducted response of large sensory axons recorded extracellularly as a potential difference between active and reference surface (or subdermal) electrodes. The electrodes are placed 4 cm apart over the nerve. Triphasic SNAPs are recorded as the wave of depolarization travels under the active surface electrodes (Fig. 5-1). Compound muscle action potentials (CMAPs) represent the extracellularly recorded potential difference between an active electrode and a muscle's motor point, recording the summated depolarization at that site of high NMJ concentration, and a

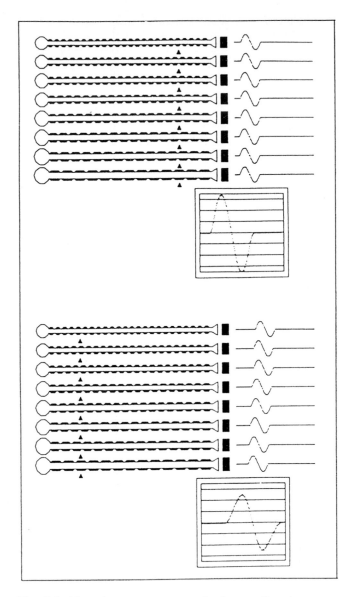

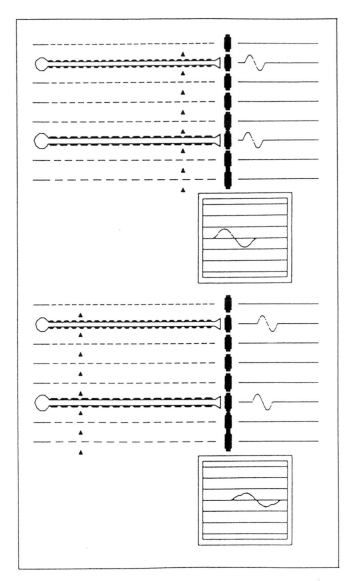

Fig. 5-2. Normal motor nerve conduction studies (computer model). Motor nerve (showing eight axons of varying size), neuromuscular junctions, and individual muscle fiber action potentials are summating to form a compound muscle action potential (CMAP). Semicircles indicate anterior horn cells *(left)*, black beads over white axons indicate myelinated internodes, solid black bars indicate muscle fibers *(right)*, and arrows indicate stimulation sites. Upper and lower traces represent distal and proximal sites of nerve stimulation, respectively. The lower CMAP trace is smaller because of physiologic arithmetic phase cancellation. (From Albers JW: Inflammatory demyelinating polyradiculoneuropathy. In Brown WF, Bolton CF, eds: *Clinical electromyography,* Boston, 1987, Butterworths.)

Fig. 5-3. Partial axon loss (axonotmesis). Six out of eight original axons have degenerated, compared with Fig. 5-2. Distal *(above)* and proximal *(below)* evoked compound motor action potential amplitudes and negative-peak areas are reduced to 25% their normal size. (From Albers JW: Inflammatory demyelinating polyradiculoneuropathy. In Brown WF, Bolton CF, eds: *Clinical electromyography,* Boston, 1987, Butterworths.)

reference electrode off the muscle, following stimulation of the nerve usually at two or more different points proximally (Fig. 5-2). The depolarization portion of recorded waveforms is the negative-peak (amplitude or area), which is directed upward on oscilloscope and printouts, reflecting the extracellular vantage point of the active electrode. *Distal*

latencies represent impulse propagation time measured in milliseconds (msec) between the most distal stimulation point and the recorded SNAP or CMAP response. *Conduction velocities* are calculated over nerve segments (e.g., the forearm), separated by discrete stimulation points, and measured in meters per second (m/sec).

Axon loss, or axonotmesis,[41] affects sensory and motor NCS in two ways: reduced waveform size (amplitude and area) and, at most, modest conduction slowing (Fig. 5-3). EMG provides correlation on acuteness, location, and severity of axon loss (see p. 40).

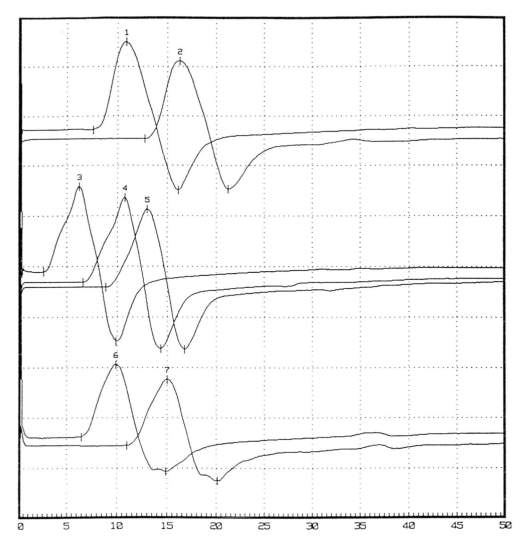

Fig. 5-4. Demyelinating-range slowing of median motor distal latencies (moderate carpal tunnel syndrome [CTS]). This 46-year-old right-handed male electronics technician with progressive knifelike pains and tingling in fingers for 3 years, left more than right, was referred for evaluation of bilateral CTS. Stimulus artifact is at left, followed by distal latency (horizontal axis), then biphasic compound motor action potentials (CMAPs). Traces are left median recording from abductor pollicus brevis muscle after stimulation at wrist (trace 1) and elbow (2); left ulnar recording from abductor digiti minimi stimulating wrist (3), below (4), and above elbow (5); and right median at wrist and elbow (6 and 7). The only abnormalities are bilaterally prolonged median distal latencies, left 7.6 msec, right 6.5 msec, each exceeding by more than 30% the upper normal of 4.4 msec. CMAPs 1, 2, 6, and 7 are shifted to the right with unaltered normal waveforms. Note that ulnar motor slowing at elbow (not shown) would shift CMAP 5 to the right relative to CMAP 4. (For all traces, gain is 5 mV between horizontal divisions; temporal sweep is 5 msec between vertical divisions.)

Demyelination may affect NCS in three possible ways: marked slowing, temporal dispersion of waveform shape, and conduction block. Marked slowing into a demyelinating range (i.e., <70% the lower limits of normal) cannot be explained by even severe loss of large, rapidly conducting axons alone. Demyelinating range slowing, measured between undistorted proximally and distally evoked waveforms, indicates synchronous slowing in all fibers in that nerve segment. Marked slowing to this degree may occur either focally on an acquired basis (e.g., chronic compression) (Fig. 5-4) or generalized and symmetric on an hereditary basis (e.g., Charcot-Marie-Tooth disease, Type I). True temporal dispersion occurs only on the basis of acquired demyelination. Proximally evoked waveforms are significantly longer in duration than distally evoked ones and may have ragged morphologies. True dispersion is the physiologic expression of asynchronous slowing among fibers within a nerve segment (Fig. 5-5). Pseudodispersion

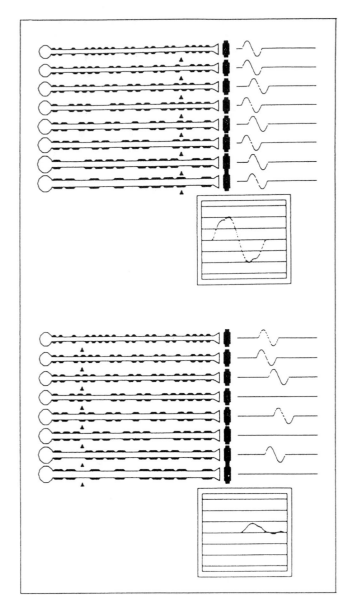

Fig. 5-5. Demyelinating temporal dispersion. Multifocal, inconsistent demyelination affects all eight axons to different degrees, compared with Fig. 5-2. The low amplitude, long duration proximally evoked waveform *(bottom)* reflects abnormal phase cancellation and conduction block among axons. Conduction block is demonstrated in the lower tracing by the 4th, 6th, and 8th axons, which do not contribute to the summated CMAP. (From Albers JW: Inflammatory demyelinating polyradiculoneuropathy. In Brown WF, Bolton CF, eds: *Clinical electromyography,* Boston, 1987, Butterworths.)

occurs on the basis of acquired severe axon loss and is confirmed by EMG demonstration of markedly reduced recruitment (see p. 41).

Conduction block, or neurapraxia,[41] also occurs on an acquired basis only and is the physiologic expression of focal myelin loss from at least several consecutive internodes along sensory or motor axons still in physical continuity. It may occur for structural reasons because of chronic

compression at common points of nerve entrapment but also for systemic reasons in autoimmune polyneuropathies in essentially random patterns (e.g., Guillain-Barré syndrome). Conduction block may be partial or complete, depending on whether some or all axons in a nerve segment are demyelinated. Conceptually, the myelin sheath is only loosely analogous to the insulation on a wire. Stripped of its insulation, a wire will still conduct electricity. Stripped of myelin from any consecutive internodes, large myelinated axons fail to propagate impulses across the gap despite continuity of axons. Distal to the point of block, sufficient stimulating current evokes depolarization and propagation of impulses in all available fibers to the recording electrodes. Proximal to the point of block, depolarization still occurs in all fibers, but only those with intact myelin propagate impulses across the gap, resulting in a smaller waveform (Fig. 5-6).

Therefore, demyelination constitutes a physiologic spectrum affecting nerve fibers, ranging from conduction block when severe, through synchronous demyelinating range slowing, to mild synchronous slowing with velocities similar to that with loss of many large, rapidly conducting axons, to asynchronous temporal dispersion. These complexities emphasize the importance that every electrophysiologic study of nerve injury reaches a well-documented and precise conclusion about the most likely principal lesion, whether axon loss or demyelination. The equivocating phrase, "mixed axon loss and demyelinating lesion," should rarely (if ever) appear as the final interpretation because it usually begs the very question it should have answered.

SENSORY NERVE CONDUCTION STUDIES

SNAPs are exquisitely sensitive indicators of the structural integrity of large myelinated axons that transmit sensory modalities including proprioception, vibration, light touch, and two-point discrimination in named nerves such as the median. SNAPs are usually recorded distally in limbs where nerves are relatively superficial and accessible for surface (or subdermal) stimulation and recording. A recorded sensory response indicates more than continuity of large sensory axons between the points of stimulation and recording. It also indicates continuity of large sensory axons between the recording point and DRG cells, including the entire course of those axons up through peripheral nerve and plexus. This is the basis for one of the most useful applications of SNAPs, their ability to distinguish preganglionic (root and CNS) from postganglionic (plexus and nerve) lesions.[6,23]

SNAPs do not measure small sensory fibers that, when injured or irritated, may underlie pain and positive symptoms arising from sensory roots, named peripheral nerves, soft tissues, and bony structures. Lesions proximal to DRG (e.g., purely sensory root compressions or avulsions, and injuries to CNS sensory tracts) may render dermatomes or limbs anesthetic. SNAPs recorded from such insensate distribu-

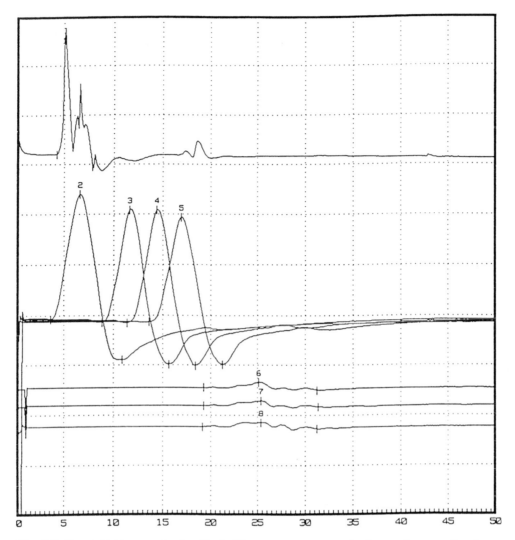

Fig. 5-6. Demyelinating conduction block. Ulnar motor nerve conduction studies recording from first dorsal interosseus muscle, showing 95% conduction block across lower brachial plexus in a 57-year-old, right-handed male dentist with progressive hand weakness for over 7 years because of multifocal motor neuropathy.[38] Clinically, there was no movement in the right first dorsal interosseus muscle (1st DIO). Tracing 1 shows an intramuscularly recorded response from 1st DIO using concentric needle electrode after stimulating ulnar nerve at the wrist. Tracings 2 to 5 show compound motor action potentials surface-recorded over muscle, after nerve stimulation at the wrist, distal to the elbow, proximal to the elbow and in axilla, respectively. Tracings 6 to 8 after stimulation at Erb's point show marked block in lower trunk or medial cord of brachial plexus. Antiganglioside antibodies were not present. Brachial plexus MRI scan showed focal gadolinium enhancement in the medial cord. Treatment with intravenous immunoglobulin resulted in prompt complete recovery. (For all traces, gain is 5 mV between horizontal divisions; temporal sweep is 5 msec between vertical divisions.) (From Parry GJ: Motorneuropathy with multifocal conduction block, *Semin Neurol* 1993; 13:269.)

tions will be normal because of continuity between affected DRGs and peripheral axons. However, normal SNAPs in weak, anesthetic limbs have ominous implications. For example, after a motorcycle accident, normal SNAPs may indicate irreparable preganglionic root avulsion. In general, reduced amplitude or absent SNAPs are generally exquisitely sensitive indicators of partial or complete lesions of plexus or nerve, especially nerve entrapment, disrupting continuity between DRG and axons. Whenever a complex partial brachial plexus injury is suspected, it is usually necessary to perform selected bilateral SNAPs representative of the C6-C8 dermatomes to detect significant relative side-to-side differences that may indicate partial postganglionic axon loss (unfortunately, the C5 dermatome has no technically measurable SNAP). Usually a two-fold side-to-side relative difference is required for sensory (and motor) amplitudes to be considered abnormal, especially when the smaller suspect amplitude is normal in absolute terms.

An important qualification is that a demonstrable post-ganglionic plexus lesion does not obviate the possibility of a concurrent root lesion, as with the hypothetical motorcyclist after sudden arm traction. Patients with preexisting nerve and plexus problems may develop superimposed root or AHC disorders, compounding the weakness and the complexity of electrophysiologic interpretation. Although challenging situations of such abnormality overload[49] are not uncommon, the key point is that reduced or absent SNAPs are not localizing in themselves, considering the distance from DRG to distal axon. Absent median SNAPs are frequently caused by median nerve entrapment in the carpal tunnel, but in isolation this finding does not prove carpal tunnel syndrome (CTS) and may actually direct attention away from other potential lesion sites such as the lateral cord of the brachial plexus.[39] CTS localization can be proved when abnormal SNAP amplitudes are supplemented by demonstrable focal slowing of sensory conduction restricted to the median nerve across the wrist, a significant discrepancy between slowed median conduction across the wrist and normal median conduction velocity in the forearm, or supportive evidence from mandatory motor NCS and EMG.

A typical CTS evaluation might start with median orthodromic sensory responses, stimulating the index and middle fingers with ring electrodes, and recording SNAPs over volar wrist 3 cm proximal to distal wrist crease using surface (or subdermal) electrodes. SNAPs can also be recorded antidromically, stimulating at the wrist and recording with ring electrodes on the fingers.[40] Regardless of the electrophysiologist's preferred technique, meticulous attention to skin preparation, temperature, and distance measurement are crucial, as is the use of norms appropriate to the technique used and the patient's age. SNAP amplitudes are measured in microvolts and have normal values but do not quantify the number of large conducting axons. If an electrophysiologist neglects to properly prepare the skin by removing excess oils or desquamated debris before applying surface recording electrodes, this will cause excessive resistance at the skin-electrode interface, causing spuriously low SNAP amplitudes that may falsely imply axon loss. Similarly, neglecting to warm the skin of the hands above 32° C or the skin of the feet above 31° C before recording SNAPs can spuriously increase and normalize abnormally low SNAP amplitudes, spuriously prolong distal latency by 0.2 msec/° C, or slow conduction by 2.4 m/sec/° C below optimal temperature.[13,17] When the only reported abnormality is conduction slowing, particularly distally in extremities, the referring physician should confirm that the limb temperature during the study is documented and appropriate before accepting the diagnosis of polyneuropathy or CTS based on those results.

SNAP waveforms are triphasic, positive-negative-positive (down-up-down), measured in microvolts (μV), with a large negative peak representing the extracellularly recorded potential difference as depolarization travels under the active electrode. The sensory distal latency, measured in milliseconds, represents the time elapsed for the wave of depolarization to propagate in large sensory axons from the point of stimulation to the recording electrodes. Returning to the CTS example, sometimes the orthodromic sensory distal latency between fingers and wrist is at upper limits of normal, measured over a distance of approximately 14 cm. Given that individual SNAPs are rarely localizing in and of themselves, the flexible electrophysiologist will apply one or several special strategies to prove focal slowing at that common, accessible site of entrapment. Such strategies include the following:

1. Measuring "short segment" latency or velocity across a segment encompassing the suspected lesion. This increases the significance of excess time contributed by a point of focal slowing as a fraction of the total conduction time. Mild focal slowing may be difficult to appreciate over a long distance such as between fingers and wrist. Using this principle, a standard method used to document subtle slowing of median sensory conduction across the wrist is the median palmar sensory response, obtained by stimulating median sensory axons in the lateral palm over thenar crease 8 cm distal to the volar wrist recording site.

2. Comparing parallel segments of adjacent, equally distal named nerves over identical distances. Conduction velocities should be similar over equal lengths of same-caliber nerves. Many electrophysiologists prefer to compare relative distal latencies between median with ulnar palmar responses, the latter recorded across the wrist over an 8-cm distance also between medial palm and volar wrist over the ulnar nerve. Other comparisons commonly used are median versus ulnar sensory distal latencies measured over identical distances between the ring finger and these nerves recorded over volar wrist or median versus radial sensory distal latencies over equal distances between the thumb and wrist.[8,21]

3. Bracketing the suspected point of slowing by comparing contiguous segments along the nerve. For example, the median sensory conduction velocity (m/sec) across the wrist calculated from palmar distance (8 cm) divided by conduction time (distal latency in msec) can be compared with the median sensory conduction velocity in the forearm (i.e., the mixed nerve response between wrist and elbow), looking for significantly different velocities confirming focal slowing at the wrist.

4. Inching the stimulator from proximal to distal across the suspected point of entrapment in very short 1-cm segments, and recording distally (e.g., from a finger), looking for an abrupt increase in intersegmental latency or a sharp decrease in amplitude, which respectively indicate focal demyelinating slowing and

conduction block.[24] Pitfalls of inching include distance measurement error caused by high currents inadvertently depolarizing the intended nerve proximal or distal to the stimulator, and unintentional costimulation of adjacent nerves.

5. Most of these localization strategies are applicable to selected motor NCS. The bracketing technique is a standard supplementary strategy for proving motor conduction slowing across certain entrapment sites such as ulnar nerve at elbow. Anatomic and technical considerations determine the situational validity of a given special strategy. For example, inching along the ulnar nerve across the elbow is problematic because of the redundant nonlinear course of that nerve segment. Similarly, bracketing motor nerve conductions across the clavicle risks not only measurement errors but also submaximal stimulation at Erb's point, both of which may spuriously suggest a demyelinating compressive lesion within the thoracic outlet.[21]

Few electrophysiologic studies are complete without some selected sensory and motor NCS and EMG. This is not to imply that every conceivable sensory and motor technique is appropriate for every patient with suspected CTS any more than a clinically oblivious cookbook protocol for all patients would be appropriate. For some patients, standard sensory NCS from the fingers is diagnostic of straightforward CTS, although full understanding of acuteness and severity requires correlation of motor NCS and EMG data. Not all CTS are created equally electrophysiologically, any more than they are clinically. Many are straightforward to prove using electrophysiologic studies, while others can be exceedingly difficult. For example, diabetic patients with tingling fingers may lack median sensory responses because of polyneuropathy alone, another common example of abnormality overload. Valid electrophysiologic proof that a diabetic patient has superimposed CTS may require sophisticated combinations of SNAPs recorded from the arms and legs, comparison of SNAP latencies between adjacent nerves of similar diameter, motor conductions, and also EMG. Flexibility is essential. If a patient's principal sensory symptoms arise from the thumb, then the electrophysiologist should not settle for borderline abnormalities among routine index or middle finger distal latencies and amplitudes but should take the time to record thumb SNAPs and to exclude a concurrent C_6 radiculopathy using EMG.

When a patient's symptoms are purely sensory, the electrophysiologist, the referring physician, and the patient must look beyond today's impressive computer-assisted technology to maintain the perspective that conventional NCS are blind to small sensory pain or c-fibers. The specialized localization methods outlined previously indicate something different, specifically, subtle conduction abnormalities in large sensory axons. Electrophysiologic proof of minimal CTS is demonstrated only by relative prolongation of median over ulnar palmar distal latencies—

even when digital and palmar latencies and amplitudes, motor NCS and EMG are normal—is not necessarily clinically relevant. There are now approximately 20 different published NCS techniques advocated for diagnosing CTS, varying in formal validation, sensitivity, specificity, and predictive value.[3] Administering numerous sensitive NCS tests can potentially be counterproductive. Selectivity by an experienced electrophysiologist is the best defense against proliferation of false positives. It is essential that the final interpretation always includes a degree of severity adjective, especially at extremes of "very mild" and "severe."

There is a loose correlation between the intensity of sensory symptoms and SNAP abnormalities. Most patients with sensory symptoms arising from named nerves show relevant sensory and sometimes motor NCS abnormalities. At the extremes, however, some patients with early CTS may have exquisite (or no) pain and no electrophysiologic abnormalities, however sensitive the methods used. Others with chronic CTS may have no pain, no sensation, and absent SNAPs. Many patients with definite CTS in their symptomatic hand and others referred for completely unrelated symptoms meet electrophysiologic criteria for CTS in their asymptomatic hands. Sensory nerve conduction studies test passive cable properties of large sensory fibers, not the sensibility content of that conduction. Small sensory fiber irritation, as by a neuroma-in-continuity, may trigger ectopic impulses (recordable investigationally using microneurography) resulting in discomfort, but unless there are large fiber abnormalities (a high probability with compression), conventional sensory NCS will be normal. The interpretation should underscore this caveat, particularly when results are indeed normal.

MOTOR NERVE CONDUCTION STUDIES

CMAPs represent summated depolarizations of individual axon-myofiber units at NMJs following stimulation of the nerve at two or more points proximally. Motor waveforms are biphasic, negative-positive (up-down) with a large negative peak measured in millivolts (mV) representing the extracellularly recorded potential difference between an active electrode over the depolarizing motor point and a reference electrode off the muscle. The large positive phase represents repolarization. Distal latencies are measured in milliseconds between a distal stimulation point (e.g., just proximal to wrist) and the motor point. Conduction velocities are calculated in meters per second between one or several proximal and distal stimulation points along the nerve. Normally, CMAPs are smooth waves, best thought of as histograms composed of the arithmetic contributions of rapidly conducting axons to the left under the negative peak (near the stimulus artifact) and slower axons to the right.

Although many principles discussed for sensory NCS also apply to motor NCS, certain differences are crucial for interpreting nerve injury. CMAPs are three orders of magnitude larger than SNAPs, making it much easier and more reliable to use CMAPs to distinguish demyelinating temporal dispersion from conduction block. Temporal dispersion of narrow SNAPs will more likely reduce their amplitudes through phase cancellation and falsely suggest axon loss, not demyelination.[25] Diagnosis of conduction block requires proximally evoked amplitude and area to be at least 20% smaller than distal ones, provided the proximal waveform's temporal duration has not spread out wider than 115% of the distal duration (many electrophysiologists prefer a more conservative definition, requiring a 50% difference between proximal and distal). When the proximal duration has spread out to more than 115%, *temporal dispersion* is present and conduction block is excluded, no matter how much the proximally evoked amplitude and area may have declined.[1] Even when motor CMAPs appear to show conduction block, there are additional pitfalls. The most common is submaximal stimulation of the nerve proximally, often caused by a combination of the depth of the nerve at that level and the patient's intolerance of necessarily high stimulating current. In some cases, severe axon loss results in straightforward arithmetic phase cancellation among surviving fibers, a distinction requiring EMG. Omitting EMG sets the stage for mistaking such pseudo-block because of axon loss for demyelination, promoting false confidence about a good outcome with conservative management, when surgical decompression of a progressively denervating lesion is the preferred procedure. Another pitfall involves common anatomic variants that may superficially mimic conduction block. In a Martin-Gruber anastomosis, axons cross over from median to ulnar nerve in the forearm. Proximally and distally evoked ulnar CMAPs resemble block between elbow and wrist and median CMAPs show the opposite, paradoxically low amplitudes at wrist versus large ones at elbow.[18]

Other important differences between motor and sensory NCS are essential to understanding electrophysiologic findings with denervation and reinnervation. Note that CMAP responses, but not SNAP responses, have NMJs interposed between points of stimulation and recording. Early NMJ failure after proximal axon transection explains the earlier decline in distally evoked CMAP amplitudes as compared with SNAP amplitudes before Wallerian degeneration affects the axons themselves.[28] Moreover, chronically after a nerve lesion, when sufficient time has passed for reinnervation, CMAPs are more likely to approach normal size than SNAPs because muscle reinnervation can occur by collateral sprouting of surviving axons still in continuity with muscle, not just by the distal regrowth of the severed axons.

LATE RESPONSES[17]

Nerve depolarization evoked by applied electrical stimuli propagates bidirectionally. Using an arrangement of recording electrodes similar to motor NCS, F-waves represent long latency round trips of single depolarizing waves elicited distally (e.g., at wrist) propagating antidromically through motor roots to the spinal cord, where they may intermittently trigger depolarization of AHCs, generating small orthodromic reflected motor responses recordable in muscles of the same myotome. Like CMAPs, F-waves require supramaximal stimulation, using current intensities 25% to 30% over that required to evoke a maximal CMAP. F-waves can be recorded from virtually any muscle that has a recordable CMAP. Normally, F-waves do not always appear after each of the 20 single stimulations recommended for valid results. Those that appear typically have different morphologies and latencies, indicating that each arises from a different axon. Prolonged latencies may indicate abnormal proximal conduction in a limb, particularly when motor conduction velocities are normal in more distal segments. Absent or delayed F-waves, while not precisely localizing, imply a lower motor neuron (LMN) disorder within that myotome somewhere between AHC and muscle. Because they traverse motor roots, F-waves provide information about both preganglionic and postganglionic axonal lesions, usually within root and plexus. Because they do not traverse the sensory root, F-waves do not solve that blind spot of electrophysiologic studies. Some patients will have normal F-waves despite dermatomal pain, motor signs, and EMG abnormalities otherwise consistent with radiculopathy. F-waves appearing after every stimulus imply hyperexcitablity in that segmental AHC pool, a sign analogous to hyperactive deep tendon reflexes, possibly indicating an upper motor neuron (UMN) lesion.

By contrast, H-reflexes can be recorded in adults only from the S_1 myotome (e.g., by stimulating the tibial nerve in popliteal fossa and recording from soleus muscle). Unlike F-waves, H-reflexes traverse true electrical reflex arcs orthodromically up sensory large fiber afferents, triggering depolarization of AHCs in the same spinal segment and propagation of orthodromic motor depolarization waves back down to muscle. Another difference is that H-reflexes are elicited using submaximal stimulation usually within a narrow current range below that required for CMAPs. In the legs absent and prolonged H-reflexes may indicate S_1 radiculopathy, but they also serve as sensitive indicators of polyneuropathy. Considering upper extremity function, recordable H-reflexes in the arms are normally seen only in infants with incomplete CNS myelination. Their generalized reappearance in adult arms implies an acquired UMN lesion.

ELECTROMYOGRAPHY[6,23]

In standard EMG, a needle electrode is inserted into the muscle of interest to record voluntary motor unit potentials (MUPs), which represent voltage potential differences generated near the needle tip by depolarizing muscle fibers. A motor unit includes a single AHC, its motor axon, and all NMJs and muscle fibers attached. MUPs, measured in millivolts, are usually triphasic (down-up-down). The amplitude of the large negative phase is the summation of synchronously firing muscle fibers very near the needle tip within several millimeters, and duration is a measure of MUP territory. With voluntary contraction, different motor units can be recognized as MUPs with different morphologies and firing patterns. Using a concentric or monopolar needle electrode, the electrophysiologist evaluates muscle electrical activity at rest, then during a gentle steady force, and finally building up to a strong steady force.

The most important abnormal spontaneous activity in the evaluation of nerve injury is regularly firing fibrillations and positive sharp waves, measured in microvolts. Normally innervated resting muscle fibers are electrically silent. Spontaneous fibrillations and positive waves in resting muscle have a similar physiologic significance, acute isolation of muscle fibers or portions thereof from trophic support by nerves. More than any other diagnostic feature, fibrillations and positive waves are what make electrophysiologic abnormalities acute. Nevertheless, fibrillations and positive waves are not specific for denervating processes. They may be seen with certain myopathies, especially inflammatory ones such as polymyositis with active muscle fiber necrosis. In denervating disorders fibrillations and positive waves appear 1 to 3 weeks after delayed Wallerian degeneration has occurred, depending on axon stump length. The fibrillations and positive waves are silenced either by reinnervation or endstage muscle fiber fibrosis after sustained denervation. Other important spontaneous activity relevant to nerve injury include complex repetitive discharges, indicating chronicity, and fasciculations, which are ectopic MUPs arising from irritable motor units, especially from their terminal arborizations.[10,29]

Graded voluntary muscle contraction with an EMG needle in place, ranging from a gentle to a strong steady force, enables assessment of voluntary MUP morphology and recruitment patterns, respectively. MUP morphologic abnormalities include increased and decreased duration and amplitude, and excess polyphasia for that particular muscle. Each of these morphologic parameters increases with normal aging in a muscle-specific manner. Each provides insight into muscle fiber innervation and structural integrity, but neither distinguishes neurogenic from myopathic processes. Large MUPs are often, but not invariably, associated with neurogenic processes, and small (especially polyphasic) MUPs are often, but not invariably, associated with myopathic ones. Normally innervated limb muscles may have approximately 15% polyphasic MUPs, while normally innervated limb girdle muscles may have 25% polyphasic MUPs. Referring physicians should be alert to overinterpretation of excess polyphasia, which, in the absence of definitely abnormal recruitment, is a nonspecific finding.

The distinction between neurogenic and myopathic processes depends on voluntary MUP recruitment patterns.[51] After partial denervation, a reduced number of available motor units (which may be larger chronically because of compensatory reinnervation) must fire faster to generate forces comparable to normally innervated muscle fibers. This is termed *reduced* or *neurogenic recruitment*. Convincing EMG localization of a denervating disorder builds on NCS to identify the anatomically most restricted exclusive structure and site (e.g., nerve, trunk, cord, root, AHC) that all abnormalities have in common. By contrast, with muscle disorders, more axons must fire sooner to generate comparable force because each motor unit delivers less than usual force as the original number of muscle fibers is depleted and surviving myofibrils are fragmented. This is termed *early, increased,* or *myopathic recruitment*.

Electrophysiology involves not just technical proficiency but also sound judgment about the proper scope of the study. Insufficient testing creates the possibility of overlooking a problem, while excessive testing unnecessarily increases costs. Among the most difficult EMG recruitment patterns to interpret are those associated with chronic myopathies such as chronic polymyositis, which can so closely resemble chronic denervation that they are commonly mistaken for motor neuron diseases.[35] Conversely, early reinnervation results in low amplitude nascent polyphasic potentials reminiscent of myopathic MUPs. It should be recalled that the combination of normal SNAPs and denervation in the same spinal segment on EMG indicates a preganglionic lesion but alone does not distinguish between root and AHC localization. Whenever multiple radiculopathies are demonstrated, the possibility of a motor neuron disorder enters the differential diagnosis. Insufficient EMG sampling in early amyotrophic lateral sclerosis (ALS) may be mistaken for acute lumbosacral radiculopathies if only the weak leg is tested, for lumbar spinal stenosis if only the symptomatic legs are tested, and for CTS if only weak median-innervated muscles are tested. Even when sensory symptoms are present, increasing the likelihood of root disorders, EMG abnormalities do not distinguish among potential etiologies. Whether an electrophysiologically demonstrable radiculopathy arises from one of the common vertebral degenerative mechanisms rather than a nonstructural cause (e.g., infection, carcinomatous meningitis) is fundamentally a clinical question to which the neurologically sophisticated electrophysiologist can and should often usefully contribute.

Skillful analysis of voluntary MUP recruitment in denervating disorders enables a semiquantitative estimate of the cumulative extent of partial denervation into approximate ordinal grades of 0%, 30%, 50%, 70%, 90%, and 100%. Subjectivity inherent in standard recruitment analysis can be minimized when an experienced electrophysiologist establishes rapport with a patient who is able and motivated to cooperate to give a smoothly graded contraction with the EMG needle in place. It is considerably more difficult to distinguish normal full recruitment from mild (30%) denervation than it is to recognize moderate (50%), moderately severe (70%), severe (90%), and complete (100%) denervation. After muscle denervation (e.g., by 70%), reinnervation mechanisms will restore strength and time will enable MUPs to mature from long-duration polyphasics toward large triphasic potentials. However, the same moderately severely reduced recruitment pattern will persist indefinitely (e.g., 30% residual innervation).

Superimposed essential and parkinsonian tremors, anxious tremulousness, and reduced consciousness levels thwart precise recruitment analysis and can render exclusion or definite diagnosis of mild denervation virtually impossible. Although EMG needle insertion is inherently but not unduly painful, sedation before the study is counterproductive if it renders the patient unable to generate smooth graded contractions. Local anesthesia is impractical and never used. The differential diagnosis of submaximal MUP firing rates includes pain (either preexisting and/or exacerbated by needle insertion), reduced effort on a volitional basis, and UMN disorders interfering with LMN activation. New computer-assisted quantitative EMG programs increase objectivity without unreasonably prolonging studies. This facilitates the direct measurement of MUP properties, including amplitude, area, duration, polyphasia, and firing rates.[15]

TIMING OF NERVE CONDUCTION STUDIES AFTER NERVE INJURY

Immediately after complete nerve injury (neurotmesis, axonotmesis, neurapraxia),[41] there is no response after attempted muscle contraction, applied touch, and electrical stimulation across the lesion. However, distal motor and sensory nerve stumps remain electrically excitable until the delayed process of Wallerian degeneration (WD) supervenes. Before WD develops, neither NCS nor EMG can distinguish neurotmesis or axonotmesis from comparable degrees of neurapraxia. The only unique immediate information that NCS and EMG studies provide about the lesion is whether there is evidence of clinically inapparent axonal continuity. Although immediate NCS can provide useful baseline information, it is usually best to wait the 10 to 12 days it takes for WD to fully develop, if practical. Evidence of subclinical continuity to acutely paralyzed muscles or numb dermatomes is demonstrated on NCS as recordable across-lesion CMAPs and SNAPs and on EMG as voluntary MUPs firing in muscle.

After WD has had time to occur, CMAP and SNAP amplitudes (and areas) elicited by electrical stimulation both proximal and distal to the lesion site decline in proportion to the amount of axon loss. With loss of all axons in a nerve, motor amplitudes remain normal or mildly reduced for 3 to 5 days and disappear by 6 to 8 days, whereas sensory amplitudes remain normal or mildly reduced for 5 to 8 days and disappear by 10 to 12 days.[9,37] Partial injuries decline and reach proportionate nadirs according to an identical timetable. For this reason, considering possible thoracic outlet syndrome (TOS), purported changes in distally evoked and recorded NCS obtained immediately after dynamic proximal arm maneuvers that transiently reproduce

symptoms are literally unbelievable. Even neurotmesis of the medial cord of the brachial plexus has no immediately measurable effect on distal NCS. CMAP amplitudes decline faster than SNAPs because biologic motor units from AHC to muscle include NMJs that fail to transmit impulses between nerves and muscles even before WD removes conduction capacity from transected motor (and sensory) axon stumps.[28] Evoked motor and sensory NCS response amplitudes, areas, and normal ranges do not quantify the actual number of conducting axons between stimulation and recording points. With neurapraxia, CMAP and SNAP amplitudes and areas elicited by stimulating distal to the lesion exceed those elicited by stimulating proximal to it in proportion to the number of axons affected by potentially reversible conduction block caused by demyelination.

Perhaps the worst time after nerve injury to obtain an electrophysiologic study is at exactly 1 week after the injury. At this time CMAP amplitudes may be absent or significantly reduced but SNAPs may still be normal, which misleadingly implies that the denervating lesion is preganglionic in root or AHC rather than in nerve or plexus. Reliable distinction of axon loss from conduction block within postganglionic nerves or plexus using NCS requires a wait of 10 to 12 days after the injury.

When there is clinical or electrophysiologic evidence of at least some continuity in motor or sensory fibers within the distribution of the injured nerve, immediate surgical nerve repair is not indicated. The reason for conservative management under these circumstances is the reasonable functional recovery that can follow reinnervation by collateral sprouting of as few as 20% of the original axon number.[11,36] It is most advantageous to wait until electrophysiologic studies can sort out with reasonable precision the relative proportions of surviving, axonotmetic, and neurapraxic fibers. On the other hand, because most patients do not typically bring premorbid baseline NCS with them to the emergency room or to the surgeon's office, it may be useful in selected cases to obtain NCS immediately after injury even when possible nerve repair will be delayed and again immediately preoperatively to establish the amount of interval axon loss and surgical baseline. Establishing a preoperative baseline is valuable for many reasons, not least of which is medicolegal. When premorbid or immediate postinjury baselines are unavailable, alternatives include side-to-side comparison of homologous nerves looking for a 50% amplitude difference and comparison with the lower limit of normal. Open, clean lacerations with clinically complete nerve transection are different. The surgeon should explore acutely, perform primary repair on grossly severed nerve trunks, but defer repair of those in physical or intraoperative electrophysiologic continuity for several months. The delay will allow time for hematomas to resolve and NCS and EMG to provide mutually complementary information about the degree of axon loss.

TIMING OF ELECTROMYOGRAPHY AFTER NERVE INJURY

Acutely denervated muscle fibers develop denervation supersensitivity, form extrajunctional acetylcholine receptors across their membranes beyond the confines of NMJs, and begin to spontaneously electrically discharge. Local tissues elaborate neurotrophic factors to attract regenerating axons toward denervated muscle, promoting formation of new NMJs. Fibrillations and positive sharp waves appear temporally according to stump length (the distance between lesion and muscle). The more proximal the lesion, the longer the stump, and the longer it takes for fibrillations and positive waves to appear in distal muscles. The time lag between axon transection and appearance of fibrillations is caused by slow axonal transport, which persists until WD supervenes, then an additional 1 to 2 weeks until intramyofibrillar mechanisms gear up to support spontaneous discharges.[6,23,37]

For example, after severe C8 root injury with axon loss, C8 paraspinal muscles begin to fibrillate at 7 to 10 days, whereas C8 (T1) innervated intrinsic hand muscles might not begin to fibrillate for 3 weeks or more. This happens even though CMAPs recorded from denervated intrinsic hand muscles may have reached nadir by 6 to 8 days. Because muscles are normally innervated by two or more roots, reduced CMAPs are seen acutely after single root injuries only when there is severe motor axon loss in that root or after multiple roots innervating that muscle are significantly denervated. By contrast, because nerves are the final common pathways to muscles for axons from two or more roots, with nerve-injury reductions in serially obtained CMAP amplitudes closely reflect the proportion (not the precise number) of axons lost. After a significant (not necessarily severe) distal axon loss lesion to a named nerve such as the median at the wrist, intrinsic hand muscles might begin to fibrillate at 7 to 10 days because of their short stump. With conduction block (neurapraxia), axonal trophic continuity persists between AHC and the muscle, so fibrillations do not develop even though EMG recruitment is reduced.[37]

EMG is the gold standard for semiquantitative determination of the cumulative extent of partial denervation of muscle, whether or not reinnervation has had time to occur. Electrophysiologic correlates of clinically detectable weakness caused by motor nerve injury are axon loss, demyelinating conduction block, and temporal dispersion, but not slowing of conduction. Whether clinical weakness develops depends on the rate of axon loss and the amount of residual innervation. With abrupt axon loss or conduction block, weakness is evident after acute interruption of only 20% to 30% of the original motor axon supply. With gradual chronic denervation compensated by ongoing reinnervation, 70% to 80% of motor axons may be lost before weakness and atrophy become detectable. Well-compensated, clinically strong muscles chronically denervated down to their last 30% axons have exhausted reserves and will weaken rapidly with additional axon loss.[23]

Immediately after nerve injury, the presence on EMG of some voluntary MUPs proves partial continuity of axons, and conservative management is indicated. Three or more weeks after nerve injury, when fibrillations signifying acute disconnection of muscle fibers from nerve develop, their density should never be confused with either the severity of denervation or residual axon supply. Profuse fibrillations and positive waves may reflect denervation that is rapid or beyond the capacity to reinnervate. By contrast, severity determinations depend entirely on voluntary MUP recruitment. When ongoing denervation is indolent and matched by the rate of reinnervation, no acute fibrillations need to be seen, but axon attrition will be reflected over time in declining recruitment. Sponaneous fibrillations and absent voluntary recruitment do not indicate whether the axon loss lesion is neurotmesis (Sunderland 5th degree, or 5°) or severe axonotmesis (Sunderland 4°).[45] Given the time element involved in WD, early exploration may be the only means of distinguishing Sunderland 4° and 5° lesions. Immediate primary repair is clearly indicated for clean neurotmesis, the mechanism of which is almost always penetrating injury such as glass, stab, or gunshot wounds.[5] Secondary repair should be delayed several months for dirty wounds and in all cases where there is clinical or electrophysiologic continuity, either routine or intraoperative. At 3 to 4 weeks after nerve injury, the recruitment pattern and the presence or absence of spontaneous activity allows for distinction between absent axonal continuity (Sunderland 4° and 5°), partial axon loss lesions for which early repair is not indicated (Sunderland 2° and 3°), and conduction block that has an excellent prognosis for recovery with conservative management by the process of remyelination (Sunderland 1° or Seddon's neurapraxia).[20,26]

MONITORING REINNERVATION AND PLANNING NERVE REPAIR

Motor reinnervation occurs in two waves: collateral sprouting of uninjured axons within muscle during the first 3 to 6 months and regeneration of severed axons growing back toward muscle at 1 to 2 mm per day or 1 in per month. By 10 to 12 days, if CMAP amplitude exceeds 20% lower limit of normal, there is a favorable prognosis for functional recovery by collateral sprouting alone, provided the mechanism of injury is not progressive.[9,37] Sensory reinnervation occurs by regeneration only. Regeneration requires a track of residual nerve structure for growth cones to follow like vines on a trellis, ideally intact endoneurium (Sunderland 2°) or perineurium (Sunderland 3°). Other factors favoring reinnervation include young age, short distance between lesion and destination (distal lesions do better), and demyelinating conduction block. Provided that the compressive lesion causing demyelination has been removed, Schwann cells can remyelinate axons in a matter of weeks to months.[6,23]

Electrophysiology has a crucial role in monitoring reinnervation. Attempted regeneration may go wrong because of scarring and high-grade Sunderland axon loss lesions, resulting in neuroma formation and aberrant regeneration.[26,44] Fibrillations and positive waves are silenced by three mechanisms. The first two, reinnervation by collateral sprouting and regeneration, represent salutary outcomes. The third, muscle fibrosis caused by sustained deprivation of nerve trophic support, follows an ill-defined phase maximally 18 to 20 months after injury when muscle fibers become unreceptive to reinnervation. Many neurologists consider 12 months as the effective cutoff. This sets a time and distance limit on how long nerve repair and grafting can be safely delayed.[27,49] When functional recovery is uncertain and delayed repair is appropriate, it is crucial that the pace of regeneration be monitored electrophysiologically to avoid missing this window of opportunity for reinnervation.[4] When expected recovery does not occur by 3 to 6 months, routine and intraoperative NCS can confirm the need for repair by showing absent conduction across the lesion site.[7,26] Electrophysiology has a well-established role in following progress after nerve repair.[16] New electrophysiologic MUNE methods, using modified NCS, long latency responses, and EMG decomposition,[14,34,43] are powerful, rapidly developing techniques ideal for future surgical outcomes research.

Electrophysiology has a role in certain aspects of planning reconstructive surgery of the hand. For example, some patients severely affected with hereditary polyneuropathies (e.g., Charcot-Marie-Tooth disease) may progressively lose useful hand function but retain enough strength in forearm muscles that those might be considered as alternative hand motors using tendon transfers. Detailed EMG of candidate muscles, using standard and quantitative techniques, can assist the surgeon in choosing muscles with an optimal combination of residual innervation, stability of innervation, and motor control.[32]

THE ELECTROPHYSIOLOGIST AS PART OF THE HAND TEAM

The purpose of electrophysiologic testing after nerve injury is to extend the diagnostic sensitivity and specificity of even the most meticulous neurologic examination. Wallerian degeneration after axon loss is a delayed process, rendering NCS most informative at 10 to 12 days after the injury and EMG most informative after 3 weeks or more. Every hand rehabilitation team should include a properly trained, board-certified, neurologically sophisticated, clinically flexible electrophysiologist-physician to assist with preoperative consultation, surgical planning, outcomes evaluation, and research. An interdisciplinary scientific partnership is now feasible and necessary between hand surgeons performing state-of-the-art repair, including some neurotrophic factors, hand therapists using objective techniques including sensibility evaluation, and electrophysiologists using increasingly quantitative and objective methods. The whole will be greater than the sum of the parts. The beneficiaries of such cooperation will be the patients with nerve injuries.

REFERENCES

1. American Academy of Neurology AIDS Task Force: Report from an Ad Hoc Subcommittee, Research criteria for the diagnosis of chronic inflammatory demyelinating polyneuropathy (CIDP), *Neurology* 1991; 41:617.
2. American Association of Electrodiagnostic Medicine: Guidelines in electrodiagnostic medicine, *Muscle Nerve* 1992; 15:229.
3. American Association of Electrodiagnostic Medicine Quality Assurance Committee: Literature review of the usefulness of nerve conduction studies and electromyography for the evaluation of patients with carpal tunnel syndrome, *Muscle Nerve* 1993; 16:1392.
4. Berry H: Traumatic peripheral nerve lesions. In Brown WF, Bolton CF, eds: *Clinical Electromyography,* ed 2, Boston, 1993, Butterworth-Heinemann.
5. Brown WF: The place of electromyography in the analysis of traumatic peripheral nerve lesions. In Brown WF, Bolton CF, eds: *Clinical electromyography,* Boston, 1987, Butterworths.
6. Brown WF, Bolton CF, eds: *Clinical electromyography,* ed 2, Boston, 1993, Butterworth-Heinemann.
7. Brown WF, Veitch J: AAEM Minimonograph #42: intraoperative monitoring of peripheral and cranial nerves, *Muscle Nerve* 1994; 17:371.
8. Carroll G: Comparison of median and radial nerve sensory latencies in the electrophysiological diagnosis of carpal tunnel syndrome, *Electroencephalogr Clin Neurophysiol* 1987; 68:101.
9. Chaudhry V, Glass JD, Griffin JW: Wallerian degeneration in peripheral nerve disease, *Neurol Clin* 1992; 10:613.
10. Daube JR: AAEM Minimonograph #11: needle examination in clinical electromyography, *Muscle Nerve* 1991; 14:685.
11. Daube JR: Electrophysiologic studies in the diagnosis and prognosis of motor neuron diseases, *Neurol Clin* 1985; 3:473.
12. Daube JR: Nerve conduction studies in the thoracic outlet syndrome, *Neurology* 1975; 25:347.
13. Denys EH: AAEM Minimonograph #14: the influence of temperature in clinical neurophysiology, *Muscle Nerve* 1991; 14:795.
14. Doherty TJ, Brown WF: The estimated numbers and relative sizes of thenar motor units as selected by multiple point stimulation in young and older adults, *Muscle Nerve* 1993; 16:355.
15. Dorfman LJ: Quantitative clinical electrophysiology in the evaluation of nerve injury and regeneration, *Muscle Nerve* 1990; 13:822.
16. Donoso RS, Ballantyne JP, Hansen S: Regeneration of sutured human peripheral nerves: an electrophysiological study, *J Neurol Neurosurg Psychiatry* 1979; 42:97.
17. Fisher MA: AAEM Minimonograph #13: H reflexes and F waves: physiology and clinical indications, *Muscle Nerve* 1992; 15:1223.
18. Gutmann L: AAEM Miminograph #2: Important anomalous innervations of the extremities, *Muscle Nerve* 1993; 16:339.
19. Hagbarth K-E, Torebjörk HE, Wallin BG: Microelectrode explorations of human peripheral nerves. In Dyck PJ, Thomas PK, et al, eds: *Peripheral neuropathy,* ed 3, Philadelphia, 1993, WB Saunders.
20. Hudson AR, Hunter D: Timing of peripheral nerve repair: important local neuropathological factors, *Clin Neurosurg* 1977; 24:391.
21. Jackson D, Clifford JC: Electrodiagnosis of mild carpal tunnel syndrome, *Arch Phys Med Rehabil* 1989; 70:199.
22. Jupiter JJ, Seiler JG, Zienowicz R: Sympathetic maintained pain (causalgia) associated with a demonstrable peripheral nerve lesion: operative treatment, *J Bone Joint Surg* 1994; 76A:1376.
23. Kimura J: *Electrodiagnosis in diseases of nerve and muscle: principles and practice,* ed 2, Philadelphia, 1989, FA Davis.
24. Kimura J: The carpal tunnel syndrome: localization of conduction abnormalities within the distal segment of the median nerve, *Brain* 1979; 102:619.

25. Kimura J, Machida M, Ishida T: Relation between size of compound sensory or muscle action potentials, and length of nerve segment, *Neurology* 1986; 36:647.

26. Kline DG: Surgical repair of peripheral nerve injury, *Muscle Nerve* 1990; 13:843.

27. Kline DG, Hudson AR: Acute injuries of peripheral nerves. In Youmans JR, ed: *Neurological surgery,* ed 3, Philadelphia, 1990, WB Saunders.

28. Landau W: The duration of neuromuscular function after nerve section in man, *J Neurosurg* 1953; 10:64.

29. Layzer RB: The origin of muscle cramps and fasciculations, *Muscle Nerve* 1994; 17:1243.

30. Low PA, ed: *Clinical autonomic disorders, evaluation and management,* Boston, 1993, Little, Brown.

31. Mackin GA: Diagnosis of patients with peripheral nerve disease, *Clin Podiatr Med Surg* 1994; 11:545.

32. Mackin GA, Gordon MJV: Restoration of useful hand function using tendon transfer surgery in severe hereditary motor sensory polyneuropathy: the role of EMG in muscle selection, *Neurology* 1996; 46(2):A318-319.

33. Maselli RA, Jaspan JB, Soliven BC, et al: Comparison of sympathetic skin response with quantitative pseudomotor axon reflex test in diabetic neuropathy, *Muscle Nerve* 1989; 12:420.

34. McComas AJ: Invited review: motor unit estimation: methods, results and present status, *Muscle Nerve* 1991; 14:585.

35. Mechler F: Changing electromyographic findings during the chronic course of polymyositis, *J Neurol Sci* 1974; 23:237.

36. Miller RG, Peterson GW, Daube JR, Albers JW: Prognostic value of electrodiagnosis in Guillain-Barré syndrome, *Muscle Nerve* 1988; 11:769.

37. Parry GJ: Electrodiagnostic studies in the evaluation of peripheral nerve and brachial plexus injuries, *Neurol Clin* 1992; 10:921.

38. Parry GJ: Motor neuropathy with multifocal conduction block, *Semin Neurol* 1993; 13:269.

39. Redmond MD, Rivner MH: False positive electrodiagnostic tests in carpal tunnel syndrome, *Muscle Nerve* 1988; 11:511.

40. Ross MA, Kimura J: AAEM Case Report #2: the carpal tunnel syndrome, *Muscle Nerve* 1995; 18:567.

41. Seddon H: Three types of nerve injury, *Brain* 1943; 66:237.

42. Shahani BT, Day TJ, Cros D, et al: R-R interval variation and the sympathetic skin response in the assessment of autonomic function in peripheral neuropathy, *Arch Neurol* 1990; 47:659.

43. Stålberg E, Bischoff C, Falck B: Outliers, a way to detect abnormality in quantitative EMG, *Muscle Nerve* 1994; 17:392.

44. Sumner AJ: Aberrant regeneration, *Muscle Nerve* 1990; 13:801.

45. Sunderland S: The anatomy and physiology of nerve injury, *Muscle Nerve* 1990; 13:771.

46. Thomas PK, Ochoa J: Symptomatology and differential diagnosis of peripheral neuropathy: clinical features and differential diagnosis. In Dyck PJ, Thomas PK, et al, eds: *Peripheral neuropathy,* ed 3, Philadelphia, 1993, WB Saunders.

47. Upton AR, McComas AJ: The double crush in nerve entrapment syndromes, *Lancet* 1973; 2:359.

48. Vinik AI, Suwanwalaikorn S, Stansberry KB, et al: Quantitative measurement of cutaneous perception in diabetic neuropathy, *Muscle Nerve* 1995; 18:574.

49. Wilbourn AJ: Brachial plexus disorders. In Dyck PJ, Thomas PK, et al, eds, *Peripheral neuropathy* ed 3, Philadelphia, 1993, WB Saunders.

50. Wilbourn AJ: How can electromyography help you? *Postgrad Med* 1983; 73:187.

51. Wilbourn AJ, Aminoff MJ: AAEM Minimonograph #32: the electrophysiologic evaluation in patients with radiculopathies, *Muscle Nerve* 1988; 11:1099.

Chapter 6

MORPHOLOGY OF THE NERVE ENDINGS IN THE SKIN OF THE HAND

Steven C. Schmidt
F. William Bora, Jr.

Sensation is one of the most crucial functions of the hand. The multitude of sensory modalities that normally function in the hand allows discrimination among objects and determination of their motion, temperature, texture, and size. Protective sensation helps to protect the hands from injury and thereby preserves their function. The sensory system of the hand aids in the detection of noxious stimuli, also protecting the hand's integrity. Recognition of the importance of intact sensation in the hand can be seen in the level of disability assigned to the loss of sensation in the hand.[1]

This diverse sensory system is accordingly complex, and not completely understood. A large number of components contribute to the normal function of sensation. Each of these components provides information to the central nervous system (CNS), which synthesizes and interprets it to form a psychophysical perception, which is used to accomplish an objective.

This chapter examines the types of receptors in the skin with respect to their histologic appearance and to the role they play in the complex sensory system of the hand.

The receptors in the skin can be categorized into three histologic types (Fig. 6-1). *Free nerve endings* terminate without any specialized structure or associated cells. In *expanded tip endings* the nerve ends in an expanded tip associated with the base of a grouping of specialized cells (e.g., the Merkel cell complex). *Encapsulated nerve endings* are marked by the termination of the nerve in a specialized capsule of connective tissue in association with connective tissue cells (e.g., Meissner corpuscles and Pacinian corpuscles).

The free nerve endings are the most abundant type of nerve ending found in the skin. They are unassociated with any type of specialized receptor organ and are derived from unmyelinated nerve fibers. In many areas of the body, a single unmyelinated nerve fiber may branch to cover a large area and overlap significantly with its neighbors. However, in the digital skin the free nerve endings have an essentially vertical pattern, each covering a minute surface area of skin with very little overlap.[2] Free nerve endings are thought to respond to displacement of the skin, painful stimuli, and temperature. In contrast, in hairy skin such as the dorsum of the hand, a single fiber may branch many times to supply hundreds of hair follicles, thus establishing a large peripheral receptive field. Each hair follicle is richly innervated, being surrounded by a meshwork of free nerve endings, so that the hair follicle can almost be considered a specialized nerve ending.

The predominant type of nerve ending with an expanded tip is the Merkel's corpuscle (Fig. 6-2). The corpuscle is composed of a Merkel cell, an epithelial cell specialized for close contact with the expanded tip of the nerve fiber (Merkel's disk), once it has penetrated the basal lamina of the epidermis. The Merkel's cell possesses dense granules near the junctions between the Merkel's cell and the underlying nerve fiber. These granules are thought to represent packets of neurotransmitters released by the

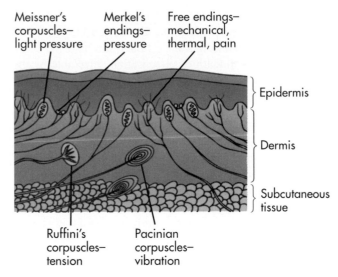

Fig. 6-1. Diagram of cross section of skin demonstrating various layers and sensory endings. (From Lindsay DT: *Functional human anatomy,* St Louis, 1996, Mosby.)

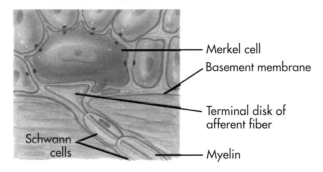

Fig. 6-2. Diagram of Merkel's corpuscle at level of basement membrane. (From Lindsay DT: *Functional human anatomy,* St Louis, 1996, Mosby.)

Merkel's cell to cause an action potential in the nerve fiber when static pressure is applied to the Merkel's cell.

A second type of expanded tip ending has been identified in which an expanded tip of a neuron comes into close contact with apparently normal epithelial cells. It is believed that these respond to cold stimuli.

The encapsulated nerve endings share a number of characteristics. They consist of a single myelinated nerve axon surrounded by a layered connective tissue sheath. Each axon is usually derived from a larger trunk that supplies a number of nerve terminals.

The Pacinian corpuscle consists of a multilayered connective tissue sheath, up to 1 mm in diameter and 3 mm in length (Fig. 6-3). This sheath consists of many lamellae of connective tissue cells separated by a low viscosity gel. The myelinated nerve fiber quickly loses its myelin sheath as it enters the Pacinian corpuscle, ending in a series of small bulbs near the other end of the capsule. They are found in many tissues but are particularly abundant in the tissue just

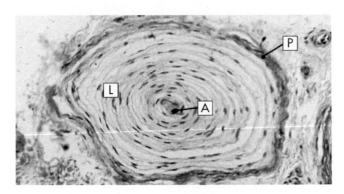

Fig. 6-3. Photomicrograph of cross section of Pacinian corpuscle. (From Stevens A, Lowe J: *Histology,* ed 2, London, 1996, Mosby-Wolfe Publishers.)

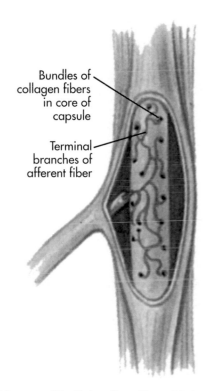

Fig. 6-4. Diagram of Ruffini ending. (From Lindsay DT: *Functional human anatomy,* St Louis, 1996, Mosby.)

below the dermis of the digits. The Pacinian corpuscle is a rapidly adapting receptor and is believed to respond to vibratory stimuli of frequencies up to 700 hertz.

Ruffini endings are small fusiform structures up to 1 mm in length with relatively few layers of surrounding connective tissue cells (Fig. 6-4). They have a fluid filled space traversed by collagen fibers that intermingle with collagen bundles in the surrounding connective tissue. A single myelinated axon enters the receptor, loses its myelin, and branches into many unmyelinated terminal fibers that closely adhere to the collagen bundles. They respond to mechanical stimuli, perhaps tensional forces on the surrounding tissues, with a sustained discharge.

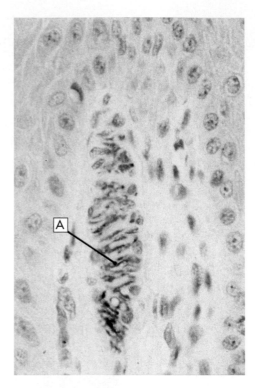

Fig. 6-5. Photomicrograph of Meissner's corpuscle. (From Stevens A, Lowe J: *Histology,* ed 2, London, 1996, Mosby-Wolfe Publishers, Ltd.)

Meissner's corpuscles are made up of modified Schwann cells in a stacked arrangement with the unmyelinated terminal segment of the nerve fiber, weaving its way through the stack of Schwann cells (Fig. 6-5). This corpuscle is surrounded by fibroblasts and a collagen network. Meissner's corpuscles are found in the glabrous skin of the palms and digits. They are rapidly adapting fibers thought to be sensitive to lower frequency stimulation such as that produced by moving the digit over a rough surface.

In 1859 Krause[3] described a new end organ in the conjunctiva distinct from the Meissner's corpuscle.[3] The Krause bulb is a small spherical ending bearing some resemblance to Pacinian corpuscles, however, they are distinct in the degree to which the axon branches. They were once believed to be responsible for the detection of cold stimuli, but this theory has since fallen into disfavor.

The numerous modalities of sensation detectable by the sensory system of the hand are equaled by the complexity and varieties of nerve endings found in the skin and subcutaneous tissues of the hand. Mechanical stimuli are detected by many different receptors, each specialized to respond to a unique range of stimuli. Because naturally occurring stimuli are rarely pure in their content, many of these specialized nerve endings respond in varying degrees to the same stimulus. The ability of the CNS to synthesize this large volume of information from many sources into a single perception allows for the interpretation of these tactile stimuli in an intelligent and useful manor. Although isolating the response of the various types of nerve endings by supplying a particular stimulus can be attempted, intact and normal sensation depends on the contribution of each of these receptors as they respond to the stimuli encountered in daily activities. A failure in the functioning of any of these components adversely alters the ability of the individual to respond appropriately to the environment. The sensory system of the hand is very complex in both its histologic structure and the physiologic synthesis of information provided by this diversity of anatomic receptors.

REFERENCES

1. *Guides to the evaluation of permanent impairment,* ed 3 rev, American Medical Association, 1990.
2. Cauna N: Fine morphological characteristics and microtopography of the free nerve endings of the human digital skin, *Ana Rec* 1980; 198:643-656.
3. Krause W: Ueber Nervenendigungen, *Z ration Med* 1859; 5:28-43.

SELECTED READINGS

Weddell G, Palmer E, Pallie W: Nerve endings in mammalian skin, *Biol Rev* 30:159-195.

Bloom, Fawcett D: *Histology,* ed 12, In Fawcett D, ed: *Bloom and Fawcett histology,* ed 12, New York, 1994, Chapman and Hall.

Weiss L, ed: *Histology,* ed 5 rev, Baltimore, 1988, Urban and Schwarzenberg.

Greenspan J, LaMotte R: Cutaneous mechanorecptors of the hand: experimental studies and their implications for clinical testing of tactile sensation, *J Hand Ther* 1993; 6:75-82.

Chapter 7

CORRELATING SENSORY MORPHOLOGY AND TESTS OF SENSIBILITY WITH FUNCTION

Judith Bell-Krotoski

Measurements of functional loss and recovery go far beyond those of first-order sensory response to touch, pressure, pain, temperature, and position.[33,41,49,56] Recognition of spatial and directional differences in objects, sizes, and shapes, and integration of these with dexterity collectively produce a quality of tactile discrimination. Moberg referred to such qualities of sensibility as *tactile gnosis.*[47,48] There are individual differences in human skills and cognitive reasoning that make precise measurement of tactile gnosis impossible. Still, test instruments used to measure sensibility need to correlate with patient function, just as treatment needs to be grounded on successful restoration of patient function.

There are measurable components of sensibility that can predict patient function. It is time that available tests of sensibility be critically reviewed and rated according to their inherent ability to predict useful patient function.[3,40,42,57,63]

One critical level of function not addressed by most tests is "protective sensation"; enough residual sensation a patient is not in danger of injury from sharp or hot objects because of impaired sensory feedback. Presence or loss of protective sensation can make a difference between hands that can be used safely around equipment and hands that are in danger of chronic injury during use without protective measures.

BACKGROUND

Too many questions remain regarding sensory loss and recovery for examiners to become complacent with the status quo. All the research and clinical studies in this area combined have yet to definitively show what is missing with a loss of sensibility, to quantify recovery, and to correlate changes in sensibility with specific treatment.[*]

When *instrument reliability* is addressed, most sensibility test instruments are found to need more refinement before their results can be depended on for accurate clinical testing.[6,25,26,34] If the type of instrument, size and shape of its stimulus, or force of its application change from one measurement to another, results of testing can vary or be invalid, even if differences in measurement groups can be shown to have statistical validity. Statistical comparisons have to be meaningful.

Once instrument reliability is established, test instruments are validated through clinical measurement. Consideration of a sensibility test's value without comparison to functional sensibility leaves much to be determined regarding the validity of a measurement. Limited comparison with function among tests currently makes it impossible to show that one measurement is more valid than another in predicting levels of loss and recovery. The skill of one patient can be different from that of another, but it is possible to minimize patient accommodation in measurements to draw meaningful correlation.

The tests most commonly used among hand surgeons and therapists for measurement of sensibility are those of two-point discrimination, light touch–deep pressure

---

*References 5, 10, 23, 32, 36, 37, 44, 59.

monofilament testing (Semmes-Weinstein monofilaments), and more recently popularized vibration–frequency recognition. These will each be discussed according to what is known regarding their correlation with patient function.

TWO-POINT DISCRIMINATION

Two-point discrimination is traditionally reported as equating with patient function.[47,48] Actual studies establishing correlation between the test and function are limited. Some authors believe two-point discrimination is a functional discrimination test because it determines the recognition between one and two points of contact on the skin surface.[27] Others believe this is more a test of proprioception. Most examiners agree it can be a test of innervation density not reproduced in the other tests.

Bell and Buford described the variations in applied force of the test in 1979, and reported that without force control of the instrument the force applied with one point is invariably heavier than two-points or vice versa.[11] LaMotte, noting this, pointed out that the test could be one of light touch–deep pressure recognition.[38] The test is more controlled if the weight of the instrument is used as the control.[45] This alone is not sufficient to call the test controlled.

Interrater reliability requires examination with controlled instruments. With uncontrolled instruments it may be possible to have agreement between two testers, particularly experienced testers, but this does not mean there is reliability among all examiners.[19] The real objective in measurements is to have agreement among all testers. The only way to establish this is with a controlled test. A force controlled two-point instrument at least needs use in clinical trials to determine what effect variations in force of application have on the test.

Moberg agrees with this need for force control and recommends at least 5 g or 10 g be used until results of controlled testing dictate otherwise.[47,48] He developed a prototype instrument applying these weights.[7] Newer computerized instruments offer the opportunity to investigate the test at consistent force to determine optimum force of application, but only to the extent these are sensitive enough to test the full range of possible application forces and are controlled enough to eliminate additional force that can be added by the examiner or patient.[16]

Weber invented the two-point discrimination test in the 1800s. Moberg popularized the test with hand surgeons.[18] Dellon introduced the moving two-point discrimination with the intent of more definitive correlation with tactile gnosis.[17] Both the static two-point discrimination test and the moving two-point discrimination test have dynamic components and are dynamic tests, one requiring relatively more movement than the other.[11,14]

Reportedly a patient with recovering nerve function can detect a moving two-point stimulus before a static two-point stimulus.[17] The moving test draws the stimulus along the finger, thus stimulates far more end organ receptors than one

of a restricted area. To compare measurements from the tests, one needs to know both that one point is not being applied more heavily than two and that one test is not being applied with a heavier application force than the other. Results can also differ with test protocol.[50] It is important that the test instrument and protocol remain consistent in study comparisons.

Normal two-point discrimination

Within the limits of current test instruments, two-point discrimination of 3 to 5 mm does, in general, positively compare to normal values of other clinical tests and is useful as a quick test to determine the presence of relatively normal sensibility in the fingertips.[2] It is important that examiners note that two-point discrimination values vary widely from distal to proximal, and current scales of interpretation are most accurate at the fingertips.[61]

Within the limits of currently used instruments, the test has been observed by more than one investigator to sometimes show a false positive (i.e., it appears normal when other sensibility tests show degrees of abnormality). This is noted particularly in patients with nerve compression.[3,54,63] Therefore, it is highly recommended that the two-point discrimination test not be depended on as the only test when a question of normality is important to diagnosis and treatment. It is possible that a controlled test may be more sensitive. It is also possible that the test will never directly correlate with other tests, even though there should be a loose correlation. If innervation density is being tested, two-point discrimination addresses a different component of sensibility from light touch–deep pressure recognition, and one test could show abnormality in earlier stages of peripheral nerve involvement when the other does not.

Neither of the two-point discrimination tests has yet been shown to have a direct correlation with a patient's graphesthesia, texture discrimination, stereognosis, propioception, or temperature and pain recognition. In concept the tests do require directional and positional discrimination, but their actual relationship to function needs definition and clarification.

Diminution in light touch epicritic sensation

Epicritic sensation is that degree of light touch that is of sufficient quality to enable recognition of textures and shapes.[63] While similar to tactile gnosis, the term is slightly different in that *epicritic sensation* refers more specifically to a general level of light touch peripheral nerve function, and *tactile gnosis* to broader patient function, which could include both light touch and deep pressure recognition.

Graduated increases of distance between the test probes of a two-point discrimination instrument are designed to demonstrate diminutions in recognition. It would be informative to know if these actually could be directly correlated with diminutions in patient discrimination of light touch and shapes.[35] Brunelli et al. demonstrated a relationship between

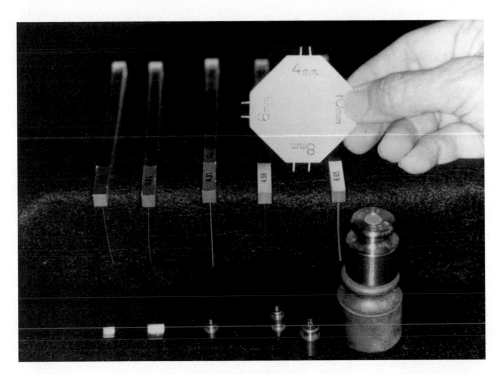

Fig. 7-1. The force of application of measurement devices is important; if instrument stimuli vary, results can vary. Shown is the Diskriminator, which varies in application force but is usually 10 g or more, and Semmes-Weinstein monofilaments with their approximate weights 2.83 50-mg, 3.61 200-mg, 4.31 2-g, 4.56 4-g, and 6.65 300-g.

decreasing moving two-point recognition and gnostic rings in a small patient sample, but this needs to be confirmed in other subjects and with force-controlled tests.[13] Force-controlled computerized instruments offer the possibility for this testing, but available instruments are not yet designed to have the sensitivity in the lighter ranges of application force (less than 1 g).[5,16] Results from two-point discrimination testing applied with 5 g of force could be quite different than testing applied with 30 g of force. The amount of application force used varies from examiner to examiner but has been measured to easily average 30 g.[9] Fig. 7-1 shows how the application force of a two-point discrimination instrument, monofilament, or any other instrument applied with 10 g of force compares with mini-kit Semmes-Weinstein monofilaments (weights are included in front of the instruments). As currently used, it is a relatively heavy stimulus and may not be sensitive enough to detect early peripheral nerve abnormality.

Loss of protective sensation

A critically important question for a patient with abnormal peripheral nerve function is if there is a danger of injury from peripheral nerve-related abnormality during use of the extremities. Is a certain recognition distance associated with redness in the fingertips for longer than 15 minutes following manipulation of objects? At what levels are there likely to be blisters or injuries under splints? What distances are associated with quick reaction to a lightbulb or microwaved cup before a burn?

There has been no study correlating two-point discrimination with presence or absence of protective sensation. Von Prince looked beyond two-point discrimination to quantify protective sensation of patients with peripheral nerve injuries because she observed that two-point discrimination testing did not provide this needed information.[57]

Von Prince observed that of two patients with absent two-point discrimination, one could feel a match that was starting to burn and one could not. This was an important observation. It is the patient who could not feel the match that is most likely to sustain injury. Von Prince determined a level of *protective sensation* using the Semmes-Weinstein monofilament test with a large series of patients having war injuries returning from Vietnam. She advocated protective sensation as a critical level of patient function and used this concept in conjunction with the two-point discrimination test and Semmes-Weinstein monofilaments. Perry later reported on protective sensation and its correlation with the ninhydrin sweat test.[52] Moberg believes that a two-point discrimination distance of greater than 12 mm is only protective, but this has not yet been established by study. Few would argue that if there is a marked decrease in recognition of two-point discrimination by either of the two-point discrimination tests, peripheral nerve abnormality exists.

VIBRATION

Vibration frequency testing has been popularized as an objective test of sensibility.[24,39] The work of Lundborg and others has recently stimulated interest in this area.[21,46,55] Lundborg has reported studies using computerized instrumentation. It is important to note his instrument does control the application force and other variables in testing. Other versions (in the United States) of this computerized instrument have not had the same control on the force of stimulus application or the force the patient can add. Some instruments do not vary the frequency of vibration but only the amplitude or the strength of the signal. The Automated Tactile Tester is an exception to this, and it does have sufficient stimulus control and range of frequency.

Current test instruments for vibration fall under the same criticism as other tests when they lack sufficient control of the actual vibration frequency produced, examiner stimulus force applied, or force added by a patient.[20] It is not enough to control only the stimulus vibration frequency. Tuning forks have the least control of any of the tests used. Their stimulus varies greatly from one examiner to another, and they are not recommended for peripheral nerve testing. It is possible for vibration testing instruments to have sufficient control, and these will become available for clinical use.[22,30,31]

Normal detection of variation frequency

Although testing of vibration has been done with normal subjects using controlled studies and the measurements may be useful diagnostically, studies do not yet address patient function. How then can one determine that a patient who falls below a theoretical norm is, in fact, abnormal? Much more investigation is required to establish the relationship between vibration frequency recognition and normal versus abnormal patient function.

Diminution in light touch epicritic sensation

If a patient has lost detection of a certain low or high frequency strength of vibration, what does this mean? Does it mean he or she will have difficulty with textures, stereognosis, or any of the other functional elements of sensation? Little if any comparison is made of vibration testing with a patient's graphesthesia, texture discrimination, stereognosis, propioception, or temperature and pain recognition. Correlation with epicritic sensation has not been established.

Loss of protective sensation

Correlation of vibration testing with presence or loss of protective sensation has not been made. It is reasonable to believe that correlation could be made with studies using sufficiently controlled instruments.

MONOFILAMENT TESTING

The Semmes-Weinstein monofilaments have been criticized as not relating to tactile gnosis, when they do correlate. Such statements are opinion more than established in study and have served to discourage use of a very good test. The monofilaments do have application force control in contrast to other sensibility test instruments, and they have been found by more than one author to correlate with defined descriptive levels of sensibility. They provide definition of a level of protective sensation.[3,57,63] Protective sensation is a critical component of sensibility rarely addressed by other tests.[15,52]

Von Frey, in the later 1800s, first described a light touch pressure test in efforts to determine organ-specific function of cutaneous end organs in the skin.[7] Using progressively sized horse hairs, he realized the value of touch pressure detection in quantitating abnormality of the mechanoreceptors. Von Frey's test was of light touch, as horse hairs can only produce the lighter range of force (less than 1 g). Semmes and Weinstein further expanded the test to include heavier detection forces that would quantify degrees of loss.

Weinstein invented the instrument device now used with the adaptation of nylon filaments set in right angles in clear plastic rods in the 1950s.[54,60] He specifically chose nylon because nylon does not have the humidity absorption of horse hairs and has optimal viscoelastic properties providing good bend recovery. He gave first authorship to Semmes in recognition of her neurophysiology contributions.

Normal monofilament detection threshold

Weinstein's psychophysic study of normal thresholds was intensive and extensive.[11,54,60-62] Threshold data in his earlier studies are confirmed by modern studies using currently available testing instruments.[8,9] Although Weinstein used the test to measure a large variety of patients with peripheral nerve abnormality, these data were not all published and available to von Prince during her studies of abnormal subjects.

Diminution in light touch epicritic sensation

Von Prince made the earliest scale of interpretation based on correlating the Semmes-Weinstein monofilaments with descriptive functional levels in patients with peripheral nerve abnormality.[57] Von Prince was an occupational therapist working with hand surgeons Omer, Curtis, and Burkhalter, among others, at Brook Army Medical Hospital.[57] Becoming disgruntled with the use of two-point discrimination in testing a large variety of peripheral nerve injuries from war wounds in Vietnam, she searched for a test that could be more predictive of function. She believed the search for another test so important, that she requested six months of leave to investigate other tests. Although not granted the full time, her search led her to the Semmes-Weinstein monofila-

Table 7-1. Von Prince scale of interpretation

	Fingertip	Thumb	Palm
Normal	2.36-2.83	2.44-2.83	2.44-2.83
Diminished two-point discrimination	3.22-3.61	3.22-3.61	3.22-3.84
Loss of two-point discrimination/ diminished protective sensation	3.84-4.17	3.84-4.17	4.07-4.31
Loss of protective sensation	4.31-6.65	4.31-6.65	4.56-6.65

Table 7-2. Werner/Omer scale of interpretation

	Point localization	Area localization
Normal	2.44-2.83	2.44-2.83
Diminished light touch	3.22-4.56	3.22-4.31
Loss of light touch	4.74-6.10	4.56-6.10

No change in scale for fingers, thumb, and palm.
Heaviest filaments omitted because they would not bend; two-point discrimination omitted and considered as a separate test; diminished two-point and loss of two-point combined to one level, diminished light touch.

Table 7-3. First Hand Rehabilitation Center scale of functional interpretation, 1976

	Fingertip	Thumb	Palm
Normal	2.36-2.83	2.44-2.83	2.44-2.83
Diminished light touch	3.22-3.61	3.22-3.61	3.22-3.84
Diminished protective sensation	3.84-4.31	3.84-4.31	4.07-4.56
Loss of protective sensation	4.56-6.65	4.56-6.65	4.74-6.65

Point localization within 1 cm required for a yes response.

ments being used at the National Institutes of Health in studies to map cortical areas of the brain in monkeys. She adapted the test for her patients with peripheral nerve injuries (Table 7-1).

Of note in the scale is the attempted correlation between decreasing detection of Semmes-Weinstein monofilaments and decreasing detection of two-point discrimination. Von Prince wanted to demonstrate a correlation between the tests so hand surgeons who primarily used two-point discrimination could readily understand the relationship.

Loss of protective sensation

Von Prince named the levels *diminished protective* and *loss of protective sensation.* She observed protective sensation was still present in slight to mild sensory impairment but was lost beyond a certain level of detection.

Omer became so convinced of the value of the Semmes-Weinstein monofilaments that following the transfer of von Prince overseas he insisted the work be continued by Werner and other therapists. Werner and Omer performed over 4000 tests in 787 patients with peripheral nerve injuries. Changes were made in the von Prince scale of interpretation based on clinical testing (Table 7-2).[63]

Importance of changes in the scale of interpretation

Werner and Omer realized the lack of direct correlation between the Semmes-Weinstein monofilaments and two-point discrimination tests. They used both of these tests but treated two-point discrimination as a separate test. The two-point discrimination test was dropped from the monofilament scale of functional interpretation. The diminished two-point and loss of two-point discrimination in the scale became diminished light touch.

Localization of a stimulus to assure recognition was an important consideration to Werner and Omer. They developed two scales of interpretation, one for point localization (covered with a dowel within 1 cm) and one for area localization (correct localization of an area touched).

The Hand Rehabilitation Center, Ltd, in Philadelphia, began using the Semmes-Weinstein monofilaments in the early 1970s. This second hand center established in the United States has served as a model for many that have followed. While the monofilament test was perceived as invaluable in following a number of patients with peripheral nerve entrapments and injuries, little was known at the time of the origin of the scale used at the center, or of the earlier works. The scale appears to contain some elements of both the von Prince, and Werner and Omer scales, omitting two-point discrimination but including protective and loss of protective sensation levels for counseling patients regarding protecting areas with sensory inpairment (Table 7-3).

I assumed responsibility for testing the large number of patients with peripheral nerve abnormalities at the center in 1976 and followed a diligent therapist by the name of Loretta Mariano, who had carefully performed evaluations there. She had used the Semmes-Weinstein monofilaments in what was then a very detailed 2-hour evaluation. (Because it was not determined which test was optimum in predicting changes in peripheral nerve function and many patients would potentially have surgery based on the results of tests, every possible test was used.) The battery included two-point discrimination, light touch–deep pressure recognition (Semmes-Weinstein monofilaments), graphesthesia, stereognosis, proprioception, vibration, temperature, pain,

Table 7-4. Current Hand Rehabilitation Center scale of interpretation, Bell, 1978

	Long kit*	Mini-kit†	Colors
Normal	1.65-2.83	2.83	Green
Diminished light touch	3.22-3.61	3.61	Blue
Diminished protective sensation	3.84-4.31	4.31	Purple
Loss of protective sensation	4.56-6.65	4.56 (high end)	Red
		6.65 (low end)	Red
Untestable		>6.65	Lined

*20-filament kit for normative study or detailed analysis.
†5-filament reduced kit sufficient for mapping or screening.
An area of normal reference is established before testing.
Point localization is not required.

object manipulation (Moberg pick up), as well as sensory and motor nerve conduction, and others.

In an earlier position at the former U.S. Public Health Service Hospital in New Orleans, I had independently come to the same conclusion as von Prince that there was additional information needed not provided by the two-point discrimination test. Some patients who had a good history of peripheral nerve neuropathy scored normal on a two-point discrimination test, performed as generally recommended by the American Society for Surgery of the Hand. A probe drawn across the hand from one nerve area to another would often demonstrate areas of diminuted detection. These patients were consistent from one day to another, among examiners, and were believed to have peripheral neuropathy not detected by the standard two-point discrimination test.

At the Hand Rehabilitation Center, I found that the Semmes-Weinstein monofilaments did detect these patients, and the test seemed a missing link—a differential probe test that offered a golden opportunity to quantify and precisely follow peripheral nerve abnormality. Using the monofilaments, an area of diminution could be established and two-point discrimination tested within and external to that area.

Despite obvious advantages of the monofilament test, there were problems with the test and use of the interpretation scale. Problems included the length of time required for the test, the absence of information and documentation for the scale, the lack of available measured forces other than the log scale, and the lack of a consistent color coding for mapping and reading abnormal nerve areas. The test needed to be shown to be repeatable and validated for use with clinical subjects tested.

Consistent color coding was introduced in the test based on the cool to warm color system used by Brand in thermography studies for degrees of temperature change.[12] This addition reduced interpretation time by making normal and abnormal areas more quickly recognizable in extent and degree.

Still, some early mappings were inconsistent and confusing. On review this was caused by (1) adjustments in the scale of interpretation for thumb and palm and (2) the requirement of point localization for a yes response.

One filament was detected by most patients at all sites, even though detection of lighter filaments varied slightly according to site. It is not usually necessary to determine if a patient can feel better than normal, but whether the patient is normal or not. The 2.83 (marking number) was detected at all sites in most patients. Where this filament was not detected, there was a specific abnormality mapped by heavier filaments. This filament was selected for screening of normal. It was used at any site with the understanding that there might be small differences in detection (to be kept in mind in data analysis).

One scale was more rational than several for various body areas. There are no arbitrary lines between fingers, thumbs, palms, and other body areas. Abitrary adjustments in the scale for site in some cases misrepresented data (a more proximal area of a returning peripheral nerve was represented as worse than a distal area of the same nerve). The accuracy of such adjustments became questionable because not enough is known or documented regarding patient response at diminuted levels of light touch–deep pressure for site adjustments to be determined so specifically. When the scale was kept constant and not changed for body site or body part, the mappings became logical and understandable.

The requirement for point localization confused results of the Semmes-Weinstein monofilament test. Results were more repeatable without point localization as a requirement. Point localization was observed to return independent in pattern from that of light touch–deep pressure after peripheral nerve laceration. Point localization was still tested, particularly in patients with nerve laceration, but it was treated as a separate test. Localization was found unnecessary to assure a patient detected a filament if an area of response was established for reference close to the part being tested. If the patient responded to the reference site, but not to a site tested, a differential in filament recognition was established (Table 7-4).

Once a consistent mapping was possible for the entire upper extremity, the Semmes-Weinstein monofilaments were used extensively in a test battery with other tests. Because a number of the patients with problems referred to the Hand Rehabilitation Center had been previously unsuccessfully treated, it was important to provide a complete evaluation. A test battery was routine for any patient referred with a history of pain, sensory abnormality, or muscle abnormality. In addition to tests for sensibility, nerve conduction testing was performed independently by another examiner for information regarding level of lesion.

After a two-year period, data from 200 tests of 150 patients with nerve lacerations and compressions were collapsed and reviewed. Data from the 20-filament Semmes-Weinstein monofilament test were found to predict perfor-

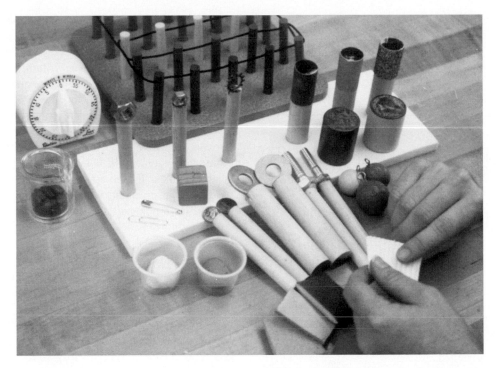

Fig. 7-2. A subject who measures normal sensibility by any test instrument should also score normal on tests of functional discrimination, including light touch textures. An early sign of functional diminution is difficulty in discerning textures.

mance on the other tests. Of the tests used, the Semmes-Weinstein monofilaments were believed to have given the most consistent and reliable results. Based on correlation with performance on the other tests used, functional descriptions were made for each functional level of the Semmes-Weinstein monofilaments for the first edition of *Rehabilitation of the Hand.*[3,7]

If the patients tested within normal limits, they had normal graphesthesia, two-point discrimination, texture discrimination, stereognosis, temperature recognition, pain, and proprioception (Fig. 7-2).

If the patients tested as having diminished light touch, they had graphesthesia and texture discrimination close to normal and adaptable, most often there was fair to good two-point discrimination, good temperature recognition and stereognosis, pain recognition, and proprioception. There was close to normal use of the hand, and the patients might not realize there had been a sensory loss.

If the patients tested as having diminished protective sensation, there was greatly reduced or lost graphesthesia and texture discrimination, usually diminution (7 to 10 mm) or loss of two-point discrimination, and decreased stereognosis and decreased temperature recognition, but there was recognition of pain and proprioception. There was often difficulty in manipulating some objects, a tendency to drop some objects, and complaint of weakness (Fig. 7-3).

If the patients tested as having loss of protective sensation, there was greatly reduced or lost graphesthesia and texture discrimination, loss of two-point discrimination,

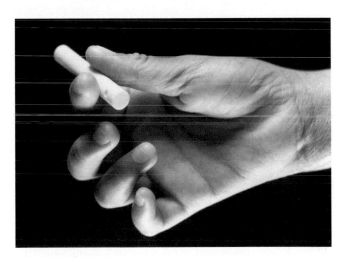

Fig. 7-3. Stereognostic discrimination is related to the use and manipulation of objects. Patients who cannot easily recognize objects by touch have difficulty manipulating some objects, particularly those outside their line of vision.

markedly reduced stereognosis, and greatly reduced if not lost temperature recognition, but the patients could still have some pain recognition (would still be able to detect a pin prick as dull and sometimes sharp) and proprioception. There was markedly reduced use of the hand and absent manipulation of objects outside line of vision. The chance for burns and other injuries from cooking, manipulating sharp objects, and using machinery was observed to be greatest at this level (Fig. 7-4).

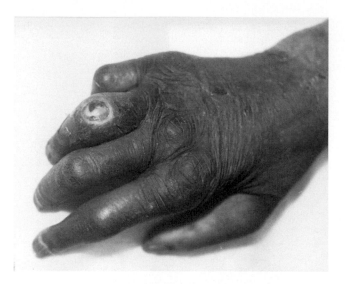

Fig. 7-4. An important component of functional discrimination rarely addressed by tests of sensibility other than the Semmes-Weinstein monofilaments is protective sensation. Shown is a patient with loss of protective sensation who has injured himself by rubbing contracted proximal interphalangeal joints against bed sheets while sleeping.

If the patients were untestable, a few of them could detect a pin prick but most could not. (Note: if a pin prick was present, the monofilament response was normal, or at any level of diminution). Proprioception tested by movement of a finger 1 cm in various directions would remain normal in most cases, even if there were complete ulnar and median nerve loss.

Mini-kit

Based on data from the monofilament and other tests, a mini-kit of 5 filaments was developed and is suitable for most testing.[3,7] Filaments within a level did not provide additional information in comparison with functional tests and required time for testing. The filaments above normal were not useful for most clinical purposes. They are important for normative studies or when a patient scores within normal limits and nerve areas are compared (e.g., ulnar and median nerve areas).

Using the last normal filament and cut-off filaments for each of the other functional levels, diminished light touch, diminished protective sensation, and loss of protective sensation, the test kit could be reduced to the most significant filaments. Two filaments were necessary for the loss of protective sensation level. In a progressive nerve loss, it is most important to determine when there first is loss of protective sensation. In a regenerating nerve that has lost response, it is most important to know when the nerve first responds to a deep pressure stimulus.

Of specific note is that the scale of interpretation (for long and mini-kits) was based in part on the first Hand

Rehabilitation Center scale, and also on correlation with functional tests, and independently from scales of von Prince, and Werner and Omer. When the first edition of the *Rehabilitation of the Hand* was written, it became important to document the origins of the scale, and the former works were revisited. The derived Hand Rehabilitation Center scale was found to be almost identical to the area localization scale of Werner and Omer if their diminished light level is divided into two divisions, and heavier and lighter filaments they omitted are replaced. It is believed that this could not have occurred unless the investigators were describing the same functional discrimination levels. In fact, there are close similarities among all the interpretation scales. The exact cut-off points may be subject to argument and changes based on controlled testing, but the relative relationship of the monofilaments to function was clear.

The specific application force values of available filament kits needed to be measured, and the relationship of available monofilament testing kits to original measurements of Semmes and Weinstein needed to be clarified. A biomedical engineer from the Rehabilitation Research Laboratory at the U.S. Public Health Service Hospital in Carville, Louisiana, was consulted regarding the need for monofilament instrument measurement during a visit he made to the Hand Rehabilitation Center in 1977. This consultation began collaborative work in sensibility research. My subsequent move to Carville allowed further investigation at that facility. Callihan assumed my position and continued studying sensibility testing at the Hand Rehabilitation Center in Philadelphia.

At the Carville facility, it was at first unknown if the testing would apply to patients with Hansen's disease. Literature then frequently described loss of sensation in such patients. Tests used at the Carville hospital were suitable for gross measurement, but not at a sensitive detection level. Clinical testing usually consisted of a pinprick examination marked on a form of the whole body (although cotton wool or a feather was sometimes used for light touch). A 1-2-g to instrument had been used experimentally. This was of nylon fishing line set in vertical fashion in a pen holder. Repeatable tests lighter than 1 g had not been used. With the Semmes-Weinstein monofilaments, it was determined that patients could be measured with nerve changes not detected by the heavier tests and that peripheral nerves could be mapped similar to any other patient with trauma and neuropathy.

Use of the monofilaments has changed the thinking of some investigators regarding the possibilities of treatment and prevention of neuropathy progression in Hansen's disease. It was thought that once a nerve was damaged, nothing could be done to improve its function other than prevention of deformity progression. When sensitive tests are possible, peripheral nerves can be detected as abnormal at an earlier stage and the status can be observed to worsen or improve over time and with treatment. Early detection became an objective in addition to identification of insensitivity for protection. Protection of insensitive limbs and the effect of stress on soft tissues had been a particular line of study and education at the Carville facility. Patients with Hausen's disease can have multiple and severe nerve involvements of both upper and lower extremities. Hand and foot screens developed using the monofilaments have now been introduced in U.S. programs and overseas for patients with Hausen's disease and any other peripheral nerve diseases, disorders, and trauma. Instrument calibration and testing protocols are still being researched.

Current interpretation scale

Over time, the monofilament test has been relied on more and more at the Hand Rehabilitation Center and other centers for definitive data both in measuring and monitoring abnormality and patient counseling regarding level of function before and after peripheral nerve surgery.[4,14,27] The derived 1978 Hand Rehabilitation Center scale of interpretation and test protocol has become standard in monofilament testing. Two-point discrimination testing has not been discouraged per se, as this is the most commonly used test and is required for some physical capacity evaluations, but it is time that the relative relationship of these tests in measuring patient function be established.

Correlations of the Semmes-Weinstein monofilaments with patient functional levels now need repeating using calibrated monofilaments and other tests of sensibility and function. More is known regarding the tests and test instruments, and there are standardized tests of function and others being developed. Weinstein has been consulted regarding his testing and recommendations for test comparisons. While most identify him with the monofilaments, his testing included two-point discrimination and localization as well as tests of function.[60] Controlled studies can add definition and understanding of stage of neuropathy and ebb and flow of peripheral nerve diminution, loss, and recovery. Sensitive tests and ability to correlate changes in the tests with treatment may directly result in improved treatment.

The protocol in which tests are compared is important and critical to the application, the generalization, and the validity of findings. Some clinical comparisons have reported little correlation of the monofilaments and other tests with function when limited numbers of subjects or groups are used, when a limited range of response is considered, or when the study has not addressed variables that can affect results.[1,22]

Besides sensitive and controlled test instruments, correlation with function is highly dependent on minimizing accommodation and eliminating patient substitution.[50] Given enough time, many patients can solve differences between rougher and smoother objects by the amount of resistance and vibration they detect from other areas.

Textures, shapes, and objects should be recognized in much less than 1 minute and should be confined to an area of the hand with a measured level of diminution. The patient needs to be given the opportunity to qualify which feels rougher or smoother, etc., just as in an examination for eye refraction. Enough numbers of subjects at specific levels of diminution needs to be included.

Studies that use uncontrolled or uncalibrated instruments, that do not eliminate substitution, and that lack control of other variables add more confusion than understanding. As with any protocol, assessment of performance on functional tests in normal subjects first needs to be established before they can be used with any degree of certainty in abnormal subjects.

Other considerations

Omer continues to believe that, in general, a patient should be able to localize the site stimulated but agrees localization can be an independent variable and inability to correctly localize should not be counted as a no response for a filament otherwise detected.[50] Motor skills vary in subjects, and some normal patients cannot localize within 1 cm.[50] Point localization, as opposed to threshold detection, is highly variable from distal to proximal.[29,60] It is now recognized that localization is highly variable in pattern of return in regenerating nerves because fascicles do not always regrow down the same nerve fascicles and there can be temporal reordering of information from cutaneous nerve endings.[18] Localization can easily be tested separately when needed.

Regarding the Semmes-Weinstein scales of interpretation that changed for fingers, thumb, and palm, we now know that adjustments in the scales were disproportionate because of unequal force increments between filaments of various sizes. Normative studies now confirm the 2.83 (filament marking number) as a good predictor of normal for the entire body, with the exception of the plantar surface of the foot, which is 3.61 (filament marking number).[8,52] Unlike tests of two-point discrimination and localization, touch-pressure detection threshold is relatively constant all over the body, supporting the use of a consistent scale.[59] Adjustments for body parts at diminuted levels of detection (diminished light touch, diminished protective sensation, and loss of protective sensation), if necessary, still require much more measurement and documentation. Adjustments in the interpretation scale need to be compared using controlled studies so that differences can be understood and the need for adjustments can be clear and substantiated.

The lighter above normal threshold Semmes-Weinstein monofilaments can be used for subjects who have a good history of peripheral nerve symptoms but who score within normal limits. The examiner can use the patient as his own control and check for differences among nerve branch areas, such as between the ulnar and median nerves. For early detection of carpal tunnel patients, Szabo now recommends including the lighter filaments from the original 20-filament set that fall above threshold and in the normal range.[53]

An area of diminished light touch can be confirmed by the patient. He or she can be asked to feel the difference between a smooth and rough surface with the affected area. Often the patient can appreciate this difference even when he or she may not have perceived there has been a sensory loss. Often at this level an area of abnormality can be mapped that demonstrates a distinct area of change—improvement or worsening with subsequent measurements. While many neuropathies are transient, early nerve involvement is not static, and it tends to become worse over time without treatment.

Dininished light touch was at first thought only to be suspect. It is so close to normal that examiners were hesitant to call it abnormal. Only after time and observation has the importance of this level been fully recognized. Peripheral nerves do not normally show diminutions unless there is underlying pathology.

Patients who present with a slight diminution can and do quickly become worse before the next visit and are then not as likely to respond to treatment. A change in this level is an early sign of change in the nerve status and a warning that should be noted. Two-point discrimination is often abnormal at this level, but in a few cases it can be normal even while Semmes-Weinstein monofilament detection is at the diminished protective sensation level.

None of the interpretation scales made adjustment for callus, but callus is always noted. Callus is an independent variable because it is a reaction of the skin to high stress, and the amount of callus a patient has when first seen can subsequently differ as use of the hand differs. Areas of callus can be present on fingertip and other contact areas of patients who have peripheral nerve diminution. Callus also occurs in patients with normal peripheral nerves if the extremities are heavily used. If a slight sensory diminution is limited to an area of callus, the examiner notes this for record but is not usually concerned regarding neuropathy. If diminution in touch-pressure detection thresholds extends inbetween callus (finger creases) or beyond callus in a specific nerve area of innervation, or is at a diminished protective sensation level or greater, it is considered abnormal and of concern regarding neuropathy. Callus can mask some early neuropathies, but the situation is usually made clear with mapping and follow up. Callus is a problem in testing mostly on the plantar contact surface of the foot where the 3.61 filament that would normally be considered diminished light touch is still within normal limits in some subjects.

TREATMENT CONSIDERATIONS

In the foot, (more than functional discrimination) a great concern regarding patient function is the level of protective sensation. Is the patient in danger of ulcers, injuries, infections, and amputations from peripheral nerve abnormality? For prevention of developing neuropathy, early detection and monitoring at lower levels of diminution are also important.

Brand correctly points out that protective sensation is no guarantee that a patient will not still be injured. This level of functional discrimination only means that from a physiologic standpoint, enough effective sensibility is still present that will usually allow a subject to recognize a noxious stimulus before there is tissue damage. For instance, a patient with a splint that is rubbing or too tight will have enough detection of possible injury that he or she will complain or remove the splint. Where protective sensation is absent, the same patient is likely to leave the splint on until a blister develops. A patient with protective sensation will recognize heat from a hot tub as noxious before keeping an extremity in long enough to cause a burn. Where protective sensation is absent there is often a time delay, and the patient is more likely to be in the hot tub long enough to sustain a burn. A patient with protective sensation is likely to recognize that a hot cup from a microwave is hot enough to burn. The patient with loss of protective sensation is better off always using gloves.

Abnormally high normal stress, repetitive stress, or shear can injure any tissue, sensate or not. Repetitive stress can cause necrotic tissue, even without breaking the skin, and is sometimes more damaging than normal stress that is perpendicular to the skin surface. Shear stress can be quickly damaging to any tissue, as when one uses a screwdriver with the palm of the hand and a blister forms. A patient with loss of protective sensation also has a greatly reduced physiologic warning system regarding these when the hands are used and is always in danger from such activities. There are often visual signs that can be seen so that damage can be minimized and protected until healed.

However, patients must be taught to look for signs of tissue damage. They need to be educated in protective care techniques and warned if they have lost protective sensation, because repetitive damage is often overlooked. This is part of the mechanism of damage to limbs in diabetic patients and others with peripheral neuropathy. Some of the damage and amputations can be prevented with education and protection from sharp objects and high concentrations of pressure in small areas (Fig. 7-5). Often elevations in temperature can be detected in tissue that has been overstressed, and temperature as well as visual examination can be used to monitor the status of tissue of an extremity after use (Fig. 7-6, *A* and *B*).

Measurement of the nerve status only at more severe levels means that patients with early developing problems may be missed at a point when they are most responsive to treatment to prevent or reverse the damage. Once there has been a loss of protective sensation, the nerve is not as likely to have the capacity to return to normal, and considerable damage to the peripheral nerve has already happened. When the lack of sensitivity of many sensibility test instruments is

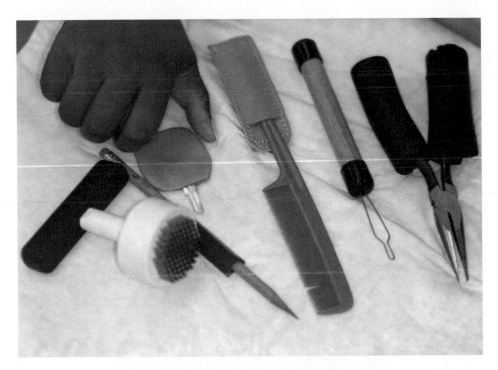

Fig. 7-5. Patients with loss of protective sensation are far more likely to have injury from normal activities; need protective care education; and modification of frequently used hot, sharp, or small objects like keys and handles.

considered, one begins to believe that with more sensitive tests and increased early intervention, there may potentially be more effective responses to treatment for peripheral nerve problems than we have yet been able to appreciate.

If there is a question of residual peripheral nerve innervation worth treating, a pinprick examination is sometimes helpful in searching for residual areas in a patient who does not respond to the Semmes-Weinstein monofilaments. If the patient responds to the pin prick as sharp, one only knows that they may be normal or abnormal at any level of detection. Some patients will not respond to a pin prick when they can detect the heaviest filament (given instructions that the pin may not feel sharp). Once this is pointed out, these patients report they detect the stimulus, but it only feels like a deep pressure or weight. (Part of the variation in the pinprick examination may be caused by the fact that the test is not yet force controlled, and application force has been measured to range from a few grams to over several hundred grams.)

Nerve conduction testing is an important adjunct to any sensibility testing. While not completely objective, nerve conduction is helpful in establishing the site of lesion.[35] There should be a loose correlation of nerve conduction with sensibility tests, but there is not always a direct correlation. Nerve conduction of a peripheral nerve can be abnormal or suspect when there is not yet a sensory or motor change. Nerve conduction can be absent when there is residual

response to deep pressure detected by the Semmes-Weinstein monofilaments.

NEED FOR CLARIFICATION IN COMPARISON STUDIES

Calibration of the Semmes-Weinstein monofilaments is critical to studies that compare instruments. Top-loading balance scales are not always accurate in monofilament measurements, because the monofilaments are a dynamic stimulus and top loading scales are designed to measure a static weight. Levin et al. measured and reported on deviation from the original log scale published by Semmes and Weinstein, but they used only three instruments. Bell and Buford reported on a system designed to measure the dynamic properties of the monofilaments and described variables in measurement.[6,11,13] Based on the mini-kit filaments, Weinstein has recently invented a newer version of the monofilament instrument with rounded tips, control of slippage during filament application, and certified calibration.[60]

CORRELATION AMONG TESTS

Definitive correlation among two-point discrimination, vibration, and monofilament light touch–deep pressure tests has not been done. Comparisons that have been made are limited by the protocol used, the lack of controlled application force, and verification of the monofilament's calibration. Where access to controlled instruments is

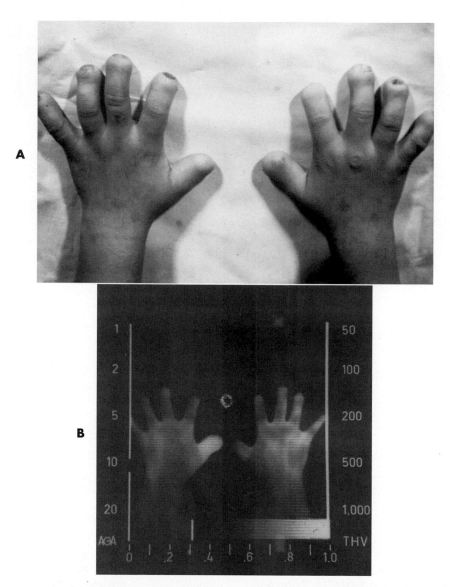

Fig. 7-6 Increasing temperature longer than 15 minutes can be a sign of too much stress in a tissue area. A 16-year-old girl with a congenital sensory radicular neuropathy, who has a loss of protective sensation is shown in **A.** Although repetitative damage can be seen at the fingertips, the left thumb was considerably higher in temperature than the surrounding areas **(B).** As seen by infared photography at the time of examination, the patient needs to minimize overuse and repetitive stress in the left thumb to prevent further tissue damage.

available, it is important for the vibration testing instruments to be used in clinical comparison studies to determine interrelation of the tests.

Increasingly, new sensibility test instruments are being developed and promoted as optimal. The advent of computerized technology has expanded the horizon of what can be developed. It is helpful for the clinician to remember that there is a need for controlled tests and that the peripheral nerve system innervating and supplying sensibility has not changed, but only attempts in its measure. All of tests need to be compared with each other and shown to have a direct correlation with function. Sensibility tests important in establishing a diagnosis are less useful in assessing outcome unless they can be associated with levels of patient function.[1]

REFERENCES

1. Amadio PC: Diagnosis, evaluation, anesthesia. In Amadio PC, Hentz VR, eds: *Year book of hand surgery,* ed 23, St Louis, 1995, Mosby.
2. American Society for Surgery of the Hand: *The hand: examination and diagnosis,* Aurora, Colo, 1978, The American Society for Surgery of the Hand.

3. Bell JA: Sensibility evaluation. In Hunter JM, Schneider LH, Mackin EJ, Bell JA, eds: *Rehabilitation of the hand,* ed 25, St Louis, 1978, Mosby.

4. Bell-Krotoski JA: A study of peripheral nerve involvement underlying disability of the hand, *J Hand Ther* 1992; July/Sept:1-10.

5. Bell-Krotoski JA: Advances in sensibility evaluation, *Hand Clin* 1991; 7(3):527-546.

6. Bell-Krotoski JA: Pocket filaments and specifications for the Semmes-Weinstein monofilaments. In Amadio PC, Hentz UR, eds: *Year book of hand surgery,* ed 18, St Louis, 1992, Mosby.

7. Bell-Krotoski JA: Sensibility testing: current concepts. In Hunter JM, Mackin EJ, Callahan AD, eds: *Rehabilitation of the hand,* ed 4, St Louis, 1995, Mosby.

8. Bell-Krotosky JA: Threshold detection and Semmes-Weinstein monofilaments: a comparison study, *J Hand Ther* (Special issue on Biomechanics) 1995; 8(2):155-162.

9. Bell-Krotoski JA, Tomancik E: Repeatability of the Semmes-Weinstein monofilaments, *J Hand Surg* 1987; 12A:155-161.

10. Bell-Krotoski JA, Weinstein W, Weinstein C: Testing sensibility, including touch pressure, two-point discrimination, point localization, and vibration, *J Hand Ther* (Special edition on Perhipheral Nerves) 1993; 6(2):114-123.

11. Bell-Krotoski JA, Buford WL: The force/time relationship of clinically used sensory testing instruments, *J Hand Ther* 1988; 1:76-85.

12. Brand PW: *Evaluation of the hand and its function,* Philadelphia, 1973, Orthopedic Clinics of North America, Saunders.

13. Brunelli G, Battiston B, Dellon AL: Gnostic rings: usefulness in sensibility evaluation and sensory reeducation, *J Reconstr Microsurg* 1992; 8(1):31-34.

14. Buford WL: Clinical assessment, objectivity, and the ubiqitous laws of instrumentation, *J Hand Ther* (Special issue on Biomechanics) 1995; 8(2):149-154.

15. Callahan AD: Sensibility assessment: prerequisites and techniques for nerve lesions in continuity and nerve lacerations. In Hunter JM, Mackin EJ, Callahan AD, eds: *Rehabilitation of the hand,* ed 4, St Louis, 1995, Mosby.

16. Dellon ES, Mourey R, Dellon AL: Human pressure perception values for constant and moving one- and two-point discrimination, *J Plast Reconstr Surg* 1992; 90:1, 112-117.

17. Dellon AL: The moving two-point discrimination test: clinical evaluation of the quickly-adapting fiber/receptor system, *J Hand Surg* 1978; 3(5):474.

18. Dellon AL: The sensational contributions of Erik Moberg, *J Hand Surg* 1990; 15B:14-24.

19. Dellon AL, Mackinnon SE, Crosby PM: Reliability of two-point discrimination measurements, *J Hand Surg* 1987; 12A:5.

20. Dyck PJ, Obrien PC, Bushek W, et al: Clinical vs quantitative evaluation of cutaneous sensation, *Arch Neurol* 1979; 33(9):651-656.

21. Dyck PJ, Zimmerman IR, O'Brien PC, et al: Introduction of automated systems to evaluate touch-pressure, vibration, and thermal cutaneous sensation in man, *Ann Neurol* 1978; 4:502-510.

22. Dyck PJ, Bushek W, Spring EM, et al: Vibratory and cooling detection thresholds compared with other tests in diagnosing and staging diabetic neuropathy, *Diabetes Care* 1979; 10(4):432-440.

23. Evans RB: Diagnosis, evaluation, anesthesia. In Amadio PC Hentz VR, eds: *Year book of hand surgery,* St Louis, 1995, Mosby.

24. Fegerr RL: Reliability of a widely used test of peripheral cutaneous vibration sensitivity and a comparison of two testing protocols. *Br J Industrial Med* 1988; 45:635-639.

25. Fess E: Clinical validation of hand rehabilitation: evaluating published research. In Hunter JM, Mackin EJ, Callahan AD, eds: *Rehabilitation of the Hand,* ed 4, St Louis, 1995, Mosby.

26. Fess E: The need for reliability and validity in hand assessment intruments, *J Hand Surg* 1986; 11A:621-623.

27. Gellis M, Pool R: Two-point discrimination distances in the normal hand and forearm, *J Plast Reconstr Surg* 1977; 59:57-63.

28. Greco RJ, Hunter JM, Schneider LH: The use of a Semmes-Weinstein sensory evaluation in CTS, Presented to the Amer Soc of Plast and Reconstruct Surg Meeting, San Francisco, 1989.

29. Halnan CRE, Wright GH: Tactile localization, *Brain* 1960; 83:677-700.

30. Horch K, Hardy M, Jimenez S, et al: An automated tactile tester for evaluation of cutaneous sensibility, *J Hand Surg* 1992; 17A(5):829-837.

31. Horch K, Hardy M, Jimenez S, et al: Evaluation of nerve compression with the automated tactile tester, *J Hand Surg* 1992; 17A(5):838-842.

32. Jabaley ME, Bryant MW: The effect of denervation and reinnervation of encapsulated receptors in digital skin. In Marchac C, Hueston JT, eds: *Transactions of the Sixth International Congress of Plastic and Reconstructive Surgery,* Paris, 1976, Masson.

33. Johansson RS, Valbo AB: Skin mechanoreceptors in the human hand: an inference of some population properties. In Zotterman Y, ed: *Sensory functions of the skin,* Oxford, 1976, Pergamon.

34. Johnston MU, Keith RA, Hinderer SR, et al: Measurement standards for interdisciplinary medical rehabilitation, *Arch Phys Med Rehabil* Saunders, Harcourt Brace Jovanovich, 1992; 73(Suppl 12):53.

35. Johnson KO, Phillips JR: Tactile spacial resolution, two-point discrimination, gap detection, grating resolution, and letter recognition, *J Neurophysiol* 1981; 46:1177-1191.

36. Kimura J: Principles and pitfalls of nerve conduction studies, *Ann Neurol* 1984; 16:415-27.

37. Koczocik-Przedpelska J, Gorski SZ, Powoerza E: Relationship between sensory nerve conduction and temperature of the hand, *Acta Physiol Pol* 1983; 34:21-28.

38. LaMotte RH: Presented in discussions at the Symposium on Assessment of Cutaneous Sensibility, Gillis W. Long Hansen's Disease Center, Carville, La, 1979.

39. LaMotte RH, Mountcastle VB: Capacities of humans and monkeys to discriminate between vibratory stimuli of different frequency and amplitude: a correlation between neural events and psychophysical measurements, *J Neurophysiol* 1975; 38:539-559.

40. LaMotte RH: Psychophysical and neurophysical studies of tactile sensibility. In Hollies N, Goldman R, eds: *Clothing comfort: interaction of thermal, ventilation, construction and assessment factors,* Ann Arbor, 1977, Ann Arbor Science.

41. LaMotte RH, Greenspan JD: Cutaneous mechanoreceptors of the hand: experimental studies and their implications for clinical tests of tactile sensation, *J Hand Ther* 1993; 6(2):75-82.

42. LaMotte RH, Srinivasan MA: Tactile discrimination of shape: response of slowly adapting mechanoreceptive afferents to a step stroked across the monkey fingerpad, *J Neuroscience* 1987; 8(6)c:1672.

43. Levin S, Pearsall G, Ruderman RJ: Von Frey's method of measuring pressure sensibility in the hand: an engineering analysis of the Weinstein-Semmes pressure aesthesiometer, *J Hand Surg* 1978; 3:211.

44. Lavine DW, Simmons BP, Koris MJ, et al: A self-administered questionnaire for the assessment of severity of symptoms and functional status in carpal tunnel syndrome, *Bone Joint Surg* 1993; 75A:11.

45. Louis DS, Green TL, Jacobson KE, et al: Evaluation of normal values for stationary and moving two-point discrimination in the hand, *J Hand Surg* 1984; 9A(4):552-555.

46. Lundborg G, Lie-Stenstrom AK, Sollerman C, et al: Digital vibrogram: a new diagnostic tool for sensory testing in compression neuropathy, *J Hand Surg* 1986; 11A:669-693.

47. Moberg E: The unsolved problem—how to test the functional value of hand sensibility, *J Hand Ther* 1991; 4(3):105-109.

48. Moberg E: Two-point discrimination test, *Scand J Rehab Med* 1990; 22:127-134.

49. Mountcastle VB, LaMotte RH, Carli C: Detection thresholds for stimuli in humans and monkeys: comparison with threshold events in mechanoreceptive afferent nerve fibers innervating the monkey hand, *J Neurophysiol* 1972; 35:122-136.

50. Nakada M: Localization of a constant-touch and moving-touch stimulus in the hand: a preliminary study, *J Hand Ther* 1993; 6:23.

51. Omer GE, Bell-Krotoski JA: Sensibility testing. In Omer GE, ed: *Management of peripheral nerve problems*, ed 2, Philadelphia, Saunders (in press).

52. Perry JF, Hamilton GF, Lachenbruch PA, Bevin AG: Protective sensation in the hand and its correlation to Ninhydrin sweat test following nerve laceration, *Am J Phys Med* 1974; 53:113.

53. Poppen NK: Clinical evaluation of the von Frey and two-point discrimination tests—correlation with a dynamic test of sensibility. In Jewett DL, McCarroll HK Jr, eds: *Nerve repair: its clinical and experimental basis,* St Louis, 1980, Mosby.

54. Semmes J, Weinstein S, Ghent L, et al: *Somatosensory changes after penetrating brain wounds in man,* Cambridge, 1960, Harvard.

55. Szabo RM, Gelberman RH, Williamson RV, et al: Vibratory testing in acute peripheral nerve compression, *J Hand Surg* 1984; 9A:104-109.

56. Vallbo AB, Johansson RS: The tactile sensory innervation of the glabrous skin of the human hand. In Gorden G, ed: *Active touch,* Elmsford, NY, 1978, Pergamon.

57. Von Prince K, Butler B: Measuring sensory function of the hand in peripheral nerve injuries, *Am J Occup Ther* 1967; 21:385-396.

58. Waylett-Rendall J: Sensibility evaluation and rehabilitation. In *Orthop Clin North Am,* Philadelphia 1988, Saunders.

59. Waylett-Rendall J: Sequence of sensory recovery: a retrospective study, *J Hand Ther* 1989; 2:4.

60. Weinstein S: Fifty-years of somatosensory research: from the Semmes-Weinstein monofilaments to the Weinstein enhanced sensory test, *J Hand Ther* 1993; 6:1, 11-28.

61. Weinstein S: Intensive and extensive aspects of tactile sensitivity as a function of body part, sex, and laterality. In Kenshalo DR, ed: *The skin senses,* New York, Springfield, Ill, Thomas, 1968, Plenum Press.

62. Weinstein S, Seren E: Tactile sensitivity as a function of handedness and laterality, *J Comp Physiol Psychol* 1961; 54:665-669.

63. Werner JL, Omer GE: Evaluating cutaneous pressure sensitivity of the hand, *Am J Occup Ther* 1970; 24:5.

EVALUATION OF SENSORY MEASURES IN NEUROPATHY

Sir Sidney Weinstein
Ronald Drozdenko
Curt Weinstein

This chapter has three purposes. First, it discusses the potential physiologic implications and interpretations of various measures of tactile sensitivity. Second, it compares the Weinstein Enhanced Sensory Test (WEST) with some other noninvasive instruments that are also used to grade tactile neuropathy or to evaluate protective sensation. Third, new noninvasive tests and procedures for evaluating neuropathy are presented.

We consider three basic views of sensory function: force sensibility, pain sensibility, and the discrimination of two points from one (two-point discrimination). We then discuss the differences among these functions of the nervous system and the problems that occur when a specific measurement procedure fails to distinguish among them.

Then we deal specifically with the noninvasive tactile sensory measurement of peripheral neuropathy. The validity and reliability of these measurement methods are presented along with data relating force thresholds to receptor density. The Rapid Threshold Procedure, a procedure for obtaining force thresholds rapidly and reliably, is also introduced. Two-point discrimination is compared with force sensibility, and a clear distinction is drawn between them, by suggesting lateral inhibition as a physiologic mechanism underlying the difference.

The WEST is presented as an instrument designed to overcome problems frequently reported with other force and pressure evaluation methods, and we directly compare the WEST with the Semmes-Weinstein and the Automatic Tactile Tester. In support of the validity of the WEST, data are presented on the relationship between age and force thresholds and on the confound of pain sensation with force thresholds.

We conclude with our prediction of future trends. Thus, we propose a potentially more valid and reliable method to measure two-point discrimination. We also propose the use of relative force thresholds to measure carpal tunnel syndrome in cases of hand callus. In general, we suggest that the future of the noninvasive measurement of sensory neuropathy will be based on the careful systematic adaptation of existing technology rather than a revolution of expensive high technology.

THREE BASIC SENSORY FUNCTIONS

A thorough and valid evaluation of afferent nerve function should minimally consider the sensations of force and pain and also the more complex perception of two-point discrimination. The two most important aspects of force sensation that clinicians must consider are (1) the loss of normal sensation, which indicates onset of neuropathy; and (2) the loss of protective sensation, which indicates that an uninformed patient may inadvertently engage in tissue-damaging behaviors.

The senior author developed the Semmes-Weinstein monofilament test in 1952. The junior authors collaborated with the senior author to develop the Weinstein Enhanced Sensory Test, which is patentd by all three authors. The third author wishes to thank K. B. Hu.

Although force sensation is relatively easy to evaluate reliably, evaluating pain sensation, even when applied noninvasively, is more troublesome. Thus, the invasive pinprick test of pain is subject to the confound of an uncontrolled manual application of force. Moreover, the use of such an invasive device is contraindicated for the evaluation of diabetic limbs, in which circulation may be greatly impaired. The pinch test may be employed instead of the pinprick test; however, those pain sensations, too, have questionable reliability (i.e., in view of the lack of control over the force applied and the area stimulated). Perhaps devices that exhibit precise control over the energy applied (e.g., a heat-conveying laser) will be found to be preferable. Assessing the presence of pain sensation, however, has limited utility in a patient with neuropathy. Certainly, in neuropathic-free individuals, pain sensation provides warning of an imminent injury. In patients with neuropathy, however, the experience of chronic pain conveys no immediately useful information. Thus, chronic pain sensations do not warn of impending injury, and, thus, pain sensations are usually not associated with any outwardly observable causation. Because neuropathic pain is not directly associated with impending danger, the patient frequently learns to ignore pain sensation as a useful warning signal.

In contrast to pain, even in patients with neuropathy, sufficient force sensation—protective sensation—warns of imminent injury. Because a major emphasis of this chapter deals with force thresholds, we discuss it in detail in subsequent sections, especially as it relates to the other measures of sensitivity.

The third means of assessing neural function is the classical determination of two-point discrimination, a cognitive, perceptual, spatial measure, that greatly depends on the integrity of basic tactual sensation and the central-nervous-system function of lateral inhibition. Lateral inhibitory function is the neurophysiologic process whereby the central nervous system (CNS) restricts the overload of multiple, simultaneously applied, neighboring stimuli from producing a singular, all-inclusive perception, thus enabling the individual to perceive the separate, neighboring stimuli. This CNS process is required to detect edges of surfaces, to recognize forms tactually, and to manipulate tools. The differentiation of two adjacent points from a single point of an applied force is necessary to evaluate the extent to which the CNS processes the spatial aspect of force stimuli adequately.

Ideally, each specific noninvasive test of nerve function should reflect only one of these three basic functions: pain sensibility, force sensibility, or two-point discrimination. Because each of these functions has a specific clinical significance, any sensory test that ambiguously overlaps any of these basic functions is less useful to the physician. Unfortunately, several commonly employed noninvasive instruments for assessing peripheral nerve function have been purported to measure similar functions. A closer consideration of the available data, however, reveals that the measures in question are not equivalent. Thus, measures of two-point discrimination, vibrotactile sensation, force sensation, and (even) pressure sensation all reflect different aspects of tactile function.

Let us briefly consider vibration sensation as an example of the unfortunate confusion among these measures. Theoretically, neurons of different diameter are differentially stimulated by different frequencies of mechanical displacement. Because the same tactile receptor system has been implicated in both the basic force detection and the more complex vibrotactile detection, the factors that affect one measure should affect the other, and, therefore, there should be a positive correlation between these two tactile thresholds. As of this publication, however, tests of vibration threshold are, unfortunately, subject to a number of errors. The most widely recognized error is that the average skin displacement during stimulation is neither known nor controlled by the vibrating device, with the unfortunate result that the vibrating displacement is added onto an unknown and usually time-varying displacement. Other problems concern the fact that vibration initiates a series of concentric traveling waves on the surface of the skin which propagate in varying degrees across the body surface. Thus, the total cutaneous area being stimulated is not well specified and may vary widely from one patient to another depending on subcutaneous fat deposits, for example. Further, the impedance of the skin to vibration varies across different body areas, a factor which adds additional error variance to the vibrotactile measures.[7,13] These errors could account for the lack of correlation across body parts between the thresholds from vibratory stimulators and the Semmes-Weinstein monofilaments.[8] This lack of correlation strongly suggests that the traditional methods currently employed for measuring vibrotactile sensation are inadequate and particularly inappropriate for use in comparing sensation across body sites. That conclusion, however, rests on the assumption that it is the simple Semmes-Weinstein monofilaments that are the valid measure for determining tactile skin sensitivity, and by implication, for detecting neuropathy. Let us examine that assumption.

DETECTION OF NEUROPATHY BY FORCE THRESHOLDS

Force thresholds may be the easiest and most reliable way to diagnose neuropathy. Bell-Krotoski reviewed methods to diagnose nerve injuries to the hand and concluded that, although not without problems, the Semmes-Weinstein monofilaments approach is an ideal objective test of cutaneous sensitivity.[3,4,16] By contrast, she found standard two-point and vibrotactile stimulation instruments too variable, because they did not control the force of application. In reviewing studies that compared the relative merit of monofilament tests and two-point discrimination tests,

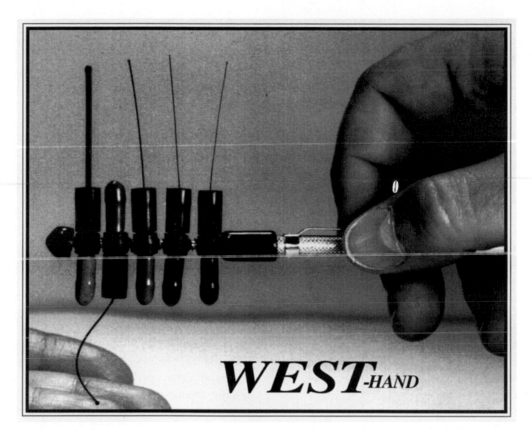

Fig. 8-1. Weinstein Enhanced Sensory Test hand instrument (WEST-hand). Closeup of a hand being tested.

Brandsma concluded that in the diagnosis and evaluation of neuropathy, monofilament tests are preferable. In studies of experimentally-induced carpal tunnel syndrome, two-point discrimination values often inappropriately demonstrated normality, whereas the thresholds obtained with the monofilaments detected the presence of severe impairment. In patients with carpal tunnel syndrome the monofilament tests were found to be 91% sensitive compared to two-point discrimination, which demonstrated only 33% sensitivity.[6] MacDermid also reported monofilament testing to be superior in the diagnosis of carpal tunnel syndrome.[14] Thus, the Semmes-Weinstein monofilaments have demonstrated comparatively good validity for testing tactile peripheral nerve function.

Monofilaments are effective in the detection of neuropathy because they control the application force automatically and continuously by virtue of their intrinsic physical qualities. The control is so fine that the monofilament automatically compensates for the vibration inherent in a tester's hand to control the applied force delivered. Experimental demonstrations of the inability, even of experienced surgeons, to keep the force of the two-point probe constant have been made by Bell-Krotoski and her associates by the use of force transducers. They also similarly studied the Semmes-Weinstein monofilaments. These demonstrations clearly reveal that the deliberately controlled and manually

applied force of the two-point probe shows considerable variability. In contrast, the manually applied force of the monofilaments remains unquestionably constant, even when the surgeons deliberately jiggled the monofilaments vertically. Uncontrolled variation of manually applied force also seriously diminishes the reliability of other sensory testing instruments. Thus, considering the clinical research, we can conclude that the thresholds of the Semmes-Weinstein monofilaments validly reflect neuropathy.

A similar force-testing instrument, the WEST, derived from the classical Semmes-Weinstein, also employs monofilaments, but, because it is new, it has not yet been extensively studied[22] (Fig. 8-1). Because the WEST uses a modified monofilament configuration, it is reasonable to ask whether the WEST monofilaments also reflect challenges to the sensory nerve. As a starting point, research showed that the thresholds obtained with the WEST monofilaments show a high correlation ($r = .99$) with the Semmes-Weinstein monofilaments across sites in neuropathic-free subjects.[22] Thus, unlike the vibrotactile measures, the WEST monofilaments have comparative validity to the Semmes-Weinstein monofilaments.

To demonstrate the basic validity of the WEST monofilaments in the detection and grading of neuropathy, an experimental case study was conducted. To detect dynamic changes in receptor integrity, ischemia was experimentally induced in one 41-year-old male volunteer subject, since reduction in the blood flow to the cutaneous receptors should affect their ability to transmit sensation. The validity of the WEST would be in question if it could not reflect the effects of ischemia. The WEST-hand, which was used for this study, employs modified monofilaments with the following factory-calibrated forces: 0.07, 0.20, 2.0, 4.0, and 200 g.[20] The test site was the ventral surface of the distal phalanx of the right index finger, and the threshold determination procedure was the Rapid Threshold Procedure.[23] Ischemia, induced by applying a tourniquet of Tygon tubing to the right arm approximately 3 cm above the elbow, was confirmed both by suppression of wrist pulse and by the drop in electronically-recorded skin temperature very near the testing site. Temperature was also electronically recorded continuously. WEST force thresholds were taken before and several times after inducing ischemia. The correlation of threshold with duration of ischemia was statistically significant ($r = .71$, $p < .01$), as was the correlation of threshold with skin temperature ($r = .69$, $p < .01$). Because the duration of ischemia correlates with thresholds measured with the WEST-hand, the modified monofilaments employed in the WEST show validity in the detection of experimentally induced neuropathy.

The high correspondence of thresholds obtained with the WEST and Semmes-Weinstein in neuropathic-free individuals, however, does not guarantee that same level of correspondence in neuropathic patients. In fact, it was hypothesized that in patients with neuropathy, the correspondence between the two instruments would be significantly reduced because stimulation with the greater force monofilaments of the Semmes-Weinstein more frequently causes pain. This potential difference between instruments is addressed in the section, "Protective Force Sensation versus Pain," p. 73.

Given advances in computer-driven technology, one might predict that such sophisticated devices are more valid than the simple monofilament tests, and indeed, one such device, the Automatic Tactile Tester (ATT), has been proclaimed superior to the Semmes-Weinstein monofilaments. The assertion was that the ATT is more valid than the Semmes-Weinstein, because the ATT pressure thresholds, but not the Semmes-Weinstein force thresholds, correlate with age.[12] In the section, "Force Thresholds and Age" (p. 73), the ATT claim is refuted by the data from both the WEST and a modified (i.e., user-calibrated-for-force) Semmes-Weinstein.

It must also be noted that although currently available computer-interfaced two-point instruments record the force of application, they do not control the force, and thus, they suffer from this major limitation. Bell-Krotoski emphasizes that controlling the application force may be the single most important aspect of peripheral nerve testing.[2,3] Certainly, by failing to calibrate the Semmes-Weinstein,

manufacturers have inadvertently impaired the validity of this simple, functional instrument and have created a disservice to those patients, physicians, and health care providers who depend on the integrity of their diagnostic instruments.

The ATT claims that it tests pressure sensitivity, whereas the WEST claims to test force sensitivity. Actually, these two measures are conceptually the same when the total area stimulated is not altered. In a study of neuropathic-free subjects, reliability of the thresholds obtained with the WEST and Semmes-Weinstein monofilaments were obtained (half-hour test-retest reliability). The Semmes-Weinstein reliability coefficient ($r = .66$) was found to be comparable to the coefficient previously reported for the ATT ($r = .66$).[12] The WEST monofilaments yielded a similar reliability coefficient ($r = .67$). It should be noted that these reliability coefficients are population dependent. For example, a population that included cases with sensory deficits (and thus, an extended range of thresholds) would increase the reliability coefficient. That is, with a more diverse population including both impaired and unimpaired subjects, the reliability coefficients are expected to increase, reflecting the extended range of data. Therefore, with respect to questioning the relative benefits of use of force or pressure thresholds, unless one is willing to accept a considerably higher expense for the advantage of having data automatically entered into a computer, there seems little to recommend computer-based pressure tests such as the ATT. To date, these computer-based tests have demonstrated neither greater reliability nor greater validity than the considerably less costly, conveniently portable, and more easily administered monofilament tests.

Bell-Krotoski reaffirmed the utility of the Semmes-Weinstein monofilaments in a review of clinical sensibility evaluation in light of computer-based tests (but before the advent of the WEST), and, in combination with electroneuromyography, concluded that the (Semmes-Weinstein) monofilaments are one of the most objective instruments for detailed mapping and screening of the extent and degree of nerve pathology.[2]

Some types of peripheral neuropathy impair the integrity of the sensory nerve by reducing the number of functioning fibers in the sensory nerve in (e.g., in contrast to complete nerve section). In these types of peripheral neuropathy, variations in receptor density may model the degree of neuropathy. Certainly, instruments that reflect normally occurring changes in receptor density are sensitive enough to grade the degree of neuropathy. Although two-point discrimination has been speculated to reflect receptor density,[10] force sensation may reflect receptor density more directly. Consideration of other sensory modalities, including loss of receptors in the visual system and loss of hair cells in the auditory system, lends support to the hypothesis that fewer receptors result in greater thresholds for the perception of the

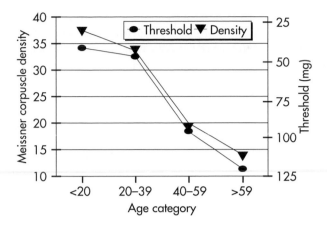

Fig. 8-2. Receptor density and WEST force thresholds as a function of age. The abscissa shows four age groupings. The left ordinate shows density of Meissner corpuscles. The right ordinate shows sensitivity by inverting the threshold scale.

intensity of the stimuli, but only marginally so for the perception of the spatial characteristics of the stimulus.

To determine whether decrease in receptor density is related to threshold changes, data previously collected by Bolton and Winkelmann[5] were correlated with data collected by the present authors. Bolton and Winkelmann took biopsies from the fifth fingers of 95 subjects of various ages and recorded the density of Meissner corpuscles. One of our research assistants, kept unaware of the working hypothesis about force thresholds and receptor density, extracted the density data from their scattergram. Using the WEST monofilaments, we then recorded force thresholds from the same anatomic site that was employed by Bolton and Winklemann in 20 normal subjects whose ages ranged 17 to 75 years (see "Force Thresholds and Age," p. 73, for a description of the subjects). The receptor density data extracted from the Bolton-Winkelmann scatter diagram were averaged into four age categories and plotted, along with the corresponding age categories for the thresholds of the same site we recorded using the WEST (Fig. 8-2). The correspondence between receptor density and the WEST thresholds is apparent. Both Meissner receptor density and sensitivity (i.e., the inverse of threshold) show a very similar pattern of decline across the age groups. This evidence provides direct support for the hypothesis that reduction in receptor density corresponds with the changes in (WEST) force sensitivity. Because receptor density is correlated with the appropriate intensity sensitivity in vision and in hearing, it should not be surprising that, for somatosensation as well, receptor density is also correlated with force sensitivity.

But how should one consider the reports that two-point discrimination correlates with receptor density? It has been reported that determining innervation density is the most critical clinical test of a fiber receptor system.[10] However, when that hypothesis was suggested, it was not known that

tests of force threshold reflect receptor density. Rather, it was hypothesized that two-point discrimination thresholds reflect receptor density. Further, citing the visual evidence in a scattergram of two-point discrimination plotted against Semmes-Weinstein monofilament thresholds, the claim was erroneously made that there was no correlation between the two measures.[10] However, a Pearson correlation of those same data (digitized by an uninformed lab assistant) convincingly shows a clear relationship between the measurements obtained with the two instruments ($r = .71$; $df = 107$, $p < .01$).[10] Thus, to the extent that two-point thresholds are impaired by loss of pressure thresholds—but only to that extent—do two-point thresholds reflect receptor density (the relationship accounts for about half the observable variance).

A misinterpretation of the work of Semmes, Weinstein, Ghent, and Teuber may have led the advocates of two-point discrimination testing astray. Using data derived from the palms of normal subjects, they found that the correlation between two-point discrimination and Semmes-Weinstein monofilament force thresholds was not statistically different from zero, but in a brain-injured group the correlation was statistically significantly greater than zero ($r = .57$; $p < .01$).[17,21] The apparent difference in reports between the correlations of 0.71 and 0.00 is undoubtedly caused by the different populations studied, and may be explained as follows. In the population with varying degrees of neuropathy, deficits in pressure sensitivity very probably influenced the correlation. That is, as pressure sensitivity is lost, eventually so is the ability to discriminate one from two points, no matter how much additional force the tester may apply to the patient's hands. Therefore, loss of sufficient pressure sensitivity invariably results in the loss of the two-point threshold. The result of Semmes, Weinstein, et al. ($r = .0$) clearly shows that, in the absence of sensory deficit, the normal variation in force threshold is totally unrelated to the normal variation in two-point discrimination. The resolution of these apparent disparities shows the importance of testing hypotheses in the relevant population. Therefore, it is reasonable to propose that two-point thresholds should be employed only in patients who first demonstrate adequate force thresholds to determine the extent of lateral inhibitory function.

SIGNIFICANCE OF INSTRUMENT AND PROCEDURE

We believe that the specific testing procedure employed is as important as the instrument used to test and suggest that various improvements to the Semmes-Weinstein (discussed below concerning the WEST) will not be fully realized unless the correct procedure is employed.

Loss of the normal force threshold is used to define the onset of neuropathy. Similarly, the inability to feel several grams of force is used to define loss of protective sensation.

Currently, 4 g is the force used to define loss of protective sensation for the hand, and the value is somewhat site specific, since, for example, 10 g is often the screening level used for the foot. Until recently, the Semmes-Weinstein monofilament test was considered the single most effective of the noninvasive tests of force threshold. In spite of its well-established reputation as an effective instrument, we responded to the need to overcome several reported problems with the Semmes-Weinstein monofilament test and developed the Weinstein Enhanced Sensory Test (WEST). The WEST incorporates modified monofilaments that were developed to increase the validity of the measurement of cutaneous tactile sensitivity, especially protective sensation. The WEST differs from the Semmes-Weinstein in several ways. First, it is factory calibrated for applied force, thereby obviating the need for the user to calibrate the stimulation forces, because calibration is essential and should result in greater interinstrument reliability. Second, the WEST employs enhanced monofilaments (U.S. patents 5316011, and 5381806, and 5492132). These enhanced monofilaments seldom slip from the test site, an improvement that speeds testing time by eliminating the need to repeat unacceptable skid-stimuli. The modified monofilaments also deliver a much less noxious stimulus even at the larger forces, which results in reduced variance in the perception of sensation for superthreshold stimuli and which may increase the validity of the force stimulus for evaluating protective sensation. Third, the WEST complete set is geometrically configured to protect the otherwise fragile lower-force monofilaments from damage. Fourth, the WEST-hand is easily portable (e.g., in a shirt pocket or purse), which may facilitate the examination of patients by their physicians.

Thus, Al-Qattan[1] recently compared the WEST with the Semmes-Weinstein in a clinical setting and studied the frequency of instrument usage (SW versus WEST) among a group of clinicians, the time required for testing using both instruments, and slippage rates on the skin for both instruments. Al-Qattan reported that three surgical residents who tested patients with median or ulnar nerve injuries increased their frequency of testing to 75% when the WEST became available, compared to only 10% when only the Semmes-Weinstein was available; indeed, as soon as the WEST became available, none of the residents selected the Semmes-Weinstein for testing. The average patient testing time also decreased while using the WEST by approximately 13% relative to using the Semmes-Weinstein. Slippage rates, the number of times the monofilament skidded along the skin during testing, were 0% with the WEST compared to 10% with the Semmes-Weinstein. Al-Qattan concluded, "the WEST has several advantages when compared with the old SW filaments and will likely encourage hand surgeons to perform pressure threshold testing more frequently in the clinic."

Scientists concerned with the relationship between the physical nature of the stimulus and its perception (psycho-physicists) have developed procedures to measure the average detection, d', of a stimulus. While there are theoretical differences between detection and threshold, a threshold may be derived from detection. Thus, psycho-physicists have determined how to estimate thresholds optimally. For the clinician, however, the optimal methods of the psychophysicist prove to be tedious and impractical in a clinical setting. On the other hand, the usual clinical alternatives (e.g., a single stimulation) are too variable except for the grossest evaluations. Even the simple ascending threshold method is more variable than an equally time-efficient method, the Rapid Threshold Procedure (RTP).[23] Although we cannot address the theory or even the rationale (beyond saving time and reducing variance) here, it is clear that the RTP has been shown to estimate thresholds in computer simulations. Further, in an experiment comparing two different psychophysical procedures with the RTP, the mean RTP threshold of a group of 30 subjects was quite comparable to the means of the psychophysical procedures employed. We have used the RTP to track the time course of rapidly acting anesthetics and, in that regard, we have repeatedly found it to be consistent. Although a complete description of the RTP can be found,[23] in brief, the RTP employs catch trials (simulated stimulation trials) and a modified descending threshold procedure, where the definition of threshold is changed from the classical descending threshold procedure. Table 8-1 defines all possibilities in generating a threshold with the RTP. Note that a threshold can be obtained in as few as three trials. Of course, if the initial (approximate) stimulus selected is much greater than the true threshold, the procedure may inadvertently be lengthened. We, therefore, suggest that the testers first use their clinical judgment to select an appropriate starting point when using the RTP.

In conclusion, because the psychophysical methods are too time consuming, and the clinical approximations are too variable, we recommend the use of the RTP with the WEST, a combination that yields consistent thresholds in a short period of time.

RELATIONSHIPS BETWEEN TWO-POINT DISCRIMINATION AND FORCE THRESHOLDS

Two-point thresholds are sometimes used (erroneously) instead of force thresholds to assess basic peripheral neuropathy. In general, we maintain that this application is unfortunate, because (the perceptual function of) two-point discrimination differs markedly from the absolute determination of the patient's ability to sense force. Thus, the threshold of two-point detection depends greatly on two separate functions. First, adequate force sensation is a necessary prerequisite to conduct this test validly. Second, lateral inhibition, which is a function of the CNS, is necessary for valid determination of two-point thresholds. Thus, the major difference between measure of force sensation and thresholds of two-point discrimination is the

Table 8-1. Rapid threshold procedure

Trial No.	Stimulus Size /Patient's Response	Comments: Stimulus Size—S1> S2 > S3, etc.; C = catch trial Patient's Response—Y = yes; N = No (Y = correct for S; N = correct for C)
		Example 1
1	S1/Y	Start with a stimulus just large enough for detection (or with a catch trial). Proceed to next lowest stimulus or a catch trial.
2	C/N	Use a catch trial in the first 3 stimulations.
3	S2/N	Failure to detect a stimulus means the next greater stimulus should be employed.
4	S1/Y	Proceed to next lowest stimulus or a catch trial. Because the patient did not feel a nonzero stimulus (S2), the necessity of a catch trial at this point in the procedure is much reduced.
5	S2/N	STOP: S2 has failed detection twice in a row (N, N), and S1 has been detected twice in a row (Y, Y). Threshold is defined as midway between the two stimuli. Threshold = $0.5 \times (S1 + S2)$.
		Example 2
1	C/N	Start with a catch trial (or with a stimulus just large enough for detection).
2	S1/Y	The first stimulus should be large enough to ensure detection.
3	S2/N	Failure to detect a stimulus means the next greater stimulus should be employed.
4	S1/N	STOP: The response pattern for S1 is (Y, N), which defines threshold. Here S1 is threshold. (Also means that S1 was probably a poor choice to start the RTP, although it worked out in this example.)
		Example 3: Case of Continuing Session
1	S1/Y	Start with a stimulus just large enough for detection (or with a catch trial).
2	C/N	Use a catch trial in the first 3 stimulations
3	S2/N	Failure to detect a stimulus means the next greater stimulus should be employed.
4	S1/Y	Detection means continue to the next smallest stimulus (or a catch trial—but when the patient fails to report a nonzero-sized stimulus, [e.g., "S2/N" above] the need for frequent catch trials diminishes).
5	S2/Y	Even though the response pattern is (N,Y), this trail was passed. *Continue* with the next smallest stimulus or a catch trial.
6	S3/any	Stops defined in examples 1 and 2 above.

introduction by the CNS of the process of lateral inhibition. Another major difference between force perception and two-point discrimination concerns a potential methodologic flaw; thus, the force of probe application is usually not controlled when two-point discrimination is determined.

A study conducted by one of us (SW) illustrates the distinction between the essentially cortically (i.e., CNS) involved test of two-point discrimination and the subcortically-mediated test of force detection.[22] During a craniotomy, the conscious patient's prestimulation two-point and force thresholds were obtained on both hands and found to be completely normal. Then, while the neurosurgeon (Dr. Mark Rayport) electrically stimulated the cortical "hand area," both force and two-point thresholds were repeated bilaterally. Although the force thresholds remained completely unchanged on both hands, the two-point threshold was totally abolished on the hand subserved by the cortical area being stimulated (the contralateral hand), while the ipsilateral hand remained unchanged. As soon as the current applied to the cortical hand area was turned off, the poststimulation thresholds were obtained: the contralateral two-point threshold returned to its normal prestimulation level, and the force thresholds on both hands remained normal and unchanged.

Thus, the "mini-seizure" experimentally induced by the electrical stimulation to the cortical hand area abolished normal lateral inhibitory function for the hand, thus causing the two points to be perceived as a single, massive stimulus affecting the entire palm. The ipsilateral (unstimulated) hand was never impaired before, during, or after the stimulation. This case study clearly emphasizes the distinction between the perceptual measure of two-point and the sensory measure of force detection.

Consider a pencil point pressed against the fingertip. In the neuropathic-free individual, the area being sensed tactually is limited approximately to the indented area of skin immediately contacting the pencil point, while the visually observable area of stimulation (i.e., the conical indentation) is considerably larger. The reason the tactual sensation is limited to the area of maximal stimulation (i.e., the punctate, restricted area directly beneath the point) is the CNS-mediated function of lateral inhibition. All nervous activity emanating from the less-indented conical areas is suppressed by the nervous response from the neighboring, more greatly indented area. Without lateral inhibitory connections within the CNS, the area of tactual sensation would correspond much more closely to the total skin area that was indented. Thus, for patients with adequate force sensation and compromised lateral inhibitory (i.e., CNS) function, the sensation resulting from contact with the pencil point corresponds more closely to the much more widespread visually observable indentation, as was seen in the craniotomy patient when his cortex was stimulated.

Because lateral inhibition, a much more complex function of the CNS, is necessary for the detection of edges in the presence of adequate force sensation, two-point thresholds can measure the sensory-component of the tactual ability to detect edges and forms. In the absence of adequate force sensation, however, deficient two-point thresholds are merely unreliable epiphenomena of the patient's simple inability to detect the presence of the two points, rather than any higher level cognitive spatial inaccuracy.

PROTECTIVE FORCE SENSATION VERSUS PAIN

One of the findings concerning the WEST monofilaments is that even the higher level forces generate little pain. As reported above, Al-Qattan supported that conclusion in a clinical setting. To test the validity of his observations and to define the statistical extent of the effect of the WEST monofilament pain-free stimulation versus the occasionally painful stimulation of the Semmes-Weinstein, we conducted an experiment. It is generally assumed that a painful stimulus excites additional neural structures in contrast to a stimulus that is perceived exclusively to evoke only the sensation of touch. In testing neuropathic-free subjects, pain is not often elicited, even when the Semmes-Weinstein monofilaments are employed, because their force thresholds are lower than in impaired patients.

Therefore, a demonstration study was designed, in which 5 subjects (4 males and 1 female), ages 20 to 46, participated. No skin conditions that might influence the results were noted in any of the subjects. Three Semmes-Weinstein monofilaments and three corresponding-force WEST monofilaments were employed. Each set of monofilaments had forces of 3.6, 15.0, and 127.0 g. Although the force of each of the stimuli is many times greater than the normal threshold forces,[21] these levels are regularly employed with patients. All stimulations were to the distal phalanx of the right index fingers and were presented randomly with each monofilament presented a minimum of ten times. Subjects were blind to the monofilament type with which they were being stimulated and were asked to rate any pain produced by the application of the monofilaments on a 0 to 10 scale (0 referred to no pain and 10 to severe finger pain). The percentages of stimulation trials with a pain rating greater than zero were recorded individually for each subject before determining the aggregate percentage of pain trials. Pain ratings for the 127-g monofilaments were averaged for each subject

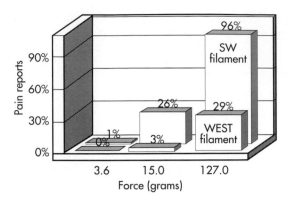

Fig. 8-3. Frequency of reported pain as a function of force applied by WEST and Semmes-Weinstein monofilaments.

individually before computing a mean of all subjects. The findings are presented in Fig. 8-3.

Note that the WEST monofilaments produced only a minimal amount of pain (1 is the lowest level of pain that could be reported) even at 127.0 g. The 3% pain report for the 15.0 g of applied force for the WEST monofilaments was caused by a minimal pain rating by one of the subjects, and none of the other subjects reported any pain for this monofilament. These results support the hypothesis that the WEST monofilaments are much less nociceptive. Moreover, in addition to the comfort level experienced by the patient, the failure to stimulate pain receptors may have clinical significance.

It was hypothesized that the ability of the WEST to reflect force sensation more uniquely (i.e., to stimulate without evoking pain) would enhance its validity to detect large-fiber neuropathy.[18] The large fibers are the last to recover following nerve resection and repair. Also, various metabolic stresses to the nervous system (e.g., diabetes mellitus) tend to affect the large fibers preferentially.

A case study was conducted, whose rationale is rooted in basic peripheral neurology. Peripheral nervous system damage usually results in increased force thresholds. Profound neuropathy of a limb leads to characteristic changes, including alteration in the physical characteristics of the skin surface (e.g., hard, smooth, discolored) and, eventually, resorption of tissue. Gradual insidious onset, for example, caused by a chronic metabolic disease or prolonged low-level intoxication, manifests with signs and symptoms gradually appearing. Initial findings are common in the lower extremities. The distal axonopathy hypothesis states that the large-diameter and long axons (historically referred to as A-fibers) are affected early. Thus, the sciatic nerve branches are especially vulnerable. At the next level, stocking-glove sensory and motor loss may be seen. Axonal degeneration commences distally and slowly proceeds toward the neuronal cell body, yielding symmetric, distal, clinical signs in the legs and arms. The earliest complaints are usually sensory—toe-tip sensations of tingling or

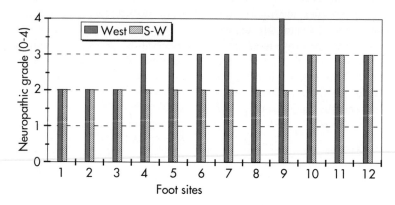

Fig. 8-4. Comparison of WEST and Semmes-Weinstein for neuropathic grades obtained in a diabetic patient. Neuropathic grade is defined as follows: 0 = normal sensitivity, 1 = reduced sensitivity, 2 = reduced protective sensation, 3 = loss of protective sensitivity, 4 = residual sensitivity, and 5 = loss of residual sensitivity.

pinprick. Paralleling the nature of the large-diameter fibers in slow-onset neuropathy is recovery from lacerations and surgical repair of nerves in which the large A-fibers are typically the slowest to recover. Note that with a slow onset of neuropathy the large-diameter fibers are affected first, and that these fibers are also the slowest to regenerate after nerve resection (e.g., surgical repair of a nerve). Conversely, the smallest fibers (historically referred to as C-fibers) are more resistant to such stress. The result is that the A-fibers, which convey sensations of force, are often affected more than the small-diameter fibers, which convey sensations of pain.

Although the WEST and Semmes-Weinstein are two ostensibly similar esthesiometers in neuropathic-free individuals, one difference between the WEST and the Semmes-Weinstein is that the WEST reduces pain associated with testing by producing both fewer painful and less intensely painful stimuli. The reason is likely a function of the type of monofilament tip. The WEST monofilament tips are more hemispheric (not sharp), whereas the Semmes-Weinstein has a contacting tip with an edge (sharp) that often presses into the skin. The differential reports of pain from stimulation with these two instruments suggest that the two instruments differentially stimulate the large-diameter fibers and the small-diameter fibers. That is, the Semmes-Weinstein stimulates the small-diameter fibers to a greater extent than the WEST, and, conversely, the WEST stimulates the large-diameter fibers solely to a greater extent than the Semmes-Weinstein.

Despite this seemingly small difference, however, there may be meaningful and practical consequences. Consider a case history of diabetes and foot neuropathy.[18] The basic axioms are (1) higher thresholds are interpreted as greater neuropathy and (2) the WEST more effectively reflects the activity of the A-fibers. A corollary of axiom 1 (the higher the force threshold, the greater the neuropathy) is that the patient with higher force thresholds is at greater risk for

ulceration. Note that pain is less important to evaluate because (for the most part) the forces for the diabetic foot that cause injury are at a level that would merely cause minor discomfort, not pain, in nondiabetic individuals. If the site is sufficiently insensitive, even low-intensity repetitive pressures may stress the skin and cause an ulcer without the patient's awareness. If one considers that sustained pressure as low as 1 g/mm^2 (conversion of units to make the comparison to monofilaments more easy) can promote ulcers,[11] it is apparent that (1) if the WEST more efficiently stimulates the large-diameter fibers solely and (2) if diabetes affects these fibers more, then testing with the WEST should result in both earlier detection and more effective grading of neuropathy. That is, WEST force thresholds on a diabetic foot should be higher than Semmes-Weinstein thresholds (Fig. 8-4).

The data presented in Fig. 8-4 are from a diabetic female patient with a long history of insulin-dependent diabetes, and of successfully, (nonsurgically) treated foot ulcers. Twelve sites on her feet were examined using the RTP, and thresholds were confirmed so that differences were not likely caused by variance associated with the testing procedure. Two instruments were compared: the Semmes-Weinstein mini-kit and the WEST-hand. Although they both nominally employ the same forces (0.07, 0.2, 2, 4, and 200/300 g),[20] the WEST monofilaments cause less pain in neuropathic-free individuals. Fig. 8-4 shows that for six (50%) of the sites there was correspondence between the thresholds (2:2 g and 4:4 g). For the remaining six (50%) sites, the WEST yielded higher thresholds, a finding consistent with the view that the WEST is more sensitive to this type of neuropathy. The lower thresholds, reflecting a relative deficiency in grading neuropathy for the Semmes-Weinstein, may be explained as follows. The Semmes-Weinstein may have stimulated the small-diameter fibers that the WEST did not, which in concert with the stimulated large-diameter fibers, caused the subject to detect stimulation, resulting in lower thresholds. Fig. 8-4 shows that for one of those six sites, testing with the WEST indicated residual sensitivity for the same site that the Semmes-Weinstein revealed only reduced protective sensation (a stepwise difference in classification of 2), a very large difference. Never did the Semmes-Weinstein yield higher thresholds than the WEST, a result consistent with the belief that the WEST is the more sensitive esthesiometer for detecting these neuropathies.

A RESPONSE TO CRITICISMS OF MONOFILAMENTS

Despite numerous studies demonstrating the consistent relative superiority of the Semmes-Weinstein over two-point tests for detecting the degree of peripheral neuropathy, the Semmes-Weinstein has come under criticism. Some of this criticism may be because of the unfortunate (and certainly indefensible) fact that Semmes-Weinstein monofilament sets are often sold uncalibrated for applied force. Unfortunately, this fact has not been generally disclosed; as a result, research has been needlessly compromised. Thus, variations in the manufacturing process of the monofilaments can cause the uncalibrated Semmes-Weinstein esthesiometer to be susceptible to undetected errors. Dellon,[10] in summarizing the concerns of some clinicians with the Semmes-Weinstein monofilaments, stated that the Semmes-Weinstein monofilaments have serious limitations, including lack of correlation with hand function, perception of pain rather than pressure with higher force monofilaments, and a lack of correspondence of thresholds with innervation density.

Let us consider each of these criticisms. The first criticism (lack of correlation with hand function) involves clearly defining the assessment capabilities of the instrument. Obviously, the Semmes-Weinstein, an instrument designed for peripheral nerve evaluation, cannot be expected to reflect the higher level, cognitive integration of sensory information (e.g., pattern recognition) or muscle recovery (e.g., grip strength). It is reasonable, however, to expect monofilament thresholds to reflect the tactile sensory aspects of peripheral neuropathies. The last two criticisms (on pain perception and innervation density) are especially cogent and have already been addressed. However, despite his earlier criticisms, Dellon,[9] in a more recent paper, conceded that monofilament testing is the most appropriate testing method early in the course of nerve regeneration.

His model states that two-point thresholds measure innervation density and are the less appropriate tests early in the process. As regeneration progresses, two-point thresholds (both static and moving) improve as nerve density increases and continue to show improvement for years after Semmes-Weinstein threshold changes have reached a plateau. Thus, according to his model, the thresholds of the Semmes-Weinstein monofilaments do not correlate with peripheral innervation density, and that innervation density increases over years following nerve resection and repair.

The present authors sharply diverge from Dellon's position on a few points. First, we equate innervation density with receptor density; otherwise it is difficult to define what innervation density is with respect to tactile sensation. Second, while we agree that monofilament force thresholds are most appropriate for monitoring early recovery from nerve repair and that two-point thresholds will recover over years, we do not attribute the ability to discriminate two points to receptor density. Rather, we attribute the change in force thresholds to changes in receptor density, and changes in two-point thresholds to the recovery of lateral-inhibitory function. We propose that receptor density is a simple function of the physiology of healing, whereas lateral inhibition, a function of the CNS, reflects more cognitive aspects (i.e., learning).

In this chapter, we present direct evidence that monofilament force thresholds reflect receptor density and also present evidence supporting the conclusion that two-point thresholds correspond only to receptor density under the very special conditions when two-point thresholds are affected by variations in force threshold, and even then, only partially so. Thus, we attribute loss of function to the simplest reason and not the more complex. We contend that the failure of patients to discriminate a single point from two points applied to their skin, when their ability to detect force is impaired, misleads the clinician. Because inability to detect force is the simpler task, impaired two-point discrimination may merely reflect this failure to detect force. Naturally, a reduced concentration of tactile receptors will result in loss of the spatial (as well as other cognitive) abilities measured by two-point discrimination. In the presence, however, of normal force sensibility, two-point discrimination conveys important information about lateral-inhibitory function and the ability to detect patterns, etc. Two-point discrimination is best employed for measuring the more complex spatial functions, and the more precise determination of the reduction of receptors is most efficiently determined by force sensitivity.

FORCE AND PRESSURE DETECTION

The most closely related of these noninvasive tests of sensitivity are force and pressure detection. Because pressure is simply force per given surface area, the relevant question concerns which method, force or pressure, is preferable for a test that best detects peripheral neuropathy.

When the contacting surface area of the stimulating probe is small, as in a monofilament, the appropriate stimulus for tactile sensation appears to be force.[15] To provide visually convincing confirmation of this fact, one need only press a pencil point against the volar surface of the fingertip. It can readily be seen that the visually observable area of skin indentation is much greater than the specifically perceived site of tactual stimulation. As a further indication, pressing two contiguous pencil points against the fingertip does not increase the area of indentation proportionally. Under those conditions, force is, thus, undoubtedly the more appropriate stimulus.

A different condition exists when the area of the probe employed for stimulation is larger. With probes of larger tip surface area, pressure seems to be the more appropriate stimulus. We might consider a functional test of a large-area stimulus to be exemplified when stimulation with two adjacent probes results in about twice the visually observable area of skin indentation. Testing a large area may be preferable for an average response of a region, whereas, conversely, pressure stimuli may be blind to very site-specific areas of insensitivity. For example, patients with reduced protective sensation may, inadvertently, induce loss of protective sensation and even ulceration at a specific site that was mechanically stressed. Thus, to test the sensibility of small, single-site, force thresholds is preferable, because, by employing force, adjacent sites cannot compensate for any sensory loss at the contiguous site.

There are other practical differences between pressure-delivering instruments versus the force-delivering Semmes-Weinstein monofilaments. Pressure stimuli usually do not confuse the sensations of pressure with pain in neuropathic-free individuals, and that has been one clear advantage of pressure stimuli over the Semmes-Weinstein monofilaments. Unquestionably, the inadvertent creation of pain has been a major deficiency of the Semmes-Weinstein. The optimal stimulus for assessing force sensation, however, is not a pressure stimulus, but rather a force stimulus that does not produce pain in the neuropathic-free individual. The advantage of the optimal force stimulus is a minimized area of stimulation for maximal differentiation between sites.

Data are presented in this chapter that describe the WEST, a new force-delivering instrument, that uses monofilaments that have been modified to result in relatively pain-free stimulation. Thus, the WEST approaches an ideal force-assessing instrument. The advantage of pain-free stimulation is not merely theoretical because pain-free force stimulation results in a more appropriate test of protective sensation and provides a more sensitive test of some common neuropathies. Conceptually, the additional, inadvertent stimulation of pain-mediating fibers lowers the validity of a test of force sensation.

Computer-controlled pressure tests are a recent innovation for testing peripheral neuropathy. As mentioned previously, Horch et al.[12] described the Automated Tactile Tester (ATT), a device that measures cutaneous sensibility, which provides six threshold measurements: touch trapezoid, two levels of vibration, temperature, two-point discrimination, and pain. They reported that the tests of the ATT have a repeatability of $r = .659$ and a correspondence of between $r = .470$ and $r = .529$ with manual measures of touch thresholds (Semmes-Weinstein monofilaments) and two point (Disk Criminator). They also reported significant correlations for five of the specific ATT tests with age. However, they did not find a significant correlation between age and both the thresholds for Semmes-Weinstein monofilaments and two-point tests. We have previously noted that manufacturers' widespread failure to calibrate the Semmes-Weinstein may have adversely affected their obtained age correlation. In light of the significant correlations for the computer-controlled ATT and the failure to find correlations for the manual tests, Horch et al. suggested that the ATT is more consistent and possibly more valid than the manual counterpart tests. Because the ATT is a computer-driven device, however, there may be some compromises in the clinical setting, such as greater expense, lower portability, and greater complexity of use. A less expensive device based on monofilaments might be more desirable if it had similar indices of validity.

FORCE THRESHOLDS AND AGE

Sensibility in all modalities generally tends to deteriorate with increasing age. Many researchers, including the present authors, have obtained that result in such diverse organs as the optic cornea, oral mucosa, and the hand. If the WEST monofilaments validly measure peripheral nerve function, then the thresholds derived by their use should reflect the effects concomitant with age.

A small study (10 males and 10 females, ages 17 to 75 years) was conducted to determine whether age affects thresholds obtained with the WEST monofilaments. All subjects were free from medical conditions that might affect cutaneous sensitivity, all were asked to refrain from taking any analgesics or anesthetics on the testing day, and all were required to report this when they arrived for testing. Informed consent was obtained from each subject in all three studies, and each study was approved by an Institutional Review Board. Two cutaneous measurement instruments were used in this study: the original Semmes-Weinstein monofilaments and its modern replacement, the WEST. A replication of thresholds on one site was obtained to evaluate simple test-retest reliability.

The characteristics of both instruments, which have been discussed previously, are summarized here. Both comprise nylon monofilaments that control the application force via diameter variation. A monofilament, when bent (buckled), delivers a constant force dependent on its geometry. There are three obvious differences between the Semmes-Weinstein and the WEST. First, the stimulation intensities of the WEST monofilaments are reported in grams of force. Second, each WEST monofilament is individually calibrated to be within 15% of the designated force. Third, because the contacting tip of the WEST monofilament is both textured and hemispheric in shape, slippage is reduced and the sharpness of the contacting tip is reduced. The stimuli used to test the neuropathic-free subjects in this study were the Semmes-Weinstein 1.65, 2.36, 2.44, 2.83, 3.22, 3.61, and 3.84, and the corresponding WEST monofilaments which were calibrated in grams: 0.0045, 0.0230, 0.0275, 0.0677, 0.166, 0.408, and 0.697. Thresholds were obtained from both instruments, in randomized testing, on the ventral surface of the distal phalanges of the fifth fingers and the palms (medial). A repeat threshold was obtained from the fifth finger at the completion of testing to assess test-retest reliability. The testing procedures for both esthesiometers were identical. Subjects extended their hand under a partition that shielded their view of the testing procedure. The RTP was used, starting with an easily detected force (0.697 g). The monofilaments were slowly pressed (not thrust) against the testing site. The duration of stimulation was about 1 second, and the monofilaments were lifted slowly from the testing site. Subjects were prompted to the occurrence of each stimulation and responded yes or no to the presence or absence of the tactile stimulus. Sham stimulations (catch trials) were randomly introduced to ensure subject compliance with the testing procedure. No subjects were eliminated as a result of responding falsely to catch trials.

To evaluate test-retest reliability, a Pearson correlation was computed for the threshold replications on the fifth finger. The coefficients for both instruments were statistically significant at better than the 0.001 level, one-tail: Semmes-Weinstein $r = .665$, and WEST monofilaments $r = .674$. The thresholds employing the WEST monofilaments showed a statistically significant correlation with age ($r = .721$; $p < .001$, one-tail). The Semmes-Weinstein thresholds showed a lower, but still statistically significant, correlation with age ($r = .543$; $p < .007$, one-tail).

Others have failed to find a statistically significant correlation with age for the Semmes-Weinstein. It is possible that a significant correlation with age for the Semmes-Weinstein was obtained in this study because we individually calibrated each Semmes-Weinstein monofilament for applied force before use. These results, therefore, suggest that the WEST monofilaments tend to be more reliable and have a higher correlation with age in neuropathic-free subjects. None of these differences was statistically significant, possibly because of the small sample size.

SEQUENTIAL VERSUS SIMULTANEOUS TWO-POINT DISCRIMINATION

In spite of our caveats, specified above, concerning the utility and potential problems inherent in the use of two-point discrimination, the measure may possess some value if, and only if, the numerous impediments to its valid use can be controlled. We, therefore, propose a solution to fulfill the objectives of a valid test. Let us consider the parameters that make for a good two-point discrimination test.

1. The application forces should be controlled. Not only should the total force when both stimulation points are simultaneously applied remain the same for repeated stimulations, but also this total force should be the same for application of the single-point versus the two-point stimulation.

2. There should be no cue to the duality or singularity of points because of inadvertent, successive application of the two points. Thus, when both points are being delivered, one point may, unintentionally, briefly proceed the other. This temporal cue is inappropriate because it translates the proposed spatial duality into a temporal duality. Both points must touch the patient at exactly the same time.

3. Both points must be applied with equal force, or else the patient may erroneously ignore the point with lesser force.

4. Temperature cues should be eliminated, perhaps by first warming the point(s) on the tester's hand before the first stimulation or, preferably, by using materials that are less heat conductive than metal.

5. It is desirable that the application force on each point be at the level of protective sensation (i.e., 4 g for the hand). If patients can perceive two-point discrimination only at force levels exceeding protective sensation, then they are at risk of applying too much (damaging) force while attempting to gain tactile information about objects (e.g., keys in their pocket).

6. The stimulus should be applied for about 1 second.

7. The points must be stationary when applied; moving stimuli create a much easier task than the stationary and should not be inadvertently moved if the stationary two-point norms are to be used.

8. The total area of cutaneous stimulation of the single point should be equal to the sum of the areas for the two points for maximal accuracy.[21]

Many of these conditions are not easy for a hand-held, two-point device to meet; however, complex instruments like an ATT are not necessary. Instead, we propose that the sequential two-point discrimination test, first described by Weinstein,[21] may be an inexpensive and valid alternative to the computer-driven tests and potentially a more valid test than the Disk Criminator or other manually applied two-point discrimination tests.

The sequential two-point discrimination test was designed by one of us and has been referred to in the literature as the point localization test.[21] The test-retest reliability of Weinstein's two-point esthesiometer is reflected by the Spearman correlation between twenty left and right body parts, which is about .99 in neuropathic-free subjects. The inter-test Spearman correlation of the Weinstein two-point esthesiometer with the Weinstein point localization across body sites test is .92. When the reliability is comparable to the interinstrument correlation, we may safely assume that these are the same test (in neuropathic-free subjects). Considering face validity, the point localization and two-point tests would not differ.

What are the expected advantages and disadvantages of using the sequential two-point discrimination test to replace the traditional, stationary, simultaneous two-point discrimi-

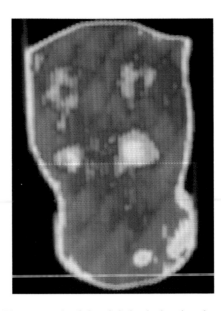

Plate 1. Thermograph of the pig's back showing the temperature contrasts some hours after removal of the applicators. The hottest spot had been under the applicator at 250 mm of mercury for 7 hours.

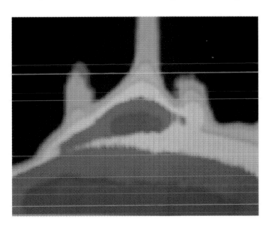

Plate 2. Thermograph of a rat footpad *before* a session of repetitive stress.

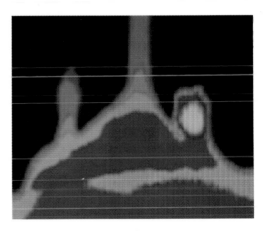

Plate 3. Thermograph of a rat footpad *after* a session of repetitive stress.

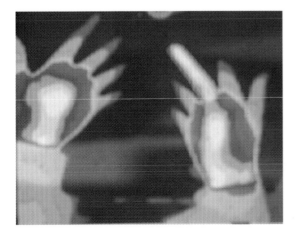

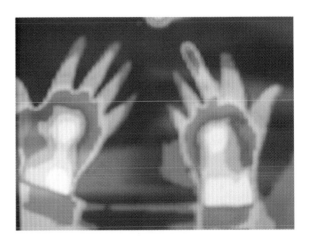

Plates 4 and 5. Thermograph of Dr. Brand's hand when it first came out of the machine (**4, at left**). The same hand after 15 minutes of rest (**5, at right**).

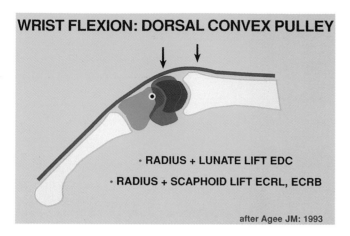

WRIST FLEXION: DORSAL CONVEX PULLEY

- RADIUS + LUNATE LIFT EDC
- RADIUS + SCAPHOID LIFT ECRL, ECRB

after Agee JM: 1993

Plate 6. Dorsal anatomical pulley. Schematic drawing illustrates the configuration of the dorsal anatomical pulley that enlarges the moments of the extensor digitorum communis, extensor carpi radialis longus and brevis when the wrist is in ulnar flexion. Arrow is moment arm for wrist extension.

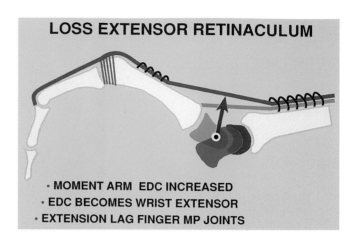

LOSS EXTENSOR RETINACULUM

- MOMENT ARM EDC INCREASED
- EDC BECOMES WRIST EXTENSOR
- EXTENSION LAG FINGER MP JOINTS

Plate 7. Loss of extensor retinaculum. Schematic drawing depicting biomechanical changes associated with loss of the extensor retinaculum.

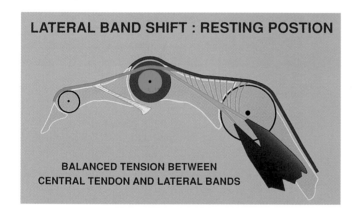

LATERAL BAND SHIFT : RESTING POSTION

BALANCED TENSION BETWEEN
CENTRAL TENDON AND LATERAL BANDS

Plate 8.

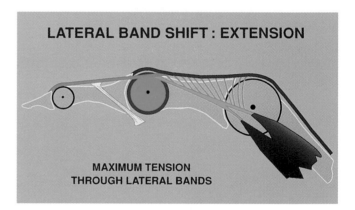

LATERAL BAND SHIFT : EXTENSION

MAXIMUM TENSION
THROUGH LATERAL BANDS

Plate 9.

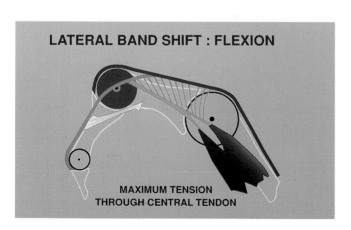

LATERAL BAND SHIFT : FLEXION

MAXIMUM TENSION
THROUGH CENTRAL TENDON

Plate 10.

Plates 8, 9, and 10. Lateral band shift. The radius of the blue circle depicts the moment arm of the extrinsic central tendon for extension of the PIP joint. The radius of the green circle depicts the moment arm of the lateral band for extension of the PIP joint. **8,** There is balanced tension between the central tendon and lateral bands in the resting position. **9,** Tension through the lateral bands increases with interphalangeal extension as their moments enlarge. Tension and the moment for extension of both IP joints is greatest in full extension. **10,** The moments of the lateral bands decrease during flexion as the moment for extension by the central increases. Only the central tendon can initiate extension of the fully flexed PIP joint normally.

Chapter 8 Evaluation of sensory measures in neuropathy 75

nation test? We expect comparable or better reliability. We note that the Pearson test-retest correlations over a period of 1 to 4 days (with three different testers—a stringent test) is .84 for the sequential two-point test but only .67 for the traditional simultaneous two-point test.[17] Consider employing the 4-g WEST monofilament as the stimulus. The total applied force is, thus, always 4 g, and because the single contacting point always has the same contacting area and same applied force, those problems no longer exist. We further note that because that test force is at the level of protective sensation, the sequential two-point test will not indicate two-point proficiency at force levels that are unsafe for the patient to apply. There can, also, never be any inappropriate sequential clue about whether the stimulus comprises one or two points because only one point is used. The heat conductivity of the probe is also no longer an issue because the WEST monofilament is a very poor conductor of heat, and there is no need to equate the total surface area of the two probes with the single probe, as in the classical simultaneous two-point test.

To evaluate the proposed replacement, the authors conducted an informal, pilot test of this sequential two-point test. We observed valid results (i.e., it seems to correlate with the subject's two-point) and retest reliability. It takes only a few seconds to complete a test (actually less than two-point), can determine protective sensation at the same time, and can be conducted with only a force-evaluation instrument. The disadvantages are minor. Thus, it takes a brief time to place a template on the skin of the patient to guide the tester's stimulation. The duration of stimulation from one point to the next may not be precisely the same, but still should be within 1 to 2 seconds, as it is for the classical two-point test.

In summary, we believe that there is a considerable potential advantage to replacing the traditional simultaneous two-point test with sequential two-point discrimination testing for diagnoses. For patient education, however, standard devices such as the Disk Criminator might still have utility because it can be used by patients to self-stimulate and monitor their progress.

RELATIVE THRESHOLDS AND CALLUS

The presence of skin callus produces a challenge to the validity of tests of peripheral nerve function. Thus, consider that callus dissipates the heat of a laser esthesiometer and increases the heat produced by surface-applied electrical stimulation. It absorbs some of the energy imparted by two-point, force, and pressure tests, and sometimes widens the effective area of indentation. Birke, of the National Foot Treatment Center, has reported (through personal communications) that being a physical laborer affects the neuropathic-free thresholds of the hand and foot when using the Semmes-Weinstein monofilaments. Presumably, the mediating variable is the presence of callus. Yet we can compensate for the effects of callus on WEST thresholds by

means of rapidly obtained measures of the hardness and thickness of the callus. A study we conducted for the National Institutes of Health indicated that measures of foot callus can be used to compensate for the effects of foot callus on WEST-generated thresholds. In comparing the relative effects of callus of the foot and hand, foot callus is usually found to be the major confound. We believe that hand callus, for the most part, is less of a confound in grading neuropathy. Hand callus, however, has been implicated in masking the mild sensory effects of carpal tunnel syndrome, for example, which makes the objective detection of the onset of carpal tunnel syndrome more dependent on interpretations of nerve-conduction velocity tests. The following discusses an alternative to compensating for callus, which does not require the callus to be measured.

Two reasons why the callus-correcting device is currently not employed are that the foot doctors claim that they can easily remove the confounding callus, and a new testing procedure may compensate for the usual levels of hand callus. The new procedure is based on the concept that a person with hand callus (e.g., a carpenter) may not be able to feel light forces (e.g., a feather) but certainly can feel the difference in weight between, a 2-pound and a 4-pound hammer, for example. Consider that the usual procedure to evaluate peripheral neuropathy with monofilaments uses absolute thresholds (e.g., 0.2 g versus 0.0 g). An equally valid method is by relative thresholds (e.g., 2 versus 4 g). The advantage of absolute thresholds is that the upper force defines the level of impairment, which is not generally true for relative thresholds. The apparent advantage of relative thresholds is that the confounding effects of common hand callus on monofilament thresholds can be circumvented. While a neuropathic-free subject could not feel 0.07 g (via WEST monofilament) on a site of hand callus, the subject could always differentiate 2 from 4 g. Further, the sensitivity of the test can be predetermined. In differentiating 2 from 4 g, apparently all neuropathic-free subjects are almost 100% correct in this task.

Experimentally induced carpal tunnel syndrome in one subject, however, showed a deficit in that relative threshold test. Thus, the concept of selecting lesser forces to try to evaluate carpal tunnel syndrome is flawed—those who are likely to get carpal tunnel syndrome are the same as those who are likely to have slightly elevated absolute thresholds because of callus. A dilemma presents itself. If the monofilament-obtained absolute threshold is slightly elevated, then should we attribute the effect to the callus or the neuropathy? The "correctly chosen" relative threshold, however, is insensitive to the effects of callus, yet still sensitive to the effects of neuropathy. Thus, the use of difference thresholds may increase the diagnostic usefulness of instruments, including the WEST. The selection of 4 g as the upper comparative force is based on the idea that 4 g is the threshold of protective sensation for the hand, and that patients who cannot differentiate 4 from 2 g have reduced protective sensation.

SUMMARY AND CONCLUSIONS

In this chapter, we have limited the discussion of the sensory evaluation of peripheral nerves to noninvasive instruments of tactile sensation, as these have been shown to be the most reliable and valid. While we agree that tactile force sensation, two-point discrimination, and pain are important to evaluate, we have discounted the perception of pain as less useful to evaluate. We have emphasized the evaluation of protective force sensation over pain evaluation because (1) force sensation can be more reliably and validly measured and (2) pain is often simply a less valid measurement for determining the status of the neuropathic patient. We have discounted the utility of the current vibrotactile instruments, which is not to say that vibration may have no use in evaluation in the future. Indeed, vibration may have great utility, if the average force level can be controlled. We have discounted the value of the usual hand-held, two-point discrimination tests from the perspectives of (1) conceptual validity (it is not a receptor density instrument) and (2) practical validity (neither force level nor true simultaneity is controlled, etc.), yet we have not discounted the spatial information that two-point discrimination tests can convey. In fact, we have proposed the sequential two-point test as a more valid and reliable (force-controlled) alternative to the traditional simultaneous two-point hand-held tests. Computer controlled noninvasive tests, also characterized by the ATT, are believed to be inappropriate because they do not control the force of application for two-point evaluations, their pain tests are no more reliable than hand-held tests, and their pressure tests are no more reliable than hand-held monofilament tests. The historically reported advantage of pressure tests over force tests (i.e., testing without stimulating pain receptors) no longer exists since the introduction of the WEST, which tests a "point" region without pain. We have argued from evidence that force thresholds reflect receptor density and that the spatial function of lateral inhibition is evaluated by two-point discrimination. A new procedure (RTP), which results in rapid, valid measurement for evaluating absolute thresholds was introduced. The potential confound of callus and two methods to circumvent its ambiguous effects were discussed.

The august history of the evaluation of somatic sensation is one of continual spiral approximation toward the goal of achieving the most valid, reliable, and precise methods and procedures. When one is also faced with the ethical and moral aspects of diagnosis and treatment of patients with neuropathy, the pragmatic considerations of ease of testing, time required for the examination, lessening of noxious and invasive stimulation, cost of the devices, etc., add to the concerns facing the clinician. In this chapter, we have elucidated our strategies and tactics to achieve some of our ultimate goals and have also pointed to several new concepts we plan to investigate in the near future.

REFERENCES

1. Al-Qattan MM: Semmes-Weinstein monofilament versus Weinstein enhanced monofilaments: their use in the hand clinic, *Can J Plastic Surg* 1995; 3(1):51-53.
2. Bell-Krotoski JA: Advances in sensibility evaluation, *Hand Clin* 1991; 7:3.
3. Bell-Krotoski JA: Sensibility testing: state of the art. In Hunter JM, Schneider LH, Mackin EJ, Callahan AD, eds: *Rehabilitation of the hand,* ed 3, St Louis, 1990, Mosby.
4. Bell-Krotoski JA, Buford WL: The force/time relationship of clinically used sensory testing instruments, *J Hand Ther* 1988; 1:76-85.
5. Bolton CF, Winkelmann RK, Dyk PJ: A quantitative study of Meissner's corpuscles in man, *Neurology* 1966; 16:1-9.
6. Brandsma J: *Intrinsic minus hand,* Amsterdam, Netherlands, 1993, Stichting voor Leprabestrijding.
7. Burgess PR, Perl ER: Cutaneous mechanoreceptors and nociceptors, vol 2, Somatosensory System. In Iggo A, ed: *Handbook of sensory physiology,* New York, 1973, Springer-Verlag.
8. Cholewiak RW, Collins AA: Sensory and physiological basis of touch. In Heller MA, Schiff W, eds: *The psychology of touch,* Hillsdale, New Jersey, 1991, Lawrence Erlbaum.
9. Dellon AL: The sensational contributions of Erik Moberg, *J Hand Ther* 1992; 15B:14-24.
10. Dellon A: *Evaluation of sensibility and re-education of sensation in the hand,* Baltimore, 1988, A Lee Dellon.
11. Duffy JC, Patout CA: Management of the insensitive foot in diabetes: lessons learned from Hansen's disease, *Military Medicine* 1990; 155:575.
12. Horch H, Hardy M, Jimenez S, Jabaley M: An automated tactile tester for evaluation of cutaneous sensibility, *J Hand Ther* 1992; 17A:829.
13. Keidel WD: The sensory detection of vibrations. In Dawson WW, Enoch JM, eds: *Foundations of sensory science,* Berlin, 1984, Springer-Verlag.
14. MacDermid J: Accuracy of clinical tests used in the detection of carpal tunnel syndrome: a literature review, *J Hand Ther* 1991; 14:169-176.
15. Posnick JC, Al-Quattan M, Pron GE, Grossman JAI: Facial sensibility in adolescents born with cleft lip after undergoing repair in infancy: *Plastic and Reconstructive Surgery* (discussion by S. Weinstein, C. Weinstein, and R. Drozdenko) 1994; 93(4):686-689.
16. Schneider LH, Mackin EJ, Bell JA, eds: *Rehabilitation of the hand,* St Louis, 1978, Mosby.
17. Semmes J, Weinstein S, Ghent L, Teuber H: *Somatosensory changes after penetrating brain wounds in man,* Cambridge, 1960, Harvard.
18. Spivak M: *Weinstein enhanced sensory test & peripheral neuropathy,* Danbury, 1994, Connecticut Bioinstruments Inc.
19. Weinstein C, Drozdenko R, Weinstein S: Evidence supporting a new model for the evaluation of skin irritation, *J Soc Cosmetic Chem* 1988; 39:315.
20. *Weinstein enhanced sensory test hand instrument: care and use manual,* Danbury, 1994, Connecticut Bioinstruments Inc.
21. Weinstein S: Intensive and extensive aspects of tactile sensitivity as a function of body part, sex, and laterality. In Kenshalo D, ed: *The skin senses,* New York, 1968, Plenum Press.
22. Weinstein S: Fifty years of somatosensory research: from the Semmes-Weinstein monofilaments to the Weinstein enhanced sensory test, *J Hand Ther* 1993; 6:11.
23. Weinstein S, Weinstein C, Drozdenko R: *WEST-body II care and use manual,* Danbury, 1994, Connecticut Bioinstruments Inc.

Chapter 9

A SUBSTITUTE FOR PAIN

Paul W. Brand

Many years ago I applied for a research grant to develop "A practical substitute for pain." The application was based on the needs of people who had lost the ability to feel pain. We had already recognized that the terrible deformities of leprosy, including the absorption of digits and the nonhealing ulcers on their hands and feet, were the result of the neuropathy that left them unable to feel pain in their limbs and eyes. If our systems were successful, it would benefit not only leprosy patients but all people who had lost sensation, including diabetics and those with nerve injuries and sensory neuropathies. Our proposal was to equip our patients with an artificial pain system, designed to warn them of danger in time to take avoiding action, as they would when feeling real pain.

METHODOLOGY

There were three parts to the study:

1. Electronic engineers would devise miniature transducers that would respond to dangerous levels of pressure as well as to high temperatures. These would be imbedded into gloves or socks or pasted onto the skin. Fine wires from these devices would lead to a hearing aid that would signal the danger by a tone, variable in pitch and in loudness, so that the patient could identify the location and the degree of danger and take avoiding action.

2. A clinical research team would study pain thresholds, to determine at what levels the transducers should be set to fire their pain signal. We did not want to set the threshold so low that the signal would inhibit safe activity, nor did we want to set the threshold so high that real damage might occur with no warning.

3. Finally we would apply the system to a group of patients who had a history of frequent injuries and burns to see how it worked in practice.

We subcontracted with the Department of Electrical Engineering at Louisiana State University to prepare the system of miniature transducers for pressure and temperature and also to lead the signals to the hearing aids.

The project really caught the imagination of the engineers. They were challenged by the need to miniaturize and also to make something rugged enough to withstand the stresses of the workplace. One of them suggested that if they made a really fine system, it might be preferred by normal people, who could then have their own pain system ablated; indeed, who would not prefer a musical signal in a hearing aid over real pain in a finger?

Having set the engineers to work, the clinical team began to study the question of thresholds. It was here that problems began. The threshold of pain is not determined by a level of pressure or on a scale of temperature. Timing and repetition make big changes in the point at which pain begins to hurt. In most cases pain becomes severe at a point just short of tissue damage.

The level of temperature is not the factor that either triggers pain or causes a burn. The threshold of pain is related to the rate and quantity of heat flow and is measured in calories, not degrees. We all know that some objects feel cold and others at the same temperature are comfortable to the touch. The ones that feel cold are made of conductive material and allow calories to flow out of one's skin into the material. The less conductive materials, usually wood, do not remove heat from the one who touches them. Thus, a temperature transducer was not enough to warn of danger from heat or cold. A heat flow meter would make sense but was impractical to miniaturize, so this approach was abandoned.

Danger thresholds for pressure were just as difficult to quantify. It was not possible to simply pick a pressure and have the engineers set their transducers to signal it by a

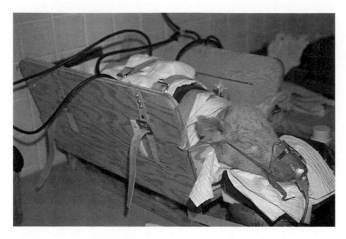

Fig. 9-1. The pig, anesthetized and in the plaster cast and supporting cradle. The tubes lead from pressure applicators each to a separate sphygmomanometer.

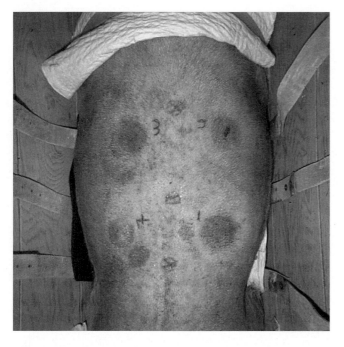

Fig. 9-2. The pig's back after having had four pressure applicators applied for 5 and 7 hours with pressures of 150 mm and 250 mm of mercury.

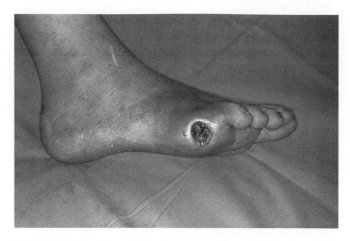

Fig. 9-3. This patient with an insensitive foot had worn a pair of new shoes for the first time since before breakfast until he went to bed that night.

warning tone. The real pain system is far more selective. It seems not to be based on the forces that impinge on the surface of the body, but rather on the earliest sign of trouble in the cells around the nerve ending.

For example, a pressure as low as 2 pounds per square inch (psi) is enough to cause immediate local ischemia, but yet is comfortable when first applied. If it is maintained continuously for some hours, it will result in necrosis of a piece of skin. Long before that time, a normal person would have felt discomfort and then increasing pain. The pain becomes intolerable just before real damage occurs.

We made a number of studies on a pig of quite low pressures applied for various periods of time (Fig. 9-1). In one experiment, under light anesthesia, the pig had four pressure applicators applied to its back, held in place by a plaster cast. Each was attached to a pressure manometer, two of which were set at 150 mm of mercury, and two at 250 mm of mercury. One of each pair was maintained at pressure for 5 hours, and the other for 7 hours.

Fig. 9-2 shows how the pig's back looked some hours after the experiment. There was no frank ulceration at any pressure site, but there was obvious inflammation, resulting in turgid swelling, sharply limited to each circle. It is worth noting that, although each pressure applicator had been prepared with rounded edges to prevent damage from shear stress at a hard edge, it was indeed the edge of each applicator that caused the most damage. We were to find that shear stress is always more damaging to tissues than normal stress. It is also more painful than normal stress.

Plate 1 (see color insert following p. 74) is a thermogram of the pig's back. This is the AGA thermovision system and each color marks a temperature change of 1° C. This gives a 10-degree spread in which blue and green are at the cold end, and orange and white are at the hot end. Note that the temperature changes follow the degrees of inflammation and tissue damage, including the circle of higher temperature that marks the areas of shear stress.

Fig. 9-3 is an insensitive foot for which the patient had bought a new pair of shoes. He wore them all day and found a discolored area of skin when he next looked at his foot. The shoe had been too tight, but he did not know it, and would not have been warned by any transducer with a threshold set above about 3 psi.

At the other extreme from the low pressures of ischemic damage is the high pressure and shear stress needed for damage from a single application of force (Fig. 9-4). It

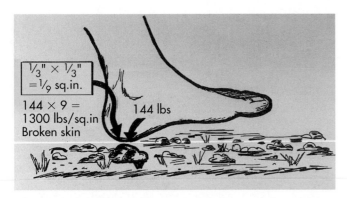

Fig. 9-4. Diagram to emphasize that to produce injury from a single step it might take a patient's whole weight to come down on an area of less than half a square inch.

takes several hundred psi before skin is broken by a single thrust. A pain transducer should sound a danger note at about 250 psi, even though direct damage might not occur for another 100 psi or higher. If this were to be the same transducer that is to sound a warning at just 2 psi after an hour of continuous pressure, it was obvious that our engineers needed more sophistication than they had anticipated.

The greatest problem of thresholds was yet to come, and it was at a level of pressure that was the most common cause of damage. Neither high nor low, but the frequent repetition of medium forces that are harmless for a few repetitions and also painless to people with normal sensibility.

Repetitive stress is a popular subject among hand therapists today and is well recognized as a cause of trouble. In the 1960s, however, we were surprised both at the low level of stress and at the number of repetitions that were required to damage and destroy the tissues of hands and feet. We determined, for example, that 20 psi was a comfortable and harmless level of pressure for normal hands and feet, and that rats (Fig. 9-5) showed no signs of discomfort when they experienced the same pressures we applied to ourselves. We then anesthetized the rats and put their footpads into a machine (Fig. 9-6) that applied exactly 20 psi repetitively for 10,000 repetitions each day for a week.

For the first day or two, we noted only a little swelling and warmth after the period of repetitive stress. We followed the histology by sacrificing one rat each day. Fig. 9-7 shows a normal footpad. Fig. 9-8 is a footpad after 2 days of repetitive moderate stress; it shows swelling and some collections of inflammatory cells. Fig. 9-9 shows a footpad after 7 days, showing gross necrosis and the histology of a neuropathic ulcer. There was no neuropathy, and at no time had this rat had more pressure than what we knew had been comfortable for a few repetitions.

We repeated the experiment with the same pressure, but only 8000 repetitions a day (and only for 5 days each week) instead of 10,000 every day. Fig. 9-10 shows the histology

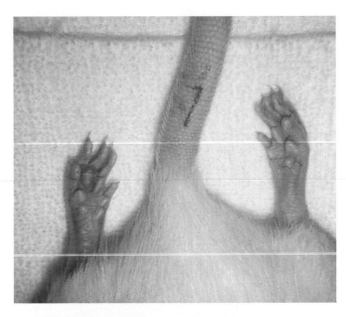

Fig. 9-5. The footpads of a Sprague Dorley rat as used for repetitive stress experiments.

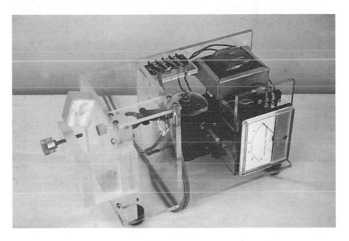

Fig. 9-6. Repetitive stress machine built for these tests. It holds the footpad against a plate through which a piston presses on the foot, giving a predetermined pressure while a counter records the number of repetitions.

of a rat after 6 weeks of that program. The tissues are normal, perhaps a little hypertrophied, but undamaged. The only difference was in the number of repetitions per week; the pressures were the same. Plates 2 and 3 (see color insert following p. 74) are thermographs of a rat footpad before and after a session of repetitive stress. We found the thermograph to be an excellent method of quantifying commencing tissue inflammation before actual damage had occurred.

Because we could not be sure how much pain would have been felt by a rat if there had been no anesthesia while undergoing repetitive stress of 20 psi, I subjected myself to exactly the same level of stress with my finger in the same machine. Because I was unwilling to biopsy my fingertips,

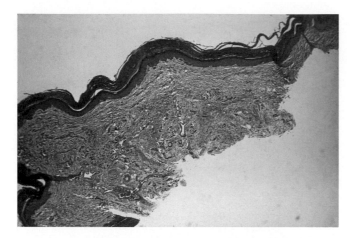

Fig. 9-7. Histology of a normal rat footpad.

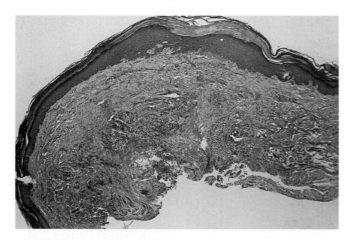

Fig. 9-8. Histology of a similar rat footpad after 20,000 repetitions, over 2 days, of 20 psi of pressure. Note increase in volume and incursion of inflammatory cells, also, hyperplasia of the epithelium at the site of the repeated stress. Note there are two areas of maximal hyperplasia side by side. These represent the edges of the applicator that, although they had been rounded off, produced more stress than the center of the applicator between them. This shows that sheer stress is more damaging to tissue than normal stress.

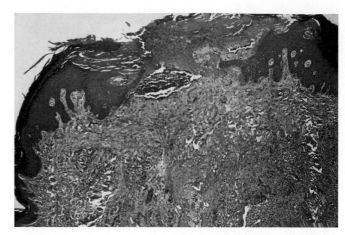

Fig. 9-9. Histology of a similar rat footpad after 7 days of the same daily program. Note gross necrosis and the histology of a neuropathic ulcer.

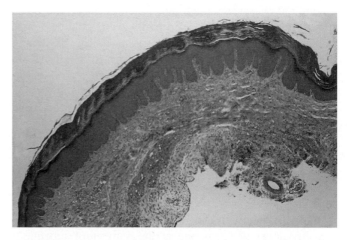

Fig. 9-10. Histology of a rat footpad after 6 weeks of a program that used the same pressures but 8000 repetitions per day instead of 10,000 repetitions and for 5 days each week instead of every day.

we judged by my subjective responses, which were confirmed by thermography.

With my finger in the machine, the little hammer felt comfortable, rather as I would feel when clapping my hands after a concert. After a few hundred beats of the hammer I was less sure that it was enjoyable. After a few thousand it became painful. Only my devotion to science kept my finger in position, and soon even that failed, and I withdrew with dignity when the pain became intolerable.

Plates 4 and 5 (see color insert following p. 74) is the thermograph of my hand when it first came out of the machine, and after fifteen minutes of rest. We had learned that only after severe trauma did a digit continue to increase its temperature during rest after removal from the source of stress.

The following day I returned to the machine and tested another finger, with similar results. On returning to the finger that had been traumatized the previous day, which was now free of pain or marked tenderness, I found that the beats of the machine produced pain much sooner than it had on the previous day and that the thermograph recorded a higher temperature sooner than it had before.

Thus, to set a threshold for repetitive stress, our engineers were challenged to develop a device that would not only register pressure, but would count the number of repetitions and would have a computer chip to plot a curve of three variables: pressure, time, and number of repetitions.

While we wrestled with thresholds, our engineers perfected small transducers and signaling devices. We began with some thresholds picked on a tentative basis. The transducers cost $450 each, so we chose subjects carefully. They kept squeezing the handles of tools and smiling when they heard the tone, relaxing their grip in response. They worked in the manual arts department. At the end of a morning of carpentry or mechanics, one or two of the transducers would be broken, or a short circuit had given a false pain signal. Manual arts was becoming an expensive department for our study.

The final problems were different and more serious. Our early success was realized because the patients had perceived it to be a sort of game. Once they were accustomed to it, they became bored. We had to turn up the volume in the hearing aid to get their attention. It got to the point that we observers could hear the tone, but the patients took no notice of it.

Finally, one of the engineers realized that to work, a signal would have to be perceived as painful. In leprosy, the warm skin of the axilla always remains sensitive, so when the engineers built a small, battery-powered shocking coil, we fitted it into the axilla where it gave a shock that was like a sting when patients ignored the audible tone.

That idea had a shorter period of success. It did indeed produce a pain, and for a while it did make people more careful in the use of their hands. But nobody *chooses* pain, and our patients were no exception. If they planned an activity they thought might take them over the threshold of pain, they would switch off the system first.

CONCLUSIONS

So far as the stated objectives of our research project were concerned, it was a failure. The patients did not perceive the transducers as a part of the body or its defenses. It was seen more as a punishment for not following the rules. They probably realized also that our thresholds were a very crude imitation of the finely graded warnings of a real pain system. As we started picking up the pieces of our broken project, we were pleased to find that some of them were really of value in their own right.

The first was what we learned about the *pathomechanics of pressure sores* in general. We had never realized that the great majority of all such ulcers do not happen suddenly or even in a day or two. Most of them take many days and sometimes weeks to develop. If the sequence of repeated stress is interrupted during the process, the tissues may return to normal without any breakdown ever taking place.

The second discovery was the *value of thermometry* as an aid to identifying areas of developing inflammation from trauma. We learned this because we thermographed the pigs, rats, and human subjects at frequent intervals through all our experiments.

We discovered that if, during a course of hand therapy, a hand is tested once a day for local temperature contrasts, there is usually time to change, in response to a new hot spot, some routine of activity or passive motion that would otherwise have resulted in real damage.

Although I appreciate thermography, more and more I take pride in the use of my own hands. They have an unerring perception of skin temperature contrasts, as they pass across a limb. Faster than I can set up a machine, I can pass my hand over the surface of a patient's hand and identify and mark one or two hot spots that need attention. My hand finds the hot spots, and then a small inexpensive thermocouple with a fast digital readout measures the actual temperature differentials for the record.

The third valuable discovery is the *effect the project had on the attitudes* of both the researchers and the patients. Many of us started off with a broad concept that pain was a bad thing. By the end of three years of attempting to imitate pain, there was no engineer, physician, or therapist on our team who did not appreciate the wonder and precision of the system with which we all come equipped. To do any good, pain must hurt; and it is essential that the "off" switch be out of reach, although we may appreciate the ability to turn it down a little, with medication.

Today, when I am trying to help patients who are frustrated with pain from injury or disease, I tell them about what I have learned about pain, and that even while I dislike it, I appreciate the wonder of the system and the way it allows me to use my body to its best advantage without crossing the threshold into danger. I love to see the gradually awakening self-respect as people recognize their own value and the wonder of their own bodies. They begin to listen to their bodies and to take charge of themselves. This is the key to real health and to happiness.

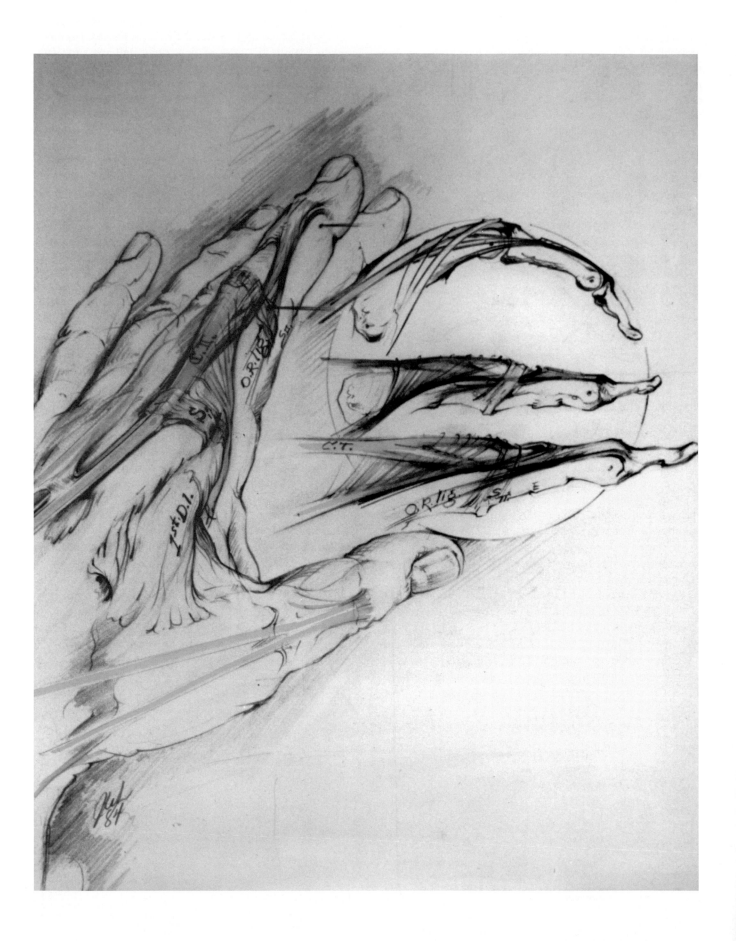

Part III

NERVE REPAIR AND REHABILITATION TECHNIQUES

Anatomic and diagrammatic exposition of the left index finger extrinsic and intrinsic extensor systems.

Chapter 10

THIRTEEN YEARS DOWN THE TRACK

Sir Sydney Sunderland

It is a little more than 13 years since this group first met at the Harrison Conference Centre of Glen Cove, Long Island, New York, on July 17 and 18, 1980. If we use the creation of this society as a useful point of reference, we are now 13 years down the track, which brings to mind the words of that enlightened British philosopher-surgeon, Wilfred Trotter, when he wrote that "even the most assiduous workman will from time to time stand back to get a more general view of his work and to contemplate its wider relations. Indeed, such intermissions are necessary if he is to escape the tyranny of detail."

As I reflect back over past events, I find that I am asking questions to which, in my autumn years and in my present circumstances, I am no longer capable of providing answers. It is perhaps not surprising that I should use the occasion of this Seattle meeting in an attempt to satisfy my curiosity. This presentation, then, has been designed solely to stimulate discussion and debate.

My first two questions relate to axon regeneration.

QUESTION 1

What is the greatest distance that a neuron, originally supporting a short axon, can be expected to regenerate a new and functionally effective axon?

(Read posthumously before the Sunderland Society, Seattle, September 1993.)
Permission to publish this address was given by Lady Gwendoline Sunderland, in 1995. From Kline DG, Hudson AR: *Nerve injuries: operative results with major nerve injuries, entrapments, and tumors,* Philadelphia, 1995, WB Saunders, pp. 593-596.

This is relevant to the planning and undertaking of some cross-innervations. Are we demanding too much of the provider neuron in these cases?

And here a note of caution. Beware of experiments on small animals, where the distances involved are too short to provide an acceptable experimental model.

QUESTION 2

My second difficulty concerns the vexing question of neurotropism as a factor assisting useful functional regeneration after nerve repair. If neurotropism, which now appears to be back in business, is doing what it is supposed to do, how are we to explain the following facts?

1. Great importance is assigned to correct axial alignment of the nerve ends during repair. Experience tells us that neurotropism does not compensate for malalignment.
2. Neuromas form at suture lines because regenerating axons grow just as readily into the interfascicular connective tissue as into fasciculi.
3. It has been demonstrated experimentally that motor regenerating axons will enter and grow down sensory endoneurial tubes, and this obviously occurs in autografting.

It seems to me that neurotropism as an aid to functional regeneration remains seriously flawed, although others may think differently.

QUESTION 3

Despite the wealth of information that has accumulated in recent years, are the results of nerve repair today consistently better and more predictable than in the past? I suspect that the answer must be only marginally so, largely because of our inability to exploit the mass of information that is now available to the surgeon. We now appear to be in an unfortunate position in which much detailed information is available on the factors adversely affecting functional regeneration but little can be done in the way of corrective measures to offset their pernicious influences.

Let us take a closer look at only three of these unfriendly factors.

1. If a length of nerve has been destroyed and the fascicular patterns at the nerve ends in no way correspond, correct alignment of the nerve ends still remains largely a matter of guesswork. Malalignment during the repair remains a potential source of error until we have a foolproof method for ensuring correct coaptation of the nerve ends. Are we any closer to a solution to this problem?

2. As yet nothing can be done to prevent the loss of those regenerating axons that enter functionally unrelated endoneurial tubes and the interfascicular epineurium. This leaves reinnervation both imperfect and incomplete.

3. Scarring at the site of coaptation of the nerve ends remains a variable and unpredictable quantity in regard to both its density and the manner in which it obstructs and misdirects the passage of regenerating axons across the nerve end interface. Will it ever be possible to control and standardize the behavior of fibroblasts and healing at that site in order to provide a framework that will facilitate the orderly passage of regenerating axons? The dilemma here, of course, is to achieve this without threatening the integrity and strength of the union.

After a searching audit of all known possible sources of error, one can only conclude that unexpected shortfalls in recovery will be inevitable and should be expected. It seems that the outcome after any nerve repair continues to carry an element of doubt and uncertainty.

QUESTION 4

We come now to the question of the plasticity of neural mechanisms within the central nervous system and the role that it plays in bringing about that further improvement that continues long after it can be attributed to any peripheral phenomena. Clearly this late improvement in response to remedial training must involve readjustments to, and the reorganization of, flexible central mechanisms, enabling the motivated patient to compensate for incomplete and imperfect patterns of peripheral reinnervation.

There is much supporting clinical evidence to favor the existence of such central mechanisms and their far greater potential in the very young than in the adult. This evidence throws no light on their nature or modus operandi.

The question then becomes, "Would knowing more about these central mechanisms inevitably lead to further and substantially improved recoveries?" Here one suspects that it will be well into the future before speculation has been replaced by reality.

QUESTION 5

My fifth and last question goes to the core of evaluating and recording motor and sensory recovery after nerve repair. Historically, the method currently in use for doing this is a continuum of that adopted and later published in 1954 in the postwar British Medical Council Report on peripheral nerve injuries. Faced with a rapid influx of war injuries in large numbers in the early 1940s, a standard method of evaluating and grading recovery was established to meet the clinicians' needs for one that was simple, clear, precise, and easily and quickly obtained; one that could be readily converted to a simple coding system; and one that could be used to quantify recovery so that, ultimately, the data collected could be used for comparing the recovery of one nerve with that of another, and the recovery of one nerve under different circumstances. All this was planned in the interest of determining management policy for the treatment of a large number of patients with the least possible delay.

To cut through the detail, there finally emerged from the deliberations an M0 to M5 grading for motor recovery and one of S0 to S5 for sensory recovery, each representing recognizable steps in recovery and with defined criteria for each of the five grades. With minor modifications over the years, this method has become entrenched in clinical practice and in the literature.

My question is, should we be satisfied with this method of recording recovery?

In response to this question, it seems to me that there are good grounds for subjecting it to a searching audit. In the first place, it lacks a useful functional basis and is, at the same time, flawed and inadequate in other respects.

When the method was introduced, it was emphasized that it was to be limited to testing and grading the power of individual muscles and that the sensory grading was to be confined exclusively to the primary sensory elements of pain (using graded pin prick and spring algesiometers), tactile sensibility (using a standardized series of Von Frey hairs), thermal sensibility (using recording techniques ranging from the simple to the complex), two-point sensory discrimination (using the points of a compass), position sense, and localization. Moving two-point discrimination and vibration sense were added at a later date. Despite the fact that the restoration of function is the central objective of nerve repair, it was specifically stated at that time that usefulness as a criterion of recovery was to be rejected, and that testing useful functional recovery was to be avoided because of the complexities involved and, presumably, because this would add to the delay in finalizing management policy.

These were serious omissions, and in their absence it is difficult to accept the claim that the results gave a clear picture of the ultimate outcome. On the contrary, because restoration of function is the name of the game, published results leave the reader with a totally inadequate picture of the ultimate outcome, limited as it is to individual movements and the primary elements of sensibility. To the patient, this information is meaningless. What is important to the patient is what can be done with, for example, the affected hand and digits when they are called upon to perform the wide range of both simple and complex tasks that are required in the course of conducting daily activities.

Again, not only does the method fall short of what is required, but it may easily lead to misleading reporting. In my own experience, repeated testing at short intervals often gave conflicting results.

Turning now to the motor grading of M0 to M5, this relates to individual reinnervated muscles acting solely as prime movers. This, however, is an oversimplistic approach to the evaluation of useful motor function. Concentrating solely on its action as a prime mover in this way neglects the muscle's important role as an antagonist, synergist, and fixator in the execution of a wide range of movements to give them refinement and precision. A residual paresis, therefore, not only impairs a muscle's function as a prime mover but also, and importantly, destabilizes the actions of other normally innervated muscles. The latter is not covered by the test for motor recovery.

Furthermore, this method of grading and recording recovery disregards the importance of sensory mechanisms in motor performance and of motor functions in sensory discrimination and stereognosis. The latter is not possible in the absence of movement. Though a variety of tests is now available for testing and evaluating tactile discrimination, the recording of sensory recovery is still based on the primary elements of sensory function.

Despite these deficiencies, the method remains entrenched in clinical practice. Persisting confidence in it is also evidenced by the reporting of new devices and techniques to facilitate testing and by the efforts taken, in the belief that measurement brings respectability, to provide, in exact numerical terms, values for each of the primary sensory components. No great accuracy can be claimed for these measurements because they relate to functions with fluctuating fortunes, and as one who has spent hours engaged in this practice, it soon became clear that it was a fruitless attempt to quantify the unquantifiable. As Trotter reminded us 52 years ago, "The affectation of scientific exactitude in circumstances where it has no meaning is perhaps the fallacy of method to which medicine is most exposed."

Finally, we return to the original claim that the method of coding recovery, as originally introduced, gave a "good picture" of the ultimate outcome. It is difficult to decide whether this is a statement of fact or just an expression of expectation because, to the best of my knowledge, the claim has never been subjected to a searching examination in an attempt to ascertain if the code did in fact equate with the restoration of useful function. Too much has to be inferred in order to make the method as decisive as some writers over the years have claimed.

In other words, when you read of a recovery grading, for example, of M4S4, what does it really tell you about the ability of the patient to use the affected digits and hand in a purposeful way to provide for a wide range of selected manual tasks and skills of a type required for the performance of his or her daily activities? End results as currently recorded are capable of grave misrepresentation.

There is, I believe, good reason for concluding that the coding system of M0 to M5 and S0 to S5 fails to cover modern requirements as these relate to complex motor and sensory functions. Despite the fact that it represents an attempt to bring objectivity into what are essentially subjective events, and no matter how useful it may be for monitoring the progress of recovery, the system is totally inadequate for recording a meaningful end result assessment. For the latter it needs to be amended and extended.

Moberg was absolutely correct in directing attention to the flaws inherent in the use of oversimplistic procedures, but even his criticism did not go far enough. Nevertheless, his "pick up" testing method represented a distinct improvement.

In recent times, the pick-up test has admittedly undergone considerable modification, elaboration, and improvement, and a variety of tests is now available for evaluating tactile discrimination. However, if the literature is any guide, much of what is currently written on the subject indicates that the main thrust of their use is to follow the progress of recovery as this occurs during a regimen of motor and sensory reeducation directed to restoring function to the hand. In this respect, it is important to distinguish between recording an end result assessment and monitoring the progress of recovery during reeducational therapy.

If medical records and published papers on this subject are to be kept within reasonable limits, then it becomes necessary to convert end result information on assessment. Needed is a coding scale that can convey to the reader, elsewhere and at a later date, a clear picture of the residual function of the hand and digits as this is reflected in the performance of the patient's daily activities. Furthermore, each grade in the scale would need to be based on clearly defined criteria, so that each grade represents clearly defined differences in the ultimate outcome of the repair, and each grade conveys to both recorder and reader the same clear and precise picture of the status of the recovery for that grade. Only in this way could the scale be used with confidence for comparing one set of results with another, one technique with another, and one management policy with another.

Briefly, this would, of course, call for the selection of suitable tasks that would need to be standardized and approved by some international body for universal acceptance and use. Clearly, there are problems in such an undertaking, but it should not be beyond the wit of man to reduce the type of tests required to achieve this to manageable proportions and to convert them to some reliable and practical coding system.

Clearly, this list of questions could be extended, but I believe I have said sufficient to indicate that the saga of nerve injury, nerve regeneration, and nerve repair is still far from complete, and it is imperative not only that research should be continued but, even more importantly, that it should be specifically directed to meeting the needs of those faced with the management of nerve injuries.

Chapter 11

TECHNIQUES IN NERVE REPAIR

Michael E. Jabaley

A description of the state of nerve repair in the mid-1990s should be viewed as only a snapshot in time because nerve repair techniques continue to evolve and the final approach is by no means settled. To fully understand the details of the techniques now in vogue, one must appreciate the background from which they have arisen and recognize those factors which determine how transected nerves are likely to be joined in the future. Against this background, this chapter reviews briefly the nature of nerve repair in the recent past and current modifications of basic nerve suture technique that have occurred. These modifications have resulted from efforts to address some of the shortcomings that were observed after the use of older methods.

All physicians have observed patients with mediocre results, both sensory and motor, after nerve suture. We have come to realize that the stumbling block to further improvement in outcomes may be the basic biology of nerve regeneration itself and that future efforts must address and try to influence this process if results are to improve. Thus, further improvement in results requires that we understand better and try to modify the biologic process of nerve regeneration.

The return of function in transected peripheral nerves is a unique process in wound healing. With bone or blood vessel, tendon, skin, or ligament, the challenge is simply to restore continuity and to permit healing to occur. Once reestablished in these tissues, structural integrity permits the part to function in a more or less normal fashion. Such is not the case with nerves. The process of Wallerian degeneration has been well described, and restoring continuity between nerve ends only sets the stage for regeneration. The actual restoration of function depends on regenerating axons

bridging the gap created by transection, finding their way down endoneurial tubes to specific end organs and beginning again the process of encoding data or transmitting motor impulses. The degree to which this process is successful depends on many factors, including the passage of time itself. We know that if axonal continuity is not restored within a reasonable period of time, motor endplates and muscle itself atrophy, distal segments constrict, and sensory reception is substantially less than it was before the injury.

The major surgical advances that have occurred in the field of nerve repair roughly span the last half century and can be considered broadly under two headings: technologic progress in nerve suture and an appreciation of the role of nerve grafting.

TECHNOLOGICAL PROGRESS

The period leading up to World War II witnessed serious attempts by surgeons to better restore continuity in transected nerves, and the Great War itself was the clinical laboratory for the treatment of patients. The large numbers of casualties provided the stimulus to examine the long-term results in nerve-injured patients. From these examinations, many conclusions were reached, all suggesting that technical limitations greatly limit the outcome of nerve repair.

After the war, there was a burst of investigative effort in peripheral nerve repair (as well as surgery in general) and there were major advances. These can be broadly grouped in three categories: (1) the availability of magnification and an appreciation of its importance (both loupe and the operating microscope), (2) refinements in instrumentation that permitted atraumatic manipulation and coaptation of nerve ends, and (3) the development of previously unavailable microsurgical suture and needle technology. None of these technical refinements altered the basic biologic processes of nerve healing in any way.

As efforts continued toward more precise nerve suture, the problems of long gaps (as well as the operative field) were magnified. It became obvious that neuroma resection back to viable and healthy nerve often resulted in substantial gaps that could only be bridged by relatively heavy sutures tied under great tension. Such repairs frequently were followed by poor functional recovery and led to some ingenious (though sometimes dubious) techniques to relieve tension. Among these were lengthy mobilizations and rerouting of nerve ends, extreme joint flexion, "bulb" suture, and bone shortening. Despite these maneuvers, ischemic nerve ends were often joined by a thick bond of scar through which axons regenerated poorly or not at all.

Nerve grafting seemed a plausible solution to the problem of the nerve gap and tension, but the results of "cable" grafting, as practiced in both Britain and the United States by Bunnell, Seddon, and Brooks were not encouraging and the technique was not widely accepted or practiced. It was not until the 1960s and 1970s that this situation changed and set the stage for the other major development in nerve repair: the development and championing of nerve grafts as a plausible alternative to suture under tension as a way to overcome nerve gaps.

NERVE GRAFTING

The efforts of Hanno Millesi and his colleagues in Vienna were significant (though not immediately accepted by everyone) in bringing nerve grafting to the attention of the surgical world and restoring credibility to a previously discredited procedure.[9] Millesi's concepts, first presented in English in 1970 at the Annual Meeting of the American Society for Surgery of the Hand, have come to be accepted as substantially correct. He demonstrated in the laboratory and stressed in his presentations the deleterious effect of tension, the need to excise epineurium (the source of scar), the importance of trimming nonviable fascicle ends, and the necessity of identifying and joining appropriate fascicles or groups of fascicles.

Millesi recognized that much of the problem with cable grafts or whole nerve grafts of large diameter was their failure to vascularize completely and the resulting ischemic necrosis. This is analogous to an overly thick skin graft, which necroses for lack of circulation. His solution was to use several small grafts (the sural nerve was the preferred, though not the only, donor source) to joint individual fascicles or bundles. This required a well-vascularized bed in which the individual lengths of graft were separated, one from another, to permit their early vascularization and survival. Thus has evolved the concept of *interfascicular nerve grafting,* whereby a conduit of viable autogenous nerve, containing the ideal substrate for regeneration, is interposed between the viable ends of appropriate fascicles.

CURRENT CONCEPTS OF REPAIR AND REGENERATION

What is our current knowledge of nerve repair? We know that a nerve contains many functioning axons, ranging from a few hundred to several thousand, depending on the diameter of the nerve trunk. These axons and their Schwann cell sheaths are surrounded, in turn, by endoneurium, perineurium, and epineurium. With transection, Wallerian degeneration occurs for a variable distance proximally and completely in the distal portion. The Schwann cells proliferate and phagocytize the axoplasm of the distal end, leaving the Schwann cell membranes and their basal lamina as the familiar endoneurial tubes. With time, these tubules collapse and constrict, but they remain at least partially patent for long periods. It is through these tubes that axon regeneration may occur.

Nerve transection produces a violent trauma to both the axons and the cell body (some of which actually die). As axon regeneration begins in the surviving nerve cells, there is increased metabolic activity in the cell body and a sprouting of axons from the proximal cut end. These sprouting axons regenerate along any available substrate, including the endoneurial tubes. Some sprouts are known to proceed along vessels, fascia, muscle, and, of course, the collagen of scar. As a consequence of this random regeneration, many axons never function. There is a subsequent "pruning" of nonfunctional axons and many sprouts simply degenerate. Those that survive proceed to their distal targets, remyelinate, and may eventually function.

Because the myriad of individual fibers in a nerve cannot even be seen, there is no likelihood that surgeons will ever be able to align individual axons successfully. Even if it were possible, the nerve would not function as such because nerve repair is not simply a physical joining of the ends but, as noted previously, it is merely the first step of the regenerative process.

Rejoining nerve ends can be accomplished in a number of ways and the type of union selected plays a role in the ultimate outcome, but it is only one of many factors at work (see the box on p. 91). Some of these are within the control of the surgeon but many others are not. Nerve ends can be rejoined in two basic ways: by direct suture or, when a distance between the nerve ends is too great, by interfascicular grafts. Whichever technique is chosen, it can be summarily stated that *the only acceptable method of repair at the present time is to physically join the ends by suture and permit the regenerative process to occur.* Whether this condition remains the choice in the future is an important question and one whose answer may change (see the following comments on tubulation).

Factors affecting outcome of nerve repair at various levels

Cell body level

Cell death
Patient age
Level of injury

Transection level

Tension
Injury to adjacent structures
Circulation
Timing of repair
Damage to remaining nerve (crush, stretch)
Trauma of repair
Foreign body (suture)
Infection

Distal segment and receptor level

Damage to remaining nerve (stretch, crush)
Timing (distal neurotubule collapse)
Atrophy of muscle
Degeneration of sensory receptors

TECHNIQUES OF NERVE REPAIR
External epineurial repair

The simplest (and still the most commonly used) method for joining nerve ends is by direct *external epineurial suture* (Fig. 11-1, *A*). In this technique, viable nerve ends are aligned as accurately as the surgeon can make them and held together by stitches placed in the external epineurium. During a period of splint immobilization, regenerating axons should bridge the interface, enter the distal trunk, and begin to proceed to appropriate sensory and motor targets. Some measure of functional recovery should occur after such a repair.

External epineurial suture is preferable when a nerve is relatively simple in cross-sectional makeup, known to have only one function, and where accurate identification of fascicles can be made. Such situations tend to occur in the proximal and most distal portions of a nerve. For example, external epineurial suture is the technique of choice for proper and common digital nerves. Similarly, a nerve of relatively few fascicles such as the radial nerve in the upper arm, can also successfully be joined in this way. The same can be said of the high brachial plexus, where specific branches cannot be identified and where function cannot be assigned to individual subunits of cords or roots.

Group fascicular repair

When a nerve is mixed (contains both sensory and motor fibers) or serves more than one function, it is preferable to identify and select those portions to which function can be

assigned and join them separately. For example, a mixed motor and sensory nerve has no hope of functional recovery if the proximal motor bundles are attached to distal sensory fascicles or vice versa.

The assignment of specific function to individual fascicles, singularly or in groups, is critical and can be made in a number of ways,[6] ranging from the use of the published maps of Sunderland to visual assessment or to electrical stimulation in either the awake or anesthetized patient (see Chapter 3 for details). Although histologic means are available for identifying motor and sensory fibers, they have not found their way into common clinical use at this time.

Once appropriate functional assignments have been made, groups of fascicles are joined by careful suture of either external or internal epineurium (Fig. 11-1, *C*). It is important to understand that in group fascicular suturing the perineurium should not be violated or injured by passing needles and sutures through it.

The purpose of sutures in this (and all other) techniques is the maintenance of alignment, not the provision of strength. For this reason, the sutures can simply be placed in the internal and external epineurium surrounding a bundle. These stitches are small and are usually few in number. In major forearm nerves where tension is not excessive, a group fascicular repair is usually the technique of choice.

Interfascicular perineurial repair

When the operating microscope and microsuture first became available, there was hope that the identification and suture of individual fascicles would result in improved clinical function.[11] Time has dispelled this notion clinically, and laboratory studies have shown no improvement when individual fascicular repair is compared with a carefully performed group fascicular or whole nerve suture. For these reasons, this technique is not presently recommended except in situations where fascicles are isolated and repair is required. In fascicular repairs, individual fascicles are identified and joined by sutures placed in their perineurium (Fig. 11-1, *B*). Although obviously more tedious and probably more traumatic, the procedure is also time-consuming and has not resulted in improved results when compared with other techniques. It was never widely accepted and has been largely abandoned except in specific circumstances. For example, a surgeon may be faced with a situation where two fascicle ends, absent any epineurium, must be joined. In this case, it should be done by one or two small diameter (10-0 or 11-0) sutures carefully placed in the perineurium, recognizing that recovery will be hampered by the foreign body and placement of a suture within the perineurial barrier.

Surgeons generally have come to appreciate the role and importance of the perineurium and have made careful effort not to incorporate it in sutures unless absolutely necessary.

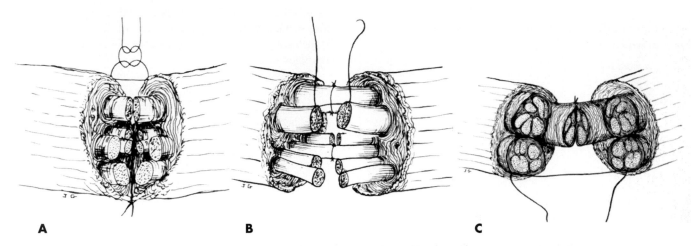

A   **B**   **C**

Fig. 11-1. Techniques of nerve suture. **(A)** External epineurial suture—most useful when nerves have few fascicles and only one function, such as a pure sensory or motor nerve. Small caliber stitches are placed in the external epineurium only, and dissection of individual fascicles is avoided. **(B)** Perineurial suture—individual fascicles are dissected, matched, and held by small caliber stitches in the perineurium. This technique is reserved for specific situations where one or more fascicles must be individually joined and where no epineurium is available. The technique damages perineurium and impairs conduction in areas where sutures are placed. **(C)** Group fascicular suture—the most commonly used technique for a mixed nerve such as the major forearm nerves. Groups of fascicles are identified, matched, and joined by individual placement in the external and internal epineurium, avoiding perineurial sutures if possible. Matching is based on specific function, either motor or sensory. (From Jabaley ME: *Plast Surg;* McCarthy JG [ed.], May JW Jr, Littler JW [sect. eds.], Philadelphia, 1990, Saunders.)

Interfascicular nerve grafting

Among the contributions of Millesi, one of the most important is the recognition of the deleterious effect of excessive tension in repairs.[9] He has shown both experimentally and clinically that a nerve graft is the only way to achieve a tension-free union and that a graft is preferable to a primary suture under excessive tension. In this technique, the fascicles are identified and function assigned to them. They are then joined by one or more segments of autogenous nerve, separately placed in such a way that each vascularizes individually. This provides a conduit along which regenerating axons may travel. By this process, tension is avoided and the problems associated with a thick barrier of scar tissue at the interface between nerve ends are fewer. The situation is analogous to the thickness of scar that forms between skin edges that have been joined primarily with no tension as opposed to edges joined with tension or even with secondary healing.

The technique of nerve grafting (Fig. 11-2) is based on the appreciation of the importance of viable nerve ends, correct identification of functioning portions, atraumatic handling of fascicles, excision of epineurium at the juncture site, and the alignment and maintenance of the coaptation by the fewest possible number of sutures of fine nonabsorbable material (usually two, or sometimes even one). To the degree that these principles are followed, the likelihood of success is increased.

In practice it is generally accepted that gaps up to 2.5 to 3 cm in major nerves can be overcome by direct suture. Greater distances are better treated by grafting, but these are guidelines only, not substitutes for sound surgical judgment. There are always exceptions. For example, much shorter distances in the hand or fingers are best treated with grafts.

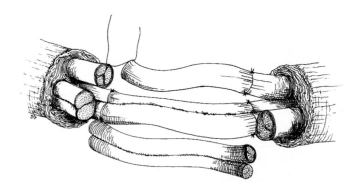

Fig. 11-2. Interfascicular nerve grafting. Individual fascicles in the proximal and distal ends of a nerve are dissected and function assigned to them as outlined in the text. External epineurium is dissected away. If tension is excessive, nerve ends are joined by individual lengths of autogenous nerve placed and separated in such a way that they may vascularize individually. Nerve grafts are usually held in position by two small sutures, placed 180° apart. Nerve grafts are the ideal conduit for regenerating axons. (From Jabaley ME: *Plast Surg;* McCarthy JG [ed.], May JW Jr, Littler JW [sect. eds.], Philadelphia, 1990, Saunders.)

The shortcomings of nerve suture with excess tension have been pointed out and are obvious. Nerve grafting has its limitations, too. It results in an anesthetic donor site, it produces two suture lines, the grafts must vascularize to function, and the technique requires intraneural dissection and identification of fascicles. For all these reasons, operating time tends to be greater. If a procedure that retained the desirable aspects of grafting without actually resorting to a nerve graft were available, it would have obvious advantages.

A MODIFICATION OF SUTURE TECHNIQUE

In an effort to relieve tension and avoid the use of grafts, many surgical investigators have proposed alternative methods for relieving tension when joining nerve ends. These alternative methods have in common a tension-relieving device that allows primary union of the transected ends without the formation of excessive scar tissue. The procedure to be described has been employed by me for the past 20 years and seems a reasonable compromise between nerve grafting and suture under excessive tension.[4]

Historically, sutures have been used for two purposes: to overcome tension and to maintain alignment. To meet the first objective, sutures are sometimes tied tightly and often produce some overlap of fascicles at the juncture. On the other hand, if sutures are tied too loosely, they may allow distraction of the fascicle ends, leaving gaps between the ends. Either condition may retard regeneration, and most surgeons have tried to avoid these ill effects by using small diameter sutures, accurately placed. Because of my frustration resulting from the inability to draw fascicles together with 9-0 to 11-0 suture, I became interested in other tension-relieving techniques. The objective was to create a nerve suture that would be analogous to the situation employed in nerve grafting, that is, with no tension between fascicle ends.

The technique is not original, and I learned that other authors had already described tension-relieving techniques. In their description of interfascicular repair, Hakstian[3] and Tsuge,[10] used epineurial sutures placed at a distance from the cut end to relieve tension. The epineurial splint technique is similar to these techniques but allows the removal of a portion of the epineurium, intraneural dissection, and internal epineurial suture placement.

It has long been Millesi's contention that the external epineurium is the primary source of fibroblasts and collagen and that it should be removed when possible. The epineurial splint is designed in such a way as to remove a portion of epineurium and use the rest as a tension-relieving device.

We have subsequently learned from the work of deMedinaceli and Seaber[2] that all these tension-relieving techniques are based on the principle of Saint Vernant. Practically speaking, this principle simply states that it is necessary to place sutures approximately 1.5 nerve diam-

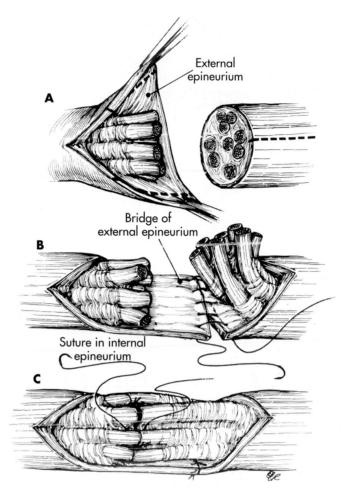

Fig. 11-3. Epineurial splint repair. (**A**) Nerve ends are dissected by incising on the dotted line and separating fascicles from epineurium. After fascicles are selected for union, excess epineurium can be trimmed away. (**B**) A splint of external epineurium is constructed with sutures placed on the deep surface of the nerve *only*. This splint serves to relieve tension on the fascicle ends. (**C**) Individual or groups of fascicles are joined by small caliber sutures placed in the internal epineurium. Closure of external epineurium on superficial surface is not necessary. (Illustration by Elizabeth Roselius, 1991. From Gelberman RH: *Operative nerve repair and reconstruction,* Philadelphia, 1991, JB Lippincott).

eters away from the cut end to relieve tension and still avoid stress on the cut end of the nerve. In so doing, the tension is taken up at a distance, allowing easy approximation of fascicles in a tension-free state (see Fig. 11-3 for details).

FUTURE DIRECTIONS

Until recently, I and many others have taught that the repair of transected nerves requires coaptation of the nerve ends and maintenance with sutures. Practically speaking, almost all repairs are still done in this way. Despite our best efforts in nerve suture, clinical outcomes today seem to have plateaued and are frequently still unsatisfactory. It is necessary that we look at new approaches and consider whether some other technique can improve results further.

In speaking on the future of nerve surgery at a meeting of the American Society for Surgery of the Hand in 1986,[5] I observed that, "it is unlikely that significant improvement would result from further technical advances in suture technique." The question that I raised was whether a transected nerve had to be sewn together for regeneration to take place. I observed that certain trends had occurred in recent years: The diameter of suture material had progressively decreased from 4-0 or 6-0 down to 10-0 or 11-0. Coincident to this, the number of sutures being placed in a repair were fewer and fewer. It seemed obvious that if these trends continued, *nerve suture would soon use no suture at all.* Thus, the challenge facing surgeons appeared to be the provision of the ideal environment for nerve regeneration, not suture technique. The remainder of this discussion deals with the ideal nerve juncture and innovative efforts to achieve it.

It was noted earlier that repairing the transected nerve is unique. The objective in nerve repair is to provide a bridge across which regenerating axons might travel to reach the opposite end and then proceed to their distal targets. Because technical aspects of suture have progressed as far as possible, we must now turn to biologic processes for alternative methods to form this bridge if we are to improve results.

Biologic factors come into play at three levels: the nerve cell body, the transection site, and the distal organs. The first and last of these factors are beyond the reach of the surgeon, and it is only at the site of nerve juncture that results can be influenced by surgery. Experimentally, pharmacologic agents have been shown to have effects on nerve cell metabolism, distal degeneration, the speed of axonal breakdown, and end organ preservation, but they are not within the scope of this discussion. Remarks here are limited only to the nerve juncture. Because nerve suture appears to have reached a point where no further improvement in clinical results seems likely, investigators have turned to other approaches. Among these is the concept of tubulation.

Tubulation was described 50 years ago by Paul Weiss,[12] but had probably been used in laboratories for some time prior to that. Weiss used veins as tubules in animals to study tropism, but the method found no use in humans until about 1980, when Lundborg,[7] Chiu,[1] MacKinnon, Dellon, Hunter, and Hunter[8] and others began a reinvestigation of the merits of tubular repairs. A variety of materials, both synthetic and autogenous, have been used for creating tubes to join nerve ends. The work can be summarized by saying that a nervelike structure can form between nerve ends joined by a tube. The length of gap which can be bridged is debatable. Whether the medium within the tube matters is not known (but it must not be blood). The structure that forms contains axons, both myelinated and unmyelinated, and is surrounded by a perineurium-like tissue. Histologically, the structure resembles nerve and is capable of conducting an impulse.

Encouraged by early results, tubular repairs have been successfully employed in animals, and clinical trials in humans are currently underway. Many questions remain about tubulation: What is the ideal material? Should it be absorbable or nonabsorbable? How long a gap can one bridge? How complex a nerve can one join? What is the best medium to place within the tube? Other questions will undoubtedly arise and these will be addressed in time. For now, surgeons must still rely on traditional suture techniques to join nerve ends.

The present state of nerve repair requires that we try to perform as careful and tension-free a juncture as possible, between viable nerve ends and in a healthy bed. This can be accomplished either by direct suture or by nerve graft. The cornerstone of this technique is accurate topographical alignment of groups or individual fascicles and the maintenance of this alignment by the careful placement of sutures in the external and internal epineurium. Whether tubulation will produce results comparable with or better than traditional methods remains to be seen.

REFERENCES

1. Chiu DTW, Janecka I, Krizek TJ, et al: Autogenous vein graft as a conduit for nerve regeneration, *Surgery* 1982; 91:226-233.
2. deMedinaceli LD, Seaber AV: Experimental nerve reconnection: importance of initial repair, *Microsurgery* 1989; 10:56-70.
3. Hakstian RW: Funicular orientation by direct stimulation, *J Bone Joint Surg* 1968; 50A:1178-1186.
4. Jabaley ME: Technical aspects of peripheral nerve repair, *J Hand Surg* 1984; 9B:14.
5. Jabaley ME: Future trends in nerve repair. Presented at American Society for Surgery of the Hand, New Orleans, 1986, J. Leonard Goldner, moderator (unpublished).
6. Jabaley ME, Wallace WH, Heckler FR: Internal topography of major nerves of the forearm and hand: a current view, *J Hand Surg* 1980; 5:1.
7. Lundborg G, Dahlin LB, Danielsen N, et al: Nerve regeneration across an extended gap: a neurological view of nerve repair and the possible involvement of neuronotrophic factors, *J Hand Surg* 1982; 7:580-587.
8. MacKinnon S, Dellon AL, Hudson AR, Mackinnon SE: Nerve regeneration through a pseudosynovial sheath in a primate model, *Plast Reconstr Surg* 1985; 75:833-839.
9. Millesi H, Meissl G, Berger A: The interfascicular nerve grafting of the median and ulnar nerves, *J Bone Joint Surg* 1972; 54A:727.
10. Tsuge K, Ikuta Y, Sakaue M: A new technique for nerve suture, *Plast Reconstr Surg* 1975; 56:496.
11. Tupper JW: Fascicular nerve repair. In Omer GE, Spinner M, eds: *Management of peripheral nerve problems,* Philadelphia, 1980, Saunders.
12. Weiss P, Taylor AC: Guides for nerve regeneration across gaps, *J Neurosurg* 1946; 3:375-389.

Chapter 12

SPLINTING PERIPHERAL NERVE INJURIES

Elaine Ewing Fess

Splinting is an integral part of rehabilitation of a peripheral nerve injury.[3,5,6,9] Depending on the level of injury and the extent of damage to the nerve, with a supple hand splinting may be used to prevent deformity or to substitute for absent active motion. If joint contractures are present, passive range of motion first must be improved before surgical intervention or functional splinting may be undertaken. Through prolonged gentle tension that encourages gradual soft tissue growth,[2] splinting is the most effective method for increasing limited passive range of motion of contracted joints. Splints also protect postoperative tendon transfers in early healing stages, or they may be used to disrupt unwanted substitution patterns or improve active range of motion during late stages of healing when resistance is permitted. Splinting is but one tool that may be employed in the rehabilitation of patients with peripheral nerve injuries. For optimum results, splinting should not be perceived as the sole rehabilitation modality, but rather as one of many integrated procedures, including, but not limited to, active and passive exercises, desensitization, sensory reeducation, functional activities, and activities of daily living and work programs. Guided by knowledge of normal and abnormal anatomy, physiology, and kinesiology; surgical information; and patient specific assessment data; rehabilitation programs are carefully adapted to meet the needs of individual patients. Data from periodic manual muscle testing and sensory evaluations provide critical indicators for determining the direction and scope of each program, indicating areas of stability and of change.[7,18]

Because injuries to peripheral nerves are not consistent in etiology or in amount of damage incurred and because patients differ in age, physiologic makeup, and inherent ability, it is important that there be close communication between surgeon, therapist, and patient during the rehabilitation process. Surgical intervention is dependent on the level of injury, extent of damage, and prognosis for recovery.[11,14,17] Before nonsurgical rehabilitation may be initiated, rehabilitation personnel must obtain specific information regarding etiology of injury, site of injury, time since injury, extent of damage, and related injuries; surgical intervention, including date of surgery, type of repair, and tension on the repair; prognosis for recovery; and specific precautions and limitations.[11] Once this information is acquired, treatment planning may be carried out in close conjunction with the surgeon and patient. If prognosis is not favorable or if recovery is anticipated to be lengthy, the surgeon may opt to do immediate tendon transfers. Postoperative treatment protocols for nerve repairs and for repaired nerves with immediate tendon transfers differ considerably.[11] It is critical that rehabilitative personnel know exactly what was done surgically and what specific course is appropriate for postoperative rehabilitation. Unfortunately, lack of communication or misunderstanding of specific requirements can present disappointing or even disastrous consequences for the patient.

Injury to a peripheral nerve results in a predictable pattern of deformity according to the nerve and level of injury. Depending on the physiologic and anatomic extent of damage, peripheral nerve injuries are classified according to Seddon[15] as neurapraxia, axonotmesis, or neurotmesis. In contrast, Sunderland describes five degrees of nerve injuries.[17] Omer and Spinner[14] clearly correlate these two classification systems regarding functional, anatomic, and

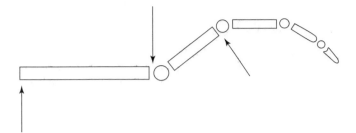

Fig. 12-1. Three-point pressure system with volar forces applied at the proximal and distal ends of the splint with a dorsal middle reciprocal force at the wrist immobilizes the wrist in a radial nerve injury.

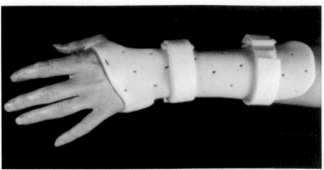

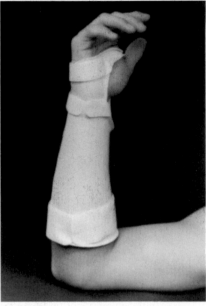

Fig. 12-2. Whether dorsally or volarly applied, a wrist immobilization splint transfers the power of the extrinsic flexors to the fingers and thumb, allowing functional use of the hand. (**A** courtesy Sharon Flinn-Wagner, M.Ed.,O.T.R./L., Cleveland.)

physiologic status. The purpose of this chapter is to briefly review the expected kinesiologic muscle imbalances attributed to compression or disruption of each of the three main upper extremity peripheral nerves and to discuss related splinting approaches used to treat these injuries. It is not within the scope of this chapter to address splinting programs as they relate to postoperative tendon transfer rehabilitation requirements. Splint terminology used in this chapter is derived from the American Society of Hand Therapists Splint Classification System.[1]

RADIAL NERVE

Arising from C6, C7, C8, and T1, the radial nerve innervates the triceps, brachioradialis, extensor carpi radialis longus and brevis, anconeus, and supinator. Its terminal motor branch, the posterior interosseous nerve (PIN), innervates the extensor digitorum communis, extensor digiti minimi, extensor carpi ulnaris, abductor pollicis longus, extensor pollicis longus, extensor pollicis brevis, and extensor indicis proprius. Functionally, the radial nerve is responsible for extension of the elbow, wrist, and metacarpophalangeal (MP) joints of the digits, and extension and abduction of the thumb. Paralysis of the triceps is unusual unless the injury is high at the level of the axilla and then, passive elbow extension is functionally compensated by gravitational pull. Supination may be substituted by the intact biceps and by shoulder movements, and active interphalangeal extension is achieved by the intact intrinsic muscles.[13] Extension of the wrist, MP joints, and thumb extension and abduction are absent in radial nerve lesions above the supinator. Loss of the posterior interosseous nerve results in dorsoradial wrist extension and loss of digital MP extension. In partial compression or injury to the PIN, loss of MP extension of one or more digits may occur.

Splinting of radial nerve injuries is primarily focused on providing wrist stability, with most authors advocating wrist immobilization in 10° to 20° dorsiflexion to enhance hand function (Fig. 12-1). Wrist stabilization allows digital flexors to transfer power to the fingers and thumb, permitting functional use of the hand. Interphalangeal (IP) extension is provided by the intrinsic muscles of the hand which are

spared in radial nerve injury. Wrist immobilization also prevents overstretching of extrinsic extensor muscles and eliminates impingement of the median nerve by avoiding prolonged wrist flexion postures.[12] Splints may be applied dorsally or volarly, depending on patient need and therapist preference. Most patients find that a simple wrist extension immobilization splint (Fig. 12-2) meets their functional needs and do not require additional MP extension splinting while awaiting radial nerve regeneration. However, on occasion, patients may need full MP extension of fingers and thumb to achieve independence in their vocational or avocational pursuits. In these instances, more extensive dynamic-assist splinting is necessary. Because this type of MP dynamic-assist splinting is designed to substitute for lost active extension rather than improve limited passive range of motion, and active flexor power is not impaired, a low profile outrigger design (Fig. 12-3) may be preferable because it is less bulky than its high profile counterpart.[8] Based on earlier work by Hollis, Colditz describes a tenodesis splint in which wrist extension is attained with active finger flexion and

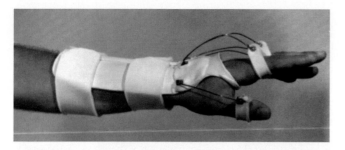

Fig. 12-3. Although more expensive, a wrist and MP mobilization splint, type O, may be required to meet the vocational or avocational needs of a specific patient who has sustained a radial nerve injury. (Courtesy Christine Heaney, B.Sc., Ottowa, Ontario.)

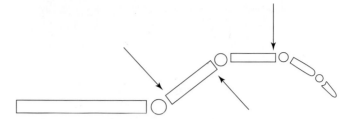

Fig. 12-4. A three-point pressure system with dorsal forces at the proximal and distal ends of the splint with a middle reciprocal volar force holds the 4th and 5th metacarpophalangeal joints in flexion in an ulnar nerve injury.

finger MP extension is accomplished with active wrist flexion.[4] These reciprocal tenodesis motions are harnessed by a dorsal static line extended from the wrist distally over a low profile outrigger fulcrum and attached to MP extension finger cuffs. A word of caution: In the current environment of managed health care, the wisdom of blanket application of dynamic-assist splints for treating radial nerve paralysis needs to be reconsidered. In terms of cost, there is considerable difference between a wrist extension immobilization splint and a dynamic MP assist splint. It may be prudent to use the simpler, less costly wrist immobilization splint for most patients, and save the more expensive dynamic-assist splint for special problems.

Splinting to correct contractures is rare in radial nerve palsy. The presence of compensatory or substitution motions coupled with gravitational pull helps maintain passive extension of involved joints. In addition, there is almost universal recognition and diagnosis of radial nerve palsy resulting in appropriate referral for therapeutic intervention. Further, when treated in a timely fashion, decompressed or repaired radial nerves may have a favorable prognosis for return of motor function.

Progressive blocking splinting may be used postoperatively to allow incremental increases in active joint extension in cases where a radial nerve has been repaired under tension and a flexed joint posture, usually of the elbow, is required to relieve the tension on the repair. Gradually, over a period of weeks, increased joint extension is allowed by the progressively applied blocking or restriction splints as the nerve undergoes physiologic adaptation and increases in length.

While injury to the sensory branch of the radial nerve does not cause motor loss, the sensory branch is important in splinting for another reason. Because of its predictable intolerance to compression, it is very important to avoid pressure on the sensory branch of the radial nerve from overlying splint components. Straps and splint edges that overlap this nerve branch often cause considerable pain that is difficult to relieve, even when the splint is removed. Splints should be designed carefully and deliberately to avoid applying pressure to this sensory nerve.

ULNAR NERVE

The C7, C8, and T1 nerve roots make up the ulnar nerve. It innervates the flexor carpi ulnaris, 4th and 5th flexor digitorum profundus, palmaris brevis, abductor digiti minimi, opponens digiti minimi, flexor digiti minimi, 4th and 5th lumbricales, interossei, deep head of the flexor pollicis brevis, and adductor pollicis muscles. Functionally, ulnar nerve paralysis results in weakened, dysfunctional pinch; weakened power grip; loss of finger abduction and adduction; and the classic claw hand deformity posture of MP joint hyperextension and IP joint flexion of the ring and small fingers. Dependent on inherent joint suppleness, clawing may not be apparent immediately after injury in the ring and small fingers of all patients. Clawing is more problematic in distal ulnar nerve lesions, where both the extrinsic finger flexors and extensors are intact, and the governing action of the intrinsic muscles on the 4th and 5th MP joints is absent. Over time, clawing becomes more apparent as joint angulation of the two ulnar digits becomes more accented. The combination of loss of thumb adductor strength, Froment's sign, thumb IP flexion during pinch, Jeanne's sign, and hyperextension of the thumb MP joint, limit the effectiveness of pinch. In addition, the claw posture interferes with functional grip by presenting the distal palm forward in conjunction with a curled finger posture, severely disrupting the hand's ability to position the fingers around an object because of zig-zag collapse of the longitudinal arch of the hand.

In supple hands, splinting ulnar nerve injuries is focused on restoring the longitudinal arch by externally reestablishing the absent intrinsic balance to the powerful extrinsic extensor muscles. Although splints may differ in design, they all provide some means of achieving passive MP flexion to the ring and small fingers (Fig. 12-4). Once MP flexion is established, the intact extrinsic finger extensors are able to actively extend the ring and small IP joints, eliminating the predisposition for development of IP flexion contractures (Fig. 12-5). Gajiwala, Sams, Pandya, and Wagh describe a lumbrical simulating splint in which two nylon threads, connected to a palmar base, pass volar to the MP joint, separate laterally, and then pass dorsal to the proximal

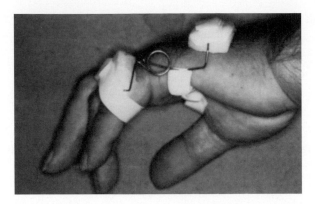

Fig. 12-5. A hand-based metacarpophalangeal extension restriction splint, type O, substitutes for lost intrinsic muscle action at the metacarpophalangeal joints and permits the extrinsic extensors to actively extend the ring and small interphalangeal joints. (From Fess EE, Philips CA: *Hand splinting: principles and methods,* St Louis, 1987, Mosby.)

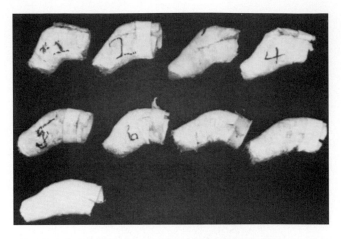

Fig. 12-6. With fixed contractures of the interphalangeal joints, passive range of motion may be improved with serial casting (proximal interphalangeal and distal interphalangeal extension mobilization splints, type O). (From Fess EE, Philips CA: *Hand splinting: principles and methods,* St Louis, 1987, Mosby.)

interphalangeal (PIP) joint and insert on an adapted finger cuff strapped to the proximal and middle phalanges.[10] Imitating lumbrical action, this splint limits active MP extension while dynamically facilitating passive IP extension. While this is an innovative approach, it may be more complicated than necessary because any splint that holds the MP in flexion allows active IP extension via the extrinsic extensor muscles making the described dynamic-assist mechanism superfluous. In addition, maintenance of the palmar arch is also important in preserving functional potential of a paralyzed hand while awaiting ulnar nerve regeneration after surgical repair.

With certain patients, positional night splints may be beneficial in alleviating nerve compression problems. For example, Seror advocates elbow night splinting as an effective nonsurgical treatment of ulnar nerve paralysis. In a study of 22 patients who were placed in night blocking splints that prevented elbow flexion beyond 60° for 6 months, all reported diminished symptoms, and electromyographic studies indicated improvement in 16 of 17 follow-up patients.[16]

If fixed joint limitations are present, normal passive range of motion must be achieved before functional splinting or tendon transfers may be undertaken. In ulnar nerve paralysis, the IP joints of the ring and small fingers are predisposed to flexion contractures. Over time, the IP joint of the thumb may also develop a flexion contracture. Splints are designed to meet the individual needs of each patient. Providing the patient can come to the clinic several times a week, serial casting is an especially effective means of improving passive range of motion of contracted IP joints (Fig. 12-6). Casts are changed every 3 to 4 days as IP extension improves. If the patient is unable to come to the clinic on a regular basis, dynamic assist mobilization splinting may be a more appropriate choice to improve passive range of motion. Because the intent of the splint is to correct joint contrac-

tures, a high profile outrigger may be a better design choice than its low profile counterpart because fewer adjustments are required as passive joint motion improves.[9,15]

As noted with radial nerve injuries repaired under tension, progressive restriction splints may be employed with repaired ulnar nerves, enabling slowly increasing joint range of motion over time as the repaired nerve increases in length. Again, it is critical that close communication exist between surgeon, therapist, and patient to achieve optimal rehabilitative results.

MEDIAN NERVE

Arising from C6, C7, C8, and T1, the median nerve innervates the pronator teres, flexor carpi radialis, flexor digitorum superficialis, palmaris longus, 2nd and 3rd flexor digitorum profundus, flexor pollicis longus, pronator quadratus, 2nd and 3rd lumbricales, opponens pollicis, superficial head of the flexor pollicis brevis, and abductor pollicis brevis. High median nerve paralysis results in loss of thumb IP flexion, and distal interphalangeal (DIP) flexion of the index and sometimes the middle finger. Elbow and wrist flexion are weak and forearm pronation is also weakened or absent, depending on how proximal the injury is. Thumb opposition is lost, and thumb flexion and abduction are weak. MP flexion and IP extension of the index and long fingers are absent. Injury to the anterior interosseous nerve produces an inability to flex the terminal joints of the thumb, index finger, and long fingers, resulting in the benediction sign, whereas more distal lesions involve only the intrinsic muscles of the thumb and radial two digits.

Splinting is often recommended as a conservative treatment for relieving compression of the median nerve at the wrist.[5,6,9,12] Kruger et al.[14] reported statistically significant improvement in sensory latency in patients who had been treated for carpal tunnel syndrome with neutral-angle

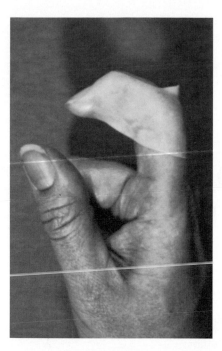

Fig. 12-7. If passive motion of the distal joints of the thumb and index fingers is limited in the end range of flexion, interphalangeal flexion splints, type O, may be used to reestablish passive range of motion. (From Fess EE, Philips CA: *Hand splinting: principles and methods,* St Louis, 1987, Mosby.)

wrist immobilization splints. They also reported a 67% rate of subjective relief of symptoms.

Many median nerve actions have substitute motions derived from overlapping ulnar and sometimes radial nerve innervations and as a result, median nerve lesions often require less intensive splinting regimens for function and maintenance of passive joint motion. Night splinting to maintain thumb carpometacarpal (CMC) motion is usually sufficient in a supple hand. Daily passive exercises are usually adequate for maintaining flexion of the thumb IP joint and DIP joints of the index and long fingers but, if stiffness occurs, simple glove band splints may be used to improve passive IP flexion (Fig. 12-7). In a rare case involving prolonged IP stiffness, it may be necessary to serially cast the distal phalanges of the thumb, index, and long fingers into IP joint flexion. If the thumb CMC web space is contracted, serial CMC web space splints may be used to increase CMC passive motion. Because the thumb CMC joint permits motion in multiple planes, it is often helpful to alternately splint the thumb in extension and in abduction.

SUMMARY

When treating peripheral nerve injuries, functional daytime splinting is often combined with nighttime maintenance splints to achieve optimum results. It is important to understand that splint "cookbooks" that rigidly designate given splints for specific diagnoses should be studiously avoided. Although similar diagnostic requirements exist, each patient must be carefully evaluated and reevaluated on an individual basis. What works for one patient may not be appropriate for another. It is the careful balancing of many factors that leads to successful rehabilitative results. Splinting is one method of improving function and joint range of motion. It is important, however, that it be used in conjunction with other treatment techniques to achieve patients' maximum rehabilitation potentials.

REFERENCES

1. The American Society of Hand Therapists: *Splint classification system,* Chicago, 1992, The American Society of Hand Therapists.
2. Brand P, Hollister A: *Clinical mechanics of the hand,* ed 2, St. Louis, 1993, Mosby.
3. Cannon NM, Foltz RW, Koepher JM, et al: *Manual of hand splinting,* New York, 1985, Churchill Livingstone.
4. Colditz JC: Splinting for radial nerve palsy, *J Hand Ther* 1987; 1:18-23.
5. Coppard BM, Lohman HL: *Introduction to splinting, a critical-thinking & problem-solving approach,* St Louis, 1996, Mosby.
6. Fess EE: Rehabilitation of the patient with peripheral nerve injury. In Mackin E, ed: *Hand clinics,* vol 2, Philadelphia, 1986, Saunders.
7. Fess EE: Documentation: essential elements of an upper extremity assessment battery. In Hunter J, Mackin E, Callahan A, eds: *Rehabilitation of the hand,* ed 4, St Louis, 1995, Mosby.
8. Fess EE: Splints: mechanics versus convention, *J Hand Ther* 1995; 8:124-130.
9. Fess EE, Philips CA: *Hand splinting principles and methods,* ed 2, St Louis, 1987, Mosby.
10. Gajiwala M, Sams S, Pandya N, Wagh A: A new dynamic lumbrical simulating splint for claw hand deformity, *Plast Reconstr Surg* 1991; 87:170-173.
11. Green DP: *Operative hand surgery,* ed 3, New York, 1993, Churchill Livingstone.
12. Kruger VL, Kraft GH, Deitz JC, et al: Carpal tunnel syndrome: objective measures and splint use, *Arch Phys Med Rehabil* 1991; 72:517-520.
13. Landsmeer J, Long C: The mechanism of finger control, based on electromyograms and location analysis, *Acta Anat* 1965; 60:330.
14. Omer GE, Spinner M: *Management of peripheral nerve problems,* Philadelphia, 1980, Saunders.
15. Seddon H: *Surgical disorders of the peripheral nerves,* ed 2, New York, 1975, Churchill Livingstone.
16. Seror P: Treatment of ulnar nerve palsy at the elbow with a night splint, *J Bone Joint Surg* 1993; 75B:322-327.
17. Sunderland S: *Nerves and nerve injuries,* ed 2, Philadelphia, 1978, Williams & Wilkins.
18. Tubiana R, Thomine J, Mackin E: *Examination of the hand and wrist,* St Louis, 1996, Mosby.

Chapter 13

DESENSITIZATION OF THE TRAUMATIZED HAND*

Janet Waylett-Rendall

Nerves traumatized by injury, amputation, and painful scar formation experience varying degrees of hyperesthesia or dysesthesia during recovery and reinnervation. Hyperesthesia, or hypersensitivity as it is more frequently termed, can be a significant deterrent to functional use of the hand and therefore must be treated by early and effective therapy intervention.[1,6]

HISTORICAL PERSPECTIVE

The term *desensitization* is relatively new, having come into popular use by hand therapists during the early 1970s; however, the techniques encompassed by this treatment descriptor have medically documented use at least since 1634 when Ambrose Pare[13] treated stump pain with massage and oils.

One of the earliest treatments of stump pain was described as pounding the stump with a wooden mallet or banging the stump against furniture, both being forms of percussion.[14] Massage, often the patient's favorite form of desensitization, has been used since 3000 BC, presumably for reduction of discomfort.

The role of desensitization at the most basic and functional level is to decrease the pain and discomfort encountered upon touch. After that is achieved, the affected area can undergo the treatment and sensory reeducation that will allow for the dexterity and the discriminatory sensation required for self-care and work activities.[1,5]

Stump pain—hand and major limb

Stump pain after amputation was the first and most widely researched diagnostic pain group with which desensitization has been successfully employed. Much has been learned by studying stump pain and its treatment and in extrapolating theories and treatment techniques from this patient group to other patients with nerve-tissue injury.[9,10,16]

Davis[3] describes six of what he believes to be the most common causes of peripherally induced stump pain: (1) improper fit of the prosthesis, usually in the lower extremity; (2) neurotemesis, related to the neuroma being "neurodesed" (tethered) in scar tissue; (3) joint pain in the area of the amputation; (4) sympathetically maintained pain; (5) referred pain, usually related to radiculopathy; and (6) bony exostoses, adherent scar, heterotrophic ossification, and ischemia.

Digital amputations

Fisher and others studied 100 patients with 144 digital amputations. Only four of these patients demonstrated painful neuromas; two were treated by surgical excision, and two with more vague complaints were treated by desensitization which decreased stump sensitivity and allowed them to return to work.[4] These authors believed the low incidence of painful neuromas in their study group was the result of early return to work. Others[3,8,12] have reported similar findings in patients who incorporated the injured extremity into their activities of daily living. Millstein and others[12] reviewed 1000 amputees in Canada and found that 51% were fully employed, 5% were employed part time, 25% were retired, and only 8% were unemployed. Outcomes were positively affected by prosthetic usage, younger age at amputation, and multidisciplinary rehabilitation.[12]

*From Waylett-Rendall J: Desensitization of the traumatized hand. In Hunter JM, Mackin EJ, Callahan AD, eds: *Rehabilitation of the hand: surgery and therapy,* St Louis, 1995, Mosby.

Phantom sensations

Phantom sensations may be felt by not only traumatic amputees, but also congenital amputees, the spinal-cord injured, and those with brachial plexus injuries.[3,9,10] Sensations experienced are varied and range from pressure, warmth, and cold to pain. It is the painful sensation, most often described as shooting, cramping, or burning, that is the greatest inhibitor of functional use.[8,14]

The painful neuroma has been most frequently blamed for the phantom pains and hypersensitivity, but recent evidence indicates that other factors may play a role as well.[8,9,10] Before we embark on a program of desensitization with our patients, we must be aware of the more recent findings concerning phantom sensations and phantom pain.

Melzack[9,10] suggests that the brain contains a neuromatrix or network of neurons that not only responds to sensory stimulation but also continuously generates a pattern of impulses he calls a *neurosignature*, indicating the body is intact.

Davis[3] states that the neuromatrix theory explains phantom sensation but not entirely phantom pain because relief of phantom pain rarely changes phantom sensation and vice versa. Davis believes phantom pain also may be caused by the loss of inhibition in the somatosensory cortex and by changes in the dorsal horn neurons secondary to peripheral injury. The injury damages the neurons, causing them to generate pain impulses, which are directed rostrally.[3]

Campbell,[2] Sachs,[15] and others[8,16] state that peripheral receptors also may fire spontaneously as an inherent pacemaker, which may give rise to a chronic, painful condition that is not stimulus mediated. There is also evidence that attempted axonal regeneration may establish areas of hyperexcitability.[15] Findings by Merzenich and others[11] with primate studies corroborate with Melzack that cortical inhibition may well play a role. This concept will be covered in greater depth in the theory section of this chapter.

Desensitization employed with other diagnostic groups

Responding to a need to provide treatment for other than stump-related pain and discomfort, hand surgeons and hand therapists expanded desensitization to encompass treatment of hypersensitivity and pain secondary to nerve injury, partial nerve injury, nerve compression, and soft-tissue injuries.[5] Clinical experience of this author has been that the commonly applied desensitization techniques used successfully with amputees, revascularization cases, burns, and complete nerve repairs are not as effective with cumulative trauma cases. Cumulative trauma injuries in my opinion respond better to pacing and other ergonomic changes at the job site, biofeedback, and psychologic intervention.

Authors such as Hochreiter and others[7] determined that vibration may be effective as a short-term desensitization technique, as seen in 24 normal subjects in their study. These individuals experienced a raised tactile threshold after 10 minutes of vibration at 80 Hz. This raised threshold lasted 10 minutes but not 15 minutes after the vibration treatment. Other investigators have demonstrated that vibration can result in an elevation of pain[1] and heat thresholds.[19]

DEFINITIONS

Before initiating evaluation and treatment of pain or hypersensitivity, one must first define and describe the condition or problem that may require desensitization. We must develop a common language when describing the discomfort we are treating with our desensitization techniques. This will facilitate research on outcome studies to determine the effectiveness of these treatment techniques, ideally through multicenter studies.

The following is a partial list of terminology based on the glossary of terms issued by the International Association for the Study of Pain.[18]

Allodynia: Pain secondary to a stimulus that is not normally painful when applied elsewhere to the body.

Anesthesia dolorosa: Pain in an insensitive area or region.

Causalgia: Severe, incapacitating pain after a traumatic nerve (median nerve in the upper extremity and the sciatic nerve in the lower extremity) lesion, associated with somatic, vasomotor, and sudomotor dysfunction.

Dysesthesia: Any unpleasant, abnormal sensation, either spontaneous or evoked. Allodynia and hyperpathia are considered examples of dysesthesia.

Hyperalgesia: Increased sensitivity to noxious stimuli.

Hyperpathia: An extreme form of hyperalgesia and allodynia characterized by the intensity of the pain, faulty localization, radiating pain, overreaction, and "after sensation."

Hyperesthesia: (Hypersensitivity is a more commonly used clinical term.) Increased sensitivity to all stimuli. Usually used to describe tactile and thermal stimuli. May be caused by scar tissue, neuromas (incontinuity and not), amputation, regenerating nerves.

Neuralgia: A nerve lesion causing intense and intermittent pain, felt maximally in the nerve distribution.

Pain: A subjective sensation recognizable to the patient but difficult to define by the therapist.

THEORIES: WHY AND HOW DESENSITIZATION MAY BE EFFECTIVE

Desensitization was reported by Barber[1] to be most effective when used early in recovery. The supposition is that it may prevent the development of permanent pain pathways in the central nervous system by manipulation of the cortical centers to inhibit their formation.[4] This occurs by having the patient use the hand in work activity, massage, and percussion. Desensitization is reported to be more effective if done during the course of work, instead of the typically prescribed three to four times per day.[3,4,12]

Using the involved hand in work results in softening scar, increasing circulation, and returning of the nerves to a normal level of activity.[4] Unlike desensitization "contact media" of corn kernels, birdshot, or stones, work also may provide the distraction from the initial discomfort, and its monetary rewards are often more motivating.

Recent research by Melzack and others[9,10,11] substantiates the need to treat the painful sequelae of amputations, brachial plexus lesions, and spinal cord injuries on at least three levels in the brain's neural circuits.

Melzack's neuromatrix or neurosignature concept contains at least three major neural circuits. The first is the classical sensory pathway that passes through the thalamus on its way to the somatosensory cortex. The second is the limbic system, which travels through the reticular formation of the brain stem and is concerned with emotion and motivation. The third system contains the cortical regions necessary for recognition of the self, cognition, memory of past experience, and evaluation of sensory inputs in relation to the self. Melzack and others postulate that this matrix is "prewired" for movement because congenital amputees also experience vivid phantoms.

This is important new information that will enhance success in desensitization programs. Knowing this, the therapist will want to capitalize on each of these three major neural circuits. Newer techniques, such as EEG biofeedback used in cognitive therapy, eventually may prove to be beneficial in chronic pain cases.

Recent findings by Merzenich and Jenkins[11] on the plasticity of cortical area 3b, representative of adult monkey hand surfaces, offer support for inhibition theories. When transected, the median nerve did not retain representational topography in the brain; instead, cutaneous receptive fields of adjacent fibers jumped in almost random order across the skin field represented cortically by the nerve. The median nerve did not recapture all of its original sensory cortex territory, possibly because the shuffled inputs provided a less effective competition against the surrounding innervated skin.[11]

DESENSITIZATION DESCRIBED

What characterizes a desensitization program? The literature describes desensitization narrowly in terms of repetitive physical stimuli applied to the injured part of the body three to four times daily.[1,5,6] More broadly, it also may encompass biofeedback to monitor and control internal tension or temperature relative to pain and discomfort. More important, it may involve return to usual and customary work or avocational activities.[12]

EVALUATION OF HYPERSENSITIVITY

To establish the level of hypersensitivity and a baseline of response to desensitization, one must conduct pretreatment evaluation of hypersensitivity. The Three Phase Hand Sensitivity Test (developed in 1980 as the Downey Hand

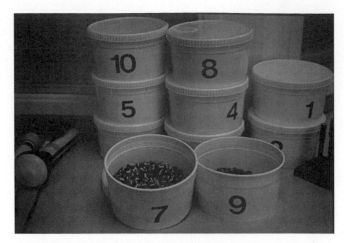

Fig. 13-1. Three Phase Hand Sensitivity Test (vibrators not shown) (North Coast Medical).

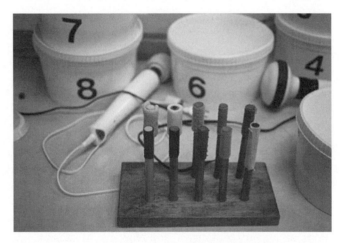

Fig. 13-2. Dowel textures of the Three Phase Hand Sensitivity Test.

Center Sensitivity Test) is the only commercially available (North Coast Medical) test to date that is specifically designed to establish a hierarchy of sensitivity (Fig. 13-1). This test, although slightly modified from the original, is the test preferred by the author but should be used in conjunction with other hand-function assessments, such as pain, touch-pressure threshold, two-point discrimination, pinch, grip, range of motion, and patient symptomatology. The Semmes-Weinstein monofilaments, most commonly used to quantify recovery of touch-pressure threshold, also may be used to establish a well-defined threshold of sensitivity.[7]

The Three Phase Hand Sensitivity Test (originally the Downey Community Hospital Hand Sensitivity Test) was tested for validity and reliability in 1981 on 40 normal subjects.[1] As indicated by the name, the test has three parts or phases. The first phase is a hierarchy of 10 textured dowels shown in Fig. 13-2. Two of the five textured dowels are randomly selected by the examiner, and the patient is

THREE PHASE DESENSITIZATION
– RECORD FORM –

1   NAME _John Doe_ _____ AGE _25_ SEX _M_

2   DIAGNOSIS _Median Nerve Laceration (Partial)_

3   SOURCE OF PAIN: AMPUTATION _____ SCAR _____ CRUSH _____ NEUROMA _____ BURN _____ OTHER _See above_

4   DESCRIPTION OF PAINFUL AREA: INITIAL: _3/7/95_

5   DISCHARGE: _____

6   DOMINANCE: RIGHT _X_ LEFT _____

7   HOW INJURY OCCURRED _____

8   DATE OF INJURY _12/5/94_ DATE OF SURGERY _12/7/94_ DATE OF 1ST RX: _12/30/94_

9   NO. OF WEEKS FROM D.O.I. OR SURGERY TO 1ST DESEN. RX: _3 weeks_

10 NO. OF WEEKS BETWEEN 1ST AND LAST RX: _____ NO. OF TREATMENTS _____ REFERRING M.D. _____

11	DOWEL TEXTURES		CONTACT PARTICLES		VIBRATION	
12	LEVEL A	DATE BEGUN/COMMENTS	LEVEL B	DATE BEGUN/COMMENTS	LEVEL	DATE BEGUN/COMMENTS
13	1 1	12/30/94	1 3	12/30 tolerated	1	1/5/95
14	2 2	"	2 2	1/17/95 "	2	
15	3 3	"	3 1		3	
16	4 4	"	4 4		4	
17	5 5	"	5 5		5	
18	6		6 6		6	
19	7		7 8		7	
20	8		8 9		8	
21	9		9 7		9	
22	10		10 10		10	

Fig. 13-3. Hypothetical patient's desensitization record.

asked to state which is the most irritating of the textures. More textured dowels are introduced one at a time, according to the specific instructions of the test. These textures range from moleskin to Velcro hook, and the patient is asked to determine which is the most irritating of the dowels. A hierarchy selected by a patient is shown in Fig. 13-3.

The second phase of this test involves the 10 contact or immersion particles, which are contained so that the patient can place the hand into the medium as shown in Fig. 13-4. These textures are placed in front of the patient in two rows. The first row includes containers one to five, and the examiner randomly selects two containers into which the patient places the involved hand (Fig. 13-5). The patient is asked to feel the particles and compare the two contact media in their level of irritation. Contact particles are introduced one at a time, with the patient asked to compare with the previously felt particles, thus developing a hierarchy of irritation of the particles.

Vibration with two vibrators of varying cycles per second is used to complete the triad of the sensitivity assessment (Fig. 13-6). The results of the initial test are used to determine the level at which the patient will begin treatment. The Three Phase Desensitization Treatment is based on the results of the Three Phase Sensitivity Test.

Pain evaluations such as the visual analog scale and the McGill Pain Questionnaire also may be indicated as part of the initial evaluation, especially if pain is the major complaint.

After treatment, one should use the same test or tests to quantify the patient's response to the desensitization program. The patient should let the therapist know that some change in sensitivity has been experienced before formal retesting is undertaken.

DESENSITIZATION: TREATMENT
Techniques

Physical modalities used in the treatment of hypersensitivity and phantom pain have been described in the literature and include, but are not limited to, percussion, vibration, massage, heat, stroking, a prosthesis in the case of an amputation, TENS (transcutaneous nerve stimulation), acupuncture, compression, distraction, graded textures, and ultrasound.[1,6]

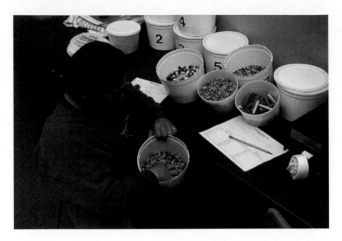

Fig. 13-4. Contact particles from the Three Phase Hand Sensitivity Test.

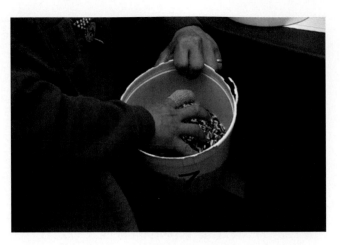

Fig. 13-5. Forced choice of irritation hierarchy of contact particles.

THREE PHASE DESENSITIZATION VIBRATION HIERARCHY

	CLINIC USE (10 minute session Electric Vibrator, except #1)	HOME USE (10 minute sessions 2 to 3 times daily, Battery-operated Vibrator)
1	Low cycle (battery-operated), no contact on area (as near as possible).	Same as clinic.
2	Low cycle, no contact (as near to area as possible).	Low cycle, no contact (as near to area as possible).
3	Low cycle, no contact (as near to area as possible).	Low cycle, intermittent contact on area.
4	Low cycle, intermittent contact on area.	Low cycle, intermittent contact on area.
5	Low cycle, intermittent contact on area.	Low cycle, continuous contact on area.
6	Low cycle, continuous contact on area.	Low cycle, continuous contact on area
7	High cycle, intermittent contact on area.	High cycle, intermittent contact on area.
8	High cycle, intermittent contact on area.	High cycle, continuous contact on area.
9	High cycle, continuous contact on area.	High cycle, continuous contact on area.
10	Vibration is not irritating.	

Fig. 13-6. Three phase desensitization hierarchy.

Recent interest in electromyographic (EMG) biofeedback at work stations may be added as a form of awareness training of internal muscle tension and give the clinician insight into how hypersensitivity increases upper extremity tension.

Desensitization should be *systematic,* sequential, structured, repetitive, and function oriented. Work or avocational activities should be included as soon as tolerated so the patient has a reality-based goal. Work simulation is used as early as possible for patients with work-related injuries and should be as close to the patient's real work situation as feasible.

Melzack's[9,10] recent findings reveal the importance of treatment directed at each level of the nervous system and delivered in a repetitive, organized, and systematic way, because this appears to be the means by which the central nervous system develops, processes, and adapts most readily to new information and learning situations.

Several stimuli have been shown to magnify pain symptoms; these include but are not limited to: exposure to cold, emotional stress, and local irritants.[8] It is best to avoid these stimuli, especially early in the desensitization treatment.

Table 13-1. Hardy, Moran, and Merritt desensitization protocol

Time	Level I	Level II	Level III	Level IV	Level V
Week 1	Tuning fork* Paraffin, massage				
(Progression to the next level requires demonstration of tolerance to a given level without signs of irritation)		Vibration, battery operated* Friction massage Constant touch/ pressure (Requires painful region to press objects into clay or intermittently press eraser onto tender site)			
			Vibration, electric* Textures, identification (rough to fine) Splints Activities		
				Vibration, electric* Object identification	
Discharge					Work and activities simulation

Adapted from Hardy MA, Moran CA, Merritt WM: Desensitization of the traumatized hands, *Va Med* 1982; 109:134-138.
*Increase from 1 to 10 minutes as tolerance improves.

Protocols

Protocols are the future of hand therapy and will be used to set a minimum standard of care. Hand therapists must develop and use the most effective protocols. The two best-known protocols for the treatment of hypersensitivity are described below.

Hardy, Moran, and Merritt protocol

Hardy and others[6] studied 16 patients functionally disabled by hypersensitivity. Patients were an average of 5 months after trauma. Their findings revealed successful outcome for 13 of these 16 patients, who returned to their previous occupations after 2 months of therapy. Two who failed treatment had surgical removal of digital neuromas. The minimum follow-up was 6 months.[6]

Hardy and others[6] used a sequential method of desensitization with five levels of treatment. The patients in this study were treated for hypersensitivity that was considered disproportionate for the injury, persisting for an average of 5 months. The Hardy protocol is shown in Table 13-1.

Used in combination with the Three Phase Desensitization Treatment, the Hardy protocol may offer the best overall treatment for hypersensitivity to date because it establishes levels of treatment and functional performance.

Three phase desensitization treatment protocol

The Three Phase Desensitization Treatment Protocol is based on a study performed in the late 1970s at the Downey Hand Center.[1] With 124 patients, this was the largest reported formal study on desensitization to date. It included 67 hand hypersensitive scars, 44 amputations, and 13 crush injuries. Treatment averaged approximately 7 weeks and was initiated 8 to 13 weeks after injury, with amputations beginning slightly later than the other diagnostic groups.

Desensitization was initiated at the level of vibration, texture, and contact media the patient could tolerate and was performed three to four times a day for 10 minutes at a time. After the completion of the program, 24 patients were randomly selected for outcome study relative to return to work. They were required to be at least 6 weeks post discharge.

Validity and reliability studies indicated that the Downey Hand Center Sensitivity Test (now known as the Three Phase Hand Sensitivity Test) could be used as both a test and a clinical tool.[1] The media from the Three Phase Hand Sensitivity Test are utilized for the Three Phase Desensitization Treatment Protocol (Table 13-2). When used as the manufacturer directs, this treatment protocol offers an excellent standardized program of graded desensitization.

Table 13-2. Three phase desensitization treatment protocol

Dowel textures	Contact particles	Vibration
1. Moleskin	1. Cotton	1. Battery/no contact
2. Felt	2. Terry cloth pieces	2. Battery/near contact
3. Quickstick	3. Dry rice	3. Low cycle/near contact
4. Velvet	4. Unpopped popcorn	4. Low cycle/intermittent contact
5. Semirough cloth	5. Pinto beans	5. Low cycle contact
6. Velcro loops	6. Macaroni	6. Low cycle continuous
7. Hard T-foam	7. Plastic wire insulation pieces	7. High cycle/intermittent
8. Burlap	8. Small pebbles	8. High cycle/intermittent
9. Rug back	9. Larger pebbles	9. High cycle/continuous
10. Velcro hook	10. Plastic squares	10. Vibration, not irritating

Adapted from Barber LM: Desensitization of the traumatized hand. In Hunter JM, Mackin EJ, Callahan AD, et al, eds: *Rehabilitation of the hand,* ed 3, St Louis, 1990, Mosby, and from North Coast Medical instruction book.

For clinics with limited space and budget, it may be attractive because the media for the test and the treatment are the same.

Hypothetical patient

Treatment of hypersensitivity can best be explained by describing the desensitization treatment of a hypothetical patient with diagnosis of midpalm crush injury. The patient indicates pain throughout the hand, the fingertips are described as feeling as if they are about to "burst open." The discomfort is experienced as tingling, burning, and shooting sensations from the palm to the finger tips. The dorsal surface of the hand displays pitting edema, the scar is adherent in the palm, and edema is present in the palm as well.

The choice of treatment modalities depends on the symptoms the patient exhibits and the findings from the sensitivity testing.

In consideration of the symptoms this hypothetical patient is demonstrating, we might best begin with retrograde massage to decrease the marked edema that may be compressing the digital nerves, to soften the adherent scar, to assist in venous return, and to begin sensory input. Often the patient has not touched the injured hand, for fear of further injury or increasing the pain and discomfort.

The massage should be light over the more painful areas and firmer in nonpainful areas where edema is marked. Psychologically, most patients enjoy massage and the contact of the therapist's hands and will tolerate some mild discomfort to obtain human touch, especially if some relief with the treatment has been offered.

The therapist may fit this patient with a compressive glove at the first visit after the retrograde massage to help control the discomfort caused by swelling. If the patient has enough motion in the fingers to make a partial fist, therapeutic putty exercises are given for the initial home program. These exercises will provide goal-directed active range of motion and help to "pump" the edema from the hand and the joint capsules; the edema also may be painful.

Testing sensitivity probably would be delayed until the second visit, when the edema may be reduced. After sensitivity is tested and the hierarchy of texture tolerance is recorded, treatment with these media would be introduced. Vibration also would be added at the second visit.

Fluidotherapy can be used at the beginning of the second treatment session to "bombard" the area with mild stimuli, at the same time increasing collagen extensibility through graded heat, allowing better motion.

The dowels from the Three Phase Hand Sensitivity Test that the patient tolerates are sent home, along with instructions to use contact particles as part of the home program. In this patient's case, rice will be used as the first contact particles for home use, because rice was at the top of the hierarchy of the contact or immersible textures. Desensitization is initiated at the level of vibration, texture, and contact media the patient can tolerate.

The dosage and frequency are three to four times a day for a minimum of 10 minutes for vibration and the same for textures. The patient continues with this treatment regimen for at least 4 to 6 weeks, and possibly longer if symptoms of hypersensitivity persist.

Vibration initially may be more uncomfortable to the patient than textures, but the patient soon prefers vibration to any other form of desensitization media in this author's opinion. Our hypothetical patient is provided with a hand-held, battery-operated vibrator for home use, applying it three to four times a day and whenever discomfort indicates.

OUTCOMES

The outcome assessment of a desensitization program should be based not only on reduction of hypersensitivity but also on functional use. Dexterity and coordination are the epitome of functional reinnervation of both sensory and motor nerves. Standardized tests such as the Purdue Peg Board could be used to evaluate median, ulnar, and combined median and ulnar nerve return because it measures recovery of fine dexterity. The Minnesota Rate of Manipulation Test can be utilized for grosser handling skills.

SUMMARY

Recent findings[9,10,12] indicate the need for a multifaceted approach for treating the hypersensitivity and pain involved in hand or upper extremity trauma. This may take the form of not only physical agents but also cognitive and psychologic techniques as well. The aim will be to enhance function by recruiting whatever neural networks will respond, either peripherally or centrally.

The literature indicates an early return to work or usual and customary activity facilitates the desensitization process. Should work simulation or work hardening begin earlier in treatment? Should desensitization treatment have specific protocols for certain diagnostic groups or should it be function related? These are questions that need to be answered in this dawning age of efficacy and outcome studies.

REFERENCES

1. Barber LM: Desensitization of the traumatized hand. In Hunter JM et al: *Rehabilitation of the hand,* ed 2, St Louis, 1990, Mosby.
2. Campbell JN, Raja SN, Cohen RH, et al: Peripheral neural mechanisms of nocioception. In Wall PD, Melzack R, eds: *Textbook of pain,* ed 2, New York, 1989, Churchill Livingstone.
3. Davis RW: Phantom sensation, phantom pain, and stump pain, *Arch Phys Med Rehabil* 1993; 74:79-91.
4. Fisher GT, Boswick JA: Neuroma formation following digital amputations, *J Trauma* 1983; V 23(2):136.
5. Carter-Wilson M: Sensory reeducation. In Gelberman RH, ed: *Operative nerve repair and reconstruction,* New York, 1991, JB Lippincott.
6. Hardy MA, Moran CA, Merritt WH: Desensitization of the traumatized hand, *Va Med* 1982; 109: 134-138.
7. Hochreiter NW: Effect of vibration on tactile sensitivity, *Phys Ther* 1983; 63(6):934.
8. Jensen TS: Phantom limb, phantom pain and stump pain in amputees during the first six months following limb amputation, *Pain* 1983; 17:243-256.
9. Melzack R: Phantom limbs, *Scientific American* 1992; April:120-126.
10. Melzack R: The John Bonica distinguished lecture. The gate control theory 25 years later: new perspectives on phantom limb pain. In Bond MR, Charlton JE, Woolf CJ, eds: *Proceedings of the VIth World Congress on Pain,* Amsterdam, 1991, Elsevier.
11. Merzenich MM, Jenkins WM: Reorganization of cortical representations of the hand following alterations of skin inputs induced by nerve injury, skin island transfers and experience, *J Hand Ther* 1993; 6(2):89-104.
12. Millstein S, Bain D, Hunter GA: A review of employment patterns of industrial amputees—factors influencing rehabilitation, *Prosthet Orthot Int* 1985; 9:69-78.
13. Paré A: *The collected works of Ambroise Pare,* London, 1634.
14. Russell WR, Spaulding JMK: Treatment of painful amputation stumps, *Br Med J* 1950; 2:68-73.
15. Sachs F: Biophysics of mechanoreceptors, *Membr Biochem* 1986; 6:173-192.
16. Sherman RA, Sherman CJ, Gall NG: A survey of current phantom limb treatment in the United States, *Pain* 1980; 8:85-99.
17. Sica RE: Changes in the N1-P1 component of the somatosensory cortical evoked response in patients with partial limb amputation, *Electromyogr Clin Neurophysio* 1984; 24:415-427.
18. Sunderland S: *Nerve injuries and their repair, a critical appraisal,* New York, 1991, Churchill Livingstone.
19. Wall PD, Cronly-Dillon JR: Pain, itch and vibration, *Arch Neurol* 1960; 2:365-375.
20. Weinstein S: Tactile sensitivity of the phalanges, *Percept Mot Skills* 1962; 14:351-354.
21. Wood W: Observations of neurons with cures and histories of the disease, *Trauma Med Chir Soc* (Edinburgh) 1829; 3:68.

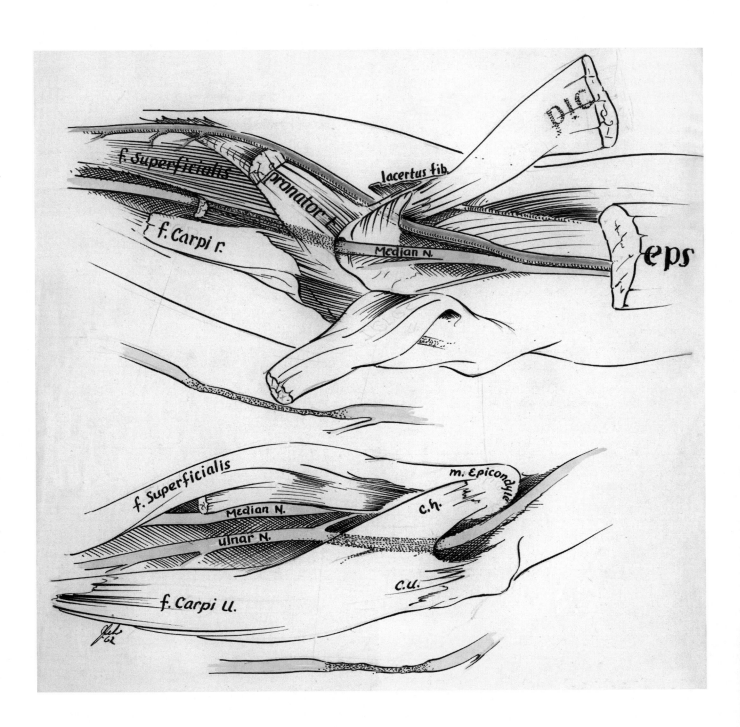

Part IV

NERVE MOBILIZATION AND GLIDING

Relationship of the median and ulnar nerves to the proximal musculature of the forearm. It is here that ischemic muscle fibrosis and contracture restricts nerve gliding and impairs nerve conduction. (From Converse JM: *Reconstructive plastic surgery: principles in correction, reconstruction and transplantation,* vol. iv, Philadelphia, 1964, Saunders.)

Chapter 14

GLIDING TISSUE OF PERIPHERAL NERVES: ITS SURGICAL SIGNIFICANCE

Hanno Millesi

Gliding tissue is a special type of loose connective tissue that provides the possibility of movement between two neighboring structures. The functional requirements for gliding tissue are different according to the magnitude of necessary motion. If the necessity for gliding passes beyond a certain limit, special structures are developed. If tendons serve as an example, one realizes that along the forearm the movement necessary for the transmission of the muscle contraction via the tendon is provided by a tissue called *paratenon* or *paratendineum.* This is a loose connective tissue in which layers of capillaries alternate with layers of elastic and collagen fibers arranged in a very loose way. These layers can be shifted against each other without losing contact. Movement within certain limits is possible with a very low friction (see p. 112). At sites where a major amount of movement is necessary, as in the fingers, tendon sheaths have been developed. In contrast to gliding tissue, the tendon sheaths consist of two synovial layers, lining a virtual space filled with synovial liquid; thus, the contact between the different layers has been lost. All this has been studied very carefully because motion, in order to transmit force from the attached muscle, is the main function of tendons.

Less well known is the passive motion that arises because structures are exposed to a different amount of passive dislocation, if they are located in a level with different distance to the level of motions of a particular joint. This difference makes the possibility of gliding against each other a necessity. This is especially true for nerves. Vessels need space for movement to allow pulsation. Nerves must be able to move against the surrounding tissue also because they have to get thicker if they slack down with flexion and they have to become thinner with elongation during extension, if the nerve is located at the flexor site of a joint.

In addition, the individual fascicles of a nerve trunk must be able to move against each other. Only if such movements at a low friction rate are possible, the nerve can adapt (e.g., to transverse compression by dislocation of the individual fascicles without rising the interfascicular pressure). A thick nerve trunk must have the possibility of gliding of the individual fascicles against each other because during flexion the fascicles of the site closer to the plane of motion experience a lesser degree of dislocation than the fascicles of the far site more distant to the plane of motion.

There is a certain amount of movement and gliding within the fascicle. It is well known that nerve fibers show an undulated course. This was originally described by Fontana[2] and rediscovered by Clarke and Bearn[1] and Sunderland.[17] By decreasing or increasing the undulated course, the nerve fibers can adapt to elongation and slacking down. The possibility for this movement is provided by the delicate structure of the endoneurial framework. Unfortunately, we do not know very much about this important relationship between an intact endoneurial framework and functional properties. We do know, however, that elongation of a fascicle causes a reduction of its diameter, which is most pronounced in the middle of the elongated segment (transverse contraction). Our studies with the thoracodorsal and the musculocutaneous nerves showed a clear relationship between the load in longitudinal and the strain in transverse direction. With increasing elongation the volume of the fascicle decreases.[10,11] Because these properties are located within the fascicle they are not a subject of this study.

TERMINOLOGY

The gliding tissue around a nerve trunk fills the space between the nerve trunk and the surrounding tissue. Such a layer of loose connective tissue on top of the epineurium was already described by Schaffer.[13] Thomas[18] described this tissue as part of the epineurium. Lang[4] provided an extensive description of this tissue and called it *conjunctiva nervorum.* Van Beek and Kleinert[19] used the term *adventitia* in analogy to the adventitia of vessels. The fact that the adventitia of the vessels merges with the gliding tissue of a peripheral nerve to form a common layer if there is a neurovascular bundle favors the use of this term.

Krstic[3] used the term *paraneurium* in analogy to the term *paratendineum.* Until a decision is made to determine which term is the proper one, I shall use *paraneurium.* This seems to be justified because of the morphologic similarity to the paratendineum and because the term *paraneurium* can be easier adopted to the terminology of surgical techniques, like paraneuriectomy. It would be more difficult to use the term *adventitiectomy.*

The gliding tissue between the fascicles is usually referred to as epineurium, because of the concept that fascicles are buried in epineurial tissue. To be able to distinguish it from the outer or epifascicular epineurium, the term *interfascicular epineurium* is used.

The gliding tissue of a peripheral nerve trunk consists of alternating layers of capillaries and loose connective tissue.[4] If a nerve is mobilized, this happens exactly in this layer. If a nerve is excised to be used as a nerve graft, one part of the paraneurium remains on top of the nerve of another part within the donor site.

The interfascicular epineurium consists of loose connective tissue and contains a different amount of fat lobules. It also carries the blood and lymph vessels. Needless to say, a monofascicular nerve segment does not contain any interfascicular tissue. A nerve trunk with only two or three major fascicles as well contains only a very limited amount of interfascicular epineurium. With an increasing number of fascicles, the percentage of so-called nonfascicular tissue increases against the fascicular tissue. The percentage of nonfascicular tissue within the nerves of the upper extremity lies at the level between 30% and 56%.[14,15,16] In the lower extremity, the percentage of nonfascicular tissue in the tibial part of the sciatic nerve lies between 18% and 42%, and in the peroneal part between 21% and 52%. In the leg the percentage of nonfascicular tissue for the tibial nerve is between 17% and 48%, and for the peroneal nerve between 32% and 70%. In a polyfascicular nerve trunk, there are fascicles

with only a small amount of interfascicular tissue between them. These fascicles are forming a fascicle group; between the individual groups there are wider spaces of interfascicular epineurium.

The paraneurium is especially developed at locations where the nerve is forced to move more than usual (e.g., the median in the carpal canal). At this site the median nerve is surrounded by a sequence of layers of paraneurium; sometimes one has the impression that a space is in the process of being formed between these layers as a way of performing some type of nerve sheath.[12]

MECHANICAL REQUIREMENTS

Shaw Wilgis[20] drew attention to the fact that the median nerve has to be able to move considerably within the carpal tunnel during flexion and extension.

The following description of events during positive and negative elongation of peripheral nerves at different sites is based on the studies of Millesi and Zöch.[8,21,22] From cadaver studies of the median and ulnar nerve, we know that the median nerve has to become elongated by 4.5% of its resting length if the joints of the upper extremity are extended. This elongation goes along with a stress of 0.5 to 0.6 newton/mm^2. The stress-strain curve of a peripheral nerve in situ is significantly influenced by branches, and for measurements of the stress situation of the nerve tissue itself segments without branches are only considered. The stress-strain curve of such a segment in situ is steeper than after excision outside the body. The difference between these two curves represents the force which is necessary to overcome the friction of the paraneurium. If we do not consider the branches of a nerve, the distribution of forces is equal over the whole segment. If, however, the gliding capacity of a nerve is locally reduced by fibrosis of the paraneurium, an equal tension distribution is impossible, and according to the site of the adhesions, the necessary elongation will be higher proximally or distally to this site. Therefore, the necessary elongation becomes for one of the two segments much higher than normal and may reach a level at which the nerve tissue reacts with fibrosis. The consequence of this situation may be called *traction fibrosis* in contrast to *compression fibrosis.* This distinction is, however, difficult to execute because it is always a combination of both. In no way is it a neuritis.

During elongation of the nerve trunk the fascicles within a nerve trunk become elongated as well and change from a relaxed state to a more stretched one. The possibility for this motion is provided by the interfascicular epineurium.

At certain levels, close to a joint, peripheral nerves are exposed to a higher amount of motion. This is especially true for the ulnar nerve in the sulcus nervi ulnaris and for the median nerve in the carpal tunnel. The fact that these two sites are frequently the localization of nerve entrapment provokes the consideration that in entrapment sites not only compression but also lack of mobility play an important role. From the studies of Millesi[8] we know very well that the median nerve moves relative to anatomic landmarks if the wrist joint is flexed or extended. These motions are dependent on the fact that the median nerve and the retinaculum flexorum are located at the flexor side of the plane of motion of the wrist joint. The relative amount of motion is dependent on the distance to this plane of motion. The relative motion is different if the distance is different. For the functional outcome, it is irrelevant whether we talk of a relative motion of the retinaculum flexorum to the median nerve or vice versa. With wrist flexion the median nerve enters the carpal tunnel from proximal distal direction, and with the wrist in dorsiflexion the median nerve moves outside of the carpal tunnel in proximal direction. Independent of this motion of the wrist joint, the median nerve is drawn by approximately 9 mm into the carpal tunnel if the fingers are extended.

As long as the paraneurium of the median nerve provides the possibility of motion, everything will be all right. What happens, however, if because of increased pressure in the carpal tunnel or for any other reason, the median nerve can not follow this movement? The answer is that in this case an increased relative motion of the fascicles inside the nerve will compensate to allow proper adaptation to the movements of the wrist joint and the fingers. In other words, if the nerve trunk of the median nerve is fixed in the carpal tunnel with the surrounding structures, the fascicles will move within the nerve trunk in a direction toward the palm if the fingers are extended. There will be no problem as long as this mechanism of compensation works well.

What will happen if the gliding capacity within the nerve deteriorates? In this case also, the fascicles cannot move; to adapt to finger extension the fascicles will be elongated. They will become thinner, and consequently, the pressure within the fascicles will rise with all the consequences to the nerve fibers.

There is another possibility of disturbance of this delicate system. If the fascicles are drawn into the palm by finger and wrist extension and the pressure in the carpal canal increases, they cannot return. The segment distal to the palmar exit of the carpal canal is now too long and will adapt a snakelike or meander-like deformity. At the same time, the segment within the carpal canal will become elongated and thinner. Such morphologic pictures can be seen in a relatively high percentage of cases of advanced carpal tunnel syndrome, if the epifascicular epineurium is split.

The nocturnal pain of patients with carpal tunnel syndrome is well known. Patients awake during the night with pain and paresthesia; the patients describe that they move the hand, massage the hand, keep the hand down, and try different motions to get relief from pain. After some time, relief occurs and patients return to sleep. So far nobody has

provided a proper explanation for this phenomenon. A consideration of a temporary entrapment of fascicles that have moved into the palm and cannot easily return may offer an explanation.

If we now consider what happens with flexion in a peripheral nerve, we have to accept the fact that with flexion of all joints the median nerve's bed becomes shorter than the resting length of the median nerve by 15%. The median nerve can adapt to this state by slacking down; this means that all the structures within the median nerve become more undulated like a harmonica. This also relates to the nerve fibers within the fascicles. Because the volume does not change without overstretching, the slacked down shorter nerve trunk needs more space. This space can be provided only by the loose connective tissue around the nerve trunk, the paraneurium and the loose connective tissue within the nerve, and the interfascicular epineurium that apparently can be displaced easily without much friction.

PATHOLOGY OF THE GLIDING TISSUE

A comprehensive pathology of the gliding tissue has yet to be written. There are good reasons to believe that some of the malformations and benign tumors of the peripheral nerves (like lipomatosis or synovial cysts) are expressions of the degeneration of the gliding tissue.

Fibrosis of the gliding tissue

The most frequent reaction of the gliding tissue caused by trauma or chronic irritation is *fibrosis,* which means collagenization and loss of elasticity and mobility—the gliding tissue loses its function. The consequences are unequal distribution of forces, which may induce further fibrosis. Fascicles that cannot move have to become elongated; they get thinner, and the volume inside the fascicles decreases with all consequences on the nerve fiber. By shrinkage the fibrotic tissue itself induces compression of the fascicles with their content. Fibrosis of the interfascicular tissue may fix the temporary meander-like deformity (as described previously). Fixation of fascicles in meander-like deformity decreases the volume inside the fascicle and, consequently, increases the pressure inside the fascicle when longitudinal forces are applied. Fortunately, in the majority of cases, the gliding tissue has a satisfactory capacity for regeneration. The success or failure of neurolysis procedures is determined by this ability.

Recurrent fibrosis of the gliding tissue

Recurrent fibrosis of the gliding tissue is the background of rare but very unpleasant conditions. Some of these patients will be discussed with case reports 1, 2, and 3. The main reason for the development of such a syndrome is the lack of regenerative capacity of the gliding tissue. This may be supported by the fact that the problem underlying the original fibrosis has not been solved properly. Another important contributing factor may be related to the one wound–one scar theory.

Tarsal tunnel syndrome may serve as an example. The plantar nerves and vessels are protected by the retinaculum tendinum flexorum at the tarsal tunnel. It is well known[10,11] that the skin over the tarsal tunnel has to move considerably to adapt to dorsi and plantar flexion. If the skin has been incised and a scar develops, this ability is reduced and the skin comes under higher tension. However, the intact retinaculum flexorum protects the neurovascular structures, and no forces are transmitted to the medial and lateral plantar nerve.

If the retinaculum was transected at the location of a tarsal tunnel syndrome, this protection has been lost and one scar will form from the skin to the tarsal tunnel. If this scar tissue becomes fibrotic, any tension of the skin or the scar in the skin, respectively, will be transmitted to the nerves in the tarsal tunnel. Fortunately the usual scar is soft, and in the majority of cases, there are no problems of this kind after tarsal tunnel operations. If, however, a recurrent fibrosis develops in the tarsal tunnel, the problems for a patient are so severe that reconsideration of the surgical approach to tarsal tunnel syndrome is justified.

The two ways to avoid such a development are as follows:

1. The incision for exploration of the tarsal tunnel should not overlie the tarsal canal. It should be on the ventral side of the malleolus internus, going down to the medial aspect of the dorsum of the foot; a wide skin flap should be raised to access the tarsal tunnel. This incision separates the skin scar from the region of the tarsal tunnel.

2. As outlined previously, dorsi and plantar flexion in the ankle joint provokes distortion of the skin, and because of the formation of scar tissue, the total circumference of the integumentum may become too tight (a situation which might be called *integumental stenosis*). The development of such an integumental stenosis can be prevented by avoiding a direct skin closure and using a split-thickness skin graft to close the incision and to achieve an enlargement of the integumentum. If this is considered in advance, it is even more important to have the skin defect at some distance to the tarsal tunnel.

A great deal of the beneficial effect of endoscopic carpal tunnel release may be because a scar overlying the carpal tunnel is avoided. This consideration is confirmed by our experience of many years with a two-portal approach, using a small incision in the thenar fold and a small incision in the rascetta. From these two incisions, the whole median nerve can be treated under direct vision and the skin and subcutaneous tissue overlying the carpal canal remain intact.

The following are other possibilities to avoid recurrent fibrosis:

1. Transposing the nerve into the site where better regeneration of the gliding tissue can be expected.

2. Covering the whole area with a skin flap well-supplied with blood.

3. Transferring gliding tissue.

CLASSIFICATION

On the basis of what has been presented so far, pathologic changes of the gliding tissue can be classified in the following categories.

Fibrosis of gliding tissue

This response develops usually as a response to any mechanical irritation (e.g., compression or chronic or acute trauma). It may also be the result of an inflammation or a local ischemia. It may be divided in three categories.

Fibrosis of type A. Fibrosis of type A involves mainly the paraneurium. The paraneurium loses its properties as loose connective tissue and becomes fibrotic. The nerve trunk loses its gliding capacity. The demarcation between paraneurium and epifascicular epineurium disappears. The whole nerve is enveloped by layers of fibrotic tissue. If the cause of the fibrosis persists, the epifascicular epineurium gets increasingly involved and, finally, fibrotic paraneurium and fibrotic epifascicular epineurium cannot be distinguished. If the fibrotic layer shrinks, the pressure within the nerve trunk increases and the fascicular tissue becomes compressed (like the contents of a too-tight stocking).

Fibrosis of type B. Fibrosis of type B involves the interfascicular tissue. The fascicles lose their ability to move against each other, an eventual meander-like deformity becomes fixed, and elongation of the nerve leads to increased compression of the fascicular tissue. Shrinkage of the fibrotic tissue contributes to the compression of the fascicles.

Fibrosis of type C. If the endoneurial framework becomes fibrotic because of chronic irritation of long-standing denervation, the properties of this delicate tissue are lost and reneurotization after decompression is unlikely to occur to a major extent. Fibrosis of type C is irreversible. The treatment is excision and restoration of continuity by nerve grafting. This condition is mentioned only to provide a complete description. It does not belong to the pathology of the gliding tissue and, therefore, is not further discussed.

Recurrent fibrosis

Under recurrent fibrosis we understand the appearance of a new fibrosis in an area that has been operated on because of deficiency of gliding tissue caused by a well-defined reason, even after this reason has been successfully removed. It usually develops after a delay of 6 months or several years. The important point in the definition is that the original reason has been successfully controlled. For instance, if a patient with thoracic outlet syndrome and a compression of the brachial plexus at the site of the scalenus muscles has been surgically treated but a new narrowing develops (maybe because of insufficient scalenotomy) and symptoms reappear, we have to deal with a recurrent thoracic outlet syndrome and not with a recurrent fibrosis. We can talk about a recurrent fibrosis if the reasons to develop a thoracic outlet syndrome have been successfully removed, but new and more severe symptoms reappear because of a fibrosis of the whole surgical field without a well-defined site of compression or irritation. The reason for a recurrent fibrosis must be suspected in the lacking regenerative ability of the patient, as far as the gliding tissue is concerned. This may be caused by local reasons (e.g., development of scar tissue in the operative field or general reasons in the patient's constitution). One is reminded of the occurrence of a keloid, which is also determined by not very well understood local and general factors.

TREATMENT

As far as the treatment is concerned, we have to differentiate between fibrosis and recurrent fibrosis. In addition, we have to consider prophylactic aspects.

Treatment of fibrosis of the gliding tissues

Surgical treatment consists basically of lysis procedures and is based on the reparative capacity of the gliding tissue. Therefore, some gliding tissue must be still available. This fortunately is usually the case. All the different types of neurolysis procedures belong to this treatment.

Obliteration. Obliteration occurs when the space between the nerve trunk and the surrounding tissue disappears because of partial fibrosis of the paraneurium. The treatment is external neurolysis. The adhesions at the site of obliteration of the paraneurium space are lysed, and the nerve trunk is mobilized from its bed. As long as the epineurium remains intact, we call this *external neurolysis*. Early mobilization of a peripheral nerve from its intact bed with intact paraneurium is not a neurolysis. A neurolysis can be performed only if part of the paraneurium is fibrotic.

Fibrosis of type A. If the paraneurium and the adjacent layers of the epineurium have become fibrotic, a *paraneuriectomy* is indicated to solve the problem of constriction of the nerve by the shrinking layers of fibrotic tissue around the nerve trunk. As long as significant parts of the external epineurial epineurial layers (epifascicular epineurium) remain intact, an external neurolysis is still done. If all the layers of the epifascicular epineurium are involved, they have to be transected as well and an *epifascicular* epineuriotomy is done. Having completed the epineuriotomy at this site, the physician exposes the fascicles. This is the first step of an internal neurolysis. Paraneuriotomy and epifascicular epineuriotomy may be performed at different locations around the circumference of a nerve to achieve complete decompression.

Fibrosis of type B. A fibrosis of type B involves the interfascicular epineurium to a lesser or greater extent. If it is on a very limited extension and the epifascicular epineuriotomy has been performed just on top of the fibrotic sector, an epifascicular epineuriotomy may be a sufficient treatment. If it is more extended in the superficial layers of the nerve trunk, the total circumference of the nerve trunk should be liberated, and in this case, an *epifascicular epineuriectomy* has to be performed. In the vast majority of cases, complete decompression of the fascicles can be achieved and no further surgery is necessary. There is enough normal interfascicular epineurium spared to serve as the origin of the regeneration of gliding tissue.

If the fibrosis is more extensive and involves larger areas between the fascicles in a polyfascicular nerve, these fibrotic elements also have to be removed to achieve decompression of the fascicular tissues. This would then be an *interfascicular epineuriectomy*. Based on my experience, this internal fibrosis never involves the total amount of interfascicular epineurium; therefore, the interfascicular epineuriectomy is always performed as a partial epineuriectomy and never as a total one. Enough interfascicular epineurium remains to serve as the origin of regeneration of gliding tissue and to provide the longitudinal blood supply. The argument that after an internal neurolysis the blood supply of the fascicular tissue is endangered is, therefore, not a valid one. The fibrotic parts do not contain vessels to a greater extent and are, therefore, insignificant to the blood supply of the nerve trunk. Removing all the interfascicular tissue and leaving the fascicles completely isolated is never performed. Only in this case might the blood supply of the fascicles be a problem. This was recommended in the past, and this may be the reason for the bad reputation internal neurolysis still has. I would confirm the bad reputation if only these very extensive procedures are summarized under the term *internal neurolysis*. If one defines internal neurolysis as any procedure within the nerve that transects the epifascicular epineurium and if one avoids these very extensive procedures, internal neurolysis has a firm place in our treatment.[6,7,9] If one is forced to do a complete isolation of all the fascicles of a peripheral nerve, which I cannot remember ever to have been indicated, I would recommend enveloping the remaining fascicles in gliding tissue provided from another area, described in the case reports.

Treatment of recurrent fibrosis (Case reports 1, 2, and 3)

In case of recurrent fibrosis a new, favorable environment for the nerve has to be created. This can be done by transposition of the nerve into an area with good gliding capacity. Learmonth's[5] procedure of transferring the ulnar nerve into the bed of the median nerve in case of irritation of the ulnar nerve in the cubital tunnel provides a new environment. In other cases gliding tissue has to be transferred in the form of a pedicled or a free-flap transfer. Sources of tissue are as follows:

Text continued on p. 120.

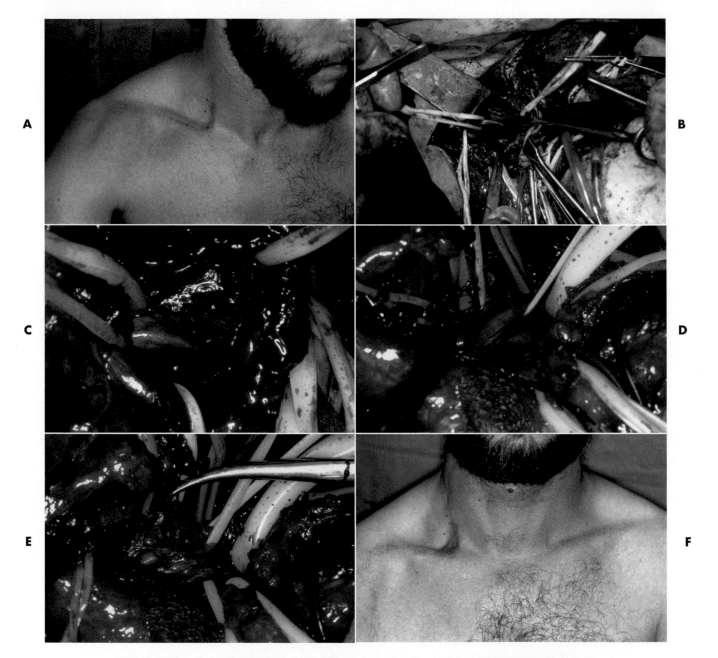

Fig. 14-1. Case 1. In 1979 surgery was performed on this 45-year-old patient because of thoracic outlet syndrome, and the original symptoms disappeared. About 1 year after the operation, the patient developed a pain syndrome involving the whole brachial plexus with functional impairment. In 1981 the patient had an operation, and an intensive neurolysis was performed (**A, B,** and **C**). After surgery the patient was free of pain. About 2 years thereafter, a new pain syndrome with similar symptoms developed. These symptoms were not associated with the original thoracic outlet syndrome. In 1983 the patient was operated on again; again neurolysis was performed with good immediate results. The patient was free of pain for more than 1 year. **D** and **E,** In 1985 the patient developed a similar pain syndrome. He presented himself for surgery but surgery was refused because he was already operated on twice without success. **F,** In 1987 the patient presented himself again for severe, unbearable pain, and with the experience of the case presented in Fig. 14-2, it was decided to perform another neurolysis with envelopment of the brachial plexus in gliding tissue.

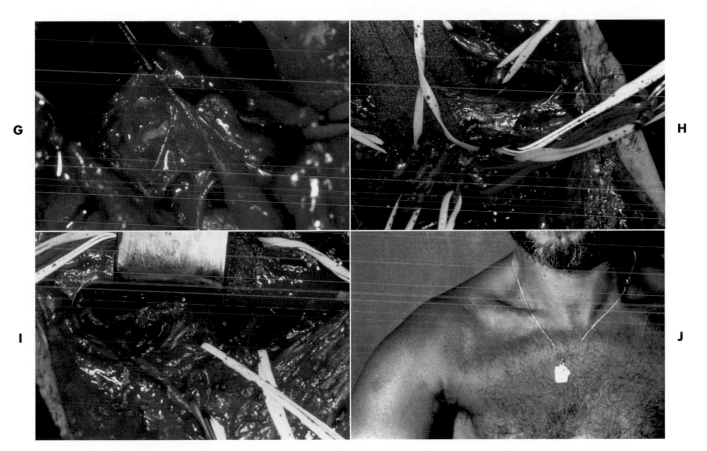

Fig. 14-1, cont'd.   An extensive neurolysis procedure was performed (**F, G, H,** and **I**), and a subpectoral gliding tissue flap was prepared and transposed to envelop the brachial plexus. Since then the patient has been free of pain. A follow-up study in 1994 shows some atrophy of the major pectoralis muscle, which functions still very well (**J**). The patient remained free of pain; the function of the right upper extremity is normal.

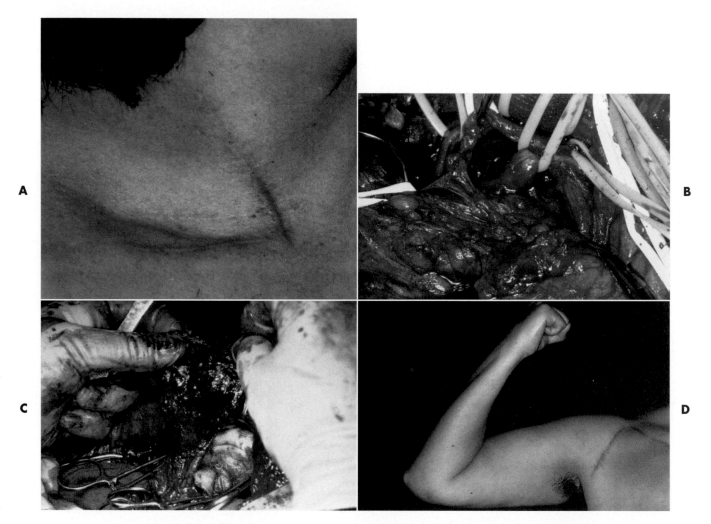

Fig. 14-2. Case 2. Surgery was performed because of thoracic outlet syndrome and recurrent pain syndrome elsewhere before 1986 (**A**). Extensive neurolysis was performed in 1986. To have a better outcome, a subpectoral gliding tissue flap was elevated for the first time (**C**) and transposed to envelop the brachial plexus. The patient recovered full function within 1 year (**A, B, C,** and **D**). The patient has been free of pain since. (With the experience of this case, the patient presented in Case 1 was successfully operated on again in 1987.)

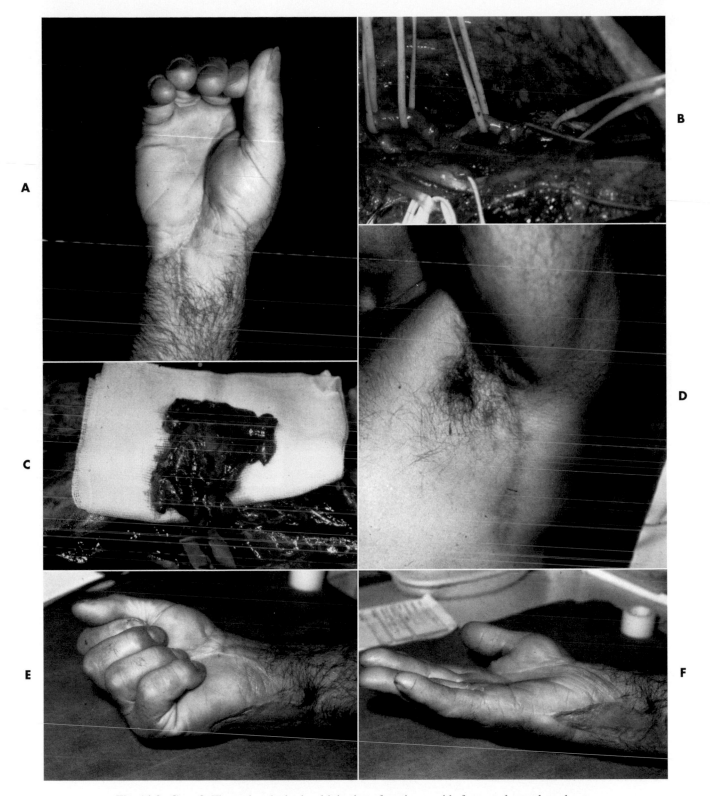

Fig. 14-3. Case 3. The patient had a local injection of corticosteroids for carpal tunnel syndrome. He developed a local infection that had to be treated surgically. As a result, severe fibrosis developed with a pain syndrome in the area of the median nerve and impairment of tendon function (**A**). The patient already had surgery three times for this pain syndrome. An external neurolysis was performed. **B** shows the median nerve during the neurolysis procedure. It was evident that if this fourth neurolysis procedure would have been performed in a classical way, a pain syndrome would have developed. Therefore, a gliding tissue flap was raised, based on the arteria thoracodorsalis and transferred by microvascular surgery to the forearm. **C** shows the donor site. The gliding tissue was used to envelop the median nerve and the flexor tendons. **E** and **F** demonstrate the result. The gliding tissue flap was inserted, using a lateral incision. The wound was covered by a split-thickness skin graft to achieve an enlargement of the integumentum.

- The gliding tissue underneath the scapula, which is supplied by the thoracodorsal vessels
- The gliding tissue underneath the pectoralis muscles, supplied by the pectoralis branch of the thoracoacromial artery
- The gliding tissue on the dorsum of the foot, supplied by the dorsalis pedis artery (more details about this artery are given in the case reports)

Prophylactic measures

It has already been mentioned that the incisions should be made in such a way so as to reduce a possible irritation of the treated nerve by the scar in the skin and to enlarge the integumentum at particular sites to avoid an integumental stenosis.

REFERENCES

1. Clarke E, Bearn JG: The spinal bands of Fontana, *Brain* 1972; 95:1.
2. Fontana F: *Traité sur le venin de la vipère et sur les poissons américains,* Firenze, 1781.
3. Krstic R: *Die Gewebe des Menschen und der Säugetiere,* Berlin-Heidelberg, 1978, Springer Verlag.
4. Lang J: Über das Bindegewebe und die Gefäße der Nerven, *Anat Embryol* 1962; 123:61-79.
5. Learmonth JR: A technique for transplanting the ulnar nerve, *Surg Gynecol Obstet* 1942; 75:792.
6. Millesi H: Eingriffe an peripheren Nerven. In Gschnitzer F, Kern E, Schweiberer L, eds: *Chirurgische Operationslehre, part* 1. Munich-Vienna-Baltimore, 1984, Urban & Schwarzenberg.
7. Millesi H: *Microsurgery of peripheral nerves: neurolysis, nerve grafts, brachial plexus injuries,* Symposium on Frontiers in Reconstructive Microsurgery, Buncke HJ, Furnas DW, eds: St Louis, 1984, Mosby.
8. Millesi H, Zöch G, Rath T: The gliding apparatus of peripheral nerve and its clinical significance, *Annales de Chirurgie de la Main et du Membre Supérieur* 1990; 9:87-97.
9. Millesi H, Rath T, Reihsner R, Zöch G: Microsurgical neurolysis, *Microsurgery* 1993; 14:430-439.
10. Millesi H, Zöch G, Reihsner R: Mechanical properties of peripheral nerves, *Clin Orthop Related Res* 1995; 314:76-83.
11. Millesi H, Eberhard D, Knabl J, Reishner R: *Integumental stenosis as a cause for pain syndrome,* Proc. 11th Congress of the International Confederation for Plastic, Reconstructive and Aesthetic Surgery, Yokohama, 1995.
12. Rath T, Millesi H: Das Gleitgewebe des N. medianus im Karpalkanal, *Handchir Mikrochir Plast Chir* 1989; 22:203-205.
13. Schaffer J: Das Bindegewebe der Nerven. In: *Lecture: Über die Histologie und Histogenese,* Berlin-Vienna, 1920, Urban & Schwarzenberg.
14. Sunderland S: The intraneural topography of the radial, median and ulnar nerve, *Brain* 1945; 68:243.
15. Sunderland S, Marshall RD, Swaney WE: The intraneural topography of the circumflex, musculocutaneous and obturatory nerve, *Brain* 1959; 82: 116.
16. Sunderland S, Ray JL: The intraneural topography of the sciatic nerve and its popliteal divisions in man, *Brain* 1948; 71:242.
17. Sunderland S: The connective tissues of peripheral nerves, *Brain* 1965; 88:841.
18. Thomas PK: The connective tissue of peripheral nerve: an electron microscopy study, *J Anat* 1963; 97:35.
19. Van Beek A, Kleinhert HR: Practical neurorrhaphy, *Orthop Clin North Am* 1977; 8:377-386.
20. Wilgis S: Paper given at the Symposium on Nerve Surgery, Montreal, 1984.
21. Zöch G, Reishner R, Beer R, Millesi H: Stress and strain in peripheral nerves, *Neuro-Orthopaedics* 1991; 10:371-382.
22. Zöch, G: Über die Anpassung der peripheren Nerven an die Bewegungen der Extremitäten durch Gleiten und Dehnung: Untersuchungen am Nervus medianus, *Acta Chir Austriaca* 1992; 96(suppl):1-16.

Chapter 15

CLINICAL ASPECTS OF NERVE GLIDING IN THE UPPER EXTREMITY

E.F. Shaw Wilgis

During limb motion, the peripheral nerve accommodates changes in the length of its bed. The longitudinal excursion of the nerve during motion has been studied recently in several ways. McLellan and Swash[3,4] recorded action potentials in the median nerve before and during active and passive motion of the limb. They found that active and passive motion had equal effects. Greatest excursions were produced by extension of the wrist and fingers and by flexion of the elbow. Extension of the wrist and fingers caused 7.4 mm of excursion, and flexion of the elbow caused 4.3 mm. The authors estimated that hyperextension of the wrist caused the median nerve to glide 10 to 15 mm. They also found that displacement of the median nerve during flexion of the wrist and fingers was two to four times greater at the wrist than in the upper arm. Dellon and co-workers[1] postulated that the radial sensory nerve had a significant excursion on radial and ulnar deviation of the wrist.

Wilgis and Murphy[8] using 15 fresh, intact adult cadaveric arms dissected the entire peripheral nervous system, focusing on longitudinal nerve excursion. They noted that the brachial plexus had an average excursion of 15 mm when moved from the frontal plane with the arm in full abduction to full adduction. The median and ulnar nerves at the elbow moved an average of 7.3 and 9.8 mm, respectively, with full motion. The greatest excursion of peripheral nerves occurred at the wrist proximal to the carpal tunnel. Here the median and ulnar nerves had 15.5 and 14.8 mm of longitudinal sliding, respectively, with the wrist ranged through a full arc of flexion and extension in the sagittal plane.

These studies are consistent with McLellan and Swash.[3,4] In the palm and digits, the excursion was considerably less.

Szabo et al.[6] in 1994, using fresh cadavers, studied the direct relationship between wrist position and displacement of the median nerve during active contraction of the flexor tendons of the wrist. The longitudinal gliding was similar to the previous findings of Wilgis and Murphy[8] and McLellan and Swash.[3,4] They also identified a displacement in an anterior-posterior direction, which was not materially affected by division of the transverse carpal ligament.

All of these studies indicate that in and around joints the nerves must have significant excursion or longitudinal gliding to accommodate joint motion.

The microcirculation of the nerves remains undisturbed during this motion because nerves are segmentally supplied by slender mobile vessels arranged in the tissue about the nerve that has been called paraneurium. Millesi[9] also describes gliding layers deeper within the nerve trunk allowing the fascicular bundles to slide in the deeper layers of the epineurium. From the microvascular point of view, each separate fascicle represents a vascular unit with its own well-defined microvascular endoneurial and perineurial vascular system. These fascicular vascular units are segmentally nourished by mobile vessels in the deep layers of the epineurium, a fact which might allow some degree of motion and longitudinal sliding of the fascicles (Fig. 15-1).

When treating the various conditions affecting nerves in the upper extremities, including compression, transection,

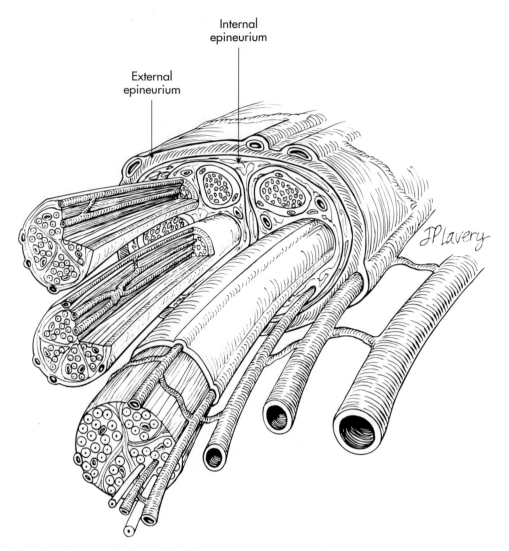

Internal
epineurium

External
epineurium

JPLavery

Fig. 15-1. Nerve showing relationship between gliding surfaces and microcirculation.

and scarring, the concept of nerve excursion must be considered.

COMPRESSION

The pathophysiologic events in chronic nerve irritation and nerve compression can be explained somewhat by the concept of peripheral nerve excursion. In the early stage of compression lesions, there is venous congestion in the nerve, which increases vascular permeability in the epineurial vessels and epineurial edema occurs. The edema then transforms into a constricting scar in the epineurium and to an adherent scar of the epineurium to the surrounding tissue.[5] This, then, limits the excursion of the nerve and increases the symptoms. When a nerve is adherent, joint motion then produces a mini-traction lesion and further internal compression occurs; thereby setting up a cycle of compression and subsequent irritation that produces adhesions and scarring, which then in and of itself produces further compression internally within the nerve.

After decompressing a compressive lesion, it is important to maintain the longitudinal excursion of the nerve in the postoperative period by therapeutic techniques described elsewhere in this chapter (see p. 123).

TRANSECTED NERVE

In facing the repair of a transected nerve, the surgeon must consider not only the internal elastic tension of the nerve, but also the necessity for longitudinal excursion during limb motion. For example, the normal retraction of the median nerve at the level of the wrist is 1.5 cm after a clean division. If one then adds the 1.5 cm of longitudinal excursion needed when taking the wrist from full flexion to full extension, the immediate demands for appropriate length of the nerve become apparent (Fig. 15-2).

In the acute situation when the nerve can be brought together and approximated under normal tension, one would expect the normal amount of longitudinal excursion to occur once the local scarring factors have subsided.

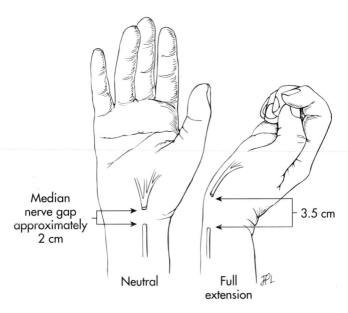

Fig. 15-2. Measurement of gap in cut nerve including excursion factor.

However, in the secondary situation, the conditions are quite different. The nerve has lost its normal elasticity because of injury and subsequent scarring. It therefore cannot be approximated under normal tension and maintain normal excursion without acute flexion of an adjacent joint. In other words, the length of the nerve substance has been shortened because of the injury. Because of this overall shortening, excursion cannot take place. If the nerve is sutured under tension with the wrist in acute flexion, there is no way the nerve can slide to its appropriate and normal distance when the adjacent joint is taken into the opposite mode of action from the position in which it was placed for the acute repair. The already existing gap between the two ends is effectively *increased* because of the excursion factor. For example, if one approaches a secondary repair of the median nerve at the wrist and the existing gap after transection of the neuroma is 2 cm, one must also consider that there is an additional 1.5 cm that must be present to accommodate the nerve's need for longitudinal excursion. This, then, makes a realistic gap of 3.5 cm, which may cause the surgeon to choose an alternative method of bridging the gap such as nerve grafting (see Fig. 15-2).

At the elbow, the excursion need can be met by transposing the ulnar nerve anteriorly, thereby reducing its need for longitudinal excursion and bridging the gap.

NERVE SCARRING

A third, and probably the most prevalent clinical problem, is nerve scarring after surgery. When a nerve is scarred to its adjacent bed and loses its excursion, a series of events is put into motion, which can produce severe symptoms of pain and nerve dysfunction. The scarred nerve tethered to its bed then suffers a chronic irritation because of distal limb motion. The distal limb motion causes the nerve to constrict at its tethered point, thereby setting up a chronic compressive lesion within the nerve and all of the inflammatory changes following that condition. When considering treatment options, one must not only free the nerve from its scarred bed, but also must provide an environmental change in the bed so that scarring will not immediately ensue during the healing phase after the operation. Neurolysis without environmental change is a worthless procedure.

There are many ways to change the environment of the neurolysed nerve. Interposing membranes such as silicone can be placed between the nerve and its bed in hopes of creating a new gliding surface. These materials must be removed at a later date and sometimes can migrate within the extremity during the postoperative period.

The nerve can be wrapped with autogenous tissues such as vein with the endothelial surface supplying the membrane between the nerve and the surrounding tissue (Fig. 15-3). The vein can be either split longitudinally and placed around the nerve or split and wrapped around the nerve in a spiral fashion.

Muscle tissue can be placed between the nerve and its surrounding structures, which may be the best solution. Local muscle flaps are particularly useful because they bring additional blood supply to the area around the nerve in addition to supplying a new environmental bed. In the distal forearm, the pronator quadratus muscle can be used as a muscle flap to cover the median nerve or the ulnar nerve; the palmaris brevis has been used in the carpal canal; the abductor digiti minimi has been used as a muscle flap to cover the median or ulnar nerve at the wrist; and one or more of the lumbrical muscles have

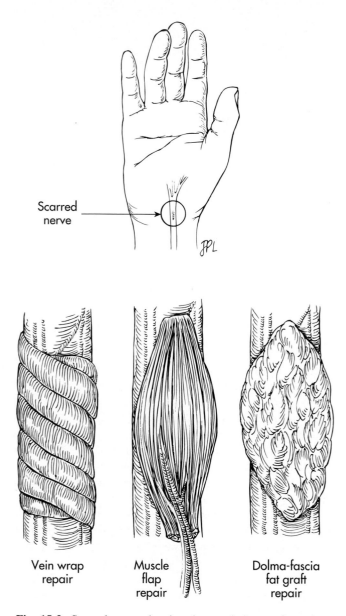

Fig. 15-3. Scarred nerve showing three techniques of coverage.

been used as a muscle flap to cover digital nerves in the palm. All of these are useful muscle flaps. In the brachial plexus region, the pectoral and latissimus dorsi muscles have been used to supply gliding surfaces for the brachial plexus.

At the elbow, the brachioradialis or a turned-over flexor carpi ulnaris muscle flap have been useful to cover the ulnar nerve.

Another tissue that has been used in our hands is a dermal fascial fat graft. This tissue has been used around nerves either as free fat grafts or vascularized fat grafts in the past.

One critique has been that the fat atrophies and disappears. Adding the dermis to the fat lessens this possibility.

We have had excellent results using this technique, particularly in and about the carpal canal.

A third technique which can be employed after neurolysis of a scarred nerve is to provide an environmental change by using a dermal fascial fat graft.[2] It may be taken and placed between the nerve and the skin. We have used this technique at the wrist level with median nerve scarring in over 100 patients with significant improvement in approximately 80% of those individuals.

A fourth method is to move a local muscle flap to surround a scarred nerve after neurolysis.[7] Local muscle flaps used include the pronator quadratus, the abductor digiti minimi, and the lumbrical muscles. Any one of these can be mobilized from its origin and insertion, kept on its vascular and nerve pedicle, and used to cover a scarred nerve in the wrist and hand.

CONCLUSION

Longitudinal excursion of the peripheral nerve is important and must be maintained when treating patients with compressed, transected, or scarred nerves.

The nerve *must* move. If a nerve is tethered by scar, symptoms will result. When considering surgery for a scarred nerve, neurolysis alone is not satisfactory, but an environmental change must be instituted to prevent further scarring of the nerve to its surrounding tissue. Nerve excursion must be considered when repairing the transected nerve so that when repaired, the nerve will again glide with joint motion.

REFERENCES

1. Dellon AL, Mackinnon SE, Pestronk A: Implantation of sensory nerve into muscle: preliminary clinical and experimental observations on neuroma formation, *Ann Plast Surg* 1984; 12:30.
2. McClinton MAM: The use of dermal-fat grafts, *Hand Clin* 1996; 12(2):357-364.
3. McLellan DL: Longitudinal sliding of the median nerve during hand movements, *Lancet* 1975; 1:633.
4. McLellan DL, Swash M: Longitudinal sliding of the median nerve during movements of the upper limb, *J Neurol Neurosurg Psychiatry* 1976; 39:566.
5. Ochoa J, Marotte L: The nature of the nerve lesion caused by chronic entrapment in the guinea pig, *J Neurol Sci* 1973; 19:491.
6. Szabo RM, et al: Median nerve displacement through the carpal canal, *J Hand Surg* 1994; 19A:901.
7. Wilgis EFSW: Local muscle flaps in the hand: anatomy as related to reconstructive surgery, *Bulletin of the Hospital for Joint Diseases Ortho Inst* 1984; 44(2):552-557.
8. Wilgis EFSW, Murphy R: The significance of longitudinal excursion in peripheral nerves, *Hand Clin* 1986; 2:761.
9. Millesi H, Terzis J: Nomenclature in peripheral nerve surgery, *Clin Plast Surg* 1984; 11:3-8.

Chapter 16

UPPER EXTREMITY NERVE GLIDING

Programs used at the Philadelphia Hand Center

Patricia M. Byron

All movement produces nerve gliding to some degree as the nerve accommodates to changes in the length of its bed produced by joint motion.[6-9] Mackinnon reports that the undulating course of the nerve fibers allows the nerve to make this accommodation.[5]

Wilgis and Murphy have provided information on the longitudinal excursion of peripheral nerves.[10] In their study of 15 cadaver arms, they stated that the brachial plexus had an average excursion of 15 mm when ranged in the frontal plane with the arm in full abduction. The median and ulnar nerves at the elbow moved an average of 7.3 and 9.8 mm, respectively, with full flexion and extension. The greatest excursion of peripheral nerves occurred at the wrist proximal to the carpal tunnel.[10]

Sunderland reported that a nerve may stretch 7% to 20% of its resting length without damage.[11]

Several factors may limit the ability of a nerve to glide as it was designed to do. These factors include anatomic anomalies, muscular imbalances, postural causes, and trauma.[2]

Nerve tension testing was developed to evaluate the ability of the nerve to glide and to help quantify limitations. In 1979 Elvey described the brachial plexus tension test also known as Elvey's test.[3] This test progressively takes up tension in the nervous system by sequential movements at the shoulder, elbow, forearm, and wrist. The test is done with the patient in the supine position to allow the individual the opportunity to relax, to improve trunk stabilization, and to improve the evaluator's control.

The possibility of tension tests for the major peripheral nerves was suggested by Kenneally et al.[4] Butler has described upper limb tension tests with median, ulnar, and radial biases.[1] "A positive test: reproduces the patient's symptoms, has responses altered by distant movement, and generally shows differences between right and left. . . ." The clearest indictment of the nervous system occurs when movement of a remote part alters the patient's symptoms."

Clearly these tests cannot be used in isolation. Complete and thorough multisystem clinical evaluations must be performed.

Because the nervous system never forgets an injury,[2] it is critical that the therapist be aware of all previous trauma, even minor ones that may be contributing to the current problem.

After injury, one goal of the therapy program must be to alter the formation of motion limiting adhesions between the nerve and the surrounding tissue. Hand therapists have attempted to prevent the development of motion-limiting adhesions in the tendon system by introducing the tendon gliding program with controlled motion soon after tendon

Special thanks to Matt Brownstein, Medical Media, Thomas Jefferson University for the illustrations included in this chapter and to Anne Simmons, original illustrator of the radial nerve gliding sequence.

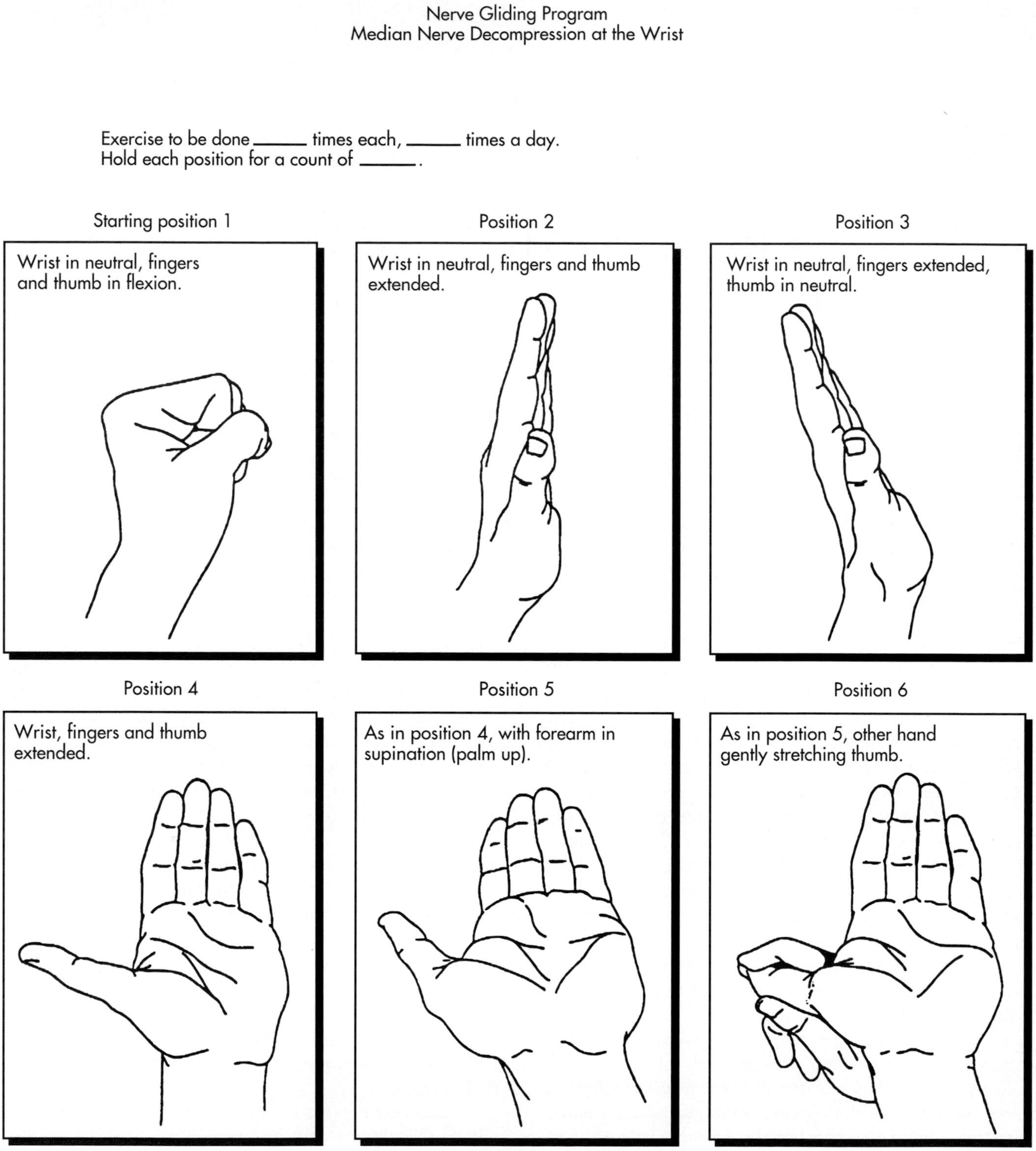

Nerve Gliding Program
Median Nerve Decompression at the Wrist

Exercise to be done _____ times each, _____ times a day.
Hold each position for a count of _____ .

Starting position 1
Wrist in neutral, fingers and thumb in flexion.

Position 2
Wrist in neutral, fingers and thumb extended.

Position 3
Wrist in neutral, fingers extended, thumb in neutral.

Position 4
Wrist, fingers and thumb extended.

Position 5
As in position 4, with forearm in supination (palm up).

Position 6
As in position 5, other hand gently stretching thumb.

Fig. 16-1. The median nerve gliding program: position 1, wrist in neutral, fingers and thumb in flexion; position 2, wrist neutral, thumb neutral, fingers extended; position 3, wrist and fingers extended, thumb neutral; position 4, wrist, fingers, and thumb neutral; position 5, forearm in supination; and, position 6, the opposite hand applies a gentle stretch to the thumb. (Redrawn with permission from Totten PA, Hunter JM: Therapeutic techniques to enhance nerve gliding in the thoracic outlet and carpal tunnel syndromes, *Hand Clin* 7[3]:505, Philadelphia, 1991, Saunders.)

repair. We attempt to prevent the development of joint stiffness through active and passive range-of-motion exercises. At the Philadelphia Hand Center, Totten and Hunter[12] proposed a series of exercises to enhance the gliding of the median nerve at the carpal tunnel and for the brachial plexus. Ulnar nerve gliding programs have been developed for patients being treated conservatively and those postanterior submuscular ulnar nerve transposition. The postoperative glide encourages movement of the nerve along its transposed route. The radial nerve gliding program was adapted from a program used at Blodgett Memorial Medical Center in Grand Rapids, Michigan. The remainder of this chapter focuses on a description of nerve gliding programs in use at the Philadelphia Hand Center. Again, these nerve gliding programs are part of a comprehensive therapy program that includes all affected tissue. It also must be emphasized that nerve gliding is an extremely powerful treatment technique that can easily produce increased symptoms and irritability if not used very carefully and with a good understanding of treatment goals.[1] The patient should not experience increased symptoms that last for an extended period.

The median nerve gliding program (Fig. 16-1) can be performed with the patient either supine or sitting, depending on the patient's ability to relax proximal musculature. The head is in midline, shoulder adducted, and the elbow in 90° of flexion. Should this starting position be altered, it must be noted so that attempts to quantify a patient's progress through the gliding program are not affected by use of different starting positions. Proximal positioning may affect distal gliding (Fig. 16-2). In position 1, the distal median nerve is in the relaxed position. In position 2, tension in the distal segment of the nerve, the digits, is increased. Wilgis and Murphy[10] report that this is the area of least excursion. In position 3, the area of greatest excursion is accessed as the wrist extends. The median nerve branch to the thumb is included in the exercise sequence at position 4. In position 5, forearm supination adds tension to the more proximal portion of the median nerve in the forearm. The addition of a gentle passive stretch is provided in position 6.

Tendon gliding is another essential part of the postoperative exercise program for the median nerve decompression patient. The flexor tendons course through the carpal tunnel and may add to postoperative restriction if they are not encouraged to glide in the carpal tunnel.

The brachial plexus gliding program (Fig. 16-3) attempts to achieve gliding for the plexus from proximal to distal. This program is used for both the postoperative brachial plexus decompression patient and for the individual being treated on the conservative program. Again, it is important to emphasize that the performance of this program should not produce tingling, numbness, or pain that requires more than several hours to resolve. The patient is attempting to move to the point of tension only. Generally, this is the point right before a slight pull or stretch or the onset of mild

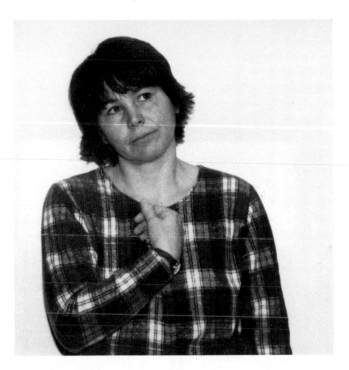

Fig. 16-2. When proximal limitation or tension reduces the ability of the nerve to glide distally, placing the nerve on slack proximally may allow for improved gliding and minimize discomfort.

alteration in sensibility is experienced. Therefore, the patient progresses in the exercise to the point where either a slight pulling or stretch or the first hint of altered sensibility is experienced and then backs off slightly from that point. Patients are instructed to move slowly and to be very conscious of changes in the involved extremity. Because this exercise sequence deals with the entire length of the nerves, it is more likely to produce an irritable response and must be initiated very slowly. The patient who presents with a very painful extremity may require a period of rest before initiating the gliding program (Fig. 16-4). It may be necessary to begin with only the proximal component of lateral cervical flexion performed toward and away from the affected side before progressing to the more distal components (Fig. 16-5). Many patients with brachial plexus problems will not experience increased symptoms during exercise performance, but rather several hours later. That this may occur can be deduced from the patient's report of their response to activity. Many patients do not connect the performance of daily activity with increased symptoms, and they require persistent questioning by the therapist to make the connection. A daily activity log may help isolate aggravating activities or activity patterns.

The ulnar nerve gliding program used in the conservative management of ulnar neuropathy at the elbow (Fig. 16-6) begins with the nerve in a position of minimal stress. The head is in midline, the shoulder forward flexed and adducted. The emphasis on the first segment of this program is on the

Nerve Gliding Program
Brachial Plexus Management

Begin with the position recommended by your therapist.

Do gliding exercises slowly and hold the position for a count of _____ .

Go through exercises to position _____ . Do not bring on pain, numbness, or tingling.

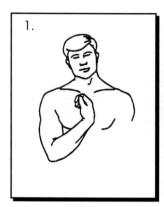
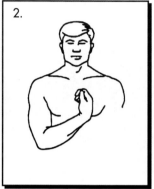
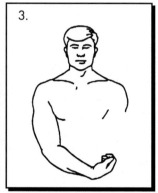
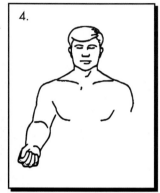

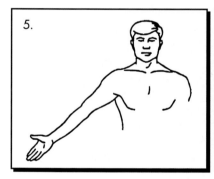
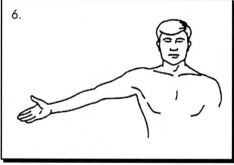
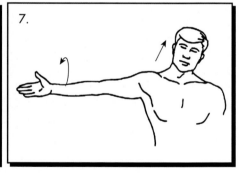

Fig. 16-3. The brachial plexus gliding program begins in position 1 with the head laterally flexed to the affected side; the fingers, wrist, and elbow are flexed. In position 2, the head comes to neutral. By position 3, the hand has moved across the chest and down to hip level. The arm gradually abducts as the patient comes to position 4 and progresses through to position 6. Lateral cervical flexion to the opposite side is the final component of this glide added in position 7. (Redrawn with permission from Totten PA, Hunter JM: Therapeutic techniques to enhance nerve gliding in thoracic outlet and carpal tunnel syndromes, *Hand Clin* 7[3]:505, Philadelphia, 1991, Saunders.)

distal ulnar nerve. In the second half of the series, the focus switches to the proximal ulnar nerve with the distal segment in a more neutral position. The patient who has progressed to this level may move from position 3 to position 4 by abducting the shoulder, extending the elbow, and bringing the wrist to neutral. For other patients, this sequence may need to be treated as two separate exercises, depending on their response to the first three positions. The elbow is a prime area of limitation in the patient with ulnar nerve pathology. It is important as we focus on nerve gliding that joints not be permitted to stiffen. We may work on a stiff joint, for example, the elbow, more safely when the positions

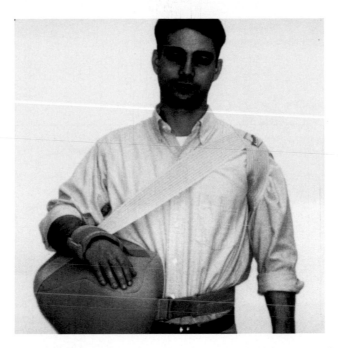

Fig. 16-4. An abduction pillow or other supportive device may be necessary to decrease pain and guarding and to reduce stress at the plexus before beginning gliding exercises.

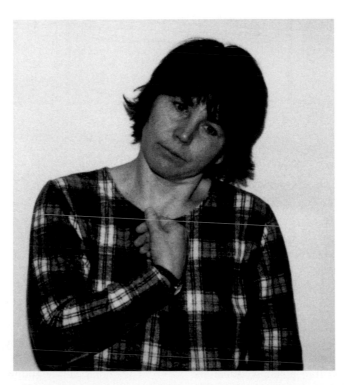

Fig. 16-5. The gliding program for this individual initially was restricted to lateral cervical flexion with the remainder of the involved extremity protected during exercise in a position of minimal stress.

Nerve Gliding Program
Conservative Management of Ulnar Neuropathy

Complete each sequence _____ times a day.

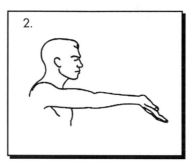 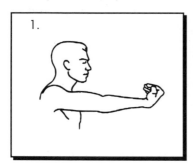 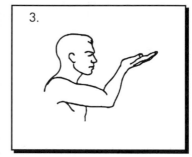

1. Assume position #1 with arm extended in front of you, elbow straight, and your wrist bent.

2. Now extend your wrist and fingers.

3. Now bend your elbow.

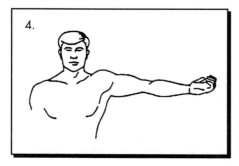 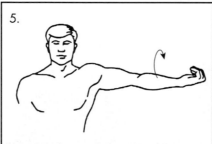 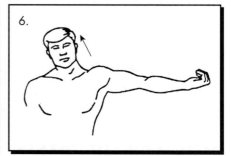

4. Move to position #4 by moving your arm to the side. Keep your wrist bent.

5. Turn your arm backward.

6. Bend your neck away from your arm (to touch your ear to the opposite shoulder).

Fig. 16-6. Conservative management of ulnar neuropathy: position 1, the arm is extended with the elbow straight and the wrist and fingers flexed; position 2, the wrist and fingers are extended; position 3, the elbow is flexed. In the second half of this sequence, position 4 begins with the arm abducted, and the wrist and fingers flexed; position 5 adds external rotation; and position 6 incorporates lateral cervical flexion to maximize tension. (From The Philadelphia Hand Center, PC, 901 Walnut Street, Philadelphia.)

of the proximal and distal joints are biased to decrease stress on the irritated nerve, thus allowing work on the joint without producing further nerve irritation.

In the postoperative ulnar nerve transposition patient, the nerve gliding program acknowledges the new anterior location of the nerve. (Fig. 16-7). Again in the initial positions, the distal segment receives prime attention. In phase two (positions 4 through 6) the proximal segment is the focus.

The radial nerve gliding program (Fig. 16-8) can be performed with the patient either standing or sitting. The sequence begins with the patient in a relaxed position

Postoperative Ulnar Nerve Gliding

Complete each sequence _____ times a day.
Go to position _____ .

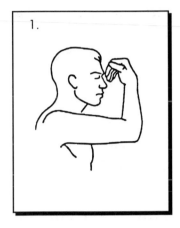
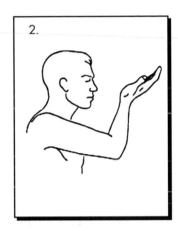
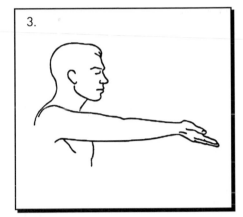

1. Assume position #1 with your elbow and wrist bent.

2. Move to position #2 by extending your wrist and fingers.

3. Now straighten your elbow.

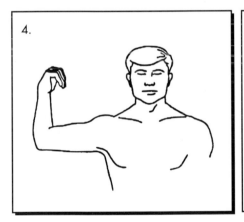
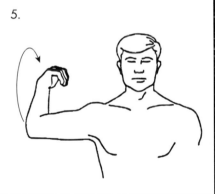
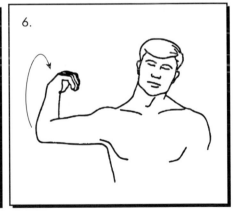

4. Assume position #4 with your elbow and wrist bent and your shoulder positioned as shown.

5. Turn your arm backward.

6. Bend your neck away from your arm (to touch your ear to the opposite shoulder).

Fig. 16-7. Postoperative ulnar nerve gliding: position 1, the arm is adducted and flexed to 90° at the shoulder, and the elbow is also flexed to 90°, the wrist and fingers are in gentle flexion; position 2, the wrist and fingers are extended; position 3, the elbow is extended. In phase 2, the arm is abducted, elbow flexed to 90°, wrist and fingers flexed; in position 5, the arm is externally rotated; and in position 6, lateral cervical flexion is added. (From The Philadelphia Hand Center, PC, 901 Walnut Street, Philadelphia.)

Radial Nerve Gliding Program

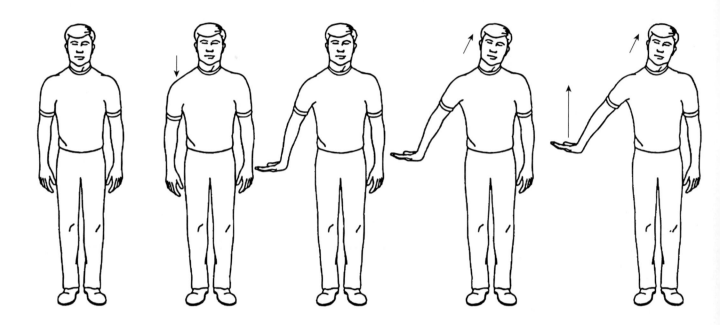

Exercise to be done _____ times each, _____ times a day.
Hold end position for count of _____ .
Move slowly.

Fig. 16-8. The radial nerve gliding program: position 1 begins with the patient standing and the body in a relaxed posture; position 2 adds shoulder depression; in position 3, the arm is internally rotated and the wrist flexed; position 4 adds lateral cervical flexion; and in position 5, the wrist is flexed as the shoulder is extended. (Redrawn from a home program form used by Blodgett Hand Rehabilitation Center, Grand Rapids, MI.)

with the arm extended and close to the body and head in midline. This program incorporates the waiter's tip position.

Again, the patient should progress through the gliding program to the point where tension is produced[2] not to the point of altered sensibility or stretch.[4] This concept stops us well before most of us would normally set the limit for exercise performance. It gives a small reinforcement as to the irritability of a nerve that has been stretched beyond acceptable limits.

Patient education is the key to successful intervention using nerve gliding techniques. Patients are generally asked to perform the exercise sequence 5 to 10 repetitions as often as each hour. Exercise frequency is determined to a large degree by the patient's report of the length of time required for any alteration in symptoms to resolve following an exercise session. The patient and therapist must understand the difference between tension and producing symptoms in

the exercise program. This is an area where harder is not better. Slow, steady exercise performance and respect for the delicate and intricate structure of the nerve provide the only hope for improvement.

REFERENCES

1. Butler DS: *Mobilization of the nervous system,* Melbourne, 1991, Churchill Livingstone.
2. Edgelow PI: *Thoracic outlet syndrome: a new approach to its treatment.* Presented at ASHT Conference on Cumulative Trauma, San Diego, 1994.
3. Elvey RL: Painful restriction of shoulder movement: a clinical observational study. In *Proceedings, disorders of the knee, ankle and shoulder,* Western Australian Institute of Technology, 1979, Perth.
4. Kenneally M, Rubenach H, Elvey R: The upperlimb tension test: the SLR test of the arm. In Grant R, ed: *Physical therapy of the cervical and thoracic spine, clinics in physical therapy 17,* Edinburgh, 1988, Churchill Livingstone.
5. Mackinnon SE, Dellon AL: *Surgery of the peripheral nerve,* New York, 1988, Thieme Medical Publishers.

6. McLellan DL: Longitudinal sliding of the median nerve during hand movements: a contributory factor in entrapment neuropathy, *Lancet* 1975; 1(7907):633.

7. McLellan DL, Swash M: Longitudinal sliding of the median nerve during movements of the upper limb, *J Neurol, Neurosurg Psychiatry* 1976; 39:566.

8. Millesi H, Zoch G, Rath T: The gliding apparatus of peripheral nerve and its clinical significance, *Ann Hand Surg* 1990; 9(2):87.

9. Millesi H: The nerve gap: theory and clinical practice, *Hand Clin* 1986; 2(4):651.

10. Shaw Wilgis EF, Murphy R: The significance of longitudinal excursion in peripheral nerves, *Hand Clin* 1986; 2(4):761.

11. Sunderland S, Bradley KC: Stress-phenomena in human peripheral nerve trunks, *Brain* 1961; 84:102.

12. Totten PA, Hunter JM: Therapeutic techniques to enhance nerve gliding in thoracic outlet and carpal tunnel syndromes, *Hand Clin* 1991; 7(3):505.

SUGGESTED READING

Barrett DS, Donell ST: Entrapment neuropathies: upper limb, *Br J Hosp Med* 1991; 46:94.

Dellon AL: Patient evaluation and management considerations in nerve compression, *Hand Clin* 1992; 8(2):229.

Hunter JM: Recurrent carpal tunnel syndrome, epineural fibrous fixation a traction neuropathy, *Hand Clin* 1991; 7(3):491.

Lundborg G, Rydevik B: Effects of stretching the tibial nerve of the rabbit, *JBJS* 1973; 55B(2):390.

Tubiana R: Carpal tunnel syndrome: some views on its management, *Ann Hand Surg,* 1990; 9(5):325.

Zoech G, Reinsure R, Beer R, Miles H: Stress and strain in peripheral nerves, *Neuro-Orthopedics* 1991; 10:73.

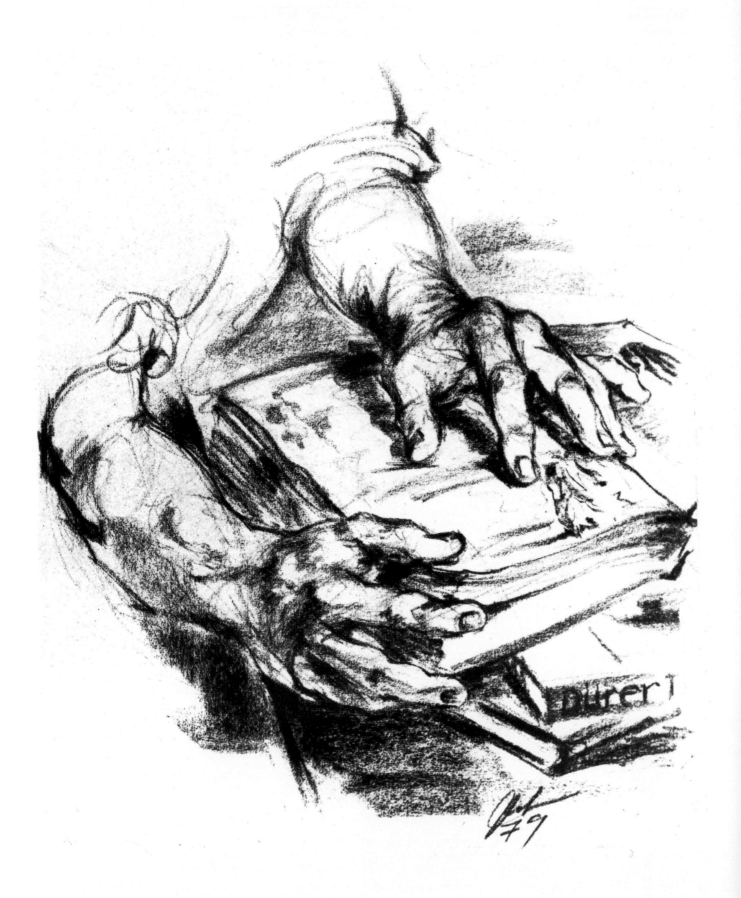

Part V

NERVE COMPRESSION

Perusing Ambroise Paré and Albrecht Durer.

Chapter 17

NERVE COMPRESSION INJURIES
The role of microvascular dysfunction

Göran Lundborg

Acute and chronic compression of peripheral nerve trunks in the upper extremity may result in neurologic dysfunction in the hand to various extents. The pathophysiology of these lesions is complex. Many factors play a role in the functional outcome of such lesions (i.e., the duration and magnitude of the compression trauma as well as the location and topography of the nerve). Because peripheral nerve trunks are anatomically complex and well-vascularized structures, an inflammatory response may be induced by compression, irritation, and stretching. Epineural edema and impaired vascular supply may result in functional disturbance long before nerve fibers per se are damaged.

Normally, nerve trunks glide with the movements of an extremity. The excursion may be as much as 15 mm, depending on location in the extremity. If there is swelling of the epineurium as a result of chronic irritation, such gliding may be impaired and a vicious circle may be induced where swelling, inflammation, impaired microcirculation, and microstretching injuries may lead to further neurologic dysfunction.

STRUCTURE AND FUNCTION OF PERIPHERAL NERVES
Microanatomy

Nerve fibers are collected in fascicles usually organized in fascicular groups (Fig. 17-1). Each fascicle is surrounded

Acknowledgment: Peripheral nerve research in our laboratory is sponsored by the Swedish Medical Research Council, project no: 5188.

by a perineurium—a mechanically strong membrane consisting of numerous lamellae composed of flattened cells possessing basement membranes on both sides.[67-70,74,75] The fascicles are embedded in loose connective tissue called the *epineurium*. The epineurium has a protective effect when a nerve is subjected to compression—several small fascicles embedded in a large amount of epineurium are less vulnerable to compression than large fascicles in a small amount of epineurium. The amount of connective tissue in the nerve trunk may vary with the level—usually it is more pronounced in nerve segments close to joints. The epineurium contains numerous microvessels.

Nerve fibers

Individual axons represent extended peripheral processes from their respective cell bodies in the dorsal root ganglion (sensory neurons) or the anterior horn of the spinal cord (motor neurons).[43] The axons together with surrounding Schwann cells constitute nerve fibers. Fibers may be myelinated or nonmyelinated. In myelinated fibers the axons are surrounded by single Schwann cells, which are arranged longitudinally along the axon. Nonmyelinated axons, on the other hand, are located in the cytoplasm of the surrounding Schwann cell.

Axonal transport

The distances between nerve cell bodies and the most peripheral part of their processes are remarkable. Because of this specific anatomy of the neuron, there is a need for an

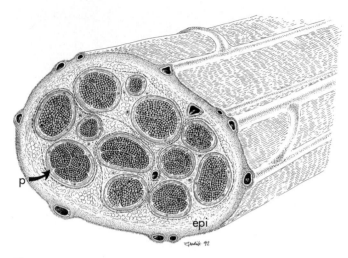

Fig. 17-1. Microanatomy of a peripheral nerve trunk and its tissue components. The axons are running in the endoneurial space of fascicles which is surrounded by a perineurium (*p*). Several fascicles constitute fascicular groups embedded in the epineurial connective tissue (*epi*).

efficient communication system between proximal and distal parts of the nerve cell. These requirements are satisfied by axonal transport systems. Most substances necessary for membrane integrity of axon membrane and cytoskeleton, as well as nerve terminals, occur in the nerve cell body. Via intraaxonal transport systems such products are constantly transported from the nerve cell body to the periphery (anterograde transport), but also in the opposite direction (retrograde transport)—the latter for transport of trophic factors synthesized in the peripheral target organs. The character and pathophysiology of the axonal transport systems have been delineated in several reports and reviews.*

Intraneural microvascular system

Impulse transmission as well as axonal transport are dependent on a continuous energy supply for their normal function. Such a nutritional supply is provided by a well-developed intraneural microvascular system comprising vessels in all layers of the nerve. Along its course, each nerve trunk segmentally receives vascular supply from the surrounding tissues via a mesoneurium, allowing a great deal of motion of the nerve trunk. In the epineurium these vessels divide into ascending and descending branches running in longitudinal direction in superficial as well as deep layers of the epineurium (Fig. 17-2, *A*). Numerous collaterals are being formed with vessels in the perineurial layer and in the endoneural space inside the fascicles (Fig. 17-2, *B*). The perineurial vessels can be seen running longitudinally between the individual lamellae

*References 1, 4-8, 19-21, 26, 27, 31, 32, 34, 35, 37, 38, 49, 55-57, 71, 78, 79, 81.

over long distances (Fig. 17-2, *C*). When they pass through the innermost layer of the perineurium, they often do this at an oblique angle (Fig. 17-2, *D*),[40,41,44] thereby setting up a critical point where these vessels are easily obliterated in association with increased intrafascicular pressure.[2,3,41,42,46]

Vital microscopic studies have demonstrated that there is, at all levels of the nerve, blood flow in proximal-distal as well as distal-proximal direction. Because of collaterals, flow direction may easily shift when a segment of the nerve is compressed.[43] Because of well-developed collaterals, peripheral nerve trunks may resist a great deal of surgical mobilization with no or minimal interference with intraneural microvascular flow.

Intraneural diffusion barriers

Vessels in the epineurium and endoneurium present different permeability properties. Injury to a nerve trunk will rapidly induce an increased permeability of epineurial vessels, resulting in edema and invasion of macrophages. The location and extent of the edema depend on the severity of the injury.[40,41,59,61] Endoneurial vessels normally do not allow passage of proteins over endothelial cells, thereby constituting a blood-nerve barrier analogous to the blood-brain barrier.[59,80] Thus, a moderate ischemic, chemical, or physical trauma may induce an epineurial edema, whereas the endoneurial vascular bed is still uneffected.

The microenvironment inside the fascicles is protected also by the perineurial sheath, acting as a diffusion barrier against macromolecules.* Because of this perineurial barrier, an epineurial edema cannot penetrate into the endoneurial space. On the other hand, because this barrier function works also from inside-out,[47] the same mechanism makes it impossible for an endoneurial edema to be drained outward through the perineurium. In this way a closed compartment syndrome in miniature may be induced inside fascicles as a result of long-standing ischemia or physical injury.[43,46]

Endoneurial fluid pressure

Normally there is a slightly positive interstitial tissue fluid pressure inside fascicles, resulting in an obvious stiffness. Because of this pressure, a small lesion to the perineurium (perineurial window) may result in herniation of the nerve fibers (Fig. 17-3). This endoneurial fluid pressure (EFP) has been estimated to about 1.5 ± 0.7 mm Hg.[51] Because surrounding tissues present a slightly negative tissue pressure (subcutaneous tissue -4.7 ± 0.8 mm Hg[9] and muscle -2 ± 2 mm Hg[28]), there may be a net pressure gradient over the perineurium of about 3 to 5 mm Hg, giving the fascicles a normal mechanical stiffness. Such a positive intrafascicular pressure may be caused by several factors (e.g., the

†References 33, 41, 48, 58, 72, 76.

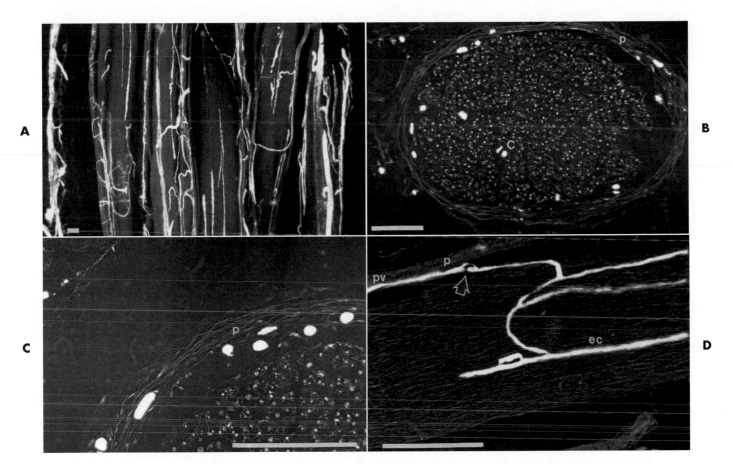

Fig. 17-2. Microvascular anatomy of a nerve trunk. **A,** Longitudinal section through a perfused median nerve from a human forearm showing endoneurial capillaries forming a longitudinally oriented pattern. Scale bar = 0.1 mm. **B,** Transverse section through single fascicle of a perfused human median nerve at wrist level. Capillaries (*c*) are seen running in the endoneurial space and in between perineurial layers (*p*). Scale bar = 0.1 mm. **C,** Transverse section through perfused median nerve showing microvessels running longitudinally between perineurial lamellae (*p*). **D,** Longitudinal section through fascicle, showing a perineurial vessel (*pv*) passing obliquely through the innermost lamellae of the perineurium (*p*) to join endoneurial capillaries *(ec)*. Arrow indicates the critical point for passage through the perineurium, constituting a "valve mechanism" where the vessel can be easily closed. (Reproduced with permission from Lundborg G: *Nerve injury and repair,* Edinburgh, 1988, Churchill Livingstone.)

hypertonicity of endoneurial fluid electrolytes compared with serum electrolytes).[52]

Physiologic excursion of peripheral nerves

Peripheral nerve trunks glide with movements of the extremities. Gliding is possible because of specific anatomic properties, including an "adventitia" around the nerve in combination with intraneural gliding layers allowing fascicles to slide in relation to surrounding intraneural tissues.[50] Restrictions in normal gliding because of local irritation and swelling are probably of considerable importance for occurrence of scarring and local entrapment situations.

In the upper arm the median and ulnar nerves may slide 7.3 mm and 9.8 mm, respectively, during full elbow flexion and extension. The corresponding figure for the brachial plexus during full abduction and adduction of the shoulder is around 15 mm.[82] In the forearm, proximal to the carpal tunnel, the excursions of the same nerves have been found to be 14.5 mm and 13.8 mm, respectively.[82] Inside the carpal tunnel, the median nerve may show a physiologic excursion up to 9.5 to 10 mm.[50] There are also movements in a peripheral nerve with flexion and extension movements.[84] Segments with branches are much stiffer compared with segments of a nerve where no branches are leaving the nerve.[83]

NERVE COMPRESSION LESIONS: STAGING AND CLASSIFICATION

Nerve compression injuries may be classified on the basis of pathophysiology, structural changes, or functional consequences (Fig. 17-4).

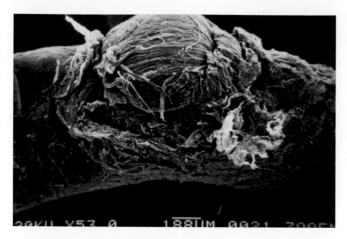

Fig. 17-3. Perineurial window resulting from a tangential cut in the perineurium. Nerve fibers can be seen herniating through the hole in the perineurium due to the positive intrafascicular pressure. (Reproduced with permission from Lundborg G: *Nerve injury and repair,* Edinburgh, 1988, Churchill Livingstone.)

Metabolic conduction block

A local metabolic conduction block may be induced when a segment of a nerve trunk is compressed and the local intraneural microvessels are obliterated (Fig. 17-4, *A*). A metabolic conduction block may be induced by an inflated tourniquet around the upper arm, resulting in complete paralysis and sensory loss in the hand within 20 to 25 minutes. Another example of such a block is the numbness of the foot when the peroneal nerve is compressed by one leg crossing over the other at knee level. When the pressure is removed, the block is immediately reversible with restitution of intraneural microvascular circulation. If there is an intraneural edema, functional restitution may need to be longer (Fig. 17-4, *B*).

Neurapraxia

Local compression at a higher magnitude may induce conduction block which last for weeks or months (Fig. 17-4, *C*). This type of long-lasting conduction block has been named *neurapraxia*.[65,66] The pathoanatomic basis is usually local damage to the myeline sheath, axonal continuity, however, being preserved. Usually, neurapraxia includes total motor paralysis, while some sensory and sympathetic function may be spared because of preserved function in the less vulnerable thin fibers.[66] The radial nerve in the upper arm may suffer from this type of reversible conduction block in association with fracture of the humerus. The situation may also occur after inflation of a tourniquet around the upper arm to too high a pressure[43] or local pressure of the radial nerve at upper arm level for other reasons (Saturday night palsy).

Axonotmesis

When there is a severe crush injury or traction injury, axons may be damaged to such an extent that their continuity

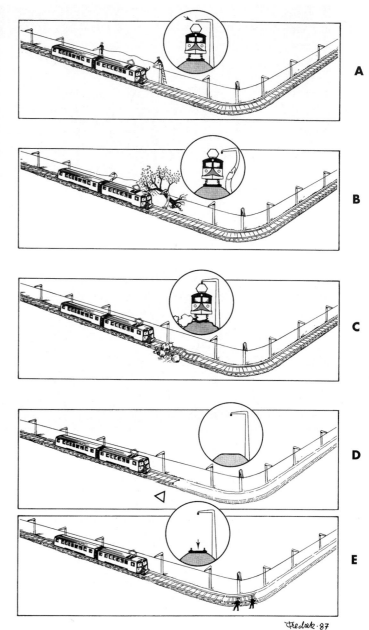

Fig. 17-4. Schematic illustration of various levels of nerve compression injury, the rails corresponding to a nerve fiber, the tracks to the endoneurial tubes, and the train to the electric impulse traveling along the nerve fiber. The electric wire corresponds to microvessels providing energy. **A,** *Metabolic conduction block.* When the local energy supply is interrupted, the train cannot move in spite of intact nerve fibers. **B,** If the electric wire system is more severely compromised (e.g., an intraneural edema), the functional recovery takes longer. **C,** *Neurapraxia* (Sunderland lesion 1). The train is stopped because of local damage to the rail (myeline damage), more distal parts of the rail as well as the energy supply still being intact. Local myeline repair may take a considerable time. **D,** *Axonotmesis* (Sunderland lesion 2). The rail is damaged and has disappeared distal to the level of injury (axonal degeneration). The track (endoneurial tube) is still intact and new rails can easily be laid down in the correct position **(E).** (Reproduced with permission from Lundborg G: *Nerve injury and repair,* Edinburgh, 1988, Churchill Livingstone.)

is broken inside the preserved endoneurial tubes (column of Schwann cells together with their basal lamina) (Fig. 17-4, *D*). In such cases functional recovery can occur only if the axons regenerate (Fig. 17-4, *E*). Because preserved endoneurial tubes in such cases may act as guidelines for the regenerating axons, correct peripheral targets are usually innervated.

Neurotmesis

Severe laceration of a nerve trunk may result in neurotmesis, implying loss of continuity together with some or all of the remaining connective tissue components of the peripheral nerve trunk. Such a lesion usually requires resection of the local scar followed by surgical repair to make it possible for axons to reinnervate the distal segment of the nerve trunk.

EFFECTS OF NERVE COMPRESSION
Distribution of pressure and redistribution of tissues

Under a compressing device, there is a pressure gradient redistributing compressed tissues toward noncompressed areas.[10,30] Under an inflated tourniquet, such pressure gradients are always greatest at the edges of the compressed segments, where severe lesions to nerves, as well as muscle tissue, may be induced if the applied pressure is very high. Such shear forces may lead to microvascular injury as well as injury to the nerve fibers.[43,54,63] It has been shown that low pressure in the inflated cuff together with limb-shaped cuffs may considerably help reduce the risk for pressure-induced injuries to underlying neuromuscular tissues.[60]

Compression at low pressure

Even low pressure, applied to a nerve trunk, may affect the microvascular flow in intraneural venules. It has been demonstrated in animal experiments that such a microvascular interference may occur even at 20 to 30 mm Hg.[62] Retrograde effects on capillary circulation in the endoneurial space may result in impaired oxygenation and nerve fiber dysfunction. The endothelial cells of endoneurial capillaries, normally providing a blood-nerve barrier, may increase their permeability as a result of long-lasting nutritional insufficiency. The result may be an edema in the endoneurial space and a compartment syndrome in miniature. Experimental studies, show that compression at a magnitude of 30 to 80 mm Hg for 2 to 4 hours may result in a threefold increase in endoneurial fluid pressure.[46] Higher pressure magnitude may result in more severe microvascular dysfunction: 60 to 80 mm Hg may lead to complete intraneural ischemia in animal experiments.[62] The critical pressure level before such an intraneural ischemia occurs depends on the systolic blood pressure of the individual.[73]

Axonal transport may also be impaired by local compression[12] because of obliteration of intraneural microvessels as well as nerve fiber deformation. A pressure of 30 mm Hg applied for 2 hours may induce a complete or partial block of intraaxonal transported proteins at the site of compression in animal experiments.[11,15,18,19,64] Also, the *retrograde* transport may be inhibited by compression because of similar mechanisms.[19] Such an inhibition of the retrograde component induces morphologic and biochemical changes in the nerve cell bodies expressed in, for example, eccentricity of the nucleus, dispersion of Nissl substance, and change in transport of tubuline.[13,14,17] Thus peripheral compression at comparatively low magnitude may have obvious consequences also for the biochemistry of centrally located nerve cell bodies.

The effect of compression on nerve fibers depends on their size and location in the nerve trunk. In general, large fibers are more susceptible to pressure than small fibers.[16,22-24,29,53] Nonmyelinated fibers are very resistant to compression and very high pressure may be needed to affect them.

Double-crush and reversed double-crush syndromes

The inhibitory effects of compression on the intraaxonal transport system helps explain why compression at one level of a nerve trunk may have effects on this structure as well as function of other segments of the same nerve. Proximal interference with anterograde axonal transport might interfere with the prevision of cytoskeletal elements to the distal axon and axolemma as well as transmittor substances required for synaptic function. The concept is important for understanding the pathophysiology of double-crush syndrome,[77] implying simultaneous entrapment of the same nerve trunk occurring at two various levels (e.g., coexistence of distal compression neuropathy and cervical neuropathy). Compression at one level of a nerve trunk may affect the whole neuron along its entire length.

One may speculate about the existence of reversed double-crush syndrome (i.e., that distal entrapment of a peripheral nerve may contribute to induction of entrapment neuropathy of the same nerve at a more proximal level).[14,43] The biologic basis of such a phenomenon may be compression-induced inhibition of retrograde axonal transport,[19] which induces changes in the nerve cell bodies.[14] This may lead to changes in anterograde transport of cytoskeletal components like tubuline,[13] thereby making more proximal parts of the neuron more vulnerable to compression trauma.

CLINICAL ASPECTS

Clinically, acute nerve compression injuries can be seen in association with blunt extremity trauma, fractures, or pressure from a tourniquet inflated to too high a pressure level.

Experiments on humans

The correlation between pressure level and nerve dysfunction has been studied in several clinical experiments.

Following inflation of a tourniquet around the upper arm to suprasystolic pressure levels, the hand usually becomes completely anaesthetic and paralytic after 20 to 25 minutes. It has been demonstrated that the anesthesia occurs at the same rate whether the cuff pressure is 150 or 300 mm Hg,[36] an observation that indicates that ischemia of the compressed segment rather than mechanical changes is the pathophysiologic basis of nerve dysfunction in these situations. This is a typical example of an immediately reversible metabolic conduction block.

In other experiments, the critical pressure levels for peripheral nerve function have been studied.[25] Gelberman et al. measured the tissue pressure inside the carpal canal of normal volunteers and with patients suffering from carpal tunnel syndrome (CTS).[25] In the control subject the tissue pressure averaged 2.5 mm Hg, while the corresponding pressure in carpal tunnel patients was 32 mm Hg. The pressure level increased with wrist flexion and wrist extension. In other experiments the pressure in the carpal tunnel was changed and monitored during controlled external compression.[45] Slight paresthesia in the hand was induced when the tissue pressure in the carpal tunnel was 30 mm Hg. When the pressure was increased to 50 to 60 mm Hg, a complete block of sensory and motor conduction occurred. The lower critical pressure at which the function of nerve fibers was jeopardized in normotensive patients was found to be 50 mm Hg. When similar experiments were carried out on hypertensive patients, 60 to 70 mm Hg were needed to induce nerve conduction block.[73]

Carpal tunnel syndrome

In CTS the clinical signs and symptoms reflect well-defined pathophysiologic stages. In this respect the syndrome constitutes an ideal model for understanding nerve dysfunction as a consequence of physiologic changes in the nerve. Because the carpal canal is a tight compartment, any process that decreases the volume of this compartment or increases the volume of its contents will cause increased tissue pressure, which might have immediate consequences for intraneural blood flow. Typical of the early stage of CTS is nocturnal paresthesia in the hand combined with relief of symptoms during the day. In CTS patients a mean pressure of 32 mm Hg has been monitored in the carpal tunnel[25]—a level which corresponds nicely to the critical pressure for impairment of intraneural venular flow[62] and axonal transport,[11,12,15,18,64] which has been observed in animals and also in compression experiments in human volunteers. In CTS patients a metabolic problem occurs in the median nerve late during the night as a result of the increased intracarpal tunnel pressure at this time.[39] The muscle pump is not working, the wrist may be flexed during sleep, and tissue fluids are redistributed into the arms because of the horizontal position. In addition, systolic blood pressure is decreased, which makes the

intraneural vessels more susceptible to external compression. The corresponding hypoxia in the nerve is expressed as paresthesia of the hand. The phenomenon has the character of a metabolic block that is immediately reversible when the patient wakes up and starts moving the hand.

More constant problems, expressed as paresthesia and numbness in the hand also during the day, are typical for the intermediate stage of CTS. At this stage a pathologic process has become manifested in the nerve—there may be an edema or perhaps local myeline disorder in some fibers. We may be dealing with a mixed lesion where some fibers suffer from metabolic disorder and others suffer from neurapraxia. Surgical decompression results in immediate functional recovery in those fibers suffering from a metabolic problem, while fibers suffering from neurapraxia may need weeks or months to recover completely.

More severe symptoms like permanent impairment of sensibility and muscle atrophy may reflect a neurapraxia or axonotmesis in the nerve, and perhaps a metabolic problem in some fiber groups. Decompression may reverse the metabolic problems, the neurapractic lesions may need longer time to recover, and those fibers that have undergone degeneration (axonotmesis) may never regain their functional properties. This may be especially true if constant intraneural edema has been invaded by fibroblasts and with time transferred to a fibrotic scar causing further constriction of the nerve trunk.

REFERENCES

1. Archer DR, Dahlin LB, Mclean WG: Changes in slow axonal transport of tubulin induced by local application of colchicine to rabbit vagus nerve, *Acta Physiol Scand* 1994; 150:57.
2. Bell MA, Weddell AGM: A descriptive study of the blood vessels of the sciatic nerve in the rat, man and other mammals, *Brain* 1984; 107:871.
3. Bell MA, Weddell AGM: A morphometric study of intrafascicular vessels of mammalian sciatic nerve, *Muscle Nerve* 1984; 7:524.
4. Bisby MA: Orthograde and retrograde axonal transport of labeled protein in motorneurons, *Exp Neurol* 1976; 50:628.
5. Bisby MA: Functions of retrograde axonal transport, *Fed Proc* 1982; 41:2307.
6. Black MM, Lasek RJ: Slow components of axonal transport to cytoskeletal networks, *J Cell Biol* 1980; 85:616.
7. Brady ST: Microtubules and the mechanism of fast axonal transport. In Weiss DG, ed: *Axoplasmic transport,* Berlin, 1982, Springer-Verlag.
8. Brady ST, Lasek RJ: The slow components of axonal transport movements, composition and organization. In Weiss DG, ed: *Axoplasmic transport,* Berlin, 1982, Springer-Verlag.
9. Chen HI, Granger HJ, Taylor AE: Interaction of capillary, interstitial and lymphatic forces in the canine hindpaw, *Circ Res* 1976; 39:245.
10. Crenshaw AG, Hargens AR, Gershuni DH, Rydevik BL: Wide tourniquet cuffs more effective at lower inflation pressure, *Acta Orthop Scand* 1987; 59:59.
11. Dahlin L, Danielsen N, McLean WG, et al: Critical pressure level for impairment of fast axonal transport during experimental compression of rabbit vagus nerve, *J Physiol* 1982; 325:84 (abstract).
12. Dahlin LB: Nerve compression and axonal transport. Sweden, 1986, Göteborg University (doctoral thesis).

13. Dahlin LB, Archer DR, McLean WG: Axonal transport and morphological changes following nerve compression: an experimental study in the rabbit vagus nerve, *J Hand Surg* 1993; 18B:106.

14. Dahlin LB, Lundborg G: The neurons and its response to peripheral nerve compression, *J Hand Surg* 1990; 15B:5.

15. Dahlin LB, McLean WG: Effects of graded experimental compression on slow and fast axonal transport in rabbit vagus nerve, *J Neurol Sci* 1986; 72:19.

16. Dahlin LB, Meiri KF, McLean WG, et al: Effects of nerve compression on fast axonal transport in streptozotocin-induced diabetes mellitus, *Diabetologia* 1986; 29:181.

17. Dahlin LB, Nordborg C, Lundborg G: Morphological changes in nerve cell bodies induced by experimental graded nerve compression, *Exp Neurol* 1987; 95:611.

18. Dahlin LB, Rydevik B, McLean WG, Sjöstrand J: Changes in fast axonal transport during experimental nerve compression at low pressures, *Exp Neurol* 1984; 84:29.

19. Dahlin LB, Sjöstrand J, McLean WG: Graded inhibition of retrograde axonal transport by compression of rabbit vagus nerve, *J Neurol Sci* 1986; 976:221.

20. Dahlström A: Axoplasmic transport (with particular respect to adrenergic neurons), *Philos Trans R Soc Lond (Biol)* 1971; 261:325.

21. de Vito JL, Clausing KW, Smith OA: Uptake and transport of horseradish peroxidase by cut end of the vagus nerve, *Brain Res* 1974; 82:269.

22. Erlanger J, Gasser H: *Electrical signs of nervous activity,* Philadelphia, 1937, University of Pennsylvania Press.

23. Fowler TJ, Ochoa J: Recovery of nerve conduction after pneumatic tourniquet observations on the hindlimb of the baboon, *J Neurol Neurosurg Psychiatry* 1975; 35:638.

24. Gasser HS, Erlanger J: The role of fiber size in the establishment of a nerve block by pressure or cocaine, *Am J Physiol* 1929; 88:581.

25. Gelberman RH, Hergenroeder PT, Hargens AR, et al: The carpal tunnel syndrome—a study of carpal canal pressure, *J Bone Joint Surg* 1981; 63A:380

26. Grafstein B, Forman DS: Intracellular transport in neurons, *Physiol Rev* 1980; 60:1167.

27. Griffin JW, Price DL, Drachman DB: Incorporation of axonally transported glycoproteins into axolemma during nerve regeneration, *J Cell Biol* 1981; 88:205.

28. Hargens AR, Akeson WH, Mubarak SJ: Fluid balance within the canine anterolateral compartment and its relationship to compartment syndromes, *J Bone Joint Surg* 1978; 60A:499.

29. Hargens AR, Rumine J, Sipe J, et al: Peripheral nerve-conduction block by muscle compartment pressure, *J Bone Joint Surg* 1979; 61A:192.

30. Hargens AR, Skyhar MJ, McClure AG, et al: Local compression patterns beneath pneumatic tourniquets applied to arms and thighs of human cadavers, *J Orthop Res* 1987; 5:247.

31. Kristensson K, Olsson Y: Retrograde transport of horseradish peroxidase in transected axons: 3. Entry into injured axons and subsequent localization in perikaryon, *Brain Res* 1976; 115:201.

32. Kristensson K, Sjöstrand J: Retrograde transport of protein tracer in the rabbit hypoglossal nerve during regeneration, *Brain Res* 1972; 45:175.

33. Larsson J, Ekblom A, Henriksson K, et al: Immunoreactive tachokinins, calciotonin gene related peptide and neuropeptide Y in human synovial fluid from inflamed knee joints, *Neurosci Lett* 1989; 100:326.

34. Lasek RJ: Protein transport in neurons, *Int Rev Neurobiol* 1970; 13:289.

35. Lasek RJ, Garner JA, Brady ST: Axonal transport of the cytoplasmic matrix, *J Cell Biol* 1984; 99:212.

36. Lewis T, Pickering GW, Rothschild P: Centripetal paralysis arising out of arrested bloodflow to the limb including notes on a form of tingling, *Heart* 1931; 16:1.

37. Lubinska L: Axoplasmic streaming in regenerating and in normal nerve fibers, *Prog Brain Res* 1964; 13:1.

38. Lubinska L: On axoplasmic flow, *Int Rev Neurobiol* 1975; 17:241.

39. Luchetti R, Schoenhuber R, Alfarano M, et al: Serial overnight recordings of intracarpal canal pressure in carpal tunnel syndrome patients with and without wrist splinting, *J Hand Surg* 1994; 19B:35.

40. Lundborg G: Ischemic nerve injury: experimental studies on intraneural microvascular pathophysiology and nerve function in a limb subjected to temporary circulatory arrest, *Scand J Plast Reconstr Surg* 1970; (suppl 6):1-113.

41. Lundborg G: Structure and function of the intraneural microvessels as related to trauma, edema formation and nerve function, *J Bone Joint Surg* 1975; 57A:938.

42. Lundborg G: The intrinsic vascularization of human peripheral nerves: structural and functional aspects, *J Hand Surg* 1979; 4:34.

43. Lundborg G: *Nerve injury and repair,* Edinburgh, 1988, Churchill Livingstone.

44. Lundborg G, Brånemark P-I: Microvascular structure and function of peripheral nerves: vital microscopic studies of the tibial nerve in the rabbit, *Adv Microscirc* 1968; 1: 66.

45. Lundborg G, Gelberman RH, Minteer-Convery M, et al: Median nerve compression in the carpal tunnel—functional response to experimentally induced controlled pressure, *J Hand Surg* 1982; 7:252.

46. Lundborg G, Myers R, Powell H: Nerve compression injury and increase in endoneurial fluid pressure: a miniature compartment syndrome, *J Neurol Neurosurg Psychiatry* 1983; 46:1119.

47. Lundborg G, Nordborg C, Rydevik B, Olsson Y: The effect of ischemia on the permeability of the perineurium to protein tracers in rabbit tibial nerve, *Acta Neurol Scand* 1973; 49:287.

48. Martin KH: Untersuchungen über die perineurale Diffusionsbarriere and gefriergetrockneten Nerven, *Zeitschrift der Zellforsch* 1964; 64:404.

49. McLean WG, McKay AL, Sjöstrand J. Electrophoretic analysis of axonally transported proteins in rabbit vagus nerve, *J Neurobiol* 1983; 14:227.

50. Millesi H, Zöch G, Rath T: The gliding apparatus of peripheral nerve and its clinical significance, *Ann Hand Surg* 1990; 9:87.

51. Myers RR, Costello ML, Powell HC: Increased endoneurial fluid pressure in galactose neuropathy, *Muscle Nerve* 1979; 2:299.

52. Myers RR, Heckman HM, Powell HC: Endoneurial fluid is hypertonic: results of microanalysis and its significance in neuropathy, *J Neuropathol Exp Neurol* 1983; 42:217.

53. Ochoa J: Nerve fiber pathology in acute and chronic compression. In Omer GE, Spinner M, eds: *Management of peripheral nerve problems,* Philadelphia, 1980, Saunders.

54. Ochoa J, Fowler TJ, Gilliatt RW: Anatomical changes in peripheral nerves compressed by a pneumatic tourniquet, *J Anat* 1972; 113:433.

55. Ochs S: Characteristics and a model for fast axoplasmic transport in nerve, *J Neurobiol* 1971; 2:331.

56. Ochs S: Axoplasmic transport. In Tower D, ed: *The nervous system I. The basic neurosciences,* vol 1, New York, 1975, Raven Press.

57. Olsson TP, Forsberg I, Kristensson K: Uptake and retrograde axonal transport of horseradish peroxidase in regenerating facial motor neurons of the mouse, *J Neurocytol* 1978; 7:323.

58. Olsson Y: Studies on vascular permeability in peripheral nerves. 1. Distribution of circulating fluorescent serum albumin in normal, crushed and sectioned rat sciatic nerve, *Acta Neuropathol Berlin* 1966; 7:1.

59. Olsson Y, Kristensson K, Klatzo I: Permeability of blood vessels and connective tissue sheaths in the peripheral nervous system to exogenous proteins, *Acta Neuropathol* 1971; 5:61.

60. Pedowitz RA: Tourniquet-induced neuromuscular injury: experimental studies on effects of pneumatic tourniquet compression and ischemia in the rabbit, and assessment of clinical techniques for facilitating the use of lower tourniquet inflation pressures, Göteborg, 1991, Göteborg University (doctoral thesis).

61. Rydevik B, Lundborg G: Permeability of intraneural microvessels and perineurium following acute, graded experimental nerve compression, *Scand J Plast Reconstr Surg* 1977; 11:179.

62. Rydevik B, Lundborg G, Bagge U: Effects of graded compression on intraneural blood flow: an in vitro study on rabbit tibial nerve, *J Hand Surg* 1981; 6A:3.

63. Rydevik B, Lundborg G, Skalak D: Biomechanics of nerves and nerve injuries—biomechanical aspects. In Frankel VF, Nordin M, eds: *Basic biomechanics of the musculo-skeletal system,* Philadelphia, 1989, Lea & Febiger.

64. Rydevik B, McLean WG, Sjöstrand J, Lundborg G: Blockage of axonal transport induced by acute graded compression of the rabbit vagus nerve, *J Neurol Neurosurg Psychiatry* 1980; 43:690.

65. Seddon H: Three types of nerve injury, *Brain* 1943; 66:237.

66. Seddon H, ed: *Surgical disorders of the peripheral nerves,* ed 2, Edinburgh, 1972, Churchill Livingstone.

67. Shantaveerappa TR, Bourne GH: The "perineurial epithelium," a metabolically active, continuous, protoplasmic cell barrier surrounding peripheral nerve fasciculi, *J Anat* 1962; 96:527.

68. Shantaveerappa TR, Bourne GH: The effects of transection of the nerve trunk on the perineural epithelium with special reference to its role in nerve degeneration and regeneration, *Anat Rec* 1964; 150:35.

69. Shantaveerappa TR, Bourne GH: The perineural epithelium of sympathetic nerves and ganglia and its relation to the pia arachnoid of the central nervous system and perineural epithelium of the peripheral nervous system, *Z Zellforsch Mikrosk Anat* 1964; 61:742.

70. Shantaveerappa TR, Bourne GH: Peripheral epithelium: a new concept of its role in the integrity of the peripheral nervous system, *Science* 1966; 154:1464.

71. Sjöstrand J, McLean WG, Frizell M: The application of axonal transport studies to peripheral nerve problems. In Omer GEJ, Spinner M, eds: *Management of peripheral nerve problems,* Philadelphia, 1980, Saunders.

72. Söderfeldt B, Olsson Y, Kristensson K: The perineurium as a diffusion barrier to protein tracers in human peripheral nerve, *Acta Neuropathol Berlin* 1973; 25:120.

73. Szabo R, Gelberman R, Williamson R, Hargens A: Effects of increased systemic blood pressure on the tissue fluid pressure: threshold of peripheral nerve, *J Orthop Res* 1983; 1:172.

74. Thomas PK: The connective tissue of peripheral nerve: an electron microscope study, *J Anat* 1963; 97:35.

75. Thomas PK: The cellular response to nerve injury. 1. The cellular outgrowth from the distal stump of transected nerve, *J Anat* 1967; 100:287.

76. Thomas PK, Olsson Y: Microscopic anatomy and function of the connective tissue components of peripheral nerve. In Dyck PJ, Thomas PK, Lambert EH, eds: *Peripheral neuropathy,* Philadelphia, 1973, Saunders.

77. Upton ARM, McComas AJ: The double crush in nerve entrapment syndromes, *Lancet* 1973; ii:359.

78. Vallee RB, Bloom GS: Mechanisms of fast and slow axonal transport, *Ann Rev Neurosci* 1991; 14:59.

79. Varon S, Adler R: Nerve growth factors and control of nerve growth, *Curr Top Dev Biol* 1980; 16:207.

80. Waksman BH: Experimental study of diphtheritic polyneuritis in the rabbit and guinea pig: III. The blood-nerve barrier in the rabbit, *J Neuropathol Exp Neurol* 1961; 20:35.

81. Weiss DG: General properties of axoplasmic transport. In Weiss DG, ed: *Axoplasmic transport,* Berlin, 1982, Springer-Verlag.

82. Wilgis S, Murphy R: The significance of longitudinal excursions in peripheral nerves, *Hand Clin* 1986; 2:761.

83. Zöch G: Über die Anpassung die peripheren Nerven an die Bewegungen der Extremitäten durch gleiten und dehnung: Untersuchungen am Nervus medianus, *Acta Chir Austria* 1992; 96 (suppl):1.

84. Zöch G, Reihsner R, Ber R: Stress and strain in peripheral nerves, *Neuroorthopaedics* 1991; 10:371.

Chapter 18

MEDIAN NERVE COMPRESSION SYNDROME AT THE WRIST

Frank D. Burke
Joe Dias
Howard Webster

THE INCIDENCE OF CARPAL TUNNEL SYNDROME

Carpal tunnel syndrome *is* the most common elective clinical condition attending the Pulvertaft Hand Centre in Derby. The local incidence of carpal tunnel syndrome was identified by reviewing the diagnoses presented to the Pulvertaft Hand Centre over a 6-month period in 1989.[2] At that time, district general hospitals had local populations formally attached to them (the advent of fund-holding general practitioners more recently has made the situation a lot more fluid). Even in 1989, though, there was an element of cross-boundary flow to other hospitals (Derby being placed at the southern end of Southern Derbyshire Health Authority's area).

Assessment technique

To calculate the incidence of carpal tunnel syndrome, it was necessary to exclude all out-of-area referrals and to calculate accurately the number of our local population served. Surgical treatment for the condition was not provided by other specialties within the hospital or elsewhere in the district.

Southern Derbyshire Health Authority is the largest nonteaching health district in the United Kingdom, and is the fourth largest district in England, providing service for a population of 527,000 people, which is 1.1% of the total population of England and Wales. Southern Derbyshire has a mixture of urban and rural population. In addition, there is a balance of industrial, agricultural, and nonmanual employ-ment. The population probably represents an average national sample.

The cross-boundary flow was estimated using the Regional Patient Information System (PIS). The records of the ten most frequent hand surgery diagnoses and treatments were extracted from the Regional PIS system for 1988 and 1989. Of 794 patients, 112 (14.1%) were diagnosed and treated in neighboring districts. We validated this cross-boundary flow by conducting a postal survey of all general practitioners in the district. The results of this assessment confirmed a 14.1% cross-boundary flow, which revealed our population to be 452,693. This figure was used to determine the incidence of carpal tunnel syndrome locally. We feel the figure does indicate a valid incidence of carpal tunnel syndrome locally in 1989, although it is accepted that milder cases, or those too ill to be considered for surgical release, may not have been referred to the Centre by other physicians.

Previous attempts have been made to identify the incidence of carpal tunnel syndrome. Stevens et al.[8] drew on records retrospectively to assess the frequency of the condition in Rochester, Minnesota, over two time periods: 1961 to 1965 and 1976 to 1980. They found the incidence to be 88 per 100,000 of population in 1961 to 1965, increasing to 125 per 100,000 of population in 1976 to 1980. Although the increased incidence could possibly be ascribed to changing patterns of work, they considered it more likely that an increased patient and physician awareness of the condition had created this effect.

Table 18–1. Statistics for carpal tunnel syndrome

Parameter	Outcome
Incidence	61 per 100,000 of population per year
Outpatient attendance	3.1 visits (normally an initial visit, a follow-up visit 2 weeks postoperatively to remove sutures, and the further final review 6 weeks later to check that all was settling well)
Inpatient stay	1.1 days (90% of the cases were day cases with some rheumatoid and long distance referrals staying 1 night postoperatively)
Operating time	0.6 of an hour from arrival in the anesthetic room to application of a dressing

A further study in 1988 identified an incidence in Santa Clara County, California, of 51 cases per 100,000 of population.[3] The authors considered that 47% of the cases were work related. No evidence of an increasing incidence was offered nor any analysis identifying clusterings of diagnoses of carpal tunnel syndrome around specific occupations felt to be at risk. The relationship of work to the development of carpal tunnel syndrome remains controversial.[4]

The attribution of clinical conditions to work-related causes varies in different countries, and is affected by the various developments in industrial legislation that have occurred in these societies. Frequently, the legal definition of a work-related injury affects clinical attitudes and to an extent confuses international debate among clinicians. In the United Kingdom, a diagnosis of a work-related injury is not readily made because of a legal requirement that there must be a proven 50% chance that the clinical condition was caused by work. The threshold for attributing clinical conditions to the work-related category in America seems a lot lower, perhaps because eligibility for workers' compensation resolves funding difficulties for the patient. Legal variations may also carry over into a clinician's assessment as to whether a clinical condition may or may not have been caused by activities at work.

Results

Our very detailed audit from first attendance through surgery to discharge permitted us to generate the statistics for carpal tunnel syndrome seen in Table 18-1.

ANALYSIS OF CASES

In the 6 months between June and November, 1989, 186 patients with a diagnosis of carpal tunnel syndrome were referred to the Pulvertaft Hand Centre. Most cases were referred by general practitioners, with others coming from rheumatologists, general physicians, and other surgeons. After initial clinical examination and review of patient history at the centre, 170 of these patients were felt to have carpal tunnel syndrome. These assessments were made without the use of electrodiagnostic studies (although a very small number had had these tests performed by physicians before referral). The other 16 referrals were felt to have diseases such as cervical spondylosis rather than carpal tunnel syndrome. Of the 170 confirmed cases, 155 patients were operated on, and of these, 121 (78%) were personally reviewed 3 years later by Howard Webster. The remainder had either died or could not be traced.

Almost all the decompression operations were performed by residents. Endoscopic techniques were not used. The procedures were 90% day cases and only 10% of the patients were in hospital overnight (rheumatoids, bilateral decompressions, or long distance referrals). The inpatients' occupancy was 1.1 days with an average of 3.7 outpatient visits for this particular group (a slightly higher figure than our overall audit average for outpatient visits). The carpal tunnel decompression procedure constituted 31% of the total number of patients operated on by the unit during the study period.

Local anesthesia

One hundred and eight of the patients' hands were operated on under local anesthesia. Bier blocks and brachial blocks were not used, simply local infiltration anesthesia to the wrist with an unanesthetized proximal tourniquet inflated for the short time required for the nerve decompression. Eleven patients (22 hands) had bilateral simultaneous release under local anesthesia, the remainder were unilateral.

Of the local anesthetic patients reviewed 3 years later, 97 were questioned about the efficacy of the procedure: 82 (85%) considered it very satisfactory; 7 (7%) had experienced some discomfort, but said they would repeat the exercise if required; and 8 (8%) had experienced some discomfort and said they would prefer a general anesthetic if further decompression was required.

Scar appearance arising from open carpal tunnel decompression

At 3 years 159 scars were evaluated: 130 (82%) were not visible to the casual glance; 28 (17.4%) were visible to the casual glance; and 1 (0.6%) was thick, broad, and hypertrophic.

Scar tenderness from open carpal tunnel syndrome

Only 3 out of 159 patients had significant symptoms of scar tenderness when reviewed at 3 years. However, 14 had minor residual tenderness to the scar that they did not consider disabling in any way. Many patients said their scar had been tender for the first 3 months after surgery, but very few had noticed problems extending beyond 6 months.

Sensibility and power on review

Detailed questioning revealed more extensive residual symptoms than had been anticipated. Of 168 hands, 114 (68%) were completely cured. However, 54 hands experienced some residual symptoms. There was often reported a period of complete relief followed by mild recurrence of symptoms months or years later, usually brought on by the use of the hand when driving or knitting, or in other activities. Symptoms, while present, were minimal and none of these patients felt the need for further surgery. They considered the operation to have all but resolved their condition completely.

In contrast, 14 of the patients did not feel that their condition had been improved by surgery. Four had nerve conduction studies postoperatively, which confirmed slowing of the median nerve conduction across the carpal tunnel, and further decompression relieved these patients' symptoms completely. Six patients were considered initially to have cervical spondylosis as well as carpal tunnel syndrome, and their continuing symptoms were thought to relate to residual proximal nerve irritation. Three patients were diabetics and may have had a diabetic neuropathy in addition to median nerve compression. No obvious cause for continuing problems was found in the final patient in this group.

OCCUPATION AND CARPAL TUNNEL SYNDROME

The data generated during our detailed audit included information on occupation. This permitted a subsequent analysis of possible effects of work on presentation of upper limb disorders. To see if there were any obvious correlations, 216 working women with conditions that could possibly be caused by work were analyzed. Congenital conditions and tumors were excluded from this group.

Derby is a city of average profile in terms of employment characteristics. The area has a broad industrial base with reasonable amounts of light-engineering and heavy-engineering companies. Based on the 1990 census, there were 157,979 women of working age within Southern Derbyshire Health Authority, of whom 31% were economically inactive. Of these women, 64.8% were employed and 4.2% were unemployed. We have estimated that the Pulvertaft Hand Centre serves 85.9% of this population with the rest being served by neighboring hospitals (14.1% cross-boundary flow). Comparison of the incidences of upper limb disorders in female workers as opposed to those among economically inactive females of working age did not support the view that work was associated with a higher incidence of hand disorders.

Carpal tunnel syndrome merited specific analysis as it was diagnosed in a large subgroup within the 216 females analyzed. Ninety-three female patients of the working age group had carpal tunnel syndrome. Of these, 53 were

Table 18–2. The results of carpal tunnel decompression

Cured	Employed	Not Working
Cured	76%	57.1%
Much better	16%	38.1%
Slightly better	8%	—
No better	—	4.8%
Worse	—	—

employed and 40 were not economically active. Nine of the working patients had desk jobs, 33 were employed in industrial jobs, 10 in moderately heavy industrial jobs, and 1 was a professional. Incidence of the disease in working females was 93.2 per 100,000 of population per year, while in those economically inactive the incidence was 147.4 per 100,000 of population per year. The mean age of the working females was 43.2 years, and the mean age for the economically inactive group was 45.4 years. This slightly earlier presentation of the disease in the working group is not statistically significant. A similar number of these patients who were not economically active (67.5%) and those who were employed (73.5%) required surgery ($P = 0.7$). We could find no evidence that carpal tunnel syndrome is more common, occurs earlier, or requires surgical decompression more often in working patients.

The inability to identify an increased incidence of carpal tunnel syndrome in working females is in agreement with Hadler's views.[4] Regrettably, our audit data did not include information on patient height and weight, so we were unable to investigate Natham and Keniston's findings[5] on the association between physical condition and carpal tunnel syndrome.

Outcome and patient satisfaction

Assessments of outcome by both patients and their doctors were also part of our audit, which permitted review of this aspect of carpal tunnel decompression. Assessments were graded on a 5 point scale from excellent to poor. We were interested in seeing if the patients' assessments of their outcomes correlated with their doctors' views, and whether workers considered their outcomes to be worse than those economically inactive. Some of the workers did believe their symptoms might have been caused by work, and we were interested to see if the frequently stated view in *Trades Union* news sheets that "work-related carpal tunnel syndrome" did badly with surgery would affect workers' perception of their surgeries' outcome. However, negative effects of outcome were not apparent in our study and the surgeon's assessment matched the patient's opinion in most cases. Overall, the economically inactive considered themselves slightly less satisfied than did the working group (but this was not statistically significant). See Table 18-2.

CONCLUSION

An in-depth study of carpal tunnel syndrome within a community was performed, revealing a local incidence of the condition in 61 per 100,000 of population per year. The employment profile of the area is likely to be the average for many cities within the United Kingdom. We found no evidence that the condition was more frequently seen in working females, nor was there any evidence that work significantly accelerates age of onset of symptoms of the disease.

Smith et al. postulated that tension on the flexor tendons could give rise to carpal tunnel syndrome through local pressure and synovitis.[7] Silverstein et al. considered that highly repetitive activities produced a risk factor for carpal tunnel syndrome.[6] While these factors may provoke carpal tunnel syndrome in a few cases, we share the view of Barton et al.[1] that the vast majority of cases of carpal tunnel syndrome are not caused by work. If it were otherwise, even this small study should have shown a significant increase in the incidence of carpal tunnel syndrome in the working female population.

The outcome following open carpal tunnel decompression under local infiltration anesthesia was considered satisfactory, although scar tenderness is a problem in the short term. Minor sensory symptoms postoperatively were more frequent than anticipated, although this was not perceived by the patients as a disability. Concomitant cervical spondylosis or diabetic neuropathy are causes of continuing symptoms following decompression. Patients were well satisfied with the outcome of surgery in most cases.

REFERENCES

1. Barton NJ, Hooper G, Noble J, Steel WM: Occupational causes of disorders in the upper limb, *British Med J* 1992; 304:309-311.
2. Burke FD, Dias JJ, Bradley MJ, Lunn PG: Providing care for hand disorders. The Derby Hand Unit experience 1989-1990, *J Hand Surg* 1991; 16B(1):13-18.
3. Carpal tunnel syndrome, *MMWR* 38:485-487, Occupational Disease Surveillance, CDC, 1989.
4. Hadler NM: Illness in the work place: a challenge of musculo-skeletal symptoms, *J Hand Surg* 1985; 10A:451-456.
5. Nathan PA, Keniston RC: Carpal tunnel syndrome and its relation to general physical condition, *Hand Clin* 1993; 9(2):253-261.
6. Silverstein BA, Fine LJ, Armstrong TJ: Occupational factors and carpal tunnel syndrome, *Am J Ind Med* 1987; 1:343-358.
7. Smith EM, Sonstegard DA, Anderson WH: Carpal tunnel syndrome: contribution of the flexor tendons, *Arch Phys Med Rehabil* 1977; 58:379-385.
8. Stevens JC, Sun S, Beard CM, et al: Carpal tunnel syndrome in Rochester, Minnesota, 1961–1980, *Neurology* 1988; 38:134-138.

Chapter 19

POSTOPERATIVE MANAGEMENT OF CARPAL TUNNEL SYNDROME

Mary C. Kasch

ETIOLOGY AND SURGICAL MANAGEMENT

Carpal tunnel syndrome, compression of the median nerve at the wrist, is the most common peripheral entrapment neuropathy in the upper extremity.[16] Symptoms of nerve compression may be vague, but usually include some combination of pain, tingling, numbness, weakness, and clumsiness. Pain may be sharp and burning with accompanying paresthesias over the area of sensory distribution.[11] First described by Sir James Paget in 1854, surgical decompression was not a common treatment for carpal tunnel syndrome until the 20th century.[15]

It is hypothesized that compression within the carpal canal results in a number of vascular responses. With mild compression, there is a slowing of interneurial blood flow, leading to pain and paresthesias.[18] More severe compression that results in nerve ischemia may induce anoxia and mechanical damage to the endothelial cells of the intraneural microvessels, resulting in increased permeability to water, various ions, and proteins. Ischemic periods may therefore be followed by intraneural edema when blood flow is restored.[11] Sustained compression can result in increased endoneurial fluid pressure and endoneurial edema, which can damage the nerve fibers.[11]

Initial nonoperative management may include splinting, steroid injection and oral antiinflammatory medication to reduce synovitis, diuretics to reduce swelling,[20] and vitamin B_6 (pyridoxine).[15] If medical management is unsuccessful, surgical decompression may be performed.

Surgical care for carpal tunnel syndrome has changed with the development of surgical endoscopes in the 1980s. Surgery may now be performed by the traditional open method or with one of a number of endoscopic devices.[1,6,12] The literature suggests that surgical results may vary depending on the surgical technique used. However, regardless of the procedure used, 80% or more of patients report relief of pain and tingling following surgery.[1,3,4]

Recent studies have found that patients undergoing endoscopic release in general returned earlier to normal activities of daily living (ADL), regained normal strength earlier, had less overall scar tenderness, and returned to work sooner.[1,3,9,14] No matter which surgical method was used, patients on workers' compensation took longer to return to work.[1,4,13] However, surgical complications of endoscopic surgery, when they occur, are significant and must be considered when selecting a surgical approach.[4,12,15]

EARLY POSTOPERATIVE CARE

Following surgery, initial postoperative care is similar for both open and closed surgical techniques. The hand should be splinted in about 20° of extension in a volar splint for 10 to 14 days following surgery until the sutures are removed. Many practitioners then splint the hand for 1 or 2 additional weeks to prevent bowstringing of the flexor tendons at the transverse carpal ligament.[10,12,15] Range of motion of the digits may start 1 or 2 days after surgery or during the week following surgery, with an emphasis on tendon gliding exercises.[23]

149

LATE POSTOPERATIVE CARE

Postoperative management after the first 2 to 3 weeks varies considerably in the literature. In some protocols, patients are seen only intermittently to update a home program for several weeks or until return to work. In others, patients are seen three times a week for 6 to 8 weeks. Work conditioning programs are also described in the literature. More formalized hand therapy is often reserved for those patients who develop one of a number of complications. Although most patients recover fully and return to regular activities quickly, problems of pain and dysfunction tend to be severe when they occur and may persist for 6 to 12 months. Pillar pain (pain in the thenar or hypothenar areas), scar tenderness, hypersensitivity, and loss of strength are the most common problems seen by the hand therapist. Reflex sympathetic dystrophy is infrequent but significant when it occurs.

EVALUATION

Evaluation of the postoperative carpal tunnel patient is usually performed after the sutures are removed. The components of the evaluation may include the following:
- Subjective symptoms such as pain, paresthesias, and hypersensitivity (a body chart of the hand and upper extremity may be helpful to record the location and nature of symptoms experienced)
- Active range of motion, including forearm rotation, wrist flexion and extension, radial and ulnar deviation, and digital motion
- Grip and pinch strength (when the patient can tolerate the pressure of the dynamometer on the palmar scar, but not before the third postoperative week)
- Hand volume using a volumeter when wound is closed or circumferential measurements
- Semmes-Weinstein monofilament test to assess current level of sensibility
- ADL assessment (Fig. 19-1)

TREATMENT

The goals of treatment should be based on the results of the evaluation. A number of treatment techniques may be used to address problems of edema, limited range of motion, scar tenderness, adhesions, tissue induration, palmar pain, and weakness.

Edema may be reduced through elevation and compressive dressings such as Isotoner gloves* or Coban wraps.† Contrast baths have also been recommended for edema.[19]

Range-of-motion exercises of the wrist can be started as soon as the splint is removed, at 2 to 3 weeks after surgery. Gentle active range of motion in all planes will usually restore range of motion of the wrist. However, some patients

require use of joint mobilization techniques to achieve full motion. Differential tendon gliding exercises[23] should be taught to the patient to promote gliding of the tendons through newly forming scar tissue.

Desensitization of the scar is often needed as the scar can be both numb and hypersensitive for some time after surgery. Desensitization is well described in the literature[2,22] and consists of rubbing a variety of textures over the scar as well as immersing the hand into graded materials such as sand or rice. The exercises should be done at least three times a day for 5 to 10 minutes each. It is important that the stimulus be mildly irritating but not noxious.

Soft supports and wraps made of Neoprene‡ or the Dura Gel Splint§ provide support and protection for sensitive tissues. The pressure of the splints may also help to soften the scar through scar anoxia. Use of Cica-Care‖ or a compressive mold made of silastic elastomer can be used with the compressive garment to apply more pressure to the scar tissue.

Strengthening can be started as pain and swelling decrease. Isometric exercises are preferred because they limit excursion of the flexor tendons through the carpal canal and decrease the likelihood of exacerbating any tenosynovitis that may have been present before surgery.

Ultrasound may be used to promote healing and scar remodeling. Electrical stimulation such as transcutaneous electrical nerve stimulation (TENS) or interferential electrical stimulation may be helpful as an adjunct to treatment for pain control. Cryotherapy using frozen ice cups, ice bags, or the Cryostim Ice Probe¶ can be applied for pain control and reduction of edema.

Continued sensory monitoring is also important. Sensory mapping using Semmes-Weinstein monofilaments is preferred.[5]

WORK CONDITIONING

Work conditioning, a progressive, structured program that uses specific work tasks and simulations designed to increase the intensity and duration of activity, may be an important component of return to work, especially for those patients with continued pain and weakness. Work conditioning should include strengthening of the entire upper extremity as well as general conditioning. Use of actual work tasks is essential to help the muscles achieve the strength and endurance required to do a specific job.

Return-to-work issues that may need to be addressed include the use of splints or supports to provide joint stability

---

*Isotoner gloves available from Aris Isotoner, Inc., 417 Fifth Avenue, New York, NY 10016.
†Coban made by 3M Medical-Surgical Division, St. Paul, MN 55144-1000.
‡Neoprene garments available from Benik Corporation, 9465 Provost Road NW, #204, Silverdale, WA 98383.
§Dura Gel Splint available from Smith & Nephew Rolyan, Inc., One Quality Drive, P.O. Box 578, Germantown, WI 53022.
‖Cica-Care Silicone Gel Sheets available from Smith & Nephew Rolyan, Inc., One Quality Drive, P.O. Box 578, Germantown, WI 53022.
¶Cryostim Ice Probe available from Pelton Shepherd Industries, 2721 Transworld Drive, P.O. Box 30218, Stockton, CA 95213.

**Hand
Rehabilitation
Center**
of Sacramento

PATIENT _____

DATE _____

Feeding
_____ Handling fork and spoon
_____ Cutting food with knife/fork
_____ Drinking from glass

Hygiene/Grooming
_____ Brushing teeth
_____ Combing/brushing hair
_____ Make-up application
_____ Shaving
_____ Grooming nails
_____ Bathing/showering
_____ Toileting

Dressing
_____ Taking clothes off hangers
_____ Putting on/taking off clothes
_____ Putting on shoes/socks
_____ Fastening (buttons, zippers, belts)
_____ Putting on bra
_____ Picking up clothes

Cooking
_____ Lifting a gallon of milk
_____ Peeling/cutting vegetables
_____ Opening bottles, jars, cans
_____ Stirring
_____ Washing/drying dishes
_____ Picking up pans and food items
_____ Grocery shopping

Homemaking
_____ Clothes in/out of washer
_____ Cleaning (dusting, scrubbing)
_____ Mopping
_____ Sweeping
_____ Vacuuming

Tool Use
_____ Using garden tools (rake, shovel, hoe)
_____ Grasping and pushing lawn mower
_____ Hammering
_____ Wrench/pliers use
_____ Sanding
_____ Using screwdriver

General
_____ Writing (how long _____)
_____ Dialing and using telephone
_____ Using scissors
_____ Keyboard use
_____ Handling wallet and money
_____ Turning on lights
_____ Shaking hands
_____ Lifting/carrying pets or children

Traveling
_____ Driving
_____ Opening doors/car doors
_____ Using keys

Recreational Activities
Previous: _____

Current: _____

Vocational Activities
Previous: _____

Current: _____

Comments
_____

_____

KEY:	
√	*Able to complete*
+	*Difficult but able to complete*
—	*Unable to complete*
NA	*Not applicable*

Fig. 19-1. The ADL checklist is one method that can be used to assess the effect injury has had on function.

when needed, instruction in proper posture, body mechanics, and adjustment of work stations and tools, including the use of ergonomic equipment where appropriate. Use of self-management techniques such as stretching and applying ice, as well as regular aerobic exercise are also important.

TREATMENT OUTCOMES

One study describes a program in which all patients undergoing endoscopic release were started on immediate wrist and finger range-of-motion exercises, functional activity as tolerated, and graded strengthening at 2 weeks postoperative. Seventy-six percent of patients returned to preoperative grip strength by 4 weeks, and 85% by 8 weeks. In that group, 57% of the workers' compensation patients returned to work by the eighth postoperative week.[7]

Another group reported a program for therapy following endoscopic release that started on the second postoperative day. The patients were instructed to wear a splint during forceful activity for 3 weeks. They were instructed in a home program and seen for a few visits to follow progress. Patients returning to heavy labor were generally treated for 3 additional weeks. When the results of this group of patients were compared with the results of patients who did not receive therapy, the authors found that preoperative grip strength was regained more quickly and patients returned to work sooner (in an average of 17 days) in the therapy group.[8]

A third study compared the results of open and closed carpal tunnel release. Patients were referred to therapy immediately if undergoing repeat surgery and at 6 weeks if they experienced weakness, stiffness, or scar sensitivity. Eighty-eight percent of patients required therapy. The endoscopic group recovered more quickly, required less therapy, and returned to work sooner than the open group. However, they also had milder preoperative symptoms.[21]

Nathan et al. found that the more frequently a patient was seen for hand therapy, the faster the patient returned to work. Stepwise regression analysis showed that the most important factor in the return to work interval was the number of hand therapy sessions per week, followed by insurance type. Overall, patients who had therapy three sessions per week returned to work 26 days sooner than those who had no therapy.[13]

Porterfield et al. described a postoperative program in which 39% of patients were placed on a work-conditioning program, beginning in the fifth week after surgery. They were treated for an average of 8 weeks. Patients who received work conditioning demonstrated greater improvement in strength (147%) than those who did not receive work conditioning (48%). Seventy-six percent of the patients who received work conditioning returned to work compared to 56% of the patients who did not participate in work conditioning. Fifty-five percent of all the patients in the study returned to their previous job; of these, 71% had received work conditioning.[17]

Only one study was found that reported no difference in range of motion and grip strength of two groups of patients treated with either a home program of warm soaks and range-of-motion exercises or with an aggressive clinical exercise program consisting of progressive resistive exercise and range of motion for 3 weeks.[10]

For many patients, recovery from carpal tunnel surgery proceeds without complication. Most patients have relief from preoperative paresthesias and usually return to work. However, many patients benefit from timely and appropriate postoperative therapy by regaining preoperative status more quickly and returning to work sooner. Therapists need to continue to study the effectiveness of their intervention and the outcomes of treatment.

REFERENCES

1. Agee JM, McCarroll HR, Tortosa RD, et al: Endoscopic release of the carpal tunnel: a randomized prospective multicenter study, *J Hand Surg* 1992; 17A:987.
2. Barber LM: Desensitization of the traumatized hand. In Hunter JM, Schneider LH, Mackin EJ, Callahan AD, eds: *Rehabilitation of the hand,* ed 3, St Louis, 1990, Mosby.
3. Brown MG, Keyser B, Rothenberg ES: Endoscopic carpal tunnel release, *J Hand Surg* 1992; 17A:1009.
4. Brown RA, Gelberman RH, Seiler JG, et al: Carpal tunnel release, a prospective, randomized assessment of open and endoscopic methods, *J Bone Joint Surg* 1993; 75A:1265.
5. Callahan AC: Sensibility assessment: prerequisites and techniques for nerve lesions in continuity and nerve lacerations. In Hunter JM, Schneider LH, Mackin EJ, Callahan AD, eds: *Rehabilitation of the hand,* ed 4, St Louis, 1995, Mosby.
6. Chow JC: Endoscopic release of the carpal ligament for carpal tunnel syndrome: 22-month clinic result, *Arthroscopy* 1990; 6:266.
7. DelaGrange L, Beribak L, DeStefan C, et al: Therapy protocol for endoscopic release of the carpal tunnel, *J Hand Ther* 1993; 6:63.
8. Garren K, Joyce J, Brown LG, Melvin L: Post-operative management of endoscopic carpal tunnel release, *J Hand Ther* 1994; 7:49 (abstract).
9. Gellman H, Kan D, Gee V, Kushner SH: Analysis of pinch and grip strength after carpal tunnel release, *J Hand Surg* 1989; 16A: 863.
10. Groves EJ, Rider BA: A comparison of treatment approaches used after carpal tunnel release surgery, *Am J Occup Ther* 1989; 43:398.
11. Lundborg G: *Nerve injury and repair,* New York, 1988, Churchill Livingstone.
12. Menon J, Etter C: Endoscopic carpal tunnel release—current status, *J Hand Ther* 1993; 6:139.
13. Nathan PA, Meadows KD, Keniston RC: Rehabilitation of carpal tunnel surgery patients using a short surgical incision and an early program of physical therapy, *J Hand Surg* 1993; 18A:1044.
14. Olson JD, Peulen VK, Palmer D, et al: Patient outcomes of Agee-3M versus Chow-Dyonics endoscopic release of the carpal tunnel versus open release (abstract), *J Hand Ther* 1994; 7:44.
15. Omer GE: Median nerve compression at the wrist, *Hand Clin* 1992; 8:317.
16. Pfeffer GB, Gelberman RH, Boyes JH, Rydevik B: The history of carpal tunnel syndrome, *J Hand Surg* 1988; 13B:28.
17. Porterfield M, Loeding L, Feely C: Outcomes of therapy following carpal tunnel release, *J Hand Ther* 1994; 7:46 (abstract).
18. Rydevik B, Lundborg G, Bagge U: Effects of graded compression on intraneural blood flow, *J Hand Surg* 1981; 6:3.

19. Swanson AB, Swanson GdG, Leonard J, Boozer J: Postoperative rehabilitation programs in flexible implant arthroplasty of the digits. In Hunter JM, Schneider LH, Mackin EJ, Callahan AD, eds: *Rehabilitation of the hand,* ed 3, St Louis, 1990, Mosby.

20. Szabo RM: *Nerve compression syndromes, diagnosis and treatment,* Thorofare, NJ, 1989, SLACK.

21. Thompson SI, Wehbe MA: Outcome study of carpal tunnel release, *J Hand Ther* 1994; 7:50 (abstract).

22. Waylett-Rendall J: Desensitization of the traumatized hand. In Hunter JM, Mackin EJ, Callahan AD, eds: *Rehabilitation of the hand,* ed 4, St Louis, 1995, Mosby.

23. Wehbé M, Hunter JM: Flexor tendon gliding in the hand, part I, *J Hand Surg* 1985; 10A:570.

Chapter 20

OUTCOME OF REOPERATION FOR CARPAL TUNNEL SYNDROME

A 20-year perspective

Peter C. Amadio

Surgical division of the flexor retinaculum is a common and successful treatment for carpal tunnel syndrome.[11,16,38,39] Reoperation for persistent or recurrent symptoms is rarely required. This chapter reviews etiology and results of reoperation for carpal tunnel syndrome based on a review of the literature and a retrospective review of a large series of cases.

In general, there are three reasons for reoperation: failure to relieve the initial symptoms, secondary to an incomplete release of the flexor retinaculum[13,15,25,37]; postoperative complications or iatrogenic injury*; and recurrence of symptoms after an initial period of relief.[21,25,41,43,49] Carpal tunnel surgery became common in the 1960s, following the pioneering work of Phalen,[38,39] who spread awareness of carpal tunnel syndrome. The first large series of primary carpal tunnel surgery began appearing at that time, and the first substantial report on reoperation was published in 1972.[25] Langloh and Linscheid reported 34 cases of reoperation, most of which had been referred for treatment after failed primary surgery elsewhere. Based on a small number of failures at their own institution, a 2% to 3% revision rate was estimated. The most common cause of failure was incomplete release of the flexor retinaculum.

Subsequent reports have covered from 2 to 50 patients each.† Although the nature of the reports does not make a true statistical comparison possible, there appears to be a trend of gradually decreasing rates of incomplete release: between 1972 and 1987, 144 patients were reported, and of these 63 had incomplete releases‡; between 1990 and 1993, an additional 137 cases were reported, with only 17 incomplete releases.[4,5,13,37,41-43]

In general, it has been held that patients with incomplete release of the flexor retinaculum are likely to have little or no improvement in symptoms after surgery, and that this sign can be useful to distinguish patients with incomplete release from those with recurrence of disease after adequate release.[6,37] If the initial procedure is done through an incision that makes adequate release of the carpal tunnel unlikely, then reoperation is more likely to be considered. Transverse incisions at the wrist crease, surgery done without the benefit of a bloodless field, and small incisions, in general, have been implicated in this regard.[25,29] However, while patients with incomplete release of the flexor retinaculum may be more likely to have no relief of symptoms following surgery, there are other possible causes of persisting symptoms, including a second site of compression, neuropathy not caused by compression, or incorrect

*References 17, 22, 27, 29, 35, 42, 49.

†References 4, 5, 13, 22, 27, 29, 37, 41-43, 47, 49.
‡References 22, 25, 27, 29, 47, 49.

diagnosis. Metabolic neuropathy may be caused by thyroid disease or diabetes and may not respond to decompression. Focal ischemia caused by small vessel disease of diabetes, lupus, polyarteritis, or some other cause, may mimic carpal tunnel syndrome, or median neuropathy may be the result of an incomplete Parsonage-Turner lesion (brachial plexopathy of unknown cause, usually temporary, and usually associated with pain).[44]

In some cases reoperation is caused by an error of treatment or judgment at the time of the initial procedure. The aphorism of C.H. Mayo to "carry out the two fundamental surgical requirements: see what you are doing and leave a dry field"[33] is still germane. Despite this age-old admonition, iatrogenic injury to the motor branch,[26] palmar cutaneous branch,[18,45] other portions of the median nerve,[34] or other carpal tunnel contents remain reported reasons for reoperation. Technical errors can even injure structures that lie beyond the confines of the carpal tunnel such as the superficial palmar arch,[34] the communicating sensory ramus between the median and ulnar nerves,[32] the ulnar nerve itself,[36,46] or even the ulnar artery. It is hard to understand how such structures could have been injured had the surgeons involved truly seen what they were doing. Befitting this exceptional status, such complications have usually been reported as isolated cases or collections from referral centers,[5,27,29] and not as findings from even large series, with the exception of those where operator experience has been in question.[47] Unfortunately, such injuries have recently been reported with increased frequency, at rates up to 1% or greater, as complications following endoscopic carpal tunnel release.[1,2,24,34] Such iatrogenic injuries appear to be caused by the advent of a new learning curve for surgeons, this time dealing with familiar anatomy in a new way. One hopes that the rates of such injuries will decrease as experience with endoscopic technique increases, and as some more recent reports suggest.

The third reason for reoperation is recurrence of symptoms after a period of initial improvement. The frequency of reoperation in this clinical situation is rather low: The literature would suggest a rate much lower than 1% and perhaps closer to 1 in 1000.[7,47] Symptoms do tend to gradually increase as one follows patients following carpal tunnel surgery.[23] The reason for the recurrence of symptoms is not particularly clear. Patients who have recurrent symptoms rather than persisting symptoms following an initial carpal tunnel procedure are less likely to have had an incomplete release of the flexor retinaculum.[6] In such patients, scarring around the median nerve and subluxation of the median nerve or other carpal tunnel contents are often observed. Hunter has suggested that previous trauma may induce fibrosis and increase the risk of recurrence following carpal tunnel surgery.[21] In a recent review from the Mayo Clinic, patients with a prior history of trauma were more likely to have had scarring noted at the time of reoperation than those patients who did not have a previous history of trauma.[6] Because it is not known how commonly scarring around the median nerve or displacement of carpal tunnel contents occurs in patients who have no symptoms after carpal tunnel surgery, it is hard to tell to what extent such findings are a cause rather than just an associated feature of reoperation surgery.

In some cases it appears that fibrosis around the nerve has developed with tethering and perhaps traction as the main cause for recurrence.[21] In other patients who have had carpal tunnel surgery, symptoms of pain, weakness, and some paresthesias develop after a return to work. In these patients the symptom categories may be the same, but the relative importance has changed: Before the first carpal tunnel release, typically, paresthesias are predominant, while postoperatively in such patients, pain and weakness are more significant.[6] Such symptoms are often called *recurrent carpal tunnel syndrome,* but the etiology may no longer include nerve compression. This is in sharp distinction to the cause of the initial carpal tunnel syndrome, which is almost always caused by compression beneath the flexor retinaculum. Because the etiology of recurrent carpal tunnel syndrome may not be the same as that of primary carpal tunnel syndrome, it may be appropriate to approach recurrent cases differently than one approaches patients with persistent symptoms caused by presumed incomplete release or iatrogenic injury. It may be wise to think of patients with recurrent symptoms not as having a recurrent carpal tunnel syndrome, but as having a postoperative median neuritis or neuropathy for which a cause needs to be identified. In some cases, as mentioned previously, this cause will be caused by fibrosis, ischemia, or traction of the nerve without additional compression. If such is found to be the case, something other than a simple rerelease of the flexor retinaculum may be appropriate to consider. It is for this reason that many surgeons advise not to do reoperations using limited exposure techniques.[5,8,21,27,31] It is appropriate to observe the full length of the median nerve across the area of previous surgery, and it is also helpful to have the patient awake so that they can actively move the fingers and wrists. In this way the surgeon can directly observe whether the nerve is being tethered to the undersurface of the remaining flexor retinaculum or to the adjacent tendons. If tethering does appear to be a significant problem, then an external neurolysis could be considered. If bowstringing or displacement of the nerve or carpal tunnel contents out of the carpal canal is observed, one may need to consider reconstruction of the flexor retinaculum.[43]

The evaluation of the patient presented for treatment of recurrent or persisting carpal tunnel syndrome must be done carefully. In a recent series, 1 in 5 reoperations for carpal tunnel syndrome required a third procedure, or resulted in a very dissatisfied patient.[6] Only one fourth of patients treated by reoperation were completely satisfied with the results of their treatment and had no residual symptoms; clearly the majority are left with some residual morbidity. Patients who present for reoperation are different than those who present for primary treatment of carpal tunnel syndrome, and they deserve a different type of evaluation.

The history should address a number of particular issues. Are the symptoms consistent with median neuropathy? If so, are they consistent with carpal tunnel syndrome? Were the initial symptoms consistent with those diagnoses? Did the symptoms change in intensity, frequency, or character after the first surgical procedure? The onset of symptoms in a new distribution should prompt a search for other etiologies or for iatrogenic injury.

All previous operative reports and electrodiagnostic studies should be reviewed. Presence or absence of certain observations may provide some clues as to potential findings at reoperation, such as partial injury to distal nerve branches.

It should go without saying that the patient's affect and motivation should also be addressed. In some cases there may be a powerful secondary gain operating. The issue may be more one of a mismatch of patient and job than of a recurrent or persistent carpal tunnel syndrome interfering with the patient's ability to perform a reasonable job. In many cases it is more appropriate to treat the patient's environment than it is to reconstruct (or just interfere with) the patient's anatomy.

Physical examination should address all the features one would consider in evaluating primary carpal tunnel syndrome, and, in addition, should always include electrodiagnostic studies. Even if these were done before the first carpal tunnel operation, it is important to document the extent of nerve involvement before reoperation. If the patient's symptoms are not supported by even minor abnormalities on electrodiagnostic studies, it is unlikely that a second operation will succeed where the first one has failed.[6]

Other diagnostic studies, not indicated for the evaluation of primary carpal tunnel surgery, may also be indicated specifically before considering reoperation, especially when the complaint may be more of pain or weakness rather than neurologic dysfunction. A number of series have documented the presence of subluxation of the median nerve or other carpal tunnel contents after carpal tunnel release and have recommended reconstruction of the flexor retinaculum as treatment.[6,22,43] This subluxation can be diagnosed preoperatively on the basis of CT or MRI cross-sectional studies, and these should definitely be considered if subluxation or displacement of the contents of the carpal canal is a possibility. Such imaging studies, particularly MRI, can also assess the flexor retinaculum and determine whether it has been completely released or not.[9,35]

The presence of persisting or recurring symptoms after carpal tunnel surgery is not sufficient reason for a second operation. Symptoms need to be significant, interfering with daily activities, and not responsive to nonoperative modalities such as activity modification, desensitization, nerve gliding exercises, splinting, steroid injections, or oral analgesics. Unless there is evidence of significant iatrogenic

injury, a reasonable period for recovery after the first operation should also be permitted; usually at least 6 months should pass before one seriously considers reoperation in the absence of iatrogenic injury.

When one considers reoperation for carpal tunnel syndrome, the question arises as to whether one should simply do a second carpal tunnel operation, exposing the median nerve in the distal forearm and palm, or whether some other procedure should be considered in association with this. Hunter has emphasized nerve gliding exercises and surgery to facilitate nerve gliding by release of perineurial adhesions.[21] This is certainly something to be considered. If the carpal tunnel contents have been displaced from the carpal canal, reconstruction of the flexor retinaculum should also be considered as an option.[43,48] This may also improve grip strength postoperatively. Although there are some experimental data to support a clinical benefit to internal neurolysis,[30] the clinical studies that have been done suggest that there is little or no benefit to be achieved from this procedure in humans.[12,16,19,20,28] This is to be distinguished from external neurolysis, or surgical mobilization of the nerve, which can be of benefit by decreasing tethering of the nerve and permitting normal nerve gliding.

A number of procedures have been described that transpose healthy vascularized tissue over the median nerve.* The palmaris brevis,[41] abductor digiti minimi,[40] hypothenar fat,[10] pronator quadratus,[14] radial fascia,[7] lumbrical muscle,[7] and synovium[48] have all been tried. Anecdotally, each of these seems to work, but the actual place of these procedures has not been tested in a scientific way, namely, in a randomized prospective clinical trial. Furthermore, these adjunctive measures may have more of a place in the multiply reoperated carpal tunnel than in the carpal tunnel syndrome being reoperated for the first time. As mentioned previously, in many if not most cases, the first reoperation for carpal tunnel syndrome will be addressing issues such as inadequate initial surgery or iatrogenic injury.

In contrast to the relatively low failure rates associated with primary carpal tunnel surgery, failure rates following reoperation for carpal tunnel syndrome have been reported to be as high as 40%.[6] Residual symptoms are common, ranging from 40% to 90%.[6] A number of factors have been found to be of important prognostic value. Short of transverse incisions for the first operation, symptoms that cause nocturnal awakening, symptoms exacerbated by activity, and a positive Phalen's sign all appear to be indicators of a more favorable outcome after reoperation.[6] Patients on workers' compensation, particularly those with normal electrodiagnostic studies, are likely to do worse.[6]

At the Mayo Clinic, from 1965 to 1995, nearly 300 patients have had a second operation for carpal tunnel syndrome and another 60 have had a third, fourth, or fifth operation. A follow-up survey 2 to 20 years postoperatively

*References 3, 7, 10, 14, 41, 48.

was performed on 250 patients who had a second operation. Many of the patients had died, had impaired mental status precluding adequate response to the questionnaire, or had had an additional surgical procedure on their hand, but a total of 116 did complete a standardized questionnaire that surveyed symptoms, functional status, and satisfaction. The results in that series reflect the concerns and observations made previously; the use of internal neurolysis, the presence of a workers' compensation claim, and the absence of abnormality on preoperative electrodiagnostic studies were all associated with poorer outcomes and satisfaction. No particular type of surgical procedure was more likely than another to be associated with improved functional status. In general, adjunctive procedures such as soft tissue flap coverage were not employed in this series, so that issue could not be addressed. As mentioned previously, these may be more relevant considerations for a third, fourth, or fifth reoperation.

The multiply reoperated carpal tunnel patient is probably a separate issue from both initial operation decisions and the decision to go ahead with a second operation. In most cases a second operation is the result of some correctable error that occurred at the time of the first procedure: either an incomplete release or iatrogenic injury. It is unusual for a first operation to fail with recurrent symptoms after an initial period of success. When such is the case, fibrosis around the nerve is often the predominant finding at the time of additional surgery. If fibrosis is found on the first reoperation, it seems reasonable to address it with mobilization of the nerve both surgically and during the postoperative rehabilitation period. If that is not successful and the symptoms recur once again, the surgeon needs to consider whether the problem is indeed amenable to a surgical solution. Recurrent or persistent nerve deficit may well be related to intraneural fibrosis, for which little if anything may be possible without jeopardizing the remaining intact nerve fibers. If pain is the major complaint, and it usually is in such cases, then two options are available to the surgeon. One option would be an additional surgical procedure involving repeat nerve mobilization combined with the introduction of a better vascularized bed around the nerve. This might take the form of a pedicled flap of muscle or even a free tissue transfer. The second alternative would be to manage the nerve pain surgically, using implantable nerve stimulators or related modalities. Finally, at some point the surgeon needs to consider whether multiple operations are in the patient's best interest. As the number of operations increases, the likelihood of success decreases.

Failure of primary carpal tunnel surgery is uncommon. When it does occur, there is a good likelihood that the reason will relate to an error at the time of initial carpal tunnel release: a wrong diagnosis, incomplete release, or iatrogenic nerve injury. Such patients are likely to have improvement after reoperation. The other large group of patients having reoperation are primarily those with symptoms of pain and difficulty returning to work. Such patients are less likely to have a good result from reoperation, particularly if there is a workers' compensation claim pending and if electrodiagnostic studies are normal. The multiply reoperated carpal tunnel patient often has problems with fibrosis within and around the median nerve. Such problems are uncommon but unfortunately are much less amenable to a surgical solution.

REFERENCES

1. Agee JM, McCarroll JR, Tortosa RD, et al: Endoscopic release of the carpal tunnel: a randomized prospective multicenter study, *J Hand Surg* 1992; 17A:987-995.
2. Brown R, Gelberman R, Seiler JG, et al: Carpal tunnel release, *J Bone Joint Surg* 1993; 75A:1265-1275.
3. Albadalejo F, Saura E, Chauarria J, et al: Vascularized ulnar flap for recurrent carpal tunnel syndrome, *Rev Esp Cir Mano* 1992; 19: 27-32.
4. Baranowski VD, Klein W, Grünert J: Revisions-operationen beim Karpaltunnelsyndrom, *Hand Chir Mikrochir Plast Chir* 1993; 25:127-132.
5. Chang R, Dellon AL: Surgical management of recurrent carpal tunnel syndrome, *J Hand Surg* 1993; 18B:467-470.
6. Cobb TK, Amadio PC, Leatherwood DF, et al: Patient outcome after reoperation for carpal tunnel syndrome, *J Hand Surg* 1996; 21A:347-356.
7. Cobb TK, Amadio PC: Reoperation for carpal tunnel syndrome, *Hand Clin* (in press).
8. Cobb TK, Cooney WP: Significance of incomplete release of the distal portion of the flexor retinaculum: implications for endoscopic carpal tunnel surgery, *J Hand Surg* 1994; 19B:283-285.
9. Cobb TK, Daley BK, Posteraro RH, Lewis RC: Establishment of carpal contents/canal ratio by means of magnetic residence imaging, *J Hand Surg* 1992; 17A:843-849.
10. Cramer LM: Local fat coverage for the median nerve, *Correspondence Newsletter* 35, ASSH, 1985.
11. Csuez KA, Thomas JE, Lambert EH, et al: Long-term results of operation for carpal tunnel syndrome, *Mayo Clin Proc* 1966; 41:232-241.
12. Curtis RM, Eversmann WW: Internal neurolysis as an adjunct to the treatment of the carpal tunnel syndrome, *J Bone Joint Surg* 1973; 55A:733-740.
13. De Smet L: Recurrent carpal tunnel syndrome: clinical testing indicating incomplete section of the flexor retinaculum, *J Hand Surg* 1993; 18B:189.
14. Dellon AL, Mackinnon SE: The transposition of the pronator quadratus, *J Hand Surg* 1984; 9:423-427.
15. Eason SY, Belsole RJ, Greene T: Carpal tunnel release: analysis of suboptimal results, *J Hand Surg* 1985; 10B:365-369.
16. Gelberman RH, Pfeffer GB, Galbraith RT, et al: Results of treatment of severe carpal tunnel syndrome without internal neurolysis of the median nerve, *J Bone Joint Surg* 1987; 69A:896-903.
17. Hanssen AD, Amadio PC, DeSilva SP, et al: Deep postoperative wound infection after carpal tunnel release, *J Hand Surg* 1989; 14A:869-873.
18. Hobbs RA, Magnussen PA, Tonkin MA: Palmar cutaneous branch of the median nerve, *J Hand Surg* 1990; 15A:38-43.
19. Holmgren H, Rabow L: Internal neurolysis or ligament division only in carpal tunnel syndrome II. A three-year followup with an evaluation of various neurophysiological parameters for diagnosis, *Acta Neurochir* 1987; 87:44-47.
20. Holmgren-Larsson H, Liezeniewski W, Linden U, et al: Internal neurolysis or ligament division only in carpal tunnel syndrome—results of a randomized study, *Acta Neurochir* 1985; 74:118-121.

21. Hunter JM: Recurrent carpal tunnel syndrome, epineural fibrosis fixation, and traction neuropathy, *Hand Clin* 1991; 7:491-504.

22. Inglis AE: Two unusual operative complications in the carpal-tunnel syndrome, *J Bone Joint Surg* 1980; 62A:1208-1209.

23. Katz JN, Gelberman RH, Wright EA, et al: Responsiveness of self-reported and objective measures of disease severity in carpal tunnel syndrome, *Medical Care* 1994; 32:1127-1133.

24. Kelly CP, Pulisetti D, Jamieson AM: Early experience with endoscopic carpal tunnel release, *J Hand Surg* 1994; 19B:18-21.

25. Langloh ND, Linscheid RL: Recurrent and unrelieved carpal tunnel syndrome, *Clin Orthop* 1972; 83:41-47.

26. Lilly CJ, Magnelli TD: Severance of the thenar branch of the median nerve as a complication of carpal tunnel release, *J Hand Surg* 1985; 10A:399-402.

27. Louis DS, Greene TL, Noellert RC: Complications of carpal tunnel surgery, *J Neurosurg* 1985; 62:352-356.

28. Lowry WE, Follender AB: Interfascicular neurolysis in the severe carpal tunnel syndrome: a prospective randomized double-blind controlled study, *Clin Orthop* 1988; 227:251-254.

29. MacDonald RI, Lichtman DM, Hanlon JJ, et al: Complications of surgical release for carpal tunnel syndrome, *J Hand Surg* 1978; 3:70-76.

30. MacKinnon SE: Secondary carpal tunnel surgery, *Neurosurg Clin North Am* 1991; 2:75-91.

31. MacKinnon SE, O'Brien JP, Dellon AL, et al: An assessment of the effects of internal neurolysis on a chronically compressed rat sciatic nerve, *Plast Reconstr Surg* 1988; 81:251-256.

32. May JW Jr, Rosen H: Division of the sensory ramus communicans between the ulnar and median nerves: a complication following carpal tunnel release, *J Bone Joint Surg* 1981; 63A:836-838.

33. Mayo CH: Splenomegaly, *Collected Papers of Mayo Clinic and Mayo Foundation* 1935; 27:555-566.

34. Murphy RX Jr, Jennings JF, Wukich DK: Major neurovascular complications of endoscopic carpal tunnel release, *J Hand Surg* 1994; 19A:114-118.

35. Murphy RX Jr, Chernofsky MA, Osborne MA, et al: Magnetic resonance imaging in the evaluation of persistent carpal tunnel syndrome, *J Hand Surg* 1993; 18A:113-120.

36. Nath RK, Mackinnon SE, Weeks PM: Ulnar nerve transection as a complication of two-portal endoscopic carpal tunnel release: a case report, *J Hand Surg* 1993; 18A:896-898.

37. O'Malley MJ, Evanoff M, Terrono AL, et al: Factors that determine re-exploration treatment of carpal tunnel syndrome, *J Hand Surg* 1992; 17A:638-641.

38. Phalen GS: Carpal tunnel syndrome: clinical evaluation of 598 hands, *Clin Orthop* 1972; 83:29-40.

39. Phalen GS: The carpal tunnel syndrome: seventeen years' experience in diagnosis and treatment of six hundred fifty-four hands, *J Bone Joint Surg* 1966; 48A:211-215.

40. Reisman NR, Dellon AL: The transposition of the abductor digiti minimi, *J Plast Reconstr Surg* 1983; 72:859-865.

41. Rose EH, Norris MS, Kowalski TA, et al: Palmaris brevis turnover flap as an adjunct to internal neurolysis of the chronically scarred median nerve in recurrent carpal tunnel syndrome, *J Hand Surg* 1991; 16A:191-201.

42. Roullet J, Morin A: Syndrome du canal carpien: plaidoyer pour un protocole opératoire: a propose de 29 réinterventions chirurgicales, *Lyon Chir* 1988; 84:54-57.

43. Sennwald G, Hagen K: La décompression du tunnel carpien: a propos de 16 reprises, *Schweiz med Wschr* 1990; 120:931-935.

44. Spinner RJ, Bachman JW, Amadio PC: The many faces of carpal tunnel syndrome, *Mayo Clinic Proc* 1989; 64:829-836.

45. Taleisnik J: The palmar cutaneous branch of the median nerve and the approach to the carpal tunnel, *J Bone Joint Surg* 1973; 55A:1212-1217.

46. Terrono AL, Belsky MR, Feldo PG, et al: Injury to the deep motor branch of the ulnar nerve during carpal tunnel release, *J Hand Surg* 1993; 18A:1038-1040.

47. Wadstroem J, Nigst H: Reoperation for carpal tunnel syndrome: a retrospective analysis of forty cases, *Ann Chir Main* 1986; 5: 54-58.

48. Wulle C: Die Synoviallappenplastik beim Rezidiv eine Medianus-Kompressions-Syndroms, *Plastische Chirurgie* 1980; 4:266-271.

49. Wulle C: Treatment of recurrence of the carpal tunnel syndrome, *Ann Chir Main* 1987; 6:203-209.

Chapter 21

CARPAL TUNNEL NEUROPATHY CAUSED BY INJURY

Reconstruction of the transverse carpal ligament for the complex carpal tunnel syndromes*

James M. Hunter
Richard L. Read
Richard Gray

To be privileged to treat the most important sensibility-endowed nerve, the median nerve, perhaps we should think like the respected conservationist Aldo Leopold, who left his mark on ecology while editor of *A Sand Country Almanac*. Before his death in 1944, Leopold formulated a deceptively simple rule for deciding whether something is good or bad for the land. "A good thing is right," he reasoned, "when it tends to preserve the integrity, stability and beauty of the biologic community. It is wrong when it tends otherwise."

Surgery for carpal tunnel syndrome (CTS) is being done more frequently than at any time in the past, and the numbers of unsatisfactory results appear to be on the increase. Rephrased, the "Aldo Leopold Rule" could be applied to hand surgery and therapy for the median nerve. A treatment is right for the hand if it tends to preserve the integrity and stability of the biologic median nerve. It is wrong if it tends otherwise.

Papers published through the 1950s, '60s, and '70s reported that the simple carpal tunnel release surgery

corrected all but the "severe type of carpal tunnel syndrome."[1,2,6,9,12–16] The simple carpal tunnel release was widely employed as the ideal solution to CTS in the 1970s and '80s. The basis of surgical treatment was that the median nerve was compressed in a tight canal and that surgical release of the transverse carpal ligament (TCL) relieved the pressure and corrected the problem. It seemed from most reports that practically all patients returned to work, and there were few indicators to suggest that patients with work related CTSs did not have good work performance after surgery.

Since the early 1980s, occupational repetitive motion injuries have seen an increase of epidemic proportion. Between 1981 and 1992, these injuries have increased from 18% to 56% of all occupational illnesses.[1,2,6] Because of a number of demographic and sociologic factors, the problem is expected to worsen during the current decade.

Carpal tunnel syndrome accounts for much of the increased incidence in repetitive trauma injuries. While surgery is successful in palliating some of the symptoms of the syndrome, it is rarely successful in returning patients to their previous levels of repetitive activity. Prevention is a key consideration to reverse this epidemic.[1,2,6]

*From Hunter JM, Read RL, Gray R: Carpal tunnel neuropathy caused by injury: reconstruction of the transverse carpal ligament for complex carpal tunnel syndromes, *J Hand Ther* 1993; 6:145-151.

When prevention fails, one must make an exacting diagnosis and then apply the proper surgical treatment to the specific median nerve problem. Unless we can differentiate alternate median nerve diagnoses, such as traction neuropathy,[4] from simple nerve compression, and apply effective nerve mobilization and nerve gliding techniques, carpal tunnel release failures will continue to plague both surgeons and therapists.

CARPAL TUNNEL SYNDROME AND DIFFERENTIAL DIAGNOSIS

There are new traumatic and work-related problems in addition to repetitive trauma that affect the peripheral nerves in the upper extremity that were not prevalent before the 1980s. To name the most obvious: the high velocity motor vehicle accident with a seatbelted driver, the use of the computer keyboard, and, finally, the shift of women to the workplace, now reported as developing CTS five to one over men.[5]

Patients are frequently seen at the Philadelphia Hand Center who have other neuropathies in the same extremity in addition to CTS, such as ulnar nerve cubital tunnel and radial nerve dorsal tunnel syndromes. These neuropathies are also being diagnosed more frequently in combination with the brachial plexus traction injury syndrome. However, to identify these neuropathies, one must have a dedicated electrodiagnostic study program available. Unfortunately, this does not prevail throughout all areas of management of hand and upper extremity problems. There are still physicians who do not order electromyography (EMG) for suspected CTS because they feel that it is costly to the patient and really not necessary in order to make the diagnosis. How wrong they must be at times when the symptoms of CTS become confused with those of a brachial plexus, C6-C7 upper trunk lateral cord neuropathy. The increasing number of brachial plexus traction injuries[13] suggests that we should require many patients with injury histories being considered for the diagnosis of CTS to have routine EMG and nerve conduction velocity (NCV) tests. These tests should include Erb's point brachial plexus screening tests and stress testing of the median nerve, as well as a complete sensibility study in therapy.

A SUGGESTED CLASSIFICATION OF CARPAL TUNNEL SYNDROMES

The following is a suggested division of CTS into three classes based on the degree of severity of the disease.
- *Class I*—The simple or typical CTS, which includes classical history, physical, and EMG/NCV findings.
- *Class II*—The complex CTS, found in a patient with a history of injury to the involved extremity and possibly other neuropathies in the same extremity. Positive EMG/NCV tests and special clinical nerve traction tests such as the Tanzer test, the Hunter test,[4,16] and the reverse Phalen's test may be found. Phalen's classical test may be negative.

This situation represents a nerve that has undergone fibrous fixation within the carpal canal and has developed a traction neuropathy from the stretching forces of joint movements applied to a now inelastic, fixed epineurium (Fig. 21-1 and Fig. 21-2).
- *Class III*—The compound median neuropathy in which traditional carpal tunnel surgery has failed and the problem is now a recurrent median neuropathy. Symptoms and EMG/NCV testing results are variable as patients reduce hand, wrist, and forearm function to protect against painful experiences with hand use. Accordingly, stress nerve conduction tests may be particularly helpful in further identifying these (traction) neuropathies. These cases represent a median nerve entrapped in the scar of wound healing after release of the TCL (Fig. 21-3). These conditions may also have led to the development of other neuropathies through compensatory misuse, entrapment of the ulnar or radial nerves, and an associated brachial plexus traction neuropathy.[4,13]

CLINICAL CORRELATION WITH EMG MOTOR AND SENSORY STRESS TESTING

All patients having a carpal tunnel neuropathy in this Philadelphia Hand Center series (300 patients) are evaluated by standardized nerve conduction and EMG testing.[7,8] These techniques are used to measure sensory and motor conduction time for the median nerve across the carpal tunnel. The same nerve conduction testing principles are applied to other peripheral nerves in the extremity to assist in ruling out radial, ulnar, and brachial plexus neuropathies.

Patients with clinical signs of carpal tunnel neuropathy caused by injury have, at times, shown normal or marginal positive motor and sensory conductions across the wrist, despite significant clinical findings and reduced work tolerance. Frustration and pondering over this problem have resulted in the median nerve traction tests described. Patients chosen for stress testing are first tested for routine and stress position baseline motor amplitude results (Fig. 21-4, *A*). A second test is repeated after 10 minutes of therapy putty gripping. Those patients who have musical instrument problems bring their instruments to the Hand Center for brief or extended practice sessions before stress testing.

The motor rather than sensory response was chosen for testing because of more secure recording electrode placement during hand grip activity.

Median motor nerve stress testing, when positive (Fig. 21-4, *B*), has shown a correlation with the patient's clinical history and examination. These results have been helpful in formulating the three classifications of CTS and the comprehensive treatment program for specific nerve pathology.

The motor nerve conduction stress testing study is part of an ongoing carpal tunnel research program at the Hand Center that will be reported in the future.

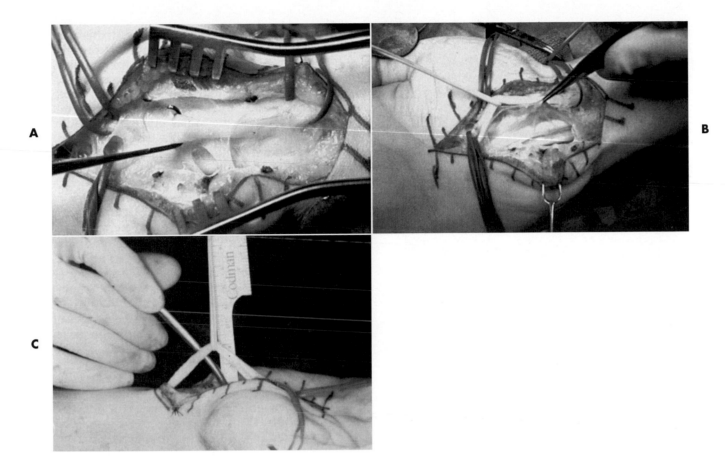

Fig. 21-1. Surgery for class II or complex carpal tunnel syndrome. The patient is a 31-year-old registered nurse with a history of motor vehicle accident in 1989. **A,** the transverse carpal ligament is opened and its corners and the hamate are marked with methylene blue. The fingers are to the left side of the illustration, and a small smooth retractor under the median nerve shows minimal elevation of the nerve due to fibrous fixations: premobilization. The median nerve is tethered to the sheaths of the flexor tendons and the wall of the carpal canal. **B,** the nerve after mobilizing mesoepineurolysis. The fibrous sheet is attached to the radial wall and the flexor sheath, encasing the median nerve. It is held on display by the forceps. (The histology of this sheet is shown in Fig. 21-2). **C,** the median nerve is elevated for vector measurements. Neutral wrist measurements show that the nerve is suspended 4.2 cm from the floor of the carpal canal at the level of the hamate, increases to 7.0 cm with wrist flexion, and decreases to 1.8 cm with wrist extension. The vascular refill of the vasonevorium on tourniquet release was 12 seconds.

CARPAL TUNNEL SURGERY COMPLICATIONS

While open carpal tunnel release or closed carpal tunnel release (endoscopic method) may be a good rule for routine CTS, it may not necessarily be good for class II CTS caused by injury or repetitive work.

In class II (see Figs. 21-1 and 21-2) CTS, the median nerve is restricted from gliding by posttraumatic epineural fibrous fixations to the flexor tendon sheaths and the wall of the carpal canal. Leaving the TCL open at surgery may weaken the hand by the bowstring effect of the flexor tendons during wrist and digit flexion,[3] widening the carpal arch, thus shortening the resting length of the thenar and hypothenar muscles. These anatomic changes reduce the excursion and contractile forces of both the extrinsic and intrinsic muscles. Magnetic resonance imaging (MRI) studies have documented volar migration of the median nerve and flexor tendons after release of the TCL.[9] Median nerve axon irritability, caused by scar entrapment and traction from wrist and digital motion, becomes painful, reducing the strength of grip and prehension.

The symptoms of a recurrent median neuropathy usually become present 6 to 9 weeks after surgery. Patients with compound or class III CTS become progressively disabled in the months that follow (see Fig. 21-3). The good rule of integrity and stability of the median nerve, now broken, may invite other neuropathies, reflex sympathetic dystrophy, and the shoulder-hand syndrome.

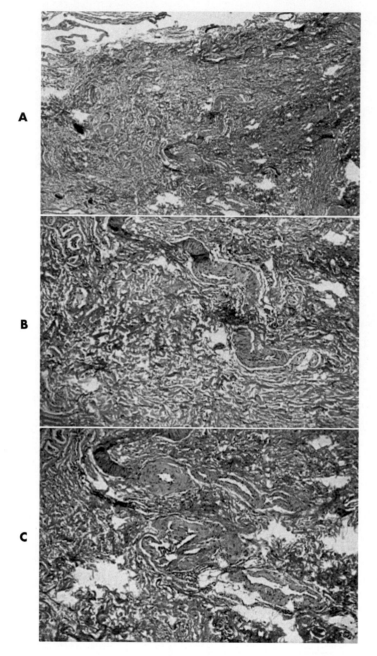

Fig. 21-2. Class II median neuropathy: typical history of epineural fibrous fixation (Fig. 21-1, *B*) under increasing magnification (from **A** to **C**). Benign fibrovascular and fibroadipose tissue with hyalinosis and chronic inflammation is present.

CLINICAL EVALUATION AND DIFFERENTIAL EMG TESTING FOR CLASS II CTS

All patients who had CTS in this series of 300 were studied by electrodiagnostic and sensibility techniques preoperatively. These patients received a clinical evaluation that included routine functional strength and sensory assess-

ments, plus stress testing for median nerve fibrous fixation, and traction neuropathy.

Three tests have become especially useful in the diagnosis of the complex (class II) CTS.
1. The wrist-finger hyperextension–forearm supination test
2. The low lateral arm external rotation (Hunter) test[16]
3. The hand grip-wrist flexion (Tanzer) test.

The *wrist and finger extension test* is similar to a reverse Phalen's test. To perform it as a traction test, pressure is exerted against the thumb and the index and middle fingers, with the wrist and forearm in supination. The site of tenderness along the nerve represents the location of nerve-deforming stress, with irritation of the nerve axonal tree. Nerve pressure sensitivity can be elicited anywhere from the wrist crease to the pronator teres level, depending on the degree and length of median nerve entrapment. Release of wrist and finger traction immediately ceases the painful irritation of the median nerve. Physicians and therapists will also note that traction neuropathy patients often prefer forearm pronation, with palms on the thigh for resting comfort. This protective position, unfortunately, begins to promote other neuropathies and a nerve-disabled limb.

The *low lateral arm abduction (Hunter) test*[16] is helpful when a more proximal neuropathy in the brachial plexus is suspected. It is performed with the arm externally rotated and abducted about 40° from the thigh. Gentle traction is accomplished by progressive wrist dorsiflexion. This position can produce painful paresthesias from C6-C7 roots over the upper trunk of the brachial plexus, then over the volar forearm, to the palm passing on the radial side of the middle finger (Schwartzman's sign).[13] This test has the potential of overriding the local conduction of the median nerve at the wrist.

The *simultaneous hand grip-wrist flexion (Tanzer) test* is the most sensitive clinical and nerve conduction stress test that helps define class II CTS. Dr. Radford Tanzer, a hand surgeon from Hanover, New Hampshire, writing in the *Journal of Bone and Joint Surgery* and *Clinical Orthopaedics*[14,15] in 1959, called attention to the problem of work failure and CTS. His research and description of this problem deserve recognition, and these are some of his comments from 1959 publications:

"One factor has failed to command the attention of virtually all writers dealing with the clinical aspects of the subject [CTS], the compressive effect on the median nerve produced by the simultaneous act of forceful flexion of the wrist and forceful grip of the fingers. The observation is based on a simple anatomic concept. When the fingers are flexed with the wrist in extension, the flexor tendons are squeezed against the posterior wall of the carpal tunnel; on the other hand, flexion of the fingers with the wrist flexed compresses the median nerve between the tight flexor tendons within the carpal canal and the transverse carpal ligament, with a force proportional to the degree of grip of the digits.''

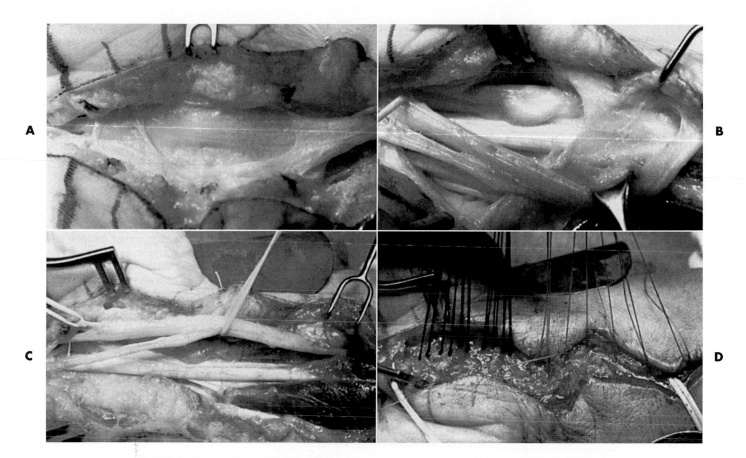

Fig. 21-3. Surgery for a 44-year-old graphic designer and schoolteacher who had previously undergone a carpal tunnel release. Because of persistent pain, a second operation for median neurolysis without ligament closure was completed one year ago. The patient, now with a class III carpal tunnel problem, is incapacitated with pain. He has been on limited duty as a schoolteacher for two years. The mildly positive electromyography/nerve conduction velocity test results are typical as the patient uses the hand and wrist minimally because of pain. **A,** With the ligament open, the corners of the transverse carpal ligament (TCL) and hamate are marked. The connective tissue surrounding the median nerve is dense and the nerve is fixed for a distance of 4 inches to the walls of the carpal canal and the fibrous flexor tendon sheaths. **B,** The median nerve, partially mobilized, reveals a fibrous sheet fixed to the radial wall of the carpal canal and the sheath of the flexor tendons at the wrist. **C,** All epineural fibrous tissue has been removed and the nerve is suspended in a rubber vessel loop. The fingers are to the left in the illustration. **D,** Anatomic reconstruction of the TCL for a recurrent median neuropathy is completed. The TCL is closed with 10 double 2-O Ethibond sutures and the antebrachial fascia is closed with six 3-O Vicryl sutures. Vascular recovery of the median nerve before TCL closure was 30 seconds. Three days postoperatively, with the nerve gliding program under way, the patient wrote a thank you note. "I am obliged to you—this is the first time I have been without pain in 2 years." Improvement continues 6 months later.

Dr. Tanzer related his experience to the reports of the frequency of CTS among patients who had a history of change to a new occupation or new avocation that required forceful grip and wrist flexion movements repeatedly. He expressed concern with hand weakness after TCL release and discussed a method he used in surgery to partly reform the divided ligament. He passed a wire suture through the long thenar muscle leaf of the TCL to a pullout button on the hypothenar eminence. This wire was removed at 4 weeks. It is important to bear in mind the philosophy of Dr. Tanzer in

the 1950s as we seek better solutions to CTS problems in the 1990s.

Dr. George Phalen wrote in 1970[11] about his 21-year experience with CTS: "The etiology of carpal tunnel syndrome has not yet been fully determined. I still believe the thickening or fibrosis of the flexor tendon synovium within the carpal tunnel is the most common cause of the syndrome." His series of histologic biopsies of the flexor tendon synovium showed either chronic inflammation or chronic fibrosis in 80% of the specimens studied. These

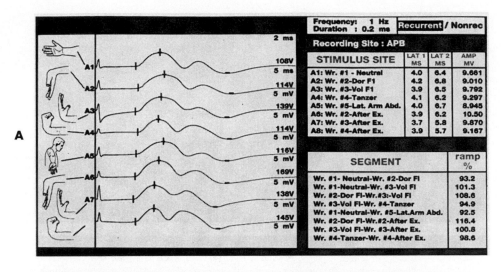

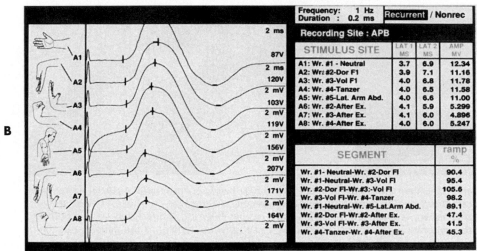

Fig. 21-4. A, Normal responses in all eight positions. **B,** Significant reduction of amplitudes in positions 6, 7, and 8 are interpreted to indicate postexercise intracompartmental median nerve compromise at the wrist, causing an activity-induced neurapraxia relative to the preexercise responses.

thoughts demonstrate Dr. Phalen's concerns about the role of the changing flexor tendon synovium in CTS. This appears to be an early description of the complex CTS that is destined to complicate the future results of simple release surgery for CTS. The course of complex carpal tunnel neuropathy is nerve entrapment.

THE RATIONALE FOR COMPREHENSIVE MOBILIZATION OF THE MEDIAN NERVE

The observations of Tanzer,[14] Phalen,[11] and Kline et al.[9] add support to mobilization of the median nerve in the hand, wrist, and forearm as a basis for closure of the flexor retinaculum of the wrist.[10,17] The normal position of the median nerve in the carpal canal is to the radial side and 1.5 to 1.8 cm above the floor. The uninjured median nerve is suspended by delicate sheets of connective tissue that

emanate from the flexor tendon ulnar and radial bursal sheaths of the fingers and thumb (clinical research done with Cmdr. Gordon Iimes, U.S. Naval Hospital, Portsmouth, Virginia). Posttraumatic synovitis and sheath remodeling convert the perineural connective tissues into fibrotic, mesoepineural thickenings that restrict longitudinal gliding of the median nerve trunk (see Figs. 21-1, *B* and 21-2). In a recurrent class III median neuropathy postoperative volar migration of the median nerve into the healing flaps of the released TCL leads to scar entrapment, the painful palm and traction neuropathy.

SURGERY FOR COMPLEX CLASS II AND COMPOUND CLASS III CTS

The senior author's goal in developing a new method of management was originally for the professional musician, artist, and heavy-duty worker, and later for the patient with a history of injury and multiple neuropathies. These patients after study were predicted to develop a weaker hand after routine surgical release of the TCL.

The brief description below acquaints the reader with the surgical approach that has been applied in over 300 consecutive cases of CTS, classes I, II, and III, seen at the Philadelphia Hand Center. Forty-two cases are considered simple or class I CTS, 94 are considered class III or recurrent carpal tunnel problems, and the remainder are, in the author's opinion, complex or class II CTSs with significant epineural fibrous fixations.

PROCEDURE

The skin incision is a gently curving line from the distal palmar crease to the first transverse crease of the wrist. The incision then makes two 60° angles and includes the antebrachial fascia, to end 1 inch proximal to the wrist crease with a triangular, radial base flap (see Fig. 21-1, *B*). The length of the incision is between 3½ and 4 inches. This length gives an ample exposure of the terminal median nerve and provides a consistent vector base for angular test measurements of the median nerve during mobilization (see Fig. 21-1, *C*). The median nerve trunk is identified and protected at the wrist while the sensory branches to the index and middle finger are isolated in the palm. A large curved Kelly hemostat is passed from distal to proximal under the TCL, over the superficial arterial palmar arch, at a radial angle of 30°. As the instrument passes the hook of the hamate, it is then straightlined against the hook to arrive along the ulnar border of the median nerve. If there are adhesions on the nerve blocking instrument passage, it should be repassed on a deeper plain. The instrument is held against the hamate in a straight line. The TCL is opened on the surface of the Kelly hemostat. It is important that all sensory branches be beneath the instrument. After the TCL is incised, the corners are marked for closure with methylene blue, and prior to mobilization (see Fig. 21-1, *A*), the median nerve excursion is ascertained by longitudinal and vector measurements (see Figs. 21-1, *B* and 21-3, *C*). Comprehensive mobilization of the median nerve results from a complete circumferential mesoepineurolysis in the palm, wrist, and distal forearm. This procedure was first described in an earlier publication.[4] The longitudinal excursion of the median nerve, in relation to the proximal border of the hamate, is measured proximal to distal and distal to proximal before and after mobilization (see Figs. 21-1, *C* and 21-3, *C*). The angular vector of the median nerve is carried out with the wrist in neutral, flexion, and extension by elevating the nerve with a small smooth retractor and measuring the vertical distance at the base of the hamate to the posterior wall of the canal (see Fig. 21-1, *B* and *C*). These measurements are also recorded before and after mobilization. The preliminary results of these measurements were previously presented in 1991 for 40 cases[9,11] and have not changed significantly as the number of cases has increased to over 300 in 1993.

Opening the entire length of the volar carpal ligament over the loge de Guyon permits protective visualization of the ulnar nerve and artery. Importantly, opening the volar carpal ligament permits the ulnar border of the TCL to lengthen 6 to 8 mm. This allows an easier closure of the TCL. The antebrachial fascia proximal to the TCL is closed separately with figure-of-8 Vicryl sutures, restoring synovial-like gliding surface for the median nerve proximal to the stress edge of the restored TCL. Following skin closure, a soft pressure dressing is applied, permitting finger-wrist motion. No splint or cast is used in the early postoperative period.

This technique, when completed, provides a restored gliding flexor retinaculum for movement and gliding of the delicate median nerve and the powerful flexor tendons of the hand.[3]

The final benefits of the procedure, complete mobilization of the median nerve and anatomic restoration of the TCL, are realized by postoperative patients who show improved precision and fist grip strengths in work therapy programs.

CONCLUSION

A new program for surgical and therapy management of CTS neuropathies has been discussed. It requires a comprehensive mobilization or a circumferential meso-epineurolysis of the median nerve in the palm, wrist, and forearm combined with a complete anatomic restoration of the TCL and antebrachial fascia over the median nerve. This is followed by immediate gliding of the median nerve and the flexor tendon system in a structured hand therapy program.

The review of results, after three years, offers the promise of consistent improvement in nerve and hand function. Class I or simple CTS generally has an acceptable outcome regardless of surgical techniques, provided that heavy workloads or demands are not in the rehabilitation picture. Patients who have problematic class II CTS or failed carpal tunnel median neuropathy class III are likely to do poorly with a simple surgical release. These patients will benefit significantly from the previously described comprehensive surgery and therapy management program.

REFERENCES

1. Delgrosso I, Boillat MA: Carpal tunnel syndrome: role of occupation, *Int Arch Occup Environ Health* 1991; 63(4):267-270.
2. Franklin GM, Haug J, Heyer N, et al: Occupational carpal tunnel syndrome in Washington State, 1984-1988, *Am J Public Health* 1991; 81(6):741-746.
3. Grant J, Boileau C: The flexor retinaculum. In *A method of anatomy*, Baltimore, 1948, Williams & Wilkins.
4. Hunter JM: Recurrent carpal tunnel syndrome, epineural fibrous fixation and traction neuropathy, *Hand Clin* 1991; 7:491-504.
5. *Proceedings of the annual meeting of the International Federation of Societies for Surgery of the Hand*, Paris, France, May 1992.

6. Jaeger SH, Spitz LK, Powell M, et al: Personal communication, 1992.

7. Johnson E: *Practical electromyography,* Baltimore, 1980, Williams & Wilkins.

8. Kimura J: *Electrodiagnosis in diseases of nerve and muscle,* Philadelphia, 1983, F. A. Davis.

9. Kline SC, Beach V, Moore JR: The transverse carpal ligament, *J Bone Joint Surg* 1992; 24A:1478-1485.

10. Millesi H, Zoch G, Rath T: The gliding apparatus of peripheral nerve and its clinical significance, *Ann Hand Surg* 1990; 9:87-97.

11. Phalen GS: Reflections on 21 years' experience with the carpal tunnel syndrome, *JAMA* 1970; 212:1365-1367.

12. Read RL: Stress testing in nerve compression, *Hand Clin* 1991; 7:521-526.

13. Schwartzman RJ: Brachial plexus traction injuries, *Hand Clin* 1991; 7:547-557.

14. Tanzer RC: The carpal tunnel syndrome: a clinical and anatomical study, *J Bone Joint Surg* 1959; 41A:626-634.

15. Tanzer RC: The carpal tunnel syndrome, *Clin Orthop* 1959; 15:171-179.

16. Totten PA, Hunter JM: Therapeutic techniques to enhance nerve gliding in thoracic outlet syndrome and carpal tunnel syndrome, *Hand Clin* 1991; 7:505-520.

17. Wilgis EFS, Murphy R. The significance of longitudinal excursion in peripheral nerves, *Hand Clin* 1987; 2:761-766.

Chapter 22

ULNAR NERVE ENTRAPMENT AT THE ELBOW

Eric R. George
Robert Lee Wilson

The ulnar nerve is vulnerable to compression as it courses around the medial aspect of the elbow. Nerve entrapment can occur secondary to direct compression, traction, scar fixation, or a combination of these factors. Surgical treatment of this entity should not be considered without careful clinical assessment, and in many instances, conservative treatment is the mainstay. This chapter reviews the historical background and carefully looks at the anatomy and pathophysiology as well as the clinical presentation and differential diagnosis of ulnar nerve compression. Various treatment options will be considered, including the indications and contraindications for each. Surgical techniques for two of the more common procedures, anterior subcutaneous transposition and submuscular transposition, are detailed, including postoperative management. The complications of operating on the ulnar nerve at the elbow are analyzed, as well as the results of surgical treatment.

HISTORY

When reviewing the history of ulnar nerve compression at the elbow, it is apparent that despite more than 100 years of clinical experience, there still remains only a personal bias for choosing one surgical technique over another. As early as 1816, Earle treated ulnar neuritis by resecting a portion of the ulnar nerve.[24] This led to the subsequent sequelae of loss of motor function and a sensory deficit.

In 1878 Panas reported on several patients with ulnar nerve compression secondary to fractures at the elbow.[24] These injuries led to bony irregularities in the condylar groove. Over the next 40 years, because of the role of trauma and the often delayed appearance of the nerve compression, the clinical syndrome became known as *posttraumatic ulnar neuritis* or *tardy ulnar palsy*. Platt reported that the mechanism of injury concerned a downward and outward stretch of the ulnar nerve.[67] Such trauma could occur with supracondylar humeral fractures, as well as with fractures through the medial humeral epicondyle. This raises the question of whether the injury occurred at the time of the trauma or was a secondary event (i.e., tardy ulnar palsy). While trauma was a recognized cause of entrapment, a small number of cases also remained for which no explanation could be determined. This type of trauma became known as the *idiopathic ulnar neuritis*.[24] Platt described an anterior intramuscular transposition for the treatment of ulnar nerve compression.[67]

In 1897 Roux of Lausanne described the first subcutaneous transpositions.[15] These were performed in heavy manual laborers, with significant callus formation about the olecranon process and cubital tunnel, thus requiring transposition of the ulnar nerve to an external position. Broca, as well as Guilleman, performed a technique to deepen the posterior condylar groove. However, this procedure was discarded when it was realized that the nerve failed to recover because of recurrent involvement with proliferative scar formation.[24]

In 1898 Curtis described a patient whose ulnar nerve was found to lay on the exposed surface of the postcondylar groove. He reported an excellent result when the nerve was placed in a more protected position.[14] In 1918 Adson described the first neurolysis for adhesions of the ulnar nerve. This included longitudinal splitting of the epineurium and perineurium in several places about the nerve's circumference.[2]

Other important techniques include Learmonth's anterior submuscular transposition in 1942.[48] Morgan and King, in 1950, presented medial epicondylectomy as a treatment of ulnar nerve compression.[44,45] Osborn, in 1957, reported his experience with a thick fibrous band running between the two heads of the flexor carpi ulnaris (FCU) as a cause of ulnar nerve compression.[63] This band, which is now known as Osborn's ligament, was originally described by Feindel and Stratford, who also coined the term *cubital tunnel syndrome*.[31] With the multiple procedures and variations in technique that have been developed, it is paramount to grasp the historical background of the condition before selecting the appropriate surgical technique to use in its treatment.

ANATOMY AND BIOMECHANICS

The ulnar nerve arises from the medial cord of the brachial plexus and contains sensory and motor fibers from the C8 and T1 nerve roots. As the nerve courses distally toward the elbow, it is accompanied by the superior ulnar collateral vessels. When it approaches the elbow, it is surrounded by the triceps muscle on its medial side and the humerus on the lateral aspect. Posteriorly, it lies in close proximity to the medial head of the triceps. Anteriorly, it is covered by the fascia that stretches from the triceps to the medial intermuscular septum. Progressing distally, the ulnar nerve then passes behind the medial humeral epicondyle, which covers it superiorly and laterally as it lies on the postcondylar groove of the olecranon. The roof of the cubital tunnel is the arcuate ligament, which is continuous with the FCU aponeurosis. The ulnar nerve then passes between the two heads of the FCU and proceeds distally.[24]

The cubital tunnel has been variably described as limited to the region between the two heads of the FCU and as extensive as its passage from the posterior compartment of the upper arm to its entrance into the flexor pronator muscle group in the forearm.[24] Currently, the cubital tunnel is referred to as the area with a fascial covering beginning proximally at the level of the medial epicondyle and olecranon and extending distally to the two heads of the FCU.

The biomechanics of the cubital tunnel, including compartment pressure, volume, and nerve dimensions, have been extensively studied.[4,21,65,75] Pressure within the tunnel is increased threefold with elbow flexion, wrist extension, and shoulder elevation in the anterior direction. Fronek also showed a sixfold increase in tunnel pressure when the hands are placed behind the head. It has been shown that with flexion of the elbow, the cubital tunnel decreases in volume as the roof of the tunnel becomes stretched. Sunderland demonstrated that the motor fibers to the intrinsic muscles were situated anteriorly and medially, and the sensory fibers were positioned superficial but more posteriorly. He also observed that the motor branches to the FCU and the flexor digitorum profundus (FDP) are positioned deepest in the cubital tunnel, being lateral and posterior.[72] This explains why a pathologic process arising in the elbow joint, such as synovitis or osteoarthritis, is more likely to initially involve the posterior fibers and thus cause problems with grip strength and wrist flexion, rather than numbness in the little and ring fingers.

Apfelberg and Larson found the ulnar nerve to elongate 4.7 mm during elbow flexion. They also noted that the nerve appeared to be larger within the postcondylar groove.[4] Later studies confirmed this and concluded that the condition was related to an increase in the amount of connective tissue present within the nerve. Further research showed that the dimension of the cubital tunnel was round in extension, but became narrowed with flexion.[10]

The ulnar nerve can be compressed at several other anatomic sites in the upper extremity. The first is the arcade of Struthers situated 5 to 7 cm proximal to the medial epicondyle. It is formed by the fascial and muscle fibers extending from the medial intramuscular septum to the medial head of the triceps. Spinner found it to be present in up to 70% of upper limbs.[43,49,51] Another possible means for compression is the anconeus epitrochlearis, which is an anomalous muscle extending from the medial border of the olecranon and triceps tendon to insert into the medial epicondyle. This muscle directly traverses the ulnar nerve posterior to the cubital tunnel, leading to neuritis.[40,46,52] A frequent site of compression is in the mid portion of the cubital tunnel, directly behind the olecranon. A fourth location is under the transverse fibrous band bridging the two heads of the FCU. The ulnar nerve also may be compressed more distally as it passes under the deep flexor pronator aponeurosis.[36]

An unusual ulnar entrapment has been reported following rupture of the biceps.[59] These patients are unique in that they will present with weakness both of grip and of elbow flexion. The mechanism for nerve compression can include the bleeding after the biceps rupture and the secondary swelling, as well as placement of the elbow in flexion for 6 to 12 weeks[58] to allow for tendon healing. When evaluating a patient, both in a clinical setting and in the operating room, all possible sites of compression must be taken into consideration.

CLINICAL FEATURES

When evaluating ulnar nerve function, it is essential to define the clinical features that are present. These include the symptoms and physical findings that lead to a diagnosis of ulnar nerve compression. Hyperesthesia in the ulnar nerve distribution, often associated with elbow flexion, is many times the initial complaint. It is usually a symptom that varies from day to day and with rest may disappear for a period of time.[24] Use of the arm, especially repetitive elbow flexion and extension, seems to exacerbate these symptoms. Patients are often awakened at night with pain at the elbow or radiating into the hand, as well as paresthesias in the ring and little finger. The symptoms usually diminish somewhat when the patient's elbow is extended. Diminished sensibility in the area supplied by the dorsal sensory branch of the ulnar nerve can help one determine the location of compression, whether it is in the cubital tunnel or at Guyon's canal.[36]

The most common symptoms of cubital tunnel syndrome include cramps, aches, and occasionally sharp pain extending down the arm into the hypothenar region in the palm. The duration of symptoms can range from several weeks to many years. Unlike carpal tunnel syndrome, the sensory loss sometimes is not bothersome. Frequently, patients will seek the care of a physician when the clinical signs of motor dysfunction, such as weakness of grasp or pinch or loss of dexterity, are the main problem. It is important to obtain an accurate history because this may allow the examiner to understand the etiology of the compression. For example, a previous elbow fracture or dislocation, acute blunt trauma, chronic repetitious elbow activities at work, or a history of arthritis may be relevant. The physical examination starts with a careful sensory examination. The sensory branches of the ulnar nerve characteristically involve the ulnar half of the palm, the volar surface of the fifth digit, and the ulnar half of the fourth digit. The dorsal sensory branch supplies the ulnar aspect of the hand posteriorly and the proximal one third of the fourth and fifth digits. There are many variations in the sensory distribution. For instance, in about 20% of the cases, the ulnar nerve may supply the entire ring and ulnar half of the middle digit.[68] To test for sensibility loss, it is preferable to evaluate those zones that are least likely to be anomalous. The most appropriate testing modalities to use are vibration and the von Frey monofilament test, which determine the threshold of lost sensibility.[24]

The motor components of the ulnar nerve play an important role in pinch, precision tasks involving the thumb and digits, symmetric finger flexion, and power grasp.

The disability associated with decreased thumb pinch is caused by weakness of the adductor pollicis, the ulnar portion of the flexor pollicis brevis (FPB), and the first dorsal interosseous. Pinch strength after a complete ulnar nerve palsy may drop by 50% to 80%.[7] The amount of pinch weakness is directly related to the degree of atrophy in the involved intrinsic muscles. The adductor pollicis and FPB function as stabilizers of the thumb metacarpophalangeal (MP) joint.

With ulnar paralysis, the loss of stability often produces MP joint hyperextension with secondary flexion of the interphalangeal (IP) joint, the posture seen in Froment's sign. As the patient pinches with more force to overcome the weakness, the deformity only gets worse. With loss of the first dorsal interosseous muscle, abduction of the index finger is impaired, which further aggravates the pinch mechanism.[24]

With a normally functioning ulnar nerve, the interosseous and lumbrical muscles coordinate digital flexion and extension, as well as abduction and adduction. MP joint flexion is initiated by the interossei, followed by flexion of the proximal and distal IP joints using the long extrinsic flexors. In ulnar nerve paralysis, with loss of the interosseous function, flexion is initiated through the long flexors, which makes an attempt to grasp objects clumsy and insufficient. Varying degrees of clawing involving the lateral two digits are seen as well, depending on the degree of muscle weakness and the laxity of the MP joints. True power grasp can be lost if there is involvement of the interosseous muscles and the FDP to the fourth and fifth digits. With ulnar nerve palsy, a 50% to 75% loss of power grasp may be seen.[16] Finally, the inability to adduct the index and fifth fingers because of weakness of the volar interossei may also be seen.

Several muscles should be selected for specific testing to gain an understanding about ulnar nerve entrapment. First, examine the FCU. This muscle may be tested by ulnar deviating the wrist in flexion or forcefully abducting the little finger. Either maneuver will tense the tendon, allowing evaluation by palpation. Mild or moderate weakness may be difficult to detect. In some cases the fibers innervating the FCU may be spared because of their lateral and posterior position within the nerve.[5,73]

The second muscles that should be tested are the FDP to the ring and small fingers. The weakness of grip in the ulnar two digits is manifested clinically when a patient reports difficulty holding a golf club or maintaining grasp on a tool (e.g., a hammer). Testing of this muscle is performed by resisting the terminal joint flexion of the patient's fourth and fifth digits or by attempting to open an individual's fully clenched fist. The examiner should be aware that variations in the innervation of the FDP by the median and ulnar nerves are frequent.[73]

The third muscle group to be evaluated includes the interossei and the lumbricals. One of the early signs of ulnar nerve entrapment is weakness of the third palmar interosseous, presenting as an abducted posture of the fifth digit. This is referred to as *Wartenberg's sign*.[76] The first dorsal interosseous also must be tested in isolation by asking the patient to resist abduction of the index finger. The muscle is easily observed, and its mass can be palpated and compared with the opposite side. One can also test the strength of digital abduction and adduction by comparing it with that of the other hand. It is important to remember that weak abduction of the fingers can also be demonstrated by contraction of the extrinsic finger extensor tendons. The lumbrical muscle's prime function is MP joint flexion. The lumbricals for the ring and little fingers are normally supplied by the ulnar nerve, and those for the index and middle finger are innervated by the median nerve. The classic claw deformity involving the fourth and fifth digits is explained by the unopposed action of the flexor tendons.

The fourth muscle group includes the hypothenar muscles. These four muscles, the palmaris brevis, abductor digiti minimi (ADM), flexor, and opponens digiti minimi are innervated soon after the nerve enters the palm from the wrist. The strength of the ADM is tested by holding both little fingers in the abducted position with resistance being provided by the opposite hand. Subtle weakness can be detected when the more powerful abductor overpowers the weaker one. The muscle bulk of the two hands should also be compared, and the opponens muscle tested by asking the patient to place the fifth digit in contact with the thumb.

Localization of the ulnar nerve entrapment to the elbow can be determined on physical examination by the presence of a paresthesias on percussion directly over the ulnar nerve. The site of apparent compression may be in the postcondylar groove or distally between the two heads of the FCU. On occasion, tenderness several centimeters proximal to the epicondyle may signal compression at the arcade of Struthers.[3,29] The elbow flexion test is an excellent diagnostic maneuver and resembles the wrist flexion test for carpal tunnel syndrome. If flexion of the elbow produces hyperesthesia or pain, it is a strong possibility that ulnar nerve compression at the elbow exists.[16] A positive Tinel's sign about the medial aspect of the elbow is less specific and each test should be compared with the opposite extremity.[22] The nerve itself can usually be palpated and the presence of nerve thickening or subluxation anterior to the medial epicondyle should be carefully evaluated. Examination of the elbow joint is also essential and may help to determine the etiology of the entrapment. A cubitus valgus deformity, elbow instability, or other joint abnormalities, as well as a flexion contracture should be noted.[16] Another provocative test for ulnar nerve dysfunction at the elbow is the inflation of a tourniquet placed proximally, which will produce numbness and tingling in the distribution of the ulnar nerve over a short period of time. Again this should be compared with the contralateral side.[24]

Ulnar nerve compression at the elbow can be divided into mild, moderate, and severe stages based on sensory, motor, and physical testing.[17,56] In the mild form, the patient will have intermittent paresthesias and vibratory perception is increased.[19,23,24] The patient may also complain of subjective weakness, clumsiness, or loss of coordination. The elbow flexion test or Tinel's sign may be positive. In the moderate stage, paresthesias are more frequent, vibratory perception is normal or decreased, and motor function is abnormal with measurable weakness in pinch and grip.[19] Physical examination may show elbow flexion and Tinel's sign to be positive and intrinsic muscle testing may be abnormal.

In the severe form, paresthesias are persistent, vibratory perception is decreased, and abnormal two-point discrimination is present. Motor examination shows measurable weakness in pinch and grip as well as muscle atrophy. A positive elbow flexion test and positive Tinel's sign are both present with abnormal intrinsic evaluation (i.e., inability to actively cross the fingers).[7,17]

The use of electrodiagnostic testing for ulnar nerve compression can be beneficial, particularly for localization. It may be specifically recommended when difficult diagnostic problems occur in the setting of multiple sites of possible nerve compression. Furthermore, some patients, even after careful clinical evaluation, may prove a diagnostic dilemma. In particular, people who have sustained work-related injuries, individuals involved in motor vehicle accidents, and those whose complaints seem disproportionate to physical findings are good candidates for electrodiagnostic testing. Furthermore, patients who have had previous ulnar nerve surgery and those who have a mixed neurologic picture should be tested as well.

Many accounts of a correlation between electrodiagnostic studies and compression have been reported.[74] However, Wilson and Krout have found that after surgery, nerve conduction studies did not correlate with the clinical improvements in their patients, and they could not distinguish between patients who had good results and patients who had bad results from surgery.[77] Some believe that the reason for this lack of correlation is the demyelination that accompanies nerve compression.[24] The delays in motor and sensory nerve conduction are related to the duration and severity of compression. In the earliest stage of entrapment, a neural ischemia occurs that immediately translates into symptoms for the patient. Yet at this stage, there may be no electrical changes. It has been shown that clinical signs are more reliable than electrical studies, which are best used as an adjunct in making the diagnosis.[12,28] There is no indication to deny surgical decompression to a patient with normal preoperative electrical studies if the history and physical examination of the patient are consistent with an established ulnar nerve compression.*

Patients with ulnar nerve compression at the elbow can be divided into five etiologic categories. The first, *external compression,* occurs after a single blow to the medial aspect of the elbow or after chronic repetitive trauma to the nerve. This can occur in the bedridden patient or through occupational trauma.[9,61]

The second cause of compression is *impingement by bone or other abnormal tissues.* The cubitus valgus deformity can produce the classic tardy ulnar nerve palsy because of chronic stretch. This deformity can occur after a supracondylar humeral fracture, following radial head resection or from progressive arthritic collapse and angulation. Synovitis from inflammation in the elbow joint, heterotopic bone, and burn scars can also produce ulnar nerve entrapment.[16]

The third category is *recurrent nerve subluxation.* Childress evaluated the ulnar nerve in 1000 asymptomatic patients and found the incidence of ulnar nerve subluxation to be 16%.[11] He divided these incidences into the category of moderate excursion, where the nerve moves out of the postcondylar groove and subluxes onto the tip of the medial

*References 8, 13, 18, 51, 54, 57, 78.

epicondyle (12%), and the category of even greater excursion showing complete dislocation when the elbow was flexed more than 90°. All of his patients were asymptomatic and the majority had the conditions bilaterally.[11] The cause of this nerve hypermobility has been attributed to an increased carrying angle of the elbow, an abnormality of the medial epicondyle or triceps insertion, or congenital laxity of the supporting tissues. Reports of symptoms related to direct trauma or chronic repetitive flexion and extension leading to subluxation have also been given.[11,16]

The fourth subdivision is *cubital tunnel syndrome,* where an aponeurotic band is responsible for nerve entrapment as described previously at four different compression points.[31,60]

The fifth and last group is labeled *idiopathic* and accounts for 30% to 50% of the patients. No specific cause for the ulnar neuropathy is discovered in spite of careful investigation, including wide surgical treatment.[9,54]

Other diagnostic methods still in the experimental stages include imaging techniques that attempt to define the parameters of the cubital tunnel. Thermography is another technique that depends on the alteration of skin temperature, which is a frequent feature of nerve injury. To date, no controlled studies have been performed using this later technique; thus it cannot be relied on as a diagnostic tool.[69]

DIFFERENTIAL DIAGNOSIS

Careful consideration must be given to the differential diagnosis of ulnar neuropathy at the elbow. Ulnar nerve compression distal to the elbow, particularly at the wrist or in the hand, can easily be missed and should come to mind when there is no weakness of the FCU or the ulnar flexor digitorum profundi. Other neurologic conditions can produce abnormalities in the hand without sensory loss and may mimic an ulnar nerve abnormality. One such condition is amyotrophic lateral sclerosis, which often starts with weakness and muscle fasciculations or atrophy in the hands.[56] Another possibility to consider, although rare, is diseases of the spinal cord, including primary nerve tumors, metastatic disease, and vascular infarctions. These lesions can be differentiated by the presence of long track signs or extensive sensory loss in the upper trunk. An infrequent lesion, but not to be forgotten, is the Pancost tumor, which may affect the medial cord of the brachial plexus. This tumor arises in the apex of the lung and is highly malignant. A common feature is Horner's syndrome with loss of sweating over the entire arm, as well as the face and head on the same side.

A third possibility to consider in the differential diagnosis is proximal compression at the level of the cervical spine. This includes degenerative changes producing cervical spondylosis and disc disease. Previously, x-ray examination was recommended to help delineate this problem. However, simple cervical x-ray evaluation showing degenerative changes in the spine cannot be correlated with cervical radiculopathy in patients over 40 years of age because degenerative disease is common with or without pathology. The patterns of muscular weakness with cervical compression that might affect different areas should be carefully tested. A confirmatory Spurling's sign or neck manipulation that exacerbates the dysesthesias will corroborate the diagnosis, and evaluation by magnetic resonance imaging or myelographic testing may be necessary. One must keep in mind the possibility of compression at a second level, the so-called double crush syndrome, when confronted with a patient having multiple areas of muscular changes.

Thoracic outlet syndrome has been a popular consideration in the differentiation for patients considered to have radiculopathy or peripheral nerve entrapment. However, it is really an uncommon condition resulting from constriction of the lower trunk of the brachial plexus. The neurologic features include atrophy of the thenar muscles and other intrinsics of the hands. Sensory loss in the C8-T1 distribution is a common feature, and this includes the medial antebrachial cutaneous nerve, which is not involved in ulnar compression neuropathy.

The last diagnostic entity to consider is the patient with a claw deformity isolated to the fourth or fifth digits. This abnormality can occur in camptodactyly, which is an unusual developmental condition most commonly found in the little finger, but sometimes the ring finger, as well. On careful examination, these patients demonstrate a proximal interphalangeal (PIP) joint flexion contracture, which is of nontraumatic origin. McFarlane has shown that the condition is caused by abnormal insertion of the lumbrical tendon in the involved digits.[55] The patients have normal sensibility and motor function in the interosseous and hypothenar muscles. Whereas other diseases and conditions can resemble ulnar compression neuropathy, the entities just discussed cover most of the problems that are encountered.

TREATMENT

Management of ulnar nerve compression at the elbow depends on the cause, the severity of the compression, and the duration of the symptoms. Although the type of surgical treatment that will give the best result remains quite controversial, most authorities agree that the best results after surgery occur in patients with mild signs and symptoms. Poor results are seen in patients with severe atrophy.[16]

Conservative management

The first consideration should be nonsurgical treatment for ulnar nerve compression. This is indicated for patients with intermittent symptoms, whether it be an acute or chronic mild neuropathy, or when the symptoms are in an early stage and without serious interference of function. The treatment entails avoidance of repetitive flexion and extension of the elbow and rest splinting of the joint in extension. For those patients with evidence of subluxation, padded splints can be placed about the elbow to avoid striking the medial aspect of the joint against a hard surface. Along with splinting, a change in the way the upper extremity is used may also improve the condition. For a mild neuropathy caused by a direct blow over the cubital tunnel, splinting of the elbow in an extended position should be continued for 2 to 3 months, especially if the symptoms are intermittent or show improvement. Lister has shown that when patients with cubital tunnel syndrome were placed in orthoplast splints with elbow flexion between 45° and 70° and the wrist supported to relax the FCU, the overall improvement for the splinted group was 86.3%.[26]

Surgical treatment

A number of treatment options have been recommended when surgical decompression of the ulnar nerve is indicated. These options include simple release or decompression, medial epicondylectomy, anterior subcutaneous transposition, anterior intermuscular transposition, and anterior submuscular transposition. The technique selected by the surgeon is often one of personal preference. Few randomized prospective studies have been performed that might give us a definitive guide.[1]

Simple decompression

Osborn[63] noted that simply dividing the band between the two heads of the FCU, compressing the nerve, and leaving the nerve in place provided a satisfactory result. In his series of 567 cases, he showed excellent results with simple decompression, with greater than 70% improvement in symptomatology. Osborn's study clearly shows that the patients who benefit the most from simple decompression technique are those with a minimal degree of nerve compression and an identifiable compressive band. In his study, 94% of the patients with a minimal degree of nerve compression achieved excellent relief of their sensory symptoms through decompression.[63,74] When the degree of compression had progressed to moderate, only 33% of the patients achieved normal strength and normal sensation; 16% had persistence of their perioperative symptoms and physical findings. When the degree of compression had progressed to the severe state, less than 25% achieved any significant functional or sensory recovery.[4,23,29,36,61] The advantages of the simple release are that it is a straightforward operation with low morbidity. The operation is not recommended for patients whose neuropathy is associated with bone or joint abnormalities, nerve subluxation, or medial epicondylitis. It is best reserved for patients who have no muscle weakness and minimal pathologic changes observed in the nerve at the time of surgery. It should be limited to those patients in which an obvious point of constriction can be identified.

The surgical technique requires a 10 to 12 cm longitudinal incision that centers slightly anterior to the medial epicondyle. The posterior branch of the medial antebrachial cutaneous nerve should be investigated and carefully protected to prevent a painful neuroma.[53] The ulnar nerve is identified proximal to the tunnel and the aponeurosis connecting the two heads of the FCU is divided. It has been recommended that the nerve should then be explored through the FCU muscle to ensure a complete nerve release.[16] This simple operation preserves the blood supply and allows for immediate remobilization to prevent scar adherence postoperatively.[30]

The disadvantages of the simple decompression include the failure to relieve symptoms (because of compression at another site) and subluxation of the nerve over the medial epicondyle, causing further traction and friction. This can be prevented by limiting decompression to the area of the aponeurosis and not releasing the nerve proximally.

Medial epicondylectomy

The technique of medial epicondylectomy was initially described by King as an alternative to a more extensive anterior transposition procedure that could result in scar constriction of the nerve and a less than optimal result.[44,45] Removing the medial epicondyle eliminates the bone block against which the nerve is compressed during elbow flexion, thus allowing the nerve to migrate anteriorly. It also eliminates the need for increased dissection and mobilization of the ulnar nerve as is required for a formal anterior transposition. With this technique, it is recommended that the nerve should not be explored, nor its branches handled.[44,45]

The elbow area is exposed by an incision similar to that previously described for the simple decompression. The nerve is exposed proximally, and the tissues overlying the nerve are incised. The nerve is only dissected sufficiently enough to allow the epicondylectomy to be performed; it is not detached from the surrounding soft tissues.[62] The medial epicondyle is then exposed by stripping the entire flexor pronator mass from the bone subperiosteally. The epicondyle is osteotomized and removed. The flexor-pronator mass is reapproximated with the elbow held in extension.* The joint is put through a range-of-motion test to check for nerve impingement. The elbow is immobilized for 10 to 14 days.

Almost all conditions known to cause ulnar nerve compression at the elbow have been mentioned as indications for medial epicondylectomy, including cubitus valgus deformities, nonunion of the medial epicondyle, bony exostoses, tumors, blood vessel aberrations, and arthritis. The major advantage of this procedure is that it requires less dissection, and therefore there is better preservation of the nerve's blood supply than anterior transpositions. It removes the compressing structures, preserves all of the small nerve branches, and allows the nerve to move freely.

The disadvantage of medial epicondylectomy is the loss of the protective effect provided by the medial epicondyle. Up to 10% of the patients have mild tenderness at the

---

*References 13, 16, 33, 35, 42, 47, 62.

incision site throughout their postoperative course.[16,24] Injury to the medial collateral ligament has been described, as well as adhesions of the nerve to the repaired muscle tendon tissue.[24,39]

Transposition

Anterior transposition of the ulnar nerve has been the most frequently performed procedure for compression at the elbow since first described by Curtis in 1898.[14]

Anterior transposition alleviates ulnar neuropathy by removing the nerve from the compressive effects of the cubital tunnel and by placing it anterior to the joint axis of motion, thus decreasing the tension on the nerve during flexion. Three methods of transposition have been described. With the first technique, the nerve is placed subcutaneously. In the second, the nerve is situated within the muscular tissue of the flexor-pronator mass. In the third technique, the nerve is placed deep to the muscles arising from the medial epicondyle. A recent review of the literature demonstrated that intramuscular transposition has shown inferior results compared with other techniques because of bleeding and muscular scarring, leading to further nerve constriction.[2,16,34]

Subcutaneous technique. Anterior subcutaneous transposition in conjunction with an external neurolysis is a procedure that has been widely reported in medical literature. The purpose is to place the nerve in a bed that is less scarred and to provide functional lengthening of the nerve, up to 3 to 4 cm. Unfortunately, a number of the articles that have been written have not made clear the technical aspects of the operation.*

The technique of Eaton, which produces a new medial fascial sling behind the transposed nerve, is the one we use.[27] With this technique, the transposed nerve is not fixed to any structure, but is protected only by the superficial fat in the region. Because no muscles are detached or sutured, the patient can begin immediate elbow motion.

Eaton's technique includes visualization and complete release of the nerve 4 cm proximal to the elbow, as well as into the forearm muscle mass. Before surgery, with the elbow in extension, the medial epicondyle is marked on the skin and a second mark is placed 1 cm anterior to this, which represents the future site for the attachment of the new fascial sling to the dermis.

The incision is centered between the olecranon and medial epicondyle for a distance of 10 cm. Cutaneous nerves are carefully dissected and retracted. The ulnar nerve is identified at the epicondyle and dissection is carried proximally. As the nerve is mobilized, the vessels accompanying it are kept in close proximity to the nerve. The dissection is continued 4 to 5 cm proximally. The medial intramuscular septum is excised from the epicondyle 4 cm proximally. A distal dissection includes

excising the fascia between the two heads of the FCU. This muscle is split for 3 to 4 cm, preserving any motor branches. The nerve should now be fully immobilized anteriorly and any remaining local areas of compression should be released. Areas of the nerve maximally compressed may require a local epineurotomy.

A fascial sling measuring 1.5 cm on each side is raised from the tissue overlying the flexor pronator muscles with the medial portion left intact. This flap is then hinged medially, placed beneath the nerve, and the three corners sutured to the dermis at the level of the previously placed mark on the skin, using 3-0 nonabsorbable sutures. With the nerve situated in this anterior position, it is supported by the muscle fascia posteriorly and surrounded by subcutaneous fat anteriorly. After the skin has been approximated, the sling is situated slightly anterior to the epicondyle, thus protecting it from this bony prominence and maintaining the nerve in this position.

To allow immediate motion, only a soft dressing is applied, and by 5 days postoperatively, the patient usually has full motion. All basic activities are allowed and only stressful activities are discouraged.

Eaton believes this operation is indicated for intractable ulnar neuritis localized to the elbow. It can also be used as an adjunct after nerve repair that has been mobilized, following open reduction of an elbow fracture after medial collateral ligament repairs, and following elbow arthroplasties. He does not mention any contraindications, but acknowledges that patients with long-standing nerve defects will have a less favorable outcome.[24]

The disadvantages of this procedure are as follows: It is more complex that either the medial epicondylectomy or the simple release. A larger skin flap is required, and thus, there is a greater likelihood for injury to the posterior branch of the medial antebrachial cutaneous nerve. There is also the potential for nerve scarring to the fascia. The subcutaneous position leaves the nerve in a more vulnerable location with the possibility of direct compression, especially in the lean individual.

Submuscular technique. With the submuscular technique (Figs. 22-1 through 22-10), the patient is supine on the operative table and after the entire arm is prepped, a sterile tourniquet is applied and the arm exsanguinated. An incision is outlined, centered between the olecranon and the medial epicondyle, the length depends on the patient's body habitus and expected location of the compression. The dissection is carried into the subcutaneous tissue, with care being taken to spare the medial antebrachial cutaneous nerve. Injury to this nerve can create enough pain to be interpreted postoperatively as incomplete ulnar nerve decompression. The ulnar nerve is first visualized above the elbow underneath the fascia, which extends from the triceps to the medial intramuscular septum. After the fascia is incised, the nerve is gently mobilized with vessel loops. The roof of the cubital tunnel is incised distally, checking

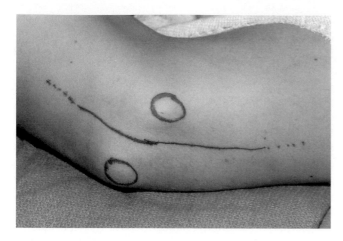

Fig. 22-1. The initial incision is made.

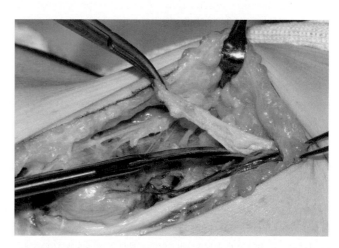

Fig. 22-4. Fascia between the two heads of the flexor carpi ulnaris are incised.

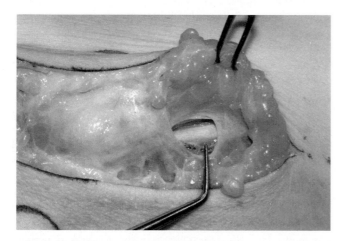

Fig. 22-2. The ulnar nerve visualized.

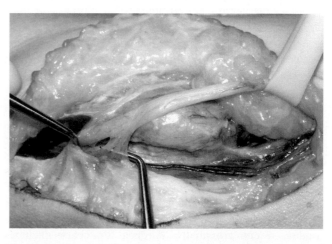

Fig. 22-5. After the nerve is completely released, it is temporarily mobilized anterior to the medial epicondyle.

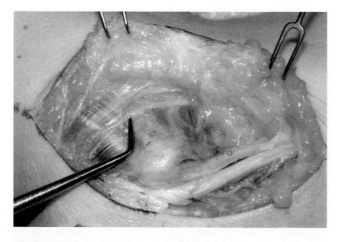

Fig. 22-3. The medial antebrachial cutaneous nerve identified.

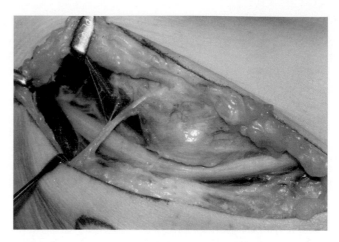

Fig. 22-6. The medial intermuscular septum is completely excised.

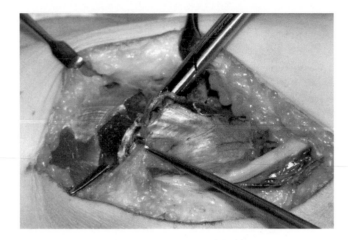

Fig. 22-7. The common flexor origin is divided.

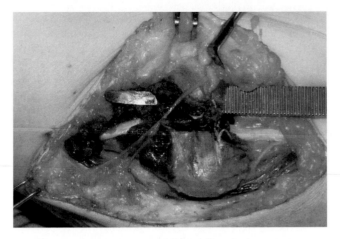

Fig. 22-9. After muscle approximation, the elevator can be passed beneath the repair confirming sufficient space.

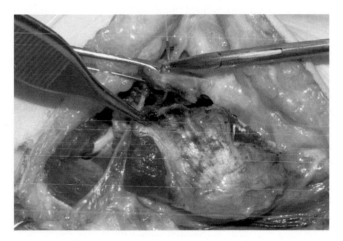

Fig. 22-8. The ulnar nerve is transposed to the submuscular position.

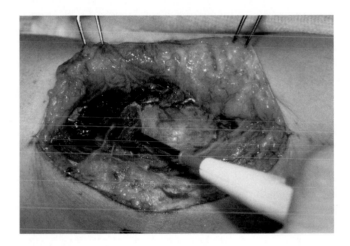

Fig. 22-10. Hemostasis is achieved and the wound is closed.

for the site of nerve compression. The fascia between the two heads of the FCU is incised. The nerve is placed anterior to the medial epicondyle to estimate whether sufficient tissue has been released proximally and distally. Small branches to the FCU must be carefully dissected and preserved. The nerve is then temporarily returned to its retrocondylar position. The medial intramuscular septum is divided down to bone from the epicondyle 6 to 8 cm proximally. Small vessels in the area need to be cauterized or ligated.[70]

A step-cut lengthening of the common flexor-pronator muscle origin is made, with length of the limbs measuring 2 cm. The muscle is divided down to the elbow joint capsule and is allowed to slide distally. The ulnar nerve is then transposed anterior to lie upon the brachialis muscle. The nerve should have a straight course, and this may require a further release of the FCU from the ulna. The muscle and fascia are reapproximated with figure of eight sutures, using 3-0 absorbable material. A sufficient passage should be left

beneath the muscle to allow a finger or an elevator to easily pass. The mobility of the nerve should be checked with gentle traction.

After hemostasis and wound closure, a splint will keep the elbow in 90° of flexion, with the forearm held in pronation. Remobilization is begun at 5 to 10 days. The patient is started on an active assistive flexion, with rest either in a posterior splint or a sling for 2 weeks after surgery. During the third and fourth weeks, active extension is initiated.

The advantages of this technique are that it removes the nerve from its pathologic location and places it in a well-vascularized bed anterior to the elbow axis. The nerve is nicely protected from external forces. The disadvantages are that it is the most complex of the operations discussed, with increased dissection allowing the potential for higher morbidity. Should a hematoma ensue, a new site for entrapment would be created. The prompt remobilization program should lead to a decrease of scarring and recurrence.

COMPLICATIONS

The goal after nerve transposition is to regain gliding function of the nerve. The concern is whether the nerve will become encased in scar tissue.[6,77] Other recognized complications after treatment of ulnar compression neuropathy include flexion contracture of the elbow, persistent common flexor origin tenderness, and medial instability of the elbow, which can occur following inadvertent release of the medial collateral ligament. Hematoma formation can be prevented by releasing the tourniquet and achieving hemostasis. Injuries to the cutaneous nerves and subsequent neuroma formation can occur with any surgical procedure on the medial aspect of the elbow. Should this occur and if the symptoms are significant, the neuroma will need to be dissected away from the area of the ulnar nerve and transposed into muscular tissue. Care should be taken so that no further traction will occur on the transposed neuroma with elbow motion. Eaton feels that tenderness over the nerve is uncommon, as is caused by fixation to the fascial sling. The early motion of the elbow precludes joint stiffness.[27]

DISCUSSION

When one concludes after a complete diagnostic workup that surgery is the necessary treatment for ulnar nerve entrapment of the elbow, it is difficult to know which operation is the most appropriate. No prospective randomized study of patients treated by different surgical techniques, that would give us guidance as to which procedure provides the best results, has been published. It is difficult to compare articles that use different staging systems, different methods to report the outcome, and different techniques. Also, many of the studies published to date have a small number of patients involved. When a universal staging system can be implemented, a true, double-blind randomized study can be performed.

Dellon[20] analyzed 50 reports from 1898 to 1988, with a total of 2000 patients. He found that with minimal symptoms, 50% responded well to nonoperative treatment, and nearly 100% of the patients improved with any of the five surgical procedures. With moderate symptoms, anterior submuscular transposition yielded the best results. Intramuscular transposition yielded the worst results and the most complications. For the severe stage, submuscular transposition gave the best overall results. We believe that surgery is indicated for ulnar nerve compression when documented abnormalities are present (motor weakness, measurable sensibility loss, or positive electrodiagnostic studies) and when conservative measures have failed. Simple decompression may be all that is required in the patient with mild symptoms where compression is localized to the area of Osborn's band. For patients with compression at other levels or with multiple areas of compression, anterior subcutaneous transposition by Eaton's technique, medial epicondylectomy, and submuscular transposition

have given us satisfactory results. For those patients with severe ulnar nerve compression or those who have failed previous nerve surgery, we believe that submuscular transposition following decompression and external neurolysis places the nerve in a well-vascularized bed and has the best chance of providing pain relief as well as return of sensory and motor abilities.

CONCLUSIONS

Ulnar nerve decompression and transposition should only be considered after careful evaluation of the condition. Nonoperative treatment is often satisfactory in patients presenting with mild cubital tunnel syndrome. The differential diagnosis to include cervical nerve decompression, thoracic outlet syndrome, and other areas of nerve compression in the arm and forearm need to be evaluated, as do systemic medical abnormalities. Subluxation of the ulnar nerve at the elbow and medial epicondylitis are conditions that need to be taken into consideration. When analyzing surgical failures, the most likely findings include entrapment of the nerve by scar tissue and failure to completely release the nerve either proximally or distally. Submuscular transposition has been found to be an effective revision technique, although internal neurolysis is rarely indicated. Patients with the worst prognosis are those with a history of multiple previous surgeries about the ulnar nerve at the elbow, when their age is greater than 50 years, or when they have had a previous submuscular transposition that failed.

REFERENCES

1. Adelaar R, Foster W, McDowell C: Treatment of cubital tunnel syndrome, *J Hand Surg* 1984; 9A(1):90-95.
2. Adson AL: The surgical treatment of progressive ulnar paralysis, *Minn Med* 1918; 1:455-460.
3. Amadio PC, Beckenbaugh RD: Entrapment of the ulnar nerve by the deep flexor-pronator aponeurosis, *J Hand Surg* 1986; 11A:83.
4. Apfelberg DB, Larson SJ: Dynamic anatomy of the ulnar nerve at the elbow, *Plast Reconstr Surg* 1973; 51:76-81.
5. Benoit BG, Preston DN, Atack DM, DaSilva VF: Neurolysis combined with the application of a Silastic envelope for ulnar nerve entrapment at the elbow, *Neurosurg* 1987; 20:594-598.
6. Brody AS, Leffert RD, Smith RJ: Technical problems with ulnar nerve transposition at the elbow: findings and results of reoperation, *J Hand Surg* 1978; 3:85.
7. Brown P: Reconstruction for pinch in ulnar intrinsic palsy, *Orthop Clin North Am* 1974; 5:323.
8. Brown WF, Yates SK: Percutaneous localization of conduction abnormalities in human extremities, *Can J Neuro Sci* 1982; 9:391-400.
9. Chan RC, Paine KW, Varghese G: Ulnar neuropathy at the elbow: comparison of simple decompression and anterior transposition, *Neurosurg* 1980; 7:545.
10. Chang KSF, Low WD, Chan ST: Enlargement of the ulnar nerve behind the medial humeral epicondyle, *Anat Rec* 1963; 145:149-153.
11. Childress HM: Recurrent ulnar nerve dislocation at the elbow, *J Bone Joint Surg* 1956; 38A:978.
12. Clark CB: Cubital tunnel syndrome, *JAMA* 1979; 241:801-802.
13. Craven PR, Green DP: Cubital tunnel syndrome: treatment by medial epicondylectomy, *J Bone Joint Surg* 1980; 62A:986.

14. Curtis BF: Traumatic ulnar neuritis-transplantation of the nerve, *J Nerve Ment Dis* 1898; 25:480-481.

15. Davidson AJ, Horowitz MT: Late or tardy ulnar paralysis, *J Bone Joint Surg* 1935; 17:844-856.

16. Dawson DM: *Entrapment neuropathies,* Boston, 1990, Little, Brown.

17. Dawson DM, Hallet M, Millender LH: *Entrapment neuropathies*, Boston, 1983, Little, Brown.

18. DeJesus PV, Stiner JC: Spontaneous recovery of ulnar neuropathy at the elbow, *Electromyogr Clin Neurophysiol* 1976; 16:239-248.

19. Dellon AL: Clinical use of vibratory stimuli to evaluate peripheral nerve injury and compression neuropathy, *Plast Reconstr Surg* 1980; 65:466-476.

20. Dellon AL: Review of treatment results for ulnar nerve entrapment at the elbow, *J Hand Surg* 1989; 14A(4):688-699.

21. Dellon AL: Musculotendinous variations about the medial humeral epicondyle, *J Hand Surg* 1986; 11(B):175-181.

22. Dellon AL: Tinel or not tinel? *J Hand Surg* 1984; 9(B):216.

23. Dellon AL: The vibrometer, *Plast Reconstr Surg* 1983; 71:42-431.

24. Dellon M, Mackinnon S: *Surgery of the peripheral nerve,* New York, 1988, Thieme.

25. Dellon AL, MacKinnon SE: Injury to the medial antebrachial cutaneous nerve during cubital tunnel surgery, *J Hand Surg* 1985; 10B:33.

26. Diamond M, Lister G: Cubital tunnel syndrome treated by long-arm splintage, *J Hand Surg* 1985; 10A:430.

27. Eaton RG, Crowe JF, Parkes JC III: Anterior transposition of the ulnar nerve with a noncompressing fasciodermal sling, *J Bone Joint Surg* 1980; 62A:820-825.

28. Eisen A: Early diagnosis of ulnar nerve palsy: an electrophysiologic study, *Neurology* (Minneap), 1974; 24:256-262.

29. Eversmann WW: Entrapment and compression neuropathies. In Green P, ed: *Operative hand surgery,* vol 2, New York, 1988, Churchill Livingstone.

30. Fannin TF: Local decompression in the treatment of ulnar nerve entrapment at the elbow, *J R Col Surg Edinb* 1978; 23:362-366.

31. Feindel W, Stratford V: Role of the cubital tunnel in tardy ulnar palsy, *Can J Surg* 1957; 1:287.

32. Foster RJ, Edshage S: Factors related to the outcome of surgically managed compressive ulnar neuropathy at the elbow level, *J Hand Surg* 1981; 6:181-192.

33. Froimson A, Zahrawi F: Treatment of compression neuropathy of the ulnar nerve at the elbow by epicondylectomy and neurolysis, *J Hand Surg* 1980; 5:391.

34. Gay J, Love J: Diagnosis and treatment of tardy paralysis of the ulnar nerve, *J Bone Joint Surg* 1947; 29B:1087-1097.

35. Gore D, Larson S: Medial epicondylectomy for subluxing ulnar nerve, *Am J Surg* 1966; 111:851.

36. Green D: *Operative hand surgery,* New York, 1988, Churchill Livingstone.

37. Hagstrom P: Ulnar nerve compression at the elbow, *Scand J Plast Reconstr Surg* 1977; 11:59-62.

38. Harrison MJG, Nurick S: Results of anterior transposition of ulnar nerve for ulnar neuritis, *Br Med J* 1970; 1:27-29.

39. Heitoff S, Millender LM, Nalebuff EA, et al.: Medial epicondylectomy for treatment of ulnar nerve compression at the elbow, *J Hand Surg* 1990; 15A:22.

40. Hirasawa Y, Sawamura H, Sakakida K: Entrapment neuropathy due to bilateral epitrochleoanconeus muscles: a case report, *J Hand Surg* 1979; 4:181.

41. Ho KC, Marmor L: Entrapment of the ulnar nerve at the elbow, *Am J Surg* 1971; 121:355-356.

42. Jones RE, Gauntt C: Medial epicondylectomy for ulnar nerve compression syndrome at the elbow, *Clin Orthop* 1979; 139:174.

43. Kane E, Kaplan EB, Spinner M: Observations on the course of the ulnar nerve in the arm, *Ann Chir* 1973; 27:470-496.

44. King T, Morgan FP: Treatment of traumatic ulnar neuritis, *Aust NZ J Surg* 1950; 20:33-42.

45. King T, Morgan FP: Later results of removing the medial humeral epicondyle for traumatic ulnar neuritis, *J Bone Joint Surg* 1959; 41B:51-55.

46. Kojima T, Kurihara K, Nagano T: A study on operative findings and pathogenic factors in ulnar neuropathy at the elbow, *Handchirurgie* 1979; 11:99.

47. Laha RK, Panchal PD: Surgical treatment of ulnar neuropathy, *Surg Neurol* 1979; 11:393.

48. Learmonth JR: A technique for transplanting the ulnar nerve, *Surg Gyn Obs* 1942; 75:792-793.

49. Leffert R: Anterior submuscular transposition of the ulnar nerves by the Learmonth technique, *J Hand Surg* 1982; 7:147-155.

50. Levy DM, Apfelberg DB: Results of anterior transposition for ulnar neuropathy at the elbow, *Am J Surg* 1972; 123:304-308.

51. Lugnegard H, Waldheim G, Wenberg G: Operative treatment of ulnar nerve neuropathy in the elbow region, *Acta Orthop Scand* 1977; 48:168-176.

52. Masear VR, Hill JJ, Cohen SM: Ulnar compression neuropathy secondary to the anconeus epitrochlearis muscle, *J Hand Surg* 1988; 13A:720.

53. Masear VR, Meyer RD, Picona D: Surgical anatomy of the medial antebrachial cutaneous nerve, *J Hand Surg* 1989; 14A:267.

54. MacNichol MF: Results of operations for ulnar neuritis, *J Bone Joint Surg* 1979; 61B:159-164.

55. McFarlane RM, Curry GJ, Evans HB: Anomalies of the intrinsic muscles in camptodactyly, *J Hand Surg* 1983; 8:531.

56. McGowan AJ: The results of transposition of the ulnar nerve for traumatic ulnar neuritis, *J Bone Joint Surg* 1950; 32B:293-301.

57. Miller RG: Cubital tunnel syndrome: diagnosis and precise localization, *Ann Neurol* 1979; 6:56-59.

58. Miller RG, Camp PE: Postoperative ulnar palsy, *JAMA* 1979; 242:1636.

59. Morrey BF, Askew LJ, An KN, Dobyns JH: Rupture of the distal tendon of the biceps brachii, *J Bone Joint Surg* 1985; 67A:418-421.

60. Mulder DW: Motor neuron disease. In Dyck PJ, Thomas PK, Lambert EH, eds: *Peripheral neuropathy*, Philadelphia, 1975, Saunders.

61. Mumemthaler M: *Die ulnarisparesen,* Stuttgart, 1961, Ferog Thieme Verlag.

62. Neblett C, Ehni G: Medial epicondylectomy for ulnar nerve palsy, *J Neurosurg* 1970; 32:55-62.

63. Osborn GV: The surgical treatment of tardy ulnar neuritis, *J Bone Joint Surg* 1957; 39B:782.

64. Paine EW: Tardy ulnar palsy, *Can J Surg* 1970; 13:255-261.

65. Payan J: Anterior transposition of the ulnar nerve: an electrophysiological study, *J Neurol Neurosurg Psychiatry* 1970; 33:157-165.

66. Pechan J, Julius I: The pressure measurement in the ulnar nerve: a contribution to the pathophysiology of the cubital tunnel syndrome, *J Biomech* 1975; 8:75-79.

67. Platt H: The pathogenesis and treatment of traumatic neuritis of the ulnar nerve in the postcondylar groove. *BR J Surg* 1926; 13:409-431.

68. Pollock LJ, Davis L: *Peripheral nerve injuries,* New York, 1933, Hoeber.

69. So YT, Olney RK, Aminoff MJ: Evaluation of thermography in the diagnosis of selected peripheral entrapment neuropathies, *Neurology* 1989; 39:1.

70. Spinner M, Kaplan ED: The relationship of the ulnar nerve to the medial intermuscular septum in the arm and its clinical significance, *Hand* 1976; 8:239-242.

71. Spinner M, Spencer PS: Nerve compression lesions of the upper extremity: a clinical and experimental review, *Clin Orthop* 1974; 104:46-68.

72. Sunderland S: The intraneural topography of the radial median and ulnar nerves, *Brain* 1945; 68:243-253.

73. Sunderland S: *Nerve and nerve injuries,* ed 2, London, 1978, Churchill Livingstone.

74. Thompson EM, Cote J: Conduction velocities in ulnar motor nerve using two separate muscles as indicators, *South Med J* 1970; 63:700.

75. Vanderpool DW, Chalmers J, Lamb DW, Whitson TB: Peripheral compression lesions of the ulnar nerve, *J Bone Joint Surg* 1968; 50B:792-802.

76. Wartenberg R: A sign of ulnar palsy, *JAMA* 1939; 112:16-88.

77. Wilson DH, Kraut R: Surgery of ulnar neuropathy at the elbow in sixteen cases treated by decompression without transposition, *J Neurosurg* 1973; 38:780-785.

78. Wright EA, McQuillen MP: Hypoexcitability of ulnar nerve in patients with normal motor and nerve conduction studies, *Neurology* (Minneap) 1973; 23:78-83.

Chapter 23

THERAPY MANAGEMENT OF ULNAR NERVE COMPRESSION AT THE ELBOW

Maureen A. Hardy

Considering the anatomical position and course of the ulnar nerve at elbow level it is apparent that this nerve is asking for trouble.

LUNDBORG[40]

Each peripheral nerve has its one most vulnerable site for compression. The elbow anatomy presents several impediments to neural health, causing it to be the most common location for ulnar nerve compression. The anatomic factors that predispose the nerve for trouble become our focus for therapeutic intervention both preoperatively and postoperatively.

PREDISPOSING FACTORS FOR TROUBLE

Superficial location. The ulnar nerve leaves its deep protected position alongside the triceps in the upper arm to become subcutaneous both proximal and distal to the medial epicondyle until it once more dives deep between the flexor carpi ulnaris (FCU) heads in the forearm. This makes the nerve easy to palpate (Fig. 23-1), but it lacks good soft tissue protection and it is susceptible to external pressure or trauma. The nerve is especially vulnerable at the postcondylar groove in the pronated position,[41] where it receives direct contact with external hard surfaces.

Largest diameter. The ulnar nerve enlarges behind the medial epicondyle as a function of age (Fig. 23-2).[10] Where nerves are vulnerable to repeated friction, the intraneural connective tissue component increases as a normal protective response.

Gliding requirement. Numerous works attest to the resting, waived course of unstretched nerves.[47,65,74] Even the blood vessels to the nerve are adapted in a coiled fashion. As traction is applied, the nerve first slides in relation to surrounding structures and then stretches. This slide and stretch phenomenon allows the nerve to elongate or unpleat with arm motion preventing neural and vascular compromise. The ulnar nerve glides 10 mm proximally with elbow flexion and elongates 4.7 mm.[3,73]

Cubital tunnel volume changes. The cubital tunnel is unique in that its volume changes with elbow position, unlike the carpal tunnel, which remains a fixed compartment at the wrist (intraneural pressure changes with respect to position, but the anatomic boundaries of the carpal tunnel remain fixed). As the elbow flexes, the olecranon moves away from the medial epicondyle. These are the bony origin and insertion for the arcuate ligament overlying the ulnar nerve (Fig. 23-3). As the arcuate ligament or roof becomes taut, the floor of the tunnel, the medial collateral ligament, relaxes and buckles inward. The combined tightening above and bulging below cause a 55% decrease in tunnel volume.[3,25]

Intraneural pressure changes. As the volume of the tunnel decreases, the intraneural pressure increases. Elbow flexion beyond 90° causes a threefold increase in pressure.[57] When wrist extension and shoulder abduction are added to a flexed elbow, the pressure increases sixfold.[44] If this posture is assumed and the FCU contracts, pressure increases twentyfold.[72] Baseball pitchers and tennis players demonstrate this traction-compression-pressure build up in their serving posture (Fig. 23-4).[28]

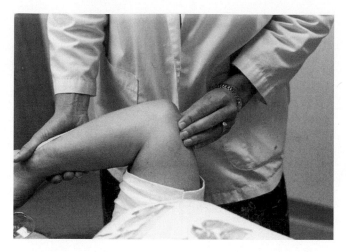

Fig. 23-1. Ease of palpation of ulnar nerve at the elbow because of its superficial location.

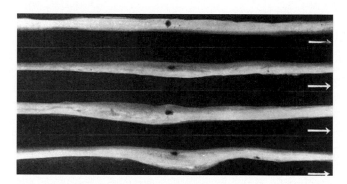

Fig. 23-2. Enlargement of ulnar nerve behind medial epicondyle as a function of age and response to friction. The nerve's location posterior to epicondyle is marked by the dot; arrow indicates the distal course of the nerve. (From Chang KSF, Low WD, Chan ST, et al: Enlargement of the ulnar nerve behind the medial epicondyle, *Anat Rec* 1963; 145:149.)

Syndrome of five. This term was coined[66] to identify the five potential areas of ulnar nerve impingement at the elbow (Fig. 23-5):

1. Medial intermuscular septum
2. Arcade of Struthers
3. Medial epicondyle
4. Osborne's arcuate ligament
5. Flexor-pronator aponeuroses

CLINICAL EVALUATION

Nerve compression is a game of millimeters.

JABALEY[33]

The popular board game CLUE requires that three mystery questions be answered correctly to win: *Who did it? Where? and With What?* These same three questions are important in diagnosing nerve compression. Our evaluation data assist in correct identification of which nerve is involved *(who),* at what location *(where),* and sometimes help

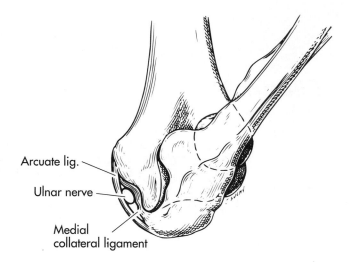

Fig. 23-3. The arcuate ligament (roof of cubital tunnel) tightens while the medial collateral ligament (floor) buckles with elbow flexion, causing decreased volume of the cubital tunnel. (From Fromison AI, Zahraui F: Treatment of compression neuropathy of the ulnar nerve at the elbow by epicondylectomy and neurolysis, *J Hand Surg* 1980; 5[4]:391.)

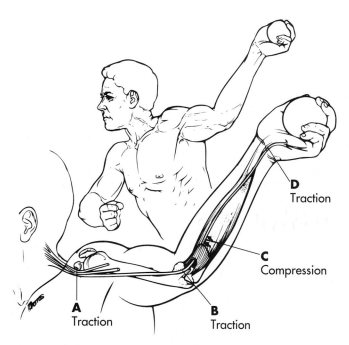

Fig. 23-4. Position of arm causing traction-compression-pressure forces along course of ulnar nerve. (From Gelberman RH: Ulnar tunnel syndrome. In *Operative nerve repair and reconstruction,* vol 2, Philadelphia, 1991, Lippincott.)

incriminate the offending structure *(what).* Unless every millimeter of compression is identified and resolved, symptoms will continue.

Evaluation data further help in the grading of compression severity and as a battery that can monitor symptom abatement or advancement.

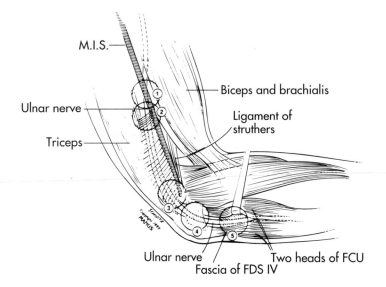

Fig. 23-5. Syndrome of five. Five potential areas of ulnar nerve impingement at the elbow: (1) medial intermuscular septum (MIS), (2) arcade of Struthers, (3) medial epicondyle, (4) Osborne's arcuate ligament, (5) flexor-pronator aponeuroses. (From Kleinman WB, Schnitz GW, and The Indiana Hand Center, Indianapolis, IN, as published in *Hand Clinics* 10(3); August 1994.)

History. The most common symptom of ulnar nerve compression is intermittent hand numbness. Patients do not often relate onset of numbness to prior activity or give precise digit involvement. Aching pain is nonlocalized about the medial elbow and is often associated with forearm cramping. Weakness is described as a clumsiness, patients often drop items. The examiner needs to question the patient for information regarding all prior trauma, especially to the neck, chest, and arm. Delayed onset of neuropraxia following childhood injuries,[55] elbow flexion contractures,[61] postanesthetic palsy,[54] gigantomastia,[16] and periods of excessive work or exercise[31] have all been described. Job activities, hobbies, sports, systemic diseases, subluxing nerves, and posture may all contribute to neural symptoms. Differential diagnosis also includes prior spinal injuries, breast surgery, medial epicondylitis, and space occupying lesions associated with ganglions, bursitis, and osteophytes, all of which can present with medial elbow pain.

Neural tension maneuvers. These are provocative tests that glide and stretch the nerve first segmentally then in a composite fashion to reproduce the symptoms of paresthesia. In effect, we choke the nerve's blood supply and look for complaints. Normal nerves can tolerate brief periods of ischemia, but damaged nerves are more susceptible.[71] This neural ischemia is a protective mechanism for the nervous system, because symptoms produced are a warning that impulse conduction is in danger.[8] The rapid onset and rapid resolution of symptoms with these tests supports the early involvement of local ischemia as the pathology. Butler[8] believes we are identifying minor yet irritating nerve injuries that are preneuropraxic, meaning that segmental demyeli-

nation has not yet occurred and nerve compression studies (NCS) are normal.

Clearing tests. Clearing tests are used to rule out proximal and distal sites of involvement that can radiate into or through the elbow.
- *Cervical Foraminal Compression Maneuvers* to rule out C8 radiculopathy[45]
- *Upper limb tension tests* to rule out brachial plexus neuritis[14,35]
- *Thoracic outlet maneuvers*[50]
- *Phalens test* to rule out compression at Guyon's canal[26]

Elbow flexion test. This test is used to stretch the ulnar nerve around the medial epicondyle and tighten the arcuate ligament. The patient should perform the maneuver with elbows off the table to avoid external pressure. Various authors describe different sensitizing posture additions, held for 1 to 5 minutes, that are used to further provoke a minimally involved nerve. Rather than viewing these prescribed positions as conflicting, it may be that the severity of the compression can be judged by time to provocation or by the number of accessory motions needed to elicit symptoms. Indeed, if paresthesias are reproduced in less than 30 seconds with simple elbow flexion, one is dealing with a more affected nerve than if a positive response is elicited only with full upper extremity ulnar nerve stretch.
- Novak[51] uses elbow flexion, supination, and a wrist-neutral position combined with pressure provocation by placing the examiner's fingers over the subject's ulnar nerve proximal to the elbow (Fig. 23-6, *A*).
- Buehler[7] uses this same posture with the addition of wrist extension to further increase intraneural pressure (Fig.

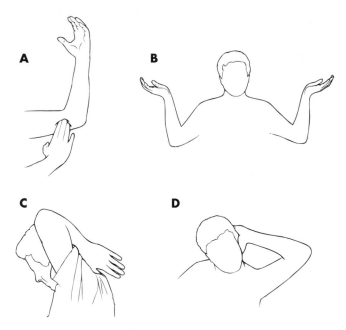

Fig. 23-6. Provocation test position for ulnar nerve at the elbow. **A,** Elbow flexion test with examiner's pressure on nerve. **B,** Elbow flexion test with wrist extension added. **C,** Elbow flexion test with shoulder flexion. **D,** Elbow flexion test with wrist extension, shoulder abduction, and cervical rotation.

23-6, *B*). The wrist position can be altered into flexion with ulnar deviation to access entrapment by the FCU.[23,72]

- Pechan[56] adds proximal positioning of shoulder flexion combined with elbow flexion to identify incipient ulnar nerve involvement (Fig. 23-6, *C*). Studies on various wrist and shoulder positions during elbow flexion showed that shoulder and wrist positions do effect the number of positive test results by sequentially raising neural pressure.[44,61]
- Butler[8] uses positioning of finger and wrist extension and supination, elbow flexion, shoulder abduction, and cervical rotation while supine to take up all slack in the ulnar nerve (Fig. 23-6, *D*). Responses of burning or tingling in the ulnar nerve distribution are indicative of early ischemic problems that precede later mechanical damage.

Tinel's sign. Gentle percussion is applied along the ulnar nerve from distal to proximal up to the paravertebral region. Tapping is omitted along the postcondylar groove and over the clavicle as this causes a positive response in normal patients due to the nerve's position adjacent to bone. A positive response is an electric shock that courses through the ulnar nerve. It is believed this represents axon sprouting as the compressed nerve attempts to repair itself.[13] A long-standing compression may no longer demonstrate a Tinel's sign, as all potential axon regeneration has occurred.

Sensibility tests. Sensory loss noted on the dorsum of the hand as well as on the volar hypothenar heel and last two digits implies involvement of the ulnar nerve (Fig. 23-7). The forearm's sensory innervation comes from

the medial cutaneous nerve and thus is not involved in sensory loss caused by ulnar nerve entrapment. The signature area or autonomous zone for ulnar nerve testing covers the distal two phalanges, volar and dorsal, of the small finger.[12]

Small myelinated and unmyelinated fibers are preferentially depleted by ischemia.[64] Because they subserve the modalities of temperature awareness and pain, these should comprise our earliest test battery for compression. Unfortunately, objective clinical tools are lacking. Studies using external compression of nerves[52] show that larger myelinated fibers are most susceptible to mechanical compression. The first change in these larger sensory perceptions occurs in threshold elevation to vibration and light touch.[17]

All testing is performed using the staircase method of adjusting stimulus intensity at each trial.[62] Supramaximal stimuli are first presented to alert the patient to the nature of the stimulus and each subsequent stimulus descends in intensity. The process continues until several reversals from detection to nondetection have occurred.

- *Vibratory threshold testing* should include both high and low frequency levels, because a debate exists over which end of the spectrum is affected first.[34,39]
- *Light touch threshold* is accessed with monofilaments in a descending mode from high to low filament pressure.
- *Two-point discrimination* is an innervation density test in which abnormal values are seen only in advanced compression. These data are helpful in gauging the degree of severity of the injury.

Muscle function

- *Flexor carpi ulnaris and flexor digitorum profundus (fourth and fifth).* These muscles are usually spared compression at the elbow because of their anatomic proximal branching within the ulnar nerve.[32] However, Fig. 23-8, *A* shows a patient with a large hematoma proximal to the elbow that resulted in complete ulnar nerve compression with loss of the flexor digitorum profundus (FDP) to the small finger (Fig. 23-8, *B*).
- *Interossei.* Subtle clawing may be observed in hand posture (Fig. 23-8, *C*) because of interossei weakness, although 50% of the population have a median to ulnar Riche-Cannieu connection in the palm that may obscure this sign.
- *1st dorsal interossei.* This muscle shows the earliest changes via electrodiagnostic studies in the cubital tunnel.[20,46] Palpation of this muscle during lateral pinch (Fig. 23-8, *D*) and comparison with the uninvolved hand is recommended.
- *Wartenberg's sign.* Persistent abduction of the small finger occurs because of intrinsic hypothenar muscle weakness and unopposed abduction pull by the ulnarly inserted extensor digiti minimi (EDM) tendon (Fig. 23-8, *E*).[70] When the patient is asked to push both small fingers isometrically against each other, the affected side is

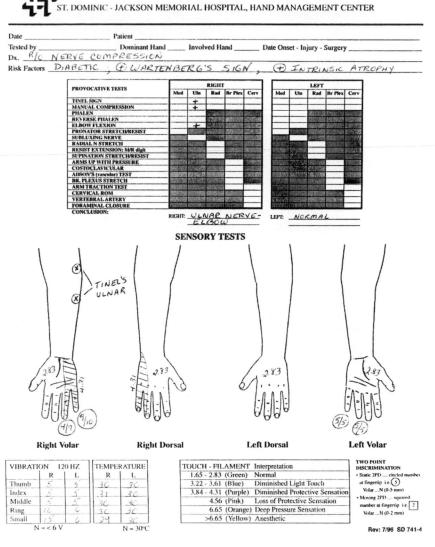

Fig. 23-7. Nerve compression form includes results of upper extremity clearing (provocative) tests, sensibility data and comments on posture, weakness, or other physical findings.

overpowered (Fig. 23-8, *F*), indicating weakness of the hypothenar muscles.

- *Lateral pinch and grip strength.* These measurements are of value to objectively document weakness and recovery.

CONSERVATIVE TREATMENT

The two general rules of conservative management are to avoid recurrent trauma and to have patience because (nerve) regrowth is slow.

TARDIF[68]

Ninety percent of patients with mild compression can recover through conservative treatment regimens.[20] Axonal regrowth may take months to occur, during which time the evaluation battery should show nonprogression of symptoms initially, followed by slow improvement.

Effective conservative management includes the following four areas of intervention:

1. *Avoid pressure on the elbow* through patient education and the use of soft heel/bow type pads during the day.[9]
2. *Make ergonomic changes* to prevent job postures of prolonged elbow flexion (computer operator), contact with hard surfaces over cubital tunnel (seamstress, assembly), repetitive supination/pronation actions (poultry workers). Also avoid forceful extension thrust from full elbow flexion (sledgehammer, press operator, throwing sports).[21,58,67]
3. *Night elbow splinting* is used to prevent prolonged elbow flexion posture during sleep. Studies on the use of nocturnal immobilization report 50% to 100% improvement when splints are used for at least 6 months.[18,29] Electromyographic improvement was also

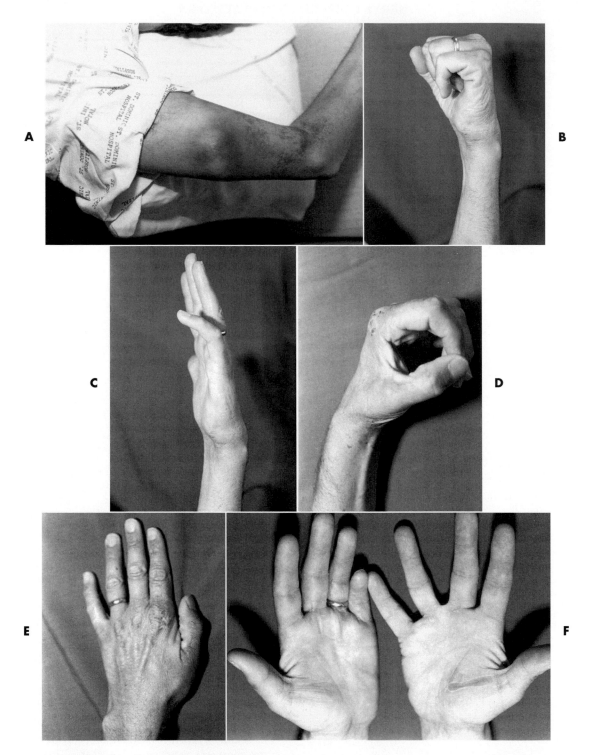

Fig. 23-8. Patient with acute onset ulnar nerve compression secondary to MVA with the following: **(A)** hematoma proximal to elbow, **(B)** loss of FDP action at the distal joint of the small finger, **(C)** subtle clawing of small finger, **(D)** first dorsal interossei atrophy noted with lateral pinch, **(E)** Wartenberg's sign of persistent abduction of the small finger, **(F)** hypothenar weakness demonstrated when the affected small finger is unable to match isometric contraction of nonaffected small finger.

noted in patients treated with splints who had previously undergone surgical decompression but failed to improve.[63] Splint designs vary from soft to semirigid thermoplastic dorsal long arm with wrist support. They all rest the elbow in a semiflexed posture to prevent elbow flexion beyond 45° to 65°.

4. *Stretching and strengthening program.* Because of the high correlation of double crush with elbow neuropathy, it is suggested that the entire upper quadrant be evaluated for sites of muscle imbalance.[43] Cervical flexors, scapula abductors, shoulder internal rotators, and forearm pronators are often shortened through poor posture. Stretching the involved muscles while using pain-free strengthening of the antagonistic muscles will help reverse multiple areas of subclinical compression.[42] Butler[8] advocates nonprovoking maneuvers of self-mobilization to address neural and nonneural restrictions to nerve gliding.

POSTOPERATIVE MANAGEMENT

The postoperative result reflects the preoperative status regardless of which procedure is used.

LUNDBORG[40]

The surgeon has three basic options for addressing recalcitrant compression at the elbow.
- Unroof the tunnel: Decompression
- Eliminate the tunnel: Medial epicondylectomy
- Remove nerve from tunnel: Transposition

Regardless of which surgical procedure is used, prolonged immobilization of the elbow is discouraged due to its deleterious effect on nerve and joint mobility.[24] Following surgical intervention, the primary goal for the therapist is to provide early, protected motion that facilitates nerve gliding. The judicial use of protective positioning will prevent disruption of soft tissue, while preventing fixation of nerve by scar tissue in the operative bed.

The conservative treatment measures previously described also become part of the postoperative regimen in order to address the cause and possible recurrence of the problem. Any preoperative positive evaluation findings are reassessed on a timely basis to ensure resolution.

Decompression

Resection of the arcuate ligament unroofs the tunnel, thus eliminating the compressive forces on the nerve. The ulnar nerve is left to glide in its good local bed (Fig. 23-9, *2*). Rapid rehabilitation and early return to work are the chief advantages of this procedure.

Postoperatively, the wound is supported with a plaster splint for 3 to 4 days. Upon removal, early active range of motion (AROM) is initiated along with distal nerve gliding exercises as described by Baxter-Petralia following carpal tunnel release (CTR).[4] In the absence of any neural discomfort, proximal nerve gliding is next encouraged with

cervical and shoulder positions added to the movement regimen.[8] By the second week, gentle strengthening exercises for the hand and wrist can be initiated.[22,48]

Complications are rare, but can be caused by prolonged immobilization with nerve-scar adherence, subluxation of the nerve without its restraining ligament, and failure to relieve symptoms because of other compressive factors.

Medial epicondylectomy

One osseous wall of the cubital tunnel is excised to eliminate this nonyielding fulcrum around which the ulnar nerve is stretched with motion (Fig. 23-9, *6*). Because the nerve is allowed to migrate over the resected bone, traction forces are diminished. Decompression of the arcuate ligament is performed concomitantly, thereby removing compressive forces. Only a portion of the flexor-pronator muscle origin is incised longitudinally for this dissection. Because the primary muscle origin remains intact, rehabilitation can progress after a brief period of immobilization.

Postoperatively, a splint is used to hold the elbow at 50° to 70° of flexion for 1 week.[28,30] Alternately, only a soft dressing and arm sling can be used to encourage early active motion.[25] Full elbow range of motion (ROM) should be achieved within a few weeks.

This procedure involves more tissue disruption as well as periosteal stripping, compared with other surgical options, which can result in increased swelling and scarring. Patients' complaints of pain often cause self-limitation when early motion is so critical for joint and nerve integrity. Elevation and intermittent use of elbow continuous passive motion (CPM) devices are often effective in pumping edema and decreasing postoperative pain.

Anterior transpositions

Transposition removes the nerve from its tunnel to escape the unhealthy factors in the old bed. In its new environment, compressive and traction forces are eliminated. Because the nerve now runs anterior to the elbow, its shorter course allows it to remain slack throughout elbow motion. The three forms of nerve transposition vary in the final resting place for the nerve and thus impact postoperative rehabilitation.

Subcutaneous transposition. The ulnar nerve is relocated from behind the medial epicondyle to a position anterior to it and is placed superficially beneath skin and fat. Various dermal-fascial slings are created to secure the nerve in its new route (Fig. 23-9, *3*). Ogata[53] showed that neural blood flow decreased significantly for up to 7 days following subcutaneous transposition compared with decompression and epicondylectomy. Postoperatively, a soft compressive dressing with an arm sling is used to support the elbow for the first week, thus preventing excessive motion of a vascular compromised nerve. AROM is encouraged and should reach 90% of normal range within

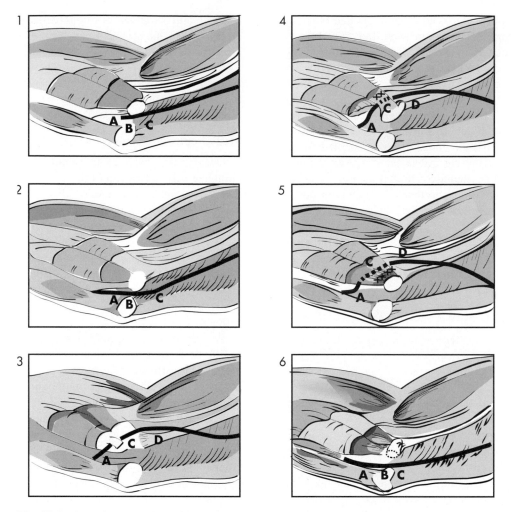

Fig. 23-9. Operative procedures for ulnar nerve at the elbow. (**1**) Normal anatomy of ulnar nerve, (**2**) decompression of arcuate ligament, (**3**) subcutaneous transposition, (**4**) intramuscular transposition, (**5**) submuscular transposition, (**6**) medial epicondylectomy. (Redrawn from Dellon Al, et al: Intraneural ulnar nerve pressure changes related to operative techniques for cubital tunnel decompression, *J Hand Surg* 1994; 19[A]6:925.)

2 weeks.[19] Ulnar nerve gliding protocol is followed as previously described.

Intramuscular transposition. The ulnar nerve is relocated from behind the medial epicondyle to a position anterior to it within a channel made in the flexor-pronator muscle bellies and is closed with a fascia repair above (Fig. 23-9, *4*). Most authors recommend splinting the elbow in a 90° flexed position and the forearm in midpronation for 3 weeks to allow soft tissue healing without disruption.[27,37] At 3 weeks, the splint is removed for AROM sessions and gradually modified into extension. Passive range of motion (PROM) and strengthening are delayed until 6 weeks. Dellon[15] suggests that 3 weeks of immobilization may be too long. In primate models, 2 weeks of splinting followed by unrestricted arm use allow allowed gliding of the nerve while protecting the tendinous-fascial repair.

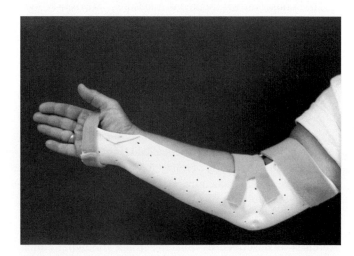

Fig. 23-10. Splint used postoperatively following submuscular transposition of the ulnar nerve.

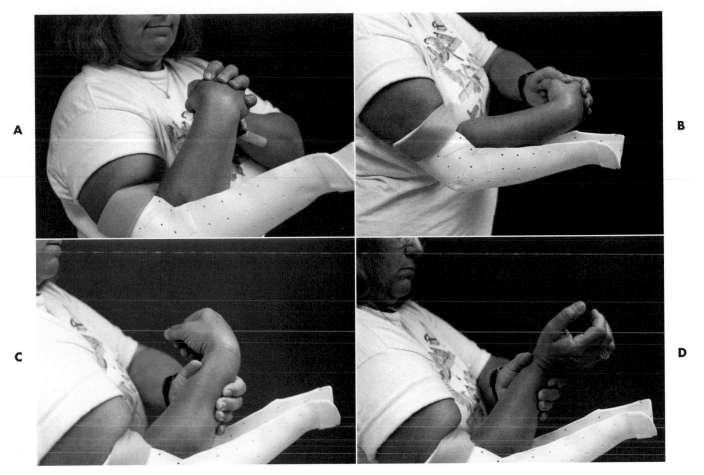

Fig. 23-11. Use of protective passive range of motion to relieve stress on the repaired flexor-pronator muscles following submuscular transposition of the ulnar nerve: (**A**) protected passive elbow flexion motion with wrist held passively flexed (**B**) and elbow extension, (**C**) protected passive wrist flexion with elbow held passively flexed, (**D**) wrist extension.

Submuscular transposition. The flexor-pronator common tendon is detached, allowing the ulnar nerve to be routed anteriorly beneath it and the muscles are reattached (Fig. 23-9, 5). It is recognized that this procedure has the longest postoperative recovery period to ensure that the muscles heal sufficiently.

Traditional protocols recommend 3 weeks immobilization in a splint holding the elbow at 90° flexion, the forearm in 45° pronation, and the wrist flexed 20° (Fig. 23-10).[6,36] Shoulder and finger ROM are encouraged during this period. The arm is then kept in a sling for an additional 2 weeks, at which time active motion is encouraged at all joints. Others advocate 2 weeks of immobilization at which time protective PROM exercises are initiated for the elbow and wrist.[60,75] Protective PROM ensures no stress on the repaired flexor pronator origin by passively flexing the wrist when elbow motion is performed (Fig. 23-11, A and B) then passively holding the elbow flexed for wrist motion (Fig. 23-11, C and D).[2]

Full elbow extension and supination are gently achieved in the following weeks. Nerve gliding protocols are gradually increased. At 3 weeks, active exercises are permitted to encourage combined wrist and elbow extension. Stretching is delayed until week six at which time strengthening exercises are also initiated.

Complications include extensor lag of 15° to 20°, which should not interfere with function,[69] cutaneous neuromas, and chronic medial epicondylitis, which is managed conservatively. Because transpositions are reserved for more severe compressions, the prognosis for full sensory and motor recovery is guarded.

THERAPY

Strengthening programs. Despite the surgical technique chosen, only one third of patients with muscle atrophy will see recovery.[16] Operative intervention can prevent further nerve damage, but nerve regrowth is limited. Adellar[1] found the presence of intrinsic atrophy to be the most significant factor in predicting final results. The challenge to prevent or reverse muscle wasting remains before us. Petterson[59] showed improved strength and endurance of the first dorsal interossei following 4 hours of daily stimulation in a patient 2 years posttransposition. Motor conduction velocity did not improve poststimulation, so it was suggested that enhanced recruitment of existing motor units led to the positive findings. The ability of partially innervated muscle to respond to electrical stimulation is caused by hypertrophy of the existing innervated muscle fibers. This treatment is not effective for the dennervated fibers.[49]

Exercise protocols for partially denervated muscles secondary to compression have been defined.[49] The duration and intensity of exercise sessions are designed to prevent muscle fatigue that leads to soft tissue overuse symptoms. Low duration of 5 to 10 minutes with resistance kept at less than 50% of maximal voluntary contraction performed several times per day should be the regimen for early rehabilitation. These parameters can be increased if soft tissue or joint inflammation does not occur. Overzealous therapy is to be avoided.

Nerve mobilization. The transition of nerve gliding principles from anatomic studies to clinical practice is our current frontier. We seek studies that direct us and confirm the appropriate intervention. Most hand therapists have incorporated segmental nerve gliding exercises for specific compression sites into their postoperative regimens. This is a good beginning. Now we need more information on composite upper extremity nerve mobilization, sequencing, duration, documentation of performance, adverse symptoms, and contraindications.

Kwan[38] reminds us that although normal nerves are flexible, with low levels of tension throughout motion, chronically injured nerves have increased stiffness secondary to long-standing intraneural edema. These stiffened nerves do not stretch the same distances as normal nerves. Lundborg[40] pleads for initial immobilization to relieve stress on the nerve and to reestablish intraneural circulation. As edema decreases, gliding increases. How do we reconcile these facts with work that shows the efficacy of immediate postoperative unrestricted motion?[11] These arguments should have a *déjà vu* quality to them. Experts on tendon healing once debated the same questions. Their discussion of these issues led to research and controlled motion protocols. Nerve mobilization techniques will be refined and better defended only through research endeavours.

Painless mobility enhancing techniques. Therapy should not hurt. There is no justification for painful stretching, splinting, or strengthening. A walk through a good hand therapy unit should show smiling faces, not tears. Brand's[5] writings present a philosophy of winning a patient's trust and cooperation through gentle, patient coaxing of tissue changes. Forceful stretching is only a temporary phenomenon, like a rubber band stretched and relaxed. True tissue lengthening requires time for the collagen matrix to biologically adjust to the new, maintained resting length. The use of simultaneous heat and stretch techniques, mobilization followed by splinting, CPM, and

endurance type exercises are all aimed at progress achieved slowly and painlessly.

REFERENCES

1. Adellar RS, Foster W, McDowell C: The treatment of the cubital tunnel syndrome, *J Hand Surg* 1984; 9A:90.
2. Amadio P, Gabel G: Treatment and complications of failed decompression of the ulnar nerve at the elbow. In Gelberman RH, ed: *Nerve repair and reconstruction,* Philadelphia, 1991, Lippincott.
3. Apfelberg DP, Larson SJ: Dynamic anatomy of the ulnar nerve at the elbow, *Plast Reconstr Surg* 1973; 51(1):76.
4. Baxter-Petralia P: Therapists' management of carpal tunnel syndrome. In Hunter, et al, eds: *Rehabilitation of the hand,* St Louis, 1990, Mosby.
5. Brand P, Yancey P: *The gift nobody wanted,* New York, 1995, Harper Perennial.
6. Broudy A, Leffert R, Smith R: Technical problems with ulnar nerve transposition at the elbow: findings and results of reoperation, *J Hand Surg* 1978; 3(1):85.
7. Buehler MJ, Thayer DT: The elbow flexion test: a clinical test for the cubital tunnel syndrome, *Cl Ortho Rel Res* 1988; 233:213.
8. Butler DS: *Mobilization of the nervous system,* New York, 1991, Churchill Livingstone.
9. Cannon N: Cubital tunnel syndrome—conservative management. In *Diagnosis and treatment manual for physicians and therapists,* Indianapolis, 1991, Hand Rehabilitation Center of Indiana.
10. Chang KSF, Low WD, Chan ST: Enlargement of the ulnar nerve behind the medial epicondyle, *Anat Rec* 1963; 145:149.
11. Cook AC, Szabo RM, Birkholz SW, King EF: Early mobilization following carpal tunnel release, *J Hand Surg* 1995; 20B(2):228.
12. Dawson D, Hallett M, Millender L: Ulnar nerve entrapment at the elbow. In *Entrapment neuropathies,* Boston, 1990, Little, Brown.
13. Dellon AL: Tinel or not tinel? *J Hand Surg* 1984; 9B:216.
14. Dellon AL, Hoaglund FT, Scheck M: Brachial neuritis, *J Bone Joint Surg* 1985; 67A:6:878.
15. Dellon AL, MacKinnon SE, Hudson AR, Hunter DA: Effect of submuscular versus intramuscular placement of ulnar nerve: experimental model in the primate, *J Hand Surg* 1986; 11B(1):117.
16. Dellon AL: Peripheral nerve injuries. In Georgiade NG, et al, eds: *Peripheral nerve injuries,* Baltimore, 1987, Williams & Wilkins.
17. Dellon AL: Sensibility testing. In Gelberman RH, ed: Nerve repair and reconstruction, Philadelphia, 1991, Lippincott.
18. Diamond M, Lister G: Cubital tunnel syndrome treated by long-arm splintage, *J Hand Surg* 1985; 10A(3):430.
19. Eaton RG: Anterior subcutaneous transposition. In Gelberman RH, ed: *Nerve repair and reconstruction,* Philadelphia, 1991, Lippincott.
20. Eisen A, Danon J: The mild cubital tunnel syndrome, *Neurol* 1974; 24:608.
21. Feldman R, Goldman R, Keyserling M: Peripheral nerve entrapment syndromes and ergonomic factors, *Am J Ind Med* 1983; 4:661.
22. Ferlic DC: In situ decompression of the ulnar nerve at the elbow. In Gelberman RH, ed: *Nerve repair and reconstruction,* Philadelphia, 1991, Lippincott.
23. Fine EJ: The ulnar flexion maneuver, *Mus and Nerve* 1985; 8:612.
24. Folberg C, Weiss A, Akelman E: Cubital tunnel syndrome, Part II: treatment, *Ortho Review* 233:March 1994.
25. Fromison AI, Zahraui F: Treatment of compression neuropathy of the ulnar nerve at the elbow by epicondylectomy and neurolysis, *J Hand Surg* 1980; 5(4):391.
26. Gelberman RH: Ulnar tunnel syndrome. In *Operative nerve repair and reconstruction,* vol 2, Philadelphia, 1991, Lippincott.
27. Gelberman RH, Eaton RC, Urbaniak JR: Peripheral nerve compression, *AAOS Inst Course Lect,* 1994; 43:31.
28. Goldberg B, Light T, Blair S: Ulnar neuropathy at the elbow: results of medial epicondylectomy, *J Hand Surg* 1989; 14A:182.

29. Harper B: The drop-out splint: an alternative to the conservative management of ulnar nerve entrapment at the elbow, *J Hand Ther* 1990; 3(4):199.

30. Heithoff S, Millender L, Nalebuff E, Petriska A: Medial epicondylectomy for the treatment of ulnar nerve compression at the elbow, *J Hand Surg* 1990; 15A:22.

31. Hodgkinson PD, McLean NR: Ulnar nerve entrapment due to epitrochleoanconeus muscle, *J Hand Surg* 1994; 19B(6):706.

32. Jabaley M, Wallace W, Heckler F: Internal topography of major nerves of the forearm and hand: a current view, *J Hand Surg* 1980; 5(1):1.

33. Jabaley M: (personal communication) 1995.

34. Jimenez S, Hardy M, Horch K, Jabaley M: A study of sensory recovery following carpal tunnel release, *J Hand Ther* 1993; 6(2):124.

35. Kenneally M, Rubenach H, Elvey R: The upper limb tension test: the SLR test of the arm. In Grant R, ed: *Physical therapy of the cervical and thoracic spine, Clinics in PT* 1988; 17:167.

36. King PB, Aulicino PL: The postoperative rehabilitation of the Learmonth submuscular transposition of the ulnar nerve at the elbow, *J Hand Ther* 1990; 3(3):149.

37. Kleinman WB: Anterior intramuscular transposition. In Gelberman RH, ed: *Operative nerve repair and reconstruction*, Philadelphia, 1991, Lippincott.

38. Kwan MK, Wall E, Massie J, Garfin S: Strain, stress and stretch of peripheral nerve, *Acta Ortho Scand* 1992; 63:267.

39. Lundborg G, Lie-Stenstrom A, Sollerman C, et al: Digital vibrogram: a new diagnostic tool for sensory testing in compression neuropathy, *J Hand Surg* 1986; 11A(5):693.

40. Lundborg G: Surgical treatment for ulnar nerve entrapment at the elbow, *J Hand Surg* 1992; 17B:245.

41. MacKinnon S, Dellon Al: Ulnar nerve entrapment at the elbow. In *Surgery of the peripheral nerve,* New York, 1988, Thieme Medical.

42. MacKinnon SE, Novak CB: Clinical commentary: pathogenesis of cumulative trauma disorder, *J Hand Surg* 1994; 19A(5):873.

43. MacKinnon SE: Double and multiple crush syndromes, *Hand Clin* 1992; 8(2):369.

44. Macnicol MF: Extraneural pressure affecting the ulnar nerve at the elbow, *The Hand* 1982; 14(1):5.

45. McKenzie RA: *The cervical and thoracic spine mechanical diagnosis and treatment,* New Zealand, 1990, Spinal Publications.

46. Miller RG: Ulnar neuropathy at the elbow (AAEM case report #1), *Muscle Nerve* 1991; 14:97.

47. Millesi H: The nerve gap theory and clinical practice, *Hand Clin* 1986; 2(4):651.

48. Nathan PA, Myers LD, Keniston RC, Meadows KD: Simple decompression of the ulnar nerve: an alternative to anterior transposition, *J Hand Surg* 1992; 17B:251.

49. Nitz AJ: Effects of acute pressure on peripheral nerve structure and function. In Currier D, Nelson R, eds: *Dynamics of human biologic tissues,* Philadelphia, 1992, Davis.

50. Novak CB, MacKinnon SE, Patterson GA: Evaluation of patients with thoracic outlet syndrome, *J Hand Surg* 1993; 18A:292.

51. Novak CB, Lee GW, MacKinnon SE, Lay L: Provocative testing in cubital tunnel syndrome, *J Hand Surg* 1994; 19A(5):817.

52. Ochoa J, Fowler TJ, Gilliatt RW: Anatomical changes in peripheral nerves compressed by a pneumatic tourniquet, *J Anat* 1972; 113:433.

53. Ogata K, Manske P, Lesker P: The effect of surgical dissection on regional blood flow to the ulnar nerve in the cubital tunnel, *Clin Ortho Rel Res* 1985; 193:195.

54. Omer GE: The cubital tunnel syndrome. In Szabo RM, ed: *Nerve compression syndromes, diagnosis and treatment*, Thorofare, New Jersey, 1989, Slack.

55. Paine KWE: Tardy ulnar palsy, *Can J Surg* 1970; 13:255.

56. Pechan J: Ulnar nerve manoeuvre as diagnostic aid in its pressure lesions in the cubital region, *Cs Neurol a Neurchir* 1973; 36(39):13.

57. Pechan J, Juluis I: The pressure measurement in the ulnar nerve: a contribution to the pathophysiology of the cubital tunnel syndrome, *J Biomech* 1975; 8:75.

58. Pechan J, Kredba J: Cubital tunnel syndrome II. Clinical aspects, *ACTA Univ Carol* (Med) 1981; 27:236.

59. Petterson T, Smith GP, Oldham A, et al: The use of patterned neuromuscular stimulation to improve hand function following surgery for ulnar neuropathy, *J Hand Surg* 1994; 19B(4):430.

60. Rayan GM: Proximal ulnar nerve compression: cubital tunnel syndrome, *Hand Clin* 1992; 8(2):325.

61. Rayan GM, Jensen C, Duke J: Elbow flexion test in the normal population, *J Hand Surg* 1992; 17A:86.

62. Rosenberger PB: Response-adjusting stimulus intensity. In Stebbins WC, ed: *Animal psychophysics,* New York, 1970, Appleton-Century-Crofts.

63. Seror P: Treatment of ulnar nerve palsy at the elbow with a night splint, *J Bone Joint Surg* 1993; 75B(2):322.

64. Shuman S, Osterman L, Bora FW: Compression neuropathies, *Semin Neurol* 1987; 7(1):76.

65. Sunderland S: *Nerve and nerve injuries,* Baltimore, 1968, Williams & Wilkins.

66. Szabo R: Pathophysiology of nerve compression syndromes. In *Comprehensive management of peripheral nerve problems,* (ASHT course notes), 1995, New Orleans.

67. Tadano P: A safety/prevention program for VDT operators: one company's approach, *J Hand Ther* 1990; 3(2):64.

68. Tardiff G: Nerve injuries: testing and treatment tactics, *Phys & Sports Med* 1995; 23(4):61.

69. Vasen A, Lacey S, Keith M, Shaffer J: Functional range of motion of the elbow, *J Hand Surg* 1995; 20A(2):288.

70. Voche P, Merle M: Wartenberg's sign, *J Hand Surg* 1995; 20B(1):49.

71. Wadsworth TG: The external compression syndrome of the ulnar nerve at the cubital tunnel, *Clin Ortho Rel Res* 1977; 124:189.

72. Werner CO, Ohlin P, Elmquist D: Pressures recorded in ulnar neuropathy, *ACTA Ortho Scand* 1985; 56:404.

73. Wilgis EFS, Murphy R: The significance of longitudinal excursion in peripheral nerves, *Hand Clin* 1986; 2(4):761.

74. Zachary LS, Dellon ES, Nicholas EM, Dellon AL: The structural basis of Felice Fontana's spiral bands and their relationship to nerve injury, *J Reconstr Microsurg* 1993; 9(2):131.

75. Zemel N, Jobe F, Yocum L: Submuscular transposition/ulnar nerve decompression in athletes. In Gelberman RH, ed: *Nerve repair and reconstruction,* Philadelphia, 1991, Lippincott.

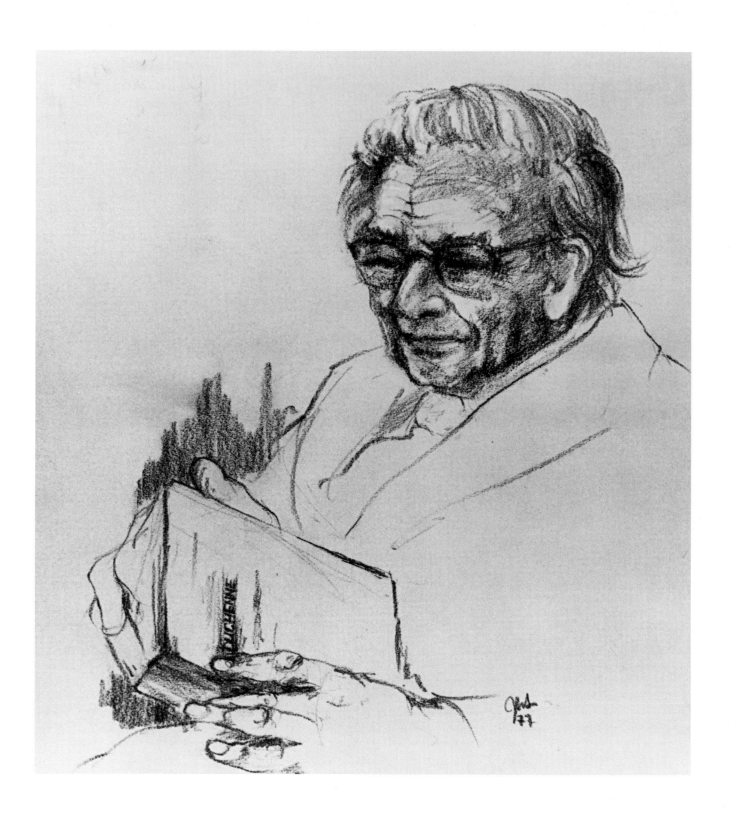

Part VI

BRACHIAL PLEXUS INJURIES

Emanuel Kaplan—a scholar of hand anatomy reflecting over his translation of Duchenne's *Physiology of Motion.*

Chapter 24

SURGICAL TREATMENT OF BRACHIAL PLEXUS LESIONS

Hanno Millesi

The brachial plexus consists of the spinal nerve C5, C6, C7, C8, and Th1. The spinal nerves are formed by the ventral root carrying motor fibers and the dorsal root carrying sensory fibers. The spinal ganglion with the neurons of the sensory fibers is located along the dorsal root. The roots unite within the intervertebral canal to form the spinal nerve. The spinal nerves C5 and C6 form the trunk portion, the spinal nerve C7 composes the medius, and trunk nerves C8 and T1 make up the inferior trunk. The nerves exchange fibers through the anterior and posterior division of the trunks, forming the lateral, dorsal, and medial cords, which give rise to the peripheral nerves.

A lesion to the brachial plexus is caused by compression of the plexus between the first rib and the clavicle, or by longitudinal traction in the case of a luxation of the shoulder joint, a fracture of the humerus, or by a combination of both compression and longitudinal traction, especially if the shoulder during an accident meets a hard object and the head still carries energy. The lesion can be an avulsion of the rootlets from the spinal cord; a rupture of the spinal nerves, trunks, or cords; or a lesion with preserved continuity and a different amount of fibrosis. The vast majority of cases are traffic accidents, mainly motorcycle accidents, followed by sport incidences. In rare cases a gunshot wound or stab wound causes a brachial plexus lesion. A brachial plexus lesion may also occur along with a fracture of the clavicle or a fracture of a transverse process of one of the cervical vertebrae.

In addition to posttraumatic lesions in adults, brachial plexus lesions occur during birth or in consequence of irradiation with the treatment of malignant tumors. This chapter is confined to posttraumatic lesions.

THE BRACHIAL PLEXUS PATIENT

Some open injuries may be in themselves indications for surgery. For example, if parts of the brachial plexus are cleanly transected by a stab wound, a neurorrhaphy is indicated. Vascular damage to the subclavian artery or vein may be part of an open or a closed injury, both cases indicate vascular surgery to repair the transected artery or vein. The question is whether at this point the brachial plexus should be explored and treated simultaneously. In my opinion this should be done only in exceptional cases. In the vast majority of cases, the patient with a hemorrhage from the subclavian artery is in a rather serious condition. The best thing to do is to deal with the vascular injury as well as possible and to avoid any additional damage to the brachial plexus, which can sometimes occur if the surgeon feels obliged to clarify the situation of the brachial plexus at the time of vascular surgery.

Initially gunshot wounds affecting the brachial plexus are treated conservatively. Frequently the lesion is the result of indirect damage and spontaneous recovery is possible.

The vast majority of patients with brachial plexus lesions present themselves as a closed injury. In a complete lesion there is a flail arm with lack of sensibility, except for the inner aspect of the upper arm. Behind this situation there might be an avulsion of all five roots without any chance of spontaneous recovery. Such a case should be operated on as soon as is suitable.

A patient with first-degree or second-degree damage (Sunderland[10]), has a good chance of spontaneous recovery within several weeks or months. It would be wrong to perform surgery in such a case. It is, therefore, the main task of our diagnostic efforts to recognize cases that have good chances of spontaneous recovery.

Patients with a first-degree damage (Sunderland)—conduction block without interruption of continuity—preserve motor conductivity beyond the first days. In cases of second-degree damage (axonotmesis) or a higher degree of damage, patients lose motor conductivity when Wallerian degeneration occurs.

Having ruled out the patient with first-degree damage, we still do not know whether there is a chance of spontaneous recovery because of the presence of a second-degree damage.

All patients in whom a proximal stump is available develop during the first weeks axon sprouts that provoke a Tinel-Hofmann sign. It must be confirmed that this Tinel-Hofmann sign includes irradiation of the paresthesias to the hand so that it is not mistaken for a Tinel-Hofmann sign caused by damage of a sensory nerve of the cervical plexus. If spontaneous recovery begins, the Tinel sign is going to move in a distal direction. In the case of second-degree damage (axonotmesis), this distal movement is rather rapid and after several weeks early signs of recovery in very proximal muscles may be detected. In all other cases surgical exploration is indicated.

Birch[1] suggested very early exploration. In this situation patients with a lesion who have good chances of spontaneous recovery would be operated on without benefit. For this reason I do not favor early operation on closed injuries. But if after 3 months no signs of recovery are apparent, the patient should be operated on. The operation should not be performed more than 6 months after the injury.

A CT myelography and MR examination may reveal a meningocelia or signs of interruption of the rootlets or the spinal nerve, respectively. A clinical sign for the presence of an avulsion is the preservation of conductivity of the sensory fibers that are still in contact with the spinal ganglion. The deep muscles of the neck and, in the case of a lesion of C5, C6, and C7, the serratus anterior muscle innervated by the long thoracic nerve, which is formed by tiny nerves leaving the spinal nerve very early, is another argument for the presence of an avulsion. A Horner syndrome is an argument for the presence of an avulsion of C8 and Th1. In case of an avulsion of all five roots, there is no Tinel sign.

These symptoms are not all completely reliable. The problem is still more complex because one root might be avulsed and the neighboring one ruptured or in continuity. A completely reliable diagnosis of the amount of damage to the spinal nerves can be established only by surgical exploration.

In contrast, if the serratus anterior muscle is working with no Horner syndrome present and the patient shows a Tinel sign in the supraclavicular fossa, it may be assumed that at least some roots are not avulsed. If the suprascapular nerve is intact and the supraspinatus muscle innervated, the site of the lesion is in a cord level.

Not all elements of the brachial plexus may suffer the same amount of damage. A pure avulsion of all five roots is represented only in 14% of our cases. In the majority of patients, avulsions and ruptures are mixed and other structures have suffered only a lesion in continuity.

Under special circumstances a partial plexus lesion may develop. We differentiate between an upper brachial plexus lesion, concerning the root C5 and C6 with loss of function of the shoulder muscles and elbow flexion but intact forearm and hand muscles; an upper brachial plexus lesion, concerning C5, C6, and C7 in which also the radialis innervated muscles are paralyzed; and a lower brachial plexus lesion, concerning the root C8 and Th1 with paralysis of the forearm and the hand muscles. An intermediate brachial plexus lesion focused on C7 is rather rare.

PROGNOSIS

A patient with an avulsion of all five roots has a very poor prognosis. Even if optimal results are achieved, the patient may only regain control of the shoulder joint and elbow flexion. We cannot expect return of function at the level of the hand. From the beginning these patients need social help in changing to a profession that can be performed with one hand. This is extremely important because the treatment of brachial plexus cases will cover a period of several years and during this time the patient has to be reintegrated into professional life. Otherwise the patient might develop depression or drug problems. In spite of the fact that objective recovery is very poor, regaining shoulder control and active elbow flexion along with an eventual arthrodesis of the wrist joint converts a useless limb that forms an obstacle into a useful limb that is not an obstacle any more. The patients are, therefore, generally happy with the result and surgery is indicated despite the fact that from a socioeconomic point of view the patient's gain will be minimal because he or she will have to change professions and will have to be compensated.

On the other hand, a patient who has a lesion with preserved continuity, maybe second-degree damage with fibrosis and compression that did not allow spontaneous recovery, will have a very good recovery after surgery.

A great problem in patients with brachial plexus lesions is pain. A high percentage of patients develop a pain syndrome, especially with root avulsions. The pain syndrome is located in the spinal cord and cannot be addressed by surgical exploration. All available treatments to control the pain should be applied. In severe cases neurosurgical procedures at the central level should be performed. From widespread statistics we know that occurrence of pain syndromes is much less frequent in patients who have undergone surgery as compared with patients who have not. There is no reason to believe that a surgical exploration of the plexus may contribute to the development of a pain syndrome.

SURGICAL APPROACH

There are two basically different ways to approach the brachial plexus.

1. *Approach from frontal direction.* The patient is in half-sitting position, and the surgeon is in front of the patient and approaches the brachial plexus from a ventral direction. Especially in this situation the clavicle forms an obstacle. For this reason, this approach frequently goes along with an osteotomy of the clavicle. The advantage of this approach is the surgeon sees the anatomic structures as he or she is used to seeing them in textbooks.

2. *Approach from cranial direction.* The patient is supine with the involved shoulder slightly elevated. The arm is scrubbed and freely moveable. The surgeon is sitting between the arm and the head of the patient and approaches the supraclavicular and infraclavicular fossa from the cranial direction. I have used this approach for many years. The big advantage is that the clavicle and other structures do not form an obstacle because they can be lifted easily, especially if the arm is adducted and lifted. The brachial plexus can be approached not only from the ventral side but from the dorsal side as well. The only disadvantage is that the surgeon must get used to the reversed anatomic picture.

INCISIONS

Again there are basically two different ways to perform the surgical incision.

1. Since the beginning of my activity in the field of brachial plexus surgery in 1963, I have used a zigzag-shaped incision, starting on the neck behind the sterno-cleidomastoideus muscle, turning laterally to follow the clavicle, turning again to traverse the pectoralis area and to meet the anterior axillary fold. If necessary the incision can be continued in a zigzag shape to the midline of the medial aspect of the forearm and then continued as long as is desired. In extreme cases, if the ulnar nerve is harvested, the incision can extend to the wrist joint. Three triangular flaps are formed by this incision: a dorsally based flap over the supraclavicular fossa, a ventrally based flap over the infraclavicular fossa, and a dorsally based flap in the pectoralis area. The dorsally based flap over the supraclavicular fossa has to be lifted to a great extent, and its base still forms an obstacle to proceeding with the dissection around the brachial plexus to its dorsal aspect. Sometimes we have had problems with the skin at the edge of the triangle and quite often the scars have become hyper-trophic and wide.

2. For several years I have used a sagittal incision to explore the supraclavicular and infraclavicular fossa. This incision was elaborated after a study of the tension and the deformity of the skin over the supraclavicular and infraclavicular fossa.[5,8] It is located in an area where the least tension and deformity occur and follows Langer's lines of cleavage. Usually, the scar is very discreet. This incision offers good access to the supraclavicular and infraclavicular fossa and especially to the dorsal aspect of the spinal nerves and their trunks.

If the C5 and C6 roots are involved, the sagittal incision has to be supplemented by a small transverse incision at the neck. The skin between the two incisions is lifted to allow sufficient exposure of C5 and C6. The sagittal incision is also supplemented on the lateral side by an incision that starts at the coracoid process, follows Langer's line to reach the axillary fold, and is then continued along the arm and forearm as desired. The advantage of this approach has been mentioned already. The only disadvantage is that there are skin flaps between the incisions that have to be lifted and pulled in different directions to allow access.

EXPLORATION OF THE BRACHIAL PLEXUS

To get sufficient access to the brachial plexus, the sulcus deltoideo pectoralis is enlarged and the minor pectoralis muscle is isolated. Then the structures of the brachial plexus can be defined laterally and medially to this muscle. At the infraclavicular level, the clavicular origin of the major pectoralis muscle is detached and the clavicle and the subclavian muscle are then isolated and lifted in different directions. Supraclavicularily, the omhyoideus muscle and the transversa colli vessels are isolated. In this way the surgeon gains different windows that can be used to access the individual parts of the brachial plexus. The main principle is to start the dissection at a level with normal structures. This is usually the level of the deltoideus pectoral sulcus lateral to the minor pectoralis muscle. From there, after the individual structures have been defined, one can easily proceed in a central direction. In the supraclavicular fossa it is often easy to define the superior trunk and follow it in a cranial and distal direction. The medius and the inferior trunks are more easily explored after the cords and divisions have been prepared coming from underneath the clavicle. After the trunks have been isolated, one can reach the dorsal aspect of the trunks and proceed to the first rib and Sibson's fascia. With root lesions, the area of the spinal nerves between the anterior and the intermedius scalenus muscle forms a mass of scar tissue and dissection becomes difficult. In this case the phrenic nerve is explored and followed to reach root C4. One then can go down from C4 to C5, and so on.

INTRAOPERATIVE FINDINGS

During the exploration the surgeon may discover the following:
1. An avulsion of a spinal nerve
2. A lesion with loss of continuity at the level of the spinal nerves, trunks, or cords with a proximal stump

3. A lesion in continuity

These three basic findings are usually combined.

Root avulsion

The extreme situation of root avulsion is an avulsion of all five roots (14% in our material). In this situation no proximal stump is available. Regeneration of muscles can be achieved only by the transfer of motor axons from other nerves to neurotisize the denervated distal stumps and muscles. It is evident that not all functions can be restored, and more important functions should have priority.

List of priorities

Elbow joint. The most important function is elbow flexion. This should be achieved by regeneration within the biceps muscle through neurotization of the musculocutaneous nerve. It is our experience that the triceps muscle frequently regenerates much better than the biceps muscle. Therefore, we neurotize the biceps and the triceps despite the fact that these two muscles are antagonists. Already at this stage we plan to perform a transfer of the triceps tendon to the biceps to have both muscles acting as elbow flexors. This gives us a second chance if the biceps muscle does not regenerate well and fails to develop sufficient force. In certain cases both muscles show only weak regeneration, but after the transfer, the combined force of the two muscles can achieve useful elbow flexion. This is an important example of how the brachial plexus reconstructive procedures are planned at the time of surgery.

Muscular extension of the elbow is not important because this feature can be provided by gravity. The patient who has a complete brachial plexus lesion with root avulsion will never have the opportunity to lift the arm so much that he or she needs the triceps function to work against gravity.

Shoulder joint. The second important function we want to restore is some movement of the shoulder joint. Control of the subluxation of the shoulder joint is needed, and we achieve this by reinnervation of the supraspinatus and the deltoideus muscle via the suprascapular and the axillary nerve. If these two muscles achieve active abduction of about 20°, the function will be useful. It is also important to establish external rotation because even the best elbow flexion does not help much if it is performed in front of the abdominal wall. The muscles that normally perform external rotation usually do not regenerate sufficient strength to do so. We must therefore plan from the beginning to do something about this. In addition to this problem, the passive range of motion in the shoulder joint becomes limited with time. To compensate for both of these factors we plan to perform, at the phase of reconstructive surgery, a rotational osteotomy of the humerus and a transfer of the major pectoralis muscle to act as an external rotator.

The major pectoralis muscle can act as an adductor as well. It is vitally important and in the case of an avulsion of all five roots, the pectoral nerves are also neurotisized.

Serratus anterior function is also desired, so the long thoracic nerve is on the priority list, too.

Forearm muscles. Neurotization of the forearm muscles is much less important than the ones of the shoulder and elbow but should be achieved if sufficient donors are available. In the case of avulsion of all five roots, this will not be possible, but for this function we may use the root C7 from the contralateral side (see below).

Sensibility. To have at least some protective sensibility, the median nerve can be neurotisized by the sensory fibers of the supraclavicular nerves. At a later stage we have, in addition, the possibility to connect the fascicles of the median nerve carrying sensory fibers for the thumb and the index finger via a long nerve graft with the intercostal brachial nerves.

If only four roots are avulsed, the remaining spinal nerve will be used to neurotisize the most important function, that is the musculocutaneous nerve. Otherwise, a nerve transfer is performed as is described for cases of avulsion of all five roots.

If only three roots are avulsed, more functions can be restored. Avulsion of only two roots is treated by nerve transfer if it concerns roots C5 and C6, but we do not treat an avulsion of C8 and Th1. In contrast, if such an avulsion is present, the ulnar nerve may be used as a nerve graft.

Axon donors in case of root avulsion

Spinal accessory nerve. This nerve can best be used to neurotisize the suprascapular nerve, the axillary nerve, or both of them. Narakas[9] developed a technique to achieve a direct coaptation between the spinal accessory nerve and the suprascapular nerve. Because the trapezius muscle is still needed and may be needed later for reconstructive surgery, this muscle should not be completely denervated. The spinal accessory nerve should be transected for a transfer only distal to the first branch to preserve innervation of the trapezius muscle.

Motor branches of the cervical plexus. Motor branches of the cervical plexus are used to innervate the medial and lateral pectoral nerve and eventually the axillary nerve. The dorsalis scapular nerve can be used to innervate the long thoracic nerve.

Intercostal nerves. The intercostal nerve II can be used to innervate the long thoracic nerve or, if this has been already achieved via the dorsalis scapular nerve, to neurotisize the thoraco dorsal nerve. The intercostal nerves III, IV, and V can be used for the musculocutaneous nerve, the intercostal nerves VI and VIIs (i.e., evt.). VIII are used for the radial nerve (mainly for the triceps branches in order to get reinnervation of the triceps muscle).

C7 from the contralateral side as suggested by Gu et al.[6] and Chuang et al.[2] It can be shown that the transection of C7 does not cause much functional loss. This is the basis for the idea to use C7 from the contralateral side to bring axons into the denervated brachial plexus. It is a difficult decision for the surgeon to choose to transect the root of a normal brachial plexus in case of a complete lesion of the contralateral plexus. Therefore, we completed the procedure in two stages. In the first stage, the C7 root was explored and ligated. After the patient awoke from anesthesia, the level of function was studied. If, due to an innervation anomaly, major loss of function would have been present, as was expected, we could have immediately opened the ligature again to prevent permanent damage. If not, the patient had the opportunity to experience the loss of function. If the patient accepted this loss of function, which in all four cases we have operated on improved after several weeks, the real transfer was performed in the second stage when the root C7 was transected and connected to the vascularized ulnar nerve. The other end was connected to the median nerve to achieve forearm muscle function. In one of the four cases, a child of 10 years, good forearm muscle function returned and the patient could use this without thinking of the contralateral arm. In the second patient, an adult, good forearm muscle function again returned; however, the patient had to think of certain movements on the contralateral side to perform movements on the paralyzed side. The two other cases were performed to prepare for free-muscle grafting.

Loss of continuity with preserved proximal stumps

In this case continuity has to be restored by nerve grafts. If the defect is confined (e.g., to the spinal nerves and part of the trunks), continuity is restored between the stumps. If, however, a longer segment is involved, it is much better to neurotisize well defined distal stumps to avoid irregular axon sprouting and dilution of the regenerated axons. In case of loss of continuity between spinal nerves and the distal end of the superior trunk, it is better to connect C5 with the dorsal division of the superior trunk and C6 with the anterior division of the superior trunk. If there is a long segment to be bridged, it is better to achieve neurotization of the elected peripheral nerves. In such a case we would connect C6 directly with the musculocutaneous nerve and not with the lateral fascicle.

Available nerve grafts
1. Sural nerve of both legs
2. Cutaneous antebrachii medialis of the ipsilateral side as free graft
3. Ramus superficialis nervi radialis of the ipsilateral side as free graft
4. Cutaneous antebrachii lateralis after preparation of the musculocutaneous nerve as free graft
5. Ulnar nerve with avulsion of C8 and Th1 as a vascularized nerve graft
6. Parts of or the total ulnar nerve with avulsion of C8 and Th1 as free grafts after preparation in individual fascicle groups without interfascicular group exchange of fibers
7. Eventually, nervous cutaneous femoris lateralis of both sides as free grafts

8. Eventually, cutaneous antebrachii medialis of the contralateral side as free graft

Lesion with preserved continuity

In this case the degree of damage has to be evaluated by microsurgical dissection. If there is fourth-degree damage (Sunderland), the segment has to be resected and the continuity restored through nerve grafts. If there is third-degree damage, the amount of fibrosis has to be evaluated. If there is a fibrosis of type C, according to Millesi,[7] with collagenization of the fascicles, the involved segment has to be resected and the continuity restored through nerve grafts. If there is a fibrosis of type B in third-degree damage, an epifascicular or interfascicular epineuriectomy has to be performed. This applies also to cases of second-degree or first-degree damage in which a fibrosis of type B has prevented the otherwise expected spontaneous recovery.

If there is a fibrosis of type A, according to Millesi,[7] an epifascicular epineuriotomy has to be performed. This also relates to the rare cases of second-degree or first-degree damage having developed a fibrosis of type A, which prevents the otherwise expected recovery. In clinical practice, of course, this is much more difficult to describe because there are transient situations (e.g., damage between the third and fourth degree). These are the cases that require an experienced surgeon.

RECONSTRUCTIVE SURGERY
Elbow flexion

It has already been mentioned that elbow flexion is the most important function and any effort is justified to achieve the goal of its return. Therefore, in very severe cases with avulsion of all five roots, we like to have a second plan. Initially we recommend neurotisizing the triceps along with the biceps to transfer the triceps to the biceps tendon during the reconstructive phase. In this way we can enforce the biceps function or replace it if the biceps did not recover well. If the two muscles recover only partially, a combined force still may be strong enough to provide useful elbow flexion.

Alternately, if there is an upper brachial plexus lesion with intact spinal roots C8 and Th1, a Steindler operation can be performed to achieve elbow flexion. The common origin of the forearm and finger flexors is detached and shifted 5 cm in proximal direction to the humerus shaft. After this procedure these muscles improve their momentum to elbow flexion.

If a latissimus dorsi muscle is available it can be transferred for use in elbow flexion.[11] Clark[3] recommended pectoralis major transfer for such cases. In inverterated cases elbow flexion can be achieved by free microvascular muscle transfer.

In the last years Doi[4] has developed a new concept. He does not explore the brachial plexus but instead starts with free microvascular muscle transfer. In the first step the gracilis muscle is transplanted to provide simultaneously elbow flexion and finger extension, using the forearm flexors as a hippomochium. The gracilis muscle is innervated by a transfer of the accessory nerve. At the same time, sensory branches of the cervical plexus are directed to the median nerve to provide it with sensibility. In the second stage the contralateral gracilis muscle is transferred by microvascular procedure to provide finger flexion. This muscle goes underneath the extensor muscles of the forearm and is innervated by intercostal nerves II, III, and IV (motor part). The sensory part of intercostal nerves II, III, and IV is directed to the ulnar nerve for sensibility. Intercostal nerves V and VI (motor part) neurotisize the triceps muscle. This is a very clever approach; the combined use of one muscle for elbow flexion and finger motion is especially interesting. There is no remark on external rotation or stabilization of the scapula.

Shoulder joint

An arthordesis of the shoulder joint provides good motion of the arm, especially if the serratus anterior muscle is normal. With a weak serratus anterior muscle, arthrodesis does not help much and many patients do not accept an arthrodesis very well in this situation. Control of the subluxation in the shoulder joint can be achieved by transferring the horizontal fibers of the trapezius muscle, including a bony segment of the acromion, to the neck of the humerus. The continuity of the acromion is restored by a bone graft. This procedure gives good stabilization and in some cases also allows active abduction to a small but important degree.

Stabilization of the scapula

To achieve stabilization of the scapula, the serratus anterior muscle should be neurotisized. This can be achieved through a nerve transfer to the long thoracic nerve. This is very important and perhaps more important than some finger flexion.

External rotation

External rotation is extremely important, but it usually does not spontaneously return because even under normal conditions the external rotators are much weaker than the internal rotators. Often the elbow joint develops stiffness so that external rotation is limited. Even if a patient has good elbow flexion and finger function, he or she can not use these functions very well without external rotation because the arm moves in front of the abdominal wall. To gain function, the patient has to be able to move the arm and the hand in space. For external rotation several muscles are available for transfer. In our method of treating complete root avulsions we perform a neurotization of the major pectoralis muscle with motor fibers coming from the cervical plexus. If the major pectoralis muscle recovers, a rotation with osteotomy is performed by about 45° to 60° and the major pectoralis muscle is transferred to the opposite side of the humerus shaft for an external rotating effect. In other cases the minor pectoralis muscle can be used for this purpose. If there is a strong teres major, this muscle also provides good external rotation.

Gripping function

After recovery has reached its peak, with or without C7 transfer, the available forearm muscles are analyzed. According to the number of muscles available, a key grip function usually can be achieved through a combination of arthrodesis procedures and muscle transfers.

Sensibility

If sensibility is lacking, one can bring it to the thumb and index finger by connecting the intercostal brachial nerves to the sensory fascicles of the thumb and index finger with long nerve grafts that are followed along the median nerve proximally as far as possible.

REFERENCES

1. Bonney G, Birch R: *Surgical aspect,* presented at Symposium on Brachial Plexus Injuries by the British Society of Surgery of the Hand, Barbicane Centre, London, November 1982.
2. Chuang Ch Ch D, Wei FC, Noordhoff MS: Cross-chest C7 nerve grafting followed by free muscle transplantation for the treatment of avulsed brachial plexus injuries: a preliminary report, *Plast Reconstr Surg* 1993; 92:717-727.
3. Clark JPM: Reconstruction of biceps brachii pectoral muscle transplantation, *Brit J Surg* 1946; 34:180.
4. Doi K: *Double free muscle transfer to reconstruct prehension following complete avulsion of brachial plexus,* video presentation at 11th Congress of the Int Soc of Plastic, Reconstructive, and Aesthetic Surgery, Yokohama, April 16-22, 1995.
5. Eberhard D, Reihsner R, Millesi H: *Optimierung der Inzisionen zur Freilegung des Plexus brachialis aufgrund von Messungen der Hautdehnung,* presented at Annual Meeting Austrian Soc of Plastic, Reconstr and Aesthetic Surgery, Zell/See Oct 14-16, 1993.
6. Gu YD, Zang GM, Yan JG, et al: Seventh cervical root transfer from the lateral healthy side for treatment of the brachial plexus, *J Hand Surg* 1992; 17B:518-521.
7. Millesi H: Eingriffe an peripheren Nerven. In Gschnitzer F, Kern E, Schweiberer L, eds: *Chirurgische Operationslehre,* Munich-Vienna-Baltimore, 1986, Urban & Schwarzenberg.
8. Millesi H, Reihsner R, Eberherd D: *Darstellung des Plexus brachialis von kranio/dorsal unter Verwendung sagittaler Hautinzisionen,* presented at Annual Meeting Austrian Soc of Plastic, Reconstr and Aesthetic Surgery, Zell/See Oct 14-16, 1993.
9. Narakas AO: Repair of brachial plexus trunks. In Brunelli G, ed: *Textbook of microsurgery,* Milano, Parigi, Barcellona, Messico, Sao Paulo, 1988, Masson.
10. Sunderland S: A classification of peripheral nerve injuries producing loss of function, *Brain* 1951; 74:491.
11. Zancolli E, Mitre H: Latissimus dorsi transfer to restore elbow flexion: an appraisal of eight cases, *J Bone Joint Surg* 1973; 55(A):1265.

Chapter 25

OBSTETRICAL BRACHIAL PALSY

*The hand therapist's role**

Judy C. Colditz

Obstetrical brachial palsy (OBP) results from stretching of the brachial plexus as the baby passes through the birth canal. If the baby's head and shoulders are pulled in opposite directions during delivery, the upper part of the brachial plexus is stretched (Erb's palsy). Breech deliveries can cause injury to the lower part of the plexus (Klumpke's palsy) when the arms of the child are hyperextended overhead. This lower cord stretch also commonly occurs when there is a face presentation and the neck is hyperextended.[3]

The reported incidence of OBP varies from 0.04 to 2.5 per 1000 live births.[11,15,22,26] This condition is associated with large-birth-weight infants and difficult deliveries.[3,22] Fortunately, sophisticated obstetrical management is decreasing the incidence of this birth-related injury.[18]

HISTORY

Smellie, in 1768, was the first to write a clinical description of this problem.[25] He documented the observation of resolution of bilateral upper extremity paralysis in a child with face presentation at birth. Danyau performed an autopsy of a newborn with brachial plexus palsy in 1851, providing the first anatomic description of this lesion.[4]

In 1872 Duchenne described traction to the arm in infants and identified the lesion as being the upper part of the brachial plexus.[5] Two years later Erb described electrical stimulation of this lesion in children and adults.[7] Although

*This chapter is dedicated to the memory of John Wesley Packer, M.D., 1939–1993.

Duchenne first described the lesion, Erb's name is commonly associated with it[22]; *Erb-Duchenne palsy* is an equally correct term for this lesion.[16]

The less common lower brachial plexus injury was described by Klumpke in 1885.[17] This lesion is an injury to the roots of C8 and T1.

DIAGNOSIS

The newborn presentation is often suggestive of absent muscle function. Absence of normal arm motor response to the startle, grasp, and Moro reflexes are observed, and deep tendon reflexes are absent.[3] A clear diagnosis of the specific muscles involved is at best difficult, because newborns cannot respond to muscle testing commands.

To further complicate an accurate diagnosis, these lesions are often partial or combinations of the classic descriptions. Frequent clinical examinations are required before muscle function can be fully and accurately observed. X-ray films must substantiate the absence of bony injury to the proximal humerus or clavicle before the diagnosis of brachial plexus injury can be confirmed.[1,14,24]

Electromyographic (EMG) examination, although technically difficult in the young child, is the most objective means of evaluation. Eng and associates state that EMGs can predict the final reinnervation outcome after the second or third examination.[6] Other authors feel that EMGs are most helpful in predicting the surgical findings and for planning operative procedures.[27] Some feel that serial clinical examination is all that is needed to determine the prognosis.[15]

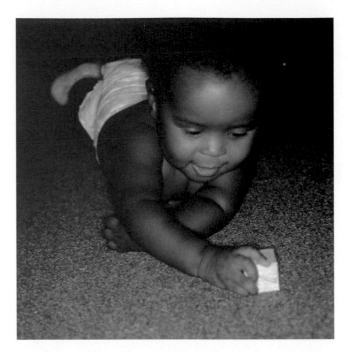

Fig. 25-1. The absence of shoulder motion prevents the child from crawling. The child may demonstrate the ability to support the weight of the upper body on the elbow.

PROGNOSIS

There is disagreement about recovery rates from obstetrical palsy.[3,10,14,15] Accuracy is clouded by the fact that many infants seen only by obstetricians spontaneously recover in the first few days or months. Those writing about long-term results are surgeons who rarely see children with early spontaneous resolution.

Determination of muscle return may be difficult to determine because the normal development of the child progresses simultaneously. The unskilled examiner may have difficulty identifying what is return and what is the appearance of normal developmental movement. Functional impairment of the upper extremity is obvious when the child is ready to crawl, as the arm simply does not work properly (Fig. 25-1). As the child begins to walk independently and begins two-handed activities, the examiner may assume there is significant progress. Although it is encouraging to the parents and examiner that the child is using the hand functionally, this use as an assist in bilateral activities may not necessarily indicate progressive muscle return[3] (Fig. 25-2).

In the earlier part of this century, because of the discouraging surgical results, most surgeons were pessimistic about operating on OBP.[13] Results from large surgical series reviewed more recently have shown improved functional results when the patients are selected for surgery according to precise criteria.[8]

Hoffer reports that all children he saw with only shoulder problems recovered completely.[15] The prognosis is worse for children with lower plexus and complete lesions.[15] The

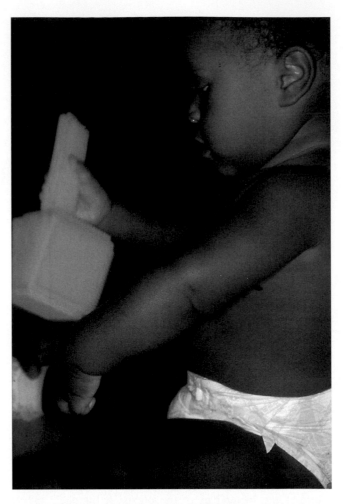

Fig. 25-2. The involved arm is used in bilateral activities that are within range of the limited shoulder flexion.

presence of Horner's syndrome carries a very poor prognosis in the children with complete lesions.[13,14] As with any nerve regeneration, the earlier and more extensive the return observed, the better the prognosis. In OBP most of the progress is seen in the first year of life and can be expected to reach maximum return by 24 months. Unlike adults, however, some children can demonstrate continued return of function up to 4 years following birth.[15]

Most authors agree that if biceps function is not seen by 3 months, then the prognosis for functional return is poor.[2,13,14,22,27] Many recommend surgery if the biceps is not active by this time.[2,13,22] Surgery can be expected to provide one grade higher of muscle function than if the child is treated conservatively.[22]

COMMON PLEXUS LESIONS
Upper plexus lesion: Erb-Duchenne palsy

Erb-Duchenne palsy is by far the most common involvement seen and has the most encouraging prognosis.[1] Many of these children undergo full spontaneous recovery within the first 3 months.[9] Classically this lesion has been described as involving the roots of C5-C6, but Terzis, Liberson, and

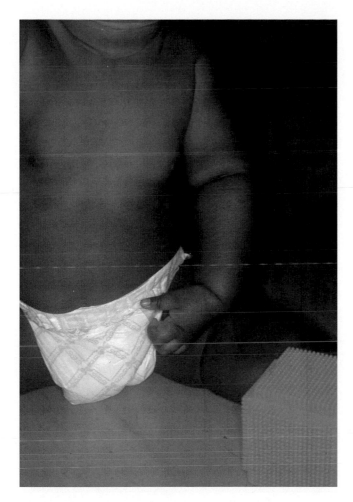

Fig. 25-3. The typical presentation of Erb-Duchenne palsy is demonstrated by the arm at the side with elbow extended and the shoulder internally rotated. The forearm is pronated and the fingers and wrist flexed.

Levine conclude that the C7 root is almost always involved.[27]

Children with Erb-Duchenne palsy present with the involved arm limp at their side, the shoulder internally rotated, the elbow positioned in full extension, the forearm pronated, and the fingers and wrist flexed[3] (Fig. 25-3). The shoulder is adducted because of the paralysis of the deltoid and supraspinatus muscles. The active pectoral and subscapularis muscles and inactive infraspinatus and teres minor keep the shoulder internally rotated.[3] Elbow extension is usually produced by gravity and paralysis of the elbow flexors: biceps, brachialis, brachioradialis. The absence of the biceps and supinator contribute to the pronated position.[3] The involvement of C7 means that the extrinsic wrist and finger extensors are absent.[27] These children have unopposed finger and wrist flexion and thus will progress to demonstrate extrinsic finger flexor tightness. Distal sensibility and vasomotor control are usually unaffected.[9]

Residual weakness is commonly seen in these patients. It is a pattern of weakness sometimes coupled with lack of a full range of motion in shoulder abduction, flexion, and external rotation, as well as elbow flexion and forearm supination. The child has the frustrating situation of being unable to position the normal hand so it can be used. In addition, the child may have weakness or absence of wrist and finger extension.[15]

Low plexus lesion: Klumpke's palsy

Klumpke's palsy or injury to C8-T1 roots also frequently includes injury to the C7 root.[27] This injury carries a poor prognosis and is rarely seen in pure form. Gilbert and Whitaker quote Wickstrom as noting that less than 10% of patients with Klumpke's palsy will recover any useful function, and thus surgical intervention should be considered at 3 months.[9]

A Klumpke's lower plexus palsy leaves the child with good proximal control but absence of intrinsic and extrinsic hand muscles. The absence of C7 function prevents return of the long extensor muscles of the hand and wrist.[27] Residual weakness of the hand always remains, usually with accompanying critical loss of sensibility in the hand.

Complete plexus lesion

Damage to the entire plexus, although rare, does occur. There is complete sensory and motor paralysis of the extremity, and the hand is clawed. The presence of Horner's syndrome is an indicator of severe involvement, worsening an already poor prognosis. Distal sensory impairment causes a vasomotor disturbance, and the hand presents with a pale marbled appearance.[9]

CLINICAL EXAMINATION OF A CHILD WITH OBSTETRICAL BRACHIAL PALSY

Piatt, Hudson, and Hoffman state that examination of an infant with OBP is "a matter of seduction; gentleness, patience, and trickery . . . "[23] The skill of the examiner is put to the ultimate test with an infant who cannot respond to requests or commands. Infants may not spontaneously exhibit certain movements when they are developmentally unable to do so.

Muscle testing

Muscle testing in the newborn is at best inaccurate because the examiner can rely only on reflex testing and observation of spontaneous movement. Direct palpation of muscles can pick up early activity, although the ability to elicit this activity is variable. EMG testing plays an early role in defining muscle activity and is helpful in determining early surgical treatment options. Keen observation during numerous visits over time is the best means to determine reliably the functional level of muscle activity. Videotaping provides objective documentation of motion on serial visits.

Many authors suggest using a simplification of the British Medical Research Council muscle testing classification

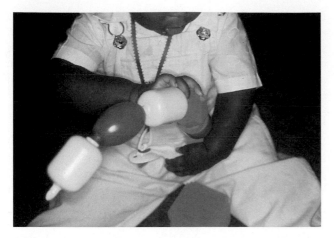

Fig. 25-4. Toys requiring bilateral skills are one of the best means to assess functional use of the extremity at an early age.

because it more easily accommodates the difficulty of muscle testing in a small child.

M0 = no contraction

M1 = contraction without movement

M2 = slight or complete movement with weight eliminated

M3 = complete movement against the weight of gravity[8,10,12-14]

Sensibility evaluation

Sensory testing in the newborn is an even greater challenge than observation of muscle activity. Intact sensory status can only be assumed as the baby withdraws from painful stimuli. In older children a reaching response to stimuli or searching for the stimulus visually assures the examiner of some level of intact sensibility. Over time, trophic changes such as nail and hair growth and changes in finger color provide additional evidence. Normal neurophysiologic development will increase the child's grasp and reaching response to stimuli. As with manual muscle testing, the therapist must be knowledgeable about the normal stages of grasp and prehension development to accurately evaluate the disability of the extremity.

THERAPIST'S ROLE IN REHABILITATION

Technology cannot replace the fundamental role of the therapist as critical observer. The therapist uses age-appropriate play activities to assess the functional and developmental disability resulting from the motor loss. An environment providing stimuli appropriate to the child's developmental level is the best means of accurate evaluation (Fig. 25-4). Observation in this group of patients is often a more critical skill than manual examination.

Even when sensory and motor return does occur, the child often ignores the arm[3] (Fig. 25-5). The key to therapy is helping the child develop an awareness of the arm and its useful potential. The focus of therapy should therefore

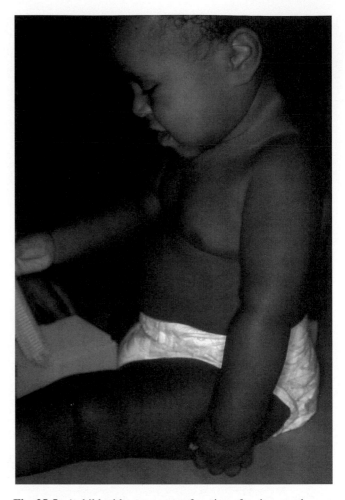

Fig. 25-5. A child with some motor function often ignores the arm if the task requires only one hand.

consist of instructions to the parents about ways they can facilitate the use of the arm while motor and sensory function returns.

The therapist's role in the treatment of a child with an OBP lesion is also vital to the parents. Parents need reassurance, answers to simple questions, practical suggestions, celebration of milestones of improvement, and frequent discussions about the expectations of functional return.

Surprisingly, I could find no reference to the role of the hand therapist in the management of OBP. In adults with brachial plexus injuries (whether treated surgically or nonsurgically), the goals are clear: prevent joint contractures, facilitate muscle return, and assist in functional use of the extremity. There is no reason why they should be different in the child. But the child's inability to communicate and participate means these goals are accomplished differently from those in the adult.

Parent education

Parents should be educated about the nature of the injury so they may better understand how to protect the healing stretched nerves and the joints with weakened muscle support and control. Immediately following birth, the child's arm should be rested against the body for the first few weeks.[22] The newborn should be handled by cradling under the head and pelvis and should not be picked up under the arms. The parents should be especially cautioned against pulling forward and upward on the arms to bring the child to a sitting position or to pick the child up. Instructing the parents to apply the child's garment sleeve to the involved arm first and remove it from the involved arm last will minimize the need to abduct or externally rotate the arm. Current precautions against placing children on their stomachs while sleeping (to reduce the risk of sudden infant death syndrome) require that the involved arm be held against the side of the body rather than be allowed to fall into external rotation while sleeping supine. Pinning the garment sleeve to the body portion of the garment will serve as a reminder to keep the child's arm against the body when sleeping, changing diapers, or handling the child.

Following the initial period of protection of the injured nerves (usually a few weeks), frequent passive range-of-motion exercises must be done by the parents to maintain normal joint motion. A routine of stretching exercises each time the diapers are changed is an excellent way to assure adequate frequency. Parents should be instructed specifically about each passive stretch position and then be able to demonstrate correct passive stretching techniques to the therapist. Full external rotation of the shoulder, for example, is difficult to maintain unless the parent understands the need to stabilize the scapula and ensure that motion is occurring at the glenohumeral joint. The most important passive stretches are full external rotation and abduction of the shoulder, full forearm supination and pronation, and concurrent wrist and finger extension (if the hand is involved).

When the child is old enough to roll over independently, the cautionary period of positional protection is long since past. Caution should remain against pulling the child up by the arm. If the child is able to crawl using the arm (some of these children skip the crawling stage), the parents should be cautious of the child bearing weight on the dorsum of a flexed wrist for prolonged periods.

Functional use of the arm is regained only as the child has both the motor ability to use the extremity and the awareness of the existence of the extremity. Without spontaneous motor ability, the hand and arm are deprived of frequent sensory input. Early rubbing and touching by the parents as well as passive motion for proprioceptive input are important. Even if the child cannot respond with motion, the arm should be stimulated each time the opposite uninvolved arm receives stimulation. Tickling of the arms simultaneously, holding the child's hands, playing pattycake, and placing the child's hand and arm on or around objects (Fig. 25-6) provide the consistent level of stimulation that can improve awareness as functional return occurs. Parents should not be allowed to

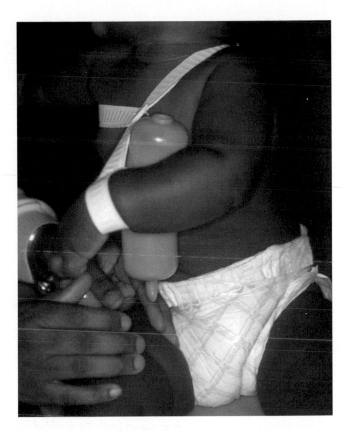

Fig. 25-6. Placing the child's arm around objects increases arm awareness. The elastic strap maintains elbow flexion.

believe that this stimulation will create return, but should understand it will enhance any naturally occurring return.

As the child reaches the developmental stage of actively bringing the arm to the midline, the parents should be instructed to bring the arm to the midline during passive play. The arm should be brought within the child's visual range. If the child with a weak shoulder can be placed in a special high chair with a high lap tray under the axilla and the food is placed so the child must reach for it, this becomes an active assistive exercise for shoulder motion. Parents should be encouraged to buy large toys such as balls that require both arms for holding (Fig. 25-7). As the child learns bilateral skills, interlocking toys, which require two hands to separate and join, should also be encouraged (see Fig. 25-4). Helping the parents with toy suggestions and play ideas to encourage reaching and manipulation maximizes the integration of sensory and motor return.

The therapist must know about developmental milestones. Therapy activities with these children can progress only as fast as their normally expected development. Therapists specializing in hand therapy may need to refer to developmental textbooks or consult with developmental colleagues to ensure accurate evaluation of functional status or to provide accurate suggestions for home therapy activities.

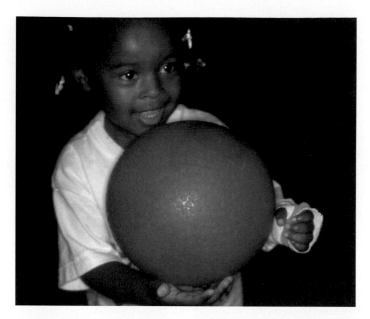

Fig. 25-7. Catching a large ball requires bilateral arm motion.

Most of all the therapist must reassure the parents. In circumstances where full return is unlikely, reassurance that the child can lead a relatively normal and healthy life despite the disability is crucial in the early years. Encouraging networking among parents of children with brachial plexus injuries, in my experience, is very positive.

Parents need to be reassured they are doing all they can to influence the progress of their child. Because they give the frequent daily stimulus, they are the primary therapy providers. Therapy sessions are only useful for documentation of progress, for solving problems, and for providing instructions to the parents about activities appropriate for the child until the next therapy visit.

Splinting

Splinting the hand can help gain and maintain passive motion of the hand; but splinting the elbow or shoulder is discouraged by some authors.[19,22] This is because of complications reported by previous authors when prolonged periods of static splinting were used to hold the arm abducted and externally rotated.

As discussed previously, children with absent wrist and finger extensors have chronic tightness of the long flexor muscles. Splinting the hand with a resting splint that concurrently extends the wrist and fingers is appropriate (Fig. 25-8). If the child is seen within the first few months of life and demonstrates significant long finger flexor tightness, splinting on a full-time basis (with removal for skin hygiene) for a short period will greatly reduce the tightness. As the child grows, the splints should be limited to sleep time use only. During this period of development the goal is to encourage use of any prehension pattern possible

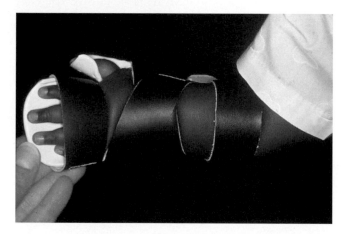

Fig. 25-8. A splint to maintain length of finger and wrist flexors requires multiple leather straps for adequate stabilization.

with the extremity. Use of a rigid hand splint during waking hours will only impede this goal.

Hand splints for children are difficult to make and to keep in place. Multiple conforming straps are necessary to keep the splint correctly positioned (Fig. 25-8). I recommend leather straps because they quickly conform to the shape of the extremity and minimize potential sharp edges or pressure areas. Because all young children have a large amount of subcutaneous fat and few defined bony prominences, prolonged pressure from the straps of a splint will deform the child's soft tissue so the strap impression may be evident long after the splint is removed. When the first hand splint is fitted, parents need reassurance that the ridging from the straps is a temporary phenomenon and not a long-term deformity.

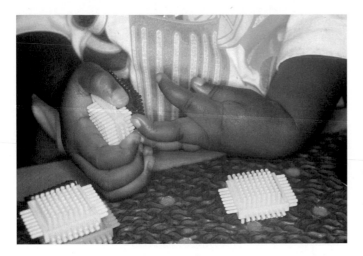

Fig. 25-9. The weak wrist extensors prevent stabilization of the wrist. The position of wrist flexion prevents opposition of the thumb to the fingers.

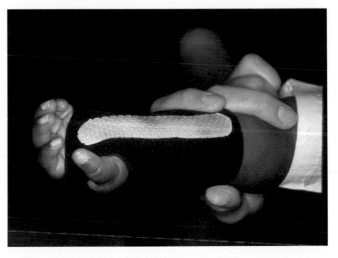

Fig. 25-10. A circumferential custom-made neoprene wrist splint with a thermoplastic stay provides wrist support but does not totally immobilize the wrist.

Children who chew or suck on the splint or remove it during sleep may require that Coban be wrapped over the splint for adequate protection. Parents must be cautioned about meticulous hygiene routines to prevent skin maceration.

In the child with active wrist and finger flexors but absent extensors, the pattern of usage is similar to the problem encountered in radial palsy. The active flexors cannot be used because of the inability of the patient to stabilize the wrist in extension while the force of the flexors is transmitted across the wrist (Fig. 25-9). These children often require long-term night splinting for the long flexor tightness and a day splint to stabilize the wrist so the child can hold objects in the hand. A small custom-made circumferential neoprene splint with a thermoplastic reinforcement may be all that is needed (Fig. 25-10). Children with stronger patterns of wrist flexion may need a molded thermoplastic splint for adequate stabilization (Fig. 25-11). The use of such a wrist splint allows for functional finger flexion, but the absence of intrinsic or extrinsic extensor muscles means that the child often cannot release objects placed in the hand. This factor is not enough, however, to suggest that the splint should not be used. The splint should be used intermittently based on the developmental age of the child and the task attempted.

Muscles undergoing nerve reinnervation should not remain stationary. It is appropriate to support a muscle so it can contract without having to first take up its fully stretched length. Simple splinting can assist muscle reinnervation. A simple elastic strap splint can be worn intermittently by the child to prevent a position of constant elbow extension (Fig. 25-12). The garment sleeve can also be pinned to the torso of the garment. This maximizes the ability to see early elbow flexion—a critical prognostic milestone for the child.

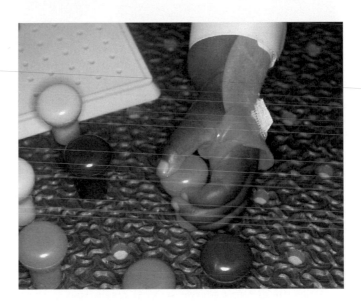

Fig. 25-11. Children who have developed strong wrist flexion need a molded thermoplastic splint to support the wrist and allow finger flexion.

Documentation of functional status

Comparison of surgical and nonsurgical results is hampered by the lack of definition of a standardized functional grading for a child's extremity.[13] Mallet[21] developed a functional classification of shoulder motion frequently referenced in the literature* (Fig. 25-13). This classification leaves much to be desired when describing hand function because it best evaluates children with upper plexus lesions where the shoulder is the site of the primary disability.[8] It is limited to demonstration of shoulder function in older

*References 8, 10, 12, 13, 18, 19, 22.

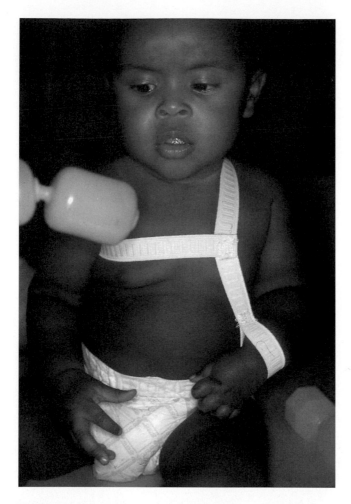

Fig. 25-12. An elastic strap supports the elbow in a flexed position.

children, as the child must be able to follow commands. Mallet's classification does not necessarily correspond with functional task ability. It is, however, a useful standard when surgeons attempt to compare surgical results and is most often used for that purpose.

Case study

B.W. is a cute, bright-eyed second child of normal gestation, who was first referred to hand therapy at the age of 10 months. Labor during her delivery was somewhat prolonged, but no specific complications were noted.

When she was first seen by an orthopedist at 3 weeks of age, no active arm motion was noted except perhaps finger flexion. At 4 months B.W. had some active shoulder flexion and elbow extension, but the critical milestone of elbow flexion was not present. Wrist and finger extension and all intrinsic hand muscles were also absent.

At 9 months wrist and finger flexion were clearly demonstrated as was the ability to stabilize the shoulder. There was still no elbow flexion or wrist and finger extension; both indicators of a poor prognosis.

At 10 months B.W. was referred to a hand surgeon who referred her to therapy. Although she had movement in her arm, she ignored her arm as if it were not part of her body (see Fig. 25-5). She held her elbow extended at all times but would initiate some shoulder flexion (see Fig. 25-2). Because she did not use her hand at all there was little reason to need the shoulder motion. She was not crawling. She would support her weight on the flexed elbow of her involved side for a short period (see Fig. 25-1) but would then roll to one side or roll over.

Her passive shoulder range was normal because of the mother's diligent stretching, but the range through which she used her shoulder was very limited (see Fig. 25-2). She used the arm to stabilize her body when sitting. The absence of wrist and finger extension prevented support on the palm of her hand. She would often bear weight on the dorsum of her flexed wrist. The functional use of the arm was limited to infrequent gross motor patterns of assist (see Fig. 25-2). She did not acknowledge objects placed in her hand but did acknowledge textured objects placed between her body and her proximal forearm area (see Fig. 25-6).

At the time of referral to therapy, tightness of the finger flexors was the only limited passive motion in the extremity (Fig. 25-14).

Initial treatment

The therapy goals were as follows:

1. To restore full passive motion (decrease long flexor tightness). This was accomplished by night and periodic day splinting to elongate the extrinsic flexors (see Fig. 25-8).
2. To protect the elbow from always being in a fully extended position to facilitate any return of elbow flexion. An elastic strap splint was fitted for periodic wear (see Figs. 25-6 and 25-12).
3. To increase self-awareness of her arm. The mother was instructed to position B.W. frequently sitting or prone with her arm positioned for support to provide a proprioceptive stimulus. The mother was asked to dress the child in short sleeves as much as possible and frequently place toys and objects between her body and the proximal forearm area. Textured objects were encouraged.

At 12 months B.W. demonstrated some active elbow flexion, but it was not full range. Her mother was instructed to put her at a tabletop level with her chest to provide support for the entire arm so the elbow could flex and extend without working against gravity. Periods in the elastic harness were continued about half of her waking day.

At 17 months B.W. was observed spontaneously using the arm for assisted holding, and when an object was placed in her hand she would hold it. The absence of active intrinsic or extrinsic extensors prevented release of objects and led to persistent long flexor tightness. Wrist extension was still not present. Splinting with a custom-made neo-

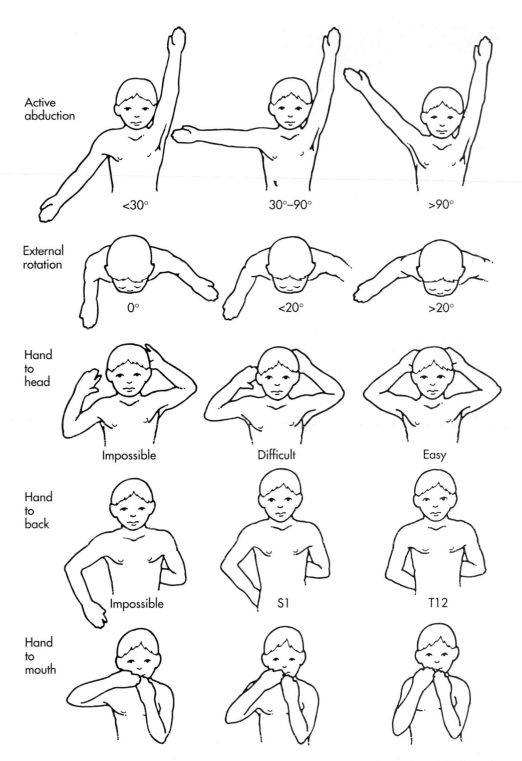

Fig. 25-13. Mallet's method of functional assessment of the shoulder. (From Hentz VR: Operative nerve repair of the brachial plexus in infants and children. In Gelberman RH, ed: *Operative nerve repair and reconstruction,* New York, 1991, Lippincott.)

prene splint with a reinforcement of thermoplastic material gave the needed support to keep the wrist out of flexion, but did not rigidly immobilize it (see Fig. 25-10). Supporting the wrist increased the spontaneous use of the palmar surface of the hand.

At 3 years she spontaneously uses the hand as an assist but cannot oppose thumb and fingertips because of the position of extreme wrist flexion (see Fig. 25-9). With a rigid wrist support, she spontaneously holds objects in her hand (see Fig. 25-11). She demonstrates about 90° of elbow

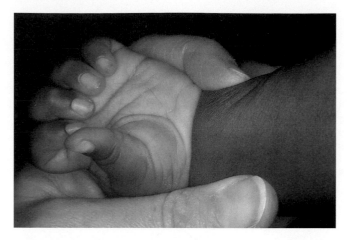

Fig. 25-14. Tightness of the finger flexor muscles is common when the wrist and finger extensors are absent.

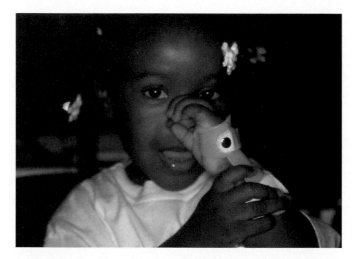

Fig. 25-15. Full elbow flexion is accomplished by assistance from the uninjured arm.

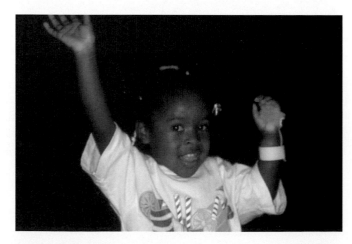

Fig. 25-16. Demonstration of limited shoulder flexion and abduction at 3 years of age.

flexion but is unable to touch her nose with her involved hand. She spontaneously brings the elbow into full flexion by assisting with the other hand when asked to touch her nose (Fig. 25-15). When reaching for the ceiling her abduction is limited to 75° (Fig. 25-16).

B.W.'s clinical picture at 3 years demonstrates the anticipated prognosis that absence of elbow flexion at 3 months means less than full return. She will likely always have limited active motion and strength in the elbow and shoulder. The extrinsic imbalance in her wrist may later be improved with a tendon transfer for wrist extension, but the likelihood of intrinsic motor return in the hand is slim.

Therapy for B.W. has consisted of parental instruction and splinting for maintenance of joint motion and periodic instructions about activities to facilitate returning function.

CONCLUSION

The pioneering work of Narakas in neurotization techniques for lesions previously thought inoperable[20] will undoubtedly be developed to a level where parents of children with brachial plexus lesions can look forward to an even more positive prognosis than at any time in the past. The current practice of surgical treatment of OBP is developing rapidly as progress is being made in microneural reconstruction.[12] Therapists in the future will have the exciting experience of working with children and parents during the return of function once previously thought to be unattainable. The skills needed by the therapist will not change. Keen observation and practical instructions for the parents will always be required to assist the child with returning muscle function and sensibility.

REFERENCES

1. Beaty JH: Paralytic conditions. In Crenshaw AH, ed: *Campbell's operative orthopedics,* St Louis, 1992, Mosby.
2. Boome RS, Kaye JC: Obstetric traction injuries of the brachial plexus, *J Bone Joint Surg* 1988; 70(B):571-576.
3. Brown KLB: Review of obstetrical palsies: nonoperative treatment. In Terzis JK, ed: *Microreconstruction of nerve injuries,* Philadelphia, 1987, Saunders.
4. Danyau M: Paralysie du membre supérieur, chez le nouveauné, *Bull Soc Chir* 1851; 2:148.
5. Duchenne GBA: *De l'electrisation localisée et de son application á la pathologie et á la thérapeutique,* ed 3, Paris, 1872, JB Balliére.
6. Eng GD, Koch B, Smokvina MD: Brachial plexus palsy in neonates and children, *Arch Phys Med Rehabil* 1978; 59:458.
7. Erb W: Über eine eigenthümliche Localisation von Lähmengen im plexus brachialis, *Verhandl Naturhist-Med* (Heidelberg) 1874; 2:130.
8. Gilbert A, Hentz VR, Tassin J-L: Brachial plexus reconstruction in obstetric palsy: operative indications and postoperative results. In Urbaniak JR, ed: *Microsurgery for major limb reconstruction,* St Louis, 1987, Mosby.
9. Gilbert A, Whitaker I: Obstetrical brachial plexus lesions, *J Hand Surg* 1991; 16(B):489-491.
10. Gilbert A, Tassin J-L: Obstetrical palsy: a clinical, pathologic, and surgical review. In Terzis JK, ed: *Microreconstruction of nerve injuries,* Philadelphia, 1987, Saunders.

11. Greenwald AG, Schute PC, Shiveley JL: Brachial plexus birth palsy: a 10-year report on the incidence and prognosis, *J Pediatr Orthop* 1984; 4(6).

12. Hentz VR: Microneural reconstruction of the brachial plexus. In Green DP, ed: *Operative hand surgery,* ed 3, New York, 1993, Churchill Livingstone.

13. Hentz VR: Operative nerve repair of the brachial plexus in infants and children. In Gelberman RH, ed: *Operative nerve repair and reconstruction,* New York, 1991, Lippincott.

14. Hentz VR, Meyer RD: Brachial plexus microsurgery in children, *Microsurg* 1991; 12:175-185.

15. Hoffer MH: Assessment and natural history of brachial plexus injury in children. In Gelberman RH, ed: *Operative nerve repair and reconstruction,* New York, 1991, Lippincott.

16. Jepson PN: Obstetrical paralysis, *Ann Surg* 1930; 91:724-730.

17. Klumpke A: Contribution à l'étude des paralysies radiculaires du plexus brachial, *Rev Méd* 1885; 5:591.

18. Leffert RD: Brachial plexus. In Green DP, ed: *Operative hand surgery,* ed 3, New York, 1993, Churchill Livingstone.

19. Leffert RD: *Brachial plexus injuries,* New York, 1985, Churchill Livingstone.

20. Narakas AO: Thoughts on neurotization or nerve transfers in irreparable nerve lesions. In Terzis JA, ed: *Microreconstruction of nerve injuries,* Philadelphia, 1987, Saunders.

21. Mallet J: Paralysie obstétricale du plexus brachial: traitement des séquelles, *Rev Clir Orthop* 1972; 58(suppl 1):166.

22. Meyer RD: Treatment of adult and obstetrical brachial plexus injuries, *Orthopaedics* 1986; 9:899-903.

23. Piatt JH, Hudson AR, Hoffman HJ: Preliminary experiences with brachial plexus exploration on children: birth injury and vehicular trauma, *Neurosurg* 1988; 22(4):715-723.

24. Scaglietti O: The obstetrical shoulder trauma, *Surg Gyn Obstet* 1938; 66:868-877.

25. Smellie W: *A collection of cases and observations in midwifery,* vol 2, ed 4, London, 1786.

26. Sunderland S: *Nerve and nerve injuries,* ed 2, New York, 1978, Churchill Livingstone.

27. Terzis JK, Liberson WT, Levine R: Obstetrical brachial plexus palsy. In Jabaley ME, Williams HB, eds: *Peripheral nerve surgery,* Philadelphia, 1986, Saunders.

Chapter 26

SALVAGE PROCEDURES FOR FAILED NERVE SURGERY

Paul W. Brown

COMMUNICATION LOOPS

The main functions of the upper extremity are to place the hand where it can function and to serve as a conduit for the nerve impulses flowing between brain and hand. Thus, a peripheral nerve problem occurring any place in the upper extremity is primarily a hand problem.

Nervous systems, whether peripheral, spinal, or central, are basically communication systems. As with any other communication system, they have transmitter and receptor elements that allow the formation of communication loops wherein a signal is transmitted and received, and its reception then triggers a return transmission and a reciprocal reception. This is a *closed loop* and represents the normal relationship between the hand and the brain (Fig. 26-1).

If either transmission or reception is blocked, the loop is deficient and would then be considered an *open loop,* which, of course, is an oxymoron.

Nerve function in the hand first has to do with the gathering of information from sensory end organs in the skin and joints of the hand then routing that information to a central processing center, the somatosensory cortex of the brain, where it is interpreted. The brain, the command center, then transmits signals to whatever muscle groups it deems appropriate. The lines of communication are the peripheral nerves. They consist of sensory (afferent) nerves carrying incoming signals from sensory end organs and motor (efferent) nerves carrying outgoing commands to motor end plates of the muscles. There is a continuous and reciprocal sending and receiving of messages between the brain and the hand (i.e., a repetitive cycle, closed communication loop) (Fig. 26-2).

If either the afferent or efferent side of the loop is disrupted by disease or trauma, a sensory or motor palsy results. Or, if both sides of the loop are broken, a combined motor-sensory palsy is the result. If the loop cannot be reconstituted by repair of the nerves, an *ancillary closed loop* can be created by substituting visual stimuli for the missing sensory input and by substituting other functional muscle-tendon units for the paralyzed muscles. Also contributing to this loop are the proprioceptive senses of the joints and muscle-tendon units acting on them (Fig. 26-3).

PRIMARY SALVAGE PROCEDURES

This chapter is concerned with surgical options for converting traumatic peripheral nerve lesions from open loops to closed loops of communication. If injured nerves are operated on without success, primary nerve salvage procedures must then be considered. If these fail, or if they are not deemed advisable, secondary salvage procedures directed at joints, muscles, and tendons may then be feasible.

Primary salvage procedures, those directed at the nerve lesion itself, fall into the following six categories:

1. Wait and see: if the lesion is simply an axonotmesis, (i.e., a neurapraxia) spontaneous recovery may occur within several months
2. Decompression: surgical release of constricting structures
3. Neurolysis: external or intraneural
4. Neuroma resection with reanastamosis or graft
5. Nerve pedicle transfer: for example, the St. Clair Strange procedure that uses the vascularized trunk of a nonsalvageable nerve to bridge the gap in an adjacent nerve
6. Neurotization: for example, spinal accessory or intercostal nerve graft with muscle microvascular transfer

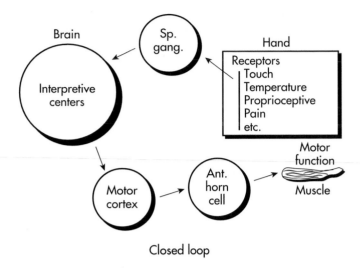

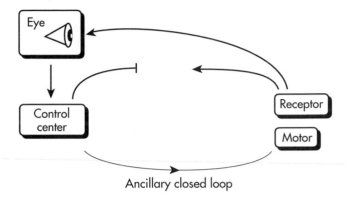

Fig. 26-3. Ancillary closed loop.

Closed loop

Fig. 26-1. Closed loop.

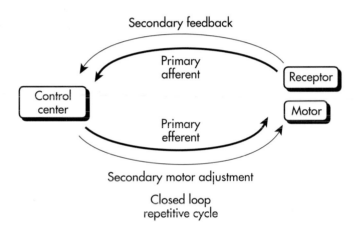

Fig. 26-2. Closed loop, repetitive cycle.

SECONDARY SALVAGE PROCEDURES

Secondary salvage procedures involve surgery on dermis, joints, tendons, or muscles.

A. Sensory loss: skin transfer, free or pedicle

B. Motor loss:
  1. Arthodesis
  2. Tenodesis
  3. Orthotic assistance
     a. Muscle driven: splint plus tenodesis
     b. Electronic or pneumatic
  4. Capsulorraphy
  5. Bone block
  6. Tendon transfer

Free or pedicle transfers of innervated skin to areas of anesthesia have proven feasible for supplying sensation to anesthetic thumbs but are fraught with complications. Neurovascular island pedicle flaps require extreme patient need for such sensation plus considerable operative skill by the surgeon. The same is true, for full thickness, sensory, revascularized skin transfers commonly referred to as *free flaps,* also an oxymoron.

Arthrodesis of a joint simplifies hand-wrist mechanics. It may be used to correct deformity, to make muscle tendon units available for transfer, or to transfer muscle power to a joint distal to the one arthrodesed.

Tenodesis affixes a tendon to bone proximal to its normal insertion or affixes one or more nonfunctional tendons to an active tendon. A passive (static) tenodesis limits the range of motion (ROM) of a joint (e.g., tenodesis of a flexor digitorum superficialis [FDS] slip to the proximal phalanx to correct a swan-neck deformity). An active (dynamic) tenodesis is motored by a muscle tendon unit and results in paradoxical motion of a joint or joints (e.g., tenodesis of denervated flexor tendons of a finger to an innervated flexor tendon).

Muscle-powered orthotic devices may be used to transmit power from a functional muscle tendon unit through a system of orthotic articulations and levers to otherwise nonfunctional digits as in the flexor-driven, flexor hinge splint used in tetraplegia. Extrinsically powered orthoses may be activated pneumatically by gas cylinders or by electricity as in myoelectric devices.

Capsulorrhaphy functions similarly to passive tenodesis by limiting the ROM of a joint as in the Zancolli capsulorrhaphy for correcting ulnar palsy clawing.

A bone block is created by affixing a bone graft in or near a joint to limit the motion of that joint. They have had a high rate of failure and are rarely used now.

Tendon transfers remain absolutely essential for salvage procedures for peripheral nerve motor palsies. The basics of tendon mechanics and the development of effective transfers were well delineated by the 1970s, and though a few refinements followed, the techniques and indications described by then are still valid; they are all well described in Green.[10] Furthermore, the tendon transfer illustrations in that text are so good that it would be fruitless for this chapter to emulate them: specifically, the chapters on radial palsy, median palsy, and the ulnar and combined palsies.[10]

Much of our understanding of tendon function and how it may be applied in tendon transfer surgery stems from the work of Paul Brand, who tells us, "There are too many books of recipes for tendon transfers in the hand. Most of us would like to believe that for every standard pattern of paralysis there is a preferred pattern of transfer. This is not so. Every hand surgeon must go through the discipline of understanding the mechanics of muscles and joints, and must know the mechanical qualities of the muscles that are available and must then apply this knowledge to each case, giving due weight to all the factors of individual need and of problems that are specific for that hand."[3]

While it is true that one should eschew cookbook surgery, there is, nevertheless, considerable merit to having a store of recipes. A competent surgeon must have the knowledge, the ability, and the judgment to select the right transfer for the patient, just as a good cook will have a file of recipes so that he or she may choose the appropriate dish for a particular meal.

The following decisive factors for tendon transfers should be considered.
1. The patient's requirements
2. What is available for transfer
3. What can be gained from the transfer
4. What will be lost from the transfer

One starts by first considering the patient's overall needs for everyday activities as well as his or her vocation and avocations, actual and potential. Next, these must be balanced against what is possible. The possibilities are assessed by evaluating the type and degree of functional loss and then considering what is available for modifying that loss. The surgeon conducts an inventory of functional tendons available for use, compares those with the paralyzed muscle-tendon units, and then decides if available procedures are up to the task proposed for the transfer. Last, knowing that transferring a tendon will always deprive the hand or wrist of some normal function, the surgeon must decide if this sacrifice is worth the cost.

It must be recognized that any motor palsy results in a weakened hand and that no tendon transfer, no matter how skillfully done, can ever restore full strength to that hand. Brand emphasizes that no tendon may be transferred without giving up something, and that the trick is to balance the weakness in the hand. We must "modify our theory and expectations to match reality."[3]

The volume, *The hand: another decade of tendon surgery,*[11] is a presentation of the faculty of the 1984 Philadelphia symposium and contains 14 chapters on tendon transfers. This chapter attempts to condense those chapters into one and reflects the teachings of the faculty of the 1994 symposium, a decade later. Two decades earlier, the publication of the 1974 symposium,[12] also presented much the same material on the same topic. At the same time (1974), another tendon symposium was published.[1] These three works plus Green's[10] cover almost all of the material

on the principles and practice of tendon transfer surgery that is known and generally accepted in the surgical world today. There have been no notable advances in the science of tendon transfer since their publication. I will reiterate much of what these works present and state some of my own preferences.

I will specifically restate the principles of tendon transfer that have been developed and described by many of the pioneers of tendon transfer surgery. Boyes, Riordan, and Curtis[2] are representative of them; their works have delineated and refined the works of Mayer, Steindler, and Bunnell.[2]

PRINCIPLES OF TENDON TRANSFERS

Tendon transfer surgery is intriguing for the surgeon; the goal of surgery is specific, the structures are discrete, and the end results are fairly predictable and are readily apparent. Its success depends on understanding and application of the following principles.

1. *The patient's needs and desires.* Variables of sex, age, vocation, and avocation must be balanced, not against what is possible but what is feasible and what serves the patient best. The results of complex operations that may be rated as excellent in the follow-up clinic, but give the patient little real functional benefit, do not represent good salvage surgery.

2. *Joint mobility.* Stiff joints and contractures will defeat both simple and sophisticated tendon transfers no matter how skilled the surgeon. Preoperative good passive ROM of any joints to be crossed are a must for the transfer to work.

3. *Joint stability.* Every joint crossed by tendon transfers must be stabilized by a balance between agonist and antagonist muscles. If any of these are nonfunctional, then the joint(s) must be stabilized by arthrodesis or external splinting.

4. *Tissue equilibrium.* Tissues traversed by the transfer must have settled down. If the transfers are done in an area of previous wounding, the early stages of wound healing must have passed: Inflammation, induration, pain, or purulence will impede or prevent excursion of a transferred tendon. If active fibroplasia is still occurring, it is certain that the fibroblasts will tightly seize the tendon placed in their realm.

5. *Timing.* This is not only related to tissue equilibrium but also to the status of the damaged nerve. If there seems a reasonable chance that the palsy is the result of a neurapraxia, then it may be best to defer the transfer(s). The guidelines are never exact. How long should one wait for signs of returning function? How much harm is done if transfers are done and nerve function then returns? How much harm is done to the patient by waiting too long? Can early transfers

facilitate functional recovery by acting as Burkhalter's internal splints?[7]

6. *Expendable donors.* No structures in the upper extremity are truly expendable; they all have a useful function. The question really is whether their sacrifice will result in a greater good in terms of overall hand function. In short, what is the trade-off?

7. *Muscle power.* The muscle-tendon unit chosen for transfer must be strong enough to do the job required of it. Better a normal muscle, but at least one that rates good.

8. *Amplitude of excursion.* The muscle-tendon unit transferred must have enough excursion to move the joint(s) through the desired ROM. These excursions, though not exact, are useful relative values: 33 mm for the wrist flexors and extensors, 50 mm for the finger extensors and extensor pollicis longus (EPL), and 70 mm for the finger flexors. Directing a monarticular tendon unit across two or three joints may increase its effective amplitude through a tenodesis effect.

9. *Line of pull.* Both strength and efficiency are conserved when the transferred tendon takes a direct (i.e., straight) course between its origin and its insertion. When a pulley is used to change the direction of pull, as in an adductorplasty and most opponensplasties, both strength and efficiency are lost.

10. *Simplicity of function.* Ideally, a transfer should perform only one function. With rare exception (e.g., the rerouted long thumb extensor for radial palsy), multiple function requirements dissipate the energy and efficiency of each component.

11. *Tension.* The tension under which the transferred tendon is placed in its suture to another tendon, capsule, or bone is critical to success. Too tight and it will result in degeneration of the muscle of the transfer; too loose and it will be ineffective in transferring power. The guideline is to suture the transfer under normal tension, but it is most difficult to determine what is normal. Transfer tension is probably the most challenging technical part of tendon transfer surgery—and it is certainly the most difficult to teach to one's students.

12. *Synergism versus antagonism.* Synergy implies co-operation: some muscles are synergistic with others (e.g., wrist extensors reinforce finger flexors). When possible, it is preferable to use transfers that are synergistic with the new function they are charged with. Though there is argument on this point, I believe its importance has been overemphasized and that no muscle-tendon unit in the upper extremity is truly antagonistic to another. Where a synergistic transfer is not possible, any other muscle can be used. With adequate training any muscle can perform the function of another. The synergy centers repose in the central nervous system, and they are amenable to reeducation.

13. *Surgical technique.* Application of Bunnell's concept of gentle handling of the tissues—atraumatic technique—is a must. The distal end of the transfer is gently pushed through anatomic lines of least resistance, using a tendon tunneler, causing as little damage (and scarring) as possible. Tissue planes should be exploited and unscarred subcutaneous tissue is generally the best. When the transfer is passed through fascia or an interosseous membrane, a large hole should be made to decrease adhesion formation.

The surgical juncture of the transfer must be strong enough to maintain its integrity before the fibroblastic activity of healing is completed. Where the recipient is another tendon, interweaving of the transfer into the other tendon gives a stronger and more reliable bond than an end-to-end suture. Insertion of the transfer to bone is best done by tunneling the tendon into the bone and affixing with a pullout suture.

14. *Sensibility.* Most peripheral nerve palsies have both motor and sensory loss. Sensory impairment may compromise the relative success of tendon transfers—the degree of compromise varying with the particular nerve involved. Loss of median sensibility is the most serious, ulnar sensory less so, and radial the least. The patient with loss of sensation in the more important parts of the hand has an open communication loop and must concentrate on visual reinforcement (an ancillary closed loop) to obtain optimum function of tendon transfers. How well patients with sensory loss learn to compensate for this loss and succeed in using their transfer depends in large part on their understanding of the problem, their motivation to make the transfer work, and the education and guidance given by the surgeon and the hand therapist.

15. *Postoperative immobilization.* All joints crossed by the transfer(s) must be stabilized throughout the early phases of healing—usually 3 to 4 weeks—after which supervised active ROM exercises are started. Depending on the strength of the transfer and the integrity of its insertion, protective splinting may be used for longer periods, removing the splint only for supervised exercise.

16. *Transfer reeducation.* How well the patient learns to use tendon transfers depends on several factors.
    a. *Motivation.* Assuming that all the foregoing criteria have been met, motivation is the most important factor. This depends, in turn on the patient's personality, the desire to return to work, and how well he or she understands the purpose of

the transfers. Children seem inherently motivated to make things work and require little or no coaching.

b. *The degree of dysfunction.* Single transfers (e.g., opponensplasty) and the least complex transfers (e.g., crossing only one joint in a straight-line pull) work the best. Of the single nerve palsies, the easiest transfers to reeducate are the radial palsy, followed by the median palsy. The transfers to restore power grip to the ulnar palsied hand are the next most difficult to retrain. Most difficult of all are the combined nerve palsies.

c. *Hand therapy.* The expertise of an experienced, empathetic, communicative, supportive, patient, and persistent hand therapist is essential and may make the difference between success and failure. The conscientious surgeon explains to the patient what he or she plans to do, and then, after the operation, what has been done; but it is the therapist who has the primary teaching responsibility, because the therapist guides the patient through the education process of teaching the tendons to perform new functions. The therapist's role, as I see it, is not that of a technician but rather of an educator and guide for the patient. The accomplished hand therapist acts as a catalyst for the patient, leading him or her from simple passive (painless) exercises through active assistive to purely active motions and then, finally, to purposeful activity as Brand puts it. Brand also emphasizes return to work, as "Work is by far the best therapy for the hand and for the spirit."[4]

MEDIAN NERVE PALSY

The major functional deficit in a median nerve paralysis is loss of sensation in the radial two thirds of the hand, particularly in the thumb, and if nerve repair fails, or is not possible, little can be done about that loss of sensibility. Motor loss, though secondary in importance, is nevertheless a significant functional handicap and much can be done about that with properly selected and executed tendon transfers.

Interruption of the median nerve in the distal forearm or wrist results in loss of opposition. If the nerve lesion is proximal to the midforearm, there is also loss of some of the extrinsic flexors of the wrist and hand. Whether the lesion is high or low, the major loss is that of opposition—the ability to oppose the tactile pad of the thumb tip to that of the index finger or to those of the index and middle fingers, or the ability to oppose the tip of the thumb to the radial side of the index finger, the so-called key pinch.

Opponensplasty

Opposition of the thumb is a composite of abduction and pronation of the first metacarpal and flexion, pronation, and radial deviation of the thumb's proximal phalanx. This complex action is the result of several force vectors from the coordinated contraction of two groups of muscles acting on the first ray. The major group, those that insert on the radial (lateral) side of the first metacarpal and proximal phalanx are the abductor pollicis brevis (APB), the opponens, and the flexor pollicis brevis (FPB). The lesser but still important group is composed of those intrinsic muscles that insert on the ulnar (medial) side of the proximal phalanx, the transverse and oblique heads of the adductor pollicis. Most commonly, the major (lateral) group is median innervated and the minor (medial) group, the two heads of the adductor, is ulnar innervated. However, variations from this nerve distribution are common, and in the most common variation—about one third of hands—the FPB is supplied wholly or in part by the ulnar nerve. Where the FPB is ulnar innervated, it can combine with the abductor pollicis longus (APL) to give a fairly effective positioning of the thumb for prehension, and median-palsied patients in this category do not need an opponensplasty.

Fibrosis or scarring in the thumb web due to trauma or long-standing disuse of the hand may cause an adduction contracture of the web or even of the trapeziometacarpal capsule. It is imperative that a reasonable passive ROM of this basal joint and of the metacarpophalangeal (MP) joint be obtained before any tendon transfer is attempted. A tendon transfer, no matter how strong or how skillfully performed, can never overcome preoperative contracture or joint stiffness.

Both extrinsic and intrinsic tendons have been used for opponensplasty. The most common extrinsics used are the FDS of the ring finger and the extensor indicis proprius (EIP). An ulnar-innervated muscle (usually the abductor digiti minimi) is preferred by some.

My own preference has been for the EIP, because it has some unique advantages. First, if detached properly from the extensor hood of the index finger, there is little or no functional loss. In this regard, it could well be considered an accessory (i.e., an expendable) tendon, and that is not the case for a finger flexor, whose loss results in some decrease in grip strength. Second, it has ample length, obviating the need for lengthening by a tendon graft. Third, its strength, though not the equal of a finger flexor, is adequate for opposition. It is easily transferred through subcutaneous tunnels that do not violate the depths of the palm. Last, it is easily trained to perform its new task, though I do not believe that synergy, or for that matter, antagonism, is a problem for any transfer in the upper extremity (Fig. 26-4).

Lacking an EIP, or where this tendon has been used for another purpose, as in a combined median and ulnar palsy where it may have been used for an adductorplasty, the ring finger superficial flexor is an excellent choice. It does weaken the grip some and it is much stronger than necessary, but it shares with the index extensor the advantage of length and ease of trainability. The classic Bunnell opponensplasty

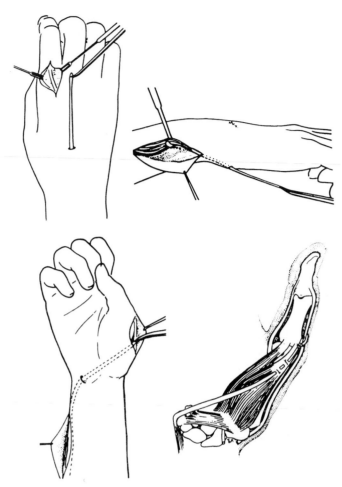

Fig. 26-4. Extensor indicis proprius opponensplasty. (Modified from Burkhalter W, Christensen RC, Brown PW: Extensor indicis proprius opponensplasty, *J Bone Joint Surg* 1973; 55[A]:725-732.)

(preceded by the Royle-Thompson transfer) uses the ring finger superficial flexor.[2]

The superficial flexor of the middle finger also may be used, but results in significant loss of grip strength. Where the EIP is not available, the extensor digiti minimi (EDM) or a wrist extensor (usually the extensor carpi ulnaris) prolonged with a tendon graft may be used. Another alternative is the palmaris longus prolonged with a strip of palmar fascia inserted into the distal adductor pollicis. This gives effective abduction of the first metacarpal but does not provide pronation or rotation.

The specifics of surgical technique for these and other transfers are described and illustrated in Green[10] and will not be duplicated here. Atraumatic handling of tissue as espoused by Bunnell[2] and the tendon tunneling techniques of Brand[3] are essential to good tendon transfer surgery. Successful postoperative management of the opponensplasty depends in large part on the patient's understanding of what was done and patient coaching by the surgeon or therapist once the thumb has been freed from its postoperative restraint, usually 3 or 4 weeks. Actually, the reeducation

of the transferred tendon can start within a few days of the surgery: The patient is instructed to frequently contract the transferred muscle tendon unit against the confines of the splint or cast. When the hand is freed the rehabilitation process is furthered by explaining to the patient that the median sensory deficit requires visual reinforcement of the function of the transfer. Once the patient understands this and has practiced it for a few days, it becomes automatic. From then on the best therapy consists of putting the hand to work performing useful functions such as arts and crafts, automobile mechanics, carpentry, kitchen work, and the like—activities with purpose that can produce predictable and concrete results.

Median extrinsic replacement

The hand with a high median palsy lacks not only thenar instrinsics but also the flexor pollicis longus (FPL), all four of the FDS muscles, the flexor digitorum profundus (FDP) of the index (and to some degree, the middle finger), the palmaris longus, the flexor carpi radialis (FCR), and the forearm pronators. The major functional loss (aside from loss of opposition) is flexion of the interphalangeal (IP) joints of the index finger and thumb and to some degree, the MP joint of the thumb. The loss of the superficial flexors of the fingers, of course, weakens overall grip strength but does not detract from finger flexion excursion.

The extrinsic loss is best made up by two transfers: the brachioradialis to the FPL and the extensor carpi radialis longus (ECRL) to the FDP of the index and middle fingers. For these transfers to work well, the wrist must have a full ROM. The brachioradialis transfer works very well as far as strength, line of pull, and ease of technique is concerned and its amplitude is fairly good, and if it is surgically freed well proximal to its musculotendinous junction. Failure to adequately free this tendon before transfer will result in a short excursion that will cause this powerful tendon to overpull the thumb extensors resulting in a thumb flexion contracture, a condition much worse than the one it was designed to correct. End-to-end suture of these transfers is preferable to side-to-side suture except where there is a fair probability that median nerve repair will be successful and that renervation of the palsied extrinsics will occur, in which case the transfers can easily be taken down.

RADIAL NERVE PALSY

A radial palsy has three significant advantages over a median or ulnar paralysis. First, it is easier to live with, and although there is significant functional loss, this can be considerably decreased with a simple wrist splint. Second, there is no concomitant sensory loss of any great importance to hand function. Last, the results of radial palsy tendon transfers are generally better and more predictable than transfers for other palsies.

Timing of tendon transfers

The one disadvantage (if it can be considered such) of radial palsies as compared with median and ulnar palsies is that unforeseen return of radial nerve function may have made them unnecessary. Of course, this may be true of any palsy, but because the most common cause of radial nerve dysfunction is a neurapraxia, unpredictable and spontaneous renervation may occur. If this does occur, the surgeon and the patient are faced with the choice of taking down the transfers or accepting the situation as it now is—a slightly weakened hand because of the transfers. If the injury has been an open one, the nerve inspected, and it is deemed that repair is not feasible, it is better to proceed promptly to tendon transfers (i.e., as soon as the wound is healed). If the injury seems not to have been severe and it is deemed probable that nerve recovery will be spontaneous, then of course it is better to wait and see. With this scenario, two questions arise: How long should one wait? and How should the hand be treated while waiting?

If a neurapraxia is the cause, early signs of muscle renervation will usually begin to appear in 3 to 4 months. If nothing has come back in 6 months, the surgeon can proceed with the transfers. This can be done with due regard to many variables: the type of injury, the validity of the history of injury, and the physical signs present at first examination. The patient should be apprised early on of the pros and cons of waiting versus early transfers. Once informed, the patient or guardians should be decision making partners of the surgeon.

Though many elaborate splints have been prescribed for radial palsy, it has been my experience that the more complex the splint for a single nerve palsy, the more it will encumber hand function and the more unlikely the patient will wear it. For the radial palsy a simple volar splint holding the wrist in 20° to 30° of extension is compatible with function, comfort, appearance, and economy. Dynamic outriggers or passive splints to maintain thumb or finger extension are commonly used, but in most cases, they are unnecessary. The patient should be instructed in simple passive exercises of the hand to maintain mobility until radial function returns or tendon transfers are done. Brand recommends a daytime wrist splint for function and a nighttime splint to hold fingers and wrist in extension to prevent a shortening of flexor muscles leading to loss of muscle fiber length,[3] though I've not found such splinting necessary.

The use of early tendon transfers such as internal splints has many advantages.[7] The best example for this is the early transfer of the pronator teres to the extensor carpi radialis brevis (ECRB), which eliminates the need of an external splint and enhances manual function by increasing power grip of the hand. If radial nerve function returns little is lost; if it does not then transfers can be done later for finger and thumb extension.

Transfers for radial palsy

The deficits are loss of wrist extension, finger and thumb extension, and usually thumb abduction. There are many possibilities for transfer: Green[10] in his section on radial palsy describes them well. Available for transfer are the superficial flexors of both index and middle fingers, the pronator teres, the palmaris longus, and both wrist flexors. Wrist or finger flexor transfers may be tunneled around either side of the wrist or may be passed through the interspace between radius and ulna. If the latter, it is important to resect a generous portion of interosseous membrane so that the transfer will slide freely through the interstice.

Peripheral nerve palsies, seen most commonly during war as gunshot and shell fragment wounds of the extremities, constitute about three quarters of all wounds incurred in combat. Most such casualties are otherwise healthy young men who are anxious to get on with their lives and are thus well motivated to make the most of whatever can be given to them to restore function to their hands. During the Vietnam war, irreparable radial nerve injuries were common: there were several hundred on my orthopedic service at Fitzsimons Army Hospital in Denver from 1966 through 1969. Where associated injury allowed, my staff found that the most effective transfers were as follows.

For wrist extension the pronator teres was transferred into the ECRB. Stripping the pronator teres free from its insertion on the distal radius, along with a generous strip of periosteum gave a transfer long enough to be tunneled obliquely around the radial aspect of the forearm and interwoven into the wrist extensor proximal to the wrist and with enough tension to maintain the wrist at about 30° of extension against gravity. Extension of the index, middle, ring, and small fingers was supplied by the flexor carpi ulnaris (FCU) tunneled around the ulnar aspect of the wrist and spliced to each of the extensor digitorum communis tendons proximal to the wrist joint. Tension of this transfer was set to hold the MP joints of the fingers at 0° against gravity with the wrist in neutral, and care was taken that the transferred tendon was set into each of the extensors with equal tension.

A single transfer, the palmaris longus tendon, was used for both thumb extension and abduction. This violated a maxim that only one tendon should be used for one function, but it was routinely demonstrated that by rerouting the EPL tendon to a position just to the radial side of the first metacarpal and suturing the rerouted palmaris longus tendon to it under moderate tension that the patient could then use the transfer as either a thumb extensor or a thumb abductor. The technique required that the long thumb extensor be severed at about the level of Lister's tubercle and then moved subcutaneously to its point of anastomosis with the detached palmaris longus just proximal to the volar aspect of the scaphoid. The patient could selectively use this transfer as either a thumb abductor or a thumb extensor by simply adducting or abducting the thumb with his thumb intrinsics, thereby moving the transfer subcutaneously over the first metacarpal. No training was required for this seemingly complex maneuver; patients picked up the technique immediately upon freeing from the postoperative splint, which was maintained for 4 weeks. Similarly, little or no reeducation of the other radial palsy transfers was necessary for most patients. Rehabilitation for these radial palsy transfer patients consisted mainly of getting them involved in some sort of meaningful activity. For these young men one of the most useful devices was the engine from a large military truck mounted on a pedestal, plus a full set of automotive mechanics' tools. Our tendon transfer patients found that dissembling and reassembling that engine was more satisfactory than basket weaving and considerably more motivating for regaining hand function than any formal exercise program.

ULNAR NERVE PALSY

The most significant deficit in an ulnar palsy is the loss of motor function of most of the intrinsic musculature of the hand. The sensory deficit, loss of sensibility along the ulnar border of the hand and in the small and ring fingers, is mostly an inconvenience and a potential hazard for burns and other injuries, but most patients learn to adjust well to this loss. The intrinsic motor loss, on the other hand, seriously compromises two of the most valuable functions of the hand, power grip and strength of pinch.

Though there is much variation in innervation of the intrinsic musculature of the hand, the usual pattern is that of ulnar supply of the seven interossei, the two ulnar lumbricals, the three hypothenars, the adductor pollicis, and the transverse head of the FPB, a total of thirteen and a half muscles that have much to do with the strength, dependability, and coordination of most manual functions. Many splints and many operations—capsulorraphy, dermodesis, tenodesis, bone blocks, arthrodesis, and tendon transfers—have been used to make up for this deficit, but only tendon transfers have produced consistently useful results, and even they have been fraught with problems. Nevertheless, static operations, such as capsulorraphy and various arthrodeses, are useful in palsies involving more than one nerve where there may be a dearth of suitable transfers or where there is associated soft tissue injury in the hand.

All of these procedures concentrate on the two basic motor deficits, those of grip and pinch, and on correcting deformity and preventing its progression. None are capable of restoring ulnar motor function to much more than half of normal strength and dexterity.

Ulnar intrinsic palsy results in a hand with a flattened transverse metacarpal arch, loss of dependable MP flexion in the ring and small fingers, and to a lesser degree in the middle and ring fingers. The loss of the interossei as MP joint flexors allows these joints to hyperextend because of the poorly opposed pull of the extrinsic extensors resulting in the classic claw deformity. The degree of deformity varies depending on the level of the nerve lesion, overlapping of intrinsic innervation by the median nerve, and variations in the basic structure of the individual hand. The deformity may be slight at first, but will invariably progress with time if ulnar renervation does not occur. Even with successful ulnar nerve repair, seldom is there better than fair to good return of intrinsic motor function. The progressive nature of the claw deformity and the generally poor results from ulnar nerve repair are arguments for early tendon transfer and against a wait-and-see approach.

Operations for grip strength

The key to enhancing the weakened grasp of the ulnar palsied hand is to provide a replacement for the paralyzed interossei as MP joint flexors. In the ulnar claw hand, flexion of these joints can only be accomplished by the extrinsic finger flexors of the four fingers, and to a slight degree by the uninvolved (usually) lumbricals of the middle and index fingers. This results in ulnar rollup, a phenomenon in which the finger flexors act first on the IP joints, and not until these joints are almost fully flexed do the MP joints begin to flex. This inefficient system not only makes for a weak grasp, but it also limits the ability of the fingers to surround wide objects preliminary to the application of grasping power.

The primary function of the interossei is to flex the MP joints of the four fingers. Their secondary function is to extend the IP joints, assisted by the lumbricals and the extrinsic extensors of the fingers. It is their flexor ability that determines most of the strength of the hand's grasp. Numerous dynamic transfers for grip strength have been developed over the years. Omer has very thoroughly catalogued and described them in Green.[10]

Numerous tendon transfers have been described to give both MP flexion and IP extension, but this dual responsibility is generally too much for a single motor, and particularly so when that motor must be extended with a complex graft tunneled through some rather complex anatomy in the depths of the hand. Brand[3,4] describes such transfers in detail and makes clear that results are dependent on a clear analysis of the problem and on exacting surgical technique. Brand's surgical technique and experience with the ulnar palsied hand are prerequisites to these complex operations—qualifications that the average hand surgeon does not have.

Looking for ways to simplify surgery and to improve results, I have discarded the more complicated operations and have concentrated on two variables. The first is to strive only for flexor power of the MP joint and to ignore extensor reinforcement of the IP joint. The second, and related, variable is to improve the insertion of the tendon grafts. In pursuing these goals I adopted Burkhalter and Strait's method, which, though not exactly simple, nevertheless

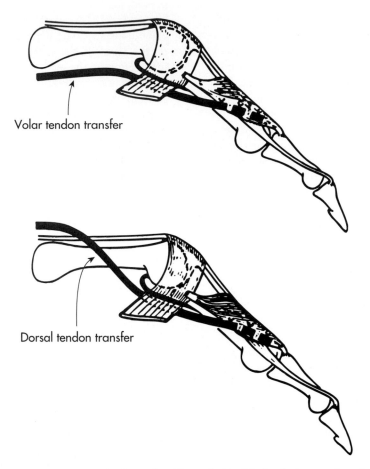

Volar tendon transfer

Dorsal tendon transfer

Fig. 26-5. Transfers for strengthening grip. (From Smith RJ: Intrinsic muscles of the fingers: function, dysfunction, and surgical reconstruction. In the American Academy of Orthopaedic Surgery, ed: *Instructional course lectures,* vol xxiv, St Louis, 1975, Mosby.)

focuses only on MP joint flexion with very secure insertion of the tendon graft into bone.[9] In this operation the motor selected depends on the level of the ulnar nerve lesion. If distal to the motor branches of the FDP, the ring finger superficialis is used, passing each slip down the lumbrical canal of the ring and small fingers and inserting the slip in a transverse drill hole in the proximal phalanx. Where the ulnar profundi are paralyzed, the ECRL (or occasionally the brachioradialis) is used, extending it with a split tendon graft passed from the dorsum of the hand through the intermetacarpal spaces with each slip passing volar to the deep intermetacarpal ligament and inserted on the radial side of the proximal phalanges of the ring and small fingers. Proper setting of the tension of the transfer is critical to success: When the wrist is held in neutral, the transfer should prevent passive hyperextension of the MP joints (Figs. 26-5 and 26-6).

Operations for pinch strength

Pinch strength is dependent on the muscles acting on the thumb and index finger as well as the integrity of the longitudinal arch of the thumb ray. The arch is maintained by a balancing of opposing forces of extrinsic and intrinsic

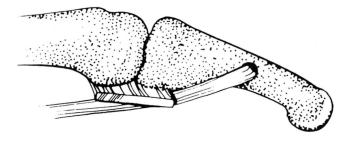

Fig. 26-6. Bony insertion of tendon graft into proximal phalanx for metacarpophalangeal flexor replacement. (From Omer GE Jr: Ulnar nerve palsy. In Green DP, ed: *Operative hand surgery,* ed 3, New York, 1993, Churchill Livingstone.)

muscles acting on the thumb. The adductor pollicis muscle not only adducts the thumb, it is also a strong flexor of the MP joint and a lesser extensor of the IP joint of the thumb. When it and the transverse head of the FPB are paralyzed, the patient attempts to compensate for the loss by increasing the pull of the FPL, which causes the IP joint to hyperflex. At the same time, the extrinsic extensors of the thumb unopposed at the MP joint create a hyperextension of that joint thus allowing the arch to collapse. The harder the patient attempts to pinch, the more pronounced becomes the deformity (i.e., MP joint hyperextension [Jeanne's sign] and hyperflexion of the IP joint [Froment's sign]).

In a key pinch the loss of the first dorsal interosseous muscle prevents the index finger from resisting the pinching force of the thumb, weak though it may be. The index is then forced into adduction unless it is buttressed by the ulnar three fingers. In pulp-to-pulp pinch the weakened index is less of a problem.

The weakened and ineffective pinch in the ulnar palsy can be effectively enhanced by an adductorplasty in which the transferred tendon is directed along the course of the adductor pollicis muscle belly and sutured into the adductor tendinous insertion. The ring finger flexor superficialis can be redirected dorsal to the flexors of the middle and index fingers and using the vertical septa of the palmar fascia as a pulley. The EIP also performs well as an adductor, though not as strong as the ring superficialis. It is directed into the palm between the third and fourth metacarpals and then along the course of the adductor muscle belly using the third metacarpal as the pulley.

Tendon transfers to substitute for the paralyzed first dorsal interosseous muscle seldom supply active abduction to the index, but they do help stabilize the finger in lateral or key pinch. Most commonly used for this is the EIP, in which case the ring superficialis would be used for the adductorplasty. At best, this transfer to the index gives only modest improvement in pinch strength.

Arthrodesis of either the IP or the MP joint of the thumb also improves strength of pinch somewhat but seldom enough to warrant the operation and the attendant loss of mobility of the arthrodesed joint.

As there are many variations of ulnar palsy depending on what intrinsics are supplied by the ulnar and by the median nerve, or in some cases, which muscles have dual innervation, the surgeon must be prepared to tailor the surgery to the particular innervation and to the special needs of the patient. Thus, Brand's warning of the dangers of recipes for tendon surgery is worth heeding, and this is especially true for ulnar palsies. In general, however, the strength of grip of the ulnar palsied hand is only about one quarter of normal and the pinch is only 10% to 20% of normal. The transfers described here will regularly bring both the grip and pinch strength to about one half of normal.[6]

COMBINED NERVE PALSIES
Low median-ulnar palsy

Injuries at the wrist and distal forearm account for this most common of the combined nerve palsies in which both sensory and motor loss result in a hand with little useful function. Not only is there loss of sensibility across the entire volar aspect of the hand, but all of the intrinsic musculature is paralyzed. This results in the most severe form of the claw hand: the hand is flattened due to the loss of the transverse palmar arch, the MP joints are hyperextended, and the IP

joints are flexed. The thumb tends to fall into an adducted position because of the unopposed secondary adduction action of the EPL, and this may progress to a fibrous adduction contracture of the thumb web. All of the wrist and finger extrinsic flexors and extensors are functional but become imbalanced as the wrist flexors overpull the extensors thereby weakening the finger flexors and allowing the finger extensors to progressively exaggerate the claw deformity.

Needed are thumb opposition, thumb adduction, and flexion of the proximal phalanges: These three basic functions can be supplied by the tendon transfers previously described and the result will be a useful hand, although seriously impaired. Anesthesia of the tactile surfaces presents not only severe functional loss but also deprives the patient of a protective pain response. Patients who are well motivated compensate for the loss of sensation by visual assistance and by enhancement of their proprioceptive senses within the joints and extrinsic muscle tendon units (i.e., by establishing an ancillary closed communication loop [p. 211]).

High median-ulnar palsy

As in the low median-ulnar palsy, the primary deficit in this combination is sensory. The motor problems are compounded by the loss of thumb, finger, and wrist flexors, leaving only radial innervated motors for transfer, and there are not enough of those to make up for the many deficits. Many combinations of tendon transfers combined with various arthrodeses and tenodeses are described,[10] but what is theoretically possible is often not reflected in functional results. It is important to temper possibilities with probabilities. The surgeon's assessment of results from multiple procedures in this complex palsy is often at odds with the patient's use of the hand.

The ECRL can be brought around the radial side of the distal forearm and sutured into the FDP of the fingers proximal to the carpal tunnel. Dependability of finger flexion with this transfer will be enhanced by arthrodesis of the distal interphalangeal (DIP) joints. Thumb opposition may be accomplished by transfer of the EIP and thumb adduction by the EDM. I prefer to preserve the ECRB for wrist extension. Arthrodesis of either of the two distal joints of the thumb will improve stability in pinch. Zancolli's capsulodesis of the MP joints of the fingers may contribute to overcoming the tendency for their progressive clawing.[5]

Ulnar-radial palsy

The ulnar-radial palsy lesion is usually located within the brachium. Lost are wrist, finger, and thumb extension, thumb adduction, and there is the usual ulnar palsy clawing due to the lack of interossei. This hand has the advantage of median sensation; normal wrist, thumb, and finger flexion, and thumb opposition, and there are enough motors available to give the hand moderately useful function. The pronator teres makes an excellent wrist extensor. Extension of the fingers and thumb can be accomplished with the middle finger superficial flexor brought through the radio-ulnar interosseous membrane and split into two slips, one going to the extensor pollicis longus and the other to the four extensor digitorum communis tendons. This makes for a rather primitive, but nevertheless effective, combined finger and thumb extension. If the palmaris longus is present it will give good thumb extension and abduction when transferred into the rerouted EPL, in which case the middle finger superficial transfer will be more effective acting only on finger extension.

Having taken care of the radial muscle-tendon deficits, there remain the two major ulnar problems—lack of thumb adduction and clawing of the ring and small fingers and sometimes of all four fingers. I prefer to furnish thumb adduction with the index finger superficial flexor and to correct the claw deformity with MP joint capsulodesis plus arthrodesis of the DIP joints.

High median-radial palsy

This is the worst of the double nerve palsies because there is not only a loss of median sensibility but also a dearth of possible motor transfers. Arthrodesis of the wrist gives needed stability to that joint and also makes available the FCU for transfer to the thumb and finger extensors. The four flexor digitorum profundi are sutured together proximal to the carpal tunnel, thus creating a tenodesis motored by the ulnar innervated finger flexors. There is no transfer available for thumb flexion or opposition: all that can be done for the thumb is to stabilize it for primitive grasp by arthrodesing the MP joint and tenodesing the APL tendon to the radius. The grasp resulting from these transfers is not much more effective than a well-fitted and functioning prosthesis, but such a hand has one significant advantage over the prosthesis in that it has some sensory feedback through its ulnar distribution.

REFERENCES

1. Boswick JA Jr, ed: *Symposium on Tendon Transfers in the Upper Extremity, Orth Clinics of North Am,* Philadelphia, 1974, Saunders.
2. Boyes JH, ed: *Bunnell's surgery of the hand,* ed 4, Philadelphia, 1964, Lippincott.
3. Brand PW: Biomechanics of tendon transfer. In Lamb DW, ed: *The Paralyzed Hand,* Edinburgh, 1987, Churchill Livingstone.
4. Brand PW: *Clinical mechanics of the hand,* St Louis, 1985, Mosby.
5. Brown PW: Zancolli capsulorraphy for ulnar claw hand: appraisal of forty-four cases, *J Bone Joint Surg* 1970; 52(A):868-877.
6. Brown PW: Reconstruction for pinch in ulnar intrinsic palsy, *Orthop Clin North Am* 1974; 5:323-324.
7. Burkhalter WE: Early tendon transfer in upper extremity peripheral nerve injury, *Clin Orthop* 1974; 104:68-79.
8. Burkhalter W, Christensen RC, Brown PW: Extensor indicis proprius opponensplasty, *J Bone Joint Surg* 1973; 55(A):725-732.
9. Burkhalter WE, Strait JL: Metacarpophalangeal flexor replacement for intrinsic-muscle paralysis, *J Bone Joint Surg* 1973; 55(A):1667-1676.
10. Green DP, ed: *Operative hand surgery,* ed 3, New York, 1993, Churchill Livingstone.
11. Hunter JM, Schneider LH, Mackin EJ, eds: *The hand: another decade of tendon surgery,* St Louis, 1984, Mosby.
12. American Academy of Orthopaedic Surgeons: *Tendon surgery in the hand* (symposium), St Louis, 1975, Mosby.

Chapter 27

DIRECT MUSCLE NEUROTIZATION

Giorgio A. Brunelli
Giorgio R. Brunelli

More and more frequently, reconstructive surgeons have to face clinical cases in which traumatic agents either have avulsed the motor nerve from the muscle(s) or have destroyed the so-called neural part of the muscle (i.e., that part in which the distal motor nerve divisions form the neuromuscular junction: the motor plates). In these cases no traditional procedure (nerve suture or nerve grafts) may be performed. In cases of surgical tumor with en block removal, a similar condition may also occur.

To overcome these problems we conducted research aiming to restore the muscular function. The goal of the research was to determine whether it was possible to achieve reinnervation of the denervated muscle by implanting into it a new nerve or grafts connected with the proximal stump of the proper nerve and divided in several artificial branches. Having obtained promising experimental results, this procedure has been successively used in patients.

HISTORY

The first experiments of direct muscular reinnervation (i.e., replanting the original or a foreign nerve into a muscle) were done by Heineke in 1914.[19] Subsequently, Erlacher, Steindler, and Elsberg reported on the technique.[10,12,13,25] Clinical applications that followed, mainly for muscle affected by poliomyelitis, had such inconsistent results that the technique was abandoned. Recently several researchers fulfilled physiologic studies on the effects of placing a nerve directly on the surface of denervated muscle.[1,17,18,21] In these experiments, the nerve was stimulated postoperatively and produced weak contractile responses from muscle. Formation of new synapses at the

contact of nerve with denervated muscle was thought to have been responsible.*

In 1970 we started experimental studies implanting a foreign nerve directly into muscle. The tibial nerve was resected and removed from the triceps and the peroneal nerve was implanted into the lateral head of this muscle, which is an aneural zone (i.e., devoid of nerve endings). Physiologic muscle responses were obtained, and formation of new motor end plates in aneural zones of muscle was noted. In 1972 Sakellarides, Sorbie, and James published similar results from experiments, performed on dogs.[24] In 1973 the experimental model was modified: The nerve was divided in several fascicles to obtain a larger area of reinnervation (Fig. 27-1).

Over the next years of animal research, more technical modifications were made, consisting mainly in the meticulous microsurgical division of the nerve in more and more numerous, artificial fascicles and in the wider distribution of these divisions both in width and depth. These technical improvements gave better results.

Histology demonstrated that these results were caused by the formation of new motor end plates between the nerve and the denervated muscular fibers.[6,22] Experimental studies have demonstrated that a denervated muscle is sensitive throughout its fibers to acetylcholine; on the contrary, normally innervated muscle is not. The wide distribution of receptors for acetylcholine in the denervated muscle allows the formation of new motor end plates even in aneural ectopic sites of muscle as a consequence of the functional

*References 2-5, 11, 14-16, 20, 23, 24.

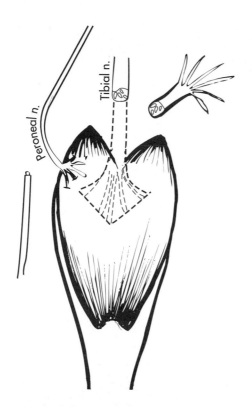

Fig. 27-1. Scheme of the experimental surgery: The tibial nerve is cut and its branches to the muscle removed from the so-called neural zone of the triceps (the zone where the nerve endings form motor end plates). The peroneal nerve is then cut, divided into thin slips, and introduced into small slits in the proximal part of the muscle, the aneural zone where normally no motor end plate exists.

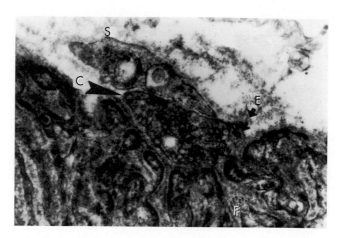

Fig. 27-2. Newly formed motor end plates after direct muscular neurotization in a previously aneural zone of the muscle. *E,* Nerve ending with synaptic vesicles; *C,* synaptic cleft; *F,* folding of the muscular membrane; *S,* cytoplasm of Schwann cell.

adaptations undergone by nerve endings and muscle membranes when in touch with one another.

MATERIAL AND METHODS

The first series of animals consisted of 21 rabbits. The distal portion of the tibial nerve with its intramuscular branches was removed to denervate the gastrocnemius muscle. The peroneal nerve was severed and implanted into the proximal portion of the lateral head of that muscle in an aneural zone. (This zone would not, under normal conditions, exhibit motor end plates.) At 1- and 2-month intervals, animals were sacrificed, and the distal end of the transplanted nerve was identified and studied by light and transmission electron microscopy. When the nerve-muscle junction was stained in an effort to detect acetylcholinesterase and motor end plates, formation of new motor end plates was noted. We think that motor end plates are functional adaptations of the nerve branches when they come into contact with the surface of the denervated muscular fibers.

A subsequent study was done on rats using a modified technique: The epineurium of the peroneal nerve was removed and artificial small branches were created under the operating microscope. These branches were implanted into muscle through small slits. The nerve branches were spread and distributed as widely and deeply as possible to both supply new innervation to the largest area of muscle and increase the number of neurotized muscle fibers. Small branches were sutured to muscle with 10-0 or 11-0 nylon suture, and the epineurium was anchored to the muscle with 6-0 suture to prevent nerve regression. A larger number of motor end plates was noted; the amount, in different microscopic fields, appeared to depend on the distance of the muscle field from the nerve implant.

Prior to sacrifice, electric stimulation of the peroneal nerve demonstrated good functional reinnervation of the triceps as early as 1 month after surgery. Muscle fibers in which new motor end plates had formed regained trophicity and showed normal morphology. On the contrary, the nonreinnervated fibers showed dystrophic appearance. Transmission electron microscopy demonstrated normal motor end plates with bare axon branches rich in presynaptic vescicles in direct contact with the membranes of muscle fibers that had normal-appearing folds. Presynaptic vesicles and mytochondria were noted in the axon branches, while only a single layer of Schwann cytoplasm was present over the axon on the opposite side of the muscle. There were no connective elements between the axon branches and the muscle (Fig. 27-2).

In subsequent research, nerve specimens were stained for acetylcholine using the technique described by Koelle and Tsuge. The fact that some of the fibers of the newly implanted nerve did not take up the stain is indirect evidence that both afferent and efferent fibers regenerated following this procedure.

Several conclusions can be drawn from this study. It appears that the sensitivity of normally innervated muscle to acetylcholine is limited and confined to the motor end plates. When new nerve fibers are inserted within normal muscle, they are not accepted. On the contrary, a denervated muscle is sensitive to acetylcholine throughout its fibers, and new nerve fibers inserted into denervated muscle *are* accepted. They provoke a functional adaptation that takes place at the point of contact of the nerve fibers with the muscle, and new motor end plates are formed.

These encouraging results may also have been caused by the adoption phenomenon, which depends on the chemotactic appeal exerted by the denervated muscle fibers on the surrounding regenerated axons. The latter send out sprouts, which become branches. They may issue from a node of Ranvier, or from the axon immediately above the motor end plate, or even from the motor end plate itself. By reinnervation of orphan muscle fibers, giant motor units are formed—two or three times bigger than normal units. They are demonstrated by electromyography (EMG). These giant motor units constitute a large part of the newly functioning muscle. A sound or regenerated axon is probably able to adopt orphan muscle fibers belonging to three or four (and possibly more) nonregenerated axons.

CLINICAL NEUROTIZATION: INDICATIONS AND OPERATIVE TECHNIQUE

After obtaining encouraging experimental results, we began clinical direct muscular neurotization in 1975.[6-9] Candidates were those patients who had sustained injuries in which the proximal nerve stump was available but the distal branches were missing because of traumatic or surgical loss of that muscle portion in which the motor nerve branches and motor end plates are located. Contraindications included a long interval of denervation such that the reparative ability of anterior horn cells were exhausted. The procedure was also inappropriate if too large a portion of muscle had been destroyed, if the remaining muscle was extremely fibrotic, or if other extramuscular limiting conditions, such as marked joint stiffness, existed. We have done 15 reinnervations of the extensor muscles of the forearm and 14 of the leg (Fig. 27-3). The procedure was also performed in seven trapezium muscles (six of which were iatrogenic); six deltoid muscles (four were caused by avulsion of C5-C6 roots of the brachial plexus, and one caused by avulsion of the muscle branches of the axillary nerve) (Fig. 27-4). Four thenar muscles, two muscles of the tongue, and one extensor pollicis longus have also been reinnervated.

The original nerve is always dissected from normal into scar tissue and up to neuroma. This is resected and the stump of the severed nerve is elongated by means of nerve grafts to muscle (Fig. 27-5). As many grafts as necessary are used to match the fascicles of the proximal stump. The grafts must be long enough to extend to a normal-appearing zone of muscle belly. (The color is of course always paler because of denervation.) The distal ends of the grafts are divided into as many thin slips as possible, which are then introduced into the muscle through longitudinal slits made as atraumatically as possible in the distal portion of the muscle. If bleeding is noted following creation of a slit, a new atraumatic slit is created in another area. Bleeding is avoided to limit the

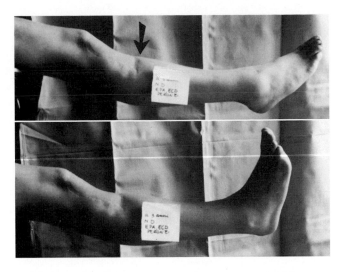

Fig. 27-3. Very good results after direct muscular neurotization of the extensor muscles of the foot due to a traumatic removal of the proximal part of the muscles. The arrow shows the loss of muscles, the stars mark the site of the skin lesion.

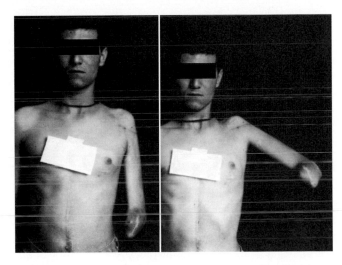

Fig. 27-4. Good results of direct neurotization of deltoid muscle by means of ulnar nerve in a young man who had sustained avulsion of C5, C6, C7, and amputation of the forearm. The neurotization allows him to wear a prosthesis.

formation of scar. The nerve branches are implanted in as wide an area as possible to increase the volume of reinnervated muscle. The epineurium is sutured to the muscle fascia with 6-0 nonabsorbable suture to avoid regression of the graft. In general, the slips stay in their slits and do not need sutures. Autogenous fibrin is sufficient to keep them in their place; if not the grafts are sewn individually with 10-0 suture. The limb is immobilized, and the reinnervated muscle is kept at rest for 15 days after surgery. Passive motion is then started and electric stimulation is begun. Other techniques, such as local radiation therapy and steroids to avoid scar formation are used routinely.

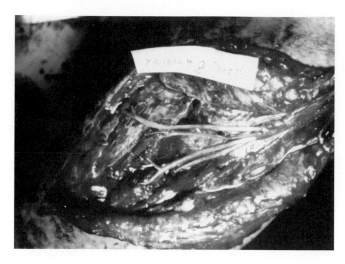

Fig. 27-5. Surgical appearance of the graft of the sural nerve proximally corrected with the nerve and distally introduced into the denervated muscles.

Table 27-1. Results of direct muscle neurotization

Muscle	Number of cases	M5*	M4*	M3+*	M3* or less
Extensor muscles, forearm	15	10	4	1	0
Extensor muscles, leg	14	11	2	1	0
Trapezius	7	4	2	1	0
Biceps	7	4	2	1	0
Thenar	4	3	1	0	0
Extensor pollicis longus	1	0	1	0	0
Deltoid	6	1	3	1	1
Tongue (hypoglosseal)	2	1	1	0	0
Total	56	34	16	5	1

*British Medical Research Council Grade: *very good* (the majority of the muscles), M5; *good*, M4; *fair*, M3+; *poor*, M3 or less.

Avulsion of the implanted grafts caused by insufficient protection during the early postoperative period must be avoided. Careful anchoring of the nerve and initial immobilization are essential. To avoid constriction of nerves and grafts, care must be taken to insure that both of them lie within as healthy and vascularized a bed as possible.

RESULTS

Results are shown in Table 27-1. They were good or very good in 50 out of the 56 cases examined.

DISCUSSION

The time needed for reinnervation to occur depends on the distance from the proximal nerve stump to the point of implantation (nerve regenerates on an average speed of 1 mm/day). In three of the cases in which the proximal stump was unavailable for reinnervation (because of avulsion of the brachial plexus from the spinal cord), a foreign donor nerve was used. In one case even an antagonist nerve (as a radial nerve branch of the triceps to the biceps) was transferred (Fig. 27-6). In all these cases functional results were good. In the reported series, 53 of the 56 cases were operated on by connecting the proper nerve with the muscle by means of sural nerve grafts.

There are no current techniques by which reinnervation can be obtained when the distal segment of the nerve has been completely destroyed. In these cases procedures such as tendon transfers and arthrodeses are commonly used.

We believe that meticulous microsurgical technique as well as the adoption phenomenon involving axonal branches, and their reinnervation of neighboring orphan motor fibers accounted for the good results achieved with direct muscular neurotization.

In a recent survey of cases using direct muscular neurotization, operated on by different surgeons using this

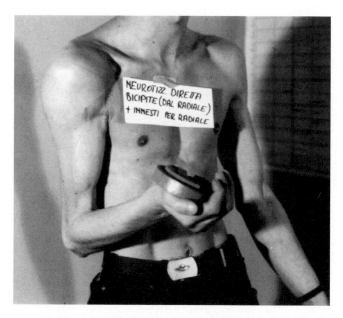

Fig. 27-6. Good result of direct neurotization of the biceps muscle after traumatic removal of part of its proximal belly and avulsion of the musculocutaneous nerve. A branch to the triceps of the radial nerve was used for neurotization.

technique, the percentage of good and very good results of those performing the procedure for the first time was not as high as that reported here. This is probably because the details of the operative technique were not rigorously and precisely carried out by the less experienced clinicians. Others, with more experience, have achieved results similar to ours.

CONCLUSION

Our experimental research and clinical applications lasting more than 25 years allow us to say that direct muscle neurotization is the only solution to the otherwise unsolvable problem of destruction of the neuromuscular junction.

REFERENCES

1. Aitken JT: Growth of nerve implants in voluntary muscle, *J Anat* 1950; 84:38.
2. Bennet MR, Pettigrew G: The formation of neuromuscular synapses, Cold Spring Harbor Symposium, *Quant Biol* 1976; 40:409.
3. Bradley R: The morphology of the normal end plate in lambs as revealed by silver impregnation and light microscopy, *Res Vet Sci* 1977; 23:250.
4. Brenner HR, Sakmann B: Gating properties of acetylcholine receptor in newly formed neuromuscular synapses, *Nature* 1978; 271:366-368.
5. Brunelli G, Monini L, Antonucci A, Maraldi N: Neurotizzazione in zona aneurale di muscoli denervati, *Il Policlinico* 1976; 83:611-616.
6. Brunelli G: Direct neurotization of severely damaged and denervated muscles. In Freilinger, et al, eds: *Muscle transplantation,* Wien, 1981, Springer Verlag.
7. Brunelli G, Monini L: Direct muscular neurotization, *J Hand Surg,* 1985; 10(A):6, 993-997.
8. Brunelli G, Monini L: Direct muscular neurotization. In Brunelli G, ed: *Textbook of microsurgery,* Milano, 1988, Masson.
9. Brunelli G: Direct muscular neurotization. In Gelbermann R, ed: *Operative nerve repair and reconstruction,* Philadelphia, 1991, Lippincott.
10. Elsberg CA: Experiments on motor nerve regeneration and the direct neurotization of paralysed muscles by their own and by foreign nerves, *Science* 1917; 45:318.
11. Engel G: Locating motor end plates for electron microscopy, *Mayo Clin Proc* 1970; 45:450.
12. Erlacher P: Ueber die motorischen nervendigungen, *Z Orthop Chir* 1914; 34:561.
13. Erlacher P: Direct and muscular neurotization of paralyzed muscles, *Amer J Orthop Surg* 1915; 13:22.
14. Fex S, Thesleft S: The time required for innervation of denervated muscles by nerve implants, *Life Sci* 1967; 6:635.
15. Frenk E, Jansen JKS, Lomo T, Westgaard RH: The interaction between foreign and original motor nerves innervating the soleus muscle of rats, *J Physiol* 1975; 247:725-742.
16. Gozenbach HR, Waser PG: Electron microscopic studies of degeneration of rat neuromuscular junctions, *Brain Res* 1973; 63:167.
17. Guth L, Zalewski AA: Disposition of cholinesterase following implantation of nerve into denervated muscle, *Exp Neurol* 1963; 7:316.
18. Gutmann E, Hanzlikova V: Effects of accessory nerve supply to muscle achieved by implantation into muscle during degeneration of its nerve, *Phisiol Bohemostaw* 1967; 16:244.
19. Heineke D: Die directs einflanzung des Nerve in den Muskel, *Zentralb Chir* 1914; 41:465.
20. Hoffman H: A study of the factors influencing innervation of muscles by nerves implanted, *Aust Exp Biol Med Sci* 1951; 29:289.
21. Katz B, Miledi R: The development of acetylcholine sensitivity in nerve free segments of skeletal muscle, *J Physiol* 1964; 170:389.
22. Korneliussen H, Sommerschild H: Ultrastructure of the new neuromuscular junctions formed during reinnervation of rat soleus muscle by a "foreign" nerve, *Cell Tissue Res* 1976; 167:439.
23. Lomo T, Slater CR: Acetylcholine sensitivity of developing junctions in adult rat soleus muscle, *J Physiol* 1980; 303:173-187.
24. Sakellarides HT, Sorbie C, James L: Reinnervation of denervated muscles by nerve transplantation, *Clin Orthop* 1972; 83:194.
25. Steindler A: The method of direct neurotization of paralyzed muscles, *Amer J Orthop Surg* 1915; 13:33.

Chapter 28

RESTORATION OF TETRAPLEGIC HAND FUNCTION USING AN FES NEUROPROSTHESIS

Michael W. Keith
FES Neuroprosthesis Multi-Center Clinical Trial Teams*

Tetraplegic patients are disadvantaged by a substantial loss of body function, the ability to work with their hands, and are thus less socially interactive and productive. American Spinal Injury Association (ASIA) class C5 and C6 cervical spinal cord injury are the most common injury levels, and yet there are few effective surgical treatments that restore hand function in the most common forms of the injury. C5 patients usually are classified O:0 or O:1 in the International Classification. C6 patients usually fall into OCu:1 or OCu:2 classification. The variance is because of the ASIA classification being based on manual muscle testing grade 3 and the International Classification requiring grade 4. The classifications are not strictly convertible, because the ASIA classification is usually referenced according to the motor level.

*Investigators of the International Multi-Center Clinical Trial of the FES Neuroprosthesis: Michael W. Keith, Hunter Peckham, Kevin Kilgore, Anne Bryden, Kathryn Wuolle, Case Western Reserve University, Cleveland Veterans Affairs Medical Center, MetroHealth Medical Center, Cleveland, Ohio; Randal R. Betz, Albert A. Weiss, M.J. Mulcahey, Shriners Hospital, Philadelphia, Pennsylvania; Andrew Egleseder, Peter Gorman, Linda Marshall, University of Maryland, Baltimore VAMC, Kernan Hospital, Baltimore, Maryland; Vincent R. Hentz, Amy Ladd, Inder Perkash, Janet Weiss, Stanford University, Palo Alto VAMC Spinal Injury Unit, Stanford, California; Gerard Sormann, Douglas J. Brown, Sara Carroll, Austin Hospital, Melbourne, Australia; John Hobby, David Grundy, Salisbury District Hospital, Salisbury, England.

Our group, a team of biomedical engineers, therapists, and hand surgeons at Case Western Reserve University, the Veterans Affairs National Center of Excellence for Functional Electrical Stimulation, and MetroHealth Medical Center, Cleveland Ohio, has developed a functional electrical stimulation (FES) neuroprosthesis that should allow high level tetraplegics to increase the number of independent activities they are able to perform.[6] They want to use unmodified objects such as public telephones or a fork in a restaurant. They want to decrease the time required for and the difficulty of performing activities of daily living and to reduce the cost of formal attendant care. We hope the neuroprosthesis will also improve self-esteem and quality of life. This is a preliminary report of early progress toward development of this new form of treatment for severe upper motor neuron paralysis during the past decade.

THE FUNCTIONAL ELECTRICAL STIMULATION NEUROPROSTHESIS (NPS-4) DESIGN

The neuroprosthesis uses eight channels of electrical stimulation under voluntary control to excite the forearm and hand muscle and to provide sensory feedback. Fig. 28-1 shows the implanted and external components of the neuroprosthesis. Voluntary movements of the contralateral shoulder are sensed by a sensor and sent to a computer program that understands muscle recruitment properties. A

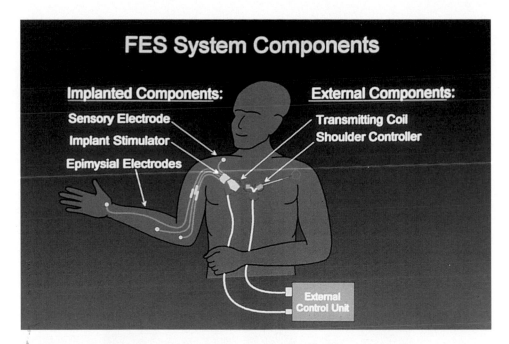

Fig. 28-1. Components of the implantable functional neuroprosthesis. External components consist of the shoulder position controller, external control unit (ECU), and the transmitting coil/antenna. Internal components are the receiver-stimulator, leads, and electrodes.

sensor detects protraction and retraction and vertical axis movements as well as the velocity of the movements. Control logic is developed with the patient to make most sensible use of the movements. Typically, the protraction-retraction axis is used for control of opening and closing of the hand, whereas vertical movements control lock and hold functions. Most patients do not have pure orthogonal control of these axes, so the software must use offsets or preferred axes for control. An external cable carries these signals to an external control unit (ECU). The ECU contains all upgradable electronic components and the program that synthesizes lateral and palmar prehension. It contains microprocessors in its memory and logs the patient's activity and hand use. The shoulder movements are converted to muscle recruitment curves and patterned to coordinate digit movement. Another cable leads to an antenna coil fixed by tape to the chest over the implanted receiver-stimulator. The commands are transmitted by encoded radio-frequency signals from the surface mounted antenna to the implanted receiver-stimulator. The carrier power of the transmitted signal is absorbed by circuitry in the receiver and stored to power the muscles. The stimulator creates wave forms of balanced charge to prevent corrosion of the electrodes. The output is of fixed constant current with modulated pulse width. The stimulation wave forms generated are carried by leads and applied by platinum electrodes to the epimysial surface, and they excite intramuscular nerve branches. Sensory feedback is applied to the subcutaneous nerves in the intact C5 sensory dermatome.[7] The stimulus is perceived as

rhythmic taps on the shoulder above the clavicle varying in rate and corresponding to the applied command. Previous research has shown that there is better perception of this stimulus when applied below the skin surface than on the surface.

SURGICAL STRATEGY

We combine standard surgical reconstructive procedures with FES neuroprosthesis implantation in a single stage to reduce cost and anesthetic risk.[1-3] Correction of contractures must be done first. In some cases where contractures are severe, they must be released or combined with serial cast immobilization and stretching before reconstructive surgery can be considered. Endpoints include full elbow extension and proximal interphalangeal (PIP) joint extension. Contractures of the fingers, especially PIP flexion contractures, are best prevented rather than released. From the first days of injury, the hands of tetraplegics must be evaluated and a program developed to prevent contractures. Some centers believe that the development of functional finger contractures is desirable. We have found finger flexion tightness and adductor tightness to be difficult to release, and they will require prolonged and expensive therapy to reverse. All patients undergo a period of surface electrical stimulation to increase the size and strength of upper extremity muscles. During this period of about 6 weeks, joint mobility and hand posture will improve because of soft tissue mobilization. Voluntary tendon transfers, such as posterior deltoid transfer for elbow extension, are always considered both to provide elbow

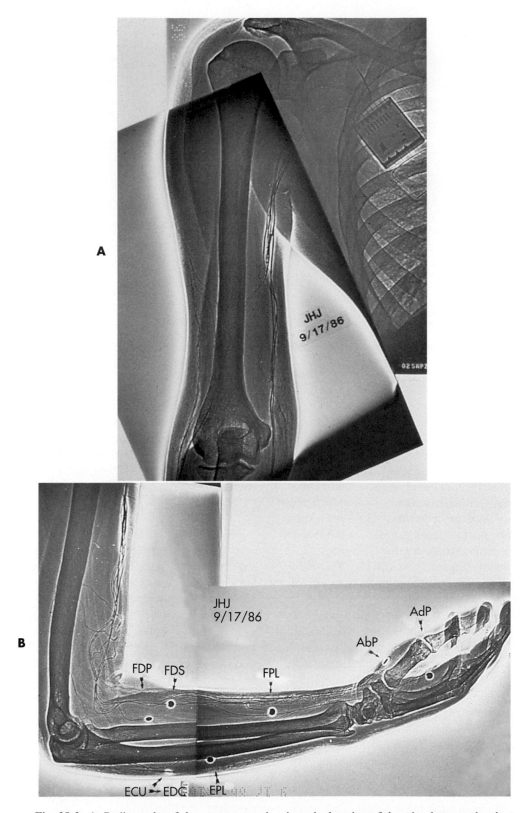

Fig. 28-2. A, Radiographs of the upper extremity show the location of the stimulator on the chest wall and electrodes dispersed at the motor points of the forearm and hand muscles. A tendon transfer of extensor digitorum communis (ECU) to extensor digitorum communin (EDC) is present. The first radiograph shows the implanted stimulator on the chest wall and leads are seen passing from connectors to the forearm. In the second radiograph, **B,** seven motor electrodes are seen on the muscles of the forearm and hand.

extension and to stabilize the elbow in the workspace. Tendon transfer and muscles crossing the elbow joint work better and their length-tension properties are optimal if the elbow can be controlled. Brachioradialis voluntary transfer to augment wrist extension in the C5 patient will allow tenodesis patterns instead of a braced wrist. In principle, FES replaces the remaining involuntary muscle groups. FES tendon transfers replace denervated muscle groups. Arthrodeses or tenodeses replace absent functional movements or simplify grasp.

The receiver-stimulator is placed on the chest wall through a transverse incision over the pectoralis fascia. The leads are tunneled to the mid upper arm where the electrode lead will be connected. Care is taken to place the leads on the neutral bending axis of the arm and to avoid tension of the electrodes. Mapping of the optimum epimysial position is done with the tourniquet released for 15 minutes to insure adequate muscle perfusion. The limb is warmed throughout the procedure with a heating blanket to maintain nerve excitability. Fig. 28-2, *A* and *B* show radiographs of the chest and arm demonstrating the location of the stimulator and electrodes on forearm muscles. The muscles chosen depend on the preoperative strength recovered, intraoperative properties, and useable patterns of grasp.

PROGRAMMING GRASP PATTERNS

Palmar prehension is created by recruiting the thenar intrinsics to position the thumb opposite the long finger. The stimulating electrode must recruit both abductor pollicis brevis and the opponens pollicis to achieve this position. The fingers start in full extension by recruiting extensor digitorum communis (EDC). The fingers move at the metacarpophalangeal (MP) and PIP joints from full extension to flex into contact with the thumb. Increasing command then increases the grasp force[4,5] (Fig. 28-3, *A* and *B*).

Lateral prehension is initiated by extending the thumb and fingers. The extensor pollicis longus (EPL) extends the thumb. If EPL is weak, extensor pollicis brevis (EPB) can be recruited but with less excursion. The EDC extends the fingers. The fingers are flexed by flexor digitorum profundus or flexor digitorum sublimis. The thumb closes against the positioned PIP joints with additional command adding more pinch force (Fig. 28-4, *A* and *B*).

Postoperative therapy consists of patterned electrical stimulation using the neuroprosthesis, much like preoperative stimulation. Stiffness that has developed during the healing process, including adhesions and joint and muscle stiffness, will relax under persistent and repeated muscle contraction and active assisted exercise. A plateau may be expected after 6 weeks. Splinting to maintain elbow extension at night is needed for 3 months as stretching of the elbow extensors is less functional.

Total active motion (TAM) improves after surgery in both lateral and palmar grasp (Figs. 28-5 and 28-6). The thumb range of motion (ROM) in palmar grasp is low because the thumb is posted in this grasp pattern. Full TAM cannot be achieved because there is yet no intrinsic muscle excitation in this version of the neuroprosthesis. In vivo experiments have shown that intrinsic replacement can increase finger extension. There is an interphalangeal extension deficit which varies with antagonist tone, flexion contracture, and extensor muscle amplitude. The degree of contracture varies from patient to patient and is a product of maintenance therapy and overall muscle stiffness. Addition of intrinsic control in the next generation may improve finger posture.

The median pinch force attainable in lateral prehension, palmar prehension, or five finger tip pinch exceeds preoperative or tenodesis pinch force and surpasses the threshold for functional pinch based on common object masses. Median pinch exceeded 5 newtons. See Figs. 28-7 and 28-8 for illustrations of this force.

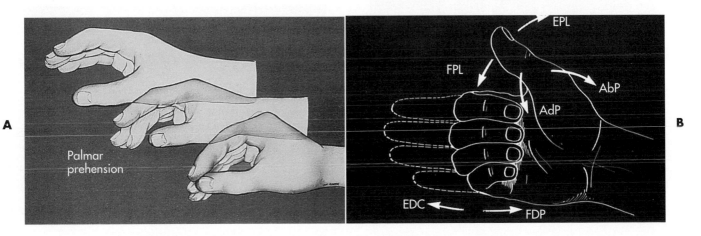

Fig. 28-3. **A** and **B** show the muscle patterns used for palmar prehension.

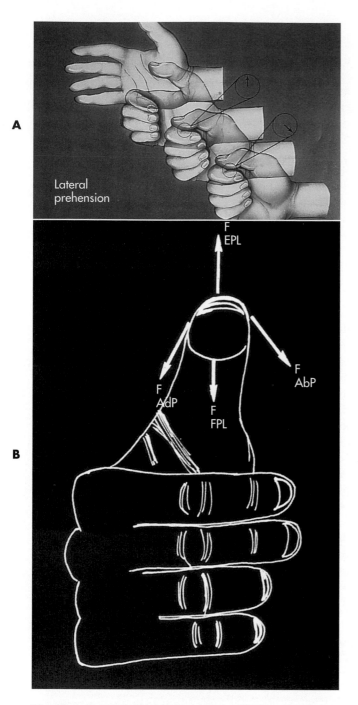

Fig. 28-4. A and **B** show the muscles used in lateral prehension.

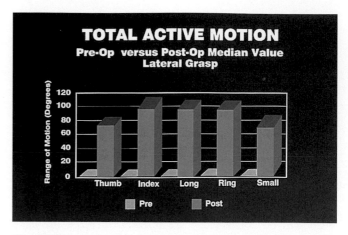

Fig. 28-5. Total active motion in lateral prehension is absent preoperatively. Each digit increases range of motion, although not to normal due to the absence of intrinsic muscle force, residual flexor tone, and adhesions present.

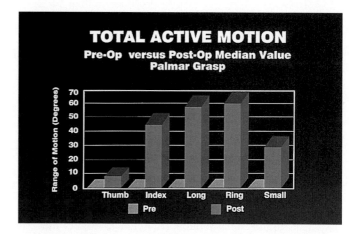

Fig. 28-6. Total active motion present in the palmar grasp pattern. There is no movement preoperatively. The thumb is posted into palmar abduction so it shows little active range of motion. Fingers flex until in contact with the thumb.

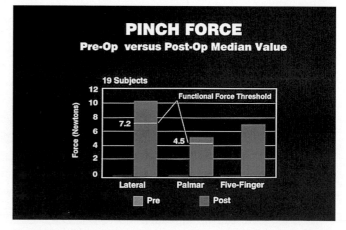

Fig. 28-7. Postoperative median pinch force in lateral prehension or palmar prehension exceeds the threshold needed for common object use.

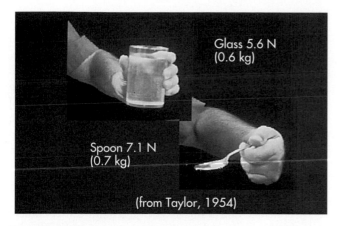

Fig. 28-8. Threshold for palmar grasp of a glass of water is 5.6 newtons. Lateral prehension force needed for lifting a spoon is 7.1 newtons.

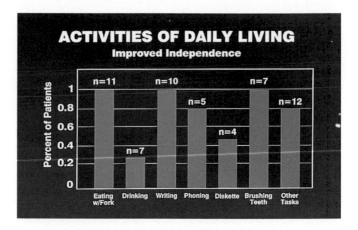

Fig. 28-10. Independence rating improved for most patients in activities of daily living.

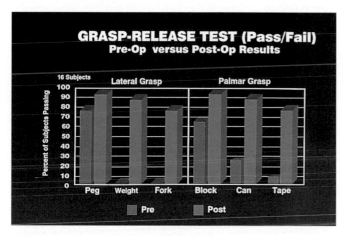

Fig. 28-9. Patients passed the grasp-release test items more often with the neuroprosthesis. Small object pinch such as peg or block can be accomplished without active motor control or force.

PRELIMINARY RESULTS OF STANDARD TESTS

The grasp-release test (GRT)[8,9] is a quantitated, standardized group of single-hand transfer and movement tests. The test emphasizes the impairment of tetraplegic patients attempting to use one hand for activities which able-bodied individuals perform with one hand. As many tetraplegics do not have a second able hand or even one with modest motor function, the second hand is often an assisting post. In addition, the patient's strategy for object acquisition and movement often involves using the mouth as a prehensile appendage with sensation and dexterity exceeding the impaired hand. The neuroprosthesis is currently provided only for one hand. Patients express a strong interest in achieving two-hand strength and ipsilateral coordination. The transfer of saliva, limitation of conversation, and awkwardness of manipulation, although functional, are quite abnormal. Although this method is acceptable among the disabled and their families by necessity, more normal

hand function is preferred. This patient group shows increases in the percentage of success in acquiring and transferring the peg, fork, and weight in the lateral prehension test (Fig. 28-9). These objects are oriented so that they can be grasped and used with slight pronation of the forearm. The weight is smooth metal and weighs 264 g. Few patients with surgical reconstruction with Moberg tenodesis or tendon transfer can lift this object or weight. All C5 patients lack sensation and sweating on the thumb and index finger so they have greater difficulty with this test than the C6 patients, because of lack of friction with dry skin and less feedback regarding slippage. There is a similar improvement in the percentage increasing the transfer of block, can, and tape using palmar prehension. These objects are larger in size and mass. The can weighs 210 g. The tape has a narrow base of support and requires arm position control to complete the task. These objects are oriented so that they can be lifted with the hand in neutral pronation-supination. Many patients can transfer the small block or peg with the passive forces and friction in the finger entirely without motor power or control. Voluntary wrist dorsiflexion control, tenodesis contracture, and adequate finger posture are needed to transfer any number of pegs or blocks with useful speed during the test period.

The Activities of Daily Living (ADL) Abilities Test contains functional models for eating, drinking, writing, using a telephone, handling a computer diskette, and brushing teeth, as well as other common tasks. Fig. 28-10 shows results in this group. Our subjects showed greatest improvement in performance during heavy object transfers and in high force tasks. ADL assessment showed a reduction in dependence on self-assistance from the mouth or opposite hand, assistive devices such as braces, or an attendant. A high percentage of patients show a strong preference for the control afforded by the neuroprosthesis compared with other methods of achieving the same function (Fig. 28-11).

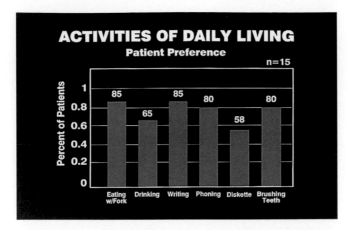

Fig. 28-11. Patients prefer the neuroprosthesis for activities of daily living.

USER SATISFACTION SURVEY

	Agree	Neutral	Disagree
Hand Appearance Improved?	7	1	1
System Reliability?	9		
Satisfied with System Function?	9		
Implant Again?	8		1
System produces benefit?	9		
Positive life impact?	7	2	
# of Activities Increased?	8	1	

Fig. 28-12. Patients rated their experience with the program in this early survey.

COMPLICATIONS

In this series of 29 patients followed through the perioperative period, one complete system was removed late because of infection after skin breakdown. Two of 232 electrodes were removed for skin erosion or infection. There were 11 examples of sensory or muscle stimulation requiring reduced stimulation level in the target muscle but with continued functional grasp patterns. This series has focused once again the concerns at the device-tissue interface. The components and devices have remained reliable.

OUTCOME SURVEY

At a 1-year interview, patients predominantly agreed with statements concerning improvement in hand appearance, system reliability, system function, repetition of the surgical procedure, personal benefit, life impact, and an increase in the number of activities performed (Fig. 28-12). The final report of the study group after longer follow-up will include results of patient reporting from the Reintegration to Normal Living, Rosenberg Self-Esteem, and other quality of life indices.

CONCLUSIONS

We conclude that at this stage of the multi-center clinical trial, a FES neuroprosthesis is effective in reducing impairment by improving hand strength and ROM. Functional outcome measures show improvement in independence and a preference for using the hand and function provided by a neuroprosthesis. The device is safe and reliable, although the problems of adhesions and potential infection are similar to those seen in tendon transfer surgery and other implantable devices.

We are grateful to our patients and co-investigators for their participation in this phase of the multi-center clinical trial.

REFERENCES

1. Keith MW, Peckham PH, Thrope GB, et al: Implantable functional neuromuscular stimulation in the tetraplegic hand, *J Hand Surg* 1989; 14(A):524.
2. Keith MW, Kilgore KL, Peckham PH, et al: Tendon transfer surgery and functional electrical stimulation, *J Hand Surg* 1996; 21(A):89.
3. Keith MW, Lacey SH: Surgical rehabilitation of the tetraplegic upper extremity, *J Neurol Rehabil* 1991; 5:75.
4. Kilgore KL, Peckham PH, Keith MW, et al: An implanted upper extremity neuroprosthesis: a five patient follow-up, *J Bone Joint Surg*(A), accepted for publication 1995.
5. Kilgore KL, Peckham PH: Grasp synthesis for upper extremity FNS, *Med Biol Eng Comput* 1993; 31:615.
6. Peckham PH, Keith MW, Freehafer AA: Restoration of functional control by electrical stimulation in the upper extremity of the quadriplegic patient, *J Bone Joint Surg Am* 1988; 70:144.
7. Riso RR, Ignagni AR, Keith MW: Cognitive feedback for use with FES upper extremity neuroprosthesis, *IEEE Trans BioMed Eng* 1991; 38:29.
8. Wuolle KS, Van Doren CL, Thrope GB, et al: Development of a quantitative hand grasp and release test for patients with tetraplegia using a hand neuroprosthesis, *J Hand Surg* 1994; 19(A):209-218.
9. Wuolle KS, et al: Assessment of hand function in tetraplegic patients using a neuroprosthesis for activities of daily living, *Am J Occup Ther*, submitted for publication, 1995.

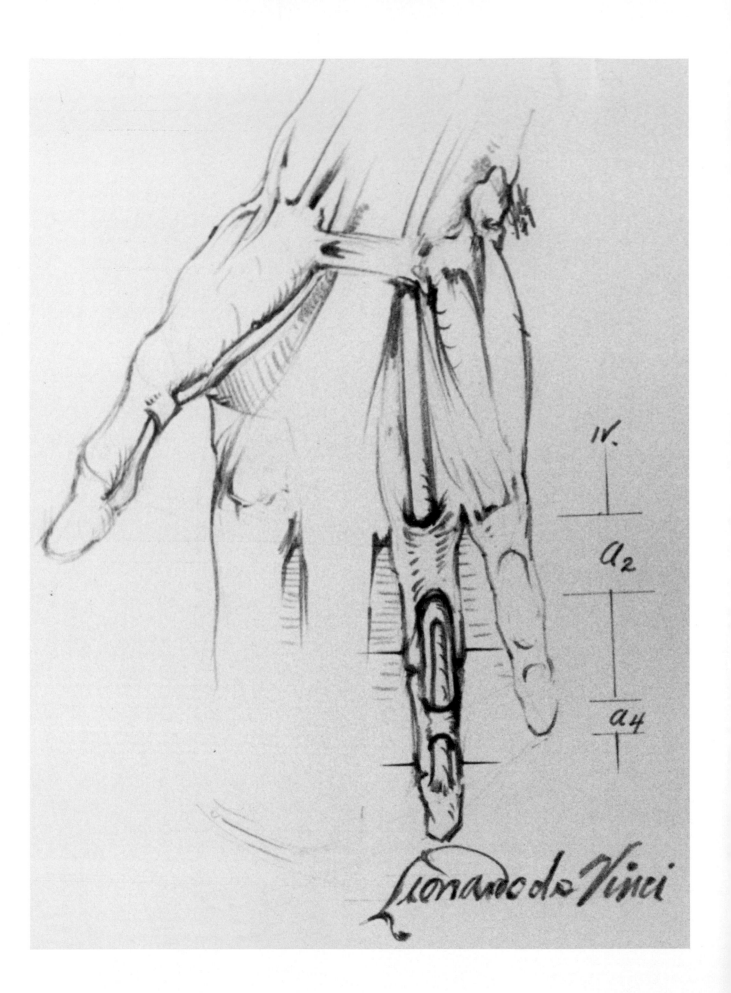

IV.

a_2

a_4

Leonardo da Vinci

Part VII

FLEXOR TENDON ANATOMY

Leonardo da Vinci, in his anatomical drawings of the hand, circa 1505, gives us a fine study of the strategic digital flexor retinacular system, free of its accessory components. The basal proximal and middle phalangeal annular fibro-osseous tunnels (pulleys) are perfectly illustrated; designated some 470 years later A_2 and A_4 by James R. Doyle—J.W. Littler, M.D., 2 June 1979. (From Littler JW, North E: *J Hand Surg* vol. 5, no. 5, Sept., St Louis, 1980, Mosby.)

Chapter 29

FUNCTIONAL ANATOMY OF THE FLEXOR TENDON SYSTEM: THE MUSCLES AND TENDON SYSTEMS OF THE FINGERS

Emanuel B. Kaplan
James M. Hunter

The muscles of the fingers are described separately from the muscles of the thumb and the wrist. The real meaning of the relationship of the muscles and the frequent variations that occur in the hand as a whole become much clearer when seen in the light of comparative anatomic and embryologic studies.

In the analysis of the muscular system it is preferable to eliminate the frequently used terms of *anomaly* for muscles that have an origin or insertion differing from accepted descriptions. It is more in line with the findings of comparative anatomy and embryology to classify all the differences as variations.

The anomalous structures fall into a different group produced by external causes: disease, exposure to radiation, or other damaging influences, either during development or in later stages. The so-called cases of developmental arrest probably also fall into the group of changes produced by abnormal chemical or physical agents.

The comparative anatomic investigations of Humphry[4] help explain a number of variations encountered in the hand. In more modern and more nearly complete studies, Straus[6]

From Spinner M, ed: *Kaplan's functional and surgical anatomy of the hand,* ed 3, Philadelphia, 1984, Lippincott.

and Haines[3] advanced the understanding of the development of the musculature. LeDouble[5] and Testut[7,8] collected a large series of muscular variations and correlated them with the findings of others. A discussion of these investigators follows.

The upper-limb girdle develops in the same way as the ribs and costal cartilages in the transverse intermuscular septum of the ventral muscles in the plane of the middle or internal oblique stratum. Essentially, they derive from the middle stratum and may be considered as serially homologous with the muscles passing from septum to septum or from rib to rib in front and behind them. It has also been shown that the external stratum of the external oblique muscle is prolonged on the limbs as a more or less complete funnel; therefore, the muscles are derivatives of the two outer strata of the ventral muscles, and they contribute largely to the muscular basis of the limbs. The muscle tissue of the limbs in the primitive form is segmented into transverse planes corresponding to the axial, cartilaginous, or osseous segments, thus resembling the disposition of the muscles in the trunk; but in the trunk, the muscle fibers, particularly the superficial fibers, are often not confined to their particular segments. The muscles of any division of a limb usually consist of three layers: the fibers of the segment itself, or the "intrinsic fibers"—of these the proximal series pass from the girdle to the first segment of the limb; the fibers derived from the distal segment, or the "extrinsic fibers"; more superficial fibers derived from the ventral muscles, or the superficial "ventral appendicular fibers." The components of these three layers are blended together in a variety of ways, making it almost impossible to define to which layer they belong.

THE PRONATOFLEXOR AND SUPINATOEXTENSOR MASSES

In vertebrates, the muscles located on the flexor surface of the forearm are segregated in an anatomic system described by Humphry[4] and called the *pronatoflexor mass.* The extensor surface was segregated into a supinatoextensor mass.

The *pronatoflexor mass,* which is undifferentiated in its area of origin at the medial epicondyle of the humerus and the corresponding parts of the ulna and radius, divides distally into separate units and distinct sections. The degree of development and differentiation varies according to the zoologic group and is subordinated to the variable functions of the forearm and the hand; thus, in certain reptiles and amphibians in which the movements of the hand are not differentiated, the muscular mass is entirely undivided. In the higher vertebrates, the functions of the hand become more nearly perfect, the needs become more multiple, and the muscles that are to accomplish those movements become more divided and more individualized. In man, out of this pronatoflexor mass we find two common flexors completely separated: an individualized flexor for the thumb and also a separate pronator. The entire mass divides into two layers: a deep layer that forms the deep flexors and the pronator quadratus and a superficial layer that divides into distinct sectors, an ulnar sector that forms the flexor carpi ulnaris, a radial sector that forms the pronator teres and the flexor carpi radialis, and an intermediary sector that forms the flexor digitorum sublimis and the palmaris longus.

In the intermediate sector, the palmaris longus expands into the palmar fascia, where it blends with the fibers of the flexor carpi ulnaris (Fig. 29-1). The flexor digitorum sublimis is a more important muscle because it absorbs a great part of the flexor carpi ulnaris and of the palmaris longus, which has a tendency to disappear.

The elements of the carpometacarpals, the metacar-pophalangeals, and the phalangeals follow the quadrate pronator in uniting or retaining their union with the flexor profundus; however, advancing distally, they often separate and attach themselves to the sides of the phalanges, forming the lumbricals from their lateral parts and the retinacula from their middle parts. The phalangeal fibers are probably included in the latter but occasionally remain separate and often disappear. The lumbricals are found chiefly on the deep surface of the angles between the tendons of the flexor profundus. In the cases of the thumb and little finger, their elements remain in part or wholly on the metacarpals and form the short flexors. For this reason, the lumbricals are not usually present on the tendons of these digits, or only one is present, lying on the radial side of the tendon to the little finger. More rarely, there is one on the ulnar side of the tendon to the little finger. In some animals, the lumbricals pass from both sides of the several tendons of the flexor profundus to both sides of the fingers with one on the ulnar side of the flexor profundus to the thumb, and one on the radial side of the little finger, making eight lumbricals. In mammals, these are usually combined into four lumbricals.

To put it another way, the lumbricals and the retinacula may be regarded as parts of the common flexor mass, which instead of becoming segmented into metacarpophalangeals and phalangeals, retain their connection with the flexor tendons and are separated with them from the metacarpus and the carpus. However, they are not detached from the phalanges to which they pass accordingly from the flexor tendon.

Their connection with the extensor tendons in man and some mammals is a reminder of the blending of antagonistic muscles into a common sheath, which is one of the features of a primitive limb (Fig. 29-2).

The flexor profundus does not only absorb or retain annexed to it these various elements of the deep stratum of the pronator flexor mass, in most animals above the salamander, the flexor profundus also retains its connection with the terminal middle portion of each digital division of the superficial stratum or superficial flexor and passes on to the terminal phalanx, while the lateral portions of the superficial flexor tendons, by disconnecting themselves from the middle terminal portion, stop at a preceding phalanx. In this way, the deep flexor perforates the superficial flexor, which splits, allowing the flexor to pass.

Tendons of this type, passing along the digit, ordinarily divide into three parts when approaching a joint. Of these, the lateral parts are attached to the phalanx immediately on the distal side of the joint; the middle part runs to the next joint, where a similar process is repeated. This is best seen in the digits of birds and reptiles where there are more than two phalanges. It is also exemplified in the usual arrange-ment of the tendons of the superficial and deep flexors of the digits; these are considered as segments of one flexor prolongation on the digit.

This flexor prolongation first detaches the lumbricals to the first phalanx from its sides, then continues to run. In a similar manner, it detaches the slips of the flexor superficialis to the middle phalanx, repeats the same process according to the number of phalanges, and finally reaches the distal phalanx.

The *supinatoextensor mass* leads to the development of the extensor muscles of the forearm. The division of the

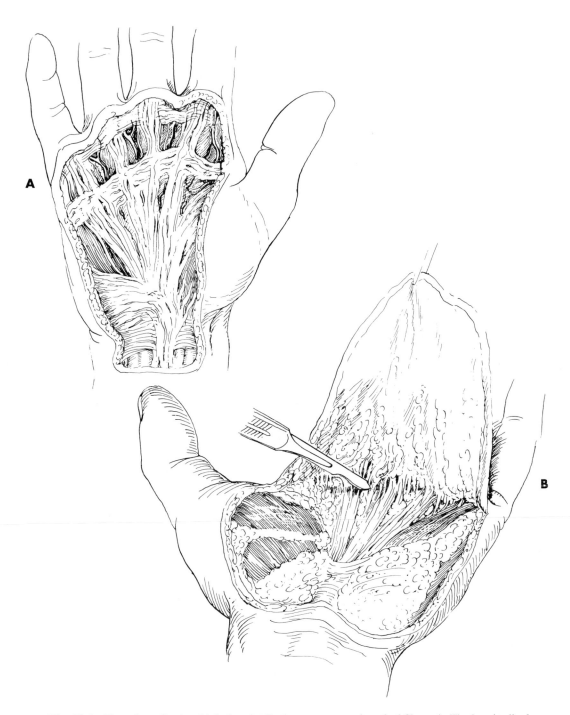

Fig. 29-1. The palmar fascia with its longitudinal, transverse, and vertical fibers. **A,** The longitudinal fibers originate in the palmaris longus (when present). Transverse fibers are concentrated in the distal palm supporting the web skin and in the midpalm are deep to the longitudinal fibers as the transverse palmar ligament. **B,** Vertical fibers extend superficially as multiple tiny tethering strands to stabilize the thick palmar skin. The deep vertical components concentrate in septa between the longitudinally oriented structures to the fingers. (From Chase RA: *Atlas of hand surgery,* Philadelphia, 1973, Saunders.)

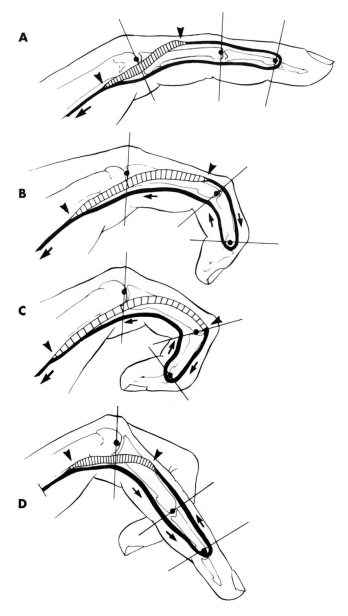

Fig. 29-2. The lumbrical muscle acts as a moderator band between the extensor and flexor mechanism in the finger. It has a moving origin from the profundus tendon and a moving insertion into the extensor mechanism through the lateral band. **A,** As the profundus tendon is pulled, the origin of the lumbrical moves proximal. **B,** Action of the profundus flexes the interphalangeal joints and moves the extensor mechanism distally, further separating the origin and insertion of the lumbrical. **C,** This becomes more exaggerated as the finger is pulled into flexion with the lumbrical relaxed. **D,** If the lumbrical muscle then contracts, its effect on the finger is to flex the metacarpophalangeal joint and extend the interphalangeal joints. This is the primary function of the lumbrical. (From Jupiter JB: *Flynn's hand surgery,* ed 4, Philadelphia, 1991, Williams & Wilkins.)

superficial stratum of this mass into three sectors (radial,middle, and ulnar) is more distinct than in the pronatoflexor masses. Because of the convexity of the elbow, they are more often cut off from the continuity of the muscles of the humerus than are the pronatoflexor masses.

Traced downward, the middle sector commonly extends on the digits forming the extensor digitorum communis. Sometimes, the radial sector reaches no farther than the lower end of the radius. In mammals, only a segment of it is inserted into the inner edge of the radius, constituting the brachioradialis. This may extend to the inner edge of the thumb or may spread over the palmar surface of the forearm. Other segments passing close to the carpus form the extensor carpi radialis; the ulnar sector (the extensor carpi ulnaris) is inserted into the other side of the metacarpus. The abductor digiti minimi is segmented from the lower end of this sector and represents a continuation of the extensor carpi ulnaris to the ulnar side of the hand. The abductor pollicis is a continuation of the more or less segmented radial section on the thumb. This shows that the three sectors of the superficial sheath of the supinatoextensor mass may be imperfectly segmented from the others, and each may be extended on the digits, or partly or wholly arrested at the more proximal points.

The deep layers of the supinatoextensor masses generally correspond to the deep pronatoflexor masses. The outer mass represents the supinator; lower down it forms the abductor pollicis longus. Still more distal, it runs in one or two portions on the pollex, forming the extensor pollicis brevis. Still more distal, it extends to the index or other fingers, forming an extensor profundus. It is evident that the muscles called extensors of the pollex, the index, and others are really derivatives of the extensor profundus. In the same way as the elements of the deep flexor stratum, the elements of the extensor stratum are usually continued further distally on the phalanges than are the elements of the superficial stratum.

In mammals, the greater part of the superficial stratum is inserted into the middle phalanx. The deeper stratum, arising from the radius and the ulna, and the still deeper stratum interossei are continued to the distal phalanges. When tendons of the superficial extensors are continued distally with prolongations of the deep stratum to the terminal phalanges, they are usually derived from the marginal parts of the digital tendons; the middle part of each tendon is inserted into the more proximal phalanx. When the tendons of the superficial extensor reach to the terminal phalanges without sagittal prolongations of the deep stratum, it is nevertheless the marginal parts of the tendon that reach the phalanges.

The disposition is reversed for the flexor tendons. The flexor tendons show that the deeper and more prolonged tendon occupies the middle position and continues its course distally to the terminal phalanx, while the superficial tendon

is inserted into one or usually both margins of a more proximal phalanx. When the superficial and deep flexors are fused into one and that one subdivides to supply the several phalanges, the middle part is usually more prolonged and never receives any marginal additions from the deeper stratum.

In higher animals in which the metacarpals admit little movement to and from one another, the interossei change their transverse direction to a course more parallel with the digits, and they extend on the phalanges and sometimes blend with the extensor tendon. In the simple limbs of some of the lower animals, the interossei are mere bands passing between the metacarpals, drawing the digits together, and antagonizing the abductors of the marginal digits.

The muscles that show differentiation of the pronatoflexor or supinatoextensor group of Humphry[4] may therefore show, in man, multiple variations, the significance of which can be grasped or interpreted from the viewpoint of the anatomist and especially the surgeon. How to interpret an additional muscle, whether to call it an atavistic reversal to the original, or whether to interpret an absent muscle as a developmental arrest is of little interest to the surgeon who must suspect what the additional or absent muscle represents anatomically and what function is connected with the structure.

The muscles that move the fingers are represented by two groups: the long extrinsic muscles originating in the forearm, and the short intrinsic muscles, originating in the hand.

Long extrinsic muscles

The long extrinsic muscles are located on the volar and the dorsal aspects of the forearm and the hand. The muscles originating from the volar surface of the forearm are flexors; the muscles originating from the dorsal aspect of the forearm are extensors.

Long flexors

The two long flexors are the flexor digitorum profundus and the flexor digitorum superficialis.

Flexor digitorum profundus

The *flexor digitorum profundus* originates in the forearm from the proximal two thirds of the volar and medial surfaces of the ulna, extending to an area just below the coronoid process of the ulna, near the fibers of insertion of the brachialis. The fibers of the flexor profundus extend toward the medial side of the ulna, where the muscle is in contact with the fibers of the supinator, situated more radially. On the medial side, more proximally, the muscle originates from the septum, which separates the flexor profundus from the flexor carpi ulnaris and occasionally from the radius, slightly distal to the bicipital tuberosity on the edge of the medial border of the radius. The origin also extends to the ulnar half of the interosseous membrane. The origin of the flexor profundus runs alongside the origin of the flexor pollicis longus, which

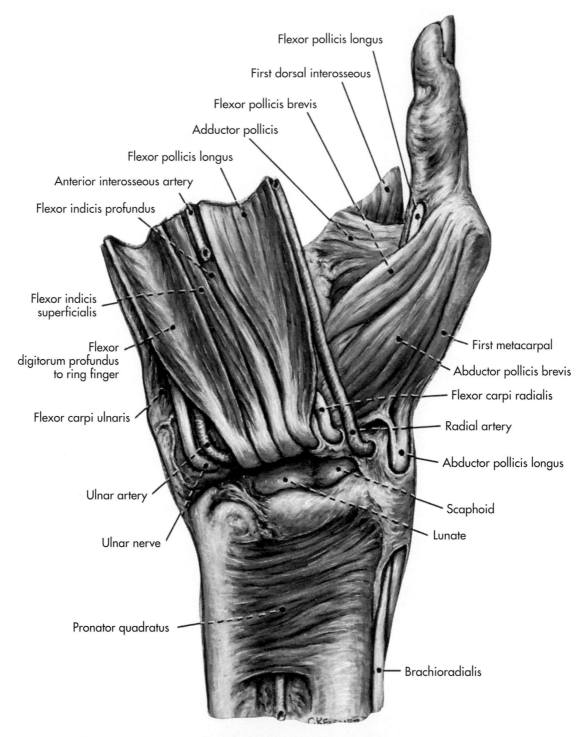

Fig. 29-3. The floor of the flexor tendon compartment of the right forearm and thumb. All the long flexors of the fingers were retracted distally to show the relation of the brachioradialis insertion, which actually forms a floor for the tunnel through which the tendons of the abductor pollicis longus and the extensor pollicis brevis pass. The additional insertion of the abductor pollicis longus into the abductor pollicis brevis is shown in this specimen. The retraction of the tendons exposes the radiocarpal joint.

is located on the radial side of the interosseous membrane, where both muscles contiguously descend almost to the origin of the pronator quadratus.

The muscular belly, which is formed by fibers running a straight distal course, finally divides into four muscular bundles in the distal third of the forearm. The most radial bundle is more widely separated and runs toward the index finger. The bundle to the little finger is sometimes separated from the bundles to the third and the fourth (middle and ring) fingers. A flattened tendon soon appears following each bundle. The fleshy fibers descend on the dorsal surface of these tendons much more distally than on the volar surface, reaching the proximal edge of the osteofibrous tunnel of the wrist (Fig. 29-3). The division between the tendon to the ring and little fingers sometimes occurs within the osteofibrous tunnel of the wrist. The relation of these tendons to the tendons of the superficialis through the wrist tunnel and in the palm of the hand will be described with the tendons of the flexor superficialis.

Flexor digitorum superficialis

The *flexor digitorum superficialis* is superficial to the flexor digitorum profundus (Fig. 29-4). It is a large, flat, fleshy muscle that originates in the forearm from the medial epicondyle of the humerus in common with the other epicondylar muscles. The fibers arise from the anterior and medial surfaces of the epicondyle, from the medial collateral ligament of the elbow, and from the medial aspect of the

coronoid process medial to the origin of the pronator teres and medial to the insertion of the tendon of the brachialis with which the flexor sublimis forms intimate connections. From here, the line of origin runs an oblique course along the oblique line of the radius—a line separating the radius into an anterosuperior supinator surface and an anterior-inferior surface for the flexor pollicis longus. The line is about 6 to 8 cm long, running from the bicipital tuberosity to the anterior border of the radius.

The origin of the flexor digitorum superficialis thus has two heads, one ulnar and the other radial with fibrous band stretching between the two heads. The median nerve and the ulnar artery pass under this band to continue their course over the more deeply situated flexor profundus muscle. Following the origin, a large, flat muscular belly descends distally, completely covering the flexor profundus muscle (see Fig. 29-3). The ulnar border is straight, and in the lowermost part of the forearm it deflects toward the radial side, thus uncovering the most ulnar part of the pronator quadratus. The radial border of the muscle is oblique toward the ulnar border of the forearm and leaves the lower half of the flexor pollicis longus muscle exposed.

Slightly distal to the middle of the forearm, the muscle belly is divided into four parts or bundles: two bundles are located more superficially and run toward the middle and the ring fingers; the other two bundles are situated deeper for the index and little fingers. The muscle fibers

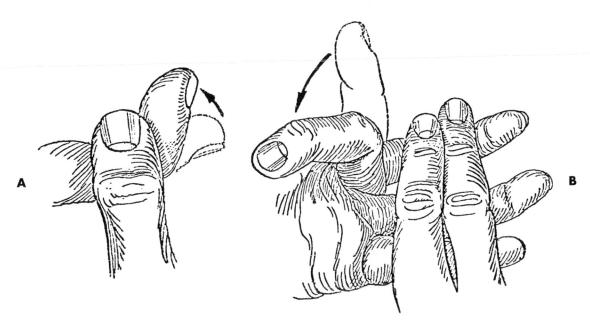

Fig. 29-4. A, The only flexor of the distal interphalangeal joint is flexor digitorum profundus. **B,** By checkreining the profundi, holding the fingers in extension, function of the superficialis muscle to the free finger may be tested. (From Chase RA: *Atlas of hand surgery,* vol 2, Philadelphia, 1984, Saunders.)

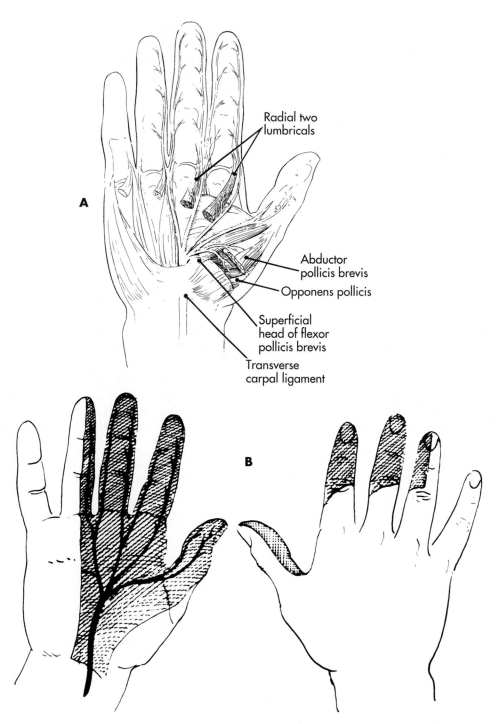

Fig. 29-5. A, The median nerve, the most superficial structure in the carpal tunnel, generally arborizes as it passes through the carpal tunnel into its terminal motor and sensory branches. The recurrent motor branches, which may actually pass through the flexor retinaculum rather than distal to it, generally innervate the two and one-half thenar muscles on the radial side of the long flexor to the thumb, the abductor pollicis brevis, the opponens pollicis, and the superficial head of the flexor pollicis brevis. In addition, there are motor branches to the two radial lumbricals from the nerve branches coursing toward the index and long fingers. **B,** Sensory branches course to the thumb, index, and long fingers and to the radial side of the ring finger. The median nerve classically lends sensibility to the palmar aspect and the distal dorsum of the thumb, index, and long fingers and the radial one-half of the ring finger. Intrinsic muscles radial to the flexor pollicis longus and the two radial lumbricals receive motor innervation from the median nerve. (From Chase RA: *Atlas of hand surgery,* vol 2, Philadelphia, 1984, Saunders.)

to the index finger are usually bipenniform. The fibers to the middle finger are unipenniform on the radial side of the tendon. The muscle fibers descend distally toward the transverse carpal ligament.

The special disposition of the fleshy fibers of the middle finger form an interesting relation to the median nerve (Fig. 29-5). The median nerve normally emerges on the radial side of the fleshy fibers of the middle finger, which cross the median nerve obliquely in a distal and ulnar direction (Fig. 29-6). This relation of the median nerve to the flexor superficialis in the distal part of the forearm may be compared with the relation of the median nerve in the proximal part of the forearm. The fibrous band of origin of the flexor superficialis crosses the median nerve in a distal and radial direction.

The tendons of the flexor superficialis reach the osteofibrous tunnel of the wrist together with the tendons of the flexor profundus. They enter the tunnel and usually retain a constant relation between themselves (Fig. 29-7). Enclosed in the synovial bursa in layers, the flexor superficialis to the middle finger—the strongest and most cylindrical—lies most superficially, alongside the flexor superficialis tendon of the ring finger, which is located on the ulnar side of the tendon superficialis to the middle finger. The tendon of the flexor superficialis to the little finger is most ulnar and at the wrist may be quite variable and can be absent or cordlike in appearance. There is always some connection to the little finger through the mesotendon system.

Variations should be noted clinically because a variety of flexion contractures of the little finger are related to shortening of the superficialis tendon system. Dissections show continuations of the synovial bursae into the palm and into the finger associated with long continuing vinculum in the finger (see Fig. 29-10). This complexity is at times correctible by tenotomy of the superficialis in the forearm or palm.

The tendon of the flexor superficialis to the index finger is found deeper and toward the tendon of the flexor superficialis of the middle finger. In the same horizontal plane with the flexor indicis superficialis, the four tendons of the flexor profundus are found. It must be mentioned that the flexor superficialis to the index finger has a tendency to shift completely under the tendon of the flexor superficialis of the middle finger; in this case, the tendon of the flexor profundus to the index finger lies immediately dorsal to the median nerve.

The tendons of the fingers. After the tendons emerge from the carpal tunnel into the palm of the hand, the superficialis and the profundus form a regular two-layer arrangement, with the superficialis occupying a superficial position and the profundus running deeper to the superficialis. The tendons diverge from the carpal tunnel radially toward the fingers. In passing in the proximal palm of the hand, the flexor profundus tendons give origin

to the lumbrical muscles. It must be noted that although the lumbrical muscles originate from the tendons of the flexor profundus, they cover the tendons of the flexor superficialis for more than half of the diameter of the superficialis tendon and sometimes conceal the superficialis completely.

Further distally, the tendons of the flexors enter the fibrous sheaths over the distal ends of the metacarpals just proximal to the metacarpophalangeal joints (Fig. 29-8). The two tendons still run in the same orders: the superficialis is the superficial and the profundus is the deep. After the tendons cross the metacarpophalangeal joint, their diameters and dispositions begin to change. The flexor profundus begins to penetrate into the flexor superficialis, which flattens out (Figs. 29-9 and 29-10). The perforation occurs through a considerable length of the superficialis tendon.

A longitudinal line appears in the middle of the tendon of the flexor superficialis at varying points in the vicinity of the metacarpophalangeal joint on the volar surface of the tendon. Approximately over the middle of the proximal phalanx, the longitudinal line over the volar surface of the tendons of the flexor sublimis becomes deeper and splits into two halves to let the tendon of the flexor profundus run through to the surface. Each half of the sublimis tendon first covers the corresponding half of the penetrating flexor profundus, then the superficialis turns around so that the anterior surface of each half becomes lateral in relation to the flexor profundus. Each half then runs posterior to the flexor profundus and emerges on the other side of the flexor profundus. In this passage, posterior to the flexor profundus, the halves cross each other. Each lateral half of the flexor sublimis, which changed from an anterior position to a lateral and then a posterior after crossing, lies in contact with the flexor profundus on its opposite side. Thus, one half of the flexor superficialis that before the penetration of the flexor profundus was, let us say for illustration, on the radial side of the flexor profundus will change its surface in contact with the profundus tendon to a posterior and then an ulnar position, producing a complete twist.

Only about half of the fibers of each half of the superficialis tendon cross posteriorly to the flexor profundus; the other half continue on the same side of the tendon and insert into the lateral crest of the volar surface of the middle phalanx where they unite intimately with the crossed fibers of the other side as far distal as the neck of the proximal phalanx. Over the proximal phalanx the posterior crossing of the superficialis tendon forms a plate that can be separated from the periosteum of the phalanx and lifted up until stopped by the insertion of the ends of the superficialis tendon into the volar crests of the middle phalanx (Figs. 29-9 to 29-11).

The opening of the superficialis tendon serves as a tunnel for the passage of the flexor profundus tendon on its
Text continued on p. 252.

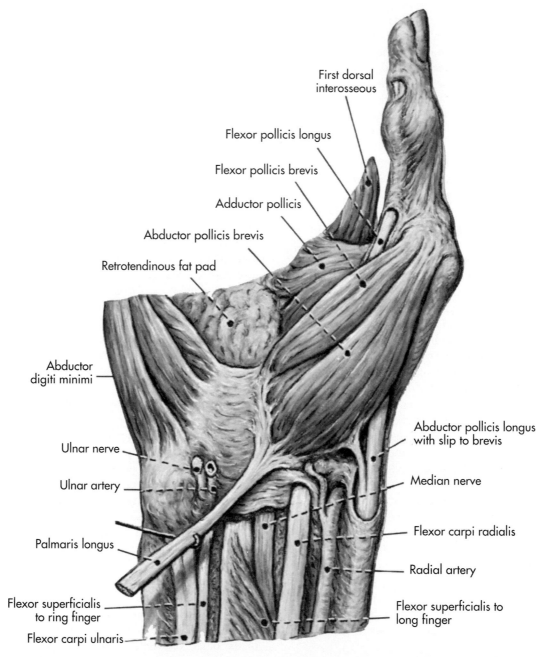

First dorsal
interosseous

Flexor pollicis longus

Flexor pollicis brevis

Adductor pollicis

Abductor pollicis brevis

Retrotendinous fat pad

Abductor
digiti minimi

Ulnar nerve

Ulnar artery

Palmaris longus

Flexor superficialis
to ring finger

Flexor carpi ulnaris

Abductor pollicis longus
with slip to brevis

Median nerve

Flexor carpi radialis

Radial artery

Flexor superficialis to
long finger

Fig. 29-6. Flexor tendons of the distal right forearm and thumb. The palmaris longus is partially inserted into the abductor pollicis brevis. The flexor carpi ulnaris is continuous through the pisiform with the abductor digiti minimi, and the fat pad of the midpalmar space is seen ulnar to the abductor pollicis.

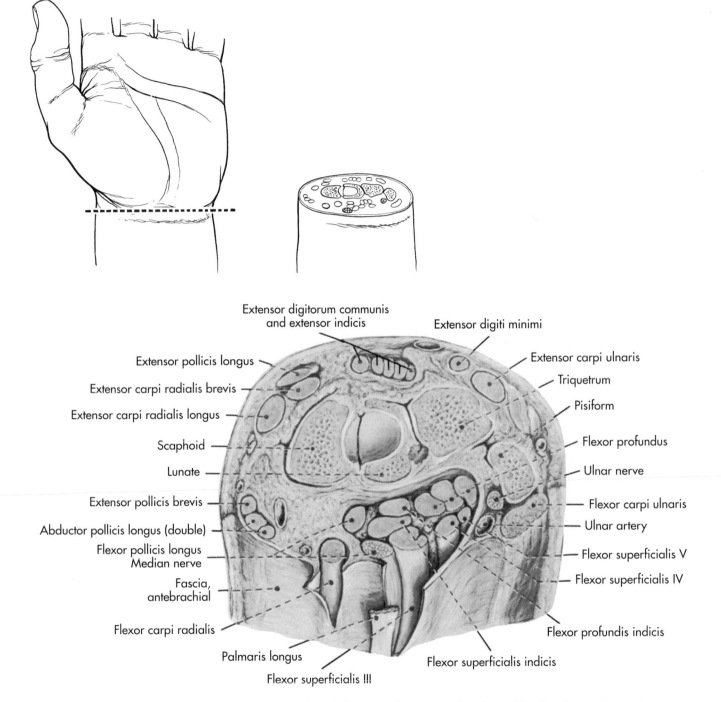

Fig. 29-7. Transverse section through the left wrist to demonstrate the relationship of tendons and bones at the wrist joint. The proximal segment was dissected, the volar skin was removed, and the palmaris longus tendon was freed from its sheath. The antebrachial fascia that encloses the median nerve and the flexor tendons and the proximal part of the carpal tunnel was opened longitudinally. The separate tunnel for the flexor carpi radialis was partially opened. Separate from the carpal tunnel, between the flexor carpi ulnaris and the transverse carpal ligament, a separate tunnel for the ulnar artery and nerve is found. It is known in the French nomenclature as the *tunnel of Guyon.*

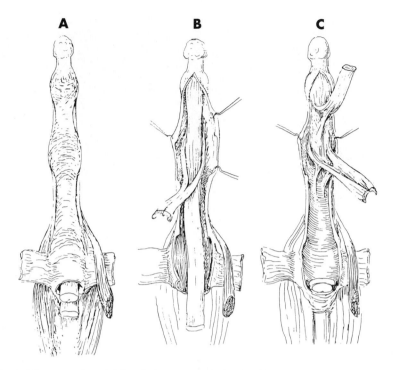

Fig. 29-8. A, Flexor tendons in the digit are surrounded by fibrous and synovial sheaths. **B,** The superficialis tendons split to allow the passage of the profundus tendon between its two tails to insert on the distal phalanx. **C,** The superficialis decussates behind the profundus tendon before inserting on the middle phalanx. (From Chase RA: *Atlas of hand surgery,* Philadelphia, 1973, Saunders.)

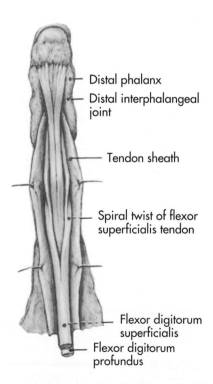

- Distal phalanx
- Distal interphalangeal joint

- Tendon sheath

- Spiral twist of flexor superficialis tendon

- Flexor digitorum superficialis
- Flexor digitorum profundus

Fig. 29-9. The flexor tendon tunnel is opened to show the flexor superficialis and the flexor profundus tendons in situ. Note division of the flexor profundus into two flat tendons as it crosses the distal interphalangeal volar plate to insert on the distal phalanx. Perforation of the flexor superficialis and the twist of the lateral slips of insertion of the superficialis are demonstrated.

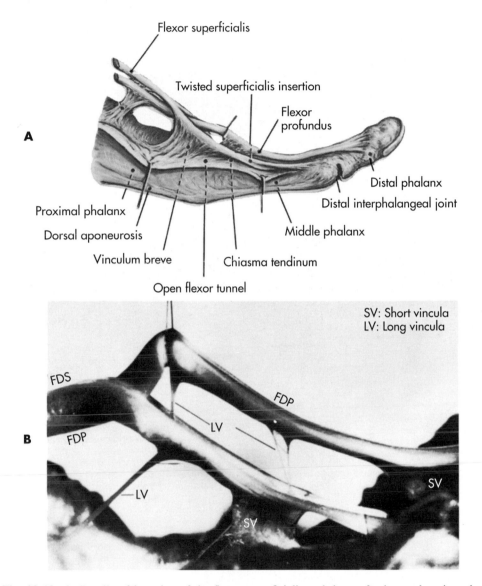

Fig. 29-10. A, Details of insertion of the flexor superficialis and the profundus tendons into the phalanges of a finger. The flexor tendon tunnel is completely open. The joint line of the distal interphalangeal joint is indicated. The perforation of the flexor superficialis by the profundus over the proximal phalanx lets the tendon of the flexor profundus pass through. The twist of the slips of the insertion of the flexor superficialis is indicated. The vincula tendinum are firmly connected with the bifurcation of the flexor superficialis at the floor of the tunnel. Another vinculum connects the flexor profundus with the floor. The insertion of the tendon of the flexor profundus into the distal phalanx occurs not only into the volar base but extends beyond the base and into the fat pad of the distal phalanx. **B,** The lateral view of the flexor digitorum profundus and the flexor digitorum superficialis. The typical anatomy of the long and short vincula is seen.

Continued.

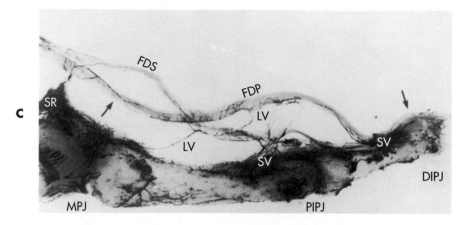

Fig. 29-10, cont'd. C, Vascular supply to vinculum and tendon. Injection-prepared specimen (Matsui). Arrows show crossover zones of the intrinsic blood of the flexor digitorum profundus.

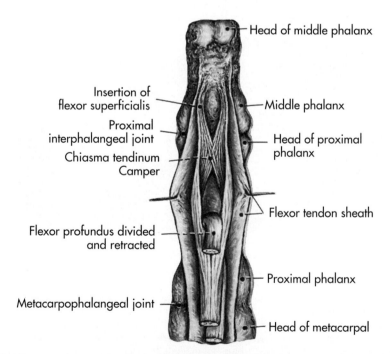

Fig. 29-11. Flexor apparatus of a finger. The distal phalanx is removed, together with the distal part of the flexor profundus. The proximal part of the flexor profundus is retracted proximally. The perforation of the flexor superficialis tendon by the tendon of the flexor profundus occurs over the volar surface of the proximal phalanx. The two lateral slips of the flexor sublimis tendon rotate completely. Part of those fibers cross to the other side of the phalanx and continue into the middle phalanx where they insert into the lateral volar crest of the middle phalanx. The other part of the rotated slip continues on the same side and inserts on the corresponding side of the phalanx into the crest of the middle phalanx. The intersection of fibers, which is similar to the intersection of the neurofibers of the chiasma opticum of the second cranial nerve, is called the *chiasma tendinum of Camper.* The chiasma tendinum forms a plate underneath the flexor profundus and can be lifted off the periosteum and the capsule of the proximal interphalangeal joint. The distal ends of the slips of the flexor superficialis usually stop a few millimeters proximal to the neck of the middle phalanx.

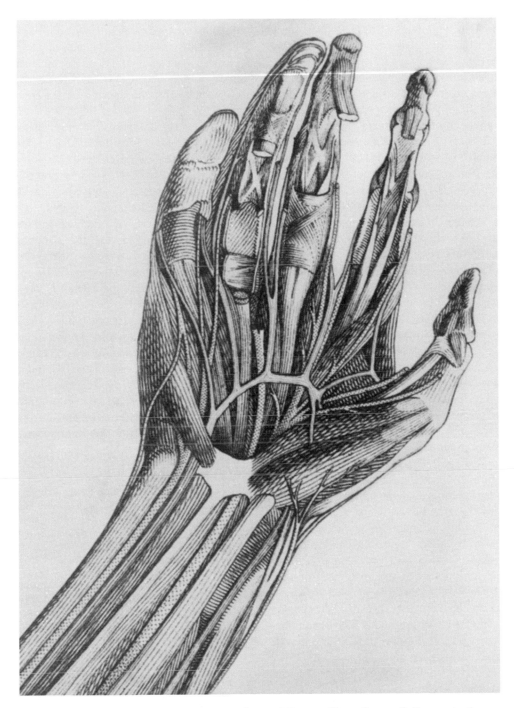

Fig. 29-12. Demonstration of the chiasma tendinum of Camper. (From Camper P: Demonstrationum Anatomico-Pathologicarum Liber Primus: Continens Brachii Humani Fabricam et Morbos, 1760, Amstelaedami.)

proximal half over the proximal phalanx. The distal half of the opening is narrowed by the passage of a constant mesotendon from the floor of the flexor tendons sheath, or rather periosteum, to the tendon of the flexor profundus. Vincula tendinum firmly connect the slips of the bifurcation of the flexor superficialis with the floor of the tunnel. Some of these vincula are slender and long; some of them are very much broader (see Fig. 29-10).

The chiasma tendinum of camper. The fibers of the flexor superficialis, which are noted distal to the perforation, form a pattern so similar to the chiasma opticum that it was called *chiasma tendinum* by Peter Camper,[2] who described it and illustrated it in his *Demonstrationum Anatomico-Pathologicarum,* published in 1760 (Fig. 29-12). It is curious to note that a similar and very beautiful illustration of the chiasma was given by Bernard Siegfried Albinus[1] in his *Historia, Musculorum Hominis* in 1774, but this intersection was not called chiasma tendinum. Camper was probably the first to call it chiasma tendinum, but he refers to the description of this structure by Albinus. Albinus gives the following names to the different parts of this apparatus:

Tendo sublimis truncatus, for the undivided sublimis tendon
Caudae duae, in quas sublimis tendo se findit, for the diversion of the tendon in two parts
Pars quam emittunt, quaque cohaerent inter se, the underlying decussation under the tendon profundus
Extrema Caudarum ultra partem illam, qua cohaerent unter se, the distal end of the decussation
Pars illa qua adjacentem tendineum Profundi contidunt, the adjacent lateral divisions of the sublimis in contact with the tendon of the profundus
Ultuma caudarum extrema, inserta ossi secunda, the insertion of the sublimis into the middle phalanx

The division of the sublimis tendon into these component parts is seldom described and may be of importance in helping to overcome failures in tendon surgery in the regions of the finger also so aptly called "no man's land." Albinus' nomenclature is quoted to show how precise and detailed were the anatomic descriptions of the anatomists of this period.

Considerable independent motion is possible between the flexor superficialis and the flexor profundus. The perforation of the superficialis serves the purpose of a most efficient pulley. The vincula normally permit sufficient motion; however, the vincula may restrict motion even in the absence of adhesions between the tendons of the superficialis and profundus, especially if fibrosis occurs in the vincula between the distal part of the perforation and the profundus tendon.

After emerging from the sublimis tendon, the distal end of the profundus tendon spreads out over the distal interphalangeal joint, occupying a wide line over the area of insertion into the distal phalanx. Frequently, the tendon is divided into two divergent bands with a longitudinal separation between them. The division of the flexor profundus tendon frequently begins just distal to the passage of the tendon through the perforation in the sublimis and is maintained until insertion takes place into the distal phalanx. The area of insertion does not stop at the base itself, but extends more distally for about one third of the phalangeal height. The tendon is intimately connected with the capsule of the distal interphalangeal joint.

It may be of interest to note that exactly the same disposition of the flexor profundus tendons was observed in the hands of the gorilla and the chimpanzee, which the author had occasion to dissect. The insertion of the profundus, the chiasma tendinum, and the splitting of the superficialis tendon were exactly similar.

The comparison of the human hand with the skeletons of hands of the gorilla and the chimpanzee shows great similarity in the configuration of the phalanges. The other bones show differences that cannot be considered too great. The general pattern of these hands is amazingly similar. The difference can be detected mostly in the enormous size of the pisiform bone, which is much more elongated and massive than is the human pisiform. The configurations of the navicular bones are somewhat different; however, the triquetral bones of the gorilla and the human are very similar. It is obvious that similar bones are usually connected with a similarity of muscles that take origin from these bones. That fact is observed in the arrangement and in the variation of the muscles with some eliminated and some added, as seen in the human hand.

REFERENCES

1. Albinus BS: Historia musculorum hominis, 1724, Leidae Batavorum, pp. 479, 639, and others. *Excellent descriptive anatomy of the muscular system with important considerations on muscular physiology, with exquisite illustrations and line drawings of the muscles of the hand. Ilustrated by Jan Wandelaer. Albinus understood the action of the intrinsic muscles of the hand. He described first the scalenus minimus, now rightfully called the muscle of Albinus.*
2. Camper P: Demonstrationum anatomico-pathologicarum liber primus: continens brachii humani fabricum et morbos, 1760, Amstelaedami, pp. 4, 19, Tab. 1, Fig. II. *Excellent atlas of anatomic drawings with precise anatomic descriptions. Not mentioned frequently. Detailed description of the insertion of the flexor superficialis tendon is given with credit to Albinus. For the first time, this insertion is called Chiasma Tendinum. This is not generally known.*
3. Haines RW: The flexor muscles of the forearm and hand in lizards and mammals, *J Anat* 1950; 84:13.
4. Humphry GM: *Observations in myology,* Cambridge, London, 1872, Macmillan. *Remarkable collection of observations of great interest and importance on the significance of muscular variations.*
5. LeDouble AF: *Traité des variations du système musculaire de l'homme et de leur signification au point de vue de l'anthropologie zoologique,* Paris, 1897, Schleicher Frères. *Most complete and valuable contribution on the variations of muscles of the human body with*

excellent comparative anatomic and bibliographic notes on the subject.

6. Straus WL: The homologies of the forearm flexors: urodeles, lizards, mammals, *Am J Anat* 1942; 70:281.

7. Testut L: *Les anomalies musculaires chez l'homme expliquée par l'anatomie comparée: leur importance en anthropologie,* Paris, 1884,

Masson. *Thorough, extensive study of the subject. Source of valuable information based on personal extensive investigations and specialized literature.*

8. Testut L, Latarget A: *Traité d'anatomie humaine,* ed 8, vol 1, Paris, 1928, Doin. *A monumental, thorough, informative, complete anatomy, probably unsurpassed in any language.*

Chapter 30

DYNAMICS OF THE FLEXOR TENDON PULLEY SYSTEM

James R. Doyle

Most tendons about the flexor side of the wrist and hand that span two or more joints are restrained by retinacular structures called, by common usage, pulleys. Pulleys maintain the flexor tendons close to the joint axis and prevent bowstringing, thus promoting efficiency and economy in wrist and finger flexion. This unique system functions under multiple constraints and requirements, including a 260° arc of motion in the fingers; incremental forces of many kilograms; and complex nutritional, circulatory, diffusion, and lubrication factors.

The system is composed of the transverse carpal ligament, the palmar aponeurosis pulley, and the digital flexor pulley system. These three components represent a unique and complex biomechanical system that provides for complete wrist and digital flexion without limiting extension. Of these three systems, the digital component is the most critical to finger flexion and must be preserved or reconstructed if satisfactory finger function is to be preserved.

These three systems maintain a constant relationship (moment arm) between the flexor tendons and the joint axis, and thereby provide for maximum joint movement within the constraints of muscle-tendon excursion. Because excursion is not a limitless factor and is directly proportional to muscle fiber length, the effectiveness of tendon excursion is dependent on maintenance of the critical relationship between the pulleys and their respective joint axes. An absent pulley results in an increased moment arm and requires increased tendon excursion to produce the same arc of motion. Because excursion is not a limitless resource, joint motion is decreased when the moment arm is increased. Even a slight increase in the moment arm

can be associated with tendon bowstringing, loss of digital flexion, or even a fixed flexion contracture. This fixed flexion contracture is caused by the contractile nature of the scar tissue which builds up along the palmar aspect of the joint. When bowstringing occurs, the angle of attack of the flexor tendon is increased, which causes greater forces on the pulleys and can lead to pulley elongation and additional bowstringing.

ANATOMIC FEATURES OF THE PULLEY SYSTEMS
Transverse carpal ligament

Kline and Moore in 1992 proposed that the transverse carpal ligament (TCL) was an important component of the digital finger flexor pulley system.[16] This broad and substantial ligament, which spans the volar side of the carpus, was sectioned in fresh-frozen cadavers and the authors noted a 25% increase in the required excursion for the profundus and a 20% increase in excursion for the superficialis. They noted that the increased excursion that was consumed after release of the transverse carpal ligament resulted in less remaining excursion for flexion of the other joints and might contribute to weakness of grip noted after carpal tunnel release. They concluded that the main purpose of the TCL was to act as a flexor pulley at the wrist. It is important to note, however, that the significant increase in flexor tendon excursion was demonstrated *only* when the wrist was in the flexed position. This could result in decreased grip strength when the wrist was flexed, although most power gripping is done with the wrist in extension. This study further serves to point out the importance of knowing the status of all three components of the system before

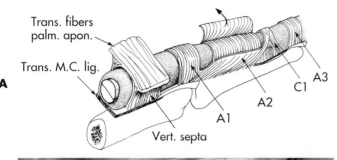

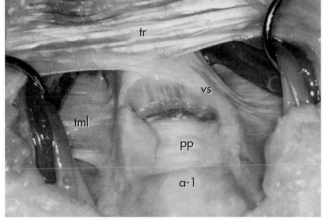

Fig. 30-1 A, Composite view of the palmar aponeurosis (PA) pulley showing its relationship to the annular pulleys and its component parts, including the transverse fibers of the PA, the transverse metacarpal ligament, and the vertical septa that span these two structures. **B,** Cadaver dissection of the PA pulley showing the transverse *(tr)* fibers of the palmar aponeurosis, the vertical septa *(vs),* transverse metacarpal ligament *(tml),* palmar plate *(pp),* and the first annular pulley *(a-1).* Note the cut ends of the flexor tendons at the distal edge of the PA pulley and the lumbrical muscles retracted on each side.

performing flexor tendon surgery throughout the system, including the wrist, palm, and finger.

Palmar aponeurosis pulley

In 1983 Manske and Lesker described the palmar aponeurosis (PA) pulley.[22] It is formed by the transverse fibers of the PA that are anchored on each side of the synovial sheath by vertical fibers or intertendinous septa, which attach to the deep transverse metacarpal ligament and thus form an archway over the flexor tendons (Fig. 30-1, *A* and *B*). Its average width is 9.3 mm, and its proximal edge begins 1 to 3 mm distal to the beginning of the membranous sheath.[10] Although it is not as closely applied to the flexor tendons as the digital pulleys, closer approximation may occur with increased tension on the palmar aponeurosis as in grasping. This proximal tension may be provided by either the palmaris longus, or the flexor carpi ulnaris, or both.[10]

Manske and Lesker established the functional significance of this structure as a pulley by noting a significant preservation of total range of finger motion if the palmar

aponeurosis (PA) pulley was intact in conjunction with section of the critical first and second annular (A₁, A₂) pulleys. Baseline total range of motion (TROM) was determined for each finger in 12 cadaver hands, and the PA, first annular (A₁), and second annular (A₂) pulleys were sequentially cut in various orders. The results of these studies indicated that functional loss associated with absence of any *one* of the three proximal pulleys is minimal. The loss of flexion associated with the absence of the A₁ or A₂ pulley is insignificant as long as the PA pulley is present. The loss of flexion increases if the absence of the A₁ or A₂ pulley is combined with absence of the PA pulley. The authors concluded that as a single functioning pulley, the A₂ pulley was the most important followed closely by the A₁ pulley. They noted that although the position of the PA pulley was the least critical of the three, its importance as a pulley was evident in the increased loss of flexion from 5.7% when it alone was present, to 12.6% when all three (PA, A₁, and A₂) pulleys were cut.

Digital flexor sheath

The digital flexor tendon sheath is composed of synovial and retinacular tissue components, which have separate and distinct functions. The *membranous* portion is a synovial tube sealed at both ends. The *retinacular* (pulley) portion is a series of transverse, annular, and cruciform fibrous tissue condensations, which begin in the distal palm and end at the distal interphalangeal (DIP) joint (Fig. 30-2). The floor or dorsal aspect of this tunnel is composed of the deep transverse metacarpal ligament, the palmar plates of the metacarpophalangeal joint (MP), the proximal interphalangeal joint (PIP), the DIP joint, and the palmar surfaces of the proximal and middle phalanges. In the index, long, and ring fingers, the membranous portion of the sheath begins at the neck of the metacarpals and continues distally to end at the DIP joint. In most instances the small finger synovial sheath continues proximally to the wrist; this is consistent with the findings of others.[11,24,25] Visceral and parietal synovial layers were identified, which agree with recent and earlier studies.[7,8,11,26,29] A prominent synovial pouch is noted proximally and represents the confluence of the visceral and parietal layers. A visceral layer reflection or pouch is also noted between the two flexors at the neck of the metacarpal, but is 4 to 5 mm distal to the more visible proximal and external portions of the synovial sheath (Fig. 30-3). The membranous or synovial portions of the sheath are most noticeable in the spaces between the pulleys, where they form plicae and pouches to accommodate flexion and extension (Fig. 30-4).

The *retinacular* (pulley) portion of the sheath is characterized by fibrous tissue bands of annular and cruciform configuration that are interposed along the synovial sheath in a segmental fashion and maintain the flexor tendons in a constant relationship to the joint axis of motion. The

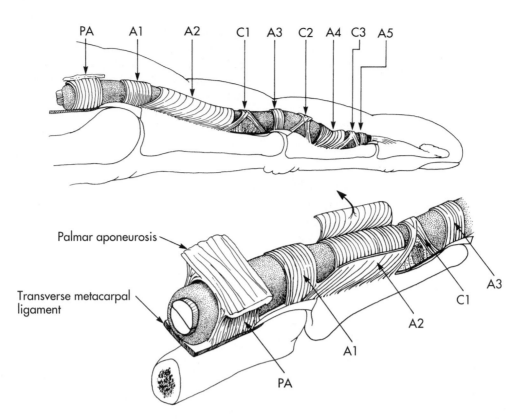

Fig. 30-2. Artist's depiction of the membranous and retinacular portions of the sheath including the palmar aponeurosis (PA) pulley, and the five annular and three cruciform pulleys.

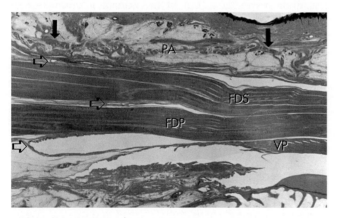

Fig. 30-3. Sagittal section of the middle finger just proximal to the metacarpophalangeal (MP) joint. The solid vertical arrows point to the proximal and distal edges of the transverse fibers of the palmar aponeurosis (PA). Note the visceral and parietal synovial layers marked by horizontal arrows which form a proximal pouch (seen palmar and dorsal to the flexor tendons—FDS, FDP).VP is the volar or palmar plate.

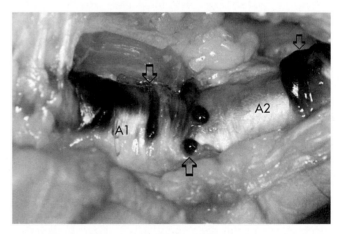

Fig. 30-4. Note the membranous (synovial) portions of the sheath *(vertical arrows)* which bulge out between the annular and cruciform retinacular components to allow motion without impingement as the metacarpophalangeal joint is flexed. *A1* is the first annular pulley, *A2* is the second annular pulley.

cruciform fibers are sometimes single oblique limbs or Y shaped.

Five annular and three cruciform pulleys have been identified (see Fig. 30-2). The first of the five annular pulleys begins in the region of the palmar plate of the MP joint. The majority of fibers (about two thirds) arise from the palmar

plate; the remainder arise from the proximal portion of the proximal phalanx (see Fig. 30-2). Although the most usual configuration of the A_1 pulley is that of a single annular pulley, which averages 7.9 mm in width, it is sometimes represented by two or three annular bands. A distinct separation between the A_1 and A_2 pulleys is the usual configuration. This separation ranges from 0.4 to 4.1 mm and is widest on the palmar aspect. In those cases that do not have a distinct separation between A_1 and A_2 pulleys, there may be a pronounced thinness to the retinacular tissue for a distance of several millimeters at the usual site of separation or large triangular-shaped openings laterally. This allows for flexion at the MP joint without any buckling of the pulley complex, and thus the potential for impingement of the tendon is avoided (see Fig. 30-4).

In contrast to the variability in configurations of the A_1 pulley, the proximal edge of the second annular pulley is constant in shape, with oblique fibers of origin beginning at the proximal and lateral base of the proximal phalanx, which join annular fibers to make a prominent and thick leading edge (see Fig. 30-2). Synovial outpouching is common in the spaces between the pulleys (see Fig. 30-4). The A_2 pulley is 16.8 mm in average width and is thickest in the distal end. The deeper annular fibers of the A_2 pulley are overlaid with oblique fibers, which at the distal end interdigitate to form the first cruciform pulley (see Fig. 30-2).

The third annular pulley (A_3) is located at the PIP joint and attaches to the palmar plate. The A_3 pulley is present in the majority of cases, and the average width is 2.8 mm (see Fig. 30-2).

The fourth annular pulley (A_4) is located in the mid portion of the middle phalanx and is overlaid with oblique fibers that form a cruciform pulley, C_3, at the distal end. The A_4 pulley is 6.7 mm in average length and thickest in its mid aspect (see Fig. 30-2).

The fifth annular pulley (A_5) is quite thin, 4.1 mm in average length, and it is attached to the underlying palmar plate at the DIP joint. The membranous synovial sheath ends at the level of the DIP joint, and no pulleys are present beyond the distal joint.

There are three cruciform pulleys in the finger. Their locations are the distal ends of the A_2 and A_4 pulleys and in the space between the A_3 and A_4 pulleys. Variation in their shape is common—some are represented by a single oblique limb and some are Y shaped (ypsiloform). The third cruciform pulley at the distal end of the A_4 pulley is formed by prominent extensions of oblique fibers overlying the A_4 pulley and is not always a separate structure.

Significant flexion in the finger is achieved without buckling of the retinacular system or impingement of the underlying tendon(s) because (1) the broader pulleys, A_2 and A_4, are located between joints, whereas the more narrow pulleys, A_1 and A_3, are over the joints; (2) the pulleys are arranged in a segmental fashion with synovial pouches and windows between them; (3) the thinner and narrower cruciform pulleys are located near joints, where they can more easily accommodate to the confined space in acute flexion (see Figs. 30-2 and 30-4). The functional adaptation of the retinacular system to the requirements of flexion is also apparent in the region of the MP joint, where some anatomic accommodation is always present between A_1 and A_2, either in the form of definite separation between A_1 and

A_2, thinning of the contiguous margins of A_1 and A_2, or triangular-shaped openings in the lateral margins of the retinaculum so that flexion can occur without buckling (see Fig. 30-4). Furthermore, compressibility of the various pulleys has been reported and may also be a factor in accommodating joint motion without buckling and impingement.[2]

Special features of the flexor sheath

Bunnell noted that a tendon sheath was an adaptation that allowed a tendon to turn a corner. He stated, "It glides around a curve on a thin film of synovial fluid between two smooth synovial-lined surfaces, just as metal surfaces in machinery glide on a thin film of oil." [7] Bunnell further noted that a tendon sheath had two layers of synovia, a visceral one investing the tendon, and a parietal layer lining the fascial (retinacular) tunnel through which the tendon glided. Lundborg and Myrhage noted a well-vascularized membrane with plicae and pouches at the margin of the pulleys that were important for flexion and stretching of the sheath.[20] They were not able to demonstrate any continuity of the synovial cell layer on the friction surface of the A_2 pulley, but they did note chondrocyte-like cells in the superficial layers of this pulley. Knott and Schmidt also observed cartilage-like tissue at the distal end of the A_2 pulley.[17] In certain avascular areas of the palmar portion of the tendons, visceral synovial tissues were absent on histologic sections. Furthermore, in some scattered areas of the palmar surface of the tendon there were areas with cartilaginous differentiation similar to the findings in the A_2 pulley. Lundborg and Myrhage concluded that the friction surface of the pulleys is devoid of vessels and that the friction and gliding in the digital sheath system takes place between two avascular structures, namely, the palmar aspect of the flexor tendons and the inner aspect of the pulleys.[20] These avascular gliding surfaces are nourished by diffusion from the synovial fluid. Histologic studies by Lundborg and Myrhage demonstrated that the vascular plexus of the synovial sheath is in continuity on the *outside* of the rigid pulleys, and by this arrangement the pulleys can meet the mechanical forces associated with finger flexion while the synovial membrane avoids vascular compression and thus the microcirculation is not compromised.[20] The well-vascularized synovial elements of the sheath represent a dialysing membrane that produces a plasma filtrate, the synovial fluid, which acts as a lubricating agent and also as a nutritional agent for the relatively avascular retinacular system and tendon.[20]

The findings of Lundborg and Myrhage are appropriately compared with the findings of Cohen and Kaplan, who in a study of the gross, microscopic, and ultrastructure (electron microscopy) of the flexor tendon sheath, noted that the sheath consists of a *noninterrupted* layer of parietal synovium reinforced externally at intervals by dense bands of collagen (the retinacular system).[8] Cohen and Kaplan further noted that the contents of the sheath were independently covered by a second similar layer of visceral synovium, and that the two layers were continuous at the proximal cul-de-sac, the vincula origins, and the tendon insertions.[8] The synovial cells lining the pulley and covering the tendons were quantitatively, but not morphologically, different from the synovial cells of the membranous (synovial) portion of the sheath. The thickness of the synovial layers was greatest at the spaces between the pulleys and thin or attenuated beneath the annular pulleys and on tendon surfaces distant from vincula and cul-de-sacs.[8]

Additional nutritional pathways were noted by Weber, who identified nonvascular channels in the flexor tendons of dogs and chickens.[27] These channels were mainly on the palmar surface, which is the least vascular. The channels appeared to be associated with nonparallel collagen fibers. Body fluid, marked by fluorescein dye was observed to penetrate the tendon in its least vascular area. Motion of the flexor tendon augmented dye penetration into the central portion of the tendon. Weber concluded that his findings supported the concept that synovial fluid nourished the flexor tendons within the digital theca.[27]

Amis and Jones focused on the interior of the flexor tendon sheath and noted that the inner aspect of the sheath was not a continuous smooth surface.[1] They noted that the thin (membranous) parts of the sheath did not attach directly to the proximal and distal borders of the pulleys in continuity, but often overlapped the superficial edges of the pulleys. Thus, on the inner aspect of the sheath, the pulleys often stood apart of their surroundings with free edges pointing both proximally and distally. The significance of these observations is that these free pulley edges may be sites for impingement or triggering of a partially cut tendon, a bulky or irregular tendon suture site, or a prominent suture knot.[1] Although the fibrous portions of the sheath become contiguous near the end of the flexion arc, it is obvious that impingement may possibly occur about any free pulley edge during the act of flexion. This anatomic finding is most noticeable about the distal end of the second annular pulley and the proximal end of the first annular pulley (Fig. 30-5, A and B).

BIOMECHANICAL PRINCIPLES

To understand this system more fully certain biomechanical principles need to be discussed including the following:
1. Muscle-tendon excursion
2. The joint motion concept called *moment arm*
3. The geometric concept of the radian
4. The concept of work of flexion
5. Lubrication factors

Excursion

Excursion of muscle is the sum of the length the muscle can be stretched from its resting length plus the length it can

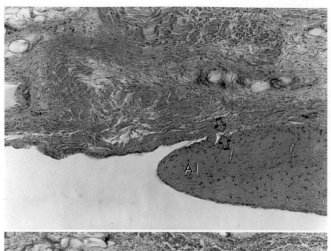

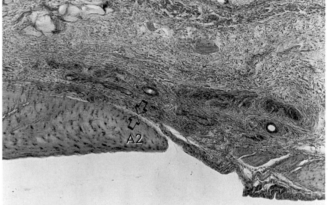

Fig. 30-5. A, Note the prominent proximal edge of the first annular *(A1)* pulley and the fact that the pulley edge stands apart of the synovial sheath which attaches well beyond its leading edge *(opposing arrows)*. **B,** Note a similar arrangement at the distal end of annular two *(A2)*. These findings illustrate the fact that the synovial membrane attaches to the *outside* of the pulley at some distance from its free edge, which could result in catching or impingement of a partial tendon laceration or bulky tendon repair. Note also the blood vessels in the sheath external to the synovial membrane.

contract from its resting state (Fig. 30-6). Muscle fibers are known to shorten by about 40% during active contraction (active excursion), and they can be passively lengthened by about 40%. Excursion is directly proportional to muscle fiber length[12] and therefore is not a limitless factor. The importance of this will be illustrated later when the relationship between excursion and moment arm is discussed. Brand has further defined excursion as potential, required, and available excursion.[5]

Potential excursion is characterized by the muscle resting fiber length without reference to the state of the connective tissue restraints. Because a muscle is never required to lengthen or shorten through a larger excursion than it takes to move the joints that it crosses through their full passive range, Brand has proposed that the term *required excursion*

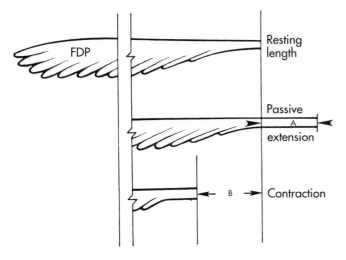

Fig. 30-6. Muscle excursion is the sum of the length that a muscle can be stretched from its resting length plus the length it can contract from its resting state. In this diagram passive extension *(A)* plus active contraction *(B)* equals excursion. Muscle fibers are known to shorten by about 40% with contraction and can be passively lengthened by about the same amount. FDP is the flexor digitorum profundus. (From Doyle JR: Dynamics of the flexor tendon pulley system. In Hunter JM, Schneider LH, Mackin EJ, eds: *Tendon surgery in the hand,* St Louis, 1987, Mosby.)

Table 30-1. Mean fiber length of the various finger flexors

Flexor	Length (cm)
Flexor digitorum profundus	
Index	6.6
Middle	6.6
Ring	6.8
Little	6.2
Flexor digitorum superficialis	
Index	7.2
Middle	7.0
Ring	7.3
Little	7.0

Data from Brand PW, Beach RB, Thompson DE: Relative excursion and potential excursion of muscles in the forearm and hand, *J Hand Surg* 1981; 6:209.

be used to define the maximum excursion that might be required of a muscle in situ. *Available excursion* (a term used by Freehafer, et al.)[13] is a measure of the maximum excursion a muscle can produce when it has been freed from its insertion. Practically speaking, the amount of available excursion is often about the same as the required excursion, but available excursion is responsive to the pattern of usage. Available excursion, according to Brand, is probably a measure of the limitation imposed by surrounding connective tissue, paratenon, paramysium, and intramuscular collagen.[5] This excursion may be increased by exercise or stretching,

Table 30-2. Flexor tendon excursions (wrist neutral)

Tendon	Mean (mm)	Range (mm)
Superficialis	24	14-37
Profundus	32	15-43

Data from Wehbé M, Hunter JM: Flexor tendon gliding in the hand, part I, in vivo excursions, *J Hand Surg* 1985; 10A:570-574.

Table 30-3. Radian, moment arm, and excursion

Joint	ROM	Radian*		Moment arm (mm)		Excursion (mm)
MP	85	1.48	×	10.0	=	14.8
PIP	110	1.92	×	7.5	=	14.4
DIP	65	1.14	×	5.0	=	5.7
						34.9 (Total)

*1 radian = 57.29°.

ROM, Range of motion; *MP,* metacarpophalangeal; *PIP,* proximal interphalangeal; *DIP,* distal interphalangeal.

Note: When the MP joint moves through its normal range of 85°, it moves through an arc equal to 1.48 radian equivalents (85 ÷ 57.29 = 1.48). Because the known moment arm of the MP joint is 10 mm, ten times 1.48 equals 14.8 mm, which is the required excursion of the flexor tendon to move the MP joint through an arc of 85°. Similar calculations may be made for the PIP and DIP joints.

but it may also be severely diminished by adhesions following injury. The implications for significant loss of motion and function in the finger are obvious when decreased muscle excursion caused by intrinsic or extrinsic factors is combined with adhesions or scarring of the sheath or joint capsule.

Some current indications of fiber length have been given by Brand, et al. (Table 30-1).[3] It is the active muscle contraction component of excursion that accounts for tendon movement and subsequent joint movement. This active component of excursion must be understood to represent approximately one half of total excursion. In a study of differential tendon gliding in the hand, Wehbé and Hunter noted a mean flexor profundus tendon active excursion of 32 mm (range 15 to 43 mm) when the finger moved from full extension to full flexion with the wrist in neutral.[28] This observed excursion range correlated with the anticipated active excursion based on muscle fiber length and the commonly accepted figures for profundus tendon excursion (Table 30-2). It also fits closely with the projected active excursion as determined by the geometry of the system (Table 30-3).

Moment Arm

Moment arm is defined as the perpendicular distance between the line of application of a force and the center of rotation (axis) of a body (joint). Stated another way, the

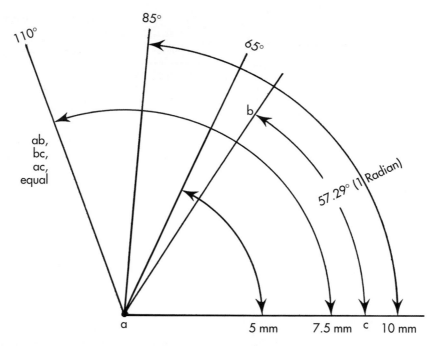

Fig. 30-7. When a radius of a circle moves through an angle of 57.29° (1 radian), any point on that radius moves through an arc equal in length to the distance between that point and the center of the circle. Note that the segments *ab, bc,* and *ac* are equidistant. The distance the flexor tendon moves while producing 1 radian of movement is equal to the perpendicular distance or moment arm between the flexor tendon and the joint axis. Any increase in the moment arm that might occur secondary to loss of a pulley results in an increase in the excursion required to achieve the same arc of motion. This graphic display demonstrates the active excursion required for complete range of motion at the distal interphalangeal (DIP, 65°), metacarpophalangeal (MP, 85°), and proximal interphalangeal (PIP, 110°) joints with their normal moment arms. For example, the normal 7.5 mm moment arm at the PIP joint requires a tendon excursion of 14.4 mm to achieve 110° of motion (see Table 30-3).

moment arm is the distance between the joint axis of motion and the central longitudinal axis of the adjacent flexor tendon. Some average and comparative figures for joint moment arm are MP, 10 mm; PIP, 7.5 mm; and DIP, 5 mm.

In reference to moment arm, a question must be raised: Does the moment arm change with motion? Evidence supporting the concept of a constant moment arm has been given by Brand, et al.[4] in a biomechanical study of the MP joint in fresh cadavers. This study demonstrated a virtual straight-line plot of joint angle change to tendon excursion, indicating that significant changes in the moment arm do not occur with motion.

Although digital moment arms probably do not change in the natural state when the normal pulley system is intact, the potential for change in the moment arm is great if significant disruption of the pulley mechanism occurs or if a disrupted pulley system is not adequately reconstructed. It must also be noted that many joints including the wrist and MP have two axes of rotation (similar to a universal joint) but in this chapter in reference to the MP joint we consider the MP joint axes to be in the coronal plane only.

Radian

A rule of geometry states that when a radius of a circle moves through an angle of 57.29° (1 radian), any point on that radius moves through an arc equal in length to the distance between that point and the center of the circle (Fig. 30-7). To state it another way, if the radius of a circle is moved 57.29° (1 radian), it will have moved a distance of 1 radian along the circumference of that circle. To state it yet another way, a radian is that distance on a circumference of a circle that is equal to the radius of that circle. A practical application immediately comes to mind in terms of the previous discussion about excursion and moment arm: When a joint moves 57°, tendon excursion and moment arm are equal. For example, when the MP joint moves through its normal range of 85° it moves through an arc equal to 1.48 radian equivalents (85° ÷ 57.29° = 1.48). The moment arm of the MP is 10 mm. Ten times 1.48 equals 14.8 mm, which is the required excursion of the flexor tendon to move the MP joint through an arc of 85°. Similar calculations may be made for the PIP and DIP joints (see Table 30-3). An increase in the moment arm because of absence or loss of integrity of a

Table 30-4. Moment arm and motion at the MP, PIP, and DIP joints

Joint	Moment arm (mm)	Lost joint motion (degrees)		
MP	2 mm increase (10 to 12)	85	to	68
PIP	1.5 mm increase (7.5 to 9)	110	to	88
DIP	1 mm increase (5 to 6)	65	to	52
		260	to	208* (Total)

*Fingertip fails palm: 2.5 cm (1 inch).
MP, Metacarpophalangeal; *PIP*, proximal interphalangeal; *DIP*, distal interphalangeal.
Note: A comparatively slight increase in the moment arm results in a significant loss of finger flexion.

Table 30-5. Range of motion (ROM), moment arm, and tendon excursions

Joint (ROM)	Moment arm (mm)	Excursion (mm)†
MP (85)	10 *	14.8*
	12	17.8
PIP (110)	7.5*	14.4*
	9.0	17.3
DIP (65)	5 *	5.7*
	6	6.8

*Normal values

$$\dagger \frac{\text{Joint ROM}}{57.29} \times \text{MA} = \text{Excursion} \qquad 34.9\text{* versus } 41.9$$

MP, Metacarpophalangeal; *PIP*, proximal interphalangeal; *DIP*, distal interphalangeal.
Note the relationship between required range of motion, normal and increased moment arm, and the resultant excursion. Joint range of motion divided by 1 radian times the moment arm yields excursion (see text).

pulley can result in significant loss of function. Table 30-4 depicts the loss of function that occurs with even a slight increase in the moment arm. Table 30-5 clearly demonstrates the relationship between normal joint range of motion (ROM), normal or increased moment arms, and the required excursion. When the required joint ROM is divided by 1 radian and multiplied by the moment arm, the result is the required excursion. Because all of the available excursion is used to achieve full finger flexion, it is obvious that an increased moment arm will result in significant loss of function.

Work of flexion

To further understand the dynamics of function of the flexor tendon pulley system, it is necessary to discuss a concept called work of flexion, first introduced in 1975,[18,19] and more recently (1985) applied to flexor pulley function.[23] Although tendon excursion can be used as a valid parameter to evaluate pulley function or efficiency, work of flexion, which represents the resistance to gliding encountered by the tendon during flexion, is a more comprehensive parameter. Practically speaking, work of flexion is probably a more useful parameter to evaluate the multiple factors that are responsible for success or failure in the management of flexor tendon injuries. This is so because it measures intrinsic as well as extrinsic factors other than the mechanical status of the pulleys such as viscoelastic forces of the skin and subcutaneous tissues, tendon adhesions, joint stiffness, and incongruity between tendon and sheath, to name a few. Peterson, et al. noted that work of flexion was found to increase to a greater extent by pulley loss than was tendon excursion. For example, loss of the A_2 pulley resulted in only an 8.5% increase in tendon excursion, but a 44% increase in work of flexion.[23] Work of flexion is therefore a more sensitive measurement of overall tendon function, because it represents the integration of all the factors that resist tendon gliding. A comparative percent difference between increased tendon excursion and increased work of flexion with excision of various pulleys is given in Table 30-6.

Lubrication factors

When a tendon or muscle moves around a bend it is constrained by some form of fibrous tissue or adjacent bone to make it efficient. The interface thus formed may develop an element of friction. In the normal state, however, significant friction does not occur because of the presence of special fluid-producing tissues called synovial membranes. These synovial tissues may be organized into special configurations such as bursae or sheaths. A prime example of a bursa is the subacromial bursa interposed between the deltoid muscle and the underlying tendons of the rotator cuff. In the finger, the flexor tendons are covered with a visceral synovial layer that interfaces with a parietal synovial layer that is most prominent in the spaces between the pulleys. The form of lubrication in the sheath is called boundary lubrication, in contrast to hydrodynamic lubrication as seen in joints.[6] Synovial fluid is a viscous fluid that exhibits resistance to flow, which is called thixotropy. This property is vital to lubrication in both joints and tendon sheaths. The smaller the radius of curvature about a joint the greater the pressure and the greater the potential for loss of function because of friction and shear stresses. A practical application of these principles would relate to width and location of reconstructed pulleys.

Discussion

The preceding comments about anatomy and biomechanical principles have provided an appropriate foundation for a practical application of these facts as they might apply to the clinical situation. Preservation of all components of the pulley system is a worthy goal, but it is not always possible. Multiple studies using sequential excision of various pulleys have demonstrated the importance of

Table 30-6. Flexor tendon biomechanics following pulley excision—skin intact

Pulley(s) excised	Intact	Percent difference	
		Tendon excursion	Work of flexion
A_1	(A_2, A_4)	-0.64 ± 2.04	10.00 ± 8.16
A_2	(A_1, A_4)	8.50 ± 1.62	44.10 ± 7.15
A_4	(A_1, A_2)	9.93 ± 3.40	19.95 ± 10.21
A_1, A_2	(A_4)	20.56 ± 3.76	62.36 ± 13.91
A_2, A_4	(A_1)	33.66 ± 4.60	107.04 ± 22.77
A_1, A_4	(A_2)	9.69 ± 1.91	39.83 ± 8.70
A_1, A_2, A_4	(none)	65.09 ± 6.21	172.35 ± 15.30

This table demonstrates that increased tendon excursion with pulley loss does not always reflect the potential functional loss that may occur because of other extrinsic factors such as tendon adhesions and joint stiffness.
Data from Peterson WW, Manske PR, Bollinger BA, et al: Effect of pulley excision on flexor tendon biomechanics, *J Orthop Res* 1986; 4:96-101.

preserving or reconstructing the second and fourth annular pulleys.[9,11,14,15,23]

In addition to the preceding comments, it must be observed that the pulley system in its normal state is ideal in all aspects, including its configuration and location, which accommodates a 260° arc of motion without impingement and with minimum friction, while at the same time using muscle-tendon excursion that is well within the natural range of the muscle-tendon unit. It must also be mentioned that the pulleys possess great strength and some typical breaking strengths have been determined that exceed most normal functional requirements.[21] Although pulley ruptures have been noted in rock climbers, these are rare occurrences that speak to the strength of the pulleys. Preservation of the pulley system is the goal throughout all phases of flexor tendon surgery. However, an intact pulley system is not always present following injury and repair. The basic principles that function in the normal system have been discussed and may serve as an introduction to the principles and techniques of pulley reconstruction, which is the subject of Chapter 32.

REFERENCES

1. Amis AA, Jones MM: The interior of the flexor tendon sheath of the finger—the functional significance of its structure, *J Bone Joint Surg* 1988; 70B:583-587.
2. Azar C, Fleegler EJ, Culver JE: *Dynamic anatomy of the flexor pulley system of the fingers and thumb,* presented at 39th annual meeting, American Society for Surgery of the Hand, Atlanta, 1984.
3. Brand PW, Beach RB, Thompson DE: Relative excursion and potential excursion of muscles in the forearm and hand, *J Hand Surg* 1981; 6:209.
4. Brand PW, Cranor KC, Ellis JC: Tendon and pulleys at the metacarpal phalangeal joint of a finger, *J Bone Joint Surg* 1975; 57A:779.
5. Brand PW, Hollister A: Muscles: the motors of the hand. In *Clinical mechanics of the hand,* ed 2, St Louis, 1993, Mosby.
6. Brand PW, Hollister A: Mechanical resistance. In *Clinical mechanics of the hand,* ed 2, St Louis, 1993, Mosby.
7. Bunnell SB: *Surgery of the hand,* Philadelphia, 1944, Lippincott.
8. Cohen MJ, Kaplan L: Histology and ultrastructure of the human flexor tendon sheath, *J Hand Surg* 1987; 12A:25-29.
9. Doyle JR: Anatomy of the finger flexor tendon sheath and pulley system, *J Hand Surg* 1988; 13A:473-484.
10. Doyle JR: Anatomy and function of the palmar aponeurosis pulley, *J Hand Surg* 1990; 15A:78-82.
11. Doyle JR, Blythe W: The finger flexor tendon sheath and pulleys: anatomy and reconstruction, *AAOS symposium on tendon surgery in the hand,* St Louis, 1975, Mosby.
12. Elftman H: Biomechanics of muscle, *J Bone Joint Surg* 1966; 48A:363.
13. Freehafer AA, Peckham H, Keith MW: Determination of muscle-tendon unit properties during tendon transfer, *J Hand Surg* 1979; 4:331.
14. Hume EL, Hutchinson DT, Jaeger SA, Hunter JM: Biomechanics of pulley reconstruction, *J Hand Surg* 1991; 16A:722-730.
15. Idler RS: Anatomy and biomechanics of the digital flexor tendons, *Hand Clin* 1985; 1:3-12.
16. Kline SC, Moore JR: The transverse carpal ligament—an important component of the digital flexor pulley system, *J Bone Joint Surg* 1992; 74A:1478-1485.
17. Knott C, Schmidt HM: The fibrous reinforcing arrangements of the digital peritenons in the human hand, *Gegenbaurs morph Jahrb* 1986; 132:1-28.
18. Lane JM, Bora FW, Black J: Cis-hydroxyproline limits work necessary to flex a digit after tendon injury, *Clin Orthop Relat Res* 1975; 109:193-200.
19. Lane JM, Black J, Bora FW: Gliding function following flexor tendon injury, *J Bone Joint Surg* 1976; 58A:985-990.
20. Lundborg G, Myrhage R: The vascularization and structure of the human digital tendon sheath as related to flexor tendon function, *Scand J Plast Reconstr Surg* 1977; 11:195-203.
21. Manske PR, Lesker PA: Strength of human pulleys, *Hand* 1977; 9:147-152.
22. Manske PR, Lesker PA: Palmar aponeurosis pulley, *J Hand Surg* 1983; 8:259-263.
23. Peterson WW, Manske PR, Bollinger BA, et al: Effect of pulley excision on flexor tendon biomechanics, *J Orthop Res* 1986; 4:96.
24. Resnick D: Roentgenographic anatomy of the tendon sheaths of the hand and wrist: tenography, *Am J Roentgenol* 1975; 124:44-51.
25. Sheldrup EW: Tendon sheath patterns in the hand, an anatomical study based on 367 hand dissections, *Surg Gynecol Obstet* 1951; 93:16-22.
26. Strauch B, de Moura W: Digital flexor tendon sheath: an anatomic study, *J Hand Surg* 1985; 10A:785-789.
27. Weber ER: Nutritional pathways for flexor tendons in the digital theca. In: Hunter JM, Schneider LH, Mackin EJ, eds: *Tendon surgery in the hand,* St Louis, 1987, Mosby.
28. Wehbé M, Hunter JM: Flexor tendon gliding in the hand, part I, in vivo excursions, *J Hand Surg* 1985; 10A:570-574.
29. Whittaker CR: The arrangement of the synovial membrane in the palmar digital sheaths, *J Anat* 1907; 41:155-157.

Chapter 31

EXCURSION OF FLEXOR TENDONS AND FRICTIONAL FORCES

S. Uchiyama
Peter C. Amadio
J.H. Coert
William P. Cooney
K-N An

The flexor pulley mechanism of the human fingers, especially A_2 and A_4 fibrous pulleys, restrains bowstringing of the tendons when crossing the joints. Because of this proper pulley constraint, coordinated finger joint motion is possible. However, when tendon excursion takes place through the pulley, drags, including friction, are encountered at the interface.[5,10] Little attention has been paid to wear or wear-through of the epitenon on the tendon surface. We examined and were able to demonstrate interesting findings of the flexor digitorum profundus (FDP) tendon surface of a 20-year-old man. Although the tendon surface looked fine macroscopically, magnification of the volar surface of the tendon often revealed that the epitenon had been worn out, perhaps as a result of friction between the tendon and the pulley, while the epitenon was intact on the dorsal surface of the tendon (Fig. 31-1).

It has been hypothesized that repetitive exposure to such friction could be detrimental. Cumulative trauma disorders in the hand and the wrist such as tenosynovitis, tendinitis, and carpal tunnel syndrome can be caused, precipitated, or aggravated by repeated tendon exertion within the hand and the wrist at certain positions, particularly in combination with increasing forceful exertions.[2,9,13] Furthermore, the friction between the pulley and the tendon has been found to be an important factor influencing the efficacy of mobiliza-

tion modalities after surgery of either pulley or tendon repair.[10]

SYSTEM FOR MEASUREMENT OF GLIDING RESISTANCE BETWEEN TENDON AND PULLEY

Previously, we have described the concept of the arc of contact for measurement of friction between a cable and a fixed mechanical pulley and its accuracy and application to the human tendon-pulley unit.[1,23] Briefly, the system consisted of a mechanical actuator with a linear potentiometer, F1 and F2 ring load transducers, a mechanical pulley (on the right of Fig. 31-2), and a weight. By changing the angle of alpha or beta, or both, the arc of contact between tendon and the pulley could be adjusted, and by changing the weights, tendon tension was also adjusted. To quantitize a pure interaction between the tendon and the pulley, a specimen to be prepared had only the FDP tendon, the A_2 pulley, and the proximal phalanx. It was mounted on the device with the volar side upward (see Fig. 31-2). When the tendon was translated toward the actuator, or proximally (2 mm/sec), there would be force difference between the two load cells because of a friction and the other force that interacted between the tendon and the pulley. We recorded F1, F2 force and corresponding excursion at the rate of 10 Hz. The average difference of F2-F1 for

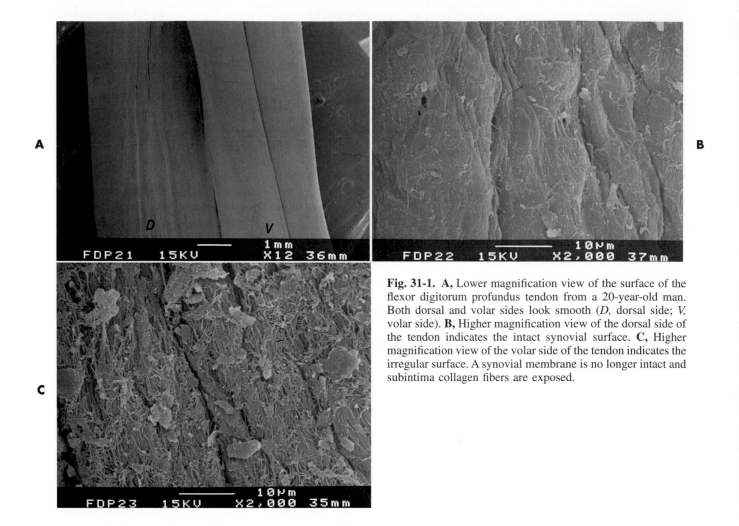

Fig. 31-1. A, Lower magnification view of the surface of the flexor digitorum profundus tendon from a 20-year-old man. Both dorsal and volar sides look smooth (*D,* dorsal side; *V,* volar side). **B,** Higher magnification view of the dorsal side of the tendon indicates the intact synovial surface. **C,** Higher magnification view of the volar side of the tendon indicates the irregular surface. A synovial membrane is no longer intact and subintima collagen fibers are exposed.

predetermined tendon excursion was defined as a gliding resistance. The force pattern of F1 and F2 as a function of excursion is shown in Fig. 31-3. F2 increased as excursion progressed. This increasing trend may come from the shape of the tendon, which varied longitudinally in the finger level. The gliding resistance varied from 0.021 N to 0.31 N with the application of 4.9 N tendon tension (weight) at various angles of alpha and beta. It was calculated that the friction coefficient between the FDP tendon and the A_2 pulley was 0.04 ± 0.014. Because a difference of F2 and F1 (gliding resistance) consisted of a friction force as well as the other forces, it should be noted that this value may not represent a real friction coefficient. However, this system would provide us with some answers to the unsolved questions, such as reaction force between tendon and pulley, gliding pattern of the repaired tendon, wear of the tendon or pulley surface, and development of tenosynovitis of the finger.

In this chapter, we discuss the difference of the gliding ability between the FDP tendon and the palmaris longus tendon, and the possible reason for the differences.

PALMARIS LONGUS TENDON VERSUS FLEXOR DIGITORUM PROFUNDUS TENDON

The palmaris longus tendon is an extrasynovial tendon and a common source for tendon graft. It is frequently used because the functional loss of the wrist is minimal, it is in the same field of surgery, and it is easily accessible.[16,25] However, after palmaris grafting, complications such as tendon adhesions and joint contractures may occur, and motion is not as good with a tendon graft as it is after tendon repair.[19] The FDP is an intrasynovial tendon within the fibro-osseous tunnel of the digit. It has both epitenon and mesotenon layers. Recently, several studies have shown differences in the biological response and healing process between intrasynovial and extrasynovial tendon grafts in vivo.[7,8,17] Adhesion to the surrounding tissue was more prominent with an extrasynovial tendon graft than with an intrasynovial tendon graft. Based on these findings, it was hypothesized that the gliding ability of the extrasynovial tendon is inferior to the intrasynovial tendon.

We compared the gliding resistance of the FDP tendon and the palmaris longus tendon at the A_2 pulley, using 14

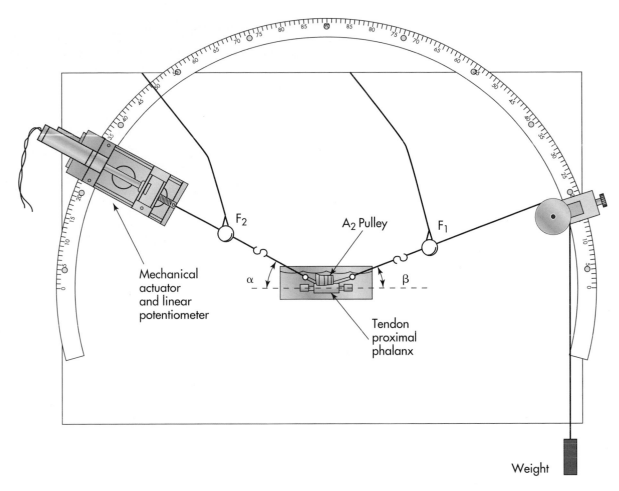

Fig. 31-2. The measurement system consisted of a mechanical actuator with a linear potentiometer, two tensile load transducers (F1 and F2), a mechanical pulley on the right of the figure, and a weight. A tendon tension could be adjusted by changing weights and arc of contact between the tendon, and the pulley could be adjusted by changing angles of alpha and beta. The tendon was translated proximally at a rate of 2 mm/sec, and F1, F2, and corresponding excursion were measured. In this movement, a friction force directed toward F1 load transducer. Because of friction and the other forces, there would be a force difference between two load transducers. This force difference for predetermined excursion was averaged and regarded as a gliding resistance.

digits, tendons, and 14 ipsilateral palmaris longus tendons.[21] For half of the specimens, the palmaris longus tendon was tested first and then the FDP tendon was tested. In the other half, the testing sequence was reversed. It was found that the gliding resistance was significantly greater when the palmaris longus tendon was tested than when the FDP tendon was tested at tendon tension of 2.45, 4.9, 9.8, and 14.7 N ($p < 0.001$). The gliding resistance of the FDP tendon was less sensitive to increasing tendon tension than was the palmaris longus tendon (Fig. 31-4).

LUBRICATION BETWEEN FLEXOR DIGITORUM PROFUNDUS TENDON AND PULLEY

To keep the tendon and pulley surface from wearing, a lubrication mechanism is assumed to be present as seen in the diarthrodial joints.[14] Several hypotheses about the

lubrication between tendon and pulley have been reported,[4,20] mainly from a biochemical prospective. In these studies, proteoglycan, fibronectin, and lipid were extracted from chicken flexor tendon synovium. However, the precise lubrication mechanisms at the tendon-pulley interface have yet to be studied. In this study, gross staining density of the tendon surface was compared visually with the human FDP tendon with and without hyaluronidase treatment and the untreated palmaris longus tendon, and strongly suggests the existence of hyaluronate or its complex on the tendon surface.[22] We found that the surface of the FDP tendon was positively stained by Alcian blue, while the palmaris longus (PL) tendon was negatively stained. After hyaluronidase treatment of the tendon, the density of staining on the FDP tendon was decreased (Fig. 31-5). It was then hypothesized that hyaluronate or its complex on the tendon

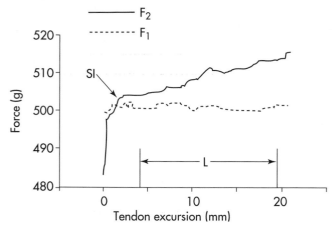

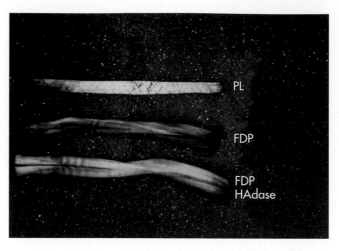

Fig. 31-3. The measurements of F1 and F2 throughout the whole excursion in the movement toward the actuator (flexion). F2 increases steeply up to the so-called status of impending motion, followed by a gradual increase in the amount of force. This increasing trend may come from the shape of the tendon. The average value of F1 and F2 for excursion of L was calculated for the analysis (SI, status of impending motion; L, excursion for calculation). (From *J Orthop Res* 1995; 13:83-89.)

Fig. 31-5. Gross staining of the surface of the tendons harvested from the same donor. *Top,* Palmaris longus tendon is negative for Alcian blue staining. *Middle,* The flexor digitorum profundus tendon is positively stained by Alcian blue. *Bottom,* Staining density of the flexor digitorum profundus tendon of the adjacent digit is now decreased after hyaluronidase treatment.

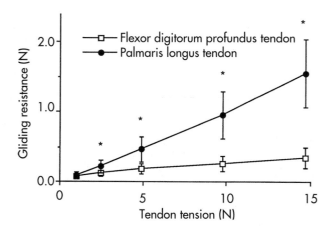

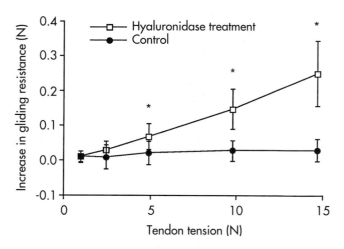

Fig. 31-4. Effect of the tendon tension and the two different tendons on the gliding resistance is shown. The gliding resistance of the palmaris longus tendon is greater than the flexor digitorum profundus tendon except at 0.98 newton load ($p < 0.001$). The gliding resistance of the flexor digitorum profundus tendon is less sensitive to the increasing load than the palmaris longus tendon.

Fig. 31-6. Effect of hyaluronidase treatment of the tendon on increase in gliding resistance is shown. The increase in gliding resistance after hyaluronidase treatment is significantly greater than that of control at tendon tensions of 4.9, 9.8, and 14.7 newtons ($p < 0.05$).

surface may play an important role in lubrication. Then we investigated the effect of hyaluronidase treatment of the FDP on the gliding resistance using 20 digits from 20 donors. Gliding resistance was measured with the FDP tendons after dissection. Then 10 tendons were treated with bovine testis hyaluronidase for 2 hours and retested. The other tendons (control) were retested without hyaluronidase treatment. The increase in gliding resistance before and

after hyaluronidase treatment was compared with that of the control group. It was found that the gliding resistance increased significantly after hyaluronidase treatment at high tendon tensions when compared with the control (Fig. 31-6).[22]

DISCUSSION

The differences of the gliding resistance between the FDP tendon and the palmaris longus tendon are the result of differences or variation within the surface structure. The PL tendon as an extrasynovial tendon does not have a synovial membrane (epitenon or mesotenon) around it. Instead, it has a paratenon of loose connective tissue. For this study, we removed the paratenon, but scanning electron microscope revealed that microscopic remnants of the paratenon remained on the surface and may have acted to resist gliding. In contrast, the FDP tendon has a synovial membrane epitenon surface that makes the gliding surface smoother.[11,18] Finding that the gliding resistance of the FDP tendon was less sensitive to lead increases than was PL tendon indicated that boundary lubrication may take place when the FDP tendon came to contact with the A_2 pulley. The FDP tendon may have fibronectins on its surface, which could bind to lipid or hyaluronic acid.[3,4] Our study showed hyaluronate and other Alcian blue positive, hyaluronidase-sensitive materials may exist on the FDP tendon surface either in a complex with fibronectin or as a part of the proteoglycans of the synovium or the tendon surface. Proteoglycan may also exist between tendon collagen fiber bundles on the volar part of the tendon as a result of adaptive differentiation of the fibrocytes into cartilaginous cells in response to repetitive compression.[12,15,24] In this study, hyaluronidase may have diffused deep into the tendon and dissolved not only the surface hyaluronate complex but also that in the tendon matrix as described previously. At lower weights, resistance did not increase significantly after hyaluronidase treatment, perhaps because a fluid film of saline solution existed between the tendon and the pulley and acted as a lubricant. As weight increased, an increase in gliding resistance became evident. We hypothesize that the fluid film may be squeezed out of the tendon-pulley interface under heavier weights, after which direct contact took place and became dominant. Under these conditions any surface lubricant, such as hyaluronate or proteoglycan, may act to reduce the frictional resistance as a boundary lubricant. Although we did not see through scanning electron microscope any obvious damage to collagen fiber structure after hyaluronidase treatment, we could not be certain that the change of viscoelasticity[6] of the tendon may have affected the gliding resistance to some extent.

Overall, we showed the superior gliding ability of the FDP tendon in comparison with the PL tendon, and we suggest that one possible reason is the difference in surface lubrication. Our observations are consistent with the finding that an intrasynovial tendon graft may heal without adhesions, whereas an extrasynovial tendon graft usually requires adhesion formation within the healing process.[17] We believe that intrasynovial tendon donors, which appear to possess a boundary lubricant on their surfaces, may result in significant improvements in tendon gliding after surgery, as compared with more traditional extrasynovial sources such as a PL tendon.

REFERENCES

1. An KN, Berglund L, Uchiyama S, Coert J: Measurement of friction between pulley and flexor tendon, *Biomed Sci Instrumentation* 1993; 29:1-7.
2. Armstrong T, Chaffin D: Some biomechanical aspects of the carpal tunnel, *J Biomech* 1979; 12:567-570.
3. Banes AJ, Donlon K, Link GW, et al: Cell populations of tendon: a simplified method for isolation of synovial cells and internal fibroblasts: confirmation of origin and biologic properties, *J Orthop Res* 1988; 6:83-94.
4. Banes AJ, Link GW, Bevin AG, et al: Tendon synovial cells secrete fibronectin in vivo and in vitro, *J Orthop Res* 1988; 6:73-82.
5. Brand PW, Thompson DE: Mechanical resistance. In Ryan JD, ed: *Clinical mechanics of the hand,* ed 2, 1993, St Louis, Mosby.
6. Cunningham KD, Frank CB, Shrive NG: Biomechanical effects of partial removal of proteoglycans from the rabbit medial collateral ligament, *Transactions of 41th Annual Meeting, ORS,* Orlando, FL, 1995; 1:160.
7. Gelberman RH, Chu CR, Williams CS, et al: Angiogenesis in healing autogenous flexor-tendon grafts, *J Bone Joint Surg* 1992; 74A:1207-1216.
8. Gelberman RH, Seiler JG, Rosenberg AE, et al: Intercalary flexor tendon grafts: a morphological study of intrasynovial and extrasynovial donor tendons, *Scand J Plast Reconstr Surg* 1992; 26(3):257-264.
9. Goldstein SA, Armstrong TJ, Chaffin DB, Matthews LS: Analysis of cumulative strain in tendons and tendon sheaths, *J Biomech* 1987; 20:1-6.
10. Horii E, Lin GT, Cooney WP, et al: Comparative flexor tendon excursion after passive mobilization, *J Hand Surg* 1992; 17A: 559-566.
11. Inoue H, Takasugi H, Akahori O: Surface study of tenosynovium in hens and humans by electron microscopy, *Hand* 1976; 8:222-227.
12. Lundborg G, Myrhage R: The vascularization and structure of human digital tendon sheath as related to flexor tendon function, *Scand J Plast Reconstr Surg* 1977; 11:195-203.
13. Moore A, Wells R, Ranney D: Quantifying exposure in occupational manual tasks with cumulative trauma disorder potential, *Ergonomics* 1991; 34:1433-1453.
14. Mow VC, Soslowsky LJ: Friction, lubrication, and wear of diarthrodial joints. In Mow VC, Hayes WC, eds: New York, 1991, Raven.
15. Okuda Y, Gorski JP, An K-N, Amadio PC: Biochemical, histological and biomechanical analysis of canine tendon, *J Orthop Res* 1987; 5:60-68.
16. Schneider LH, Hunter JM: Flexor tendons-late reconstruction. In Green DP, ed: *Operative hand surgery,* New York, 1988, Churchill Livingstone.
17. Seiler JG, Gelberman RH, Williams CS, et al: Autogenous flexor tendon grafts: a biomechanical and morphological study in dogs, *J Bone Joint Surg* 1993; 75A:1004-1014.
18. Steinberg PG, Hodde KC: The morphology of synovial lining of various structures in several species as observed with scanning electron microscopy, *Scanning Microscopy* 1990; 4:987-1020.
19. Strickland JW: Flexor tendon surgery, *J Hand Surg* 1989; 14B:261-272, 268-382.
20. Tsuzaki M, Yamauchi M, Banes AJ: Tendon collagens: extracellular matrix composition in shear stress and tensile components of flexor tendons, *Connective Tissue Res* 1993; 29:141-152.
21. Uchiyama S, Amadio PC, Berglund L, An K-N: Gliding characteristics of human intrasynovial and extrasynovial tendons. In Blankervoort L,

Kooloos JGM, eds: *Abstract of Second World Congress of Biomechanics,* Amsterdam, The Netherlands, 1994.

22. Uchiyama S, Amadio PC, Ishikawa J, An K-N: Effect of hyaluronidase treatment on the gliding resistance between the tendon and the pulley, *Transactions of the 41st Annual Meeting, ORS,* Orlando, FL, 1995.

23. Uchiyama S, Coert JH, Berglund L, et al: Method for the measurement of friction between tendon and pulley, *J Orthop Res* 1995; 13:83-89.

24. Vogel KG, Ordog A, Pogany G, Olah J: Proteoglycans in the compressed region of human tibialis posterior tendon and in ligaments, *J Orthop Res* 1993; 11:68-77.

25. Wehbé MA: Tendon graft donor sites, *J Hand Surg* 1992; 17A:1130-1132.

Chapter 32

RECONSTRUCTION OF THE FLEXOR PULLEY MECHANISM

William P. Cooney

In the treatment of flexor tendon injuries, that is, both tendon repair and tendon grafts, reconstruction of the flexor fibro-osseous pulley system can be necessary. Anatomic studies have demonstrated that the fibro-osseous pulleys are critical to the function of flexor tendon in providing both excursion and strength for normal finger function. In this chapter, I examine the recent studies of both the anatomy and the mechanics of the flexor pulley system and describe the methods in use today for pulley reconstruction.

ANATOMY

The fibro-osseous pulley system is made up of a series of bony and fibrous connections between the flexor tendon sheath and the phalanges or the volar plate (Figs. 32-1 and 32-2). Beginning proximal, the pulleys are numbered as the A_1, A_2, A_3, A_4, and A_5.[6,14] The A_1 pulley is just proximal to the metacarpophalangeal (MP) joint. The A_1 pulley combined with pulleys of the flexor retinacular system help maintain normal gliding, excursion, and force transmission at the MP joint. Release of the A_1 pulley can be performed provided that the palmar pulleys are maintained to prevent bowstringing.

The A_2 pulley is just distal to the A_1 pulley with a small cruciate component between the two, which is a common source of a palmar retinacular ganglion cyst. It is a bony pulley that extends almost the entire length of the proximal phalanx. It is the strongest and most important pulley with respect to proximal interphalangeal (PIP) joint motion (Fig. 32-3). Loss of the A_2 pulley leads to significant loss of potential motion at the PIP joint. Reconstruction is generally recommended when it is deficient.

The A_3 pulley is a volar plate pulley similar to the A_1 pulley in that it moves with flexion of the respective joint (see Fig. 32-2). It is separated from the A_2 pulley by the second cruciate (C_2) pulley. It is second in importance in preventing bowstringing at the PIP joint but is relatively weak (Figs. 32-4 and 32-5). Reconstruction is indicated in the absence of the A_2 pulley.

The A_4 pulley is the second bony pulley taking origin from the middle phalanx. It is second in importance to the A_2 pulley in maintaining full motion of the finger. It is most important for full motion at the distal interphalangeal (DIP) joint. Reconstruction of the A_4 pulley is recommended when it is absent. When both the A_2 and A_4 pulleys are absent, they should be reconstructed for best return of flexor tendon excursion and digital flexion.

The A_5 pulley is the final volar plate-type pulley. Its importance at the DIP is minor and reconstruction is not required. It is commonly released in flexor tendon repair and tendon grafts, and is rarely reconstructed because it might interfere with tendon excursion. It also is not a very strong pulley with respect to mechanical force resistance (see Figs. 32-4 and 32-5) and is not required if strong pinch or grip is anticipated from the patient.

In the thumb, the pulley anatomy is different than the finger pulley system. The thumb has a primary or A_1 pulley just proximal to the MP joint and an oblique pulley overlying the proximal phalanx. There is a distal or A_2 pulley at the volar plate of the DIP joint. In surgery on the thumb, it is essential to protect or reconstruct the oblique pulley but not necessarily the A_1 and A_2 pulleys.

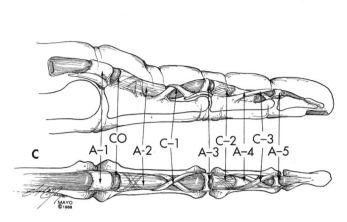

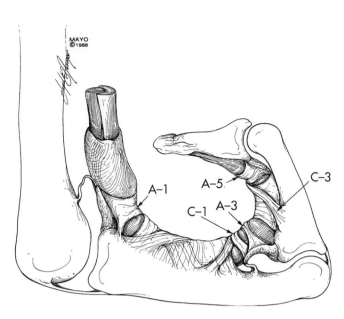

Fig. 32-1. Anatomy of human pulleys: fibro-osseous annular pulleys (A_2, A_4), volar plate annular pulleys (A_1, A_3, A_5), cruciate or condensable pulleys (C_1, C_2, C_3). (From Lin GT, Cooney WP, Amadio PC, An K-N: Mechanical properties of human pulleys, *J Hand Surg* 1990; 15B:428.)

Fig. 32-2. The cruciate pulleys have one fixed attachment to bone and one moveable attachment to volar plate. (By permission of Mayo Foundation.)

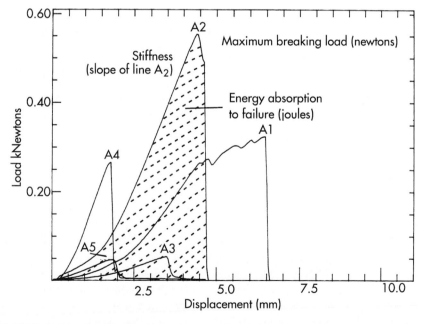

Fig. 32-3. Parameters from the load-displacement curve are used to define the mechanical property of the normal and reconstructed pulley. A_1, A_3, A_5 are volar plate pulleys; A_2, A_4 are bone pulleys. (From Lin GT, Cooney WP, Amadio PC, An K-N: Mechanical properties of human pulleys, *J Hand Surg* 1990; 15B:429.)

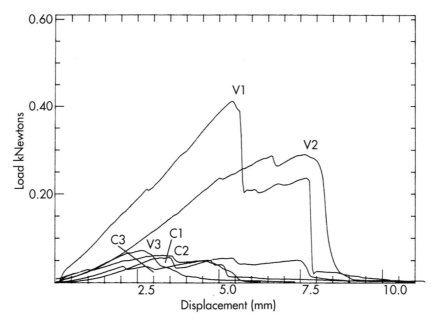

Fig. 32-4. Typical force-displacement curves for C_1-C_3 pulley and volar plate "belt loop" pulley, V_1-V_3. (From Lin GT, Cooney WP, Amadio PC, An K-N: Mechanical properties of human pulleys, *J Hand Surg* 1990; 15B:429.)

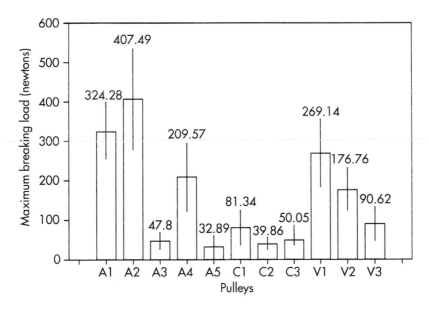

Fig. 32-5. Maximum breaking load of the pulley. (From Lin GT, Cooney WP, Amadio PC, An K-N: Mechanical properties of human pulleys, *J Hand Surg* 1990; 15B:428.)

PULLEY INJURY

Pulley injuries are most commonly associated with lacerations to the flexor tendons in which there is scarring from improper tendon repair.[2,13,23] On reexploration for tenolysis, the flexor tendon sheath system either cannot be freed of the scarred tendon repair or is injured in the process of performing the tenolysis. Occasionally, a tendon avulsion injury[5,25] will of itself damage the flexor tendon sheath and rupture one or more of the pulleys. At the time of surgical exploration, damage to the flexor pulley mechanism, more properly called the fibro-osseous sheath, should be assessed. To free up a scarred tendon bed from a previous flexor tendon repair, emphasis has been properly directed to preserve the A_2 and A_4 pulleys.[6] I recommend preserving the A_1 and A_3

pulleys,[12] if possible; when dissecting in the palm, I would also make an effort to retain the distal portion of the palmar pulleys.[18]

In some pulley injuries, it is reasonable and necessary to dilate the pulley system by use of urethral dilators or uterine sounds. Pulley dilation may be necessary prior to placement of silicone tendon spacers such as the Hunter tendon graft.[2,13,23] Pulley dilation often allows for a primary tendon graft, but only if the tendon glides easily within the fibro-osseous tendon sheath. Reconstruction of the pulley mechanism should almost always be performed around a silicone (or similar inert material) tendon graft so that a gliding mechanism for tendon excursion can be maintained. With the recent recognition that tendon reconstruction should be performed using tissues with intrinsic tenosynovium[1,8,24] (i.e., extensor retinaculum or a toe or finger flexor tendon) rather than extrinsic tenosynovium, as found with palmaris longus, plantaris, and extra retinacular portions of extensor tendons, primary tendon graft and pulley reconstruction may be considered.[2,25,26]

PULLEY BIOMECHANICS

There has been considerable interest in the biomechanics of pulleys as they relate to both the forces that pulleys need to resist as well as the resistance to tendon gliding that must occur at the tendon pulley interface.* In Chapter 31, there are the recent reports of frictional forces that occur with tendon gliding. Suffice to say that frictional forces can be measured within the fibro-osseous pulley system[26] and that efforts are under way to better understand the methods by which the friction forces can be minimized. It is now well known, for example, that the tendons and pulleys both have areas of fibrocartilage that have developed in response to both compressive and frictional forces[21] and that tendon anatomic areas vary with postnatal age.[20] Pulleys, like tendons, are also covered with epitenon cells that respond to injury and repair in a similar fashion. These epitenon cells may produce a type of hyaluronic acid lubricant that helps maintain tendon gliding and reduce frictional forces. In tendon or pulley reconstruction, efforts to replace such a lubricant mechanism must be considered.

With respect to the biomechanics themselves, my colleagues and I have performed a number of studies that examine the length and breadth of the pulley, the breaking strength and minimal strength needed for repair, and the ideal parameters for pulley repair (see Fig. 32-3).[15-17] Pulleys function more than just as a sling placed proximal to a joint; they bear force throughout their length, distributing the force of tendons during grip and pinch in a physiologic manner. The reconstruction of a pulley of near normal length and strength is important in the redistribution of tendon forces to not only be mechanically efficient but also to

*References 3, 4, 10, 11, 16, 18, 19, 26, 28.

maintain a well-lenitive surface for smooth, unfettered, tendon gliding.[17]

In measurement of pulley mechanics, we have observed that the bony pulleys have greater inherent strength than the volar plate pulleys (see Fig. 32-5). They are longer and distribute forces more broadly with less potential bowstringing effect. The bony pulleys are more important in the initiation of joint motion because they are fixed, whereas the volar plate pulleys have the advantage of dynamic action because they move forward in flexion with the joint, changing the moment arm effect in response to joint flexion. With flexion, for example, the volar plate pulley becomes farther away from the joint center of rotation making the tendon force component greater with increasing flexion. Without the volar plate pulley, the tendon moment arm becomes more affected by the length of the bony pulley because there would be greater bowstringing effect with a short A_2 or A_4 pulley than with one of normal length.

METHODS OF PULLEY RECONSTRUCTION

Pulley reconstruction can be divided into three basic techniques. The first technique attempts to use the remaining peripheral rim of pulley (Fig. 32-6)[13,27] in which one could weave a tendon graft to replace the lost pulley system. This technique has the advantage of replacing the entire length of the pulley and adjusting the tension within the system. It has the disadvantage of relative weakness of the remaining pulley rim and the potential of over tightening the repair and narrowing the tendon space with the effect of increasing tendon adhesions and friction. It is also mechanically the weakest of the pulley reconstruction techniques (Figs. 32-7 and 32-8).

The second method of pulley reconstruction involves a peripheral or extrinsic wrapping of a tendon graft around the digit.[9,15,22] Both flexor tendon, extensor tendon, and extensor retinaculum have been used for such a reconstruction. Most commonly this method is used for reconstruction of the A_2 or A_4 pulleys. The tendon graft can be placed through bone, but most commonly it is wrapped dorsal or above the extensor tendon mechanism. This method has the greatest strength of the pulley reconstruction techniques when two or three loops are placed around the bone (see Fig. 32-8) but does not provide the potential for an "anatomic" pulley because its length is limited to 4 to 5 mm. This may result in loss of tendon excursion (Fig. 32-9). Studies have demonstrated that the multiple loops of tendon can carry force equal to the normal pulley and greater than the other forms of pulley reconstruction. Therefore it may be more desirable when high tendon force in grasps is anticipated or desired. Current techniques using multiple strands of tendon have provided good clinical results.

The third technique involves the relatively ingenious use of the volar plate itself for the pulley reconstruction.[12] Both

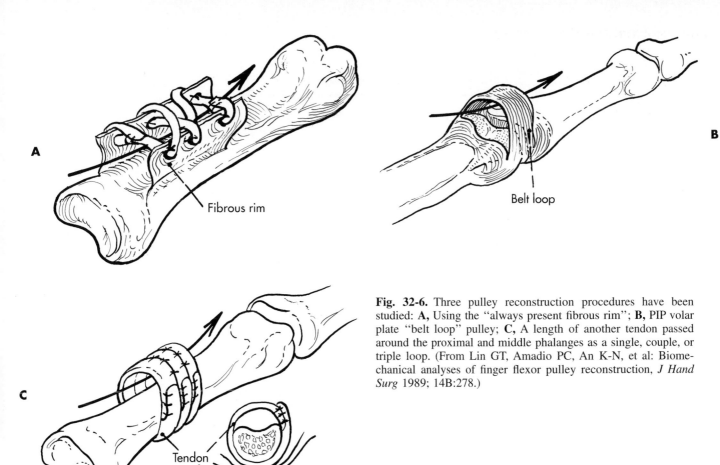

A Fibrous rim

B Belt loop

C Tendon graft

Extensor tendon

3 loops

Fig. 32-6. Three pulley reconstruction procedures have been studied: **A,** Using the "always present fibrous rim"; **B,** PIP volar plate "belt loop" pulley; **C,** A length of another tendon passed around the proximal and middle phalanges as a single, couple, or triple loop. (From Lin GT, Amadio PC, An K-N, et al: Biomechanical analyses of finger flexor pulley reconstruction, *J Hand Surg* 1989; 14B:278.)

Range of motion

Injured or repaired pulley

Intact pulley

Effective motion

Relative Absolute

Range of excursion

Bowstringing laxity

Tendon excursion (cm)

Joint flexion angle (degree)

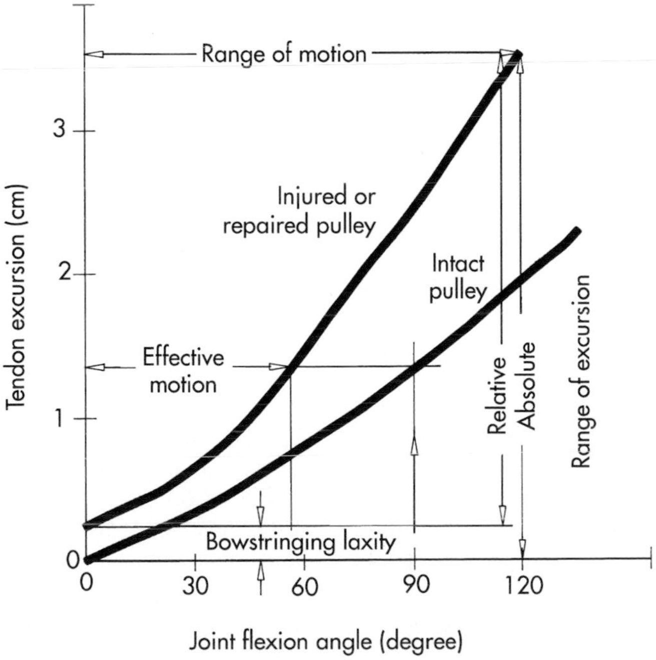

Fig. 32-7. Definition of the parameters used for assessing tendon excursion and joint displaced relationship. (From Lin GT, Amadio PC, An K-N, et al: Biomechanical analyses of finger flexor pulley reconstruction, *J Hand Surg* 1989; 14B:278.)

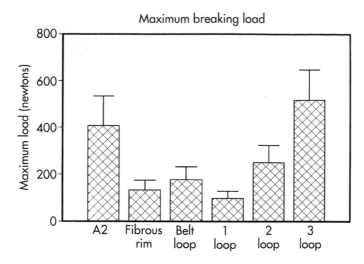

Fig. 32-8. Maximum breaking load of the intact and reconstructed A$_2$ pulley. (From Lin GT, Amadio PC, An K-N, et al: Biomechanical analyses of finger flexor pulley reconstruction, *J Hand Surg* 1989; 14B:278.)

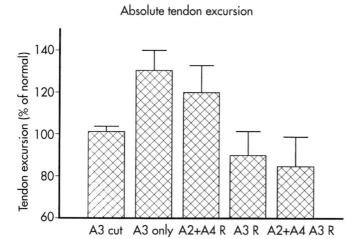

Fig. 32-9. Effect of pulley conditions on proximal interphalangeal absolute tendon excursion. (From Lin GT, Amadio PC, An K-N, et al: Biomechanical analyses of finger flexor pulley reconstruction, *J Hand Surg* 1989; 14B:278.)

experimentally and clinically it has been used for A$_1$ and A$_3$ pulley reconstruction, either alone or in combination with A$_2$ and A$_4$ pulley repairs. Mechanically, it improves tendon gliding by keeping the tendon close to the joint center of rotation. Frictional forces may increase, however, with this method of reconstruction[7] but have not been studied. They would be expected to be higher because the pulley length is no more than 2 to 3 mm. This method is best used with a Hunter tendon graft or other inert material. Use of silicone or dacron artificial tendon improves the tendon gliding and appears to provide a gliding environment.[2,23]

SUMMARY

Tendon pulley (fibro-osseous sheath system) reconstruction may be required to restore normal mechanics and tendon excursion following injuries to the flexor tendon system. Tendon sheath injury can occur in association with acute lacerations or more commonly late during tenolysis or tendon graft reconstruction. Biomechanical studies have confirmed that the A$_2$ and A$_4$ pulleys are the most important and without them excessive tendon bowstringing would occur that would ultimately limit full finger flexion into the palm.

Tendon bowstringing, while increasing the potential force across a joint, ultimately leads to reduced tendon excursion, altered tendon gliding, and increased frictional forces, which would limit both motion and tendon force transmission. This would result in decreased pinch and grasp force. Every effort should be made, therefore, to maximize the accuracy and precision of the tendon and tendon sheath repair and to have tendon pulley reconstruction that duplicates normal anatomy. The biomechanics of the pulley system do not provide for much variance in tendon moment arms or compliance within the fibro-osseous tunnel. Subsequently, failure to reconstruct the entire pulley system may have consequences on normal tendon excursion, gliding, and the ability to overcome frictional forces. On the other hand, tendon forces can be quite high, for example, in the manual laborer, and some loss of excursion for a stronger pulley repair may be desirable in that it would hold up better over time. As in many areas of hand surgery, pulley reconstruction should be tailored to the special needs of the patient, degree of tendon pulley injury, and the potential for a successful result, as may be dictated by the original trauma. With newer understanding of the biomechanics of tendon sheath reconstruction and information on the frictional forces that different types of reconstruction may produce, improved methods of tendon sheath repair should be forthcoming.

REFERENCES

1. Abrahamsson SO, Gelberman R: Maintenance of the gliding surface of tendon autografts in dogs, *Acta Orthop Scand* 1994; 65(5):548-552.
2. Amadio PC, Wood MB, Cooney WPd, Bogard SD: Staged flexor tendon reconstruction in the fingers and hand, *J Hand Surg* 1988; 13A(4):559-562.
3. An KN, Ueba Y, Chao EY, et al: Tendon excursion and moment arm of index finger muscles, *J Biomech* 1983; 16(6):419-425.
4. Bartle BK, Telepun GM, Goldberg NH: Development of a synthetic replacement for flexor tendon pulleys using expanded polytetrafluoroethylene membrane, *Ann Plastic Surg* 1992; 28(3):266-270.
5. Bowers WH, Kuzma GR, Bynum DK: Closed traumatic rupture of finger flexor pulleys, *J Hand Surg* 1994; 19A(5):782-787.
6. Doyle JR, Blythe W: The finger flexor tendon sheath and pulleys: anatomy and reconstruction. In American Academy of Orthopaedic Surgeons: *Symposium on tendon surgery in the hand,* St Louis, 1985, Mosby.
7. Eaton CJ: Possible complication of belt loop pulley reconstruction, *J Hand Surg* 1993; 18A(1):169-170 (letter, comment).
8. Gelberman RH, Seiler JGd, Rosenberg AE, et al: Intercalary flexor tendon grafts: a morphological study of intrasynovial and extrasynovial donor tendons, *Scand J Plastic Reconstr Surg Hand Surg* 1992; 26(3):257-264.
9. Hanff G, Dahlin LB, Lundborg G: Reconstruction of flexor tendon pulley with expanded polytetrafluoroethylene (E-PTFE): an experimental study in rabbits, *Scand J Plastic Reconstr Surg Hand Surg* 1991; 25(1):25-30.
10. Hume EL, Hutchinson DT, Jaeger SA, Hunter JM: Biomechanics of pulley reconstruction, *J Hand Surg* 1991; 16A(4):722-730.
11. Idler RS: Anatomy and biomechanics of the digital flexor tendons, *Hand Clin* 1985; 1(1):3-11.
12. Karev A, Stahl S, Taran A: The mechanical efficiency of the pulley system in normal digits compared with a reconstructed system using the "belt loop" technique, *J Hand Surg* 1987; 12A(4):596-601 (see comments).
13. Kleinert HE, Bennett JB: Digital pulley reconstruction employing the always present rim of the previous pulley, *J Hand Surg* 1978; 3A(3):297-298.
14. Landsmeer JMF: *Atlas of Anatomy of the Hand,* Edinburgh, 1976, Churchill Livingstone.
15. Lin GT, Amadio PC, An KN, Cooney WP: Functional anatomy of the human digital flexor pulley system, *J Hand Surg* 1989; 14A(6):949-956.
16. Lin GT, Amadio PC, An KN, et al: Biomechanical analysis of finger flexor pulley reconstruction, *J Hand Surg* 1989; 14B(3):278-282.
17. Lin GT, Cooney WP, Amadio PC, An KN: Mechanical properties of human pulleys, *J Hand Surg* 1990; 15B(4):429-434.
18. Manske PR, Lesker PA: Palmar aponeurosis pulley, *J Hand Surg* 1983; 8A(3):259-263.
19. Manske PR, Lesker PA: Strength of human pulleys, *Hand* 1977; 9(2):147-152.
20. Okuda Y, Gorski JP, Amadio PC: Effect of postnatal age on the ultrastructure of six anatomic areas of canine flexor digitorum profundus, *J Orthop Res* 1987b; 5:231-241.
21. Okuda Y, Gorski JP, An KN, Amadio PC: Biochemical, histological, and biomechanical analyses of canine tendon, *J Orthop Res* 1987a; 5(1):60-68.
22. Okutsu L, Ninomiya S, Hiraki S, et al: Three-loop technique for A_2 pulley reconstruction, *J Hand Surg* 1987; 12A(5 Pt 1):790-794.
23. Schneider LH, Hunter JM: Flexor tendons—late reconstruction. In Green DP, ed: *Operative Hand Surgery,* New York, 1988, Churchill Livingstone.
24. Seiler JG, Reddy AS, Simpson LE, et al: The flexor digitorum longus: an anatomic and microscopic study for use as a tendon graft, *J Hand Surg* 1995; 20A(3):492-495.
25. Tropet Y, Menez D, Balmat P, et al: Closed traumatic rupture of the ring finger flexor tendon pulley, *J Hand Surg* 1990; 15A(5):745-747.
26. Uchiyama S, Coert JH, Berglund L, et al: Method for the measurement of friction between tendon and pulley, *J Orthop Res* 1995; 13(1):83-89.
27. Weilby A: Referenced in the paper of Kleinert and Bennett, 1978 (reference 13).
28. Widstrom CJ, Johnson G, Doyle JR, et al: A mechanical study of six digital pulley reconstruction techniques: part I. mechanical effectiveness, *J Hand Surg* 1989; 14A(5):821-825.

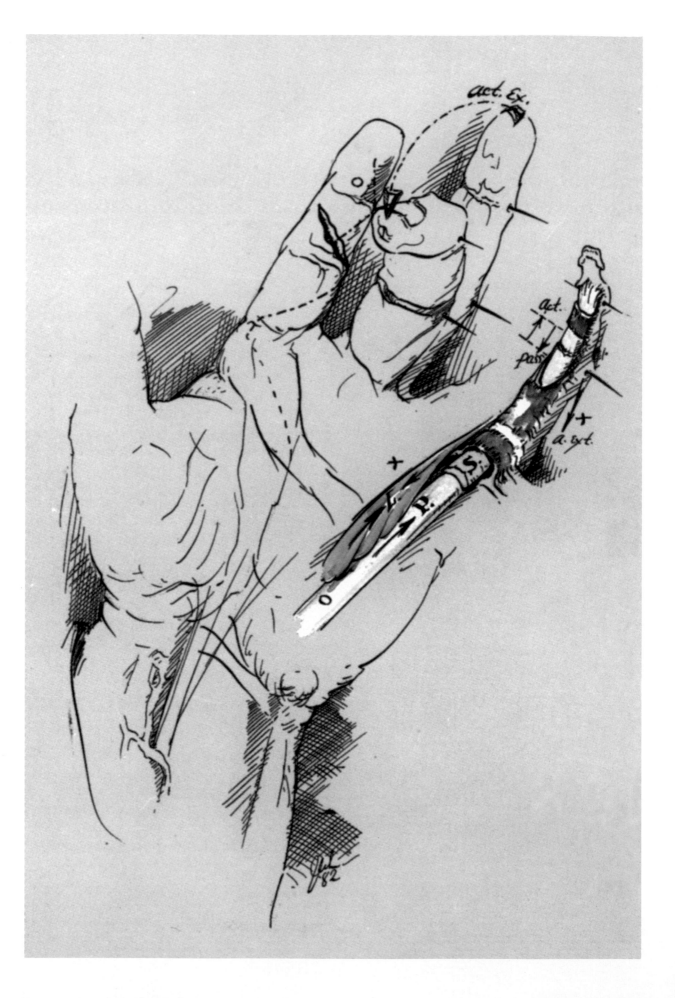

Part VIII

TENDON HEALING AND NUTRITION

Passive elastic band flexion and active extension movement for the guarded finger is critical to the hand therapy regimen following primary intrathecal tendon repair. Reflex contraction of the lumbrical muscle, initiated by the extrinsic extensor, advances the profundus tendon and reduces excursion tension at the more distal site. (From *J Hand Ther,* vol. 2, no. 2, April/June, 1989, Hanley & Belfus [cover drawing].)

Chapter 33

INJURY TO THE VASCULAR SYSTEM AND ITS EFFECT ON TENDON INJURY IN NO MAN'S LAND

Takeshi Matsui
James M. Hunter

This chapter investigates the distribution of blood vessels in the flexor tendons of human fingers and the effect of injuries to tendons and vincula on blood vessel distribution in the tendons. With the advances in operative procedures and postoperative management using early passive motion for flexor tendon injuries in no man's land, excellent results of primary tendon repair have been reported.[5,15] The prevailing view on the process of repair of injured tendons in the past was that an injured tendon in the digital fibrous sheath would not heal without participation of the surrounding tissue. It is now, however, demonstrated that the flexor tendon has intrinsic repair potential with the recent advances in clinical and experimental studies. Many authors place emphasis on the role of the synovial fluid in the process of nutrition or repair of injury to tendons.[3,4,6,8,9] There is also evidence of profuse vascularization of the human digital flexor tendons in no man's land,[1,2,7,10-14] it seems important for surgical improvement in the treatment of tendon injuries, especially primary tendon repair, to investigate the distribution pattern of blood vessels in tendons.

MATERIALS AND METHODS

Thirty-eight specimens taken from autopsy and traumatic amputation were examined. The age of the subjects ranged from newborn 10 hours old to 88 years (Table 33-1). After irrigation, diluted India ink–Latex solution was injected using hand syringes and angiocaths, which were inserted into the major arteries (Fig. 33-1). Following formalin fixation, the specimens were dissected under magnification (Fig. 33-2). They were dehydrated in ethanol, cleared in a solution of tricresyl phosphate and tributyl phosphate. Vascular patterns of the tendons were studied and photographed by transillumination (Fig. 33-3). Injuries to the tendons were made with a wire before irrigation.[10,11]

RESULTS

In the flexor digitorum profundus tendon, two separate vascular systems are confirmed. The proximal vascular system, which is supplied by palmar longitudinal channels and vessels of synovial reflection, runs proximal to the base of the proximal phalanx. Distal to the base of the proximal phalanx, the distal vascular system is observed, which is derived from long and short vincula. The distal vascular system is mainly located at the dorsal portion of the flexor profundus tendon, although the proximal system is mainly situated at the volar-central portion of the tendon. In addition, volar portion was avascular in the distal vascular system. Therefore shifting of vessels between these longitudinal vascular systems is recognized at the base of the proximal phalanx (Fig. 33-4). Fig. 33-5 shows the scheme of

Table 33-1. Age distribution of specimens: 38 hands (Jefferson Medical College and Shinshu University School of Medicine)

Age	No. of specimens
0-10	7
11-20	1
21-30	3
31-40	1
41-50	2
51-60	7
61-88	17

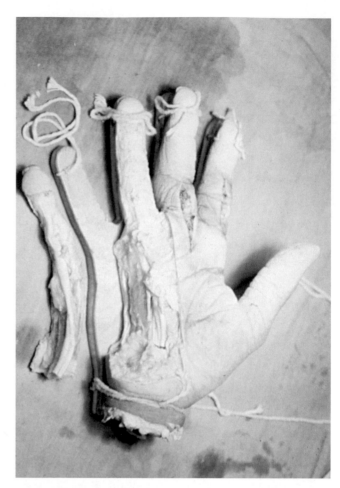

Fig. 33-2. Dissection under magnification.

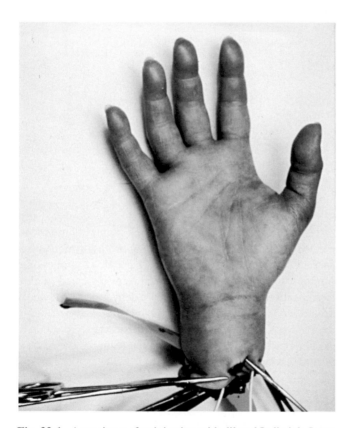

Fig. 33-1. A specimen after injection with diluted India ink–Latex solution.

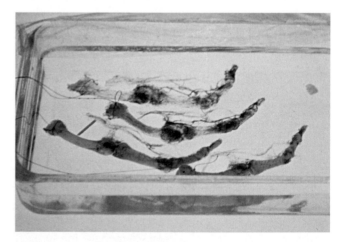

Fig. 33-3. Specimens in the clear solution.

profundus tendon blood vessel arrangement; shifting of the vessels is seen. In the distal vascular system, the volar portion is avascular.

Following ligation of the short vinculum of the superficialis tendon with a wire, a pronounced avascular change is noticed in the profundus tendon (Fig. 33-6). Ligation of both superficialis tendon slips proximal to Camper's chiasm, however, does not affect vessels in the long vincula of the profundus tendon, and consequently no vascular change occurs in the profundus tendon (Fig. 33-7). These findings indicate that an optimal level of excision of the superficialis

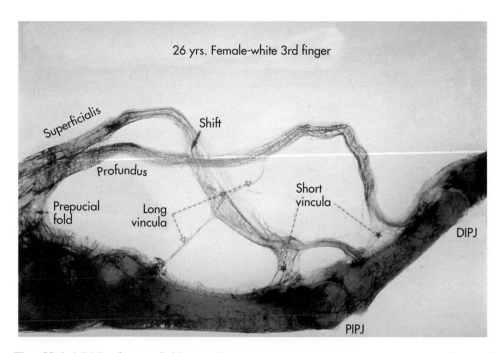

Fig. 33-4. Middle finger of 26-year-old woman. An arrow shows crossover (shifting) of intratendinous longitudinal blood vessels of profundus tendon.

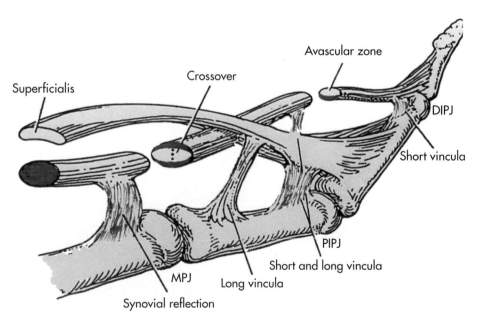

Fig. 33-5. Blood vessel arrangement of profundus tendon.

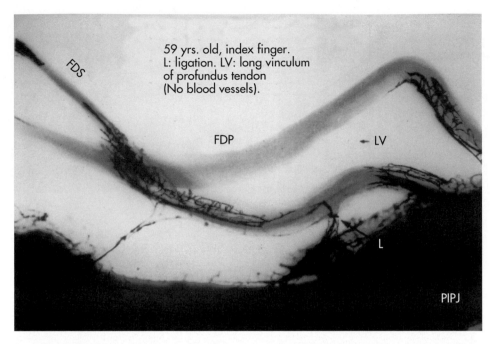

Fig. 33-6. Index finger of 59-year-old man. *L*, Ligation of short vinculum of profundus tendon.

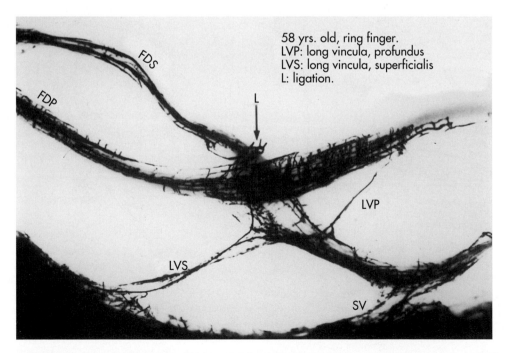

Fig. 33-7. Ring finger of 58-year-old man. *L*, Ligation of superficialis tendon near bifurcation; *LVS,* long vinculum of superficialis tendon; *LVP,* long vinculum of profundus tendon.

88 yrs. Female-white 5th finger

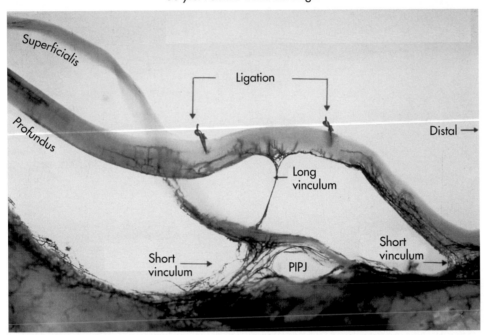

Fig. 33-8. Little finger of 88-year-old woman. *L,* Ligation of profundus tendon at volar portion.

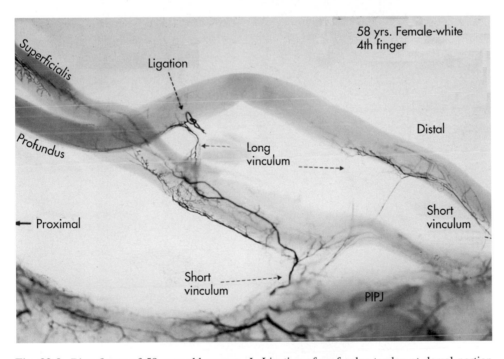

Fig. 33-9. Ring finger of 58-year-old woman. *L,* Ligation of profundus tendon at dorsal portion.

tendon, if necessary, should be proximal to Camper's chiasm to preserve blood vessels of the profundus tendon.

Volarly placed partial ligation of the profundus tendon has the minimum effect on blood vessels, which are mainly situated dorsally in the distal vascular system of the tendon (Fig. 33-8). Dorsally placed ligation interrupts vascular channels of the tendon and produces avascular segment of the tendon (Fig. 33-9). Therefore a main suture should be placed volarly in the profundus tendon when an end-to-end suture is attempted in clinical practice.

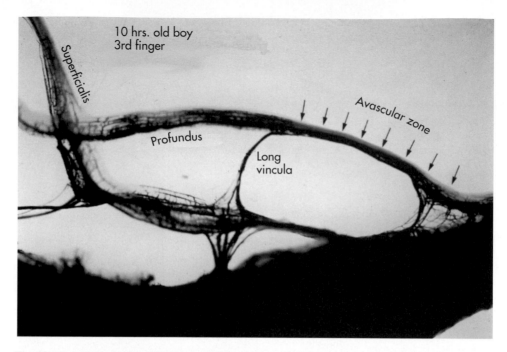

Fig. 33-10. Middle finger of 10-hours-old boy. Arrows indicate avascular zone of profundus tendon.

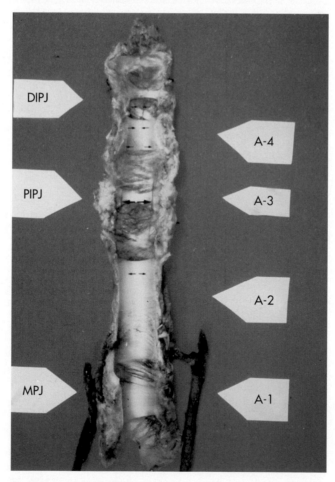

Fig. 33-11. Digital fibrous tendon sheaths observed from dorsal aspect. A-1 to A-4: pulleys. *MPJ,* Metacarpophalangeal joint; *PIPJ,* proximal interphalangeal joint; *DIPJ,* distal interphalangeal joint. Arrows on pulleys show linear impression of profundus tendon in fibrous tendon sheath.

DISCUSSION AND SUMMARY

According to previous reports, an avascular zone was uniformly recognized at the volar portion of the long flexor tendons in the fibrous tendon sheath.[1,7] On the other hand, our study demonstrated that the volar avascular zone is confined to the distal vascular system (Fig. 33-10). Now, when one views a fibrous tendon sheath from its dorsal aspect, distinct striae are seen running longitudinally from the distal interphalangeal joint up to the middle of the proximal phalanx. These striae are notches caused by the flexor profundus tendon, and they coincide quite well with the avascular zone of the tendon (Fig. 33-11). These facts are considered to provide a mechanical basis for avascularity at the volar portion of the tendon. As to the optimal level at which the flexor digitorum superficialis tendon is to be excised, the level proximal to Camper's chiasm is recommended for excision in order to not disturb vascular distribution of the profundus tendon.

Volarly placed partial ligation of the flexor profundus tendon at a point between the base of the proximal phalanx and the short vinculum had no significant influence on the intratendinous vascularization of the tendon, because this area is supplied by dorsally located longitudinal vessels. Therefore a core suture should be placed on the volar side of the profundus tendon when an end-to-end suture is attempted in clinical practice.

REFERENCES

1. Brockies JG: The blood supply of the flexor and extensor tendons of the fingers in man, *J Bone Joint Surg* 1953; 35B:131.
2. Caplan HS, Hunter JM, Merklin RJ: Intrinsic vascularization of flexor tendons. In American Academy of Orthopaedic Surgeons: *Symposium on tendon surgery in the hand*, St Louis, 1975, Mosby.
3. Garner WL, McDonald JA, Kuhn III C, Weeks PM: Autonomous healing of chicken flexor tendons *in vitro*, *J Hand Surg* 1988; 13A:697.
4. Gelberman RH, Manske PR, Vande Berg JS, et al: Flexor tendon repair *in vitro*: a comparative histologic study of the rabbit, chicken, dog, and monkey, *J Orthop Res* 1984; 2:39.
5. Lister GD, Kleinert HE, Kutz JE, Atasoy E: Primary flexor tendon repair followed by immediate controlled mobilization, *J Hand Surg* 1977; 2:441.
6. Lundborg G, Rank F: Experimental intrinsic healing of flexor tendons based upon synovial fluid nutrition, *J Hand Surg* 1978; 3:21.
7. Lundborg G, Myrhage R, Rydevik B: The vascularization of human flexor tendons within the digital synovial sheath region: structural and functional aspects, *J Hand Surg* 1977; 2:417.
8. Mass DP, Tuel RJ: Intrinsic healing of the laceration site in human superficialis flexor tendon *in vitro*, *J Hand Surg* 1991; 16A:24.
9. Matsuda S: A study on cell proliferation in cultured human tendons: time dependence, and labeling of 5-bromodeoxyuridine, *J Jpn Orthop Assoc* 1994; 68:961.
10. Matsui T, Merklin RJ, Hunter JM: A microvascular study of the human flexor tendons in the digital fibrous sheath: normal blood vessel arrangement of tendons and the effects of injuries to tendon and vincula on distribution of tendon blood vessels, *J Jpn Orthop Assoc* 1979; 53:307.
11. Matsui T, Jaeger SH, Merklin RJ, Hunter JM: Effect of injury to tendons and vincula on the vascular system of flexor tendons. In Hunter JM, Schneider LH, Mackin EJ, eds: *Tendon surgery in the hand,* St Louis, 1987, Mosby.
12. Matsui T, Hunter JM: The effects of aging and variations in vincula on flexor tendon vascularization. In Tubiana R, ed: *The hand,* vol 3, Philadelphia, 1988, Saunders.
13. Ochiai N, Matsui T, Miyaji N, et al: Vascular anatomy of flexor tendons. 1. Vincular system and blood supply of the profundus tendon in the digital sheath, *J Hand Surg* 1979; 4:321.
14. Smith JW: Blood supply of tendons, *Am J Surg* 1965; 109:272.
15. Verdan CE: Half a century of flexor tendon surgery, *J Bone Joint Surg* 1972; 54A:472.

Chapter 34

TENDON HEALING
Molecular and cellular regulation

Michael E. Joyce
Jueren Lou
Paul R. Manske

Flexor tendon injury is common and often results in disability. Improvements in operative and rehabilitation techniques have advanced treatment; however, many repairs continue to fail from either a rupture at the tendon anastomosis site or by the formation of restrictive adhesions. Gene therapy, cellular biology, molecular biology, and genetic engineering are the tools that will be used in the decades ahead to advance tendon healing and to improve hand function in our patients with this devastating injury.

In comparison with chapters discussing the clinical and surgical management of tendon healing, this chapter provides a scientific foundation for tendon healing. An in-depth understanding of the complex cascade of cellular and molecular events that govern tendon healing is essential in the design and implementation of any clinical program. After decades of progress in surgery and rehabilitation, this advanced scientific foundation will lead to new treatments of injured tendons in the decades ahead.

This chapter explores both tendon healing and adhesion formation, the two principal biologic responses comprising tendon repair. For each process, significant molecular and cellular events are described in detail. In addition, the role of a powerful group of regulatory proteins called growth factors is discussed. These peptides regulate cellular proliferation and differentiation, inflammation, and matrix synthesis during tendon healing. In addition to understanding the role of growth factors during tendon healing, genetic engineering can synthesize growth factors for potential pharmacologic use in the treatment of tendon

healing. To comprehend how growth factors could be used to improve tendon healing and to prevent adhesion formation, a scientific understanding of molecular and cellular regulation is essential.

MOLECULAR AND CELLULAR REGULATION

Injury to a tendon results in a predictable and inevitable cascade of cellular and molecular events that are initiated by the release of platelet alpha granule regulatory proteins into the injury hematoma. Cellular events that characterize an injury response are similar for all injured tissues and include cellular proliferation and migration, the synthesis of a new matrix, and the organization of that matrix into complete specialized tissue. The cellular and molecular regulation of adhesion formation is governed by the same fundamental concepts as the regulation of tendon healing. Understanding these fundamental cellular and molecular pathways is the first step toward understanding tendon healing.

Tendon healing is composed of a limited number of different cell types: tenocytes, epitenocytes, tendon sheath fibroblasts, capillary endothelial cells, and inflammatory cells. Whereas most cells have specialized roles that contribute to the overall repair process, some cells can contribute to pathologic healing responses. For example, when tendon sheath fibroblasts are stimulated by the same regulatory proteins that control the repair process, they respond with adhesion formation, which hinders the repair process. Other cells, such as inflammatory cells, are beneficial at the initiation of the repair process, but if they

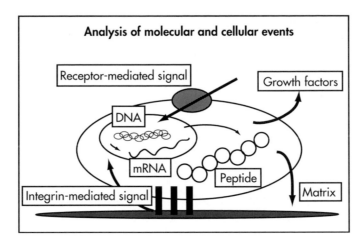

Fig. 34-1. Analysis of molecular and cellular events. Cellular function is regulated by several mechanisms including receptor-mediated and integrin-mediated signals. The cell responds to these signals with the transcription of specific genes into mRNA, which can be measured experimentally by northern analysis. This newly synthesized mRNA is then translated into its corresponding polypeptide, which can be measured and localized with polyclonal or monoclonal antibody immunohistochemistry.

persist too long after the initial injury, they become detrimental to successful tendon healing.

The molecules involved in the repair process can be divided into three general categories. *Adhesion molecules,* termed *integrins,* are polypeptides that allow cells to bind and interact with their extracellular matrix. In addition to attaching cells to their matrix, integrins also transduce cellular regulatory signals that can alter cellular function. The second category is *matrix molecules,* such as type I collagen, in combination with many other proteins and proteoglycans, these molecules form the actual substance of the tendon itself. The third group is *growth factors.* These polypeptides are synthesized in situ by tendon cells, released from the injury hematoma, and secreted from surrounding inflammatory cells. Growth factors are extremely potent polypeptides that regulate all cellular function and thereby control the entire healing process.

There are more than 100 known growth factors; however, the number that are important in tendon healing is limited. While the entire list of pertinent growth factors is still incomplete, this chapter focuses on three specific factors that are central to tendon healing. These are transforming growth factor-β (TGF-β), basic fibroblast growth factor (bFGF), and platelet-derived growth factor (PDGF). More important than the specific growth factors discussed here are the actual principles that govern how growth factors regulate complex processes such as tendon healing.

ANALYSIS OF MOLECULAR AND CELLULAR EVENTS

The study of molecular and cellular regulation has advanced greatly during the past decade. A multitude of new investigative tools allows for a more specific analysis of

molecular and cellular events. To understand how these tools are used to study tendon healing, some background on genetic regulation is essential. Cell function is regulated by signals received from either cell-surface receptors or from the integrins that bind the cell to its surrounding extracellular matrix (Fig. 34-1). Extracellular growth factors bind these receptors and stimulate the cell to carry out specific functions. This is accomplished within the cell by the regulation of specific genes.

The turning on and off of different genes is how complex cascades, such as tendon healing, are regulated. For example, a growth factor will bind to a cell-surface receptor stimulating the cell to make collagen. In response to this receptor the cell will "turn on" the gene for collagen through a process called transcription. Here, the cell transcribes collagen DNA into mRNA. It is the mRNA that is translated through a separate process into the actual collagen polypeptide. Individual collagen peptides are subsequently assembled into large and complex collagen matrix molecules. This process of gene regulation is identical for every new protein that is made during the tendon healing process.

Experimentally, the mRNA for important proteins can be measured during tendon healing with a process called *northern analysis.* This technique allows one to see when different genes for various proteins are turned on during tendon repair. Using an animal model for tendon healing, we used northern analysis to determine how the genes for collagen, integrin, and various growth factors are regulated during the repair process. In experiments described later, immunohistochemistry was used to localize the proteins made by these genes to specific cells, at specific time points, during tendon repair.

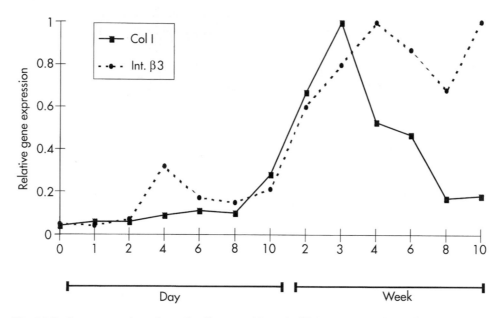

Fig. 34-2. Gene expression of type I collagen and integrin-β3. Northern analysis of type I collagen and integrin-β3 during the course of in vivo tendon healing. Each time point is the pooled mRNA from at least six separate specimens. Quantification was determined by densimetric scanning of the exposed radiograph.

THE REGULATION OF GROWTH FACTORS, COLLAGEN, AND INTEGRIN DURING TENDON HEALING

An initial series of experiments were designed to determine the gene expression of several proteins essential to tendon healing. Using an established in vivo tendon healing model, the following study was undertaken. White Leghorn chickens sustained a surgical 50% laceration of their flexor tendon in zone II of their long limb. Their injured leg was placed in a soft dressing, and the animals were allowed unrestricted cage activity. Beginning with 1 noninjured tendon, then injured tendons daily for 2 weeks, and weekly for 3 months, 6 chickens at each time point were killed for analysis. The injured tendon and 5 mm of surrounding tendon callus were harvested and underwent mRNA extraction and subsequent northern analysis.

The gene expression of type I collagen increased 7 to 10 days after tendon injury, peaked at 3 weeks, and continued at high levels for a total of 6 weeks after injury (Fig. 34-2). It is interesting to compare the gene expression of collagen with the cell membrane adhesion protein integrin-β3. An important function of this protein is to attach tendon cells to their surrounding extracellular matrix. Integrin transmits regulatory information from the surrounding extracellular matrix to the cell. This essential regulatory pathway controls the organization of newly synthesized collagen into the complex tertiary matrix found in mature tendons. Integrin gene expression increased after collagen, with a peak at 4 weeks and continued high levels of expression for 3 months

after injury, long after collagen gene expression had decreased.

TGF-β is a family of four related peptides where TGF-β2 and TGF-β4 have similar function in the regulation of cellular proliferation and differentiation, and the stimulation of matrix synthesis. In contrast, TGF-β3 acts as an antagonist of TGF-β2 and TGF-β4, often fulfilling the function of an "off switch" to the many functions of these growth factors. Understanding the gene regulation of the TGF-βs during tendon healing gives insight into the regulatory mechanisms that govern the repair process.

We found a similar gene expression pattern for TGF-β2 and TGF-β4 with 2 peaks, the first at day 6 and a second larger and longer peak at 2 to 3 weeks (Fig. 34-3). This suggests a role for TGF-β in both the inflammation and matrix synthesis stages of tendon healing. In contrast, TGF-β3 gene expression peaks at a later point, suggesting that its role is down-regulating the functions of TGF-β2 and TGF-β4 and allowing the tendon repair process to come to completion. Whereas gene expression during normal tendon healing is understood, similar studies of abnormal tendon healing, such as in cases with excessive adhesion formation, are currently under way. Here we hope to determine if excessive gene expression of TGF-β4 or decreased gene expression of TGF-β3 is responsible for the excessive matrix synthesis that characterizes adhesion formation.

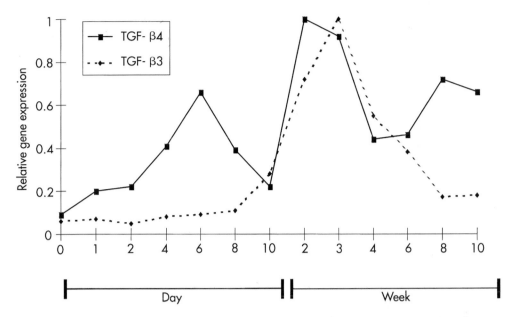

Fig. 34-3. Gene expression of transforming growth factor-β. Northern analysis of TGF-β3 and TGF-β4 during the course of in vivo tendon healing. Each time point is the pooled mRNA from at least six separate specimens. Quantification was determined by densimetric scanning of the exposed radiograph.

CELLULAR LOCALIZATION OF GROWTH FACTORS AND COLLAGEN DURING TENDON HEALING

Following gene expression, the newly synthesized mRNA is translated into its corresponding protein. This processes is controlled by further regulatory mechanisms; therefore, in addition to gene expression, it is also necessary to understand the location of protein synthesis during tendon healing. An in vivo chicken tendon laceration model was designed for this purpose. Here, a 50% surgical laceration of the flexor tendon was made and not repaired. Six animals were harvested for analysis daily for 4 weeks, then 4 animals were harvested weekly for 3 months, for a total of 104 animals. After injury the limbs were immobilized in a soft dressing until the animal was sacrificed for histology and immunohistology. The localization of TGF-β, bFGF, PDGF, and type I collagen was completed with specific polyclonal and monoclonal antibodies and a standard detection system.

A summary of these data gives additional insight into the complex regulation of tendon repair. Growth factor localization was both site and time specific. Immunolocalization of each growth factor showed specific intracellular, extracellular, or matrix patterns. Furthermore, during the repair processes, each growth factor was identified during a restricted time period. These data support the long-contended concept of an intrinsic tendon repair mechanism.

Polyclonal antibody localization of TGF-β showed tremendous amounts of the protein being released from the injury hematoma. This was not restricted to the immediate laceration, but extended for several centimeters along the tendon sheath. Hematoma TGF-β has a likely role in the initiation of the tendon repair process, because it is known to stimulate both cellular proliferation, and the differentiation of epitenon mesenchymal cells into tendon cells. TGF-β is also a potent inducer of matrix synthesis. The presence of TGF-β within the hematoma, away from the immediate tendon laceration, suggests the possibility that TGF-β could also initiate tendon adhesion formation.

Within 4 days of injury, TGF-β2 and TGF-β4 are localized to intracellular tendon cells at the site of repair (Fig. 34-4). Early in the repair process, intrinsic regulation of tendon healing is suggested by the intracellular staining of cells for an important regulatory protein. PDGF was localized within 48 hours of injury, again with an intracellular pattern, but in comparison to TGF-β, PDGF was found mostly within the epitenocytes. Because this protein controls cellular proliferation, it may be working synergistically with TGF-β to initiate the repair process. These findings were in contrast to bFGF, which was localized later in the repair process and always with an extracellular pattern. This peptide was found to accumulate within the newly synthesized tendon matrix for weeks after the injury. The well-described role of bFGF in the regulation of matrix synthesis suggests a similar function in tendon healing with this model.

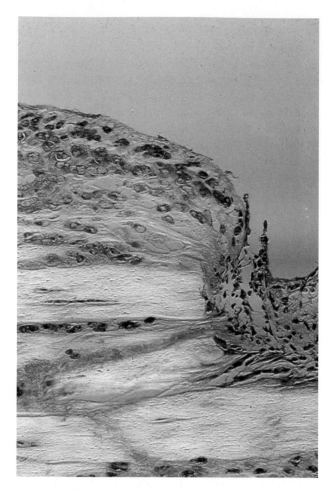

Fig. 34-4. Immunolocalization of transforming growth factor-β during tendon healing. Black stained cells show the polyclonal antibody intracellular localization of TGF-β2 to both tenocytes and epitenocytes at the site of a tendon laceration seven days after injury (original magnification 200×).

SUMMARY
Regulation of tendon healing

The first step in tendon healing (the injury and inflammation stage) is characterized by the formation of an injury hematoma that contains large amounts of TGF-β (Fig. 34-5). Epitenocytes synthesize PDGF, whereas all tenocytes synthesize TGF-β. This stage sees the initiation of cellular proliferation and differentiation but little matrix synthesis. The second step in tendon healing is the matrix synthesis stage. Here there is increased gene expression and synthesis of TGF-β as well as the beginning of bFGF accumulation within the extracellular matrix. Collagen gene expression is rapidly rising, and its synthesis is demonstrated with immunohistology to the injury gap. The gene expression of integrin is just starting in the later part of this stage. Finally, the third step of tendon healing (matrix remodeling) begins. Increased gene expression of the TGF-β antongonist, TGF-β3, initiates the reversal of TGF-β regulatory functions. Increasing expression of integrin corresponds to the

characteristic feature of the stage in the repair process, matrix remodeling. There is decreased gene expression and synthesis of collagen as the new matrix production slows. This final stage continues for months and maybe years after injury.

Regulation of tendon adhesion formation

Having discussed many of the mechanisms that regulate tendon healing, we now ask the question: Do similar mechanisms govern the principal problem faced during tendon repair—the formation of tendon adhesions? The same growth factors that stimulate tendon cells to initiate healing may also be stimulating the tendon sheath fibroblast to follow a similar cascade of cellular proliferation and matrix synthesis, the only difference now being that this process results in the formation of restrictive adhesion. To test this hypothesis we performed a series of in vitro and in vivo experiments analyzing the role of growth factors in tendon adhesion formation.

Previously we showed both the gene expression and local synthesis of several growth factors at both the site of tendon repair and within the tendon sheath. The first hint of the role of growth factors in adhesion formation was found in a series of in vitro tendon sheath experiments that demonstrated a dose dependent stimulation of cellular proliferation and matrix synthesis by TGF-β, bFGF, and PDGF. Taken together, these data suggest that growth factors may stimulate adhesion formation following tendon injury. The need for an in vivo study, designed to show the ability of growth factors to stimulate adhesion formation in the absence of any tendon injury, became apparent. The following experiments were then performed to investigate the effect of exogenous growth factors on the formation of tendon adhesion formation by both histologic and biomechanic analysis.

In the first experiment, 54 white Leghorn chickens were anesthetized before a nontraumatic blunt 27-gauge needle was inserted distal to the distal interphalangeal (DIP) joint and gently advanced, in a retrograde fashion, within the tendon sheath to zone II. Five microliters of growth factor or buffered saline was injected and the limbs were immobilized in a soft dressing. A single 5.0 μl injection distributed along the entire tendon sheath from the metacarpophalangeal (MP) to the DIP joint. Injected limbs were randomized to one of several groups: group I: buffered saline controls, group II: PDGF, group III: TGF-β1, group IV: TGF-β2, group V: TGF-β3, and group VI: bFGF at doses of 100 ng to 10 μg. Animals were killed for histologic analysis 2 or 4 weeks after injection. In the second experiment, 36 chickens were randomized to 4 groups (right limb = experimental, left = sham): group I: TGF-β2 harvested at 2 weeks, group II: TGF-β2 harvested at 6 weeks, group III and group IV were sutured without laceration at 2 and 6 weeks, respectively. At harvest the limbs were tested for work of flexion in a tensile testing machine.

Tendon healing

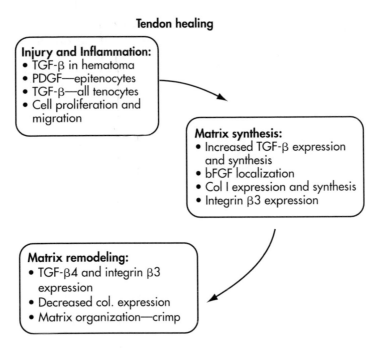

Fig. 34-5. Growth factors and tendon healing. Tendon healing progresses through three principle stages: injury and inflammation, matrix synthesis, and matrix remodeling. During each process growth factors regulate specific cellular function, and the synthesis and remodeling of new tendon extracellular matrix.

In the first experiment, the saline-injected controls demonstrated a varied morphology with only minor areas of epitenon thickening and no adhesions. PDGF injection stimulated mild synovial hyperplasia at low dose, but marked hyperplasia at high dose, whereas a 5.0 μg dose resulted in both the proliferation of tenocytes and mild extracellular matrix synthesis. No adhesions formed as a result of PDGF injection. bFGF injections had a minor effect on the tendon and tendon sheath, and only at higher doses did it stimulate proliferation of epitenocytes and cells lining the tendon sheath; no adhesions were identified. TGF-β1 and TGF-β2, but not TGF-β3 stimulated synovial cell proliferation within the tendon sheath and a moderate thickening of the epitenon cell layer at very low doses (50 ng and 200 ng). At high doses, TGF-β1 and TGF-β2 (1 μg and 5 μg) stimulated tremendous cellular proliferation, throughout the tendon sheath and tendon proper, that was associated with a loss of normal morphology. All TGF-β1 and TGF-β2 injected specimens demonstrated areas of adhesion formation between the tendon and its surrounding sheath, whereas TGF-β3 did not stimulate any adhesion formation. In the second experiment, TGF-β2 injections stimulated time-dependent adhesion formation in nontraumatized tendons. At 2 weeks the work of flexion increased 26%, and at 6 weeks 46% ($p < 0.005$ for both), which compares with a sutured tendon that has a 3- and 2.5-fold increase at 2 and 6 weeks, respectively (Fig. 34-6).

This study was the first to describe a molecular mechanism for the formation of tendon adhesions and builds upon our previous studies that localized the production of endogenous growth factors during tendon healing. The effect of exogenous growth factors, when applied within the tendon sheath, is the specific stimulation of cellular responses that lead to pathologic adhesion formation. While bFGF and PDGF had effects on tendon and synovial cell regulation, they did not stimulate adhesion formation. In contrast, TGF-β1 and TGF-β2, but not TGF-β3 (a known in vivo inhibitor of TGF-β1 and TGF-β2), stimulated the formation of adhesions between the tendon and its surrounding sheath. This effect was dose dependent and specific for TGF-β, suggesting that TGF-β synthesis, following tendon laceration, is an important mechanism for tendon adhesion formation.

Gene therapy in tendon healing

Tendon healing and adhesion formation are the result of a complex cascade of cellular and molecular mechanisms. We demonstrated many of these specific growth factor dependent pathways earlier in this chapter. Having this information is of little practical value unless this knowledge is used to manipulate and improve the healing process or inhibit the formation of adhesions. Through surgery, the direct manipulation of tissue has been possible for decades, however, the biologic response of the tissue to surgery has been beyond our control. Through the rapidly evolving field of gene therapy, this may no longer be the case. For the first time, gene therapy will permit the direct manipulation of cellular and molecular events

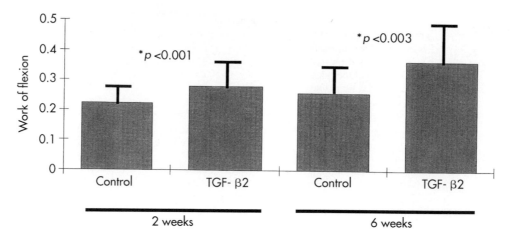

Fig. 34-6. Growth factor stimulation of adhesion formation. Chickens underwent atraumatic injection of 1 μg of TGF-β2 or control into their flexor tendon sheath. The flexor tendons were not injured. Two and six weeks after injection the limbs were harvested and the work of flexion was tested in a tensile testing machine. TGF-β2 stimulated a significant ($p < 0.1$) increase in the work of flexion suggesting the formation of an adhesion.

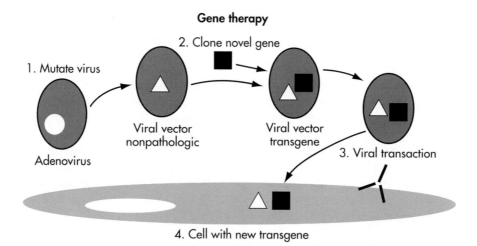

Fig. 34-7. Genetic engineering of a gene therapy vector. *1,* The adenovirus is mutated to delete its pathologic capacity but retain its ability to infect host cells. *2,* A novel gene (or transgene) is cloned into the adenoviral vector. *3,* adenoviral "infection" is allowed to take place within host tissue. The transgene is then transferred to the host cell along with the viral genome. *4,* The host cell will express the transgene and synthesize the coded protein.

the same as surgery permits the direct manipulation of whole tissues.

Gene therapy is defined as the in vivo introduction of genes into the cells that comprise specific tissue. This definition broadly defines many different strategies for inserting the genes into the cells, as well as the very wide range of genes that can be used. As the term *gene therapy* implies, the purpose of transferring genes into the host tissue is to achieve a specific biologic response. Most often the goal is to alter the physiology of the host in a specific way. For example, if a patient is unable to make a certain necessary protein, then the gene for this protein can be

transferred to the appropriate cells, thereby allowing the cells to synthesize the missing protein. In a similar fashion, if a patient produces an abnormal protein that results in a specific disease, gene therapy can allow an inhibitor of this gene to be transferred to the specific tissue, thereby inhibiting the synthesis of the abnormal gene and reversing the disease process.

While many methodologies exist for transferring genes into cells, the method that appears most promising is one that uses a genetically altered virus to infect the host tissue, bind to specific cells, and inject the treatment gene into the target cells. Our laboratory has been using this strategy

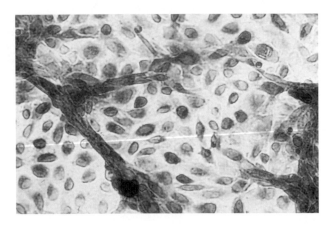

Fig. 34-8. Gene therapy in vitro infection of tendon sheath fibroblasts. Tendon fibroblast cell culture after exposure to an adenoviral gene therapy vector. The transgene b-galactosidase was successfully transferred to 100% of the cells after a single exposure. The black staining indicates cells expressing the transgene after exposure to the enzyme substrate.

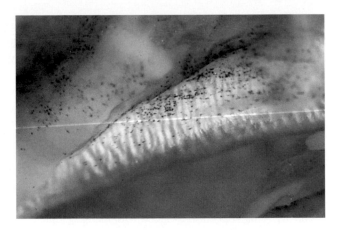

Fig. 34-9. Gene therapy in vivo infection of tendon cells. Whole mount of a chicken flexor tendon and surrounding tendon sheath 4 days after a single in vivo exposure to an adenoviral gene therapy vector with the b-galactosidase transgene. That vector was introduced into the chicken tendon in a single injection beneath the tendon sheath. Black staining indicates cells that are expressing the transgene after exposure to the enzyme substrate.

to develop a gene therapy vector for use in treating tendon injuries. It turns out that the virus of the common cold, adenovirus, is well-suited for gene therapy in tendon tissues. Fig. 34-7 shows the methods used in the construction of an adenovirus gene therapy vector system. First, we mutate the virus to remove its pathologic capacity, but leave its ability to infect unaffected cells. This genetically altered virus does not divide in cells, nor does it kill the cells that it infects; it simply inserts any genes within the virus into the cell.

In the second step, the gene of interest is cloned into the mutated adenovirus vector. That gene could be a new growth factor; it could be the inhibitor of a growth factor; or it could be a matrix protein such as collagen. There are few restrictions on the type of genes used for gene therapy. The gene cloned into the vector virus is called a *transgene*. With the third step, the viral vector is allowed to infect the host or target cells using its normal viral infection mechanisms. The potential host cell range, for treatment with a particular gene therapy virus, is not unlimited; for each vector the target cells must be determined empirically. When the virus infects a cell, the transgene is inserted along with the other viral genes into the host cell, and the forth and final step in the process is complete. The host cell, in our case a tenocyte, will turn on the new gene and synthesize the protein it codes for, thereby allowing the cells to have the new genetically engineered molecular function.

The newly constructed viral vector can then be used in both in vitro experimental tissue culture systems and in vivo animal models of tendon healing and adhesion formation. This ability, to use the same gene therapy vector system when advancing from in vitro to in vivo experimental systems, dramatically enhances the speed and accuracy with which novel gene therapy treatment regimens can be developed.

Our development of a gene therapy vector system for tendon healing began with the construction of an adenoviral vector system with an easily detectable transgene. This necessary first step allows for the determination of the several important parameters in gene therapy. First, it can establish the host range for the vector. Second, the penetration of the vector can be determined. For example, does the vector infect 1% or 90% of the cells in the host tissue? Finally, the detector gene can be used to estimate the stability of the transgene in the host cells. Whether the transgene remains stable for 1 day or 100 days has important implications on how the gene therapy vector can be used therapeutically. In our tendon healing models we used the b-galactosidase transgene, because it turns cells a brilliant blue color when exposed to the substrate. Fig. 34-8 shows the successful in vitro infection of tendon sheath fibroblasts. We then injected 5 µl of this adenoviral vector between the tendon and the tendon sheath, in the same fashion used in earlier experiments. Fig. 34-9 shows stained tendon cells and demonstrates the successful infection of tendon cells with the gene therapy vector. We have determined that this construct remains stable for at least 75 days after a single infection of the gene therapy vector.

This series of experiments opens the door for "molecular surgery." Once important cellular and molecular events during tendon healing are identified, gene therapy gives us the power to intervene and improve the process. We can increase some growth factors or decrease other growth factors. As our knowledge of tendon healing expands, we may soon have the ability to inhibit scar formation and stimulate true tendon regeneration. Gene therapy goes beyond traditional surgery to cellular and molecular surgery and the ability to restore injured tendons to normal.

CONCLUSION

Tendon healing is a complex cascade of cellular proliferation and differentiation, matrix synthesis, and eventual tenocyte-regulated remodeling to complete tendon structure. This process is regulated by growth factors that are released from the hematoma at the time of injury and are then synthesized by local cells during the repair process. In a similar fashion, growth factors also regulate the formation of pathologic tendon adhesions.

As our understanding of the molecular events regulating tendon repair evolves, the ability to manipulate gene expression becomes important both scientifically and therapeutically. This goal was advanced with the development of a genetically engineered adenoviral gene therapy vector. Using a prototype gene, we have successfully performed in vitro and in vivo gene transfer to tenocytes and tendon sheath fibroblasts, and we have demonstrated the retention of a functional gene product for 75 days. The potential to genetically manipulate the molecular regulation of tendon healing and adhesion formation is at hand; advances in our understanding of tendon healing and new treatment options will soon follow.

ACKNOWLEDGMENTS

This work was supported by a grant from Shriner's Hospital.

BIBLIOGRAPHY

Abidi N, Scully SP, Regan J, et al: Acidic FGF gene expression during rat fracture healing determined by quantitative polymerase chain reaction, Transactions of 37th annual meeting of the Orthopedic Research Society, 1991; 438.

Amadio PC, Hunter JM, Jaeger SH, et al: The effect of vincular injury on the results of flexor tendon surgery in zone 2, J Hand Surg 1985; 10A(5):626-632.

Assoian RK, Sporn MB: Type-b transforming growth factor in human platelets: release during platelet degranulation and action on vascular smooth muscle cells, J Cell Biol 1986; 102:1217-1223.

Baird A, Esch F, Mormede P, et al: Molecular characterization of fibroblast growth factor: distribution and biological activities in various tissues, Recent Prog Horm Res 1986; 42:143-205.

Banes AJ, Enterline D, Bevin AG, Salisbury RE: Effects of trauma and partial devascularization on protein synthesis in the avian flexor profundus tendon, J Trauma 1981; 21:505-512.

Braithwaite F, Browckis JG: The vascularization of tendon of the fingers in man, J Bone Joint Surg 1951; 35B:131-138.

Brown GL, Nanney LB, Griffen J, et al: Enhancement of wound healing by topical treatment with epidermal growth factor, N Engl J Med 1989; 321:76-79.

Caplan HS, Hunter JM, Merklin RJ: Intrinsic vascularization of flexor tendons. In Symposium on tendon surgery in the hand, St Louis, 1975, Mosby.

Chirgwin JM, Przybyla RJ, MacDonald RJ, Rutter WJ: Isolation of biologically active ribonucleic acid from sources enriched in ribonuclease, Biochemistry 1979; 18:5294-5299.

Davidson JM, Klagsbrun M, Hill KE, et al: Accelerated wound repair, cell proliferation, and collagen accumulation are produced by a cartilage-derived growth factor, J Cell Bio 1985; 100:1219-1227.

Deuel TF, Huang JS, Huang SS, et al: Expression of a platelet-derived growth factor-like protein in a simian sarcoma virus transformed cells, Science 1983; 221:1348-1352.

Deuel TF, Semior RM, Huang JS, Griffin GL: Chemotaxis of monocytes and neutrophils to platelet-derived growth factor, J Clinical Invest 1982; 69:1046-1049.

Deuel TF: Polypeptide growth factors: roles in normal and abnormal cell growth, Annu Rev Cell Biol 1987; 3:443-492.

Esch R, Baird N, Gospodarowicz D, et al: Primary structure of bovine pituitary bFGF and comparison with the amino-terminal sequence of bovine brain aFGF, Proc Natl Aca Sci USA 1985; 82:6507-6511.

Flanders KC, Thompson NL, Cissel DS, et al: Epitope-dependent immunohistochemical localization of transforming growth factor-b, J Cell Biol 1989; 108:653-660.

Folkman J, Klagsbrun M, Sasse J, et al: A heparin-binding angiogenic protein, basic fibroblast growth factor, is stored within basement membrane, Am J Pathol 1988; 130:393-400.

Folkman J, Klagsbrun M: Angiogenic factors, Science 1987; 235:442-447.

Froger-Gaillard B, Charrier AM, Thenet S, et al: Growth-promoting effects of acidic and basic fibroblast growth factor on rabbit articular chondrocytes aging in culture, Exper Cell Res 1989; 183:388-398.

Furlow LT: The role of tendon tissues in tendon healing, Plastic Reconst Surg 1976; 57:39-49.

Gelberman RH, Manske PR, Vande Berg JS, Lesker PA: Flexor tendon repair in vitro: a comparative histologic study of the rabbit, chicken, dog, and monkey, J Orthop Res 1984; 2:39-48.

Grotendorst GR, Martin GR, Pancev E, et al: Stimulation granulation tissue formation by platelet-derived growth factor in normal and diabetic rats, J Clin Invest 1985; 76:2323-2329.

Heine UI, Munos EF, Flanders KC, et al: Role of transforming growth factor-b in the development of the mouse embryo, J Cell Biol 1987; 105:2861-2876.

Heldin CH, Johnsson A, Wennergren S, et al: A human osteosarcoma cell line secretes a growth factor structurally related to a homodimer of PDGF A-chains, Nature 1986; 319:511-514.

Hooper G, Davies R, Tuthill P: Blood flow and clearance in tendons, J Bone Joint Surg 1984; 66B:441-443.

Ingber DE, Folkman J: Mechanochemical switching between growth and differentiation during fibroblast growth factor-stimulated angiogenesis in vitro: role of extracellular matrix, J Cell Biol 1990; 109:317-330.

Joyce ME, Terek RM, Jingushi S, Bolander ME: Role of transforming growth factor-b in fracture repair. In Transforming growth factor-b's chemistry, biology, therapeutics, Ann New York Acad Sci 1990; 593:107-123.

Joyce ME, Jingushi S, Scully SP, Bolander ME: Role of growth factors in fracture repair. In Clinical and experimental approaches to dermal and epidermal repair: normal and chronic wounds, New York, 1991, Wiley-Liss.

Joyce ME, Heydemann A, Bolander ME: Platelet-derived growth factor regulates the initiation of fracture repair, Ortho Trans 1990; 14(2):460-462.

Joyce ME, Jingushi S, Bolander ME: Transforming growth factor-b in the regulation of fracture repair. In Lane J, ed: Orthopaedic clinics of North America—pathologic fractures in metabolic bone disease, Philadelphia, 1990, Saunders.

Joyce ME, Roberts AB, Sporn MB, Bolander ME: Transforming growth factor-b gb and the initiation of chondrogenesis and osteogenesis in the rat femur, J Cell Biol 1990; 110:2195-2207.

Joyce ME, Scully SP, Flanders K, et al: Differential expression and synthesis of TGF-β1 and TGF-β2 in human and rat fracture healing, Anaheim, CA, 1991, Orthop Res Soc.

Kleinert HE, Kutz JE, Ashbell TS, Martinez E: Primary repair of lacerated flexor tendons in "No Man's Land," J Bone Joint Surg 1967; 49A:577.

Katsumi M, Tajima T: Experimental investigation of healing process of tendons with or without synovial coverage in or outside of the synovial cavity, J Niigata Med Assoc 1981; 95:532-567.

Labarka A, Paigen K: A simple, rapid, and sensitive DNA assay procedure, Ann Biochem 1980; 102:344-352.

Landi A, Elves M, Piagge W: The blood flow of rabbits' tendons: variation with age, activity and hypoxia, *Acta Orthop Scand* 1983; 54:832-835.

Landi AP, Altman FP, Pringle J, et al: Oxidative enzyme metabolism in rabbit intrasynovial flexor tendons, II, studies of nutritional pathways, *J Surg Res* 1980; 29:281-286.

Leffert RD, Weiss C, Athanasoulis CA: The vincula: with particular reference to their vessels and nerves, *J Bone Joint Surg* 1974; 56A:1191-1198.

Lindsay WK, Thomson HG: Digital flexor tendons: an experimental study, part I, the significance of each component of the flexor mechanism in tendon healing, *Brit J Plastic Surg* 1960; 12:289-319.

Lindsay WK, Thomson HG, Walker FG: Digital flexor tendons: an experimental study, part II, the significance of a gap occurring at the line of suture, *Brit J Plastic Surg* 1960; 13(1):1-9.

Lindsay WK, McDougall EP: Digital flexor tendons: an experimental study, part III, the fate of autogenous digital flexor tendon grafts, *Brit J Plastic Surg* 1961; 13(4):293-304.

Lindsay WK, Birch JR: The fibroblast in flexor tendon healing, *Plastic Reconst Surg* 1964; 34:223-232.

Lundborg G, Rank F: Experimental intrinsic healing of flexor tendons based upon synovial fluid nutrition, *J Hand Surg* 1978; 3(1):21-31.

Lundborg F, Holm S, Myrhage R: The role of the synovial fluid and tendon sheath for flexor tendon nutrition: an experimental tracer study on diffusional pathways in dogs, *Scand J Plastic Reconst Surg* 1980; 14:99-107.

Lundborg G: Experimental flexor tendon healing without adhesion formation—a new concept of tendon nutrition and intrinsic healing mechanisms, a preliminary report, *Hand* 1975; 8(3):235-238.

Lundborg G, Hansson HA, Rank F, Rydevik B: Superficial repair of severed flexor tendons in synovial environment—an experimental study on cellular mechanisms, *J Hand Surg* 1980; 5(5):451-461.

Manske PR, Bridwell K, Lesker PA: Nutrient pathways to flexor tendons of chickens using tritiated proline, *J Hand Surg* 1978; 3(4):352-357.

Manske PR, Bridwell K, Whiteside LA, Lesker PA: Nutrition of flexor tendon in monkeys, *Clin Orthop Rel Res* 1978; 136:294-298.

Manske PR, Lesker PA, Bridwell K: Experimental studies in chickens on the initial nutrition of tendon grafts, *J Hand Surg* 1979; 4(6):565-575.

Manske PR, Lesker PA: Nutrient pathways of flexor tendons in primates, *J Hand Surg* 1982; 7(5):436-447.

Manske PR, Gelberman RH, Vandeberg JS, Lesker PA: Intrinsic flexor tendon repair: a morphological study in vitro, *J Bone Joint Surg* 1984; 66A:385-396.

Manske PR, Lesker PA: Histologic evidence of intrinsic flexor tendon repair in various experimental animals: an in vitro study, *Clin Orthop Rel Res* 1984; 182:297-304.

Manske PR, Lesker PA, Gelberman RH, Rucinsky TE: Intrinsic restoration of the flexor tendon surface in the non-human primate, *J Hand Surg* 1985; 10A(5):620-637.

Manske PR, Lesker PA: Comparative nutrient pathways to the flexor profundus tendons in zone II of various experimental animals, *J Surg Res* 1983; 34:83-93.

Matthews P: The fate of isolated segments of flexor tendons within the digital sheath: a study in synovial nutrition, *Brit J Plastic Surg* 1976; 29:216-224.

Matthews P, Richards H: The repair potential of digital flexor tendons: an experimental study, *J Bone Joint Surg* 1974; 56B:618-625.

Matthews P, Richards H: The repair of flexor tendons within the digital sheath, *Hand* 1975; 7:27-29.

McDowell CL, Snyder DM: Tendon healing: an experimental model in the dog, *J Hand Surg* 1977; 2:122-126.

Morales TI, Joyce ME, Sobel ME, et al: Transforming growth factor-b in calf articular cartilage organ cultures: synthesis and distribution, *J Biophysiol Biochem* 1991; 288(2):397-405.

Morales TI, Wahl LM, Hascal VC: Correlated metabolism of proteoglycan and hyaluronic acid in bovine cartilage explant cultures, *J Biol Chem* 1989; 263:3632-3638.

Mustoe TA, Pierce GF, Thomason A, et al: Accelerated healing on incisional wounds in rats induced by transforming growth factor-b, *Science* 1987; 234:1333-1335.

Nemeth GG, Bolander ME: Isolation and analysis of ribonucleic acids from skeletal tissues, *Anal Biochem* 1990; 183:301-305.

Peacock EE: A study of the circulation in normal tendons and healing grafts, *Ann Surg* 1959; 149:415-428.

Peacock EE: Fundamental aspects of wound healing relating to the restoration of gliding function after tendon repair, *Surg Gyn Obst* 1964; 119:241-250.

Peacock EE: Biological principles in the healing of long tendons, *Surg Clin N Am* 1965; 45(2):461-476.

Peterson WW, Manske PR, Bollinger BA, et al: Effect of pulley excision on flexor tendon biomechanics, *J Ortho Res* 1986; 4:96-101.

Peterson WW, Manske PR, Dunlap J, et al: The effect of various methods of restoring flexor sheath integrity on the formation of adhesions following tendon injury, *J Hand Surg* 1990; 15A:48-56.

Peterson WW, Manske PR, Kain CC, Lesker PA: Effect of flexor sheath integrity on tendon gliding—a biomechanical and histologic study, *J Orthop Res* 1986; 4:458-465.

Pierce GF, Mustoe TA, Senior RM, et al: In vivo incisional wound healing augmented by platelet-derived growth factor and recombinant c-sis gene homodimeric proteins, *J Exp Med* 1988; 167:874-987.

Pierce GF, Mustoe TA, Lingelbach J, Masakowsk VRI, Griffin GL, Senior RM, Deuel TF: Platelet-derived growth factor and transforming growth factor-b enhance tissue repair activities by a unique mechanism, *J Cell Biol* 1989; 109:429-440.

Postletwaite AE, Keski-Oja J, Moses HL, et al: Stimulation of the chemotactic migration of human fibroblasts by transforming growth factor-β, *J Exp Med* 1987; 165:251-256.

Potenza AD: Critical evaluation of flexor tendon healing and adhesion formation within artificial digital sheaths, *J Bone Joint Surg* 1963; 45A:1217-1233.

Potenza AD: Tendon healing within the flexor digital sheath in dog, *J Bone Joint Surg* 1962; 44A:49-64.

Potenza AD: Prevention of adhesions to healing digital flexor tendons, *JAMA* 1964; 187(3):99-103.

Potenza AD: Mechanisms of healing of digital flexor tendons, *Hand* 1969; 1(1):40-41.

Rifkin DB, Moscatelli D: Recent developments in the cell biology of basic fibroblast growth factor, *J Cell Biol* 1989; 109:1-6.

Roberts AB, Sporn MB: The transforming growth factor-bs. In Sporn MB, Roberts AB, eds: *Peptide growth factors and their receptors,* Heidelberg, 1991, Springer-Verlag.

Roberts AB, Sporn MB, Assoian RK, et al: Transforming growth factor type b: rapid induction of fibrosis and angiogenesis in vivo and stimulation of collagen formation in vitro, *Proc Natl Acad Sci USA* 1986; 83:4167-4171.

Roberts AB, Anzano MA, Smith JM, et al: Transforming growth factor-b, *Proc Natl Acad Sci USA* 1990; 78:5339-5343.

Rosen DM, Stempien SA, Thompson AY, Seyedin SM: Transforming growth factor-b modulates the expression of osteoblast and chondrocyte phenotypes in vitro, *J Cell Physiol* 1988; 134:337-346.

Rosen DM, Stempien SA, Seyedin SM: Differentiation of rat mesenchymal cells by cartilage-inducing factor, *Exper Cell Res* 1986; 165:127-138.

Ross R, Raines EW, Bowen-Pope DF: The biology of platelet-derived growth factor, *Cell* 1986; 46:155-169.

Ross R: Peptide regulatory factors: platelet-derived growth factor, *Lancet* 1989; May:1179-1182.

Russell JE, Manske PR: Biochemical evaluation of organ cultures from primate flexor tendons, *Con Tissue Res* 1989; 23:51-64.

Russell JE, Manske PR: Collagen synthesis during primate flexor tendon repair in vitro, *J Orthop Res* 1990; 8:13-20.

Saike RK, Gelfand DH, Stoffel S, et al: Primer-directed enzymatic amplification of DNA with a thermostable DNA polymerase, *Science* 1988; 239:487-491.

Schepel SJ: Intrinsic healing flexor tendons in primates. In Hunter JM, Scheider LH, Mackin E, eds: *Tendon surgery of the hand,* St Louis, 1987, Mosby.

Scully SP, Joyce ME, Abidi N, Bolander ME: The use of polymerase chain reaction generated nucleotide sequences as probes for hybridization, *Molecular and Cellular Probes,* 1990; 4:485-495.

Senior RM, Griffin GL, Huang JS, et al: Chemotactic activity of platelet alpha granule proteins for fibroblasts, *J Cell Bio* 1983; 96:382-385.

Seyedin PR, Segarini PR, Rosen DM, et al: Cartilage-inducing factor-b is a unique protein structurally and functionally related to transforming growth factor-b, *J Bio Chem* 1987; 262:1946-1949.

Seyedin SM, Thomas TC, Thompson AY, et al: Purification and characterization of two cartilage-inducing factors from bovine demineralized bone, *Proc Natl Acad Sci USA* 1985; 82:2267-2271.

Seyedin SM, Thompson AY, Bentz H, et al: Cartilage-inducing factor-A, *J Bio Chem* 1986; 261:5693-5695.

Sporn MB, Roberts AB, Wakefield LM, Assoian RK: Transforming growth factor-b: biological function and chemical structure, *Science* 1986; 233:532-534.

Sporn MB, Roberts AB, Wakefield LM, de Crombrugghe B: Some recent advances in the chemistry and biology of transforming growth factor-b, *J Cell Bio* 1987; 105:1039-1045.

Sporn MB, Roberts AB: Peptide growth factors are multifunctional, *Nature* 1988; 332:217-219.

Sporn MB, Roberts AB, Wakefield IM: Some recent advances in the chemistry and biology of transforming growth factor-b, *J Cell Bio* 1987; 105:1039-1045.

Sprugel KH, McPherson JM, Clowes AW, Ross R: Effects of growth factors in vivo, I, cell ingrowth into porous subcutaneous chambers, *Am J Pathol* 1987; 129:601-613.

Thompson NL, Flanders KC, Smith JM, et al: Cell type specific expression of transforming growth factor-b1 in adult and neonatal mouse tissue, *J Cell Bio* 1989; 108:661-669.

Verdan C: Primary repair of flexor tendons, *J Bone Joint Surg* 1960; 42A:647-657.

Vigny M, Ollier-Hartmann MP, Lavigne M, et al: Specific binding of basic fibroblast growth factor to basement membrane-like structures and to purified heparin sulfate proteoglycans of the EHS tumor, *J Cell Physiol* 1988; 137:321-328.

Wahl SM, Hunt DA, Wakefield IM, et al: Transforming growth factor-b induces monocyte chemotaxis and growth factor production, *Proc Natl Acad Sci USA* 1987; 84:5788-5792.

Young L, Weeks PM: Profundus tendon blood supply within the digital sheath, *Surg Forum* 1971; 21:504.

Chapter 35

TENDON HEALING
Cellular turnover and matrix metabolism

Sven-Olof Abrahamsson

The movement and nutrition of the flexor tendons within the phalanges of the hand is made possible by an intricate arrangement of the tendons and the surrounding tissues. From the level of the metacarpophalangeal (MP) joints to the insertions on the distal phalanges, the flexor tendons are enveloped by a thin and double-walled tendon sheath, creating a synovial cavity. The intrasynovial part of the flexor tendon is partly nourished by a dorsal vascular arrangement, the vincular system, and partly by diffusion from the synovial fluid. Injuries within this region create major problems, because adhesions form between the tendon and its surrounding tissues. This process adversely affects the functional results of surgical repair but has nevertheless been claimed to be essential for a successful healing of the tendon injury.

Flexor tendons may also, however, be nourished by diffusion from the surrounding synovial fluid, and they have been suggested to possess an intrinsic capability for healing. This would, in principle, make it possible for the tendon to heal without the usual invasion by vessels and connective tissue cells via adhesions, thereby avoiding the detrimental effects of the latter.

The matrix of tendons is composed of collagens, proteoglycans, and glycoproteins. These matrix components are synthesized by the resident tendon cells, both under normal conditions and during the healing process. During healing, tendon cells proliferate, differentiate, and migrate. Growth factors, either circulating or locally produced, could affect cell proliferation and matrix metabolism, as has been shown for cartilage and other connective tissues.

To improve the clinical outcome of tendon surgery, we need to better understand the regulation of the cellular and metabolic events involved in tendon healing. Since 1987 I have performed a series of experiments in vivo and in vitro designed to illuminate the following questions:

1. Can flexor tendon segments be cultured in vivo in a chamber where nutrition is based only on diffusion of interstitial tissue fluid, and do such segments show signs of intrinsic healing under these conditions?
2. Can endotenon cells proliferate and restore the smooth surface of a flexor tendon segment during culture in a diffusion chamber?
3. What are the morphologic, biochemical, and metabolic differences between the various segments of the synovial flexor tendon?
4. What is the response of cultured flexor tendon segments to serum, insulin, and recombinant insulin-like growth factor-I (rhIGF-I) with respect to matrix synthesis and cell proliferation?
5. What are the consequences on flexor tendon metabolism of long-term culture in medium supplemented with rhIGF-I? Can serum be replaced by rhIGF-I?
6. What are the effects of brief dehydration of the flexor tendon on matrix metabolism and cell proliferation?

EXPERIMENTAL MODELS

New Zealand white rabbits of both sexes, weighing 2.5 to 3.5 kg, were used as experimental animals. Intrasynovial flexor tendon segments between the MP and proximal interphalangeal (PIP) joints and of the forepaws or back paws were harvested for culture in vivo or in vitro.

In vivo, one tendon segment was placed in a chamber, with a plastic ring with Millipore-membranes (pore size 0.3 μm) pasted with silicon glue on both sides.[2] After closure,

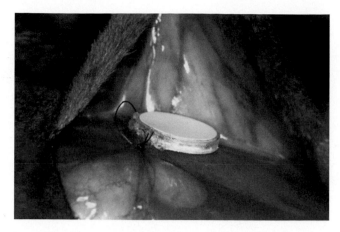

Fig. 35-1. The diffusion chamber, a plastic ring (14 mm in diameter, 2 mm in height) covered on both sides with a Millipore membrane (pore size 0.3 μm) pasted with silicone glue, sutured subcutaneously on the back of a rabbit.

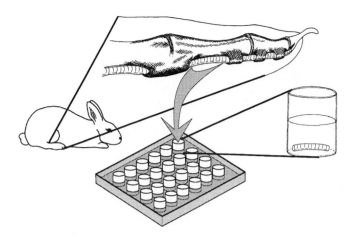

Fig. 35-2. Tendon segments, placed one segment per well, in a 24-dish plate.

the chambers were sutured subcutaneously on the back of the rabbit and tendons were cultured for various periods of time (Fig. 35-1).

In vitro, the tendon segments were placed, one segment per well, in multidish plates and cultured in gentamicin, ascorbic acid, and bovine serum albumin supplemented MCDB 105 medium (Fig. 35-2).[1] Following 1 day of culture, the medium was replaced by fresh, supplemented medium containing serum or a stimulating factor. Tendons were labeled on the third day with ^{3}H-proline and ^{35}S-sulfate or ^{3}H-thymidine. On the fourth day, tendon segments were rinsed once and chase incubated twice. In long-term cultures, the supplemented medium was replaced by fresh medium every second day, and degradation or new synthesis of matrix components of cultured tendon segments was studied after different times in culture and by using different labeling techniques.

Determination of incorporation rates

Dry weight was determined after lyophilization. Dried tendons labeled with ^{3}H-proline or ^{35}S-sulfate were dissolved and then separated on a column of Aminex A6 eluted with sodium citrate buffer.[1] Radioactivity in peaks corresponding to ^{35}S-sulfate, ^{3}H-hydroxyproline, and ^{3}H-proline were measured with a radioactivity flow detector. The macromolecular content of ^{35}S-sulfate and ^{3}H-hydroxyproline was used as a measure of the new synthesis of proteoglycan and collagen, respectively. The incorporation of ^{3}H-proline was corrected for the known relative ratio of proline to hydroxyproline in collagen to represent the de novo synthesis of noncollagen protein. Following extraction, DNA of tendons labeled with ^{3}H-thymidine was mixed with liquid scintillator and counted in a scintillation counter.

Quantification of collagen, noncollagen protein, and hexosamines

The hydroxyproline content was determined colorimetrically by the chloramine-T method.[9] The noncollagen protein (α-amino acid) content was determined colorimetrically by the ninhydrin procedure.[8] The glycosaminoglycans were extracted and separated on an Aminex A9 column eluted with a phosphate buffer. The hexosamine content was assayed by the 2-cyanoacetamide procedure with glucosamine and galactosamine standards.[7]

Histologic examination

For light microscopy, tendon sections were stained with hematoxylin-eosin, and for scanning electron microscopy, the prepared tendon explants were covered with gold or palladium.

STUDIES
Intrinsic tendon healing in vivo

The ability of tendon segments to survive and heal in vivo was studied by using Millipore chambers where nutrition is based on diffusion of interstitial tissue fluid.[2] Divided and sutured tendons were incubated for up to 6 weeks in subcutaneous chambers, and their morphology and healing process were examined by light microscopy. Tendon segments frozen in liquid nitrogen were incubated to detect any entry of foreign cells (cell seeding) into the chamber, and intact tendon segments were cultured in chambers with defects in the membrane to simulate leakage into the chamber. Collagen and protein synthesis and cell proliferation were also examined in intact and frozen tendons and in native tendons of the same rabbits.

After 6 weeks of incubation, the tendon segments were white and the ends rounded off and covered with a soft and grayish tissue. This tissue corresponded to proliferated epitenon cells that covered the tendon ends and bridged the

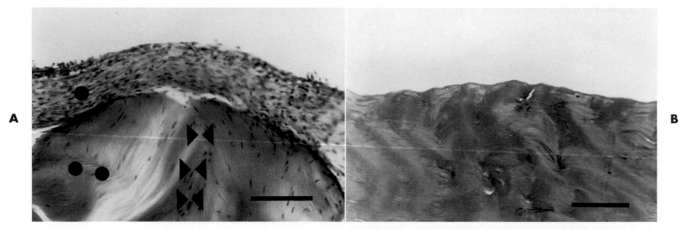

Fig. 35-3. A, Tendon segments incubated 6 weeks in diffusion chamber illustrating slightly stained endotenon cells (●●) and heavily stained and proliferating epitenon cells (●) covering the tendon repair *(arrow),* bar 200 μm. **B,** Frozen tendon segment incubated 6 weeks in the diffusion chamber showing no stained endotenon or epitenon cells, bar 400 μm. (From Abrahamsson S-O, Lundborg G, Lohmander LS: *Scand J Plast Reconstr Surg and Hand Surg* 1989; 23:199-206.)

sutured tendon gap (Fig. 35-3, *A*). Within endotenon, collagen fibers with a wavelike pattern and stained cells were observed. In some cases the number of cells within the central parts of the tendon was reduced. In no cases were collagen fibers observed bridging the gap. Explants frozen in liquid nitrogen before incubation showed no morphologic signs of cell proliferation (Fig. 35-3, *B*). On the contrary, tendons incubated in perforated chambers were richly invaded by blood cells. Biochemical measurements demonstrated that new collagen synthesis in incubated tendons was reduced by 50% compared with that of native tendons, whereas protein synthesis did not differ between the two groups. In contrast, cell proliferation was increased by a factor of 15 in the incubated group. As expected, frozen tendons showed little or no traces of cellular activity.

These histologic and biochemical studies show that tendon explants, cultured in a diffusion chamber where nutrition exclusively is based on nutrition, survive and exhibit an intrinsic capacity for healing.

Restoration of tendon surface by endotenon cells

The ability of endotenon cells to proliferate and restore the smooth surface of a "peeled" flexor tendon segment was investigated by using the diffusion chamber.[3] Epitenon, including the most superficial collagen fibers, was carefully removed from tendon segments under the microscope. The peeled tendons were then divided, sutured, rinsed in saline solution, and placed in chambers. Some of the tendons were used as controls, whereas most of them were cultured in the subcutaneous chambers for 2 to 11 weeks. All tendons were examined by light or scanning electron microscopy (SEM).

I found that longitudinally oriented and parallel collagen fibers appeared underneath the regular, smooth, and cobblestone-like surface of the native tendons and that the epitenon completely had been removed from all control tendons (Fig. 35-4, *A*). After 2 weeks of incubation, most of the tendons were covered by elongated, fibroblast-like cells, covering the ends and bridging the gap. The surface mainly showed a dense network of fibers that was covered by slightly elongated, flattened, and interconnected cells (Fig. 35-4, *B*). After 5 and 11 weeks of incubation, the tendons were covered by the former type of surface, containing flattened cells in multiple layers (Fig. 35-4, *C*).

Thus, a tendon deprived of its epitenon layer still contains multipotent cells capable of producing collagen, bridging the gap, and restoring the surface. These findings are not consistent with the hypothesis that the epitenon is an indispensable source for cell migration and matrix production during tendon healing.

Segmental variation of microstructure, matrix synthesis, and cell proliferation in intrasynovial deep flexor tendons

In the following experiment, the morphologic, biochemical, and metabolic differences between various segments of the intrasynovial region of the deep flexor tendon were investigated.[1] Digital deep flexor tendons from the region of the synovial sheath were divided into macroscopically well-defined segments: proximal, intermediate, and distal (Fig. 35-5). The tendon segments were examined with light microscopy or incubated and labeled for analysis of new matrix synthesis or cell proliferation. The contents of collagen and protein of the incubated tendons were also determined.

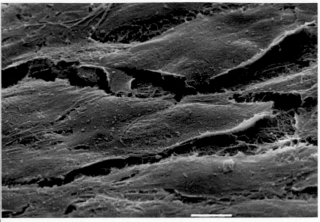

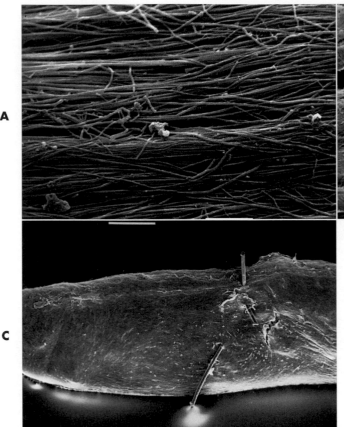

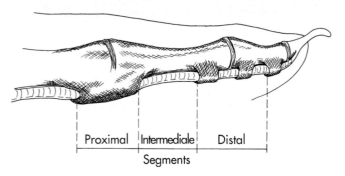

Fig. 35-4. Scanning electron microscopy (SEM) of flexor tendon segments. **A,** Peeled tendon surface; bundles of parallel collagen fibers (× 3500), bar 5 μm. **B,** The surface of peeled tendons after 2 weeks of incubation in a chamber, showing elongated and partly interconnected cells, covering a network of fibers (× 1500), bar 10 μm. **C,** SEM of a peeled tendon after 5 weeks of incubation, illustrating the reconstructed smooth and cobblestone-like surface (× 25), bar 1 μm. (From Abrahamsson S-O, Lundborg G, Lohmander LS: *J Hand Surg* 1991; 17B[5]:553-560.)

Fig. 35-5. Schematic drawing of the deep flexor tendon within the tendon sheath region of rabbit; illustrating the three morphologically and biochemically different regions. *1,* Proximal, located volar to the metacarpophalangeal joint, passes underneath a pully. *2,* Intermediate, volar to the proximal phalanx, passes between two pulleys. *3,* Distal, volar to the middle and inserts on the distal phalanx, passes underneath two pulleys.

The dorsal aspect of the proximal segment and a smaller volar part of the distal segment contained areas with a cartilage-like appearance, whereas the remaining parts of the tendon, including the intermediate segment, appeared as normal tendon tissue. Proteoglycan synthesis was elevated in the proximal and distal segments, whereas collagen and protein synthesis were elevated in the intermediate, and cell

proliferation in the intermediate and distal segments (Fig. 35-6). I also found a slightly lower collagen and protein content in the distal segments.

These results show that the rabbit deep flexor tendon within the synovial sheath contains two segments with fibrocartilage-like areas. These segments have a higher proteoglycan and a lower collagen and noncollagen protein synthesis compared with the segment with true tendon tissue. Cell proliferation is also lower within the proximal segment than in the intermediate and distal segments. These biochemical characteristics correlate well with the morphologic variations and may reflect an adaptation of tendon metabolism to different mechanical forces. These segmental variations may also be of importance for the healing capacity of the deep flexor tendon.

Recombinant human insulin-like growth factor-I stimulation of matrix synthesis and cell proliferation in short-term explant culture

As flexor tendon cells are metabolically active and morphologically and biochemically adapted to environmental requirements, circulating factors may be recognized as capable of influencing the activity of the tendon cells. In the following experiments, dose response effects of rhIGF-I (10

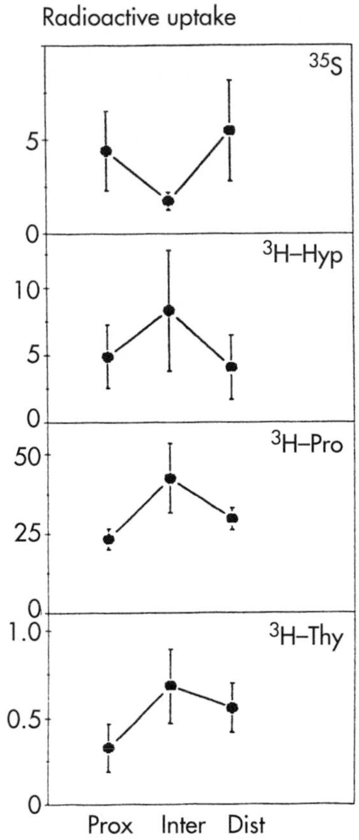

Radioactive uptake

Radioactive incorporation

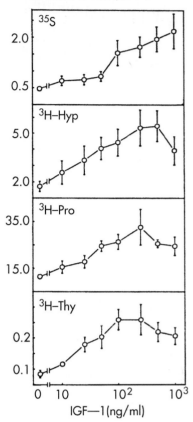

Fig. 35-6. Segmental variation in matrix synthesis and cell proliferation in the deep flexor tendon within the tendon sheath region. Values are presented as mean radioactive uptake (10^3 dpm/mg dwt) $\pm$ SD (n = 8) of ^{35}S-sulfate, ^{3}H-hydroxyproline, ^{3}H-proline, and ^{3}H-thymidine, respectively, in the proximal, intermediate, and distal segments. (From Abrahamsson S-O, Lundborg G, Lohmander LS: *Scand J Plast Reconstr Surg Hand Surg* 1989; 23:191-198.)

Fig. 35-7. Log-dose response effects of rhIGF-I (ng/ml) on proteoglycan, collagen, noncollagen protein, and cell proliferation in intermediate segments of rabbit tendon. Values are presented as mean radioactive uptake (10^3 dpm/mg dwt) $\pm$ SEM (n = 6) of ^{35}S-sulfate, ^{3}H-hydroxyproline, ^{3}H-proline, and ^{3}H-thymidine, respectively. (From Abrahamsson S-O, Lundborg G, Lohmander LS: *J Orthop Res* 1991; 9:495-502.)

to 1000 ng/ml), insulin (50 to 50,000 ng/ml), and fetal calf serum (FCS) (2% to 20%) on the synthesis of matrix components, and cell proliferation were investigated in short-term explant cultures of intermediate flexor tendon segments.[4]

I found that rhIGF-I stimulated matrix synthesis in a dose dependent manner in the interval of 10 to 250 ng/ml and cell proliferation at 10 to 100 ng/ml (Fig. 35-7). Insulin, however, stimulated matrix synthesis and cell proliferation in the dose interval of 250 to 5000 ng/ml, and FCS stimulated the collagen synthesis and cell proliferation at a concentration of 2% to 15%. I also observed that the stimulation of matrix synthesis by insulin had an apparent biphasic pattern, with maxima for collagen synthesis at 50 and 5000 ng/ml. In contrast, the rhIGF-I and FCS stimulation was monophasic, with maximal stimulation by rhIGF-I at 250 ng/ml and by FCS at 15%.

Thus these experiments illustrate that synthesis of matrix components and cell proliferation in deep flexor tendon

explants may be stimulated by recombinant human insulin-like growth factor, insulin, and fetal calf serum, further emphasizing the intrinsic cellular activity within tendons and suggesting a role for growth factors in regulating tendon metabolism.

Recombinant human insulin-like growth factor-I and serum effects on matrix metabolism in long-term explant culture

The effects of serum and rhIGF-I on tendon metabolism were investigated and compared in long-term explant culture in vitro.[5] In one experiment, segments of forepaw deep flexor tendons were cultured for 3 weeks in medium with FCS and then examined by light microscopy. In two experiments, degradation of matrix components during 12 days in culture was compared with matching pairs of tendon segments cultured in medium either with rhIGF-I or without rhIGF-I (BSA) and with tendon segments cultured in medium either with rhIGF-I or FCS. In

Radioactive uptake

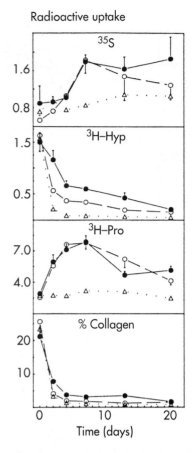

Weight

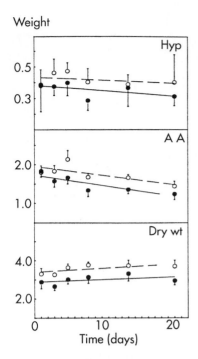

Fig. 35-8. Matrix synthesis in matched pairs of intermediate segments of rabbit flexor tendons incubated in medium supplemented with 10% FCS (O--O) and 50 ng/ml rhIGF-I (•—•) and the relative matrix synthesis of those cultured in unsupplemented medium (△••△). Values are presented as mean radioactive uptake (10^4 dpm/mg dwt) $\pm$ SEM (n = 6) of ^{35}S-sulfate, ^{3}H-hydroxyproline, ^{3}H-proline, and percent collagen of total protein, respectively, in explants on day 0 to 21. (From Abrahamsson S-O, Lundborg G, Lohmander LS: *J Orthop Res* 1991; 9:503-515.)

Fig. 35-9. Hydroxyproline (HYP) and amino acid (AA) content and tendon dry weight in intermediate segments of rabbit tendons incubated in medium supplemented with 10% FCS (O--O) or 50 ng/ml rhIGF-I (•—•). Values are expressed as mean weight per tendon (mg/tendon) $\pm$ SEM (n = 6) on day 0 to 21. (From Abrahamsson S-O, Lundborg G, Lohmander LS: *J Orthop Res* 1991; 9:503-515.)

additional experiments, new synthesis of matrix components, over a period of 20 days, was compared with tendons cultured either in medium with BSA or FCS and in medium either with BSA or rhIGF-I. Dry weight, hydroxyproline, amino acid, and hexosamine content were also determined.

The endotenon cells from the tendons cultured for 3 weeks stained well and the epitenon cells showed signs of proliferation. The estimated half-time (t½) for elimination of newly labeled proteoglycans ranged from 5 to 9 days and for noncollagenous protein from 5 to 7 days in either medium. In tendons cultured in medium with additions, synthesis of proteoglycan and noncollagenous protein increased threefold during the first week and then stabilized (Fig. 35-8). The mean glucosamine and galactosamine content of tendons harvested on day 0 was 0.058 ± 0.004 and 0.270 ± 0.060 µg/mg wet weight tendon, respectively. The total hexosamine content per tendon did not change by time. The amino acid content on day 0 was 0.6 ± 0.2 mg/mg dry

weight, but decreased by about 25% during culture (Fig. 35-9). There was no measurable elimination of collagen in explants cultured in either medium, and new collagen synthesis decreased to 10% of control when cultured with additions and to 3% without additions. The total hydroxyproline content of all harvested tendons on day 0 was 0.12 ± 0.05 mg/mg dry weight and remained at this same level in both complemented media (see Fig. 35-9).

In summary, our results show that in long-term culture of flexor tendon explants, the addition of rhIGF-I or serum to the culture medium stimulates matrix synthesis but does not influence turnover rates. The total hexosamine and collagen contents in tendons cultured in medium with rhIGF-I remain at the same level, while noncollagen protein content decreases slightly. Because there are no major differences in matrix metabolism between tendons cultured in medium supplemented with FCS or with rhIGF-I and because tendon metabolism is maintained during culture in either of the two media, our results show that rhIGF-I may be used as a growth factor supplement in serum-free culture of tendon tissue.

Inhibition of matrix synthesis and cell proliferation by dehydration

The intrinsic cellular activity of flexor tendons is continuously modified by the status of the environment and

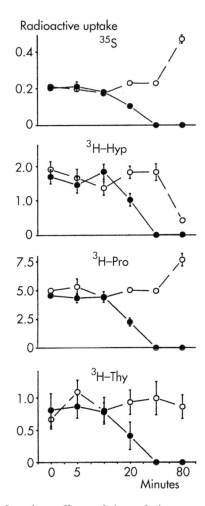

Fig. 35-10. Log-dose effects of time of air exposure (min) on proteoglycan, collagen, noncollagen protein synthesis, and cell proliferation in split intermediate segments of rabbit flexor tendon that were not irrigated (•) or were irrigated (O) with physiologic saline solution. Values are presented as mean radioactive uptake (10^4 dpm/mg dwt) $\pm$ SEM (n = 6) of ^{35}S-sulfate, ^{3}H-hydroxyproline, ^{3}H-proline, and ^{3}H-thymidine, respectively. (From Abrahamsson S-O, Lundborg G, Lohmander LS: *Acta Orthop Res* 1991; 62(2):159-162.)

may be affected by circulating growth factors and hormones. Any manipulation of the environment (e.g., by trauma, pharmaceuticals, or altered load) might affect primarily the cellular activity and metabolism within tendons and secondarily the healing capacity, adhesion formation, and mechanical properties. In the following experiments, we investigated the metabolic effects of external manipulation, by exposing tendon segments to dehydration, without or with simultaneous irrigation.[6] The tendon segments were exposed to air (0 to 80 min) in a laminar flow hood at 23° C and a relative air humidity of 63%. The effects of dehydration on matrix synthesis and cell proliferation were compared with matching groups of tendon segments, which were kept moist with physiologic saline (2 drops/5 min), and measured following radioactive labeling in short-term explant culture.

After 20 minutes of exposure to air, the tendons lost half of their ability to synthesize matrix components and DNA and lost all their ability after 40 minutes. Tendons irrigated with saline remained viable (Fig. 35-10).

These results show that dehydration inhibits in vitro matrix synthesis and cell proliferation in tendon explants and that the effects may be counteracted by keeping the exposed tendon segments moist with physiologic saline solution. These results also show that tendon tissue is sensitive to external manipulation, which should be considered during tendon surgery.

SUMMARY

Since 1987 we have developed methods for the culture of tendon segments in vivo and in vitro and have performed morphologic examinations and quantitative determinations of metabolism of matrix components and DNA. We have demonstrated that the tendon is a living, heterogenous, and metabolically active tissue with intrinsic capacities for cellular repair that vary between anatomic sites and types of tendons and may be influenced by growth factors and external manipulation.

The possible clinical implications of these results are obvious: Healing may vary between anatomic sites of deep flexor tendons, tendons do not need adhesions to heal and may be mobilized during repair, early load should be favorable in stimulating tendon cells to proper and adequate reorganization of the repair site, and tendons should be kept moist during repair.

REFERENCES

1. Abrahamsson S-O, Lundborg G, Lohmander LS: Segmental variation in microstructure, matrix synthesis and cell proliferation in rabbit flexor tendon, *Scand J Plast Reconstr Surg and Hand Surg* 1989; 23: 191-198.
2. Abrahamsson S-O, Lundborg G, Lohmander LS: Tendon healing in vivo: an experimental model, *Scand J Plast Reconstr Surg and Hand Surg* 1989; 23:199-206.
3. Abrahamsson S-O, Lundborg G, Lohmander LS: Restoration of the injured flexor tendon surface: a possible role for endotenon cells, a morphological study of the rabbit tendon in vivo, *J Hand Surg* 1991; 17B(5):553-560.
4. Abrahamsson S-O, Lundborg G, Lohmander LS: Recombinant human insulin-like growth factor-I stimulates in vitro matrix synthesis and cell proliferation in rabbit flexor tendon, *J Orthop Res* 1991; 9:495-502.
5. Abrahamsson S-O, Lundborg G, Lohmander LS: Long term explant culture of rabbit flexor tendon: effects of recombinant human insulin-like growth factor-I and serum on matrix metabolism, *J Orthop Res* 1991; 9:503-515.
6. Abrahamsson S-O, Lundborg G, Lohmander LS: Dehydration inhibits matrix synthesis and cell proliferation: an in vitro study of rabbit flexor tendons, *Acta Orthop Res* 1991; 62(2):159-162.
7. Moore S, Stein WH: Photometric ninhydrin method for use in the chromatography of amino acids, *J Biol Chem* 1948; 176:367-388.
8. Lohmander LS: Analysis by high-performance liquid chromatography of radioactively labeled carbohydrate components of proteoglycans, *Anal Biochem* 1986; 154:75-84.
9. Stegemann H, Stalder KH: Determination of hydroxyproline, *Clin Chim Acta* 1967; 18:267-273.

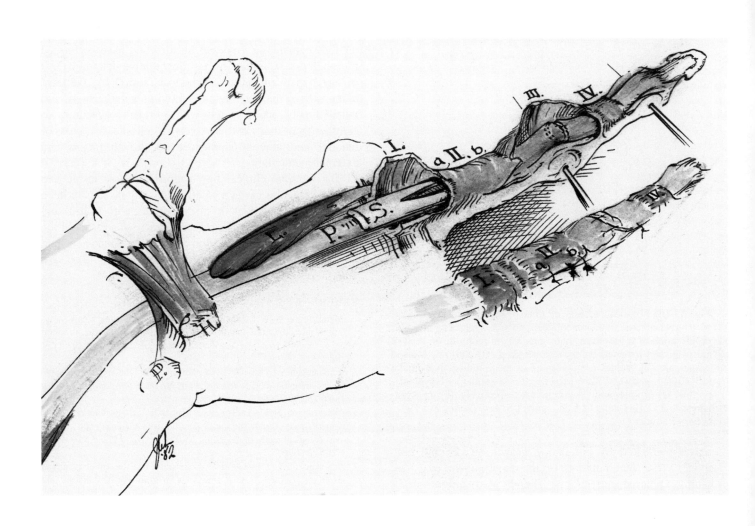

Part IX

MANAGEMENT OF ACUTE FLEXOR TENDON INJURIES

Sheath exposure of third digital lumbrical-profundus system, with tendon severed at extended PIP level: sheath closed over suture. Strategic II and IV fibro-osseous annuli demonstrated.

Chapter 36

CONCEPTS THAT CHANGED FLEXOR TENDON SURGERY

Harold E. Kleinert
Fergal M. McGoldrick
Nicholas H. Papas

To address concepts that changed flexor tendon surgery we must first go back and look at surgical evolution.[1,16] (Table 36-1). Flexor tendon surgery is, relatively speaking, a recent art. Galen, in the second century AD, did not recommend repair. Instead, he believed nerves and tendons were of similar origin, suggesting a strong risk of convulsions following surgery to repair these structures. Paracelsus reinforced this theory and said, "nature is horrified at the barbarians who sew up wounds." Even as late as the eighteenth century, the French surgeons Louis and Pibrac vehemently objected to surgery. However, Avicenna, the famed Arabian surgeon from the tenth century, advocated that every time a nerve (meaning tendon) is cut through or ruptured, it must be sewn together. This prophetic teaching was largely ignored because of Galen's influence until the fourteenth and seventeenth centuries when Roger of Parma, William of Salicet, and others advocated tenorrhaphy.

Tendon surgery flourished in the seventeenth century. Surgical concepts, however, remained primitive and confusing. For example, the eminent surgeon, Gargenot, following the example of Petit, included the skin in the tendon suture. Other surgeons (Sharpe, in London, for example) regularly sutured divided tendons. By the middle of the nineteenth century, tendon surgery had become accepted; Syme reported several successful cases in the 1850s. In the 1880s, Nicoladoni described techniques of tendon repair, and Codovilla, in 1889, was the first to recognize the importance of preserving the tendon sheath to minimize adhesion formation.

Toward the end of the nineteenth century, reports appeared of tendon transfer for correction of poliomyelitic deformity. Kirschner, in 1909, and Louis and Davis in 1911 in the United States published experimental studies concerning direct transplantation of both tendons and fasciae. Graft thickening and scarring presented a major problem. In 1910, Biesalski successfully used the autogenous sheaths of paralyzed tendons to prevent adhesions. Lexer of Jena, in 1912, first emphasized the importance of preventing adhesions by careful suturing and early motion 6 days after an operation. This formed the basis for the work of Leo Mayer. He published three articles that outlined the fundamental tenets of modern flexor tendon surgery. He elaborated on tendon blood supply, the role of mesotenon and paratenon, and the digital sheath in tendon function. He emphasized three basic rules for operative care:

1. The operation should never be undertaken unless the surgeon personally can perform effective postoperative care.
2. Early motion should be instituted at the right time.
3. Graded exercises should be used with protective splints.

In 1918, Sterling Bunnell[8] elaborated in his classic article how scar formation developed after tendon transfer. He outlined his philosophy on atraumatic technique, emphasized the need to preserve the pulley system, and established a plan for postoperative immobilization and active motion starting at 3 weeks postsurgery. In subsequent articles,[9-11] published between 1922 and 1928, he drew attention to many of the now commonly accepted

Table 36-1. Evolution of flexor tendon surgery

Date	Name	Comments
131-201 AD	Galen	Described tendons and nerves as single entity; strongly discouraged repair (convulsions)
980-1037 AD	Avicenna	Described direct tendon repair; teaching forgotten due to prominance of Galenian doctrine
14th century	Guy de Chauliac	Defended tenorrhaphy (only partially succeeded)
16th century	Ambroise Pare, Felix Wurtz of Bale, Andre della Croce	Incidentally described cases of tenorrhaphy; described in detail cases of primary tenorrhaphy
17th century	Roger of Parma, Roland Lanfranchi of Milan, William of Salicet	Advocated tenorrhaphy following Avicenna's teachings
	Moinichen	(*Medico-Surgical Observations,* 1665) Described successful cases of tenorrhaphy
	Landzweerde	Detailed successful tendon repair in canine model (in Scultet's *Armamentarium Chirurg.*)
	Meekren	(*Observ. med. chirurg.,* 1682) first demonstrated insensibility of tendons
	Job Baster of Zeland	Three instances of successful tendon repair using a single silk suture to reapproximate the tendon ends in 1677 (reported by Van der Wiell, *Observat. rares de medicine et de chirurgie,* 1789)
	Gauthier, Boevoaert, Maynaert	Successful cases of tenorrhaphy (according to Meekren, *Observ. med. chirurg.,* 1682)
	La Vauguion	In his treatise of surgical operations (1698), performed not only primary tendon repair but also tenorrhaphy in long-standing cases; described scar excision, freshening up divided tendon ends which had become "callous," and direct repair
	Bienaise	Additional skin incision to expose tendon ends; reapproximated ends by tying silk suture around each tendon end and pulling them together (*avoided* direct suturing on tendon ends)
	Kisner	(*De laesione tendinum,* 1699) preferred direct suturing of tendon ends
	Purman	Army surgeon in wars of Brandenbourg; enthusiastically supported and described 12 cases of successful primary tenorrhaphy
18th century	Jean Louis Petit	(*Traite des Operations de Chirurgie,* Paris, 1720, vol II) included skin in tendon suture to avoid direct contact with tendon ends
	Nuck	(Quoted by Van der Wiell, *Observat. rares de medicine et de chirurgie,* 1789, vol II, p 429) successful division and repair of canine external flexor
	Samuel Sharp	(1739) Regularly sutured divided tendons
	von Haller	(1752) Conclusively demonstrated insensibility of tendons
	Marc Anthony Petit	(Mid-to-late 1700s) Successful repair in immediate and delayed cases of tenorrhaphy using silk suture
19th century	Gensoul, Acher, Blaindin, Sanson	(1830s) Successful cases of tenorrhaphy
	Rognetta, Mondiere	(1837) Attacked tenorrhaphy (despite previous successes!)
	Syme of England	(1850) Several successful repairs; tenorrhaphy now becomes accepted procedure
	Nicoladoni	(1880s) Described techniques of tendon repair (localization procedure)
	Codivilla of Bologna	(1889) First recognized importance of preserving digital sheath
20th century	Biesalski	(1910) Also recognized importance of preserving digital sheath to prevent adhesion formation
	Lexer of Jena	(1912) Palmaris longus used as flexor tendon graft; also emphasized careful suturing and early motion
	Mayer	(1916) Described blood supply of tendons, tendon sheath motion, importance of peritenon, tendon transfer (i.e., formed basis of present-day concepts of reconstructive flexor tendon surgery)
	Kirchmayr of Vienna	(1917) First described "grasping" method of tendon suturing
	Sterling Bunnell	(1918, 1922, etc.) Reviewed anatomy and physiology of tendons; achieved excellent results in flexor tendon grafting; described importance of pulley system, atraumatic technique, good instrumentation, postoperative rehabilitation
	Mason, Shearon, Allen	(1932, 1940, 1941, etc.) Experimental and clinical work on tendon repair and tendon healing
	Graham, Littler, Boyes	(1940s and 1950s) Authorities on tendon surgery in US
	Pulvertaft	(1940s and 1950s) Authority on tendon surgery in UK; advocated more objective evaluation of postoperative function
	Siler	(1950) Reported on primary tenorrhaphy of flexor tendons

Table 36-1. Evolution of flexor tendon surgery—cont'd

Date	Name	Comments
	Verdan	(1950s) Reverted to primary repair of flexor tendons
	Kelly	(1958) Reported on primary tendon repair
	Young, Harmon	(1960) 5-0 Running chromic catgut suture; rubberband traction
	Kleinert, Kutz, et al.	(1950s, 1960s) Primary repair in zone II; used modified Bunnell core suture, running epitenon suture; described protected active postoperative mobilization using rubberband traction
	Bruner	(1960s) Zigzag volar digital incision for flexor tendon surgery
	Peacock, Potenza, Matthews, Richards	(1960s, 1970s) Furthered understanding of flexor tendon physiology
	Hunter	(1960s, 1970s, 1980) Use of artificial tendons and gliding artificial implants for tendon sheath reconstruction; further described anatomy of flexor tendons (pulley, vincular, synovial, and vascular structures)
	Kessler, Tajima, Tsuge	(1970s) Described methods of intratendinous suturing; techniques remain popular today
	Duran, House	(1970s) Controlled *passive* motion postoperatively
	Lundborg	(1970s, 1980s) Role of tendon sheath and synovium in healing and tendon nutrition
	Matev, et al.	(1980) Delayed primary suture of flexor tendons cut in digital theca
	Lister	(1980s) Importance of sheath closure in primary tendon repair
	Manske	(1980s) Flexor tendon nutrition

hand surgical principles. These included comfortable seating, relaxed and "light-fingered" assistants, sharp instruments, and good lighting. Careful attention to handling of soft tissues and meticulous hemostasis, augmented by the use of magnification loupes and more refined suture material and instrumentation, is necessary to ensure that these important aspects of tendon repair are not overlooked. Today, these points are discussed rarely, but they always deserve consideration. Bunnell also developed the concept of "no man's land." This may have retarded conceptual progress by thirty years because primary repair was abandoned in favor of tendon grafting.* Pulvertaft, in agreement with this, stated that it was not difficult to suture tendons and prepare the ground for sound union—the real problem was to obtain a freely sliding tendon capable of restoring good function. Beginning in the 1950s, however, others recognized their own less-than-satisfactory results with primary tendon grafting for repair of zone II flexor tendon lacerations and reverted to primary tendon repair. Careful technique, improved suture materials, and increased emphasis on postoperative rehabilitation led to improved results.

It can thus be seen, historically, that several central themes permeate the literature: (1) tendon healing, (2) suture technique, (3) postoperative splintage and rehabilitation, and (4) evaluation of results. These will now be conceptually reviewed; we will examine how each of these issues has evolved to the present day.

*References 2, 4-6, 14, 18, 32, 33, 36, 43, 44, 75.

TENDON HEALING

Several accounts of animal experimentation have been written that describe tendon healing. Beginning with those in the seventeenth century, they detailed healing and complete recovery in a canine model after sectioning and repair of the Achilles tendon and later the external flexor of the canine carpus.[16] Principles of tendon healing, previously stated many times in the literature,[45,46,48] were summarized by Potenza: Tendons heal by the fibroplastic response of the surrounding tissues whose own integrity has been violated.[54-56] Deductions immediately followed: The greater the tissue trauma, the greater the fibroplastic response and hence the greater the resultant adhesions. Therefore, any surgically imposed trauma must be kept to a minimum. Following reports by Siler,[60] Kelly,[24] Verdan,[70] Young and Harmon,[76] and the senior author's report of his ten-year experience with favorable results with primary repair for acute zone II flexor tendon injury,[27] several others began investigating new areas of tendon physiology. New, more correct concepts of tendon healing arose from these studies.[22,37-42,47,52] Sheath excision was abandoned. Matthews and Richards investigated the effects of splinting, suture, and excision of the tendon sheath on the healing of incompletely transected flexor tendons in a rabbit model, both separately and in various combinations. When all procedures were performed together, the repair was accompanied by dense adhesion formation with little evidence of any healing activity by the tendon cells.[47] Their experiments suggested that the adhesions were the result not of any single factor studied but of all three, contributing in various degrees. Suturing (Bunnell's technique) produced the most adhesions, but synovial sheath excision and immobilization also contributed.[27]

Tendons receive their nutrition through at least two pathways. In 1916, Leo Mayer described the blood supply of tendons.[48] In the 1970s, Hunter established that blood supply is provided directly through the vincular system.[22] Synovial fluid within an intact tendon sheath was shown to provide an additional pathway of nutrition through diffusion of metabolites across the synovial space. Indeed, Lundborg demonstrated the potential of flexor tendon healing without any adhesion formation and postulated that tendons possess an intrinsic capacity for healing without any adhesion formation and postulated that tendons possess an intrinsic capacity for healing with nutrients obtained solely from diffusion from within the synovial sheath.[37-40] Manske and Lesker[42] in 1985, and Manske[41] in 1988, used tracer materials to compare the role of vascular perfusion and synovial diffusion in supplying the nutritional needs of the flexor tendon within its sheath. They concluded that there is a dual source of nutrients, but that diffusion is a more effective pathway than perfusion. Other authors have confirmed this.[38]

SUTURE MATERIAL AND TECHNIQUES

The rapid acceleration in manufacturing technology in this century has permitted surgeons to address biomechanical concepts that hitherto limited progress for hundreds of years. The early pioneers in hand surgery were limited to natural fibers such as silk, linen, cotton, catgut, and steel wire as their main suture materials. Today, several newer synthetic suture materials are readily available for use in tendon surgery. These include the nonabsorbable sutures Ethilon (monofilament nylon), Prolene (monofilament polypropylene), Ethibond (braided polyester suture coated with polybutilate), Ticron (braided polyester fiber), and Supramid (braided nylon loop suture), and the absorbable sutures Maxon (monofilament polyglyconate) and PDS (monofilament polydioxanone). Trail[67] has shown that monofilament polyglyconate and stainless steel wire each possess high tensile strength and provide good knot security, whereas braided polyester and polypropylene offer a reasonable compromise.

In 1917, Kirchmayr, a Vienese surgeon, published a method of "locking" sutures in tendon repair.[26] This technique remained buried in the literature until its reintroduction in the late 1960s as the Kessler suture.[25] Bunnell described his crisscross weave in 1918, and Mason and Allen described their technique in 1941.[45] Bunnell realized the importance of early mobilization in flexor tendon repair, but the lack of adequate suture materials and techniques led to failure of primary repair. This resulted in abandonment of primary repair in acute flexor tendon injury in favor of wound debridement and primary closure as an initial stage. This was to be followed by delayed tendon grafting.

Claude Verdan initially subscribed to Bunnell's teachings on delayed tendon grafting for repair of zone II injuries. He performed more than 60 tendon grafting procedures. However, in his book *Chirurgie reparatrice et fonctionnelle des tendons de la main,* he came to the conclusion that primary repair of injured zone II flexor tendons is not only possible but also advisable.[71] He described a technique of coaptation and immobilization using transfixion pins across the proximal and distal tendon ends. He later included the use of four 6-0 ophthalmic silk epitenon quadrant sutures to better coapt the tendon ends. In following the prevalent thinking at the time, namely, that one should excise the tendon sheath around the area of repair to allow neovascularization (as promoted by Mason, Boyes, and others), Verdan excised approximately 1 inch of digital tendon sheath around the repair site.[70] Ironically, the importance of the flexor tendon sheath in preventing adhesions had been recognized by Codivilla of Bologna in 1889 and Konrad Biesalski of Berlin in 1910.

James Hunter, beginning in the 1960s, refined techniques of flexor tendon grafting, describing the use of artificial tendons and artificial gliding implants for tendon sheath reconstruction.[19-21,23] He also elaborated on the anatomy of flexor tendons with respect to the pulley system, the vincular system, and the synovial and vascular structures.[22]

In the last 25 years, there have been many modifications in suture technique. Surgeons, now armed with new stronger synthetic materials, have sought new apposition of tendon ends to permit aggressive mobilization without gapping or rupture.[12,15,49,57,58] Modifications of the original Kirchmayr-Kessler technique include the locking suture of Pennington and Tajima's double-ended technique.[53] Wade showed that an epitenon suture offered greater strength.[72] Halstead's mattress epitenon suture[51] represents another variation. Tsuge[68] published his experience with a loop suture in 1977. In the same year Becker described the beveled repair, which converted mechanical tendon forces from longitudinal to transverse. More recently, Savage reported his experience with a crisscross six-strand method.[59] Lee[34] described his double loop (DOLL) in 1990. Messina[50] reported in 1992 his double-armed suture (DAS) technique of a Bunnell tenorrhaphy and running epitenon suture, augmented by a second pullout suture. In 1993, Silfverskiold described his epitendinal cross-stitch,[61,62] which appears to be much a stronger configuration than the conventional running epitendinal repair. Strickland[64] evaluated a new technique of a four-strand Tajima and horizontal mattress repair with a running, locking, peripheral epitendinous suture.

Biomechanical research has flourished as technology has permitted us to evaluate our techniques. Urbaniak showed in his excellent research[69] that the load to failure was equivalent for Bunnell's and Kessler's techniques. Greenwald demonstrated that an augmented Becker suture was stronger than the Kessler method.[17] Wagner compared the locking suture (Kirchmayr-Kessler), Kessler-Tajima, and

Savage techniques; the Savage repair was significantly stronger than either Kessler variation.[73] Trail has also shown that the Becker and Savage techniques demonstrate, in the laboratory setting, superior loads to failure than either the Kessler or Bunnell sutures.[66] The tried and proven Kirchmayr-Kessler suture may, therefore, have significantly enhanced strength if a crisscross technique, as advocated by Silfverskiold, is used as an epitenon suture.

However, it is difficult to translate conflicting biomechanical findings to help clarify clinical questions. To date, much of the research is not sufficiently applicable clinically to be of any value other than to give us a possible range of stress-loading values for flexor tendons. The underlying concept is to create a suture technique that has sufficient strength to withstand forces applied at a very early stage (i.e., early motion [active or passive]). What has propelled this change in philosophy has been the evolution of rehabilitation programs in the last 30 years, notably beginning with the program of passive assist–active extension begun by the senior author.

POSTOPERATIVE MANAGEMENT

Mayer's three guidelines for postoperative care, outlined earlier in this chapter, hold remarkably true to this day. Bunnell, in 1918, outlined his postoperative plan for immobilization and active motion beginning at approximately 3 weeks after the operation.[8] Such was the influence of Bunnell and others that for 30 years no other concepts were considered or described. Littler[36] reinforced this concept in 1947 when he emphasized that early motion had no place in tendon grafting, because the tendon junctures did not unite.

Even in 1955, in reports by both Boyes,[4] and Allen,[2] splinting was still advocated for up to 3 weeks, with no attempt made at early mobilization. However, Mason,[44] in an editorial in 1959, signaled the end of this attitude by noting an undue pessimistic approach that had been adopted in primary tendon repair. Siler[60] had reported in 1949 active flexion beginning at 12 days. The splint was adjusted as needed, then completely removed at 28 days. Verdan[70] advocated early mobilization, but still did not mobilize for 3 weeks. He mentioned the role of systematic active exercises and documented the probable benefit of passive motion at releasing adhesions. The senior author developed, beginning in 1954, his now-established technique of protected mobilization.[27] Rubber bands were fixed to the nails and coupled to the use of active extension against a limiting dorsal block splint. Interestingly, Young and Harmon[76] had independently reported on the use of a silk suture passed through the nail and tied to a rubber band, whose opposite end was fixed to a wrist band of adhesive tape. No splintage or dressing was used. Passive extension was performed on the first postoperative day. The true outcome of this technique is difficult to evaluate, because the postoperative ratings were based on amounts of workers' compensation awards.

When Kleinert's long-term clinical findings were presented in 1967, they were met with mixed skepticism. Fortunately, the conclusions were verified when evaluated independently heralding the modern era of tendon rehabilitation. Since then, there has been an explosion of interest in tendon surgery and postoperative care. In the last 25 years, many ideas have evolved from the active extension–passive flexion mode of Kleinert,[28,29,31,35,74] from the Duran and Houser modification of controlled passive motion (extension)[13] to the controlled active motion regimen. This latter technique has been popularized in the British Isles with a notable paper by Small from Belfast in 1989.[63] However, his tendon rupture rate of 9.4% is far greater than that of the Kleinert regimen (3.3%). This may be because the Kleinert model is based on the finding that contraction against resistance of one group of muscles results in synergistic relaxation of its antagonists. In 1994, Bainbridge and Elliott[3] recorded a rupture rate of 7.14%, indicating that the continued higher morbidity of this regimen suggested that active motion is not as controlled as it seems. Silfverskiöld[62] rightly cautioned us in this regard by noting that resisted gripping, even if not confirmed by the patient, may well account for unexpected ruptures. He wrote, "Having all four digits kept in the flexed position by rubber bands provides some measure of safety in this respect, insofar as it makes it difficult to use the hand actively for gripping." It must be noted that these changes in rehabilitation have been often linked to new suture techniques. This makes it difficult to evaluate the respective role of each change in treatment. Although the path to total success remains strewn with obstacles, enormous strides have been made thus far in our conceptual thinking and will continue into the future.

EVALUATION OF RESULTS

Guy Pulvertaft was the first to suggest that "it is unsatisfactory to classify results as good, fair, and poor because these terms convey little meaning. A method of classification is needed which is accurate, does not contain excessive detail, and can be readily understood." Pulvertaft further stated that the Boyes method (distance of fingertip pulp to distal palmar crease) was not useful in measuring the functional results of isolated profundus tendon repair. He was the first to promote actual measurements of the distal interphalangeal joint as an objective measure of results.[57,58] Although there have been many different classifications suggested over the last 20 years, three remain most popular. The Louisville classification, described in 1977 by Lister,[35] and the Buck-Gramcko classification of 1976[7] were quickly superseded by the *Report of the Committee on Tendon Injuries* published in 1980.[30] This formed the first basis of a logical classification system and introduced the concept of total active motion (TAM). Strickland modified this classification in 1985 by excluding metacarpal-phalangeal joint (MCPJ) motion.[65] While this has been popularized and even modified again, it is deficient because it ignores the MCPJ arc of motion. It would seem appropriate that this issue be readdressed with a new report that takes into account recent research and gained experience. This has become mandatory because of the rapid worldwide expansion and acceptance of hand surgery as a distinct specialty, with its resultant plethora of diverse publications. If conceived in harmony by the respective national and international bodies, it will enable a universally acceptable classification to become the framework for reporting surgical outcomes.

CONCLUSION

Changing concepts in research and clinical care have, in the last 30 years, shaped our thinking such that Bunnell's concept of no man's land now appears to represent a historical curiosity. Perhaps of most significance is the development of hand surgery as a separate, recognized specialty. Formal training fellowships, notably in the United States, but now spreading worldwide, have created and continue to train a new generation of highly qualified surgeons. These clinicians have the requisite skills, understanding, and clinical acumen to ensure much better outcomes in flexor tendon surgery. We can look ahead with renewed optimism provided we remain openminded to new techniques and ideas, even though at times they will conflict sharply with accepted dogma. Only then will real progress be made.

REFERENCES

1. Adamson JE, Wilson JN: The history of flexor tendon grafting, *J Bone Joint Surg* 1961; 43A:709-716.
2. Allen HS: Management of laceration of the flexor tendons within the digits, *Surg Clin North Am* 1955; 35:189-194.
3. Bainbridge LC, Robertson C, Gillies D, Elliot D: A comparison of post-operative mobilization with passive flexion-active extension and controlled active motion techniques, *J Hand Surg* 1994; 19B:517-521.
4. Boyes JH: Evaluation of results of digital flexor tendon grafts, *Am J Surg* 1955; 89:1116-1119.
5. Boyes JH: Immediate vs. delayed repair of the digital flexor tendons, *Ann Western Med and Surg* 1947; 1(4):145-152.
6. Boyes JH: Why tendon repair? *J Bone Joint Surg* 1959; 41A:577-579 (editorial).
7. Buck-Gramcko D: A new method for evaluation of results in flexor tendon repair, *Handchirurgie* 1976; 8:65-69.
8. Bunnell S: Repair of tendons in the fingers and description of two new instruments, *Surg Gyn Obstet* 1918; 26:103-110.
9. Bunnell S: Repair of tendons in the fingers, *Surg Gyn Obstet* 1922; 35:88-97.
10. Bunnell S: Reconstructive surgery of the hand, *Surg Gyn Obstet* 1924; 39:259-274.
11. Bunnell S: Repair of nerves and tendons of the hand, *J Bone Joint Surg* 1928; 10:1.
12. Bunnell S: Gig pull-out suture for tendons, *J Bone Joint Surg* 1954; 36A:850-851.
13. Duran RJ, Houser RG: Controlled passive motion following flexor tendon repair in zones 2 and 3, American Academy of Orthopaedic Surgeons, *Symposium on tendon surgery in the hand*, St Louis, 1975, Mosby.
14. Fowler SB: The management of tendon injuries, *J Bone Joint Surg* 1959; 41A:579-580 (editorial).
15. Graham WC: Flexor tendon grafts to the finger and thumb, *J Bone Joint Surg* 1947; 29:553-559.
16. Gratz CM: The history of tendon suture, *Med J Record* 1928; 127:Feb 1 and 15:156-157, 213-215.
17. Greenwald DP, Hong HZ, May JM: Mechanical analysis of tendon suture techniques, *J Hand Surg* 1994; 19A:641-647.
18. Holm CL, Embick RP: Anatomical considerations in the primary treatment of tendon injuries of the hand, *J Bone Joint Surg* 1959; 41A:599-608.
19. Hunter JM: Artificial tendons, early development and application, *Am J Surg* 1965; 109:325-338.
20. Hunter JM, Salisbury RE: Use of gliding artificial implants to produce tendon sheaths. Techniques and results in children, *Plast Reconstr Surg* 1970; 45:564-572.
21. Hunter JM, Salisbury RE: Flexor tendon reconstruction in severely damaged hands, *J Bone Joint Surg* 1971; 53A:829-858.
22. Hunter JM: Anatomy of flexor tendons—pulley, vincular, synovia, and vascular structures. In Spinner M, ed: *Kaplan's functional and surgical anatomy of the hand*, ed 3, Philadelphia, 1984, Lippincott.
23. Hunter JM, Singer DI, Jaeger SH, et al: Active tendon implants in flexor tendon reconstruction, *J Hand Surg* 1988; 13A:849-859.
24. Kelly AP Jr: A study of 789 consecutive tendon severances, *J Bone Joint Surg* 1959; 41A:581-598.
25. Kessler I: The "grasping technique" for tendon repair, *Hand* 1973; 5:253-255.
26. Kirchmayr L: Zur technik der sehnennaht. In Garre K, Perthes G, Borchard A, eds: *Zentralblaff fur Chirurgie* 44. Jahrgang Nr. 27-52 Juli-Dezember, Verlag von Johann Ambrosius Barth, Leipzig, Germany, 1917.
27. Kleinert HE, Kutz JE, Ashbell TS, et al: Primary repair of lacerated flexor tendon in no man's land, *J Bone Joint Surg* 1967; 49A:577 (abstract).
28. Kleinert HE, Kutz JE, Atasoy E, et al: Primary repair of flexor tendons, *Orth Clin North Am* 1973; 4:865-876.
29. Kleinert HE, Kutz JE, Cohen MJ: Primary repair of zone 2 flexor tendon lacerations, American Academy of Orthopaedic Surgeons, *Symposium on tendon surgery in the hand*, St Louis, 1975, Mosby.
30. Kleinert HE, Verdan CE: Report of the committee on tendon injuries, *J Hand Surg* 1983; 8:794-798.
31. Kleinert HE, Schepel S, Gill T: Flexor tendon injuries, *Surg Clin North Am* 1981; 61:267-286.
32. Koch SL: Division of the flexor tendons within the digital sheath, *Surg Gyn Obstet* 1944; 78:9-22.
33. Kyle JB, Eyre-Brook AL: The surgical treatment of flexor tendon injuries in the hand, *Br J Surg* 1954; 41:502-511.
34. Lee H: Double-loop locking suture: a technique of tendon repair for early active mobilization, part 1, evolution of technique and experimental study, *J Hand Surg* 1990; 15A:945-952.
35. Lister GD, Kleinert HE, Kutz JE, et al: Primary flexor tendon repair followed by immediate controlled mobilization, *J Hand Surg* 1977; 2A:441-451.
36. Littler JW: Free tendon grafts in secondary flexor tendon repair, *Am J Surg* 1947; 74:315-321.
37. Lundborg G: Experimental flexor tendon healing without adhesion formation—a new concept of tendon nutrition and intrinsic healing mechanisms, *Hand* 1976; 8:235-238.
38. Lundborg G, Holm S, Myrhage R: The role of the synovial fluid and tendon sheath for flexor tendon nutrition, *Scand J Plast Reconstr Surg* 1980; 14(1):99-107.
39. Lundborg G, Rank F: Experimental intrinsic healing of flexor tendons based upon synovial fluid nutrition, *J Hand Surg* 1978; 3(A):21-31.
40. Lundborg G, Rydevik B: The vascularization of human flexor tendons within the digital synovial sheath region—structural and functional aspects, *J Hand Surg* 1977; 2(A):417-427.

41. Manske PR: Flexor tendon healing, *J Hand Surg* 1988; 13B:237-245.
42. Manske PR, Lesker PA: Flexor tendon nutrition, *Hand Clin* 1985; 1(1):13-24.
43. Mason ML: Primary and secondary tendon suture: a discussion of the significance of technique in tendon surgery, *Surg Gyn Obstet* 1940; 70:392-402.
44. Mason ML: Primary tendon repair, *J Bone Joint Surg* 1959; 41A:575-577 (editorial).
45. Mason ML, Allen HS: The rate of healing of tendons. An experimental study of tensile strength, *Ann Surg* 1941; 113:424-459.
46. Mason ML, Shearon CG: The process of tendon repair: an experimental study of tendon suture and tendon graft, *Arch Surg* 1932; 25:615-692.
47. Matthews P, Richards H: The repair potential of digital flexor tendons: an experimental study, *J Bone Joint Surg* 1974; 56B:618-625.
48. Mayer L: The physiological method of tendon transplantation, *Surg Gyn Obstet* 1916; 22:182-192.
49. Mayer L: Repair of severed tendons, *Am J Surg* 1938; 12:714.
50. Messina A: The double-armed suture. Tendon repair with immediate mobilization of the fingers, *J Hand Surg* 1992; 17A:137-142.
51. Nealon TF, ed: *Fundamental skills in surgery,* ed 3 Philadelphia, 1979, Saunders.
52. Peacock EE Jr: Biological principles in the healing of long tendons, *Surg Clin North Am* 1965; 45(2):461-476.
53. Pennington D: The locking loop tendon suture, *Plast Recon Surg* 1979;63:648-652.
54. Potenza AD: Tendon healing within the flexor digital sheath in the dog, *J Bone Joint Surg* 1962; 44A:49-64.
55. Potenza AD: Critical evaluation of flexor tendon healing and adhesion formation without artificial digital sheaths: an experimental study, *J Bone Joint Surg* 1963; 45A:1217-1233.
56. Potenza AD: The healing process in wounds of the digital flexor tendons and tendon grafts: an experimental study. In Verdan C, ed: *Tendon surgery of the hand,* Edinburgh, 1979, Churchill Livingstone.
57. Pulvertaft RG: Tendon grafts for flexor tendon injuries in the fingers and thumb, *J Bone Joint Surg* 1956; 38B:175-194.
58. Pulvertaft RG: Suture materials and tendon junctures, *Am J Surg* 1965;109:346-352.
59. Savage R, Risitano G: Flexor tendon repair using a six strand method of repair and early active mobilisation, *J Hand Surg* 1989; 14B:396-399.
60. Siler VE: Primary tenorrhaphy of the flexor tendons in the hand, *J Bone Joint Surg* 1950; 32A:218-225.
61. Silfverskiold KL, Anderson C: Two new methods of tendon repair: an in-vitro evaluation of tensile strength and gap formation, *J Hand Surg* 1993; 18A:58-65.
62. Silfverskiold KL, May EJ: Flexor tendon repair in zone II with a new suture technique and an early mobilization program combining passive and active flexion, *J Hand Surg* 1994; 19A:53-60.
63. Small J, Brennen M, Colville J: Early active mobilisation following flexor tendon repair in zone 2, *J Hand Surg* 1989; 14B:383-391.
64. Strickland JW, Cannon NM, Gettle KH: *Indiana Hand Center Education Newsletter* 1993; 1:1.
65. Strickland JW: Results of flexor tendon surgery in zone II, *Hand Clin* 1985; 1(1):167-179.
66. Trail IA, Powell ES, Noble J: The mechanical strengths of various techniques, *J Hand Surg* 1991; 17B:89-91.
67. Trail IA, Powell ES, Noble J: An evaluation of suture materials used in tendon surgery, *J Hand Surg* 1989; 14B(4):422-427.
68. Tsuge K, Hoshikazu I, Matsuishi Y: Repair of flexor tendons by intratendinous suture, *J Hand Surg* 1977; 2(6):436-440.
69. Urbaniak JR, Cahill JD, Mortensen RA: Tendon suturing methods: analysis of suture strengths. In American Academy of Orthopaedic Surgeons: *Symposium on tendon surgery in the hand,* St Louis, 1975, Mosby.
70. Verdan CE: Primary repair of flexor tendons, *J Bone Joint Surg* 1960; 42A:647-657.
71. Verdan CE: Half a century of flexor tendon surgery, *J Bone Joint Surg* 1972; 54:472-491.
72. Wade PJF, Wetherell RG, Amis AA: Flexor tendon repair: significant gain in strength from the Halstead peripheral suture technique, *J Hand Surg* 1989; 14B:232-235.
73. Wagner WF, Carroll C, Strickland JW, et al: A biomechanical comparison of techniques of flexor tendon repair, *J Hand Surg* 1994; 19A(6):979-982.
74. Werntz JR, Chesher SP, Breidenbach WC, et al: A new dynamic splint for postoperative treatment of flexor tendon injury, *J Hand Surg* 1989; 14A(3):559-566.
75. White WL: Secondary restoration of finger flexion by digital tendon grafts, *Am J Surg* 1956; 91:662-668.
76. Young RES, Harmon JM: Repair of tendon injuries of the hand, *Ann Surg* 1960; 151:562-566.

Chapter 37

EVALUATION OF SUTURE CALIBER IN FLEXOR TENDON REPAIR

Applications for active motion

John S. Taras
James S. Raphael
Stanley D. Marczyk
Wayne Bauerle
Randall W. Culp

In the pursuit of improving the results of flexor tendon repair, a great body of knowledge regarding the healing of tendons, repair strengths of various suture techniques,[31] and the value of postoperative tendon mobilization[7,16] has been amassed. The sum of this research has led to wide acceptance of the practice of atraumatic repair, use of synthetic braided or synthetic monofilament core suture of 4-0 caliber with a running epitendinous stitch, and postoperative passive mobilization as gleaned from Strickland's survey of the members of the American Society for Surgery of the Hand.[28] In searching for a method that limits tendon adhesions, a variety of tendon repair techniques have been applied to a program of controlled active mobilization.* The focus of the repair techniques designed to withstand the increased stresses of active mobilization has centered around increasing the strength of the repair. Despite numerous reports on the mechanical strengths of repair techniques, little attention has been paid to the effect of the suture caliber used for repair. In this study, we sought to determine in a biomechanical model: (a) the effect of suture caliber on core suture strength of the commonly used

modified Kessler and modified Bunnell techniques along with a new double-grasping technique (Fig. 37-1), (b) to compare the strength of the standard running epitendinous suture with the cross-stitch epitendinous technique (Fig. 37-2), (c) to evaluate the combined double-grasping and cross-stitch technique comparing the results with theoretical models of the forces necessary for active mobilization after flexor tendon repair and to review the early clinical experience with flexor tendon repairs using the double-grasping and cross-stitch techniques.

MATERIALS AND METHODS

Two hundred fresh frozen flexor tendons were harvested from cadavers, transected, repaired, and stressed to tensile failure as measured in newtons with an Instron-1000 materials testing machine. The modified Kessler, modified Bunnell, and double-grasping core suture[4,11,30] techniques were evaluated with synthetic braided (Ethibond) suture of 5-0, 4-0, 3-0, and 2-0 caliber. Running and cross-stitch epitendinous techniques[22] were tested with 6-0 and 5-0 caliber monofilament (Prolene) suture without a core suture. Finally, the combined double-grasping core suture (5-0 to 2-0) and cross-stitch (6-0) tendon repairs were assessed. Ten

*References 1-3, 6, 8, 10, 13, 20, 24, 25, 29.

314

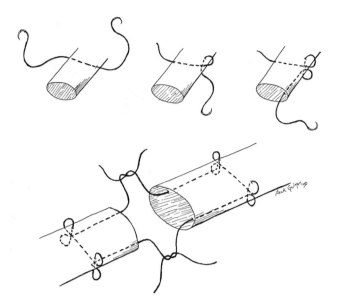

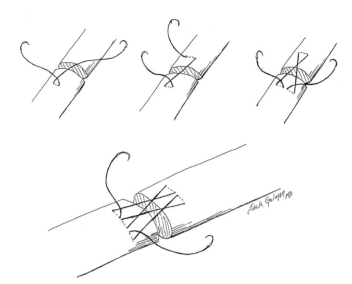

Fig. 37-1. Double-grasping core suture technique. This core suture technique provides an extra throw at the corners of the suture fixation, thereby increasing the grasping quality of the suture.

Fig. 37-2. Cross-stitch epitendinous technique. The cross-stitch creates an external weave similar to a Chinese finger trap.

Table 37-1. Tensile strength of tendon repairs (in newtons)

	Suture Technique					
Suture Size	Running Epitendinous	Cross-stitch Epitendinous	Kessler	Bunnell	Double-grasping	Double-grasping + 6-0 Cross-stitch
6-0	11	27				
5-0	14	32	15	12	14	27
4-0			22	24	23	62
3-0			28	34	37	73
2-0			41	59	61	73

tests were performed for each technique's suture caliber arrangement.

All repaired tendons were mounted on the materials testing machine and stressed to tensile failure at 20 mm/min cross-head speed. Failure was defined as either suture pullout or suture breakage. Gap formation was not measured as a precursor to repair failure.

The clinical results of 21 flexor tendon repairs in 14 digits using the combined double-grasping and cross-stitch technique were reviewed. There were 3 flexor pollicis longus (FPL), 4 flexor digitorum profundus (FDP) zone I, and 14 flexor digitorum superficialis (FDS) FDP zone II repairs performed.

RESULTS

The average tensile strength of each type of tendon repair tested is summarized in Table 37-1. The strength of core suture repairs using modified Kessler, modified Bunnell, and the double-grasping techniques were equivalent for all 5-0 and 4-0 suture calibers, averaging 14 and 23 newtons,

respectively (Fig. 37-3). The mode of failure for all 5-0 and 4-0 core sutures was by suture rupture in all but three of the 4-0 modified Kessler repairs (Fig. 37-4). When 2-0 and 3-0 sutures were used for the core repair, the Bunnell and double-grasping techniques were stronger than the modified Kessler. Failures in this subgroup revealed 6 of 10 of the 3-0 and 10 of 10 of the 2-0 modified Kessler repairs failed due to suture pullout, while only 4 of 20 of the failures with the Bunnell or double-grasping techniques were caused by suture pullout (see Fig. 37-4). Increasing suture caliber notably affected core suture strength for all techniques tested with 4-0 being 64% stronger than 5-0 (23/14 newtons), 3-0 43% stronger than 4-0 (33/23 newtons), and 2-0 63% stronger than 3-0 (54/33 newtons) when assessed as the average of all techniques.

In comparing running versus cross-stitch epitendinous repairs, we found the cross-stitch to be about 2.5 times stronger for both 6-0 and 5-0 caliber sutures. Using 5-0 or 6-0 monofilament suture, the cross-stitch technique was also stronger than all 4-0 and 5-0 core repair techniques used

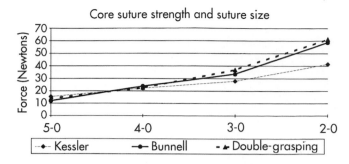

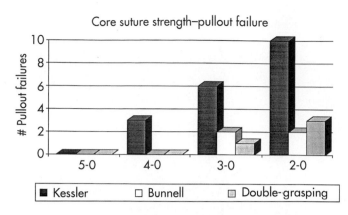

Fig. 37-3. Core suture strength and suture size. A significant increase in core suture strength is gained by increasing the core suture caliber.

Fig. 37-4. Core suture strength pullout failure. The Kessler core suture proved to have a lesser grasping strength with failure occurring by pullout of the suture with larger diameter sutures.

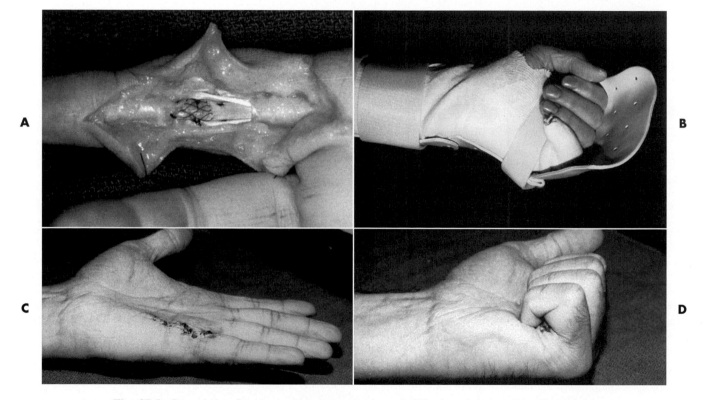

Fig. 37-5. Case study of active motion postoperative rehabilitation program. This 32-year-old professional guitarist sustained a zone II flexor tendon laceration of his small finger. **A,** the tendons were repaired with a 3-0 double-grasping core suture and a 6-0 cross-stitch epitendinous suture. **B,** active motion was initiated on postoperative day 1. **C** and **D,** full motion is restored by 3 weeks after repair.

alone. The 6-0 cross-stitch averaged 27 newtons of tensile strength compared to the 4-0 core suture modified Kessler, Bunnell, and double-grasping techniques, which averaged 22, 24, and 23 newtons, respectively.

When used in combination with a 6-0 cross-stitch epitendinous repair, the double-grasping core suture peaked at 73 newtons of tensile strength when the core suture size was 2-0 or 3-0.

The clinical results of flexor tendon repair using the 3-0 double-grasping and 6-0 cross-stitch technique combined with an active motion postoperative therapy protocol were graded by the Strickland method.[27] Overall recovery of digital motion was graded as excellent in 12 and good in 2, with 8 (57%) recovering normal or nearly normal (over 90%) of motion (Fig. 37-5). The average percent return of motion in the series was 87%. The 3 cases of FPL repair averaged 92% recovery of motion. The 4 cases of zone I FDP repair averaged 91% recovery of motion. The 7 digits with FDP and FDS repairs in zone II averaged 83% recovery of motion.

DISCUSSION

Urbaniak's[32] 1975 report analyzing the tensile strengths of tendon suturing methods detailed the mechanical properties of flexor tendon repair techniques and the forces imparted on the tendons during both passive and active digital motion. In Urbaniak's immobilized canine model, significant initial repair strength was lost during the early phase of healing. The initial repair strength was not recovered until 3 weeks postoperatively. During this period of tendon weakening, tensile strength dipped perilously close to that within an actively flexing digit. Savage[20] followed this study a decade later with an analysis of the mechanical properties of tendon repair noting that a significant increase in the repair strength could be gained by increasing the number of suture strands crossing the repair site. By using a technique that tripled the suture material fixing the tendons together and allowing a sufficient grasping hold of the tendon, the repair strength could theoretically be tripled. Using a porcine in vitro model, Savage demonstrated a repair strength of 67 newtons using his six strands of 4-0 braided polyester technique. His technique could support active mobilization of the digit and was used with apparent success in a limited clinical series. Trail[31] studied the Savage technique in a human cadaver model using 4-0 braided polyester and found the tensile strength to be about half (32 newtons) that reported by Savage, but greater than twice as strong as standard two-strand repairs. Notwithstanding the gain in repair strength, the acceptance of Savage's technique appears to be limited by the technical difficulty in clinical application.

Repair techniques that were experimentally demonstrated to be stronger than the standard two-strand repairs were presented by Ketchum (52 newtons, 4-0 polyester),[12] Robertson (51.6 newtons, 3-0 monofilament),[19] and Lee (45 newtons, 4-0 polyester)[13] using four strands of suture. In each experiment the repair strength was about twice the strength of standard repairs that used half the suture material. Lee[14] followed his experimental work with a clinical study using active mobilization for 11 Zone II flexor repairs noting 1 rupture and excellent clinical outcomes in the series.

In our study, using an in vitro cadaver model, we found that core suture caliber has a significant effect on repair strength. Looking at mode of failure for standard two strand repairs using 5-0 or 4-0 core sutures, the strength of repair was dependent upon the strength of the suture itself, not the technique. When the suture caliber is increased to 3-0 or 2-0, a significant gain in repair strength can be achieved without

adding to the technical difficulty of the repair. When using 3-0 or 2-0 core sutures, the grasping quality of the technique appears to play a significant role in the repair strength. The modified Kessler suture proved to have the weakest grasp in this regard with failure occurring by suture pullout in a majority of the tests when 3-0 or 2-0 suture was used. The Bunnell and double-grasping core suture techniques had better grasping power with failure primarily dependent on the strength of the suture itself.

Translating this to the clinical setting, our data support other studies that have shown that the two-strand 4-0 repair should provide sufficient strength to permit a passive mobilization therapy regimen in which it is estimated that forces of about 9 newtons[21,32] are encountered. Despite this, rupture of the repair occurs in up to 7% of clinical trials with close postoperative therapy supervision.[5,26] It is likely that even under controlled circumstances inadvertent active tendon stress occurs and exceeds the repair strength leading to rupture. Our report supports using a larger caliber suture to increase the margin of safety by increasing the repair strength even when a passive mobilization program is to be followed. One limitation met in increasing the suture caliber is the addition of bulk to the repair because of increased knot size. The effect on the microcirculation of the tendon may likewise be affected by increasing the suture caliber, and is not addressed by our study.

Recent attention has been directed to the role of epitendinous suture in preventing gap formation and adding to the core suture repair strength, as greater strength is found in those techniques designed to grasp the tendon ends.[15,17,18,22,33] In our study, the cross-stitch technique reported by Silfverskiöld proved to be about 2.5 times stronger than the running epitendinous suture. Increasing the suture caliber from 6-0 to 5-0 added a modest amount of strength to the epitendinous repair (3 newtons for running, 5 newtons for cross-stitch). Our findings differed from Silfverskiöld's study on bovine flexor tendons, where we found the strength of the cross-stitch using 6-0 monofilament suture (27 newtons) to be less than half the 63 newtons Silfverskiöld found using 6-0 braided polyester. Although not measured in our study, gap formation was not observed until near failure in most specimens using the cross-stitch with and without core suture. This may be attributable to the Chinese finger trap weave pattern of the cross-stitch technique in which a squeeze is placed upon the repair site with tension. The effect on the microcirculation of the tendon could be affected by this squeezing, but it was not addressed by our study.

The final series of tests performed in our study assessed the combined double-grasping and cross-stitch techniques. Strength peaked at 73 newtons for both 3-0 and 2-0 core suture calibers using a 6-0 monofilament epitendinous cross-stitch. This compares favorably with the reported tensile demands of active unresisted flexion of the digit which range up to 35 newtons,[21,32] but insufficient to resist forceful resisted flexion and pinch, which average 50 to 80 newtons and range up to 120 newtons with forceful pinch.[12,21,32] The precise tensile resistance requirements of the repaired tendon in the clinical setting are unknown. Many factors likely act to increase the resistance of the tendon in the injured digit and repaired tendon, such as swelling of the digit and increased drag of the tendon. Also unknown are the effects of repair strength during passive and active mobilization programs in the clinical setting. With concern about repair site weakening as demonstrated in Urbaniak's[32] immobilized canine model, active motion in the early postoperative period has largely been avoided. On the other hand, Gelberman[9] has demonstrated that stressed tendons will heal and gain tensile strength faster than unstressed repairs. Thus the repair strength necessary to safely permit active digital flexion after flexor tendon repair remains unknown.

While passive mobilization techniques can produce tendon excursion approaching that of active flexion, individual variation is great.[23] Given a repair technique that safely tolerates the added strain of an active mobilization program, more predictable and potentially greater tendon excursion may ensue. Strickland[29] recently presented a rationale for determining the initial repair strength required for active mobilization after flexor tendon repair and concluded that a repair of 42 newtons should provide sufficient safety for such a regimen. The combined double-grasping 3-0 core and cross-stitch 6-0 epitendinous suture with a strength of 73 newtons on theoretical grounds should provide repair strength sufficient to support an active mobilization regimen.

Reports by Small,[25] Cullen,[6] and Elliot[8] have shown that early active mobilization can also be achieved, with rupture rates only marginally higher than those of passive mobilization programs, using standard repair techniques. The results of the series using early active mobilization programs using standard repair techniques[6,8,25] have not, however, demonstrated results better than those achieved with passive programs.

Although the information collected in this study was used as a basis to determine a suture repair technique of sufficient strength to permit active motion of repaired flexor tendons, it does not compare the standard or alternative core suture techniques with stronger epitendinous techniques with that of our preferred technique. Therefore it is not our intention to demonstrate the advantage of the double-grasping cross-stitch combination over other methods of tendon repair, which provide an increase in repair strength.

Currently, we are applying the technique of the combined double-grasping and cross-stitch repair in the clinical setting using an active mobilization program and are encouraged by the early results. At this point, however, we believe that further clinical study must be undertaken to assess the efficacy of this technique.

REFERENCES

1. Becker H, Orac F, Durnselle E: Early active motion following a beveled technique of flexor tendon repair: report on fifty cases, *J Hand Surg* 1979; 4(5):454-460.
2. Becker H: Primary repair of flexor tendons in the hand without immobilization—preliminary report, *Hand* 1978; 10(1):37-47.
3. Brunelli G, Vigasio A, Brunelli F: Slip-knot flexor tendon suture in zone II allowing immediate mobilization, *Hand* 1983; 15(3):352-358.
4. Bunnell S: Repair of tendons in the fingers, *Surg Gynecol Obstet* 1922; 35:88-97.
5. Chow JA, Thomes LJ, Dovelle S, et al: A combined regimen of controlled motion following flexor tendon repair in "no man's land," *Plast Reconstr Surg* 1987; 79(3):447-453.
6. Cullen V, Tolhurst P, Urb D, Page R: Flexor tendon repair followed by controlled active mobilization, *J Hand Surg* 1989; 14B:392-395.
7. Duran J, Huber R: Controlled passive motion following flexor tendon repair in zones 2 and 3. In *AAOS symposium on tendon surgery of the hand*, St Louis, 1975, Mosby.
8. Elliot D, Moiemen NS, Flemming AFS, et al: The rupture rate of acute flexor tendon repairs mobilized by the controlled active motion regimen, *J Hand Surg* 1994; 19B(5):607-612.
9. Gelberman RH, Woo SL, Lothringer K, et al: Effects of early intermittent passive mobilization on healing canine flexor tendons, *J Hand Surg* 1982; 7A:170-175.
10. Hester TR, Hill L, Nahai F: Early mobilization of repaired flexor tendons within digital sheath using an internal profundus splint: experimental and clinical data, *Ann Plast Surg* 1984; 12(2):187-198.
11. Kessler I, Nissim F: Primary repair without immobilization of flexor tendon division within the digital sheath, *Acta Orthop Scand* 1969; 40:587-601.
12. Ketchum LD, Martin NL, Kappel DA: Experimental evaluation of factors affecting the strength of tendon repairs, *Plast Reconstr Surg* 1977; 59(5):708-719.
13. Lee H: Double loop locking suture: a technique of tendon repair for early active mobilization, part I, evolution of technique and experimental study, *J Hand Surg* 1990; 15A:945-952.
14. Lee H: Double loop locking suture: a technique of tendon repair for early active mobilization, part II, clinical experience, *J Hand Surg* 1990; 15A:953-958.
15. Lin GT, An K-N, Amadio PC, Cooney WP: Biomechanical studies of running suture for flexor tendon repair in dogs, *J Hand Surg* 1988; 13A:553-558.
16. Lister G, Kleinert H, Kutz J, Atasoy E: Primary flexor tendon repair followed by immediate controlled mobilization, *J Hand Surg* 1977; 2:441-451.
17. Mashadi ZB, Amis AA: Strength of the suture in the epitenon and within the tendon fibres: development of stronger peripheral suture technique, *J Hand Surg* 1992; 17B:171-175.
18. Pruitt DL, Manske PR, Fink B: Cyclic stress analysis of flexor tendon repair, *J Hand Surg* 1991; 16A:701-707.
19. Robertson GA, Al-Qattan MM: A biomechanical analysis of a new interlock suture technique for flexor tendon repair, *J Hand Surg* 1992; 17B:92-93.
20. Savage R: In vitro studies of a new method of flexor tendon repair, *J Hand Surg* 1985; 10B:135-141.
21. Schuind F, Garcia-Elias M, Cooney W III, An KN: Flexor tendon forces in vivo measurements, *J Hand Surg* 1992; 17A:291-292.
22. Silfverskiöld KL, Anderson CH: Two new methods of tendon repair: an in vitro evaluation of tensile strength and gap formation, *J Hand Surg* 1993; 18A:58-65.
23. Silfverskiöld KL, May E, Tornwall A: Tendon excursion after flexor tendon repair in zone II: results with a new controlled motion program, *J Hand Surg* 1993; 18A:403-410.
24. Silfverskiöld KL, May EJ: Flexor tendon repair in zone II with a new suture technique and an early mobilization program combining passive and active motion, *J Hand Surg* 1994; 19A:53-60.

25. Small JO, Brennen MD, Colville J: Early active mobilization following flexor tendon repair in zone 2, *J Hand Surg* 1989; 14B(4):383-391.

26. Strickland J, Glogovac SV: Digital function following flexor tendon repair, zone II, comparison of immobilization and controlled passive motion techniques, *J Hand Surg* 1980; 5:537-543.

27. Strickland JW: Results of flexor tendon surgery in zone II, *Hand Clin* 1985; 1:167-179.

28. Strickland JW: Opinions and preferences in flexor tendon surgery, *Hand Clin* 1985; 1(1):187-191.

29. Strickland JW, ed: Flexor tendon repair—Indiana method, *Indiana Hand Center Newsletter* 1993; 1(1):1-19.

30. Taras JS, Hunter JM: Acute flexor tendon injuries. In Cohen M, ed: *Mastery of surgery,* Boston, 1994, Little, Brown.

31. Trail IA, Powell ES, Noble J: The mechanical strength of various suture techniques, *J Hand Surg* 1992; 17B:89-91.

32. Urbaniak JR, Cahill JD, Mortenson RA: Tendon suturing methods: analysis of tensile strengths. In *AAOS symposium of tendon surgery of the hand,* St Louis, 1975, Mosby.

33. Wade PJF, Wetherell RG, Amis AA: Flexor tendon repair: significant gain in strength from the Halsted peripheral suture technique, *J Hand Surg* 1989; 14B:232-235.

Chapter 38

THE ROLE OF EPITENON PERIPHERAL REPAIR ON THE STRENGTH AND FUNCTION OF FLEXOR TENDON LACERATIONS

John M. Bednar

The relationship between early tendon motion and improved clinical results after flexor tendon repair in zone II has been clearly shown.[1,3,7,9,16] The most commonly used protocols use early passive motion of the digit to achieve improved tendon motion and decreased tendon adhesion.[3,7,9,14-16] Early active motion would be superior in achieving improved motion after tendon repair, if a tendon suture was used that was strong enough to prevent gap formation or rupture at the tendon repair site.

A repair performed using a core suture does not have sufficient strength to reliably allow early active motion. The addition of an epitenon suture to the core suture adds significant strength to the repair site. This added strength approaches the level at which early active tendon motion can be considered safe.

FLEXOR TENDON FORCES

Tendon forces have been measured by several authors[2,11] to determine the force that a flexor tendon repair would be subjected to during active and passive finger and wrist motion. Passive motion of the wrist generates 0.1 to 0.6 kgf (0.98 to 5.88 newtons), while passive finger motion generates 0.1 to 0.9 kgf (0.98 to 8.82 newtons) (Fig. 38-1, A). Active wrist motion generates 0.2 to 0.4 kgf (1.96 to 3.92 newtons). Active finger motion generates 0.1 to 3.5 kgf (0.98 to 34.3 newtons) and grasp produces 1.9 to 6.4 kgf (18.6 to 62.7 newtons) (Fig. 38-1, B). Any suture repair technique to be used in a patient in which early active motion is planned in the postoperative period would have to be strong enough to withstand at least these forces.

SUTURE TECHNIQUE TENSILE STRENGTH

The breaking strength of the commonly used suture techniques for flexor tendon repair has been measured by Urbaniak.[17] The repair techniques measured involved the use of only a core suture. Breaking strength ranged from 1.68 kgf (1683 gmf, 16.5 newtons) for an interrupted repair to 3.97 kgf (38.9 newtons) for a Kessler repair. This level of tensile strength of a core suture is below the force generated at the repair site during active finger motion and grasp.

The addition of a running epitenon suture was first proposed to invert the tendon edges to decrease tendon adhesion and improve gliding. Wade and associates[18] demonstrated that the epitenon suture not only improved tendon gliding but also contributed to the strength of the repair and decreased gap formation under load. Lin and associates[8] have shown that the additional strength provided by an epitenon suture varys according to the method used. A simple running epitenon suture had an average breaking

Passive motion

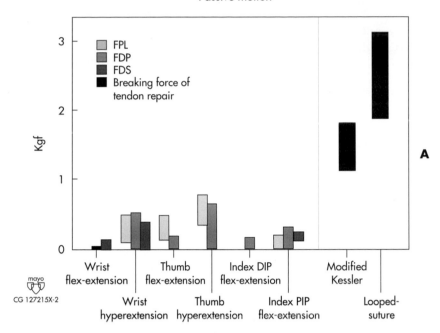

Active motion

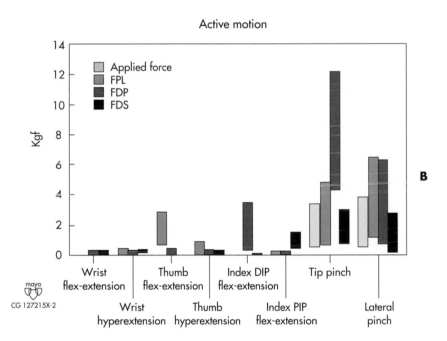

Fig. 38-1. A, The forces generated in the flexor tendons during passive motion. **B,** The forces generated in the flexor tendons during active motion. (From Schuind F, Garcias-Elias M, Cooney WP II, An K-N, *J Hand Surg* 17A[2]:297, 1992.)

strength of 6.48 newtons, a Lembert-type suture 14.55 newtons, and a locking type suture 24.43 newtons. These measurements were for a tendon repaired using only an epitenon suture without a core suture.

The combination of a core suture and an epitenon suture will further increase the tensile strength of a tendon repair. Silfverskiöld and associates[13] measured this effect. They found the breaking strength for a modified Kessler suture performed with a 4-0 polyester suture to be 27.4 newtons. The addition of a 6-0 epitenon suture along the volar half of the tendon increased the strength of the repair to 37.6 newtons and the addition of a circumferential epitenon suture increased the strength to 47.8 newtons. A modified transverse mattress suture (cross-stitch, Fig. 38-2) developed by Silfverskiöld was also tested in this model and found to increase tensile strength to 62.8 newtons.

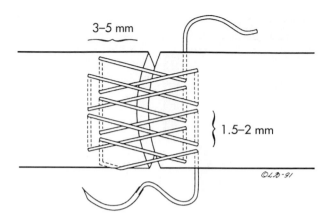

Fig. 38-2. Modified transverse mattress suture. (From Silverskiöld KL, Anderson CH, *J Hand Surg* 18A[1]:59, 1993.)

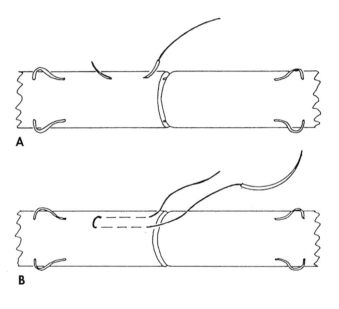

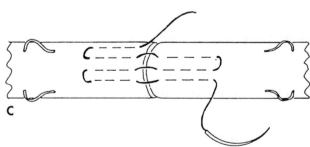

Fig. 38-3. Technique for Halsted tendon suture. (From Wade PJF, Wetherell RG, Amis AA, *J Hand Surg* 14B[2]:233, 1989.)

An alternative technique described by Wade[19] involved the use of a Halsted suture technique (Fig. 38-3). This core suture epitenon combination had a measured breaking strength of 79.2 newtons. The strength of these suture techniques is well beyond that level which would be required to withstand the force of early active motion postoperatively.

SUMMARY

Early active motion after zone II flexor tendon repair would decrease tendon adhesion and result in a greater arc of total active motion. Active motion places forces on the repair site, which are greater than that which a repair with only a core suture can withstand without gap formation and rupture. The addition of a running epitenon suture significantly increases the tensile strength of the repair site. A grasping type of locked epitenon suture produces tendon-breaking strengths that are sufficiently high to withstand the forces generated by early active motion postoperatively.

These data, however, were generated from cadaver tendons and do not account for the decreased pullout strength of the tendon ends, which occurs 4 to 10 days postinjury.[4-6] The effect of cyclic stress[10-12] and gap formation or the effect of the increased tendon sheath dissection required to place these sutures on tendon adhesion were not studied.

REFERENCES

1. Becker H, Orak F, Duponselle E: Early active motion following a beveled technique of flexor tendon repair, report on fifty cases, *J Hand Surg* 1979; 4:454.
2. Bright DS, Urbaniak JS: Direct measurements of flexor tendon tension during active and passive digit motion and its application to flexor tendon surgery, *Trans Orthop Res Soc* 1976; 240.
3. Duran RJ, Houser RG, Coleman CR, Postlewaite DS: A preliminary report in the use of controlled passive motion following flexor tendon repair in zones II and III, *J Hand Surg* 1976; 1:79.
4. Gelberman RH, VandeBerg JS, Manske PR, Akeson WH: The early stages of flexor tendon healing: a morphologic study of the first fourteen days, *J Hand Surg* 1985; 10A:766.
5. Ketchum LD: Suture materials and suture techniques used in tendon repair, *Hand Clin* 1985; 1:43.
6. Ketchum LD, Martin NL, Kappel DA: Experimental evaluation of factors affecting the strength of tendon repairs, *Plast Reconstr Surg* 1977; 59:708.
7. Kleinert HE, Kutz JE, Ashbell S, Martinez E: Primary repair of lacerated flexor tendons in "no man's land," *J Bone Joint Surg* 1967; 49A:557.
8. Lin GT, Amadio PC, Cooney WP III: Biomechanical studies of running suture for flexor tendon repair in dogs, *J Hand Surg* 1988; 13A(4):553.
9. Lister GD, Kleinert HE, Kutz JE, Atasoy E: Primary flexor tendon repair followed by immediate controlled mobilization, *J Hand Surg* 1977; 2:441.
10. Pruitt DL, Manske MD, Fink B: Cyclic stress analysis of flexor tendon repair, *J Hand Surg* 1991; 16A(4):701.
11. Schuind F, Garcias-Elias M, Cooney WP III, An K: Flexor tendon forces: in vivo measurements, *J Hand Surg* 1992; 17A(2):291.
12. Seradge H: Elongation of the repair configuration following flexor tendon repair, *J Hand Surg* 1983; 8:182.
13. Silfverskiöld KL, Anderson CH: Two new methods of tendon repair: an in vitro evaluation of tensile strength and gap formation, *J Hand Surg* 1993; 18A(1):58.
14. Silfverskiöld KL, May EJ, Tornvall AH: Gap formation during controlled motion after flexor tendon repair in zone II, a prospective clinical study, *J Hand Surg* 1992; 17A(3):539.
15. Strickland JW: Flexor tendon repair, *Hand Clin North Am* 1985; 1:55.

16. Strickland JW, Glogovac SV: Digital function following flexor tendon repair in zone II, a comparison of immobilization and controlled passive motion techniques, *J Hand Surg* 1980; 5:537.

17. Urbaniak JR, Cahill JD, Mortenson RA: Tendon suturing methods: analysis of tensile strength. In *AAOS symposium on tendon surgery in the hand,* St Louis, 1978, Mosby.

18. Wade PJF, Muir IFK, Hutcheon LL: Primary flexor tendon repair: the mechanical limitations of the modified Kessler technique, *J Hand Surg* 1986; 11B(1):71.

19. Wade PJF, Wetherell RG, Amis AA: Flexor tendon repair: significant gain in strength from the Halsted peripheral suture technique, *J Hand Surg* 1989; 14B(2):232.

Chapter 39

INDICATION AND TECHNIQUES FOR EARLY POSTOPERATIVE MOTION AFTER REPAIR OF DIGITAL FLEXOR TENDON PARTICULARLY IN ZONE II

Tatsuya Tajima

In the present era of advanced surgery of the hand, the treatment of lacerated or ruptured digital flexor tendons, particularly in zone II, is still problematic, because no one obtains an absolutely excellent result. The main problem is how to prevent adhesion and disruption of the sutured site.

Although Lindsay,[7] Matthews,[10] Manske,[9] Lundborg,[8] and others[14] proved intrinsic healing of the digital flexor tendons experimentally, laceration of the tendon is usually accompanied with laceration of tendon sheath and other tissues surrounding the tendons. The reparative process takes place simultaneously at the same level, which inevitably causes adhesions of the healing tendon with surrounding tissues, as Peacock[6] aptly pointed out with the phrase, "one wound one scar" (Fig. 39-1). So far the only practical means to minimize adhesion is early postoperative movement of the sutured site.

Kleinert[5] and Duran[3] proposed practical methods of early motion. Kleinert's method seems more popular, because appropriate placement of his splint is regarded to ensure safe early motion of the operated digit; this technique seems easier than Duran's passive movement, which has to be done very carefully. The reason Kleinert's method is considered safe is that passive flexion of the interphalangeal (IP) joints is done by rubber band traction and limited active extension by active contraction of the lumbricals, which stretches the flexor digitorum profundus (FDP) distally and makes its active contraction impossible (Fig. 39-2). This prevents a sudden strong pull being exerted on the suture site, which can cause disruption. However, some hand surgeons were concerned about danger of disruption caused by early motion. As a result we asked our hand therapists to induce electromyography (EMG) from the FDP in every case in which this operation had been performed, and often found active contraction of the FDP taking place simultaneously with active contraction of the lumbricals (Fig. 39-3). Perhaps this takes place because if the origins of the lumbricals do not shift distally simultaneously with contraction of the lumbricals, the power of extension of IP joints will be stronger. Therefore if resistance of limited active IP joints' extension is stronger (e.g., with friction by edema or too strong a pull of rubber band), the FDP may automatically contract to a certain extent not to shift the origins of lumbricals distally (Fig. 39-4). Simultaneous contraction of the FDP with contraction of the lumbricals has been proved not only by our group but also by Cition and Forster,[2] who published their data in 1987.

MODIFIED SPLINTS

Wolff,[15] one of Kleinert's associates, published a modified type of the original Louisville type of splint in 1986. It

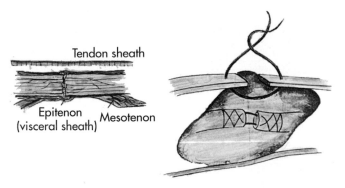

Fig. 39-1. Why postoperative early motion is necessary despite experimentally proved intrinsic healing of the tendon. In a clinical situation, laceration of a flexor tendon usually is accompanied by laceration of tissues surrounding the tendon; and the reparative process takes place at the same site; therefore extrinsic healing is inevitable. Surrounding tissues are simultaneously lacerated and reparative process takes place in a common space "One wound one scar" after E. Peacock 1970.

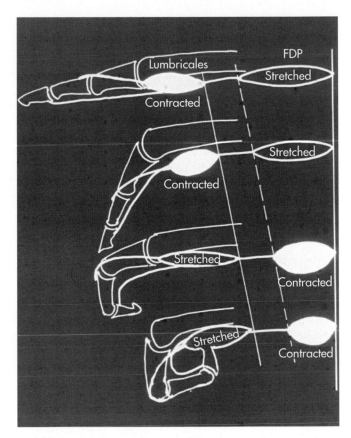

Fig. 39-2. Active extension of interphalangeal joints, regardless of the position of metacarpophalangeal joints, is made by active contraction of lumbricals, which pull the flexor digitorum profundus (FDP) distally and makes its active contraction weaker.

T.O. 26 yrs, M.   '89.8.23: Laceration of FDP and FDS little, Rt.   H.M. 18 yrs, M.   '89.9.7: Laceration of FDP long and ring, FDS
'89.8.24: Repaired   ring, rad. prop. dig.N. long and ring
                                                                                             '89.9.8: Repaired
Early motion: uneventful   '89.9.21: FDP long ruptured

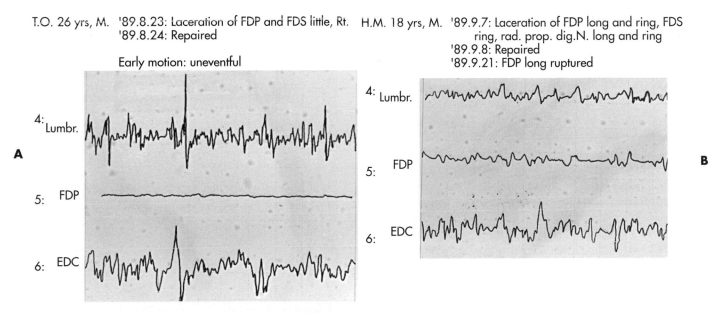

Fig. 39-3. A, Limited active extension of the interphalangeal (IP) joints does not usually cause active contraction of the flexor digitorum profundus (FDP), as pointed out by Kleinert. **B,** However, active extension of the IP joints occasionally causes active contraction of the FDP, which tends to disrupt the sutured site of the digital flexor tendon when the rubber band is too tight or there is edema.

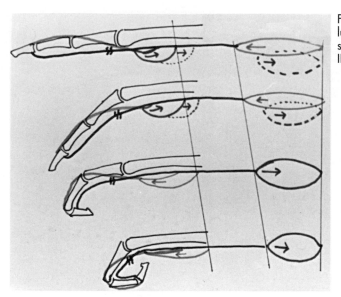

FDP can contract while lumbrical contracts for stronger extension of IP joints.

Fig. 39-4. If the resistance to active extension of interphalangeal (IP) joints is strong, the flexor digitorum profundus (FDP) may actively contract to prevent the distal migration of the origins of lumbricals, which may strengthen the power of active extension of IP joints.

has a roller bar at the metacarpophalangeal (MP) joint level to increase passive flexion of IP joints. Attachment of a safety pin at the MP joint level can fulfill this purpose (Fig. 39-5), but the modified splint has another important mechanism, that is, a spring coil that does not increase tension of the rubber band when the operated finger is more extended. One of my co-workers in the Niigata University Hospital made the tape-measure type of splint, which is attached at the level of MP joints with velcro adhesive tape and also a spring coil that supresses the increase of rubber-band tension when the operated digit extends more (Fig. 39-6), possessing nearly the same mechanism as the modified Louisville type. In 1989 I moved from the University Hospital to the Niigata Hand Surgery Foundation, where another modified type of splint was being used for early postoperative motion, which was designed by Dr. Yoshizu, one of my former trainees. This splint has a transverse bar at the level of the MP joints to increase passive IP joint flexion, but has no spring coil that supresses the increase of rubber-band tension when the IP joint is more extended. Therefore the hand therapist has to grasp the fishing line or rubber band and move the grasping point distally during limited active extension of IP joints so that no increased tension is exerted on the suture site. Instead, another fishing line connected to another rubber band is hooked to the adjacent digit with a little more tension than to the operated digit, so that less power can be exerted on the suture site than the adjacent digit (Fig. 39-7). This may make limited active extension of the operated digit smoother and prevent disruption of the suture site. It is ideal to hook the rubber band to all four digits (i.e., index to little fingers) and let them extend

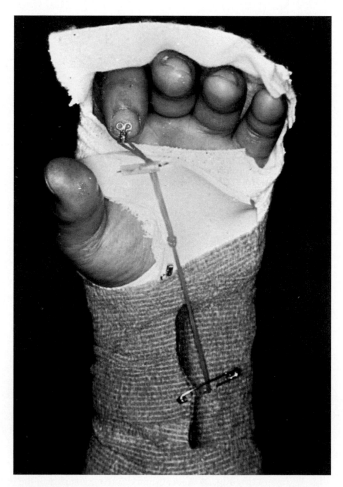

Fig. 39-5. A safety pin placed at the metacarpophalangeal joint level as a pulley can increase passive flexion of interphalangeal joints.

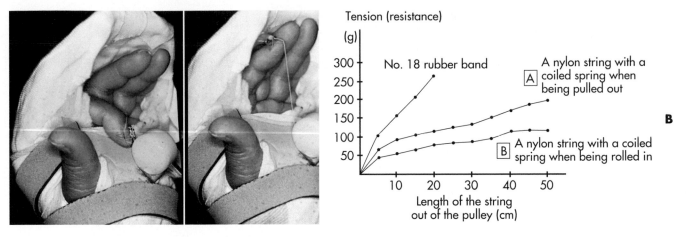

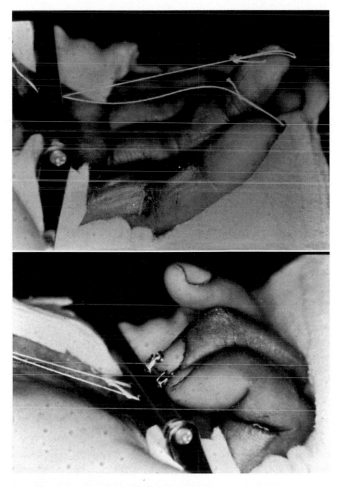

Fig. 39-6. **A,** Handy, tape-measure type of splint made by Dr. Tanaka, which can be attached at metacarpophalangeal joint level. **B,** The tension of the fish line does not increase much when interphalangeal (IP) joints are extended (compare tension of *A* when the IP joints are extended and *B* when the IP joints are passively flexed).

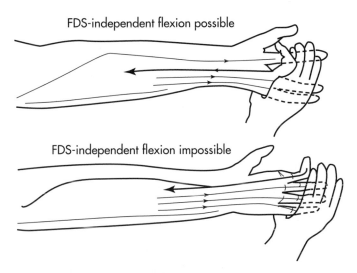

Fig. 39-7. Another type of splint now used in our institute. A fish line with more tension is anchored to the adjacent digit, so that less power of passive flexion and active extension is exerted on the operated digit (i.e., on the suture site of the flexor tendon).

Fig. 39-8. In the flexor digitorum superficialis (FDS), muscle fibers to flex each digit are fairly independent, so that a certain muscle fiber can be stretched distally, but other muscle fibers can actively contract, while in the flexor digitorum profundus (FDP) muscle, certain muscle fibers for a digit cannot independently contract or be stretched.

Table 39-1. Early mobilization versus immobilization in unfavorable group (39 fingers)*

	E	G	F	P
Kleinert method (29 fingers)	6 (21%)	10 (34%)	2 (7%)	11 (38%)
	55%			
Immobilization (10)	1 (10%)	1 (10%)	1 (10%)	7 (70%)
	20%			

*Follow-up study shows that the results of cases with Kleinert's original splint were better than those with postoperative immobilization for 3 weeks.

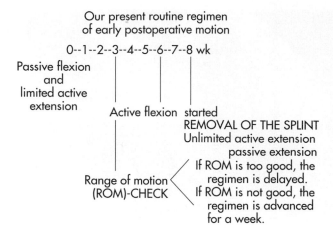

Fig. 39-9. Our present routine regimen of early postoperative motion.

Table 39-2. Original Kleinert method versus our method*

	Original Kleinert method				Our method			
	E	G	F	P	E	G	F	P
Total	13 (31%)	12 (29%)	3 (7%)	14 (33%)	11 (73%)	2 (13%)	2 (13%)	0 (0)
	60%				86%			
Favorable G.	7 (54%)	2 (15%)	1 (8%)	3 (23%)	11 (79%)	2 (14%)	1 (7%)	0 (0)
	69%				93%			
Unfavorable G.	6 (21%)	10 (34%)	2 (7%)	11 (38%)	0 (0)	0 (0)	1 (100%)	0 (0)
	55%							

*Follow-up study shows that the results of cases with modified splint are better than those cases with Kleinert's original splint.

or flex together, because an FDP muscle does not allow opposite movement of each independent digit as a flexor digitorum superficialis (FDS) can (Fig. 39-8). At the Niigata Hand Surgery Foundation, except in cases in which immobilization was indicated, the original Kleinert splint had been used until 1987, then the modified splint described previously was used.

RESULTS

Three years ago, we did a follow-up examination of 42 fingers of 37 cases, in which both lacerated digital flexor tendons in zone II were repaired. The average follow-up period was 29 months so we could compare the results of (1) immobilization for 3 weeks, (2) the original Kleinert method, and (3) the Tajima modified splints. Cases were classified into favorable and unfavorable cases in which other tissues were also injured. Cases treated with Kleinert's original splint gave better results than cases treated with immobilization (Table 39-1) for 3 weeks; better results were obtained in cases treated with the Tajima splint than in those treated with the Louisville splint (Table 39-2).

Our present regimen of early postoperative motion is placement of the Tajima splint the day after surgery, passive flexion, and limited active extension for 3 weeks. The splint is kept on for another 2 weeks, but during this period careful active flexion is started. The splint is removed at 6 weeks when unlimited active extension is started. Allow passive extension at 8 weeks. If contracture is marked at the end of the third week or at the beginning of the fourth week, our regimen is advanced a week. If movement is very smooth, the regimen is delayed for 1 week, considering the possibility of disruption (Fig. 39-9).

Chow[1] obtained the best results we know of by combining Kleinert's method with Duran's passive movement in the first 2 weeks after flexor tendon repair. The reason for his excellent results could have been because of excellent material (i.e., young soldiers as Strickland[13] pointed out). However, our present results are as good as Chow's. I would like to mention briefly that we leave the flexor sheath open except at A_2 and A_4 and do not try to close the sheath completely. We do this because this procedure may have an advantage, as Lister described, but also a drawback of

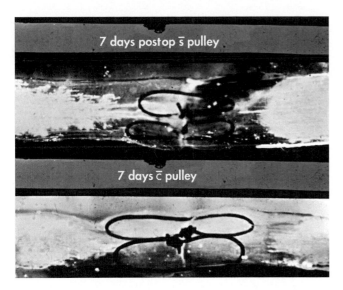

Fig. 39-10. Completely closing the flexor tendon sheath may have certain advantages, but simultaneous disadvantages (e.g., squeezing the blood circulation of the sutured site), as this experiment shows. (Result of our experimental study, with chicken's digital flexor tendon, a week after suturing its laceration, melcox, a molding resin is injected into ulnar artery.)

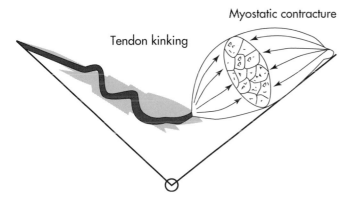

Fig. 39-11. There are two kinds of shortening of tendons, after a certain interval between time of laceration and repair. One is *myostatic contracture* and the other is *kinking of the proximal tendon,* surrounding which a connective tissue scar is formed, which can be released by a strong distal pull intraoperatively.

squeezing the blood supply to the suture site, which our experiment proved (Fig. 39-10). I repair the lacerated flexor tendon whenever reasonably possible, regardless of the interval since the injury. The term *delayed primary repair* is often used, but its definition is not unanimously agreed on. The definition of the Committee of the International Federation of Societies for Surgery of the Hand (IFSSH) is within 2 weeks,[13] but that of Kessler[4] is within a month. In zone II laceration of digital flexor tendon, approximation of lacerated tendon stumps is often possible by a strong distal pull of the proximal tendon segment, which releases kinking of the tendon segment falling into shortening by scarring the

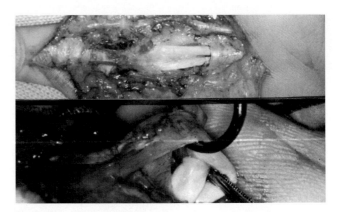

Fig. 39-12. The lacerated proximal stump of the flexor digitorum profundus (FDP) tendon, although invisible at the chiasma, did not retract too far by still connecting lumbricals and vincula. In this case the proximal stump of the lacerated FDP tendon was located just beneath or dorsal to the chiasma, which made direct repair possible, although the interval between laceration and repair was 6 months.

connective tissues surrounding the tendon (Fig. 39-11), but the reason approximation of both stumps is possible is that a proximal stump does not retract too far by still connecting lumbricals and vincula (Fig. 39-12).

DISCUSSION

Kessler pointed out that the postoperative early motion with the Louisville type of splint does not necessarily move the suture site of the digital flexor tendon. His conclusion was based on his observation that passive flexion and limited active extension do not necessarily move the stainless steel wire used for tendon suture visualized in x-ray film (Fig. 39-13).

This can theoretically happen, with the distal tendon segment being kinked during passive flexion and stretched during limited active extension (Fig. 39-14). The securest method to move the sutured site is to actively flex the operated digit,[4] which absolutely needs active contraction of the FDP with inevitable movement of the sutured site. However, this movement can disrupt the suture site, particularly during the first 10 days when tensile strength becomes weakest. However, very strong sutures can tolerate the early active motion. With this idea, our group is tentatively trying a very strong suture by hooking modified Tsuge's intratendinous suture at three places on the volar aspect of the flexor tendon, which must be theoretically nearly as strong as Savage's six-strand suture[12] (Fig. 39-15). This suture has been tried so far in three patients who were admitted for very careful active flexion of the operated digit under supervision of a hand therapist. Results were all excellent, without disruption of the suture site. Our group is doing experimental study on whether Tsuge's suture can be replaced with the Kessler-Tajima suture (Fig. 39-16) and evaluating which suture will be stronger during the postoperative period.

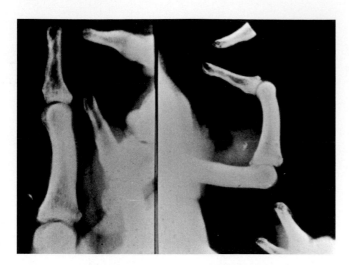

Fig. 39-13. Kessler pointed out that passive flexion and limited active extension of interphalangeal joints do not necessarily move the suture site of the digital flexor tendon, proved by an x-ray film with a stainless steel marker.

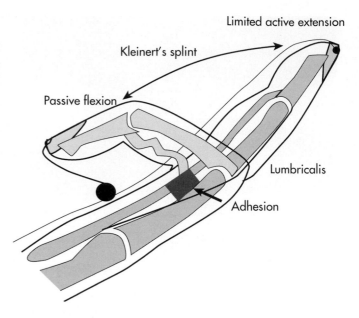

Fig. 39-14. Theoretical basis of passive flexion and limited active motion of interphalangeal (IP) joints do not always move the suture site of the digital flexor tendon. Passive flexion makes the distal segment of the tendon kink, which can be stretched by active extension of IP joints, without moving the sutured site.

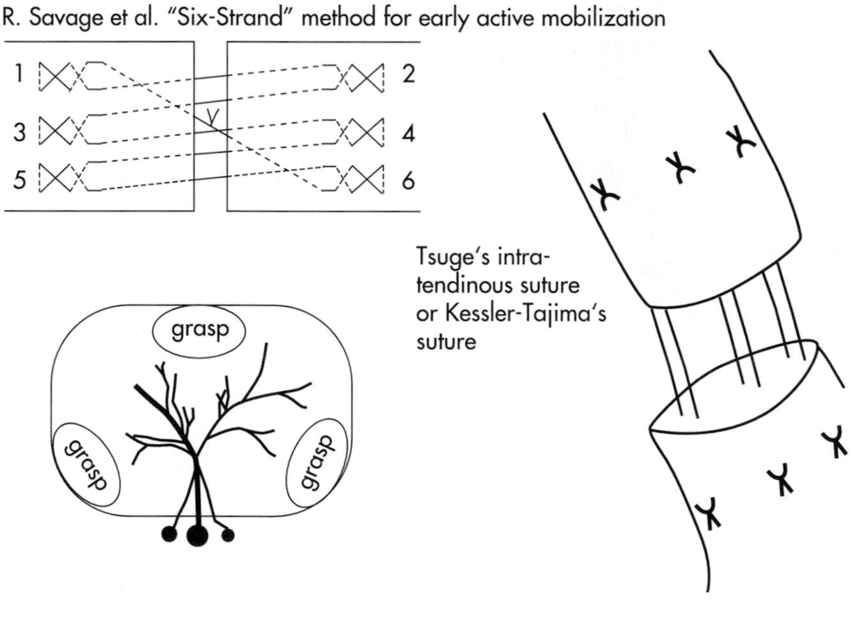

R. Savage et al. "Six-Strand" method for early active mobilization

Tsuge's intra-tendinous suture or Kessler-Tajima's suture

grasp grasp grasp

Fig. 39-15. A kind of six-strand suture being used tentatively in our institute, is considered very strong, because it is similar to Savage's suture, using three Tsuge's sutures with looped thread or the Kessler-Tajima suture. Circumferential sutures are added after the core stitches.

We consider early postoperative motion inappropriate in the following cases:

1. Children in which a plaster cast keeps the operated finger in flexion and nonoperated fingers in extension (i.e., pulling the FDP muscle fibers distally so that they cannot contract)
2. Cases in which bilateral volar proper digital arteries are lacerated and have to be microsurgically anastomosed
3. Patients who are unable to observe our strict instructions
4. Adults with EMG signs of FDP contraction during limited active extension of the operated digit, in which very careful negative feedback training can be done under supervision of a hand therapist

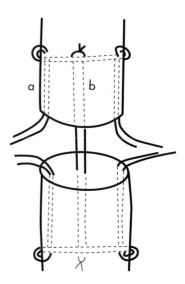

Fig. 39-16. In tentative use of Kessler-Tajima suture, a double 4-0 nylon thread with curved needles at both extremities are used, *a;* Tsuge's suture can be used as the third suture, *b.*

SUMMARY

Although Lindsay,[1] Manske,[3] Lundborg,[4] and others, proved intrinsic healing of digital flexor tendons exists, extrinsic healing is inevitable in most clinical cases, because laceration of the digital flexor tendon is accompanied by laceration of tissues surrounding the tendon, and the reparative process takes place in the same level as pointed out by Peacock.[6] Therefore the only practical means of preventing adhesion is early postoperative movement. Limited active extension with a Louisville type splint is often accompanied with simultaneous contraction of the FDP, which is proved by EMG study of the FDP and which can be an important factor in disruption of the suture site. As Kessler pointed out, gliding of the suture site takes place securely only by active flexion of the operated digit. The early postoperative active flexion may need a very strong suture to prevent the disruption of the sutured site, but it should not squeeze circulation too much or cause over-

reaction, and its technique should not be difficult. We are trying two of Tsuge's sutures at the volar aspect of a flexor tendon, which may be theoretically as strong as Savage's six-strand suture, with excellent results. We are experimentally testing whether Tsuge's suture can be replaced by the Kessler-Tajima suture.

REFERENCES

1. Chow JA, Thomes LJ, Dovelle S, et al: A combined regimen of controlled motion following flexor tendon repair in no man's land, *Plast Reconstr Surg* 1987; 79:447-453.
2. Citron ND, Forster A: Dynamic splinting following flexor tendon repair, *J Hand Surg* 1987; 12B:96-100.
3. Duran R, Houser RG: Controlled passive motion following flexor tendon repair in zone 2 and 3. In *AAOS symposium on tendon surgery in the hand,* St Louis, 1975, Mosby.
4. Kessler I, Nissim F: Primary repair without immobilization of flexor tendon division within the digital flexor sheath, *Acta Orthop Scand* 1969; 40:587-601.
5. Kleinert HE, Kutz JE, Cohen MJ: Primary repair of zone 2 flexor tendon laceration, *AAOS symposium on tendon surgery in the hand,* St Louis, 1975, Mosby.
6. Kleinert HE, Verdan C: Report of committee on tendon injuries, *J Hand Surg* 1983; 8:794-798.
7. Lindsay WK, Thompson HG: Digital flexor tendons: an experimental study, part I, the significance of each component of the flexor mechanism in tendon healing, *Brit J Plast Surg* 1960; 12:289-316.
8. Lundborg G, Rank F: Experimental intrinsic healing of flexor tendons based upon synovial fluid nutrition, *J Hand Surg* 1978; 3:21-31.
9. Manske PR, Gelberman RH, VandeBerg JS, Lesker PA: Intrinsic flexor-tendon repair: a morphological study in vitro, *J Bone Joint Surg* 1984; 66A:385-396.
10. Matthews P, Richards H: The repair potential of digital flexor tendons: an experimental study, *J Bone Joint Surg* 1974; 56B:618-625.
11. Peacock EE Jr, Van Winkle W Jr: Repair of tendons and restoration of gliding function. In Peacock EE Jr, Van Winkle W Jr, eds: *Surgery and biology of wound repair,* Philadelphia, 1970, Saunders.
12. Savage R, Risitano G: Flexor tendon repair using a "six-strand" method of repair and early active mobilization, *J Hand Surg* 1989; 14B:396-399.
13. Strickland JW: Discussion of the paper cited in reference 12, *Plast Reconstr Surg* 1987; 73:454-455.
14. Tokita Y, Yamaya A: An experimental study on the repair and restoration of gliding function after digital flexor tendon injury, part I, repair of the sutured digital flexor tendon within the digital sheath, *J Jpn Orthop Assoc* 1964; 48:107-127.
15. Wolff TW: *Modification of Louisville dynamic splint for flexor tendon injury,* Abstract of the 3rd Congress of IFSSH, Tokyo, 1986.

Chapter 40

POSTOPERATIVE THERAPY CONCEPTS IN MANAGEMENT OF FLEXOR TENDON INJURIES
Early mobilization

Karen Stewart Pettengill

Postoperative management of tendon injuries has changed tremendously over the last 20 years with the development of new surgical and therapeutic techniques and growing understanding of the mechanisms of tendon healing and nutrition. Today most hand specialists appreciate the benefits of early mobilization of the healing tendon, although there remain many instances in which tendons are immobilized routinely (e.g., zone I and II extensor tendon injuries). There are also a number of gray areas, such as the choice between active and passive mobilization, the method of mobilization, and the timing and progression of the therapy program. This chapter discusses some of the current trends in early postoperative mobilization of flexor tendons and the rationale behind each.

The various approaches to postoperative tendon management can be divided into three categories: *immobilization, early passive mobilization,* and *early active mobilization.* These categories are based on how the tendon is managed during the initial protective stage (the first 3 to 6 weeks after tendon repair, when the repair is going through the crucial early phases of healing). After this protective stage, the various therapy programs do not differ widely.

In *immobilization programs,* the repaired tendon is completely immobilized during the protective stage: a postoperative splint or cast holds the forearm and hand in a protected position to keep the tendons in a shortened position with no tension on the repair—wrist neutral or flexed,

metacarpophalangeal (MP) joints flexed, interphalangeal (IP) joints usually in full extension. Passive and active range of motion wait until 3 or 4 weeks after surgery, when the repair is theoretically strong enough to withstand the stress of motion.

For *passive mobilization programs* a similar dorsal splint or cast is applied, with the wrist again in a neutral or flexed position, MP joints in flexion, and IP joints allowed to extend fully. However, during the protective stage of therapy, tendons are mobilized through *passive* flexion and active or passive extension (e.g., rubber-band traction into flexion followed by active extension). The splint prevents composite wrist and finger extension and thus protects against excessive stress to the tendon juncture. Active contraction of the involved flexor begins 3 to 6 weeks after surgery.

In contrast, *active* mobilization means mobilization through controlled *active* flexion exercises in the protective stage of therapy, usually starting by 24 to 48 hours after repair. The tendon is protected by a splint or cast similar to that used for passive mobilization protocols.

The differences between the three approaches are defined by the factors that influence tendon healing during the crucial early weeks after repair.

HISTORICAL PERSPECTIVE

Although early mobilization of tendon injuries is not a new idea,[30-32] the road to our contemporary view has been tortuous. The actual mechanism of tendon healing and nutrition has long been the subject of debate. The prevailing wisdom for many years was that tendon repairs must be immobilized for the first few weeks, because they relied on the ingrowth of adhesions from surrounding tissues to provide both nutrition and a healing response.[60,61] In 1941 Mason and Allen[55] published a study demonstrating that the immobilized tendon repair underwent a decrease in strength within the first 5 days of repair, followed by a gradual increase in strength, with two plateaus, at 14 to 16 days and at 21 days. They noted that "function" or stress to the repair caused a rise in tensile strength, but that if such stress were not carefully controlled (e.g., if unrestricted use of the tendon were allowed) an unacceptable inflammatory reaction and adhesion formation would result. They also concluded that controlled stress was not directly related to increased strength unless applied after 14 days. Their study found the best results (strongest repairs with less separation at the repair site) in tendons immobilized initially for at least 2 weeks and then subjected to restricted mobilization. Mason and Allen's work has been used by many to support immobilization of tendon repairs for the first 3 weeks before initiating active motion (based on their findings of a second plateau in strength at 21 days). However, it is generally recognized that immobilization allows uninhibited proliferation of adhesions that result in unacceptably poor gliding function in many patients. Proponents of early passive mobilization use Mason and Allen's time frame to delineate an initial period of protected *controlled* stress to the repair.[26,73]

In 1960 Young and Harmon published results of their early passive mobilization program,[87] but it was not until the 1970s that this approach gained wide acceptance. Kleinert and associates[37,38] and Duran and Houser[17,18] demonstrated improved recovery of gliding function using two different approaches to early passive mobilization of flexor tendons. Strickland and Glogovac's 1980 publication compared immobilized repairs with those treated by early passive mobilization and found clear superiority in the group mobilized early.[76] In the meantime, evidence was accumulating to support the importance of both intrinsic tendon nutrition and intrinsic healing mechanisms to the recovery of function in the repaired tendon.* In particular, the work of Gelberman and associates[21,22,24,25,27] indicated that not only do tendons possess an intrinsic healing capacity, but early controlled mobilization increases the intrinsic contribution to healing, controls formation of restrictive adhesions, and increases the strength of the repair. Hitchcock in 1987[33] demonstrated in a chicken tendon model that whereas immobilized repairs did undergo the decline in strength noted in the first 5 days by Mason and Allen,[5] immediate *controlled* mobilization of the repaired tendon *reversed* that

process and actually was associated with an immediate *increase* in repair strength. This observation has been confirmed in other studies.[78]

In conjunction with all of these developments, there have been two crucial trends. One is the improvement in surgical technique in a number of ways, from atraumatic handling of tendons to the evolution of stronger suture designs and materials. Sutures now in use withstand greater stress, are less traumatic to the tendon and its intrinsic circulation, and possess improved flexibility and gliding characteristics. The second important trend is the growth of hand and upper extremity rehabilitation as a specialty. Without a knowledgeable hand therapist, the more demanding and complex postoperative protocols would be impossible. In fact, the surgeon and the therapist must understand each other's level of expertise and knowledge and must communicate clearly and often about the injury, surgery, and postoperative therapy to achieve the most desirable results.

EARLY PASSIVE MOBILIZATION
Original Kleinert and Duran programs

In the original Kleinert[37,38] passive mobilization program, the postoperative splint or cast held the wrist in 45° of flexion, with MP joints flexed 10° to 20°. The Duran and Houser[17,18] approach held the wrist at 20° of flexion with the MP and IP joints in a relaxed position of flexion (maintained by rubber-band traction). Duran and Houser mobilized the tendons using manual passive exercises to push the tendons proximally and to pull them distally, and they used the rubber bands for protective positioning in flexion between exercise sessions. Kleinert used rubber bands to resist extension. An EMG study by Lister and others[41] supported Kleinert's proposition that resistance to extension would induce relaxation in the antagonist flexors, thus reducing stress to the repair during passive tendon glide distally. Therefore the patient would extend the fingers to the limit of the splint 10 times hourly, allowing the rubber bands to flex the fingers passively between repetitions. In both programs, the fingers rested in flexion under rubber-band traction when not exercising, and rubber-band traction was directed from the fingernails to a point proximal to the wrist. Fig. 40-1 illustrates a splint used for a modified version of the original Kleinert protocol.

Further evolution of early passive mobilization programs

Preventing proximal interphalangeal joint flexion contractures

An unfortunate drawback to rubber-band traction is the high risk of proximal interphalangeal (PIP) joint flexion contractures caused by one or both of two factors. First is the resting position in flexion between exercises. In the zone II injury, for which early mobilization is used most often, the palmar laceration often crosses the PIP flexion crease. The

*References 2, 3, 21, 22, 24-27, 33, 45-52, 83-85.

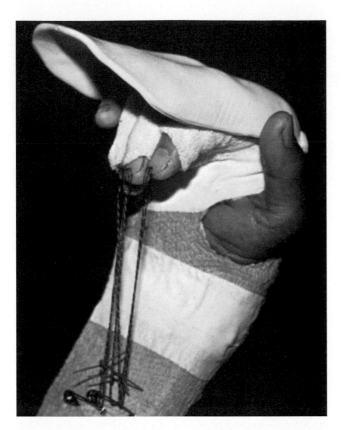

Fig. 40-1. In this splint for a version of the original Kleinert protocol, the metacarpophalangeal and proximal interphalangeal joints are held in flexion by rubber-band traction, but the distal interphalangeal joint rests in almost complete extension. (From Stewart KM, van Strien Gwendolyn: Postoperative management of flexor tendon injuries. In Hunter JM, Mackin EF, Callahan AD, eds: *Rehabilitation of the hand: surgery and therapy,* ed 4, St Louis, 1995, Mosby.)

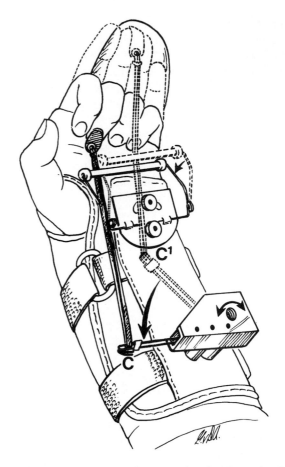

Fig. 40-2. The postoperative flexor tendon (PFT) traction brace used with a modified version of the Kleinert protocol. The rubber band is attached to a lever *C* that swings distally to decrease resistance during active digit extension. (From Werntz J, Chesher S, Breidenbach W, et al: A new dynamic splint for postoperative treatment of flexor tendon injury, *J Hand Surg* 1989; 14A:561, Churchill Livingstone on behalf of the *J Hand Surg*, New York.)

effects of scar shortening and adherence of peritendinous tissues compounds the PIP joint's predisposition toward flexion contractures. To counteract this tendency, many therapists now immobilize the fingers in IP joint extension at night, between exercise sessions, or both; some use PIP joint extension splints inserted between the finger and the dorsal protective splint. In addition, experienced therapists and particularly reliable patients can perform protected passive PIP extension, with the distal interphalangeal (DIP) and MP joints flexed.

The other major contributor to PIP flexion contractures is the difficulty of achieving full extension against excessive rubber-band traction. Citron and Forster[13] performed an EMG study to determine the difference in relaxation of flexors with varying amounts of resistance to extension. Not only did they find no greater relaxation with greater resistance, but they also discovered that their subjects' flexors did not always synergistically relax with resistance to extension. This threw some unexpected doubt on the earlier findings by Lister.[41]

Werntz and others[86] studied the amount of resistance offered to extension by an ordinary rubber band in a typical dorsal protective splint. They found that the resistance to extension increased substantially in the final degrees of extension, making it measurably more difficult to achieve full extension. On the basis of these findings, they proposed use of a splint that decreased resistance to extension as the finger neared the full extension allowed by the splint (Fig. 40-2). Others have controlled resistance to extension by manually releasing rubber-band tension[56] or by using two sets of rubber bands: one for exercise and one to maintain a flexed resting position.[16]

Achieving maximum tendon excursion

Although one can logically see that passive flexion of the digits will passively push the flexor tendons proximally, and passive or active extension will pull the tendons distally, the actual amplitude of passive tendon excursion will vary with the joints flexed, the degree to which they are flexed, and the

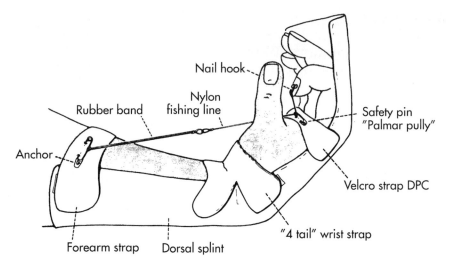

Fig. 40-3. This splint, designed by Linwood Thomes, incorporates a palmar pulley to redirect the line of pull for more complete flexion. Although not shown in this illustration, two separate sources of traction may be used: a complete rubber band for rest and a rubber band cut in half to provide decreased resistance during extension exercise. (From Chow J, Thomes L, Dovelle S, et al: A combined regimen of controlled motion following flexor tendon repair in "no man's land," *Plast Reconstr Surg* 1987; 79:447-453.)

condition of the peritendinous tissues. A number of studies have examined this question, both in cadaver models and in living subjects following tendon repair.* These studies have produced a combined body of evidence demonstrating several fundamental facts.

First, the ultimate gain in *active* flexor tendon glide depends on the *passive* tendon excursion attained during the first phase of early passive mobilization programs. Although there appears to be a point beyond which increasing the amplitude of passive excursion does not further increase active glide, it appears also, for both flexor digitorum profundus (FDP) and flexor digitorum superficialis (FDS) that if more than 3 to 5 mm of passive excursion (as recommended by Duran and Houser[18]) can be attained, active excursion will be correspondingly better.[68,69]

Second, to attain maximum passive flexor tendon excursion, both IP joints must be taken through their full passive range of flexion and extension. PIP joint range of motion has a greater effect on passive FDP glide than does DIP range of motion, but both contribute significantly.† Third, if synergistic wrist flexion and extension are added to the mobilization program, even greater excursion will be attained in both extrinsic flexor tendons.[14,35]

Based on these studies as well as clinical observation, various splints have been designed with the goal of improving passive excursion. The original splints use rubber-band traction to direct the traction from the distal forearm to the fingernail. This line of pull flexes the MP joint more than the

IP joints, and the PIP joint more than the DIP joint (see Fig. 40-1). In 1984 Slattery and McGrouther[70] proposed redirecting the traction by passing it through a palmar pulley. Pulling the fingertips in toward the distal palmar crease flexes the IP joints far more effectively than pulling toward a point proximal to the wrist. Others have proposed similar splint adaptations. Werntz and others[86] and Chow and others[11,12,16] proposed splints that incorporate not only control of resistance to extension, as mentioned previously, but also redirection of flexion force toward the palm (Figs. 40-2 and 40-3). Brown and McGrouther proposed a similar splint for flexor pollicis longus (FPL) lacerations, immobilizing the proximal phalanx to passively flex the thumb IP joint more effectively and thus attain better passive FPL gliding.[8]

Based on the studies cited earlier,[14,35] Cooney and associates have used a splint (still in the prototype stage) that incorporates synergistic wrist extension with finger flexion and wrist flexion with finger extension to maximize passive flexor mobilization.

Studies by Silfverskiöld and associates[68,69] convinced them that to achieve ultimately the best possible active tendon gliding, the early passive mobilization program must incorporate full passive IP flexion and extension. Toward that end they designed a protocol,[56] the "Four-Finger protocol," that includes several key elements. First, the flexion force is directed toward the palm by use of a palmar pulley. Second, they ensure full active extension against the elastic traction by teaching the patient to use the uninvolved hand to manually release elastic tension during active extension. Third, when the finger is returned to the flexed position by the elastic traction, the patient adds a manual push into

*References 8, 14, 34, 35, 57, 68, 69.
†References 14, 34, 35, 57, 68, 69.

complete flexion (it is very difficult to passively flex the fingertips all the way to the palm through elastic traction alone). Fourth, all four fingers are included in the splint even if not injured, on the principle that better passive excursion is attained if all four FDP tendons are pushed proximally at the same time. Finally, at night, the patient wears an additional volar splint component holding the IP joints in extension.

Duration and frequency of exercise

Gelberman and others[23] examined the effects of increasing the duration and frequency of passive mobilization, through use of continuous passive mobilization (CPM) in treatment of flexor tendon repairs. Their results clearly showed improvement in the CPM group, which appears to indicate that increasing the number of repetitions and frequency of exercise sessions improves the effectiveness of early passive mobilization. A companion study[77] looked at the effect of frequency compared with the effect of duration of passive mobilization (12 cycles/min for 5 minutes versus 1 cycle/min for 60 minutes). Frequency (rate) of mobilization had a greater effect on tensile properties of the healing tendon. This supports those early passive mobilization programs that incorporate exercise hourly rather than two or three times a day.

Initiation of passive mobilization: How early should motion begin?

Feehan and Beauchene, in 1990, asked why many hand specialists continued to delay active mobilization until 4 to 6 weeks with repairs that had undergone an early passive mobilization program, whereas immobilized repairs were moved actively at 3 weeks.[20] The common explanation is that early mobilized repairs lack the support of peritendinous adhesions, and may be more subject to rupture. However, experimental evidence has shown that the immobilized repair undergoes an initial *decrease in strength,* compared with an *increase in strength* in the repair mobilized early.[33,55,78]

Feehan and Beauchene's theory was that the increase in strength should outweigh the risk posed by lack of peritendinous adhesions. Because previous studies had not used a model approximating that used in human patients, their study of canine flexor tendon repairs used a mobilization program similar to that used in humans. They found that the mobilized repairs, indeed, increased in resistance to rupture, and early mobilization appeared to improve efficiency of healing.

More recently, Tottenham and associates[79] looked further into the timing of passive mobilization programs. They compared results when zone II flexor tendon repairs were mobilized passively within the first postoperative week with results when mobilization was delayed until between 1 and 3 weeks postoperatively. Although this retrospective study used a small number of patients (22 total) and did not find a statistically significant difference, there was a clinically significant difference in that the early interven-

tion group had no fair or poor results, and the delayed intervention group had a total of 25% fair or poor results. Experienced hand specialists have observed this clinical difference for years; this is the first attempt to scientifically study the question.

Questioning the efficacy of early passive mobilization

Many have questioned how effectively passive motion mobilizes flexor tendons. Passive proximal gliding has been compared to pushing a cooked noodle down a tube: One would expect it to bunch up and fold on itself, and indeed, surgeons have observed this intraoperatively. Not only is the tendon a flexible structure, which therefore could be expected to behave like a cooked noodle, but it is also an injured structure. With the increased bulk of edema and suture, wouldn't one expect the tendon to "catch" and move with difficulty through the surrounding injured, edematous tissues? In fact, Lane and associates[39] in 1976 found that when a suture was placed in an otherwise uninjured rat tendon, the resultant hematoma and edema formation caused a rapid decrease in normal gliding function and an increase in the work of flexion. This trend continued until day 14. Unfortunately, by day 14 adhesion formation is well under way in the injured tendon, so when we mobilize a tendon early, we must carefully balance the known factors hindering gliding (edema, hematoma) with the potential for adhesion formation and the ability of the repair to withstand the stress of mobilization without gap formation.

So why do passive mobilization programs work? The radiographic studies of Silfverskiöld and associates[68,69] have shown that particularly with PIP flexion and extension, passive motion does mobilize the tendon, although with variations from one patient to another depending on factors such as type and extent of injury and local inflammation. In addition, hand specialists have observed that a great number of patients "cheat" on their passive mobilization programs by actively flexing either during the passive flexion exercise or inadvertently between exercises. If only the involved fingers are included in dynamic flexion traction, for example, the patient might use the unsplinted fingers, provoking a synergistic contraction of the involved muscle-tendon unit. Contrary to our fears, many of these patients do exceedingly well, raising the question as to whether a light active flexor contraction might be not only harmless but possibly even beneficial.

EARLY ACTIVE MOBILIZATION
Rationale and definitions

Observations of successful "cheating" are partly responsible for the recent interest in *active mobilization* of flexor tendon repairs. Although flexor tendons had been mobilized actively in previous years,[30-32] the repairs had been bulky and traumatic to the tendon tissue, and results were poor, leading experts to back away from such aggressive early treatment. Today we have at our disposal atraumatic grasping sutures with superior strength and gliding characteristics, allowing a greater margin of safety in active mobilization.

Early active mobilization programs can be divided into two categories: *place-hold* (or active-hold) flexion and true *active* flexion programs. In place-hold mobilization programs, the digits are moved into flexion passively and the patient is asked to maintain the position actively with a very gentle muscle contraction. Active flexion programs require that the patient actively flex without passive assistance.

Many active and place-hold active mobilization programs have been proposed, most depending on use of a specific suture with superior strength.* Examination of specific suture techniques goes beyond the scope of this chapter; a few pertinent points should suffice. Taking into account comparative studies of suture strength by a number of authors,† and studies of the force a suture must withstand during active flexion,‡ we now know that a well-placed core suture of the types most commonly used today, when combined with a strong peripheral suture, can withstand light active motions. The strength of the suture appears to increase in direct proportion to the number of strands crossing the repair, and running lock peripheral sutures appear to be stronger than interrupted or simple running sutures. The sutures most commonly used today by hand surgeons are some version of a modified Kessler in conjunction with a running or running lock peripheral suture, so we can assume that given a sound repair performed without unusual complications, and a cooperative, intelligent patient, a repaired flexor tendon theoretically could benefit from active mobilization within 24 to 48 hours of repair.

Representative early active mobilization programs

The following is an overview of four recent publications. Among them they represent varying views on major issues in active mobilization of flexor tendons: What type of repair is appropriate for early active mobilization? What wrist position is the most favorable for early active digit flexion? How can one control the strength of the contraction adequately?

In 1993 Gratton described a modification of the protocol first described in 1989 by Cullen and associates and by Small and associates.[15,28,71] Following FDP repair with a modified Kessler core suture and an unspecified circumferential suture, a dorsal postoperative plaster slab is applied. The wrist is held at 20° of flexion and the MP joints at 80° to 90° flexion, allowing full IP joint extension. Exercise begins 24 to 48 hours after repair and continues every 4 hours during the day. Two repetitions of full passive finger flexion are

*References 1, 5-7, 9, 10, 15, 19, 28, 29, 58, 63, 67, 72, 75.
†References 4, 19, 36, 40, 53, 54, 59, 62, 66, 75, 78, 80-82.
‡References 4, 19, 62, 64, 65, 72, 74.

followed by two repetitions each of active flexion and active extension. By the end of the first week the patient is expected to achieve full composite passive flexion, active extension of IP joints and active flexion of the PIP joint to 30° and the DIP joint to 5° or 10°. The expected range of active flexion increases each week, reaching 80° to 90° at the PIP joint and 50° to 60° at the DIP joint by the fourth postoperative week. The protective phase of exercise (controlled active flexion, as described) continues until 4 to 6 weeks, depending on how quickly the patient recovers active tendon glide.

Also in 1993, Evans and Thompson[19] calculated the internal and external forces acting on the repaired flexor tendon during active flexion. They theoretically analyzed those forces in varying positions and also examined the literature regarding suture strength. They found that place-hold flexion in a partial fist (MP joints 83°, PIP joints 75°, and DIP joints 40°) with the wrist in 20° extension imposed a safe amplitude of force on a repair performed with a sound core and peripheral suture, while still adequately mobilizing the tendon. Furthermore, they use a strain gauge to measure the actual force exerted by the patient in maintaining the flexed digit posture, and limit the force of flexion to <50 g. In Chapter 43, Evans discusses the calculation of force placed on the healing tendon.

In recommending that the wrist be extended during digit flexion, Evans and Thompson drew on a study by Savage[64] that calculated the work of tendons in varying positions of the wrist and digits. Savage found that in 45° of wrist extension and 90° of MP flexion, the work of finger flexion was considerably less than in alternative positions. According to the work of Cooney and associates[14] and of Horii and associates,[35] simultaneous wrist extension and finger flexion elicits greater FDP and FDS glide passively. It is logical to assume that wrist extension would therefore aid in active proximal glide of finger flexors.

Strickland[72,74,75] and Cannon[10] also drew on the work of Savage, Cooney, and Horii in developing their place-hold active flexion protocol, which involves synergistic wrist extension and digit flexion. This program is intended for use following repair with a 4-strand core suture (a Tajima plus a horizontal mattress) with a running lock peripheral suture. The patient performs passive mobilization exercises (modified Duran—passive digit flexion and extension) within the confines of a dorsal protective splint (wrist and MP joints flexed, IP joints allowed full extension) and then replaces that splint with an exercise splint to perform the place-hold mobilization exercises. This second splint (Figs. 40-4, 40-5, and 40-6), hinged at the wrist, allows full wrist and digit flexion and 30° of wrist extension, and blocks the MP joints at 60° of flexion, while allowing full IP joint extension. The patient simultaneously flexes the fingers passively and extends the wrist actively to the limits of the splint, and then actively holds the fist, before relaxing and allowing the wrist to drop into flexion and the digits to extend. At 4 weeks the exercise splint is discontinued.

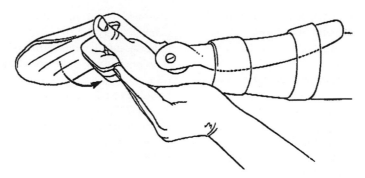

Fig. 40-4. The patient extends the wrist actively with simultaneous *passive* digit flexion. (From Cannon N: Post flexor tendon repair motion protocol, *Indiana Hand Center Newsletter* 1993; 1:13.)

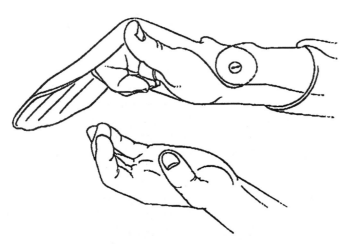

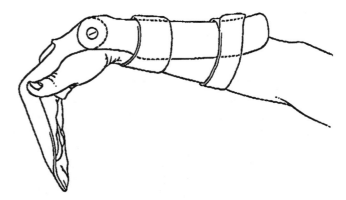

Fig. 40-5. The patient then maintains digit flexion with a gentle active muscle contraction. (From Cannon N: Post flexor tendon repair motion protocol, *Indiana Hand Center Newsletter* 1993; 1:13.)

Fig. 40-6. The wrist is allowed to relax into flexion with simultaneous digit extension (limited to 60° at the metacarpophalangeal joints). (From Cannon N: Post flexor tendon repair motion protocol, *Indiana Hand Center Newsletter* 1993; 1:13.)

Based on the four-finger passive mobilization program described earlier,[56] Silfverskiöld and May[67] have developed another active place-hold program. The splint is identical to that used for their four-finger program, except that the wrist is held at neutral instead of in flexion to decrease the work of digit flexion. Following passive mobilization exercises, the digits are fully flexed passively and flexion is maintained with an active flexor contraction. This program is intended for use with a specific repair: a modified Kessler core suture and a cross-stitch peripheral suture.

Comparisons and questions

In reviewing the representative active mobilization protocols, one can see several key differences among them. First, while all involve use of a standard dorsal protective splint, the wrist position varies from flexion in the Gratton, Strickland/Cannon, and Evans and Thompson approaches to neutral in the Silfverskiöld approach. However, it should be noted that in both the Strickland/Cannon and the Evans and Thompson approaches the dorsal protective splint is removed for the place-hold active flexion exercise, using the exercise splint (which allows 30° of wrist extension) for the

Strickland/Cannon approach and performing exercises in 20° of wrist extension without a splint for the Evans and Thompson approach. In contrast, for the Silfverskiöld and May approach the splint stays on for place-hold flexion, keeping the wrist at neutral, while the Gratton approach holds the wrist in 20° of flexion during active digit flexion exercise. In light of the work of Savage, it would seem best to keep the wrist at least at neutral if not in extension to decrease the required force of flexion during active or place-hold contraction. However, Gratton argues that the wrist should be held in flexion to *increase* the difficulty of flexing the digits, thus discouraging excessive active motion by patients when they are unsupervised.

Another difference lies in the means of controlling the strength of flexor contraction. Gratton sets a goal for a limited number of degrees of flexion for each week, raising that goal gradually week by week. While this does not control precisely the strength of the contraction, it does communicate to the patient that expectations are modest, and thus presumably only modest outputs of force are needed. Evans and Thompson use several means to control the strength of contraction. First, they assume that place-hold flexion requires less force than active flexion. Second, their biomechanical calculations show that partial finger flexion requires less force than full flexion. Third, they use a strain gauge to measure the force of flexion: Patients are to exert no more than 50 g of force.

Strickland/Cannon also use place-hold flexion to control force. As "insurance," before attempting place-hold flexion with the involved hand, the patient uses the other hand to practice maintaining a fist with the least possible force. Strickland/Cannon also suggest using EMG biofeedback to help the patient control the contraction. Silfverskiöld and May also use place-hold flexion as a means of controlling the strength of the contraction. Their patients, like those of Gratton, are hospitalized for several days after surgery, and their compliance can be monitored closely.

The four programs have certain features in common. All of the authors select compliant, intelligent patients, and begin therapy within 24 to 48 hours after repair. All expect the digits to be passively ranged before exercise to reduce the resistance imposed by joint stiffness; they also presume that careful edema control will reduce the additional resistance imposed by excessive bulk of the digit.

Each protocol has its limitations. As already noted, the Gratton protocol may require excessive work of the flexors because the wrist remains in flexion during digit flexion. The Evans and Thompson approach involves place-hold active flexion exercises that can be performed only in the clinic. The Strickland/Cannon protocol can be performed only by patients who can be relied on to correctly change splints at home. Both the Gratton and the Silfverskiöld and May programs depend on hospitalizing patients for several days after surgery to monitor compliance. This would be difficult in many cases, at least in the United States.

Finally, a basic assumption of the place-hold protocols is open to question. If, as has been suggested, passive flexion of the digits during passive mobilization exercises causes tendons to fold and bunch up, surely the same is true of the passive flexion phase of place-hold exercises. In other words, when the digit is passively flexed, the tendon folds on itself, and when we ask the patient to hold the position with an active contraction, we expect the muscle to contract strongly enough to *unfold* the tendon and pull it out of its bunched up position. If this is indeed the case, then those place-hold protocols involving wrist extension (Evans and Thompson, Strickland/Cannon) are theoretically both most effective and safest, because wrist extension assists flexor glide by pulling proximally on the tendon during the passive digit flexion–active wrist extension phase of exercise. Therefore, at least theoretically, the tendon will not bunch up, and a gentle flexor contraction will suffice to hold the position actively.

SUMMARY

This is an exciting time for tendon rehabilitation. We now know that mobilizing a flexor tendon within the first few days of repair controls adhesion formation, stimulates intrinsic healing, and increases the strength of tendon repairs. The evidence indicates that given current and developing surgical and therapeutic techniques, early active flexion may be the most effective method of mobilizing repaired tendons in appropriately selected patients. However, we must not be so carried away by our enthusiasm that we forget the needs of the individual patient. There will always be patients who simply cannot follow an early mobilization program. There will always be some repairs performed under poor conditions, increasing excessively the risks of early mobilization. These tendons must be immobilized initially. The surgeon and therapist must take all factors into account in planning postoperative management.

REFERENCES

1. Allen BN, Frykman AK, Unsell RS, Wood VE: Ruptured flexor tendon tenorrhaphies in zone II: repair and rehabilitation, *J Hand Surg* 1987; 12A:18.
2. Amadio P, Jaeger S, Hunter J: Nutritional aspects of tendon healing. In Hunter J, Schneider L, Mackin E, Callahan A, eds: *Rehabilitation of the hand,* St Louis, 1990, Mosby.
3. Amadio PC, Hunter JM: Prognostic factors in flexor tendon surgery in zone 2. In Hunter JM, Schneider LH, Mackin EM, eds: *Tendon surgery in the hand,* St Louis, 1987, Mosby.
4. Aoki M, Manske PR, Pruitt DL, Larson BJ: Work of flexion after tendon repair with various suture methods: a human cadaveric study, *J Hand Surg* 1995; 20B:310.
5. Becker H: Primary repair of flexor tendons in the hand without immobilization, preliminary report, *Hand* 1978; 10:37.
6. Becker H, Orak F, Duponselle E: Early active motion following a beveled technique of flexor tendon repair: report on fifty cases, *J Hand Surg* 1979; 4:454.
7. Boulas HJ, Strickland JW: Strength and functional recovery following repair of flexor digitorum superficialis in zone 2, *J Hand Surg* 1993; 18B:22.
8. Brown CP, McGrouther DA: The excursion of the tendon of flexor pollicis longus and its relation to dynamic splintage, *J Hand Surg* 1984; 9A:787.
9. Brunelli G, Vigasio A, Brunelli F: Slip-knot flexor tendon suture in zone II allowing immediate mobilization, *Hand* 1983; 15:352.
10. Cannon N: Post flexor tendon repair motion protocol, *Indiana Hand Center Newsletter* 1993; 1:13.
11. Chow J, Stephens M, Ngai W, et al: A splint for controlled active motion after flexor tendon repair: design, mechanical testing and preliminary clinical results, *J Hand Surg* 1990; 15A:645.
12. Chow J, Thomes L, Dovelle S, et al: A combined regimen of controlled motion following flexor tendon repair in "no man's land," *Plast Reconstr Surg* 1987; 79:447.
13. Citron N, Forster A: Dynamic splinting following flexor tendon repair, *J Hand Surg* 1987; 12B:96.
14. Cooney WP, Lin GT, An K-N: Improved tendon excursion following flexor tendon repair, *J Hand Therapy* 1989; 2:102.
15. Cullen K, Tolhurst P, Land D, et al: Flexor tendon repair in zone 2 followed by controlled active mobilization, *J Hand Surg* 1989; 14B:392.
16. Dovelle S, Heeter P: The Washington regimen: rehabilitation of the hand following flexor tendon injuries, *Physical Therapy* 1989; 69:1034.
17. Duran R, Coleman C, Nappi J, et al: Management of flexor tendon lacerations in zone 2 using controlled passive motion postoperatively. In Hunter J, Schneider L, Mackin E, Callahan A, eds: *Rehabilitation of the hand,* St Louis, 1990, Mosby.
18. Duran R, Houser R: Controlled passive motion following flexor tendon repair in zones 2 and 3. *AAOS symposium on tendon surgery in the hand,* St Louis, 1975, Mosby.

19. Evans RB, Thompson DE: The application of force to the healing tendon, *J Hand Therapy* 1993; 6:266.
20. Feehan LM, Beauchene JG: Early tensile properties of healing chicken flexor tendons: early controlled passive motion versus postoperative immobilization, *J Hand Surg* 1990; 15A:63.
21. Gelberman RH, Amiel D, Gonsalves M, et al: The influence of protected passive mobilization on the healing of flexor tendons: a biochemical and microangiographic study, *Hand* 1981; 13:120.
22. Gelberman RH, Menon J, Gonsalves M, et al: The effects of mobilization on the vascularization of healing flexor tendons in dogs, *Clin Orthop* 1980; 153:283.
23. Gelberman RH, Nunley JA, Osterman AL, et al: Influences of the protected passive mobilization interval on flexor tendon healing: a prospective randomized clinical study, *Clin Orthop* 1991; 264:189.
24. Gelberman RH, VandeBerg JS, Lundborg GN, Akeson WH: Flexor tendon healing and restoration of the gliding surface: an ultrastructural study in dogs, *J Bone Joint Surg* 1983; 65A:70.
25. Gelberman RH, VandeBerg JS, Manske PR, Akeson WH: The early stages of flexor tendon healing: a morphological study of the first fourteen days, *J Hand Surg* 1985; 10A:776.
26. Gelberman RH, Woo SL-Y: The physiological basis for application of controlled stress in the rehabilitation of flexor tendon injuries, *J Hand Therapy* 1989; 2:66.
27. Gelberman RH, Woo SL-Y, Lothringer K, et al: Effects of early intermittent passive mobilization on healing canine flexor tendons, *J Hand Surg* 1982; 7:170.
28. Gratton P: Early active mobilization after flexor tendon repairs, *J Hand Therapy* 1993; 6:285.
29. Groth GN, Loeding LA, Young VL: Early active mobilization of flexor tendon repairs utilizing the double loop locking suture technique, *American Society of Hand Therapists Annual Meeting,* Orlando, 1991.
30. Harmer TW: Tendon suture, *Boston Med Surg J* 1917; 177:808.
31. Harmer TW: Certain aspects of hand surgery, *N Engl J Med* 1936; 214:613.
32. Harmer TW: Injuries to the hand, *Am J Surg* 1938; 42:638.
33. Hitchcock TF, Light TR, Bunch WH, et al: The effect of immediate constrained digital motion on the strength of flexor tendon repairs in chickens, *J Hand Surg* 1987; 12A:590.
34. Horibe S, Woo SL-Y, Spiegelman J, et al: Excursion of the flexor digitorum profundus tendon: a kinematic study of the human and canine digits, *J Orthop Res* 1990; 8: 167.
35. Horii E, Lin GT, Cooney WP, et al: Comparative flexor tendon excursion after passive mobilization: an in vitro study, *J Hand Surg* 1992; 17A:559.
36. Ketchum LD, Martin N, Kappel D: Experimental evaluation of factors affecting the strength of tendon repairs, *J Hand Surg* 1991; 16B:135.
37. Kleinert HE, Kutz JE, Ashbell S, Martinez E: Primary repair of lacerated flexor tendons in no man's land, *J Bone Joint Surg* 1967; 49A:577.
38. Kleinert HE, Kutz JE, Cohen MJ: Primary repair of zone 2 flexor tendon lacerations. *AAOS symposium on tendon surgery in the hand,* St Louis, 1975, Mosby.
39. Lane JM, Black J, Bora FW: Gliding function following flexor tendon injury, *J Bone Joint Surg* 1976; 58A:985.
40. Lin GT, An K-N, Amadio PC, Cooney WP: Biomechanical studies of running suture for flexor tendon repair in dogs, *J Hand Surg* 1988; 13A:553.
41. Lister GD, Kleinert HE, Kutz JE, Erdogan A: Primary flexor tendon repair followed by immediate controlled mobilization, *J Hand Surg* 1977; 2:441.
42. Lundborg G: Experimental flexor tendon healing without adhesion formation: a new concept of tendon nutrition and intrinsic healing mechanisms, a preliminary report, *Hand* 1976; 8:235.
43. Lundborg G, Holm S, Myrhage R: The role of synovial fluid and tendon sheath for flexor tendon nutrition, *Scand J Plast Reconstr Surg* 1980; 14:99.
44. Lundborg G, Myrhage R, Rydevik B: The vascularization of human flexor tendons within the digital synovial sheath region: structural and functional aspects, *J Hand Surg* 1977; 2:417.
45. Lundborg G, Rank F: Experimental intrinsic healing of flexor tendons based upon synovial fluid nutrition, *J Hand Surg* 1978; 3:21.
46. Lundborg G, Rank F: Experimental studies on cellular mechanisms involved in healing of animal and human flexor tendon in synovial environment, *Hand* 1980; 12:3.
47. Manske P, Bridwell K, Lesker P: Nutrient pathways to flexor tendons of chickens using tritiated proline, *J Hand Surg* 1978; 3:352.
48. Manske P, et al: Nutrition of flexor tendons in monkeys, *Clin Orthop* 1978; 136:294.
49. Manske PR: Flexor tendon healing, *J Hand Surg* 1988; 13B:237.
50. Manske PR, Lesker PA: Nutrient pathways of flexor tendons in primates, *J Hand Surg* 1982; 7:436.
51. Manske PR, Lesker PA: Diffusion as a nutrient pathway to the flexor tendon. In Hunter JM, Schneider LH, Mackin EJ, eds: *Tendon surgery in the hand,* St Louis, 1987, Mosby.
52. Manske PR, Whiteside AL, Lesker PA: Nutrient pathways to flexor tendons using hydrogen washout technique, *J Hand Surg* 1978; 3:32.
53. Mashadi ZB, Amis AA: The effect of locking loops on the strength of tendon repair, *J Hand Surg* 1991; 16B:35.
54. Mashadi ZB, Amis AA: Strength of the suture in the epitenon and within the tendon fibres: development of stronger peripheral suture technique, *J Hand Surg* 1992; 17B:172.
55. Mason J, Allen H: The rate of healing of tendons: an experimental study of tensile strength, *Ann Surg* 1941; 113:424.
56. May EJ, Silfverskiöld KL, Sollerman CJ: Controlled mobilization after flexor tendon repair in zone II: a prospective comparison of three methods, *J Hand Surg* 1992; 17A:942.
57. McGrouther DA, Ahmed M: Flexor tendon excursions in "no man's land," *Hand* 1981; 13:129.
58. Messina A: The double armed suture: tendon repair with immediate mobilization of the fingers, *J Hand Surg* 1992; 17A:137.
59. Noguchi M, Seiler JG, Gelberman RH, et al: In vitro biomechanical analysis of suture methods for flexor tendon repair, *J Orthop Res* 1993; 11:603.
60. Potenza A: Critical evaluation of flexor tendon healing and adhesion formation within artificial digital sheaths: an experimental study, *J Bone Joint Surg* 1963; 45A:1217.
61. Potenza AD: Tendon healing within the flexor digital sheath in the dog: an experimental study, *J Bone Joint Surg* 1962; 44A:49.
62. Pruitt DL, Manske PR, Fink B: Cyclic stress analysis of flexor tendon repair, *J Hand Surg* 1991; 16A:701.
63. Savage R: In vitro studies of a new method of flexor tendon repair, *J Hand Surg* 1985; 10B:135.
64. Savage R: The influence of wrist position on the minimum force required for active movement of the interphalangeal joints, *J Hand Surg* 1988; 13B:262.
65. Schuind F, Garcia-Elias M, Cooney WP, An K-N: Flexor tendon forces: in vivo measurements, *J Hand Surg* 1992; 17A:291.
66. Silfverskiöld KL, Andersson CH: Two new methods of tendon repair: an in vitro evaluation of tensile strength and gap formation, *J Hand Surg* 1993; 18A:58.
67. Silfverskiöld KL, May EJ: Flexor tendon repair in zone II with a new suture technique and an early mobilization program combining passive and active flexion, *J Hand Surg* 1994; 19A:53.
68. Silfverskiöld KL, May EJ, Tornvall A: Flexor digitorum profundus excursions during controlled motion after flexor tendon repair in zone II: a prospective clinical study, *J Hand Surg* 1992; 17A:122.
69. Silfverskiöld KL, May EJ, Tornvall AH: Tendon excursions after flexor tendon repair in zone II: results with a new controlled-motion program, *J Hand Surg* 1993; 18A:403.
70. Slattery P, McGrouther D: A modified Kleinert controlled mobilization splint following flexor tendon repair, *J Hand Surg* 1984; 9B:34.

71. Small J, Brennen M, Colville J: Early active mobilisation following flexor tendon repair in zone 2, *J Hand Surg* 1989; 14B:383.

72. Strickland J: Flexor tendon repair: Indiana method, *Indiana Hand Center Newsletter* 1993; 1:1.

73. Strickland JW: Biologic rationale, clinical application, and results of early motion following flexor tendon repair, *J Hand Therapy* 1989; 2:71.

74. Strickland JW: Flexor tendon injuries: I. foundations of treatment, *J Am Acad Orthop Surg* 1995; 3:44.

75. Strickland JW: Flexor tendon injuries: II. operative technique, *J Am Acad Orthop Surg* 1995; 3:55.

76. Strickland JW, Glogovac SV: Digital function following flexor tendon repair in zone 2: a comparison study of immobilization and controlled passive motion, *J Hand Surg* 1980; 5A:537.

77. Takai S, Woo SL-Y, Horibe S, et al: The effects of frequency and duration of controlled passive mobilization on tendon healing, *J Orthop Res* 1991; 9:705.

78. Tanaka H, Manske PR, Pruitt DL, Larson BJ: Effect of cyclic tension on lacerated flexor tendons in vitro, *J Hand Surg* 1995; 20A:467.

79. Tottenham VM, Wilton-Bennett K, Jeffrey J: Effects of delayed therapeutic intervention following zone II flexor tendon repair, *J Hand Therapy* 1995; 8:23.

80. Trail IA, Powell ES, Noble J: The mechanical strength of various suture techniques, *J Hand Surg* 1992; 17B:89.

81. Urbaniak JR, Cahill JD, Mortenson RA: Tendon suturing methods: analysis of tensile strengths. *AAOS symposium on tendon surgery in the hand,* St Louis, 1975, Mosby.

82. Wade PJF, Wetherell RG, Amis AA: Flexor tendon repair: significant gain in strength from the Halsted peripheral suture technique, *J Hand Surg* 1989; 14B:232.

83. Weber E, Hardin G, Haynes D: Synovial fluid nutrition of flexor tendons. 36th Annual Meeting, American Society for Surgery of the Hand, 1981.

84. Weber ER: Synovial fluid nutrition of flexor tendons, *Orthop Res Soc* 1979; 4:227.

85. Weber ER: Nutritional pathways for flexor tendons in the digital theca. In Hunter JM, Schneider LH, Mackin EJ, eds: *Tendon surgery in the hand,* St Louis, 1987, Mosby.

86. Werntz J, Chesher S, Breidenbach W, et al: A new dynamic splint for postoperative treatment of flexor tendon injury, *J Hand Surg* 1989; 14A:559.

87. Young R, Harmon J: Repair of tendon injuries of the hand, *Ann Surg* 1960; 151:562.

Chapter 41

FLEXOR TENDON REPAIR WITH ACTIVE MOBILIZATION
The Gothenburg experience

Krister L. Silfverskiöld
Esther J. May

Early active mobilization after tendon reconstruction is not a new concept. By the 1920s and 1930s several of the pioneers of modern hand surgery recommended that active movements should begin a few days after tendon repair to minimize adhesion formation.[9,23,32,41] This approach never gained widespread popularity, probably because of the disappointing results obtained by other surgeons, and experimental evidence that seemed to indicate that optimal healing was best achieved by a few weeks of postoperative immobilization.[47,54,60,61,75] Most surgeons, therefore, preferred to immobilize the hand for at least 3 to 4 weeks after repair, before active movements were begun. Adhesions were accepted as an inevitable part of the early healing process, and only in the secondary stages of healing could these be modified by active exercises.

During the 1960s early controlled motion programs based on passive flexion techniques were introduced.[13,39,48,91] Since then clinical experience with various modifications of these techniques has shown that controlled motion with passive flexion does produce better results than previously obtained with postoperative immobilization.* Experimental studies have also shown that early passive motion has a beneficial effect on the repair process itself, including an increase in tensile strength and less restrictive adhesion formation.[22,28,29,34,87] With the increasing awareness that adhesions are not a prerequisite for tendon healing, more and more emphasis has been placed on techniques and exercises

intended to increase early tendon glide through a large controlled range of motion.†

The recent renewed interest in early mobilization programs incorporating active flexion as well as active extension‡ represents the next step in our efforts to improve results.§ With these developments the evolution of treatment for flexor tendon injuries has completed a full circle. In this chapter, we describe the experience at the Gothenburg Hand Surgery Unit in developing and evaluating a postoperative program incorporating active flexion as well as a repair technique able to tolerate the strain placed on the repair by such a program.

SUTURE TECHNIQUES
Tensile strength

The initial strength of a tendon repair depends on two main factors: the amount of suture material bridging the repair site and the holding power of the tissue grasps. There is a linear relationship between the cross-sectional surface area of the suture material, or in other words, the number (and thickness) of strands bridging the repair, and its breaking strength. The maximum possible breaking strength

---

*References 7, 10, 13, 14, 17, 24, 43, 48, 59, 79, 82.

†References 10, 16, 40, 49, 56, 77, 88.
†References 1, 11, 19, 44, 57, 63, 66, 78.
§Although the recent, more widespread interest in early active motion can be traced to the late 1980s, a number of authors, including Murray,[58] Hernandez,[33] Emery,[20] Becker,[4] and Brunelli[5] have previously reported on the use of early active motion.

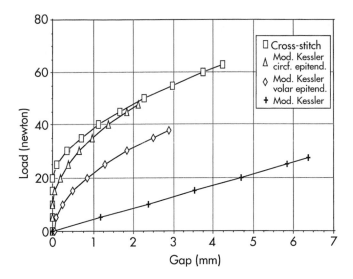

Fig. 41-1. Load versus gap during in vitro tensile strength testing of suture techniques performed on sheep tendons. Each curve represents a mean regression line obtained from 10 repairs. The end point of each curve represents the mean ultimate breaking strength.

of most traditional suture techniques such as those described by Bunnell,[8] Mason and Allen,[54] Kessler,[35] Brunelli,[6] Tajima,[80] and Tsuge[83] are, therefore, all defined by the two suture strands bridging the repair.

As a baseline for subsequent comparisons we tested the tensile strength of the modified Kessler repair, performed with a 4-0 braided polyester suture, on cadaver tendons from sheep[69] and found, as others have also found, that the repair starts gapping immediately[2,53,65,85] and eventually ruptures with a gap between 5 and 10 mm.[2,65] In our trials the mean final gap was 6.4 mm (Fig. 41-1). The repair usually ruptures when the suture material breaks[38,84,95] at a maximum load of between 14 and 30 newtons.* In our studies the mean breaking strength was 27 newtons. Adding more complicated grasps such as varying kinds of locking loops cannot increase the ultimate breaking strength, and in many cases it probably only increases the tendency to gap formation by additional unraveling of the grasps as shown by Mashadi and Amis.[53] Some strength can be added by using a 3-0 suture, but a further increase in the gauge would be prohibitive because of bulkiness. The type of suture material used will have some effect on tensile strength, but in practice the variations in strength of most knotted modern suture materials are not great and have proved of minor importance for the overall strength of repairs.[30,62,86]

If we increase the amount of suture material bridging the repair, by adding a running 6-0 conventional over and over peripheral stitch, the dynamics of the repair improve (see Fig. 41-1). Gap formation decreases, and ultimate tensile strength increases. The repair ruptures when the peripheral

*References 2, 30, 44, 53, 65, 84, 85.

suture grasps pull through the tendon tissue at a mean load of 38 newtons with a two-thirds circumferential peripheral suture and at a mean of 48 newtons with a fully circumferential peripheral suture. Although a 6-0 suture was used, the limiting factor was not the suture material but the poor holding power of the simple over and over tissue grasps. For an optimal result it is thus necessary to increase both the number of suture strands and the holding power of the tissue grasps in such a way that the strength of each component is evenly matched. This can be done by either increasing the number of grasps and strands used in various modifications of core sutures,[15,32,44,64,65] or by using more sophisticated peripheral suture techniques.[2,36,45,52,86] If the technique is to be of general practical use in the clinical situation, it must, however, also be simple and quick to perform.

Tendon forces

The question of how strong a tendon repair needs to be to tolerate active movements is still unanswered. In experiments by Urbaniak et al.[84] and Schuind et al.,[67] the force on *uninjured* flexor digitorum profundus (FDP) tendons during unresisted active flexion varied between approximately 1 and 29 newtons. These results were obtained in small groups of patients. In larger materials the forces are likely to vary even more. In the clinical situation after tendon repair the forces are also likely to increase because of factors such as an increase in friction, swelling, and stiffness. Lane et al.[42] in a study on rats, showed that, compared with an uninjured tendon, work of flexion increased significantly as early as 1 hour after tendon suture. Another problem is that patients cannot be expected to always follow postoperative instructions. It is likely that some may sometimes inadvertently use the hand for at least light gripping in awkward daily activities. Even with appropriate screening of suitable patients, it is also probable that a small percentage frankly disregard instructions without our knowledge. Mean forces of 60 to 80 newtons have been recorded during active gripping with individual values ranging up to approximately 120 newtons.[37,67] Although tendon repairs cannot be expected to tolerate such forces, a good suture technique should ideally provide some additional safety margins in terms of tolerating the forces of at least light active gripping.

We need more information before we can define the strength of a tendon suture suitable for active motion. Until then the search for an optimal method is largely a matter of trial and error. In our experience the commonly used two-strand core techniques are not strong enough, even if combined with a conventional peripheral suture.

The cross-stitch

Our solution to this problem is a modified horizontal mattress stitch in which each suture strand crosses over two other strands as it bridges the repair site (Fig. 41-2, *A*). Each grasp is approximately 1.5 to 2 mm wide and just deep enough to get a secure hold in the peripheral surface layer of

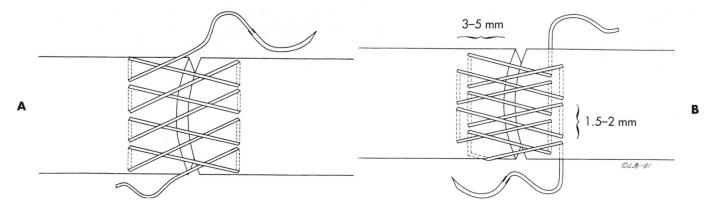

Fig. 41-2. Two versions of the cross-stitch. **A,** When suturing starts on the near side of the repair (close to the operator), the weave pattern is obtained by simply moving obliquely across the repair. **B,** When suturing starts on the far side of the repair (opposite the operator), the weave pattern is obtained by letting each tissue grasp overlap the preceding by approximately 50%. No special needle passages are necessary to produce the intricate patterns illustrated schematically here. The symmetric placement of grasps used here for the sake of clarity is not necessary in actual practice. Grasp size, overlap, and distance to tendon edge can be adapted to needs as the suture is performed. In both versions, suturing usually starts and ends with a knot on the dorsolateral aspects of the tendon in order to obtain a nearly fully circumferential suture line. (From Silfverskiöld K, Andersson C: Two new methods of tendon repair: an in vitro evaluation of tensile strength and gap formation, *J Hand Surg* 1993; 18A:58.)

the tendon. This technique is called the cross-stitch.[69] By moving obliquely across the repair site instead of in a parallel fashion, as in a conventional mattress suture, a series of half-closed, self-tightening suture loops are formed without any special needle maneuvers. When the suturing starts on the far side of the repair and proceeds toward the operator, the same weave pattern is obtained by letting each suture grasp overlap the preceding by approximately 50% (Fig. 41-2, *B*). In both versions, suturing begins and ends on the dorsolateral aspects of the tendon to obtain an almost fully circumferential suture.

We initially called the cross-stitch epitendinal technique to emphasize the peripheral and relatively superficial placement of the sutures. Unfortunately, this has led to some confusion regarding the correct application of the technique and to varying results in terms of its tensile strength in experimental studies. In practice, purely epitendinal suture grasps are difficult and time consuming to place; in addition, they are weaker than sutures grasping some of the superficial tendon fibers.[52] The cross-stitch, as used in clinical practice with grasps placed within the superifical fibers, should, therefore not be described as an epitendinal techique, but simply as a peripheral running stitch.

There are several advantages to the cross-stitch technique. It fulfills the criteria of simplicity and speed. The circumferential placement of many continuous grasps distributes the tension evenly around the circumference of the tendon. Deformation and strangulation are avoided. The use of only one transverse tissue grasp for each loop of suture bridging the repair prevents the unravelling and

elongation seen in more complicated designs.[53] Lin et al.[45] have discussed the possibility that poor gliding ability of the suture may prevent the suture strands bridging the repair from obtaining equal length as the load increases, a phenomenon that may cause uneven distribution of tension on the suture line and weaken the repair significantly. By avoiding locking elements, the cross-stitch minimizes this problem. For the same reason we prefer to use a low friction monofilament suture such as nylon or prolene. The external placement of sutures away from the cut ends of the tendon avoids any potential zone of devascularization and softening and minimizes further trauma and fraying of the tendon. On increasing tension this suture configuration also tends to act as a Chinese finger trap, gently compressing the tendon ends and actually decreasing the volume of the repair, thus ensuring smooth gliding. In the otherwise difficult situation when the tendon ends are severely frayed and further trimming is not possible, the collecting and compressive effects of this design are particularly helpful.

In vitro tensile strength testing[69] showed that the breaking strength of the cross-stitch performed with a 6-0 suture, on its own, without any core suture, is around 63 newtons or 6 kg, which is 133% stronger than the 27 newtons recorded for the modified Kessler alone and 33% stronger than the 48 newtons recorded for the modified Kessler combined with a fully circumferential conventional peripheral suture (see Fig. 41-1). Breaking strength per cross-stitch grasp was 6.3 newtons, which was more than double the simple over and over grasp even though it was reinforced with a modified Kessler core suture.

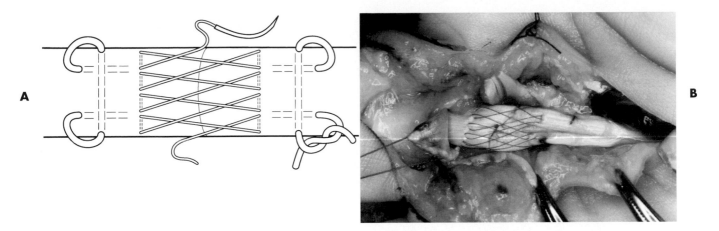

Fig. 41-3. The cross-stitch combined with a modified Kessler core stitch. **A,** Schematically, without overlap. **B,** In vivo, with overlap. (From Silfverskiöld K, Andersson C: Two new methods of tendon repair: an in vitro evaluation of tensile strength and gap formation, *J Hand Surg* 1993; 18A:58.)

Although experimentally the mean breaking strength of the cross-stitch was more than twice the maximum forces registered during unresisted active movements by Urbaniak et al.[84] and Schuind et al.,[67] we presently prefer to use it together with a conventional modified Kessler core suture, mainly because of the added safety of two independent systems should one fail for technical reasons, such as poor knotting or breakage of the suture caused by mechanical damage during suturing. A thicker suture (5-0) would have decreased the risk of damage and further increased the strength of the repair, but the added bulk would have increased the risk of the repair not gliding freely under pulleys. Our initial clinical experience also showed that the cross-stitch is easier to insert if the tendon ends are first stabilized with some kind of core stitch (Fig. 41-3).

The adequacy of a tendon repair is of course not only dependent on its initial mechanical strength but also on how the repair technique interacts biologically with the healing processes. Comparative in vivo studies in animals have not identified any significant differences between a number of conventional core suture techniques, neither in terms of rupture rates, tensile strength, and gliding function, nor in terms of various histologic parameters.[12,90] The role of the cross-stitch in this context is discussed later.

POSTOPERATIVE MOBILIZATION
Rationale

An optimal postoperative mobilization program following flexor tendon repair restricts or prevents adhesion formation, promotes healing of the repaired tendons, and minimizes complications. The widespread popularity of postoperative programs based on passive flexion techniques is to a large extent based on their ability to fulfill, at least partly, these criteria. Clinical results are, however, still far from optimal. Poor results caused by adhesions are still frequent, and ruptures are not uncommon. The mechanisms

by which passive motion affects adhesion formation, to what extent the repaired tendon actually moves, and what effect such movement has on subsequent results were also largely unknown at the time when we began our studies. The increasing emphasis on producing as large a controlled range of motion as possible* is based on the previously unproven assumption that the resulting tendon excursions would increase in a similar fashion and that adhesion formation and clinical results are correlated to the magnitude of the excursions obtained during the early healing period. The rationale for programs incorporating early active flexion, is, of course, also based on this assumption. Gelberman et al.[26,27] have discussed another possibility, namely, that adhesion formation could be affected on a cellular level, by tension alone, without much movement of the tendon. Intermittent stress and small movements could be enough to induce a cellular response that promotes a differentiation between the sheath and the tendon itself. Another problem is the role of adhesions in the healing process itself. Although there now exists ample experimental evidence showing that tendons possess an intrinsic healing capability, we still do not know whether healing based on intrinsic capabilities alone is of the same quality and proceeds at the same rate as when augmented by adhesions. If not, then our attempts to minimize or prevent adhesions altogether may lead to an increase in gap formation, an increased rupture rate, or at least a need for protecting the repair over a prolonged period.

Studies of tendon excursions and gap formation

Patients and methods. To clarify these issues metal markers were placed in the FDP on each side of the repair during operation.[70,72-74] Postoperatively, tendon excursions and gap formation were measured on x-ray films. Linear regression analysis was used to examine the relationships

*References 10, 16, 40, 49, 56, 77, 88.

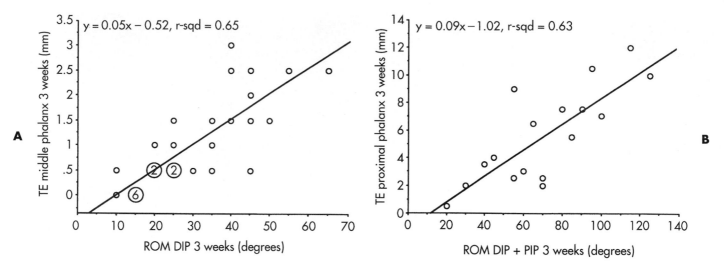

Fig. 41-4. The relationship between controlled range of motion (ROM) and the corresponding tendon excursion (TE) 3 weeks after the operation. Coinciding values indicated by larger circles with the number of digits within. **A,** distal interphalangeal (DIP) joint: $n = 29$, $r = 0.81$, $p = 0.0001$. **B,** DIP + proximal interphalangeal (PIP) joint: $n = 17$, $r = 0.79$, $p = 0.0002$. (From Silfverskiöld K, May E, Törnvall A: Flexor digitorum profundus tendon excursions during controlled motion after flexor tendon repair in zone II: a prospective clinical study, *J Hand Surg* 1992; 17A:122.)

between excursions, gap formation, and subsequent active interphalangeal (IP) joint range of motion recorded during a 1-year follow-up in two consecutive groups of patients with approximately 40 to 45 zone II FDP repairs (with or without concomitant FDS lacerations) in each group. Conventional methods of repair (modified Kessler and a simple over and over peripheral suture) were used in conjunction with early mobilization based on passive flexion (dynamic traction), of one digit in the first group,[72] and of all four digits in the second group.[74] In the second group the patients also increased their passive flexion range by pushing down the tips of the digits with their healthy hand.

Tendon excursions. The results showed that there was in fact a roughly linear correlation between early controlled IP joint range of motion and the magnitude of the resulting tendon excursions during the early mobilization period (Fig. 41-4) and that the size of these excursions did have a significant influence on final results in terms of active IP joint range of motion 1 year postoperatively (Fig. 41-5). We also found that with early passive flexion of the proximal interphalangeal (PIP) joint, mean tendon excursions along the proximal phalanx, per 10° of flexion, varied between 76% and 90% (depending on the program) of what was subsequently obtained with normal active flexion in the same digit and joint. Passive flexion of the distal interphalangeal (DIP) joint was much less efficient, resulting in excursions along the middle phalanx, per 10° of joint motion, of only between 39% and 63% of the corresponding excursions recorded during active flexion.

Gap formation. We also found that there was no clinically significant negative relationship between gap formation and tendon excursions (Fig. 41-6, *A*) or between

gap formation and clinical results in terms of subsequent active IP joint range of motion (up to 1 year postoperatively). Gaps up to between 8 and 9 mm were compatible with good results (Fig. 41-6, *B*). On the contrary there was a slight tendency for an increase in gap size to be associated with better results. Hagberg and Selvik[31] made the same observation in a smaller number of patients ($n = 10$). The most likely explanation is that more aggressive mobilization, in terms of controlled range of motion and the resulting tendon excursions, does cause an increase in gap formation through an added strain on the repair, but as long as rupture does not occur, the dominating effect is an improved gliding function and better clinical results. In view of the more or less generally accepted view that gaps of more than a few millimeters have a definite negative effect in terms of adhesion formation and clinical results, these findings were surprising. Most of our previous knowledge concerning the negative effect of gap formation was, however, based on animal studies, in which the digit was immobilized postoperatively.[46,47,54,81] In terms of the few existing previous clinical studies, our results differ from the findings of Seradge,[68] but are in accordance with those of Hagberg and Selvik[31] and Ejeskär and Irstam.[18] Our results indicate that the functional borderline between gap formation and rupture lies somewhere around 10 mm. Scar remodeling by a controlled amount of stress and movement thus seems to be effective in both building a scar of high tensile strength and restricting or modifying the adhesions connected with gap formation during postoperative immobilization.

In summary, the findings in these two groups of patients treated with passive flexion programs indicated that overall clinical results could be expected to improve if tendon

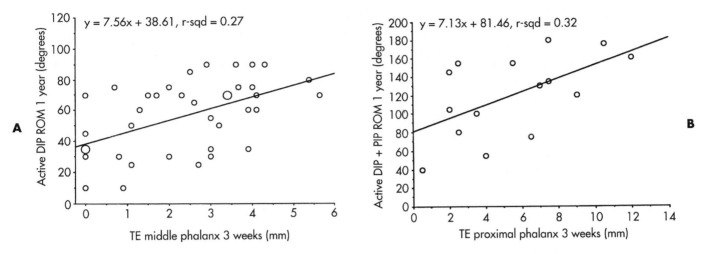

Fig. 41-5. The relationship between tendon excursions (TE) during controlled motion 3 weeks after operation and active range of motion (ROM) in the corresponding joints 1 year after operation. **A,** DIP joint: $n = 38$, $r = 0.52$, $p = 0.0009$. **B,** DIP + PIP strengths: $p = 15$, $r = 0.56$, $p = 0.03$. (From Silfverskiöld K, May E, Törnvall A: Tendon excursions after flexor tendon repair in zone II: results with a new controlled motion program, *J Hand Surg* 1993; 18A:403.)

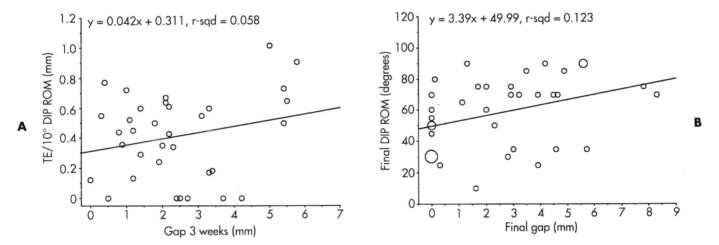

Fig. 41-6 A, The relationship between gap formation and tendon excursions (TE) along the middle phalanx per 10° of distal interphalangeal (DIP) joint motion during controlled motion 3 weeks after the operation ($n = 34$, $r = 0.24$, $p = 0.2$). **B,** The relationship between final gap formation and active DIP range of motion (ROM) 1 year after the operation ($n = 36$, $r = 0.35$, $p = 0.04$). (From Silfverskiöld K, May E: Gap formation after flexor tendon repair in zone II: results with a new controlled motion programme, *Scand J Plast Reconstr Surg* 1993; 27:263.)

excursions during the early controlled motion period (in particular those related to DIP joint motion) could be increased. The use of an early mobilization program incorporating active flexion seemed to be the most obvious way to achieve this.

Active flexion program

Patients and methods. In a third group of 46 patients with 55 zone II injuries (FDP or FDP and FDS combined), the FDP laceration was repaired with a combination of the cross-stitch described previously and a modified Kessler core stitch.[71] On the first to third postoperative day a program was begun, in which, apart from dynamic flexion traction to all four digits (Fig. 41-7, *A*) and additional passive flexion with the help of the other hand, the patients also flexed their fingers actively while simultaneously maintaining maximum passive flexion (Fig. 41-7, *B*).[71]

The strength and effect of these active contractions were checked and adjusted by a therapist or a doctor so as to produce an active flexion, without any passive help from rubber bands or the other hand, of at least 80° in the PIP joint and at least 40° to 45° in the DIP joint, before discharge on

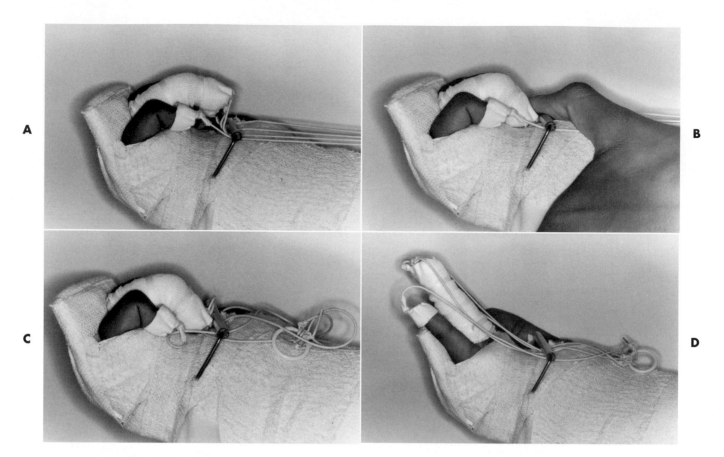

Fig. 41-7. Active flexion program. **A,** Passive flexion with only rubber bands. **B,** Flexing actively while ensuring maximum passive flexion with the other hand. **C,** Supervised testing of active flexion with rubber bands uncoupled. **D,** Active extension with rubber bands uncoupled. (From Silfverskiöld K, May E: Flexor tendon repair in zone II with a new suture technique and an early mobilization program combining passive and active flexion, *J Hand Surg* 1994; 19A:53.)

the third to fourth postoperative day (Fig. 41-7, *C*). Such checks of the unassisted active range of motion (without simultaneous passive flexion) were thereafter only done by the surgeon or a therapist, once weekly at routine outpatient reviews. The patients were carefully instructed that, when performing the exercises on their own, they should not flex actively without simultaneous passive flexion.

Full active extension was ensured by the patients unloading the tension of the rubber bands by uncoupling or drawing them distally with the other hand during the active extension phase (Fig. 41-7, *D*). At night, the rubber bands were released from their attachment on the forearm and the digits were held in full extension with the help of a volar splint attached with a velcro strap. This program was maintained for 4 weeks before unassisted active movements without any splinting were commenced. It will henceforth be referred to as the *active program*.[71] These patients were followed at regular intervals for at least 6 months.

Because early tendon excursions have such a significant influence on results, we believe that it is important that a large range of controlled motion is established soon after the operation (probably within a week). In preliminary trials we

found that it was difficult to obtain such a range with active flexion alone. Pain, swelling, and stiffness tended to inhibit voluntary active flexion and increase the tendency for cocontraction of extensor muscles. With the program described here active flexion is always combined with as much simultaneous passive flexion as possible. In addition to preventing passive joint stiffness and optimizing the quite substantial excursions available with passive motion alone, this procedure minimizes the power necessary to actively further mobilize the tendon.

In our experience, it is also difficult to consistently obtain a large passive range of digital flexion if the program relies solely on the patient using his or her other hand, especially if all four digits are to be mobilized. The use of heavy rubber bands and a palmar pulley provides a continuous bending force that gently and very efficiently overcomes any initial passive stiffness. As a protective measure, preventing the patient from using the hand for gripping, the rubber bands are also much less cumbersome than palmar splint extensions.[19]

Tendon excursions. Three weeks postoperatively, controlled IP joint range of motion, tendon excursions at both

Table 41-1. Tendon excursions, the corresponding joint range of motion, and tendon excursions per 10° of joint motion (TE/10°) recorded during controlled motion 3 weeks after the operation

	DIP		PIP	
	Active $n = 30$	Passive $n = 39$	Active $n = 19$	Passive $n = 21$
Tendon excursion (mm)	5.3	2.4	14.6	9.1
Joint motion (degrees)	65	57	89	75
TE/10°	0.8	0.4	1.6	1.2

A comparison between patients treated with our active flexion program (active) and a previous group of patients treated with the same program but without the active flexion component (passive). The differences between the active and passive groups were all significant (Mann Whitney U; $p < 0.05$). *DIP*, Distal interphalangeal; *PIP*, proximal interphalangeal.

Table 41-2. The mean size of gaps in millimeter during the early controlled mobilization period (3 weeks postoperative) and 3 or more months after the operation

	3 Weeks Postoperative	Final (≥3 Months Postoperative)
Active ($n = 42$)	1.6*	2.8
Passive ($n = 36$)	2.5	2.6

A comparison between patients treated with the active flexion program (active) and a previous group of patients treated with the same program but without the active flexion component (passive).

*Significantly smaller than in the passive group (Mann Whitney U; $p < 0.05$).

middle and proximal phalanx level, and tendon excursions per 10° of joint motion were all significantly larger than in the preceding group of patients treated with the same postoperative program but without the active flexion component (Table 41-1). Excursions per 10° of controlled DIP joint motion increased from 54% (with only passive flexion) to 82% (with active program) of the optimal (i.e., excursions per 10° of normal active motion) and similarly from 74% to 88% for PIP joint motion.

Gap formation. The mean gap size 3 weeks postoperatively was significantly smaller than in previous patients treated with only passive flexion (Table 41-2), which also confirms the in vivo strength of the cross-stitch. The finding that the difference in gap size was not retained throughout the follow-up period was probably because the patients in the active group had a significantly better early active range of motion, lost less muscle bulk, and were much more inclined to use the hand normally on coming out of the splint 4 weeks postoperatively. The faster return of normal function thus brought with it an added strain on the repair during the second and third postoperative months.

Table 41-3. Mean active IP joint range of motion in degrees 6 weeks and 6 months after operation—a comparison of the active ($n = 53$) and passive ($n = 49$) treatment programs*

	6 Weeks Postoperative		6 Months Postoperative	
	Active	Passive	Active	Passive
DIP	50	30	63	50
PIP	83	77	94	95
DIP + PIP	132	106	157	144

*Two ruptures in each treatment group are not included.
DIP, Distal interphalangeal; *PIP*, proximal interphalangeal.

Table 41-4. Results in the active group ($n = 55$) according to Strickland's original classification system

	Range of Motion (Degrees)	No. of Digits	%
Excellent	≥150	39	71
Good	125-149	14	25
Fair	90-124	0	0
Poor	<90	0	0
Ruptures		2	4

Clinical results. As a result of the improvements in controlled motion excursions, clinical results in terms of subsequent active IP joint range of motion also improved (Table 41-3). Results according to Strickland's original classification are shown in Table 41-4. The mean composite IP joint range of motion 6 months postoperatively was 157° (excluding 2 ruptures). Using Strickland's[79] definition of normal function (175° of composite IP joint range of motion), this corresponds to an average return of function equal to 90% of normal function. Excluding the two ruptures, no patient obtained less than a 70% return of normal function.

Despite the added strain of active flexion, the rupture rate was the same as with only passive flexion. In the two ruptures that occurred (both were reoperated on within a few days), the suture materials of both the cross-stitch and the modified Kessler suture had broken with the knots intact. The tendon stumps were firm and well vascularized, and there were no signs of the sutures pulling through the tendon tissue. The mode of failure was thus the same as in the majority of specimens tested in vitro. Therefore, it is likely that the load that caused these ruptures was in the vicinity of, or higher than, the breaking strength recorded in vitro for the cross-stitch alone (mean of 63 newtons) and probably the result of active gripping.

Effects on healing. The possibility that the combination of two suture methods, and the fairly extensive suturing involved, could have a detrimental effect on the vascular perfusion and the healing of the tendon stumps was not supported by the findings of this study. By off-loading the core suture and distributing the tension around the circumference of the tendon, the cross-stitch could, instead, have decreased any strangulatory effect attributable to the core suture. By applying the cross-stitch only to the palmar three quarters of the tendon circumference, the dorsal vascular axis was avoided and thus also any potential strangulatory effect from the cross-stitch itself.

The use of early active flexion may also have had a beneficial effect on synovial diffusion by increasing pressure gradients within the tendon (both through intermittent axial tension and by lateral tension against pulleys) in a manner analogous to the diffusion of nutrients in cartilage. Such an effect is supported by studies by Lundborg[50,51] who in dogs found that synovial diffusion was promoted by active motion but not by passive motion. Many studies have shown that a controlled amount of stress can induce a faster return of tensile strength.* Others have shown that stress enhances fibroblast proliferation,[3] the synthesis of DNA,[25,76] protein,[76] and collagen.[3,28,60] It seems likely that the stress provided by active motion is more consistent and physiologic, as long as it does not exceed the strength of the repair.

Complications. In view of the traditional principles of early wound treatment, the aggressive therapeutic approach necessary to obtain optimal tendon excursions was initially of some concern in terms of swelling and possible wound complications. As could be expected, the push for a large controlled range of motion within a few days after the operation did result in some additional swelling during the first postoperative week. In most cases this resolved quickly and by the third postoperative week the swelling, as measured by the mean circumference of the basal phalanx, was actually less in the patients treated with the active program compared with patients in our first group treated with a Kleinert traction program. There were no wound complications that prevented completion of the treatment program.

Flexion contractures are probably a multifactorial problem at least partly caused by swelling and shortening of ligaments and other capsular structures. This process is very likely compounded by not obtaining full extension during daily exercises and keeping the digits in the flexed position during the night. In our studies we found that the frequency of flexion contractures can be decreased by using a shorter dorsal splint, extending only to the level of the PIP joints and extension splinting during the night.[55] Full active extension during exercises was also ensured by unloading the rubber bands during the active extension phase. The fear of increasing the rupture rate by involuntary nightly contractions against the volar splint was not substantiated in our studies.

*References 21, 22, 29, 34, 36, 54, 87, 89.

SUMMARY AND CONCLUSIONS

The overall purpose of our studies was to learn more about the effects of early postoperative mobilization after flexor tendon repair in the clinical situation, in particular in terms of tendon excursions and gap formation and, ultimately, to use this information to improve results. Our findings indicate the following:

- There is a positive correlation between the magnitude of tendon excursions obtained during the early mobilization period and subsequent clinical results in terms of active IP joint range of motion.
- There is a roughly linear relationship between early controlled IP joint range of motion and the size of the resulting excursions of the FDP tendon.
- As long as the tendon is kept moving and frank rupture does not occur, the influence of gap formation is not clinically significant.
- If a strong enough suture technique is used, results can be improved by using an early mobilization program that optimizes tendon excursions through a combination of passive and active flexion of all four digits.
- The in vitro strength of the cross-stitch, a new peripheral suture technique described and evaluated in our studies, is significantly greater than the strength of conventional repair methods.
- The in vivo strength of the cross-stitch used in conjunction with a modified Kessler repair is sufficient for early postoperative mobilization with a combination of passive and active flexion.

Approximately 50 to 70 patients with zone II injuries are treated at the hand surgery unit in Gothenburg yearly. The suture technique and the active flexion program described here have now been used on a routine basis by residents in training and staff specialists alike for more than 4 years with continuing good results. With increasing experience, exchange of ideas, and research, operative techniques and postoperative treatment programs will continue to evolve and improve. Although the basic technique of suturing tendons (as well as other tissues) has survived for a long time, it seems likely that with further developments in biotechnology new techniques will eventually replace sutures. The concept of early active mobilization, on the other hand, is probably here to stay. Being the most physiologic approach it seems hard to improve on, if safely applied. Even if, in the future, pharmacologic agents and other treatment modalities will be available to influence adhesion formation and promote healing, it seems likely that these will be used in conjunction with early active mobilization rather than replace it. The more general effects of early mobilization, such as prevention of muscular atrophy, swelling, and stiffness seem difficult (or desirable) to achieve in any other way.

REFERENCES

1. Bainbridge L, Robertson C, Gillies D, Elliot D: A comparison of postoperative mobilization of flexor tendon repairs with "passive

flexion-active extension" and "controlled active motion" techniques, *J Hand Surg* 1994; 19B:517.

2. Becker H: Primary repair of flexor tendons in the hand without immobilisation, preliminary report, *Hand* 1978; 10:37.
3. Becker H, Diegelmann R: The influence of tension on intrinsic tendon fibroplasia, *Orthop Rev* 1984; 13:153.
4. Becker H, Orak F, Duponselle E: Early active motion following a beveled technique of flexor tendon repair: report on fifty cases, *J Hand Surg* 1979; 4:454.
5. Brunelli G, Monini L: Technique personnelle de suture des tendons fléchisseurs des doigts avec mobilisation immédiate, *Ann Chir Main* 1982; 1:92.
6. Brunelli G, Vigasio A, Brunelli F: Slip-knot flexor tendon suture in zone II allowing immediate mobilization, *Hand* 1983; 15:352.
7. Bullon A, Novo A: Primary repair of flexor tendons in the hand with early passive mobilization, *Int Orthop* 1988; 12:61.
8. Bunnell S: Repair of tendons in the fingers and description of two new instruments, *Surg Gynecol Obstet* 1918; 26:103.
9. Bunnell S: Repair of tendons in the fingers, *Surg Gynecol Obstet* 1922; 35:88.
10. Chow J, Thomes L, Dovelle S, et al: A combined regimen of controlled motion following flexor tendon repair in "no man's land," *Plast Reconstr Surg* 1987; 79:447.
11. Cullen K, Tolhurst P, Lang D, Page R: Flexor tendon repair in zone 2 followed by controlled active mobilization, *J Hand Surg* 1989; 14B:392.
12. Defino H, Barbieri C, Goncalves R, Paulin J: Studies on tendon healing: a comparison between suturing techniques, *J Hand Surg* 1986; 11B:444.
13. Duran J, Houser R: Controlled passive motion following flexor tendon repair in zones 2 and 3. In *AAOS symposium on tendon surgery in the hand*, St Louis, 1975, Mosby.
14. Earley M, Milward T: The primary repair of digital flexor tendons, *Br J Plast Surg* 1982; 35:133.
15. Easley K, Stashak T, Smith F, Van Slyke G: Mechanical properties of four suture patterns for transected equine tendon repair, *Vet Surg* 1990; 19:102.
16. Edinburg M, Widgerow A, Biddulph S: Early postoperative mobilization of flexor tendon injuries using a modification of the Kleinert technique, *J Hand Surg* 1987; 12A:34.
17. Ejeskär A: Flexor tendon repair in no man's land: results of primary repair with controlled mobilization, *J Hand Surg* 1984; 9A:171.
18. Ejeskär A, Irstam L: Elongation in profundus tendon repair, *Scand J Plast Reconstr Surg* 1981; 15:61.
19. Elliot D, Moiemen N, Flemming A, et al: The rupture of acute flexor tendon repairs mobilized by the controlled active motion regimen, *J Hand Surg* 1994; 19B:607.
20. Emery F: Immediate mobilization following flexor tendon repair: a preliminary report, *J Trauma* 1977; 17:1.
21. Enwemeka C: Functional loading augments the initial tensile strength and energy absorption capacity of regenerating rabbit achilles tendons, *Am J Phys Med Rehabil* 1992; 71:31.
22. Feehan L, Beauchene J: Early tensile properties of healing chicken flexor tendons: early controlled passive motion versus postoperative immobilization, *J Hand Surg* 1990; 15A:63.
23. Garlock J: The repair processes in wounds of tendons and in tendon grafts, *Ann Surg* 1927; 85:92.
24. Gault D: A review of repaired flexor tendons, *J Hand Surg* 1987; 12B:321.
25. Gelberman R, Amiel D, Gonsalves M, et al: The influence of protected passive mobilization on the healing of flexor tendons: a biochemical and microangiographic study, *Hand* 1981; 13:120.
26. Gelberman R, Manske P: Factors influencing flexor tendon adhesions, *Hand Clin* 1985; 1:35.
27. Gelberman R, Nunley J II, Osterman A, et al: Influences of the protected passive mobilization interval on flexor tendon healing: a prospective randomized clinical study, *Clin Orthop* 1991; 264:189.
28. Gelberman R, VandeBerg J, Lundborg G, Akeson W: Flexor tendon healing and restoration of the gliding surface, *J Bone Joint Surg* 1983; 65A:70.
29. Gelberman R, Woo S, Lothinger K, Akeson W, Amiel D: Effects of early intermittent passive mobilization on healing canine flexor tendons, *J Hand Surg* 1982; 7:170.
30. Haddad R, Kester M, McCluskey G, et al: Comparative mechanical analysis of a looped-suture tendon repair, *J Hand Surg* 1988; 13A:709.
31. Hagberg L, Selvik G: Tendon excursion and dehiscence during early controlled mobilization after flexor tendon repair in zone II: an x-ray stereophotogrammetric analysis, *J Hand Surg* 1991; 16A:669.
32. Harmer T: Certain aspects of hand surgery, *N Engl J Med* 1936; 214:613.
33. Hernandez A, Velasco F, Rivas A, Preciado A: Preliminary report on early mobilization for the rehabilitation of flexor tendons, *Plast Reconstr Surg* 1967; 40:354.
34. Hitchcock T, Light T, Bunch W, et al: The effect of immediate constrained digital motion on the strength of flexor tendon repairs in chickens, *J Hand Surg* 1987; 12A:590.
35. Kessler I: The "grasping" technique for tendon repair, *Hand* 1973; 5:253.
36. Ketchum L, Martin N, Kappel D: Experimental evaluation of factors affecting the strength of tendon repairs, *Plast Reconstr Surg* 1977; 59:708.
37. Ketchum L, Thompson D, Pocock G, Wallingford D: A clinical study of the forces generated by the intrinsic muscles of the index finger and the extrinsic flexor and extensor muscles of the hand, *J Hand Surg* 1978; 3:571.
38. Kim S: Further evolution of the grasping technique for tendon repair, *Ann Plast Surg* 1981; 7:113.
39. Kleinert H, Kutz J, Atasoy E, Stormo A: Primary repair of flexor tendons, *Orthop Clin North Am* 1973; 4:865.
40. Knight S: A modification of the Kleinert splint for mobilization of digital flexor tendons, *J Hand Surg* 1987; 12B:179.
41. Lahey F: A tendon suture which permits immediate motion, *Boston Med Surg J* 1923; 188:851.
42. Lane J, Black J, Bora F: Gliding function following flexor tendon injury, *J Bone Joint Surg* 1976; 58A:985.
43. Langlais F, Gibbon J, Canciani J, Thomine J: Sutures primitives des tendons fléchisseurs en zone II (103 doigts): resultats et limites du "Kleinert," *Ann Chir Main* 1986; 5:301.
44. Lee H: Double loop locking suture: a technique of tendon repair for early active mobilization, part 1: evolution of technique and experimental study, *J Hand Surg* 1990; 15A:945.
45. Lin GT, An KN, Amadio PC, Cooney W III: Biomechanical studies of running suture for flexor tendon repair in dogs, *J Hand Surg* 1988; 13A:553.
46. Lindsay W, Thompson H: Digital flexor tendons: an experimental study. part 1: the significance of each component of the flexor mechanism in tendon healing, *Br J Plast Surg* 1960; 12:289.
47. Lindsay W, Thompson H, Walker F: Digital flexor tendons: an experimental study, part II: the significance of a gap occurring at the line of suture, *Br J Plast Surg* 1960; 13:1.
48. Lister G, Kleinert H, Kutz J, Atasoy E: Primary flexor tendon repair followed by immediate controlled mobilization, *J Hand Surg* 1977; 2:441.
49. Lopez M, Hanley K: Splint modification for flexor tendon repairs, *Am J Occup Ther* 1984; 38:398.
50. Lundborg G, Holm S, Myrhage R: The role of the synovial fluid and tendon sheath for flexor tendon nutrition, *Scand J Plast Reconstr Surg* 1980; 14:99.

51. Lundborg G, Myrhage R, Rydevik B: The vascularization of human flexor tendons within the digital synovial sheath region—structural and functional aspects, *J Hand Surg* 1977; 2:417.

52. Mashadi ZB, Amis AA: Strength of the suture in the epitenon and within the tendon fibres: development of stronger peripheral suture techniques, *J Hand Surg* 1992; 17b:172.

53. Mashadi ZB, Amis AA: The effect of locking loops on the strength of tendon repair, *J Hand Surg* 1991; 16B:35.

54. Mason M, Allen H: The rate of healing of tendons, *Ann Surg* 1941; 113:424.

55. May E, Silfverskiöld K, Sollerman C: Controlled mobilization after flexor tendon repair in zone II: a prospective comparison of three methods, *J Hand Surg* 1992; 17A:942.

56. McLean N: Some observations on controlled mobilization following flexor tendon injury, *J Hand Surg* 1987; 12B:101.

57. Messina A: The double armed suture: tendon repair with immediate mobilization of the fingers, *J Hand Surg* 1992; 17A:137.

58. Murray G: A method of tendon repair, *Am J Surg* 1960; 99:334.

59. Nielsen A, Jensen P: Primary flexor tendon repair in "no man's land," *J Hand Surg* 1984; 9B:279.

60. Peacock E: Fundamental aspects of wound healing relating to the restoration of gliding function after tendon repair, *Surg Gynecol Obstet* 1964; 119: 241.

61. Potenza A: Tendon healing within the flexor digital sheath in the dog, *J Bone Joint Surg* 1962; 44A:49.

62. Powell E, Trail I, Noble J: Non-suture repair of tendons, *J Biomed Eng* 1989; 11:215.

63. Pribaz J, Morrison W, Macleod A: Primary repair of flexor tendons in no man's land using the Becker repair, *J Hand Surg* 1989; 14B:400.

64. Robertson G, Al-Qattan M: A biomechanical analysis of a new interlock suture technique for flexor tendon repair, *J Hand Surg* 1992; 17B:92.

65. Savage R: In vitro studies of a new method of flexor tendon repair, *J Hand Surg* 1985; 10B:135.

66. Savage R, Risitano G: Flexor tendon repair using a "six strand" method of repair and early active mobilisation, *J Hand Surg* 1989; 14B:396.

67. Schuind F, Garcia-Elias M, Cooney W III, An KN: Flexor tendon forces: in vivo measurements, *J Hand Surg* 1992; 17A:291.

68. Seradge H: Elongation of the repair configuration following flexor tendon repair, *J Hand Surg* 1983; 8:182.

69. Silfverskiöld K, Andersson C: Two new methods of tendon repair: an in vitro evaluation of tensile strength and gap formation, *J Hand Surg* 1993; 18A:58.

70. Silfverskiöld K, May E: Gap formation after flexor tendon repair in zone II: results with a new controlled motion programme, *Scand J Plast Reconstr Surg Hand Surg* 1993; 27:263.

71. Silfverskiöld K, May E: Flexor tendon repair in zone II with a new suture technique and an early mobilization program combining passive and active flexion, *J Hand Surg* 1994; 19A:53.

72. Silfverskiöld K, May E, Törnvall A: Flexor digitorum profundus tendon excursions during controlled motion after flexor tendon repair in zone II: a prospective clinical study, *J Hand Surg* 1992; 17A:122.

73. Silfverskiöld K, May E, Törnvall A: Gap formation during controlled motion after flexor tendon repair in zone II: a prospective clinical study, *J Hand Surg* 1992; 17A:539.

74. Silfverskiöld K, May E, Törnvall A: Tendon excursions after flexor tendon repair in zone II: results with a new controlled motion program, *J Hand Surg* 1993; 18A:403.

75. Skoog T, Persson B: An experimental study of the early healing of tendons, *Scand J Plast Reconstr Surg* 1954; 13:384.

76. Slack C, Flint M, Thompson B: The effect of tensional load on isolated embryonic chick tendons in organ culture, *Conn Tissue Res* 1984; 12:229.

77. Slattery P: The modified Kleinert splint in zone II flexor tendon injuries, *J Hand Surg* 1988; 13B:273.

78. Small J, Brennen M, Colville J: Early active mobilisation following flexor tendon repair in zone 2, *J Hand Surg* 1989; 14B:383.

79. Strickland J, Glogovac S: Digital function following flexor tendon repair in zone II: a comparison of immobilization and controlled passive motion techniques, *J Hand Surg* 1980; 5:537.

80. Tajima T: History, current status, and aspects of hand surgery in Japan, *Clin Orthop* 1984; 184:41.

81. Tokita Y, Yamaya A, Ito Y, et al: An experimental study of the repair and gliding function of digital flexor tendon following injury, *Int Orthop* 1977; 1:179.

82. Tropet Y, Menez D, Dreyfus-Schmidt G, Vichard P: Recent simple flexor tendon injuries in zone I, II, III of Verdan: results of tendon repairs concerning 115 fingers in 99 patients, *Ann Chir Main* 1988; 7:109.

83. Tsuge K, Ikuta Y, Matsuichi Y: Intra-tendinous tendon suture in the hand, *Hand* 1975; 7:250.

84. Urbaniak J, Cahill J, Mortenson R: Tendon suturing methods: analysis of tensile strengths. In *AAOS symposium on tendon surgery in the hand*, St Louis, 1975, Mosby.

85. Wade P, Muir I, Hutcheon L: Primary flexor tendon repair: the mechanical limitations of the modified Kessler technique, *J Hand Surg* 1986; 11B:71.

86. Wade P, Wetherell R, Amis A: Flexor tendon repair: significant gain in strength from the Halsted peripheral suture technique, *J Hand Surg* 1989; 14B:232.

87. Weeks P, Wray R: Tendon gliding and repair. In *Management of acute hand injuries: a biological approach*, St Louis, 1978, Mosby.

88. Werntz J, Chesher S, Breidenbach W, et al: A new dynamic splint for postoperative treatment of flexor tendon injury, *J Hand Surg* 1989; 14A:559.

89. Woo S, Gelberman R, Cobb N, et al: The importance of controlled passive mobilization on flexor tendon healing, *Acta Orthop Scand* 1981; 52:615.

90. Wray R, Weeks P: Experimental comparison of technics of tendon repair, *J Hand Surg* 1980; 5:144.

91. Young R, Harmon J: Repair of tendon injuries of the hand, *Ann Surg* 1960; 151:562.

Chapter 42

FLEXOR TENDON REPAIR
The Indianapolis method

James W. Strickland
Karan H. Gettle

The ability to return normal flexor tendon excursion after severance within the digital sheath has proven to be a formidable task. It may be the ultimate challenge for the hand surgeon; drawing on all of his or her anatomic, biomechanic, biologic, and physiologic knowledge and demanding the utmost in surgical perfection. Despite the numerous innovative flexor tendon repair techniques and the introduction of a succession of aggressive postrepair rehabilitation protocols, the results of flexor tendon repairs in zone II appear to have leveled off short of the recovery of near normal digital performance that surgeons have historically tried to achieve. While this failure to accomplish the same predictable success that other upper extremity operations achieve may be secondary to uncontrollable factors such as age, the nature of the injury, and the particular patient's healing capacity,[39] the quest goes on to find just the right combination of repair and rehabilitation techniques to break the biologic barrier and return good digital function following almost all such injuries.

This chapter describes a flexor tendon repair method and postrepair rehabilitation program that has been used at the Indiana Hand Center for several years. The combined protocol is based on available scientific information and the rationale for both the suture technique and the protocol for the application of early passive and active motion stress is provided. We by no means suggest that this is the ultimate answer to the difficult problem of predictably returning excellent finger motion after all zone II flexor tendon injuries, but, in our hands, it has provided results that are significantly better than we have achieved with any other methods.

SCIENTIFIC RATIONALE
Historical information and research

The techniques of flexor tendon repair and the protocols for postoperative mobilization of the repaired tendon were, for many years, based on anecdotes, hearsay, and published papers, many of which were woefully lacking in scientific credibility. As a result of the conflicting and confusing information available to the surgeon, flexor tendon repair methods evolved from trial and error. Although there appears to have been slow improvement in the functional recovery following such repairs, it would be safe to say that the results were mediocre at best.[44]

In recent years there has been a plethora of laboratory and clinical information published in various hand, orthopedic, and plastic surgery journals that offer assessments of the strongest methods of flexor tendon repair and the best postrepair motion protocols. These investigations stem from the consensus that the greater the increments of stress imparted to the repair site and the greater the excursion of the healing tendon, the quicker the tendon will achieve normal tensile strength with the fewest motion restricting adhesions. Trying to interpret these reports and compare them with other studies has been almost impossible given the different laboratory models, in vivo versus in vitro investigations, different testing methods, and diverse definitions of failure. We have studied almost all of these reports and have tried to correlate their findings to each other and to the clinical setting. Although we admit to having taken considerable scientific liberty in doing so, we can now offer a few supportable conclusions, a few reasonably accurate suppositions, a few speculative pos-

Table 42-1. Tensile stresses on normal flexor tendon

Passive motion	500 g
Light grip	1500 g
Strong grip	5000 g
Tip pinch – index FDP	9000 g
FDS repairs = <30% of these values	

These numbers fail to recognize the increased demands resulting from digital swelling and tissue drag.
FDS, Flexor digitorum superficialis; *FDP,* flexor digitorum profundus.

sibilities, and, finally, some conjectures with regard to the best method for returning satisfactory excursion to repaired flexor tendons. We have incorporated these thoughts into a scheme for the management of such injuries, and the results of this protocol have returned what are easily the best we have experienced in our practice in the difficult area of flexor tendon repair.

While we make no attempt to review the long list of laboratory studies that were summarized for our current protocol, we present some facts and assumptions that provide the biologic rationale for the method. To simplify an understanding of this information, it is categorized, summarized, and presented in the following sections.

Tendon healing

- Tendons heal by a combination of extrinsic and intrinsic cellular activity. The more intrinsic, the less the adhesions.[45]
- If the repair is not stressed, the healing process may take up to 8 weeks, and repaired tendons will have minimal tensile strength throughout the healing process.
- Stressed tendons will heal faster, gain tensile strength faster, and have less adhesions and better excursions than unstressed tendons.[45]
- Repair strength usually decreases by 10% to 50% between 5 and 21 days postrepair (unstressed).[29]
- The tensile stresses on a normal flexor tendon in an unswollen finger are shown roughly (conservative working numbers)[49] in Table 42-1.

Repair strength

- 3-0 or 4-0 synthetic braided sutures are probably the best for tendon repair. Each larger caliber increases the repair strength somewhat.[1]
- The strength of a tendon repair is roughly proportional to the number of suture strands that cross the repair site.[37,47]
- Increasing the number of suture strands increases repair strength, but adds to the technical difficulty and increases the volume of suture material in the repair site.[44]
- The estimated strengths for unstressed 2-, 4-, and 6-strand flexor tendon repairs (without an epitendinous suture) at 0, 1, 3, and 6 weeks are shown in Table 42-2.[44,47]
- Gap formation at the repair site becomes the weakest part of the tendon, unfavorably alters tendon mechanics, and

Table 42-2. Estimated repair strength, no epitendinous suture

	0 Week	1 Week (−50%)	3 Weeks (−33%)	6 Weeks (+20%)
Two strands	1800 g	900 g	1200 g	2200 g
Four strands	3600 g	1800 g	2400 g	4200 g
Six strands	5400 g	2700 g	3600 g	6500 g

may attract adhesions resulting in decreased tendon excursion.[48]
- Repaired tendons rupture through the suture or knot.[37,53]
- Locking loops contribute little to strength and may actually collapse and lead to gap formation at moderate loads.[43]
- A peripheral epitendinous suture results in an increase in repair strength and a significant reduction in the tendency for gap formation at the repair site. This improved strength and decreased gap formation are maintained with cyclic stress.[7,30,38]
- Horizontal mattress or running locked peripheral epitendinous sutures have been shown to add the greatest strength and resistance to gap formation.[30,50]

A number of publications indicate that it is a safe assumption that these sutures add at least 40% to the repair strength or about 700 g. The addition of 700 g to all repairs throughout the healing process would change the repair strength as shown in Table 42-3.[44,47]

The data in Table 42-3 indicate that 4- and 6-strand flexor tendon repairs with a horizontal mattress or running lock peripheral epitendinous suture enjoy relative safety for both passive and light active digital motion during the entire healing process in the unswollen digit.

Sheath repair

- Repairing the sheath following tendon suture would seem to have theoretical advantages of providing a barrier for adhesion formation, restoring synovial fluid nutrition, and restoring the sheath mechanics[23,24,33,41,51]; however, the sheath is often technically difficult to reestablish and there are little valid data (clinical or experimental) to substantiate that it improves the results of flexor tendon repair.[10,25,26,35]

Postflexor repair motion

- Averaged from several articles,[10,13] flexor tendon excursion for 10° increment of joint motion equals

  FDP* = 1.5 mm per 10° DIP joint flexion

  FDP + FDS = 1.5 mm per 10° PIP joint flexion

- Clinically (from radiographs of repairs tagged with metal markers), this excursion decreases as follows[39]:

*FDP, Flexor digitorum profundus; DIP, distal interphalangeal; FDS, flexor digitorum superficialis; PIP, proximal interphalangeal.

Table 42-3. Repair strength with epitendinous suture with horizontal mattress or running lock

	0 Week	1 Week (−50%)	3 Weeks (−33%)	6 Weeks (+20%)
Two strands	2500 g	1200 g	1700 g	2700 g
Four strands	4300 g	2150 g	2800 g	5200 g
Six strands	6000 g	3000 g	4000 g	7200 g

$$FDP = 0.3 \text{ mm per } 10° \text{ DIP flexion} = 36\%$$

$$FDP + FDS = 1.2 \text{ mm per } 10° \text{ PIP flexion} = 90\%$$

- Tendon excursion in the most commonly used postrepair splints varies depending on the range of wrist and composite digital motion permitted by the splint.[13] The ability to synergistically bring the wrist into extension provides the greatest excursion of repaired flexor tendons.[4]
- The least tensile demand on a zone II repair during *active* digital flexion occurs when the wrist is in 45° extension and the metacarpophalangeal (MP) joints are fully flexed.[5]
- Based on this information, the best postoperative protocol probably has the following components[44,47]:
  - Compensates for a swollen finger
  - Keeps the wrist and MP joints flexed at rest
  - Keeps PIP and DIP joints extended at rest
  - Passively flexes the digit before wrist extension
  - Permits active maintenance of passively achieved digital flexion with the wrist in extension
  - Uses frequent application of motion stress

Pharmacologic adhesion-retarding agents

The oral administration of ibuprofen or indomethacin have been shown to modestly improve functional recovery.[6,31]

FLEXOR TENDON REPAIR
Anesthesia

We prefer to carry out flexor tendon repairs on an outpatient basis under axillary block anesthetic. The blocks are administered by an anesthesiologist and most use 0.5% bupivacaine so that the patient will experience prolonged postoperative anesthesia, permitting them to return home comfortably before experiencing any postoperative discomfort. The block is carried out in a separate area with additional sedation provided depending on the desires of the patient.

Surgical technique[44,47]

It is always necessary to extend the wound of injury in both proximal and distal directions to provide wide visibility of the area of injury. Whenever possible, we prefer midaxial wound extensions in an effort to return well-nourished subcutaneous tissue over the repair site and minimize the proximity of skin scarring to the underlying tendon repairs.

An adequate view of the surgical field must be created to avoid the need to carry out delicate tendon repairs within the constraints of a small surgical wound. Although T extensions of transverse lacerations should generally be avoided, there are occasions where we may use them to gain access to digital nerves or vessels.

Zone I

In zone I (distal to the superficialis insertion over the middle phalanx) when only the FDP has been severed, there is usually little difficulty finding the proximal tendon end, which is at least temporarily retained in the finger by its vinculum and can usually be located in the distal portion of the proximal phalanx or at the level of the PIP joint. Careful dissection exposes the entire distal half of the flexor tendon sheath, and the entire A_4 annular pulley should be preserved. If the DIP joint was flexed at the time of injury, the tendon will probably have a short distal stump over the base of the distal phalanx and can be exposed by opening the C_3-A_5 pulley complex. It will also be necessary to open the C_2 or C_1 cruciate-synovial segments proximal to the A_4 pulley to retrieve the proximal stump of the divided profundus tendon. After the proximal profundus is delivered into the appropriate cruciate-synovial interval, a core suture is placed in the tendon allowing it to be passed distally under the A_4 annular pulley without the need for further instrumentation of the tendon. The proximal tendon is usually maintained in position by the passage of a transversely oriented 25 gauge hypodermic needle, and the repair is completed distal to the A_4 pulley by an end-to-end tendon suture, if enough distal tendon remains to accept a suture. If the distal stump is short or nonexistent, the profundus stump may be reattached by first elevating an osteoperiosteal flap from the base of the distal phalanx and then drilling an oblique hole beneath the flap, directed so as to penetrate the dorsal cortex just beneath the proximal fingernail. A double-armed (straight needles) 3-0 suture is placed in the proximal tendon stump and passed through the bone hole. In this instance, it is better to use a synthetic monofilament suture placed in a criss-cross (unlocked) fashion so that the suture can be easily pulled and extracted after bone and tendon healing has occurred. The sutures are then used to pull the tendon beneath the periosteal flap and are tied over a cotton pad–button combination over the nail. In our view, pullout wires are now unnecessary for any type of tendon repair. An alternative method is to use a commercial bone-anchor suture to reattach the profundus to the distal phalanx. When possible, the tendon attachment should be supplemented by sutures through some adjacent sheath or periosteum.

Zone II

For zone II (from the origin of the flexor tendon sheath to the insertion of the superficialis tendon over the midportion of the middle phalanx) flexor tendon repairs, it is again necessary to make proximal and distal extending incisions that provide satisfactory exposure of the repair site. Dissection proceeds with identification and protection of the digital nerves and arteries and, if they have been severed, the ends are mobilized and brought into proximity for suturing.

At this point, we gently clear off the flexor sheath, which allows an assessment of the level and extent of sheath injury and the position of the tendon ends. Depending on the level of injury, we will open either the C_1 (between A_2 and A_3) or C_2 (between A_3 and A_4) cruciate-synovial windows using connecting incisions along one end and one side.

When opening the intact components of the sheath, every attempt must be made to preserve the annular components (A_1, A_2, A_3, A_4) that are almost impossible to repair. Tendon suture should be performed in the cruciate synovial sheath windows, which can usually be restored following tendon suture. By acutely flexing the DIP joint and, to some extent, the PIP joint, it is usually possible to deliver the profundus and superficialis stumps into a cruciate window, and if at least one centimeter of the distal tendons can be exposed in this manner, core sutures can be placed in the profundus tendon and two superficial slips without great difficulty. If a lesser length of distal tendon is present in the window, then the next most distal cruciate-synovial interval must be opened for core suture placement.

The actual joining of the tendon ends can then be carried out in either window, depending on the most distal point that can be achieved for the proximal tendon stumps, the length of the distal tendons, and their most proximal position during DIP joint flexion.

Tendon retrieval

Retrieval of the proximal tendon ends may be difficult, but there are several techniques that can facilitate their delivery into the repair site. We emphasize that repeated blind grasps down the sheath with an instrument will often fail to retrieve the proximal stumps and may, in fact, damage the delicate synovial lining of the pulleys and provoke adhesions. Such efforts are permissible only if the tendon(s) can be visualized in the sheath and is sufficiently close to the cruciate-synovial window to assure that an end can be atraumatically pinched with forceps and delivered distally.

Many tactics have been suggested to facilitate tendon capture and repositioning when the proximal ends have retracted farther down the proximal sheath. These methods include proximal to distal "milking" of the tendons toward the repair site and the use of various types of catheters or silicone rods, which are sutured to the ends of the tendon stumps in the palm and passed through the sheath in an effort to pull the tendons back into their distal position.[6,21,36] We have had little success with the milking method and rarely rely on the catheter technique because of the difficulty in correctly restoring the anatomic relationship between the

superficialis and profundus tendons and delivering them through the narrow A_1 orifice for passage from the palm to the digit. Two clever techniques have made this dilemma easier.

1. If the tendon end is visible in the sheath, a skin hook can be employed.[36] The hooked end is slid along the surface of the sheath until it is past the tendons, and the hook is then turned toward the tendons and pressed into the most superficial one. When the hook engages a tendon, the instrument is pulled distally and both tendons will usually follow. They can then be held in position by a 25-gauge hypodermic needle.

2. More frequently, the following method is employed.[44,45,47] A small catheter is passed from the distal wound into the palm (or vice versa) beneath the annular pulleys. An important feature of this method is that the flexor tendons are left in situ in the sheath, and through a midpalmar incision, the catheter is sutured to both tendons several centimeters proximal to the A_1 pulley. The catheter is then pulled distally and will easily deliver the tendon stumps into the distal repair site. A transversely oriented needle will secure the tendons for repair and the connecting suture can be severed in the palm and the catheter withdrawn. Core sutures can then be placed in the proximal profundus stump and the superficialis slips and the tendons can usually be brought into juxtaposition with the distal stumps for repair.

When the proximal tendon ends have retracted into the palm, it is extremely important to reestablish the proper anatomic relationship of the profundus and superficialis tendons. To accomplish this, the profundus has to be passed back through the hiatus created by the superficialis slips, so that it lies palmar to Camper's chiasma and recreates the relative positioning that was present at the level of tendon laceration. Failure to restore the correct relationship will create an impediment to unrestricted tendon gliding following repair. Once the proper tendon anatomy has been reestablished, a catheter passed retrograde from the cruciate window is attached to the tendons, and, usually with some difficulty, the tendons are entered into the sheath and delivered distally where they can be maintained with a transversely oriented hypodermic needle.

Flexor tendon suture

Although several methods of 4-strand flexor tendon repair have been described, most are somewhat complicated or require a double suture.[41] The method that we use consists of a simple 2-strand core stitch that enters and exits through the tendon ends and has locking grasps on the side of the tendon.[44,47] For the repair, we usually employ 3-0 braided synthetic suture material for the core sutures and may elect to use the 4-0 for children's tendons. An additional horizontal mattress suture is inserted across the tendon ends to complete a 4-strand repair. A running horizontal lock stitch is used as a peripheral epitendinous stitch, and we have found it to be easier than some of the more complicated methods described in recent articles.

At the conclusion of the tendon repair, the flexor sheath is repaired using 6-0 nylon suture on a small needle and, at this point, the DIP joint can be extended, a maneuver that delivers the repair distally.[42] The repaired sheath usually serves as a smooth conduit for the repair site as it moves under an annular pulley. When the flexor tendon sheath cannot be repaired, we usually elect to leave it open, although no more than 1.5 cm of sheath should be excised.

On occasion the tendon suture process is complicated by the need to use two adjacent windows (usually C_1 and C_2) for core suture placement, and the final repair is carried out in the most appropriate window after the proximal or distal stumps have been delivered into position by passing their core suture ends under the intervening annular pulley (usually A_3) and pulling the tendon ends into position. Flexor sheath repair is facilitated if the bulk of the tendon juncture can be minimized and careful sheath incisions have been used. To facilitate the passage of tendon repair beneath the annular pulleys, we usually elect to close the overlying cruciate-synovial sheath before extending the interphalangeal (IP) joints.

At the conclusion of the repair, digital nerves and occasionally digital arteries are repaired, and the skin is then sutured using fine nonabsorbable sutures. A large, bulky, compressive dressing immobilizing all the digits and the thumb is used postoperatively with the wrist in midflexion and the fingers in a balanced position of moderate flexion of the MP, PIP, and DIP joint levels. The use of antibiotics depends on the personal philosophy and discretion of the surgeon. Our preference is to use them in both the acute and delayed setting.

POSTOPERATIVE MANAGEMENT
Rationale

Following the publication of numerous papers demonstrating the superior results that followed flexor tendon repairs managed by one of several mobilization programs, almost all hand surgeons already employed some type of early motion protocol.* Experimental confirmation of the biologic efficacy of these methods has been provided by the excellent laboratory studies of Gelberman et al.,[12,15,16] which indicate that, in the canine model, early passive motion increases the tensile strength of flexor tendon repairs at an earlier stage in the healing process, while lessening adhesions and improving angular joint motion.[9,14,20,28,46] As the development of these methods has evolved, emphasis has been placed on techniques that employ not only a greater amount of composite digital motion but also the use of synergistic wrist extension in an effort to gain the greatest amount of excursion of the repaired tendon.

*References 8, 11, 17-19, 22, 27, 32, 34, 40, 44.

It now appears that light active digital flexion carried out with the wrist in extension should be relatively safe for those flexor tendons repaired with a 4-strand core suture technique augmented by some type of running lock peripheral epitendinous suture. Because this repair protocol uses such a tendon repair method, this postoperative program should permit the active maintenance of full composite digital flexion once the wrist is brought from flexion to extension.

Indiana post flexor tendon repair protocol

The details of this method have been worked out by Nancy Cannon and Karen Harmon Gettle, therapists at the Indiana Hand Center, and have worked extremely well for those patients who are well motivated and demonstrate a serious desire to maximize their recovery.[2,44,47] The therapists spend a great deal of time with the patient explaining the details of the therapy program and ensuring that the patient comprehends all the details of the somewhat rigorous regimen. The program can be summarized as follows.

Two splints are fabricated. The first is a traditional dorsal blocking splint that positions the wrist in 20° palmar flexion, the MPs in 50° of flexion, and the IPs in neutral. The second splint is a new tenodesis splint patterned in a manner somewhat similar to the synergistic splint described by the Mayo Clinic.[4] The splint is designed so that it allows full flexion of the wrist but incorporates either a hinged component or a dorsal, removable section, which allows the wrist to be brought into 30° of dorsiflexion. When restricting velcro straps are removed, the digits are permitted a full range of motion with the exception of the MP joints, which are immobilized so that they will not extend beyond 60°. The hinge component of the splint is simply a binder screw post that is readily available through office supply stores.

The formal therapy program consists of efforts to maximize independent and combined gliding of the FDS and FDP tendons during each exercise session. Fifteen repetitions of passive flexion and extension of the PIP joint, the DIP joint, and the entire digit are carried out during each hour, and these exercises are performed within the restraints of the dorsal blocking splint, which immobilizes the wrist and MP joints in flexion. The hinge wrist splint is then applied, and within the restraints of the tenodesis splint, the patient passively flexes the digits completely and then extends the wrist. The patient is then asked to gently contract the long flexor muscles and hold the position achieved by passive flexion for at least 5 seconds. After 5 seconds, the patient relaxes the muscle contraction and allows the wrist to drop back into flexion. This will automatically allow the digits to straighten within the confines of the splint. This exercise sequence is performed for 25 repetitions each hour throughout the day.

This protocol is followed for 4 weeks with adjustments made depending on problems that the patient may experience, particularly with regard to digital edema and joint stiffness. The development of any flexion contractures at either the PIP or DIP joint is closely monitored, and appropriate splinting and exercise programs are designed to ensure the recovery of full digital extension. At 4 weeks, the tendons should have regained sufficient strength to allow the splints to be removed for gentle active and passive exercises. The dorsal block splint is worn between exercises, and the program continues to emphasize passive digital flexion with the wrist flexed, followed by active maintenance of that flexion with the wrist extended. The patient then drops the wrist into flexion and extends the digits to complete the tenodesis sequence. Active flexion and extension exercises of the digits and wrist are performed with a light muscle contraction and the patient is instructed not to simultaneously extend the wrist and digits.

At 5 to 6 weeks, more vigorous exercises are permitted including isolated tendon excursion exercises, blocking exercises, and passive extension exercises. Strengthening is initiated at 8 weeks in a gradual, progressive manner.

It should be emphasized that this protocol will not work for everyone. It is important for the surgeon to spend some hours in the cadaver laboratory to develop the technical skills for the 4-strand repair and the running lock peripheral epitendinous stitch. Success also requires a well-trained therapist who thoroughly understands the rationale for the rehabilitation program and its pitfalls. Finally, the method cannot succeed without an intelligent, motivated, and cooperative patient.

Complications

Rupture of one or both flexor tendon repairs is a significant complication, and the preferred treatment is prompt reexploration and repair. In our cases, there have been ruptures, and (almost without exception) they have occurred in patients who were doing so well with their rehabilitation program that they elected to use their hands in an extremely strong manner (such as heavy lifting) well before the tendons had returned to sufficient strength to tolerate the extremely high tensile demands of such activity.

The most frequent late complication following early postoperative mobilization programs is the development of flexion contractures at the PIP or DIP joints, or both. Prompt recognition of the development of contractures, modification of the motion program to permit greater extension, and the judicious use of dynamic splints can help prevent or overcome those deformities before they progress too far.

Occasionally, despite the best possible repair and strong cooperation from the patient, the tendons may become adherent and fail to glide sufficiently to return adequate digital function. The decision to carry out a secondary tenolysis procedure is based on serial joint measurements, which indicate that there has been no appreciable improvement for several months despite a vigorous therapy program

and the conscientious efforts of the patient. The procedure should not be considered until all wounds have reached equilibrium with soft pliable skin and subcutaneous tissues and minimal reaction around the scars. Joint contractures must have been mobilized and a normal or near normal passive range of digital motion achieved.

Considerations

The restoration of function to a digit following flexor tendon interruption and repair may be a long and tedious process. Strong rapport must be developed between surgeon, patient, and therapist. When initiating the care of a patient with such an injury, the surgeon should spend considerable time explaining the problems related to a particular injury, the likelihood of achieving success, and include the fact that several procedures may be necessary to maximize the recovery of digital function.

We continue to employ a 4-strand core stitch flexor tendon repair combined with a continuous running lock suture to impart sufficient strength to the repair to permit a vigorous postrepair motion protocol that would appear to maximize the excursion of the repaired tendon while minimizing the possibility of rupture. Although the results of this technique have been encouraging, the rapid advances currently occurring in flexor tendon surgery will unquestionably lead to even better techniques and results in the future.

STUDY METHODS AND RESULTS

This section analyzes the early results of the controlled early active motion program for zone I and zone II flexor tendon repairs developed at the Indiana Hand Center.

Between 1992 and 1995, 40 patients with zone I and zone II flexor tendon division in 44 digits were managed by a controlled early active motion program. Twenty-one digits required repair of both the profundus and superficialis, while 23 needed only the profundus repaired. Fourteen subjects had 18 associated lacerations of one or both digital nerves. No patient included in the study sustained injury to more than two digits.

Procedure

Using standard goniometers, active range of motion was measured at initial, final, and long-term follow-up visits. The Strickland formula and classification system for zones I and II flexor tendon injuries was used to compute total active motion (TAM) of the involved digits. Grip strength was assessed at the long-term evaluation using 3 Jamar dynamometers that had been checked for calibration every 6 months.

Results

The time between injury and surgical repair ranged from the same day to 31 days postinjury, with a mean of 3.78 days.

Mean time from surgery to initiation of therapy was 2.95 days, with a range of 1 to 7 days. Time from the initial therapy visit to discharge from therapy ranged from 0 (three patients did not return after the initial visit) to 1162 days, with a mean therapy time of 81.76 days. Time from repair to long-term follow-up visit ranged from 0.52 to 2.38 years, with a mean of 1.4 years.

Total active motion

Initial evaluation. All 40 patients were measured at the time of their first postrepair therapy visit. TAM measurements ranged from 70° to 150° with a mean of 118.41°. According to the Strickland classification system for zone I and zone II flexor tendon repairs, 1 finger was ranked as excellent, 20 were good, 18 were fair, and 5 were poor at the time of initial evaluation.

Final evaluation. Thirty-four patients (37 digits) had final TAM measurements taken at the time of release from therapy. Six of the original 40 patients were not evaluated for a final TAM. Three of these individuals (four repairs), were not seen in therapy after the initial visit and three ruptured. Final TAM scores ranged from 40° to 195° with a mean of 129.59°. No statistical difference was found between the other finger TAMs, and no statistical difference was found between FDP and FDS repairs and FDP repairs alone. According to the Strickland classification system, at the time of discharge from therapy, 9 digits had an excellent result, 17 were good, 9 were fair, and 2 were poor.

Time from injury to repair for patients in the excellent TAM category ranged from repair done on the same day to 13 days postinjury. All the patients with excellent TAMs began therapy between 1 and 3 days postoperative (67% at 2 days).

Long-term follow-up evaluation. A total of 17 patients (19 digits) returned for the long-term follow-up assessment. Long-term TAM ranged from 100° to 185° with a mean of 149.47°. This represented a statistically significant mean increase in TAM of 18.89° since the discharge evaluation ($p <0.0052$). No significant differences were found for subject sex, hand of injury, between the FDP and FDS repair and the FDP repair, or the surgeon who did the repair. At the long-term follow-up, 11 digits were ranked excellent, 5 good, and 3 fair, according to the Strickland classification.

Grip strength

Handle position 2, grip strengths were assessed for 13 subjects at the time of discharge from therapy and for 15 subjects at the long-term evaluation using a calibrated Jamar dynamometer. Comparison of injured with normal side grip strengths ranged from 48% to 125% with a mean of 79% at the discharge evaluation. At the long-term follow-up, percent of injury to normal side grip improved to a range of 53% to 131% with a mean of 94%.

Complications

Ruptures. Three patients (6.8%) sustained ruptures of the repaired flexor tendons. One patient's repair that was done at 31 days postinjury ruptured on the twelfth postoperative day. A second patient's repair also ruptured on the twelfth day. Both ruptures were the result of unauthorized removal of the splint and concomitant active use of the hand. The third patient was 58 days postoperative, and the repair ruptured while exercising with the DIP blocked. Before the rupture, this patient had a Strickland TAM classification of good.

Triggering. It has been noted that patients who tend to be more active than the program requires may develop mild triggering with active flexion. With approval of the referring surgeon, these patients have continued with the normal protocol without increasing the severity of symptoms. One patient did receive a steroid injection, resulting in decreased symptoms and improved motion.

Limited therapy. One patient belonged to a health maintenance organization (HMO) plan that limited therapy to 6 visits. The patient was not seen for a period of 6 weeks and returned with a loss of 100° and a fixed flexion contraction.

Fixed flexion contraction. Two patients developed a fixed flexion contracture at the PIP between final and long-term follow-up. Both had a FDP laceration to the small finger and required a sustained flexed posture in their profession.

DISCUSSION

Using final TAMs in the excellent category as a standard, success does not appear dependent on the repair being done the day of injury. Results appear to improve when therapy is initiated between 48 to 72 hours postsurgery. The mean change in TAM of 12.3° from the initial therapy visit to the final therapy visit indicates the importance of achieving an excellent TAM during the first weeks of therapy.

To avoid rupturing, blocking exercises should not be included for patients with high, fair, or better TAM. Caution must be taken by modifying the program when increased risk factors such as edema, joint stiffness, or wound problems are present.

Therapists also need to be aware of substitution patterns such as trapping with normal fingers, which often lead to poor active muscle contraction. It is important that a full, digitally independent, composite fist be achieved with the place and hold exercises.

ACKNOWLEDGMENTS

We acknowledge Nancy Cannon OTR, CHT for her contribution to the development of the hand therapy program and Elaine E. Fess, MS, OTR, CHT for her contribution to the statistical computations.

REFERENCES

1. Bright DS, Urbaniak JS: Direct measurements of flexor tendon tension during active and passive digit motion and its application to flexor tendon surgery, *Trans Orthop Res Soc* 1976; 6:240.
2. Cannon NM: Post flexor tendon repair motion protocol, *Indiana Hand Center Newsletter* 1993; 1(1):13-17.
3. Carstadt CA, Madsen K, Wredmark T: The influence of indomethacin on biomechanical and biochemical properties of the plantaris longus tendon in the rabbit, *Arch Orthop Trauma Surg* 1987; 106:157-160.
4. Chow JA, Thomes LJ, Dovelle SW, et al: A combined regimen of controlled motion following flexor tendon repair in "no man's land," *Plast Reconstr Surg* 1981; 79(3):447-453.
5. Chow JA, Thomes LJ, Dovelle SW, et al: Controlled motion rehabilitation after flexor tendon repair and grafting, a multi-centre study, *J Bone Joint Surg* 1980; 70B(4):591-595.
6. Cooney WP: In Lin GT, An K-N: Improved tendon excursion following flexor tendon repair, *J Hand Surg* 1989; 2:102-106.
7. Delfino HLA, Barbieri CH, Goncalves RP, Paulin JBP: Studies on tendon healing, a comparison between suturing techniques, *J Hand Surg* 1986; 11B(3):444-450.
8. Duran RH, Hauser RG: Controlled passive motion following flexor tendon repair in zones 2 and 3. In *AAOS symposium on flexor tendon surgery in the hand,* St Louis, 1975, Mosby.
9. Duran RH, Hauser RG, Stover MG: Management of flexor lacerations in zone 2 using controlled passive motion postoperatively. In Hunter JM, Schneider LH, Mackin EJ, Bell JA, eds: *Rehabilitation of the hand,* St Louis, 1978, Mosby.
10. Eiken O, Holmberg J, Ekerot L, Salgeback S: Restoration of the digital tendon sheath, a new concept of tendon grafting, *Scand J Plast Reconstr Surg* 1980; 14:89-97.
11. Garlock JM: The repair process in wounds of tendons and in tendon grafts, *Ann Surg* 1980; 85:92.
12. Gelberman RH, Amiel D, Gonsalves M, et al: The influence of protected passive mobilization on the healing of flexor tendons: a biochemical and microangiographic study, *Hand* 1981; 13(2):120-128.
13. Gelberman RH, Botte MJ, Spiegelman JH, Akeson WH: The excursion and deformation of repaired flexor tendons treated with protected early motion, *J Hand Surg* 1986; 11A:106-110.
14. Gelberman RH, Jayasanker M, Gonsalves M, Akeson WH: The effects of mobilization on the vascularization of healing flexor tendons in dogs, *Clin Orthop Rel Res* 1980; 153:283-289.
15. Gelberman RH, VandeBerg JS, Lundborg GN, Akeson WH: Flexor tendon healing and restoration of the gliding surface, *J Bone Joint Surg* 1983; 65A:70-80.
16. Gelberman RH, Woo SLY, Lothringer K, et al: Effects of early intermittent passive mobilization on healing canine flexor tendons, *J Hand Surg* 1982; 7A:170-175.
17. Harmer TW: Tendon suture, *Boston Med Surg J* 1917; 177:808-810.
18. Harmer TW: Injuries to the hand, *Am J Surg* 1938; 42:638-658.
19. Harmer TW: Cases of tendon and nerve repair, *Boston Med Surg J* 1926; 194(16):739-747.
20. Kleinert HE, Kutz JE, Ashbell TS, Martinez E: Primary repair of flexor tendons in "no man's land," *J Bone Joint Surg* 1967; 49A(3):577.
21. Kulick MI, Smith HS, Hadler K: Oral ibuprofen: evaluation of its effect on peritendinous adhesions and the breaking strength of a tenorrhaphy, *J Hand Surg* 1986; 11A:110-120.
22. Lee H: Double loop locking suture: a technique of tendon repair for early active mobilization: part I, evolution of technique and experimental study, *J Hand Surg* 1990; 15A:945-952.
23. Lin GT, An K-N, Amadio PC, Cooney WP: Biomechanical studies of running suture for flexor tendon repair in dogs, *J Hand Surg* 1988; 13A:553-558.
24. Reference deleted in proofs.
25. Lister GD: Incision and closure of the flexor tendon sheath during tendon repair, *Hand* 1983; 14:123-155.
26. Lister GD: Pitfalls and complications of flexor tendon surgery, *Hand Clin* 1985; 1(1):133-146.
27. Lister GD: Personal communication, 1988.
28. Lister GD, Kleinert HE, Kutz JE, Atasoy E: Primary flexor tendon repair followed by immediate controlled mobilization, *J Hand Surg* 1977; 2(6):441-451.
29. Manske PR: Flexor tendon healing, *J Hand Surg* 1988; 13B(3):237-245 (review).
30. Mashida ZB, Amis AA: Strength of the suture in the epitenon and within the tendon fibres: development of stronger peripheral suture technique, *J Hand Surg* 1992; 17B:172-175.
31. McGrouther DA, Ahmed MR: Flexor tendon excursions in "no man's land," *Hand* 1981; 13:129-141.
32. Morris RJ, Martin DL: The use of skin hooks and hypodermic needles in tendon surgery, *J Hand Surg* 1993; 18B:33-34.
33. Peterson WW, Manske PR, Dunlap J, et al: Effect of various methods of restoring flexor sheath integrity on the formation of adhesions after tendon injury, *J Hand Surg* 1990; 15A:48-56.
34. Robertson GA, Al-Quattan MM: A biomechanical analysis of a new interlock suture technique for flexor tendon repair, *J Hand Surg* 1992; 17B:92-93.
35. Saldana MJ, Ho PK, Lichtman DM, et al: Flexor tendon repair and rehabilitation in zone II open sheath technique versus closed sheath technique, *J Hand Surg* 1987; 12A(6):1110-1113.
36. Savage R: The influence of wrist position on the minimum force required for active movement of the interphalangeal joints, *J Hand Surg* 1988; 13B:262-268.
37. Schuind F, Garcia-Elias M, Cooney WP, An K-N: Flexor tendon forces: in vivo measurements, *J Hand Surg* 1992; 17A:291-298.
38. Seradge H: Elongation of the repair configuration following flexor tendon repair, *J Hand Surg* 1986; 11A:106-110.
39. Silfverskiöld KL, May EJ, Tornvall AH: Flexor digitorum profundus tendon excursions during controlled motion after flexor tendon repair in zone II: a prospective clinical study, *J Hand Surg* 1992; 17A:122-131.
40. Sourmelis SG, McGrouther DA: Retrieval of the retracted flexor tendon, *J Hand Surg* 1987; 12B(1):109-111.
41. Strickland JW: Flexor tendon repair, Hand Clinics Symposium on flexor tendon surgery, *Hand Clin* 1(1):55-68. Philadelphia, 1985, Saunders.
42. Strickland JW: Flexor tendon surgery, part 2: flexor tendon repair, *Orthop Rev* 1986; 11(11):701-721.
43. Strickland JW: Flexor tendon repair: Indiana method, *Indiana Hand Center Newsletter* 1993; 1:1-12.
44. Strickland JW: Flexor tendon injuries: I. foundations of treatment, *JAAOS* 1995; 3(1):44-62.
45. Strickland JW: Flexor tendon injuries: II. operative technique, *JAAOS* 1995; 3(1):44-62.
46. Strickland JW, Glogovac SV: Digital function following flexor tendon repair in zone II: a comparison of immobilization and controlled passive motion techniques, *J Hand Surg* 1980; 5(6):537-543.
47. Strickland JW: Management of acute flexor tendon injuries—symposium on rehabilitation after reconstructive hand surgery, *Orthop Clin North Am* 1983; 14(4):827-849.
48. Trail IA, Powell ES, Noble J: The mechanical strength of various suture techniques, *J Hand Surg* 1992; 17B:1:89-91.
49. Urbaniak JR: Replantation in children. In Serafin D, Georgiade NG, eds: *Pediatric plastic surgery,* St Louis, 1984, Mosby.

50. Urbaniak JR, Cahill JD, Mortenson RA: Tendon suturing methods: analysis of tensile strengths. In *AAOS symposium on tendon surgery in the hand,* St Louis, 1975, Mosby.

51. Wade PJF, Muir IFK, Hutchenon LL: Primary flexor tendon repair: the mechanical limitations of the modified Kessler technique, *J Hand Surg* 1986; 11B:71-76.

52. Wade PJF, Wetherall RG, Amis AA: Flexor tendon repair: significant gain in strength from the Halsted peripheral suture technique, *J Hand Surg* 1989; 14B:232-235.

53. Wagner WF, Carroll C, Strickland JW, et al: A biomechanical comparison of techniques of flexor tendon repair, *J Hand Surg* 1994; 19A(6):1-5.

Chapter 43

IMMEDIATE ACTIVE SHORT ARC MOTION FOLLOWING TENDON REPAIR

Roslyn B. Evans
David E. Thompson

Postoperative management of the repaired tendon with immobilization, passive motion, and active motion continues to be controversial, but the trend in current experimental and clinical research is moving toward some degree of active motion in the immediate postrepair phase of tendon healing. After 80 years of research dedicated to the problems of tendon healing and tendon gliding, we are returning to the solutions suggested in 1912,[75] 1917,[58] and 1923[71] for maintaining tendon glide with active motion in the healing phase.

The positive influence of early controlled stress at a tendon repair site has been demonstrated with numerous experimental and clinical studies for both flexor and extensor tendon. Questions concerning timing of stress application,[2,47,52,59,86] duration of exercise,[51,121] tendon excursion,* internal tendon forces as they relate to joint angle and external load,[41,45,46,68] resistance or drag imposed by viscoelastic changes associated with injury,† splint geometry,‡ and patterns of passive movement[21,30,64,99,108] have been explored. Each study offers new insight into the biochemical and biomechanical effects of early controlled motion bringing us closer to the answers to our questions regarding the application of controlled stress to the healing tendon: Why? When? How often? How far? How much?

The most critical question as stress is applied to a repaired tendon in the first two stages of wound healing concerns the tensile strength of the tendon repair as it relates to the internal tendon forces transmitted to that repair site with controlled motion. Force application must be less than the tensile strength of the specific tendon repair to prevent gapping or rupture at the repair site.

Numerous investigations have focused on methods of tendon suture in the search for a repair that will tolerate the forces of controlled motion and increased excursion. The characteristics and performance of various repairs have become even more critical as the shift from passive to light active motions has taken place in postoperative therapy protocols.

In contrast, there has been little focus on the application of force to the healing tendon, and the therapist has been placed in the unfortunate position of mobilizing a healing tendon "by feel" or by uncontrolled parameters defined by terms such as "light active motion," "place and hold," or "light resistance." Until recently[46] there has been no definition of the term *active motion* as it relates to postoperative tendon programs with respect to defined external force application and joint angle. Without carefully defined parameters, it is not possible for a therapist or patient to consistently reproduce internal tendon forces in the desired range.

This chapter focuses the attention of the hand clinician on the tensile strength of and applied forces to the healing tendon by providing the following:

---

*References 34, 39, 44, 45, 50, 60, 61, 87, 91.
†References 3, 5, 16, 17, 72, 79, 98, 124, 131, 135.
‡References 19, 22, 26, 29, 44, 61, 112, 134.

1. A rationale for the use of a limited degree of active motion to a tendon repair site to supplement passive motion protocols as a means of maintaining functional tendon glide during the early phases of tendon healing
2. An explanation for the calculation of estimated tensile strengths of various repairs and for the calculation of internal tendon forces as they relate to joint position and applied external load, so that the hand clinician will have a reasonable estimate of the balance between tensile strength and force application
3. A description of techniques of clinical application of active tension for the flexor and extensor system
4. A summary of results to support the use of active tension to supplement passive programs

DEFINING PROBLEMS

Inconsistent clinical results with postoperative passive motion programs[49,111,117] and questions regarding actual tendon excursion with passive motion programs[57,60,61,82,87] have inspired the shift from passive-only motion to some degree of active motion to ensure true proximal migration of a tendon repair site with early motion programs.

Most recently developed active motion programs for flexor tendon repair have been dependent on stronger repair techniques,* and some promising results have been reported. These suture techniques specifically designed for active motion have not been widely accepted, because many surgeons complain that they are too bulky and technically difficult. The increase in resistance to gliding, which results from the use of increased suture material, or the effect on tendon edema from increased handling with the more complex repair techniques has not been determined in vivo.

Using controlled active motion with conventional suture not specifically designed for active motion, such as the modified Kessler with an epitenon suture[66,70,127,128] has not been recommended, because it is generally felt by most tendon experts that these repairs do not have enough tensile strength to tolerate the forces of active motion.[82,87,107,108] Several problems exist with this assumption.

1. References in the literature that discuss internal tendon forces as they relate to the tensile strength of a repair all refer to two in vivo studies of flexor tendon forces, both of which measured intact tendon in the carpal tunnel while the patients were under local anesthesia.[105,125] The measurements of internal tendon forces in these two studies are widely variable with both passive and active motion, because that motion was produced in both studies[105,125] by an undefined force, yet these measurements of internal tendon forces are cited almost without exception by those who feel that conventional suture will not tolerate active tension.[82,87,105,109]

2. Until recently[46] there has been no definition of the term *active motion* as it applies to postoperative management of flexor or extensor programs, specifically with respect to joint angle and external force application. Without a strict definition there has been no repeatable and reliable technique for applying stress to a tendon repair site with internal forces that are in a range compatible with standard repair technique.
3. A high percentage of excellent and good results have been achieved by some clinical researchers, who have described active protocols in association with tendons repaired with conventional suture.†
4. Many of us have observed clinically that it is the patients who cheat within their passive motion programs by applying some active tension to the repaired tendon with conventional repair who often enjoy the best functional outcome.

These factors suggest that there may be a safe range for controlled active motion that is compatible with currently available popular suture technique not specifically designed for active motion protocols.

In the clinical situation, applying active tension to a healing tendon repair site requires that the hand clinician has specific information concerning the tendon repair technique and the suture material used for the repair in question, understands how internal forces are transmitted to that repair site with respect to external loads and joint position, and understands the variables associated with healing and drag. The next two sections address these issues.

ESTIMATING TENSILE STRENGTH AT A REPAIR SITE
Variables

Repair strength depends on the size of the tendon, mechanical properties of the suture material,[67,76] technique of repair,[4,13,125] number of strands crossing the repair,[67,73,76,97,103,122] number and location of suture knots,[6] the tendon-suture interface,[76] the addition of a circumferential suture to the core suture,[95,128] the order of core and epitenon suture,[94] surgical skill, and, theoretically, the timing of stress application.[2,47,52,59,86]

It has been demonstrated that the ultimate tensile strength of a tendon repair increases linearly as the number of suture strands crossing the laceration site increases.[6,103] The addition of a circumferential or epitendinous suture to the core suture will improve tensile strength as well as add significant resistance to gap formation.[76,95,128] Aoki, et al.[6] have concluded that the number and location of suture knots affect gap strength. They have demonstrated that locating the knots outside rather than within the tendon repair site will increase the tensile strength for 2-, 4-, and 6-strand repairs and that tensile strength will be greater in 1-knot than in

---

*References 12, 20, 73, 90, 103, 107, 120, 128.

†References 8, 32, 36, 41, 43, 54, 114.

2-knot sutures.[6] The advantages of the *epitenon-first* suture placement in flexor tendon repair has been studied,[94,100] and it has been demonstrated that the epitenon-first technique is 22% stronger than the modified Kessler and allows more of the opposing ends to be in direct contact.[94]

Stronger repair techniques have been designed to withstand the internal tendon forces generated by early active mobilization programs,* but the effect of these techniques on tendon gliding, tendon nutrition, passage through the pulley system, and on the repair process is unknown.[4,5]

Comparative analysis of reported tensile strengths

Table 43-1 provides a comparative analysis of reported tensile strengths of the various tendon repairs at gapping and failure with some variables defined. Tensile strengths reported in the literature are difficult to compare because of the large number of variables that exist within each study (subject, suture material, suture technique, and method of study) and because most studies are performed in vitro and do not consider the healing properties of tendon at the laceration site.[4,53] Reports that describe force in newtons (N) are converted to grams to simplify calculations for early motion programs. Newtons (N) are converted to grams (g), and kilograms (kg) to grams with the following formulas:

$$\frac{Newtons}{9.8} \times 1000 = Grams$$

$$Kilograms \times 1000 = Grams$$

Load to gapping

The differences between load to gapping and load to failure are significant with most repair techniques and are important clinically.[94,95] The load to which a tendon gaps is the number that must be respected with all active motion programs when considering the tensile strength of each individual repair. Gap formation has been associated with increased adhesion formation, poor gliding function, and poor clinical results.[53,77,106] While most surgeons feel that gapping above 1 to 3 mm is incompatible with a good result, it has been demonstrated by one group of investigators in an in vivo study that gaps of up to 10 mm in repaired flexor digitorum profundus (FDP) tendons are compatible with good functional range of motion.[108]

To estimate the tensile strength of any given repair, the clinician should consider the load to gapping of the core suture, add the load to gapping of the peripheral suture, and then adjust the numbers to account for the decrease in tensile strength thought to be associated with early tendon healing.[86,125] Repair strength should be considered to be decreased by 50% the end of the first postoperative week, 33% the end of the third postoperative week, and increased by 20% by the end of the sixth postoperative week.[119,120,125]

If two tendons are repaired within one digit, then the tensile strength of each tendon should be considered separately. Tendons do not share load as suggested by some investigators. Rather, each tendon is subjected to the full external load. This point is important particularly in zone II where the FDP and flexor digitorum superficialis (FDS) may be repaired with different suture techniques, and thus the tensile strength of the two tendons may vary considerably. The FDS, which is typically repaired with weaker suture, experiences more tension than the FDP with applied external load.[46]

Examples of calculation

Examples of estimated tensile strength of several repairs are given to clarify the preceding points.

Conventional repair

The modified Kessler repair with an epitendinous suture is considered to be a standard flexor tendon repair and is used by some investigators in clinical studies of immediate active motion protocols.† This repair is a proven technique, technically reproducible, and widely accepted.[94] The addition of a peripheral tendon suture to the core suture adds significant tensile strength to the repair[76,95,107,128] and is essential if active tension is to be applied to the modified Kessler core suture.

Flexor digitorum profundus. A number of researchers have measured the tensile strength of the modified Kessler (see Table 43-1), but for this example we will use the numbers produced in a cadaver study of FDP tendon with cyclic testing. The load to gapping with cyclic stress for the FDP has been measured at 2280 g if repaired with a modified Kessler (3-0 silk) with the addition of a circumferential epitenon suture (6-0 prolene).[95] This number, reduced by 50% to factor the anticipated drop in tensile strength the end of the first week, will equal 1140 g.

Flexor digitorum superficialis. The FDS repaired with a horizontal mattress suture (both slips repaired) was found to gap 2 mm with loads of 1100 g for the index finger, 2708 g for the long finger, 1045 g for the ring finger, and 1011 g for the small finger.[15] These numbers become dangerously low when reduced by 50% to account for the anticipated drop in tensile strength associated with healing by the end of the first week, becoming 550 g for the index, 1354 g for the long, 523 g for the ring, and 505 g for the small finger. However, the FDS repaired with a Tajima suture that has been measured at load to 2-mm gapping at 2722 g for the index finger (1361 g when reduced by 50%), 2690 g (1345 g) for the long, 1334 g (667 g) for the ring, and 1681 g (841 g) for the small finger has tensile strength in a range that may tolerate some controlled active motion.[15]

Text continued on p. 371.

---

*References 4, 9-12, 73, 74, 103, 107, 109, 120.

†References 8, 32, 36, 41, 43, 54, 114.

Table 43-1. Comparative analyses of reported tensile strengths of tendon repair

Repair Technique	Study*	Subject	Suture Material Core	Suture Material Circumferential	Gapping†	Failure†	Comments
Modified Kessler	Silverskiöld et al. 1993[107]	Sheep tendon	4-0 polyester	6-0		(4080 g) **48 N**	
	Trail et al. 1992[122]	Human cadaver	4-0 braided polyester	6-0	(1730 g) **17.0 N, 1 mm**	(2140 g) **21 N**	
	Robertson and Al-Quattan 1992[97]	Porcine tendon	3-0 monofilament polypropylene	6-0	(22.90 g) **22.4 (2.4) N**	**34.9 (2.3) N**	
	Newport and Williams 1992[93]	Human cadaver	4-0 prolene		**1353 g, 2 mm**	**1830 g**	Study of extensor tendons
	Pruitt et al. 1991[95]	Human cadaver	3-0 silk	6-0 Prolene	(890 g) **0.89 ± 0.18 kg** (core only) (2280 g) **2.28 ± 0.47 kg** (core and epitenon)	(2280 g) **2.28 ± 0.25 kg** (core only) (2710 g) **2.71 ± 0.42 kg** (core and epitenon)	
	Wade et al. 1989[128]	Human cadaver	5-0 stainless steel	5-0 braided polyester (Halstead)	(4300 g) **42.1 ± 10.0 N**	(8080 g) **79.2 ± 13.7 N**	Halstead peripheral
	Wade et al. 1989[128]	Human cadaver	5-0 stainless steel	5-0 braided polyester (circumferential)	(2220 g) **21.8 ± 13.3 N**	(4270 g) **41.8 ± 13.5 N**	Circumferential
	Haddad et al. 1988[56]	Porcine tendon	4-0 polyester		(220 g) **2.2 N, 1 mm**	(1360 g) **13.3 N**	
			4-0 braided nylon		(310 g) **4.0 N, 1 mm**	(1470 g) **14.4 N**	
	Cieslik et al. 1986[27]	Human cadaver	3-0 stainless steel	5-0 stainless steel	(660 g) **6.44 ± 2.06 N**	(2260 g) **22.17 ± 3.14 N**	
	Savage 1985[101]		4-0 polyester			(1330 g) **13 N**	
	Urbaniak et al. 1975[125]	Canine tendon	4-0 stainless steel			**3970** immediate; **1830 g** at 5 days	
Modified Kessler	Papandrea et al. 1995[94]	Canine FDP	4-0 braided polyester	6-0 braided polyester		Average (1600 g) **1.6 kg** to (4800 g) **4.8 kg** (n = 13)	Modified Kessler and epitendinous running
Modified Kessler Epitenon-first	Papandrea et al. 1995[94]	Canine FDP	4-0 braided polyester	6-0 braided polyester		Average (2500 g) **2.5 kg** to (6100 g) **6.1 kg**	Modified Kessler with epitenon-first technique Epitenon-first found 22% stronger than modified Kessler with epitendinous

Continued

Revised from Evans RB, Thompson DE: The application of force to the healing tendon, *J Hand Ther* 1993; 6(4):272-274.

*For complete reference citations, see the reference list.

†Conversion of newtons to grams: N/9.8 × 1,000 = g. Conversion of kilograms to grams: kg × 1,000 = g. Original calculations for tendon tensile strength with load to gapping or failure set in boldface; author's conversion are set in italic. Standard deviations are not converted.

FDP, Flexor digitorum profundus; *FDS,* flexor digitorum superficialis.

Table 43-1. Comparative analyses of reported tensile strengths of tendon repair—cont'd

Repair Technique	Study*	Subject	Suture Material Core	Suture Material Circumferential	Gapping†	Failure†	Comments
Modified Kessler	Aoki et al. 1994[4]	Human cadaver	4-0 braided polyester	6-0 prolene	(1440 g) **1.44 kgf**	(2550 g) **2.55 kgf**	Cyclic testing
	Barmakian et al. 1994[9]	Canine FDP	4-0 monofilament nylon	6-0 prolene Lembert epitendinous	2-mm gap (2550 g) **25 N**	(3370 g) **33 N**	
Modified Kessler with central wire loop	Barmakian et al. 1994[9]	Canine FDP	4-0 monofilament nylon	6-0 prolene Lembert epitendinous	2-mm gap (3980 g) **39 N**	(3980 g) **39 N**	Central wire loop connects the two transverse limbs of modified Kessler
Kessler	Wray and Weeks 1980[136]	White leghorn chicken	5-0 polyester coated with tetrafluoroethylene			**53.8 ± 8.6 kg/cm²**	In vivo after 1 month immobilization
	Bhatia et al. 1992[13]	Human cadaver	4-0 ethibond	6-0 prolene		(1270 g) **12.4 ± 1.6** N with direct load (2500 g) **24.5 ± 4.7** N with cyclic load	6-0 circumferential added 86% tensile strength
Kessler Suture locking modification	Wagner et al. 1994[129]	Canine FDP	4-0 braided nylon		2-mm gap In vitro: (1120 g) **11 N** In vivo: Week 1 (1120 g) 11 N Week 3 (1220 g) 12 N Week 6 (1530 g) 15 N		2-mm gap defined as failure
Kessler plus "deep biting peripheral suture"	Williams et al. 1995[135]	Human cadaver	4-0 polypropylene	5-0 polypropylene	2-mm gap (3060 g) 30 N	(5100 g) 50 N	Cyclic loading active motion
Kessler/Tajima	Wagner et al. 194[129]	Canine FDP	4-0 braided nylon		2-mm gap in vitro: (1120 g) **11 N** In vivo: Week 1 (1730 g) 17 N Week 3 (920 g) 9 N Week 6 (1530 g) 15 N		2-mm gap defined as failure

Name	Reference	Tissue	Suture material	Additional suture	Value 1	Value 2	Comments
Tajima	Boulas and Strickland 1993[15]	Human cadaver	3-0 braided nylon 3-0 braided nylon 4-0 braided nylon		(At 2 mm): Index, **2,722 ± 456 g** Long, **2690 ± 735 g** Small, **1681 ± 397 g**		Study for FDS, note difference with tendon size; strong FDS may allow active motion
Kirchmyer/Kessler	Lee 1990[73]	Human cadaver, lower extremity	4-0 dacron		**1000 g, 3-5 mm**	**2252 g**	
Bunnell	Newport and Williams 1992[93]	Human cadaver	4-0 prolene		**1425 g, 2 mm**	**1985 g**	Study on extensor tendon repair
	Trail et al. 1992[122]	Human cadaver	4-0 braided polyester		*(360 g)* **3.5 N, 1 mm**	*(1790 g)* **17.5 N**	Poor suture to prevent gapping
	Pruitt et al. 1991[95]	Human cadaver	3-0 silk	6-0 prolene	*(1060 g)* **1.06 ± 0.40 kg** (core only) *(2790 g)* **2.79 ± 0.54 kg** (core and epitenon)	*(1610 g)* **1.61 ± 0.28 kg** (core only) *(3080 g)* **3.08 ± 0.33 kg** (core and epitenon)	
	Haddad et al. 1988[56]	Porcine tendon	4-0 polyester		*(450 g)* **4.4 N, mm**	*(2860 g)* **28.0 N**	
			4-0 braided nylon		*(560 g)* **5.5 N, 1 mm**		
	Cieslik et al. 1986[27]	Human cadaver	3-0 stainless steel	5-0 stainless steel	*(520 g)* **5.10 ± 5 N**	*(1680 g)* **16.49 ± 6.08 N**	Immobilized 1 month in vivo
	Wray and Weeks 1980[136]	White leghorn chicken	5-0 polyester coated with tetrafluoroethylene			**62.6 ± 9.7 kg/cm²**	
	Ketchum et al. 1977[67]	Canine tendon	4-0 Teflon			*(3200 g)* **31.39 ± 2.55 N**	
	Schink and Gersbach 1961[104]	Human cadaver	Stainless steel, no gauge given			*(4000 g)* **39.24 N**	
	Urbaniak et al. 1975[125]	Canine tendon	4-0 stainless steel		**3930 g immediate; 630 g at 5 days**		
Mason-Allen	Urbaniak et al. 1975[125]	Canine tendon	4-0 stainless steel			**4030 g**	
Strickland	Robertson and Al-Qattan 1992[97]	Porcine tendon	3-0 prolene		*(1700 g)* **16.7 (4.3) N**	*(3100 g)* **30.4 (3.0) N**	
Kleinert	Wray and Weeks 1980[136]	White leghorn chicken	5-0 polyester coated with tetrafluoroethylene			**66.8 + 12.0 kg/cm²**	In vivo with 1 month immobilization
Becker	Trail et al. 1992[122]	Cadaver tendon	4-0 braided polyester		*(1939 g)* **19 N**	*(3570 g)* **35 N**	Best at preventing gap formation

Continued

Table 43-1. Comparative analyses of reported tensile strengths of tendon repair—cont'd

Repair Technique	Study*	Subject	Suture Material Core	Suture Material Circumferential	Gapping†	Failure†	Comments
	Becker and Davidoff 1977[11]	Cadaver tendon	6-0 polypropylene		(2000-3000 g) **19.6 + 29.4 N**	(3450 g) **33.8 N**	For active motion
	Cieslik et al. 1986[27]	Cadaver tendon	3-0 stainless steel	5-0 stainless steel	(1190 g) **11.69 ± 5.20 N**	(8840 g) **86.62 ± 25.41 N**	Cyclic testing
	Aoki et al. 1994[4]	Human cadaver	4-0 braided polyester	6-0 prolene	(2220 g) **2.22 kgf**	(3000 g) **3.00 kgf**	Cyclic testing
Ketchum	Pruitt et al. 1991[95]	Cadaver tendon	3-0 silk	6-0 prolene		(400 g) **3.92 ± 0.33 kg** (core only) (460 g) **4.49 ± 0.33 kg** (core and epitenon)	Cyclic testing
Savage	Trail et al. 1992[122]	Cadaver tendon	4-0 braided polyester		(560 g) **5.5 N**	(3420 g) **33.5 N**	
Savage	Savage 1985[101]	Porcine tendon	4-0 braided polyester		(2000 g) **19.62 N**	(6860 g) **67.20 N**	
Savage	Aoki et al. 1994[4]	Human cadaver	4-0 braided polyester	6-0 prolene	(2450 g) **2.45 kgf**	(8290 g) **8.29 kgf**	Cyclic testing
Interrupted Savage-type core sutures	Aoki et al. 1995[6]	Canine FDP tendon	5-0 coated braided polyester	7-0 prolene			Defining number and location of suture knots on mechanical properties
				2 strands, 2 knots outside	(950 g) **0.95 kgf**	(160 g) **1.60 kgf**	Increased gap strength with one knot outside technique
				4 strands, 4 knots outside	(1050 g) **1.05 kgf**	(2880 g) **2.88 kgf**	
				6 strands, 6 knots outside	(1250 g) **1.25 kgf**	(3810 g) **3.81 kgf**	
				6 strands, 3 knots outside	(1890 g) **1.89 kgf**	(4840 g) **4.84 kgf**	
Savage	Wagner et al. 1994[129]	Canine FDP	4-0 braided nylon		2-mm gapping In vitro: (4080 g) 40 N In vivo: Week 1 (3470 g) 34 N Week 3 (2450 g) 24 N Week 6 (4390 g) 43 N		2-mm gap defined as failure Savage technique significantly stronger that suture locking modification of modified Kessler

Technique	Author	Model	Suture material	Suture material	Force	Force	Comments
Tsuge	Pruitt et al. 1991[95]	Human cadaver	3-0 silk	6-0 prolene	(890 g) 0.89 ± 0.18 kg (core only) (2490 g) 2.49 ± 0.35 kg (core and epitenon)	(1650) 1.65 ± 0.33 kg (core only) (2810 g) 2.81 ± 0.42 kg (core and epitenon) 65.0 ± 104. kg/cm²	In vivo, tested at 1 month after immobilization
	Ways and Weeks 1980[136]	White leghorn chicken					
Mesh sleeve with new epitendinal cross-stitch	Silfverskiöld and Anderson 1993[107]	Sheep tendon	Mersilene mesh	6-0		(10,510 g) 103 N, mesh repair; (6430 g) 63 N cross-stitch	For immediate active motion
Double loop locking suture (DOLLS)	Lee 1990[73]	Human cadaver	4-0 dacron			4400 g	For immediate active motion
Double-armed suture	Messina 1992[90]		Standard Bunnell with 6-0 prolene 2-0, 3-0 nylon for pull-out				For immediate active motion
Internal tendon splint	Aoki et al. 1994[4]	Human cadaver	4-0 braided polyester	6-0 prolene	(2050 g) 2.05 kgf	(8460 g) 8.46 kgf	Cyclic testing; may allow active motion
Dorsal tendon splint	Aoki et al. 1994[4]	Human cadaver	4-0 braided polyester	6-0 prolene	(3150 g) 3.15 kgf	(8100 g) 8.10 kgf	Improved gap strength; cyclic testing active motion
Interlocked	Robertson and Al-Qattan 1992[97]	Porcine tendon	3-0 prolene		(4710 g) 46.2 (5.8) N	(5270 g) 51.6 (5.6) N	
Looped suture repair	Haddad et al. 1988[56]	Porcine tendon	4-0 nylon		(410 g) 4 N, 1 mm	(2500 g) 24.5 N	
Interrupted	Trail et al. 1992[122]	Human cadaver	4-0 braided polyester		(1530 g) 15 N	(1840 g) 18 N	
	Ketchum et al. 1977[67]	Canine tendon	4-0 teflon		(1660 g) 16.31 ± 6.87 N	(2160 g) 21.20 ± 8.34 N	
	Urbaniak et al. 1975[125]	Canine tendon	4-0 stainless steel			(1683 g)	
	Schink and Gersbach 1961[104]	Human cadaver	Stainless steel, no gauge given			(500-1000 g) 4.91-9.81 N	

Continued

Table 43-1. Comparative analyses of reported tensile strengths of tendon repair—cont'd

Repair Technique	Study*	Subject	Suture Material Core	Suture Material Circumferential	Gapping†	Failure†	Comments
Over and over peripheral suture	Mashadi and Amis 1991[85]	Human cadaver		5-0 stainless steel	(1940 g) **19 N, 1 mm** (3060 g) **30 N, 2 mm**	(4590 g) **45 N**	Peripheral suture within tendon fibers 83% stronger than in epitenon
Halstead peripheral	Wade et al. 1986[127]			5-0 braided polyester			
Lembert running suture	Lin et al. 1988[76]	Canine tendon	None	6-0 polydioxanone		(1480 g) **14.55 ± 2.58 N**	Peripheral with no core
Running locking peripheral suture	Lin et al. 1988[76]	Canine tendon	None	6-0 polydioanone		(2490 g) **24.43 ± 4.14 N**	Peripheral with no core
Simple peripheral	Lin et al. 1988[76]	Canine tendon	None	6-0 polydioxanone		(710 g) **6.98 ± 1.74 N**	Peripheral with no core
Figure-of-8	Newport and Williams 1992[93]	Human cadaver	4-0 prolene		**587 g, 2 mm**	**696 g**	Study on extensor tendons
Side-to-side	Urbaniak et al. 1975[125]	Canine tendon	4-0 stainless steel			**3230 g**	Immediate strength
Mattress suture	Newport and Williams 1992[93]	Human cadaver	4-0 prolene		**488 g, 2 mm**	**840 g**	Study on extensor tendons
Horizontal mattress	Boulas and Strickland 1993[15]	Human cadaver	3-0 braided nylon 4-0 braided nylon		Index, 1100 ± 176 g; ring, 1134 ± 332 g; small, 1011 ± 240 g		Study of FDS repair
Nicoladoni	Urbaniak et al. 1975[125]	Canine tendon	4-0 stainless steel			2683 g, immediate; **560 g,** at 5 days	

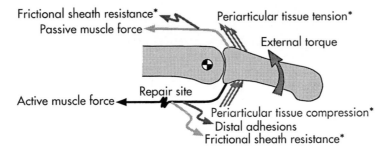

Fig. 43-1. The many forces that act to produce loading on a repaired tendon. *Those forces which are enhanced by edema are noted with an asterisk.*

Repair designed for early active motion

Increasing repair strength requires an increase in the amount of suture material bridging the repair site and the use of more powerful and stable tissue grasps.[107] A number of repair techniques that may provide the additional strength required to better tolerate the forces of active motion have been described. Again, these numbers must be adjusted for tendon softening associated with early healing, so the following numbers should be reduced by 50% by the end of the first postoperative week. The 6-strand repair described by Savage gaps 2 mm at 4080 g and fails between 6000 and 7000 g.[103] The 4-strand double loop locking repair of Lee fails at 4400 g.[73] The 4-strand Tajima and horizontal mattress repair with supplementary peripheral running lock suture utilized by Strickland in his early motion program fails at 4300 g.[120] The mesh sleeve (epitendinal suture) described by Silverskiöld and Andersson has a mean breaking strength of 10,510 g.[107] The internal tendon splint and dorsal tendon splint described by Aoki et al. gaps at 2050 g and 3150 g, and fails at 8460 g and 8100 g, respectively.[5] A new design for the modified Kessler with a Lembert running epitendinous suture gaps 2 mm at 3980 g.[9]

Extensor tendon repairs

The tensile strength of extensor tendon repairs has not received much attention in the literature. Newport et al. found that the mattress suture gapped 2 mm at 488 g, failed at 840 g; figure-of-eight gapped at 587 g, failed at 696 g; Kessler gapped at 1353 g, failed at 1830 g; and Bunnell gapped at 1425 g, failed at 1985 g.[93]

The numbers of load to gapping provided by these studies on the tensile strength of the various repairs provide the therapist with a working knowledge of repair strength at the various stages of healing. The force applied to the repair site must be less than the tensile strength of the repair at its lowest point (the end of the first week) with an adequate safety margin.

ESTIMATING INTERNAL TENDON FORCES WITH ACTIVE MOTION

This section defines internal tendon forces as they relate to various joint angles and applied external loads and discusses the variables that would alter these internal tendon forces. Guidelines for loading (i.e., protocols for exercise and splinting) at a tendon repair site can be formulated based on the estimated transmission of force to the repair site as it relates to the estimated tensile strength of any given repair.

Internal tendon forces in the digital flexor or extensor system are determined by the following:
1. Joint angles of the wrist and digital joints that alter the resistance of the antagonistic muscle-tendon units
2. The applied external load
3. The resistance of edema, hematoma, periarticular tissues, suture bulk, and bandaging
4. The speed of motion

The following concepts are important to the understanding of internal tendon tension:
1. All external torques must be balanced by torques produced internally by muscles and other tissues.
2. The internal force at the repair site is always greater than the external force or load applied at the fingertip.
3. Internal tendon tension is equal throughout the length of the tendon unless limited by adhesion.[46]

Mathematic modeling of internal tendon forces

Internal tendon forces for active motion programs following tendon repair have been calculated in a mathematical model for both the flexor and extensor system.[45,46]

As can be seen in the idealized joint shown in Fig. 43-1, there is a balance between the internal and external forces and moments around the joint. The active force of the muscle (see the bottom left of Fig. 43-1) is counterbalanced by the effects of *all* the other effects. The agonist force acts directly through the tendon repair site. Even when there is no external load, the repair must bear the burden of frictional effects both within the sheath and arising from the antagonist muscle(s), as well as compression and tension of the soft tissues around the joint, and distal adhesions. By studying this simple abstract joint, an appreciation can be gained for all of the mechanical elements that affect the force transmitted to the repair. For a given external force, increasing its distance from the joint increases the moment and thus the force to the repair. An increase in frictional sheath resistance directly

Table 43-2. Mathematic calculation of internal tendon forces

Variable	Relaxed Position		MAMTT (SAM)		Composite Fist	
Wrist position	45° E		45° E		45° E	
MP position	40° F		83° F		85° F	
PIP position	54° F		75° F		95° F	
DIP position	45° F		40° F		75° F	
External load	50 g		50 g		50 g	
Internal force FDP	41 g[1]	(82 g)[2]	41 g[1]	(82 g)[2]	2050 g[1]	(4100 g)[2]
Internal force FDS	0 g[1]	(0 g)[2]	605 g[1]	(1210 g)[2]	1650 g[1]	(3300 g)[2]

From Evans RB: Immediate active short arc motion for the repaired zone I and II flexor tendon, *J Hand Surg Am,* submitted May 1995.
[1]Drag eliminated.
[2]Drag considered.
MP, Metacarpophalangeal; *PIP,* proximal interphalangeal; *DIP,* distal interphalangeal; *FDP,* flexor digitorum profundus; *FDS,* flexor digitorum superficialis.

increases the force through the repair. Increases in the spasticity of the antagonist muscle add to this force, as do an increased tissue rigidity caused by edema or adhesions.

Flexor system. In the flexor system, internal tendon forces were calculated in a mathematic model with drag eliminated.[46] The wrist was positioned at 45° of extension to reduce the resistance of the antagonistic extensors,[46,102] while the digital joints were positioned in (1) the relaxed position, (2) the position of immediate active short arc motion (SAM), and (3) the full fist position. An external load of 50 g was applied to the mid portion of the distal phalanx for all three positions in the mathematic model. A summary of internal tendon forces for the FDP and FDS in these three positions is provided in Table 43-2. The results of that study suggest that active motion with a 50-g external load in the position of SAM (wrist extension modified to 20° to 30°, metacarpophalangeal (MP) flexion 80°, proximal interphalangeal (PIP) flexion 75°, and distal interphalangeal (DIP) flexion 40° is compatible with a standard modified Kessler with an epitendinal repair, but that the position of full flexion is not, and forces in this position exceed the tensile strength of conventional repair.

Extensor system. The resistance applied to the central slip with active motion of 30° flexion to 0° of extension was analyzed.[45] Joint angle versus tendon force for the PIP joint was calculated mathematically with a simple model that assumes that the flexors are inhibited and exert no torque on the PIP joint (clinically the flexors are inhibited by placing the wrist in 20° to 30° of flexion while the PIP is actively moved from 0° to 30° of flexion and back to 0° extension). In this model, the only torques on the joint are caused by the weight of the finger, the tension of the central extensor tendon, and an elastic torque arising from the surrounding tissues. A constant moment arm is assumed based on the work of Brand,[16] and the finger is modeled as a simple weight acting downward at the center of mass. The force analysis both with and without gravity, affects predicted tendon forces that are 291 g and 286 g of force, respectively.[45]

Internal tendon forces for the extensor digitorum communis (EDC) were defined for zones V, VI, and VII[46] in a similar fashion with resistance from the antagonistic muscle-tendon group and any other drag eliminated. With the wrist positioned at approximately 20° of flexion, and with only the weight of the finger as external load, active motion at the MP joint from 30° of flexion to 0° of extension will transmit 300 g of internal tendon tension to repairs in zones V, VI, and VII. However, as the wrist is extended and tension in the flexor system is increased, these forces rise dramatically to 1200 g if the wrist is neutral and digital joints extended.[46]

The clinical implication is clear. For all early active motion programs, wrist position is critical. Force transmission is reduced in the flexor system if the wrist is in mild extension to decrease resistance from the extensor system, and likewise internal tendon tension is reduced in the extensor system by placing the wrist in mild flexion for the place and hold component of the active exercise component.

Internal tendon forces measured in vivo

Internal tendon forces following repair have not been measured in the human hand. Huge variations must exist dependent on suture technique, edema, hematoma, status of periarticular tissues, and timing of stress application. The following studies provide some insight into these variables, but the data will not be complete until internal tendon tensions can be measured in vivo with a force transducer[33] that is placed at the tendon repair site throughout the healing phase in a substantial number of patients.

Internal tendon forces with active and passive motion have been measured in two in vivo studies.[105,125] Both studies measured tendon forces on intact tendons at the level of the carpal tunnel while the patients were under local anesthesia. Although the information that they provide is important, the numbers of internal force provide us with limited information, because in both studies external forces were undefined (the end point of terminal flexion and applied external load) and because the intact tendons were not subject to the increase in forces from suture and wound reaction.

Urbaniak et al.[125] measured tension in the flexor tendons under several conditions. They found in their investigation that the stress of digital passive flexion-extension ranged from 200 to 300 g, that flexion against mild resistance did not impose more than 900 g of internal tendon tension, and that flexion against moderate resistance imposed approximately 1500 g of internal tendon tension. The authors give no definition of "active motion," "active motion against mild resistance," or "active motion against moderate resistance," and no definition of force with these motions except to mention that in one instance tension in the FDP of a ring finger in one patient measured 1250 g with a pull of 2 pounds on a grip meter. They comment on the effect of the tourniquet stating that it reduced the maximum force of contraction, but that the patients were able to produce tensions of approximately 5000 g with maximum effort.

Schuind et al. measured flexor tendon forces up to 900 g with passive motion and 3500 g with "active unrestricted motion."[105] Their measurements of active unrestricted flexion (otherwise undefined) range from 400 to 3500 g for the flexor pollicis longus (FPL), 100 to 2900 g for the FDP, and 300 to 1300 g for the FDS, even under testing conditions. The wide variation in these numbers in a group of patients who were given the same instructions for motion probably is representative of what happens in the clinical situation. Reproducing specific forces with active motion in unsupervised situations without specific guidelines for joint angle and external load may result in forces that are either below those needed for minimal therapeutic tendon excursion, or worse, forces that may exceed the tensile strength of the repair resulting in gap or rupture.

The numbers of internal tendon forces in these two studies are cited frequently with reference to early motion programs. It is important to recognize that external force application was not controlled in either study.

Resistance to tendon gliding

The numbers of internal tendon tension provided by mathematic modeling[45,46] represent tendon forces that have not been increased by resistance from suture material, the antagonistic muscle tendon system, periarticular soft tissues, pulleys, or wound healing. The numbers provided by the two in vivo studies[105,125] do not reflect the resistance of suture material or wound healing. Internal tendon forces will be increased when those variables are considered. The following studies provide some information regarding the increase in tendon forces from drag.

Work of flexion. The resistance to flexor tendon gliding or excursion in the flexor system has been referred to as the work of flexion (WOF).[5,31,55] The term has been used to describe the summation of forces necessary to move a tendon along its excursion distance reflecting the biomechanical work that the tendon produces during finger flexion.[5] Work

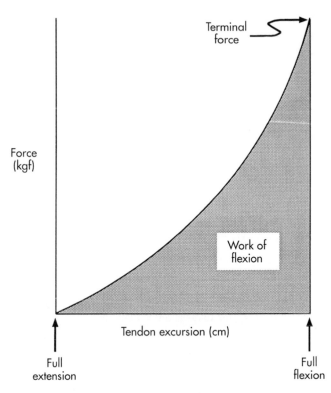

Fig. 43-2. This schematic represents the biomechanical indices of tendon gliding. Terminal force is the force that is exerted with complete digital flexion and is expressed as kilograms force (kgf). Tendon excursion is the excursion from full extension to full composite flexion and is expressed as centimeters (cm). The integrated shaded area under the force-excursion curve represents the work of flexion or resistance to tendon gliding and is expressed as kilograms force per centimeter (kgf/cm). (From Lane JM, Black J, Bora FW: Gliding function following flexor-tendon injury: a biomechanical study of rat tendon function, *J Bone Joint Surg* 1976; 58A[7]:986.)

of flexion has been calculated[5,72] as the area under the force-excursion curve (Fig. 43-2) and expressed as kilograms force-centimeter (kgf-cm)[72] and kilogram force-meter (kg fm).[5] *Terminal force* represents the tendon force recorded at full digital flexion, and excursion represents the total tendon excursion at full flexion. Resistance to tendon gliding or WOF is increased by the effect of edema, hematoma, adhesion, periarticular stiffness, joint position, and the speed of exercise.

Resistance of wound healing. In an experimental study of the effects of early wound healing on terminal force, excursion, and work of flexion, Lane et al.[72] examined the changes in gliding function of flexor tendons in rat digits from 1 hour to 8 weeks after a standard injury. They demonstrated that all three indices were affected within 1 hour of surgery, indicating that postoperative edema and hematoma will restrict tendon glide and WOF well before collagenous adhesion has been deposited. *Terminal force* on the experimental side had increased (when compared

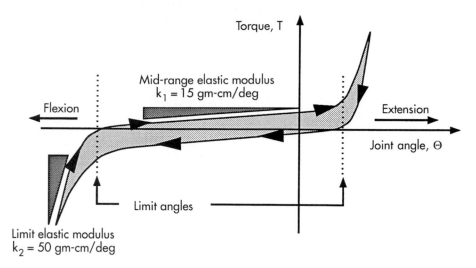

Fig. 43-3. The passive elastic torque necessary to move the joint. The area inside the curve represents the resistance from edema or drag, which can be equal to or greater than the resistance of joint motion. Edema could double the force at the repair site with active motion. (From Evans RB, Thompson DE: The application of force to the healing tendon, *J Hand Ther* 1993; 6[4]:269.)

with control limbs) an average of 0.216 (±0.08) kgf 1 hour after surgery, 0.553 (±0.08) kgf at 1 week, and then declined to 0.308 (±0.06) kgf at 8 weeks. *Relative excursion* was immediately altered in the repaired digit, increasing immediately after surgery by 13% and a further increase of 15% at 1 week, but thereafter decreasing. The work of flexion was increased between the experimental and control limbs from 0.002 (±0.06) to 0.188 (±0.06) kgf-cm 1 hour after operation, with an increase of WOF by 300% (0.508) kgf-cm 2 weeks after surgery, thereafter decreasing at 8 weeks to 0.230 (± 0.04) kgf-cm.

The authors[72] point out that the force applied by the muscle in vivo depends on several factors including the speed or rate of flexion and its resting position at the time flexion is initiated.

Canine flexor tendon adhesion formation was studied in an experimental model with crush-abrasion injury combined with 3 weeks of immobilization.[98] The production of visible adhesions limited toe motion and work. Biomechanical testing demonstrated that with a force of 8 N (820 g), tendon excursion and flexion were each reduced a minimum of 41% in all of the experimental digits. Achieving 10 mm of excursion in the lateral experimental toes required 118% more work than in the control group.[98]

The WOF in the complex tendon injury or tendon treated with immobilization will be greater than with simple tendon injury treated with early motion.

Brand, Llorens, and Thompson[16,17,79] do not use the term WOF, but refer to the restraints of friction and the elastic resistance of soft tissues as *drag*. Muscle fibers, tendons, ligaments, fascia, and peritenon have been categorized as *elastic* components that contribute to joint stiffness, whereas the movement of fluid within the synovial capsule and the compression of tissues are categorized as *viscous* components.[16,17,79] The passive elastic torque necessary to move a joint is depicted in Fig. 43-3[46] which represents a typical hysteresis curve showing the torque required to move a joint passively through its range of motion. Through the mid range of the hysteresis curve, the torque required to move the joint passively is minimal. In this range, few structures are being stretched or displaced resulting in few forces to act on a joint. However, a sharp rise in torque occurs at the end ranges of joint motion as resistance increases from the antagonistic muscle and compression of the soft tissues.

Llorens points out that the peritenon is a limiting factor at the end ranges of motion. He observes that during the mid range of motion the peritenon uncoils and allows for movement, but that once a tendon has traveled a certain distance through a tendon sheath, the peritenon begins to stretch and resist movement in ever-increasing amounts.[79] This general behavior can be felt in one's own hand. If one passively moves the MP joint from extension to flexion, little torque is required until it reaches approximately 80°, but at this point resistance to further finger flexion rises dramatically.[46] This resistance is caused by the elongation of the agonist-antagonist muscle groups, as well as the distension and compression of the periarticular tissues.[17]

Llorens has measured the resistance to motion in the mid range of motion for the finger joints in normal hands and has estimated that the resistance from edema can be equal to or greater than the resistance of joint motion ($k_1 = 15$ g-cm/degree).[79] Thompson has adopted a much stiffer elastic modulus value of $k_2 = 50$ g-cm/degree at flexion angles greater than the limiting angle (see Fig. 43-3).[46] These limit angles at the ends of both flexion and extension motion are highly dependent on wrist position. This relationship is stronger for individuals with lax tissues than for those with stiffer, less compliant tissues.

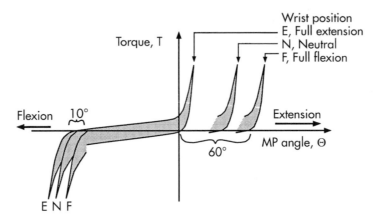

Fig. 43-4. Influence of wrist position on torque-angle behavior at the metacarpophalangeal (MP) joint.

Clinically this means that we should assume that internal tendon forces in a repaired tendon are double or more than those in the unoperated digit because of the effects of edema and that internal tendon forces can be expected to rise dramatically as the digital joints move from moderate flexion to the end ranges of flexion.[46] Other investigators have also concluded that tendon forces are the greatest at the end ranges of flexion.[5,7,72,131] Aoki et al.[5] produced force-tendon excursion curves of the digits in cadaver hands, which are similar to the mathematic modeling.[46,79] The curve demonstrated an initial gradual elevation as finger flexion was initiated, plateauing throughout the mid range of flexion, and increasing in what they describe as "logarithmic fashion" as terminal flexion was reached.[5]

Influence of wrist position. The effect of wrist position is portrayed in a general fashion in Fig. 43-4. The extension limit angle of the MP joint may drop as much as 60° as the wrist moves from full flexion to full extension. The flexion limit angle changes only about one-fifth as much as the extension limit angle. The following generalizations may be drawn from this behavior of normal MP joints:
- The limitation of MP flexion is generally within the joint itself and is not caused by the passive elastic forces arising from stretching the extensor.
- The limitation of MP extension is principally caused by the passive stretch of the flexors.
- At full wrist flexion, the range of motion of the MP joints is greater than at full wrist extension.
- To avoid the torques arising from the elastic forces at the limit angles while still eliciting motion of the tendons, one should position the wrist at neutral or in slight flexion.

Clinically this means that positioning the wrist in neutral or slight flexion during digital joint exercise will minimize torque from the periarticular tissues of the MP joint and will thus decrease internal tendon forces within the digit. The clinician must consider that increased wrist extension will increase flexor tendon excursion. How much flexor tendon excursion is necessary to limit peritendinous adhesion? The

clinical questions for each tendon repair are as follows: Are the internal tendon forces generated by the joint angles and external load used for the active component exercise compatible with the tensile strength of that particular repair, and do they provide the excursion necessary to prevent limiting adhesion? Internal tendon forces will be the least in the middle ranges of wrist and digital joint motion.

Resistance of suture material. Aoki et al.[5] found that WOF increased in direct proportion to the amount of suture material at a tendon repair site. In a laboratory study of 33 FDP tendons from 9 fresh-frozen cadaver hands, the mechanical work of flexion before and after tendon repair using 6 different repair techniques was investigated. The average increase in WOF was found to be lowest for the 2-strand modified Kessler[63] (4.8%) and the lateral margin Becker[11] (6.5%). The 6-strand Savage repair[101] increased WOF by 10.9%, dorsal tendon splint by 16.2%, and the internal tendon splint by 19.3%.[4] The greatest increase in WOF (44.3%) was for the external nylon mesh sleeve.[107] The authors note that of the methods of repair tested, the Savage[101] and tendon splint techniques[4] provide the initial tensile strength (8.1 to 8.4 kg fc)[4] to tolerate the forces of active motion, while only increasing WOF by 10% to 20%, and that although the mesh sleeve[107] provides good tensile strength (10.3 kg fc), WOF with this repair is increased by 44%.

These numbers from a cadaver study do not account for the resistance of edema, hematoma, and adhesion, but they add important information regarding the internal tendon forces applied with active motion. The authors point out that the more complex tendon repairs, which require more surgical manipulation, may result in increased postsurgical edema and thus may add to WOF in the early healing phases. Stronger repairs with increased suture material designed for active motion programs will have an effect on the resistance applied to that repair.

Frictional resistance to FDP from FDS. Walbeehm and McGrouther[131] have investigated the mechanical interactions of tendon loading and motion between FDS and FDP tendons and the distal edge of the A_2 pulley (DEA_2) in cadaver hands. Their work indicates that there is a narrowing of the tunnel formed by the FDS through which the FDP passes if the FDS tendon is loaded proximally. They liken the FDS decussation to the Chinese finger trap, creating a gripping tendency of the FDS on the FDP. They point out that this narrowing with load is not sufficient to prevent motion in the normal system and that this increased frictional resistance between the tendons and sheath may be important to tendon nutrition and synovial fluid circulation. A second intriguing finding of this study concerns the changing shape of the FDP. The FDP tendon has a two-stranded contrarotational spiral of tendon fibers; their course is parallel to the FDS fibers. They demonstrate how, with loading, the FDP changes cross-sectional shape resulting in a slight decrease in volume allowing the tendon to adjust its shape as it moves through the bifurcation.[131] They conclude that their work supports that of Martin.[83]

Clinically, these findings would seem to raise some questions regarding suture bulk and the effect of suture on the ability of both the FDP and the decussation to change shape as they interact at Camper's chiasma. Resistance to gliding or WOF could be affected by changes in volume from suture or edema. The gripping mechanism of the FDP by the FDS may be a factor in tendon rupture at this level.[96] Adhesion between the FDS and FDP at this level is a common cause of PIP flexion contracture and poor functional motion following flexor tendon repair in zone II; it is critical that the two tendons glide relative to each other at this level.

Frictional forces of the digital pulleys. The forces imposed on a tendon repair site by the digital pulley system in vivo are unknown,[29] although it seems clear that frictional forces at the tendon-pulley interface would be elevated by the increase in tendon volume from suture, edema, or adhesion. The following studies have measured resistance at the tendon-pulley interface.

The normal kinematics of friction[124] and its quantification[3,124] as it occurs at the tendon-pulley interface have recently been studied. The same investigators have examined the effect of flexor tendon repair on the gliding resistance between the FDP and the A_2 pulley in 10 cadaver ring fingers.[29] The gliding resistance was measured for the intact FDP tendon and for the same tendon after it was transected and repaired with a 4-0 ticron core suture and a 6-0 running epitendinous nylon suture. The tendons were tested passively with 2.45 N (250 g) based on the work of Schuind.[105] These investigators found that resistance to tendon gliding was altered significantly through the A_2 pulley after repair; the friction coefficient and resistance to gliding were approximately doubled ($p < 0.005$).[29] The difference in resistance between normal and repaired tendons was greatest at 0% to 40% excursion but was statistically significant to 80% excursion. The resistance to

motion at a 60° arc of contact in the repaired group was a mean of 0.432 N (40 g) with a standard deviation of 0.183 N (20 g).

It is interesting to note that the first three specimens tested in this study were repaired only with a core suture and that all ruptured at the suture line because of *hooking* at the edge of the A_2 pulley but that none of the tendons repaired with both core and epitendinal sutures ruptured. The authors[29] suggest that because the pattern of the coefficient of friction throughout the excursion changed after repair, then the gliding surface and the shape of the tendon were changed with repair.

Williams and Amis[135] recorded the increased forces generated by in vitro tendon repaired with the Kleinert technique,[70] and that of a deep biting peripheral suture (DBPS)[84] used alone or in conjunction with a square or modified Kessler core suture with the technique of Coert.[29] With load of 30 N (3060 g), 50% of the standard repairs had failed, but all of the new combined repairs (DBPS) plus Kessler core suture were intact with a mean gap formation of 2.03 mm. The increased load as the repair was pulled through the A_2 pulley was measured. The force caused by the repair increased from 0 to 4.5 N (460 g).[135] The repair site was subjected to increased resistance at the prominent edge of the A_2 pulley, but those forces tended to decrease as the repair was remodeled by cyclic flexion. One limitation of this study was that the repaired tendon was not necessarily tested in its own finger, so it would seem that the variation in pulley and tendon size would influence the results.

Resistance from the speed of exercise. The speed of motion contributes to viscous resistance.[17,72,79,130] Thompson has determined that the effect of speed is identical to the effect of edema; the increase in resistance is directly proportional to the increase in either. Fig. 43-3 demonstrates that torque increases as joint angles increase and as the speed of motion increases.[46] Wainwright et al.[130] demonstrated that fast excursion rates approach the threshold between linear elastic and viscoelastic behavior. Lane et al.[72] make the point that WOF is related to the energy required for flexion and the rate of flexion. A slower rate of flexion allows for greater relaxation of the tissues and thus lower peak forces are generated.[72]

The obvious clinical implication with the early motion programs is that slower motions are safer. The active hold for the SAM programs described in the next section are all preceded by slow passive motions to reduce the drag of tight joint and edema, and the active exercise components are all performed with specific joint angles, controlled external load, and slow speed of exercise.

CLINICAL APPLICATION OF SAM PROGRAMS
Flexor zones I and II

On the basis of clinical experience, theoretical work,[46] and review of the work of others on internal tendon forces

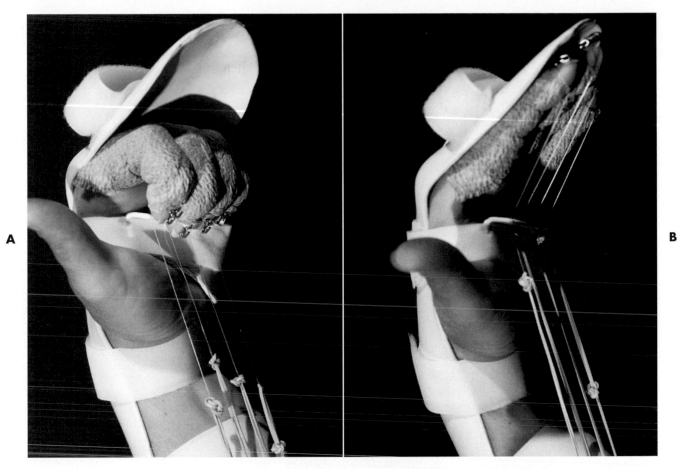

Fig. 43-5. A, The zone II repaired flexor tendon is protected in a dorsal splint which positions the wrist at 30° to 40° of flexion, metacarpophalangeal (MP) joints at 45° of flexion. The dorsal hood extends to the fingertip level allowing the proximal interphalangeal (PIP) and distal interphalangeal (DIP) joint extension to 0°. Four finger traction with a palmar pulley holds the digits into the distal palmar crease between the active extension-passive flexion exercise. **B,** Active extension of the digits against the dynamic traction must bring the PIP and DIP joints to absolute 0° extension to avoid flexion contracture and limiting adhesion between the flexor digitorum superficialis and flexor digitorum profundus. (**A** and **B** from Evans RB: Immediate active short arc motion for the repaired zone I and II flexor tendons, *J Hand Surg* [submitted for publication].)   *Continued.*

and repair strength, the senior author developed an active motion program for the flexor tendon with standard repair (modified Kessler with epitenon suture). Zone II will be described before zone I to minimize description needed for the zone I technique.

Technique of rehabilitation. Repaired tendons in zones II and proximal are treated with a standard rehabilitation program,[23,88,115,118] supplemented with a component of immediate active motion. The standard protocol includes a dorsal protective splint which positions the wrist at 30° to 40° of flexion, MP joints at 45° of flexion, with the dorsal hood extending to the fingertip to allow PIP and DIP extension to 0°. Four-finger traction[88] is set up with monofilament and rubber bands originating on the proximal forearm with a pulley in the palm, so that the digits are held into the distal palmar crease in between exercise sessions (Fig. 43-5, *A*). The patient is instructed to actively

extend the digits against the rubber-band traction extending the interphalangeal (IP) joints to 0° (Fig. 43-5, *B*) and to allow the traction to return the digits to their flexed position. These exercises are supplemented by 10 to 20 repetitions of passive finger flexion exercises, which bring the digits passively into the distal palmar crease, and active PIP and DIP joint extension to 0° for all digits simultaneously, while the MP joints are held in full flexion by the contralateral hand to ensure that the PIP joints are extending completely. At night the traction is removed and the fingers are strapped to the dorsal hood with the PIP joints resting in extension.

This patient routine is supplemented in supervised therapy sessions with immediate active SAM to the injured and uninjured digits. The active hold component is preceded with slow, repetitive passive motions from the relaxed position to composite flexion by the therapist to reduce the

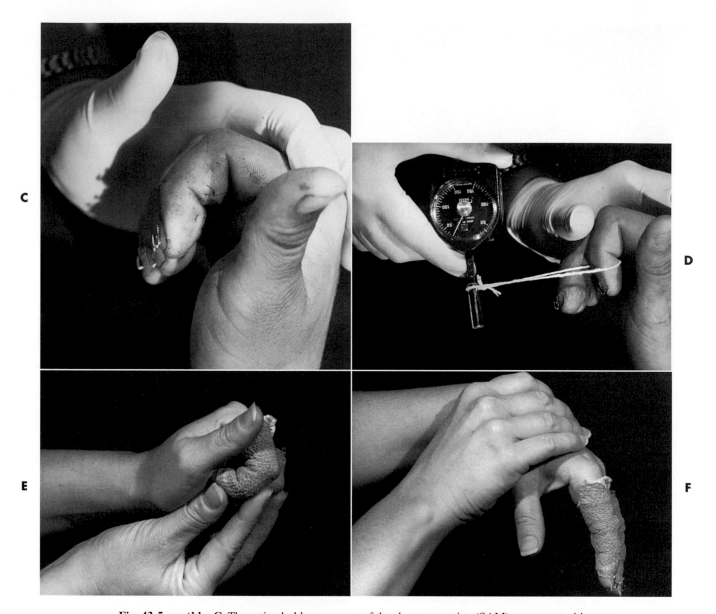

Fig. 43-5, cont'd.   C, The active hold component of the short arc motion (SAM) program positions the digits in moderate flexion (MP 80°, PIP 75°, DIP 30° to 40°) under therapist supervision. **D,** External force is measured with the Haldex pinch meter as the patient applies 15 to 20 g of force at the mid portion of the distal phalanx in the active hold position of SAM. (**C** and **D** from Evans RB, Thompson DE: The application of force to the healing tendon, *J Hand Ther* 1993; 6[4]:276.) **E,** The wrist and finger tenodesis exercise is performed under therapist supervision. The therapist passively holds all fingers of the injured hand into the palm and simultaneously extends the wrist to 30° to 40° of extension. **F,** The wrist is then passively flexed to full flexion while the fingers are allowed to position in extension through a natural tenodesis action. (**E** and **F** from Evans RB: Immediate active short arc motion for the repaired zone I and II repaired flexor tendon, *J Hand Surg* [submitted for publication].)

drag or resistance from edema and tight joint until the passive torque[18] is estimated to be <300 g. The active hold component is then employed to theoretically create some true proximal migration of the repair site with joint angles of 20° to 30° of wrist extension, 80° of MP flexion, 75° of PIP flexion, and 30° to 40° of DIP flexion. The hand is placed in this position by the therapist and the patient is asked to gently maintain this position to create some active tension in the flexor system (Fig. 43-5, *C*). To control the amount of external load applied to the tendon repair site, a small calibrated Haldex* pinch meter (<150 g) is used to measure the force of flexion. That force is measured and observed by both patient and therapist during the active exercise. A string is applied to the gauge arm of the pinch meter at a 90° angle and then around the middle portion of the distal phalanx at a 90° angle as the patient applies 15 to 20 g of force with the active hold exercise (Fig. 43-5, *D*). These exercises are then followed by wrist tenodesis exercise[30] in which the therapist passively holds all fingers of the injured hand into the palm and extends the wrist to approximately 30° to 40° (Fig. 43-5, *E*), followed by passive wrist flexion to approximately 60°, while the fingers are allowed to position in extension through a natural tenodesis action (Fig. 43-5, *F*). At 21 days the patient begins unsupervised active hold exercises, and therapy proceeds according to the usual protocols.[23,88,115,118]

Repaired tendons in zone I are treated with a combination of the *limited zone I protocol*[39] and the SAM protocol for zone II.[42] A dorsal static protective splint positions the wrist at 30° to 40° of flexion, the MP joints at 30°, the PIP joints at 0°, with dorsal protection to the fingertips. The affected DIP joint(s) is splinted at 45° of flexion with a second dorsal digital splint that extends from the proximal portion of the middle phalanx to the tip of the finger (Fig. 43-6, *A*). The digital splint is taped only at the middle phalanx. Dynamic traction is not employed. The patient is instructed to perform the following exercise regimen within the confines of the two splints with an empirical 10 to 20 repetitions every waking hour. The distal joint is passively flexed from the 40° to 45° flexion angle to 75° (or full flexion) (Fig. 43-6, *B*); the digits are passively placed in a full fist position (Fig. 43-6, *C*) and a modified hook fist position (Fig. 43-6, *D*), which is made possible by the modest position of MP flexion within the dorsal splint. The MP joints are passively hyperflexed by the uninvolved hand, and the patient extends the PIP joint in the affected digit to absolute 0° extension (Fig. 43-6, *E*). The distal strap is then used to position the unaffected fingers in extension, and a gentle place and hold active exercise for the FDS is performed (Fig. 43-6, *F*). During structured therapy sessions, the therapist performs these same exercises, but in addition, removes the hand from both splints for controlled wrist tenodesis exercises (Fig. 43-5, *E* and *F*)[30] and the SAM component of active flexion described for zone II (Fig. 43-5, *D*).[41] The distal joint is not allowed to extend beyond the 40° to 45° flexion angle during the first 3 weeks. At 21 days the patient is allowed to initiate active flexion independent of the therapist, and at 25 to 28 days the dorsal digital splint is removed and the usual active tendon gliding exercises well described in the literature are initiated.[132,133]

Active hold for the repaired FPL will not be endorsed or described in this chapter, although the senior author has used

this technique in eight cases, with good results in seven. Internal tendon forces with specific joint angles have not been measured for the FPL, and other investigators have noted an 11% rupture rate for the FPL with active motion programs.[36]

Clinical experience. A comparison study of zone I and zone II flexor tendon injuries treated with standard passive rehabilitation protocol and the SAM technique has been presented† and submitted for publication.[41] All patients were treated by the senior author in a 4-year period, and were referred by 38 different plastic or orthopedic surgeons. Surgical technique was not controlled, but most repairs were the standard modified Kessler[69,70] with an epitendinous suture, with the exception of tendon to bone repair in some zone I injuries. Each patient in both groups was categorized as having either a simple or complex injury. A simple injury was one to skin, tendon, vessel, and nerve. Complex injuries included the preceding plus associated injury to cartilage, ligament, bone, or a crush component. Patients were excluded for insufficient follow-up or concomitant extensor tendon injury.

All digits were evaluated in regard to functional outcome as determined by active IP motion. The results for each digit were calculated as a percentage of normal (excluding the MP joint) according to the following formula.[116]

$$\frac{TAM\ (PIP + DIP\ flexion) - extensor\ lag \times 100}{175} =$$

% normal combined PIP and DIP flexion

Results were classified[51] by strict criteria. An excellent result was 85% to 100% normal motion (>150°), good 70% to 84% (125° to 149°), fair 50% to 69% (90° to 124°), poor less than 50% (<90°). Detailed demographic information was recorded and is available.[41]

Zone II flexor tendon injuries were analyzed prospectively as two groups. Forty-four digits were treated with immediate active SAM protocol[41] and compared to 32 digits treated with passive motion‡ and a component of wrist tenodesis.[30] Final results for zone II are summarized in Tables 43-3 and 43-4. Group IIA refers to patients treated with the SAM protocol, and group IIB to standard flexor tendon rehabilitation protocol with passive motion only techniques, both described previously.

Each category was considered separately for statistical analysis.§ No statistical significance was noted between groups IIA and IIB with regards to sex, day motion was initiated, day of discharge, PIP extension deficit, or complexity of injury. Active range of motion was significantly

*JIL Tools, J.D. Mard Industries, Truckhoe, NY.

†Evans RB: Immediate active short arc motion for the zone I and II repaired flexor tendon, American Society for Surgery of the Hand, scientific session, annual meeting, Cincinnati, October 28, 1994 (in press).
‡References 24, 25, 34, 35, 69, 78, 113, 118.
§Statistical analysis was performed by Isadore Enger, M.A., M.S., statistician, Department of Orthopaedics and Rehabilitation, University of Miami, School of Medicine, Miami, Florida.

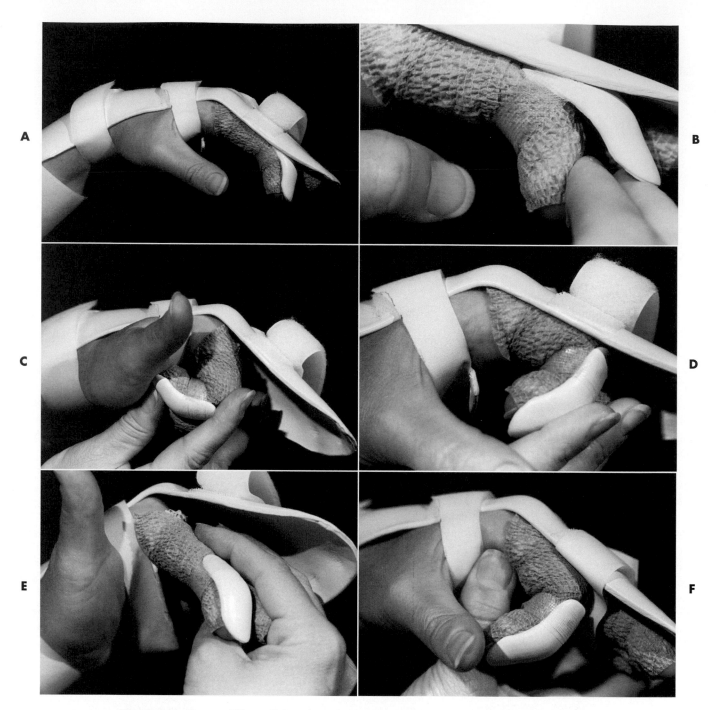

Fig. 43-6. A, The zone I flexor digitorum profundus repair is protected for the first 21 days postrepair with a dorsal static protective splint, which positions the wrist at 30° to 40° of flexion, the metacarpophalangeal (MP) joints at 30°, the proximal interphalangeal (PIP) joints at 0°, with dorsal protection to the fingertips. The affected distal interphalangeal (DIP) joint is splinted at 45° of flexion with a second dorsal digital splint that extends from the proximal portion of the middle phalanx to the tip of the finger. (From Evans RB: A study of the zone I flexor tendon injury and implications for treatment, *J Hand Ther* 1990; 3:137.) **B,** The DIP joint is flexed passively from the 40° to 45° flexion angle within the two protective splints to full flexion, theoretically providing some mechanical stress at the repair site without causing gap formation. **C,** The digits are passively placed in the full fist position to provide passive excursion of the flexor digitorum profundus (FDP) and flexor digitorum superficialis (FDS) and to reduce drag in preparation of the active exercise. **D,** The digits are passively placed in a modified hook fist position made possible by the modest position of MP flexion to encourage differential excursion between the FDP and FDS. **E,** The MP joints are passively hyperflexed by the uninvolved hand while the PIP joints are actively extended to absolute 0° to prevent PIP joint flexion contracture. (**C, D,** and **E** from Evans RB: A study of the zone I flexor tendon injury and implications for treatment, *J Hand Ther* 1990; 3:138.) **F,** The distal strap is used to position the unaffected digits in extension while a gentle place and hold exercise for the FDS is performed. This position will decrease internal tendon tension in the flexor digitorum profundus.

Table 43-3. Final results and statistical analysis zone II flexor tendon injuries

Criteria Compared	Group IIA (SAM)		Group IIB (Passive)		Statistical Analysis	
	Mean	Std. Dev.	Mean	Standard deviation	Student *t* Test	Chi Square
Number of digits	44		32			
Mean age	30	12.0	38.9	17.10	0.009	
% Male sex	64%		75%			0.293
PIP flexion	92.46°	7.08	86.06°	9.20	0.001	
DIP flexion	48°	16.72	28.94°	11.91	0.0005	
PIP extension lag	5.43°	8.09	8.97°	10.43	0.10	
TAM	135.59°	29.87	106.50°	24.80	0.0005	
% Normal	77.36%	17.10	60.81%	14.24	0.0005	
Grade	Good		Fair			0.0005
% Complex	23%		22%			
Day motion	3.66	2.48	4.22	2.06	0.301	
Day discharge	54.43	17.12	59.47	14.82	0.185	

From Evans RB: Immediate active short arc motion for the repaired zone I and II flexor tendon, *J Hand Surg Am,* submitted May 1995.

PIP, Proximal interphalangeal; *DIP,* distal interphalangeal; *TAM,* total active motion.

Table 43-4. Classification of results zone II*

Grade	Group IIA (Short Arc Motion)	Group IIB (Passive)
Excellent: 85% to 100%, ≥150°	19 (43%)	1 (3%)
Good: 70% to 84%, 125° to 149°	14 (32%)	8 (25%)
Fair: 50% to 69%, 90° to 124°	6 (14%)	16 (50%)
Poor: 0% to 49%, >90°	5 (11%)	7 (22%)
	44 digits	32 digits

From Evans RB: Immediate active short arc motion for the repaired zone I and II flexor tendon, *J Hand Surg,* submitted May 1995.

*Tendon injuries evaluated by the Strickland-Glogovac formula and classification according to criteria established by Gelberman et al.

improved in regard to PIP, DIP, TAM, and percentage of normal in the SAM group (IIA), as compared with the passive only group (IIB).

When evaluated separately, simple injuries demonstrated better results overall. Within the simple subcategory, sex, day motion started, and PIP extension deficit were not significant, but all other categories were highly significant in favor of group IIA over group IIB (*p* <0.0005).

Complex injuries in group IIA demonstrated no statistically significant improvement over complex injuries in group IIB; however, there was a trend in all motion categories for improved range of motion in the complex SAM group over the complex passive group. Group IIA averaged PIP flexion of 87°, group IIB 82°. Group IIA averaged DIP flexion of 34°, group IIB 28°. Group IIA averaged PIP extension deficit of 11°, group IIB 16°. Group IIA averaged TAM of 111°, group IIB 94°. Group IIA

averaged a total of 64% of normal (fair) and Group IIB 54% of normal (fair).

Two ruptures occurred in the zone II groups (1 in group IIA and 1 in group IIB). The rupture in group IIA occurred at 7½ weeks postoperative while working with the senior author as the PIP was manually blocked and the patient was asked to flex the DIP joint independently. Prior to rupture, active flexion in this digit was MP 90°, PIP 90°, and DIP 50°. Both tendons had been repaired, but only the FDP ruptured. This incident raises concern regarding external support during blocking exercise and its effect on tendon glide. Of interest also in this particular case was that on reoperation the surgeon found no adhesion at the FDP repair site. The tendon was repaired at 48 hours postrupture, the SAM protocol was again utilized, and final results at 9 weeks were MP 90°, PIP 100°, and DIP 60°, with no extension deficit. The rupture in zone II was excluded as it occurred in a noncompliant patient who removed the splint prematurely.

Zone I repairs (107 digits) were analyzed as 3 groups dependent on postoperative management.[41] The 29 digits in group IA were treated with a combination of the limited zone I protocol[39] and the SAM protocol and were evaluated prospectively; the 38 digits in group IB were treated with the limited zone I protocol only[39] and were evaluated prospectively; the 40 digits in group IC were treated with passive motion[34,69,118] using dynamic traction and were evaluated both retrospectively and prospectively in a previous study on the zone I tendon injury.[39]

Final results for zone I injuries are summarized in Table 43-5. Each category (age, sex, final active range of motion for PIP flexion, DIP flexion, TAM, and percent of normal) was considered separately for statistical analysis.* Results for the limited zone I (group IB) and passive group (group

*Statistical analysis was performed by Isadore Enger, M.A., M.S., Statistician, Department of Orthopaedics and Rehabilitation, University of Miami, School of Medicine, Miami, Florida.

Table 43-5. Final results and statistical analysis zone I

Criteria Compared	Group IA (SAM)[1]	Group IB (Limited Zone I)[2]	Group IC (Passive)
Number of digits	29	38	40
Mean age	36	43 ($p = 0.106$)[3]	31 ($p = 0.294$)[3]
% Male sex	83%	71%	65%
PIP flexion	96°	89° ($p = 0.001$)[3]	76° ($p = 0.0005$)[3]
DIP flexion	48°	41° ($p = 0.080$)[3]	25° ($p = 0.00005$)[3]
TAM	144°	130° ($p = 0.016$)[3]	101° ($p = 0.00005$)[3]
% Normal	82%	74% ($p = 0.016$)[3]	58% ($p = 0.0005$)[3]
Grade	Good+	Good ($p = 0.002$)[3]	Fair ($p = 0.0005$)[3]
% Complex	34%	Not calculated	Not calculated
Day motion	3	Not calculated	Not calculated
Day discharge	49	Not calculated	Not calculated

From Evans RB: Immediate active short arc motion for the repaired zone I and II flexor tendon, *J Hand Surg,* submitted May 1995.
[1]Immediate active short arc motion.
[2]Limited zone I flexor tendon protocol.
[3]Comparison to SAM criteria, student *t* test.
PIP, Proximal interphalangeal; *DIP,* distal interphalangeal; *TAM,* total active motive.

IC) were each compared with the SAM (group IA) protocol individually for statistical analysis, but not with each other. The active group was significantly improved over the passive group in all regards, and over the limited group I with regards to all categories except DIP flexion. The similarity between the SAM and limited zone I group is probably due to the fact that even with the limited zone I protocol, the patient is probably applying some active tension to the repair site within the passive program.

Within the SAM group (group IA) 19 simple injuries were studied in comparison to 10 complex injuries. As would be expected, simple injuries produced the best results, but only the day of discharge was significant in favor of the simple injuries (45 versus 57 days) ($p <0.004$). The simple injuries averaged 149° of TAM, complex 136° ($p = 0.286$); DIP motion 51° simple versus 42° complex ($p = 0.627$); percent of normal 85% simple (excellent) versus 77% complex (good).

Two ruptures occurred in Zone I, one in group IA when a patient attempted to lift a laundry basket within the confines of his splint, and one in group IC in a nonexercise-related incident in which the splint was removed and normal motions were attempted.

Discussion. The use of immediate active motion as a means of limiting adhesion and improving tendon gliding is neither new,[58,65,71,75] nor widely accepted in clinical practice, but it is the subject of renewed interest in flexor tendon management. Several investigators have reported improved results with early motion programs that include a component of active motion with conventional repair* over treatment with passive motion alone. Other investigators have described active motion programs with stronger suture tech-

nique designed to tolerate the increased forces of active motion.†

The shift from passive only to active motion protocols is a result of inconsistent clinical results with passive protocols and questions regarding true tendon migration with passive motion. Many tendon experts now believe that a component of active motion may be necessary to move the repair site proximally.[57,60,61,82,87] Passive motion, especially if the tendon is swollen, may only cause the tendon to buckle, fold, or roll up at the repair site. Experimentally, passive motion in flexor tendons has been demonstrated to be as little as half that of theoretically predicted values under conditions of low tension.[61] Actual tendon excursion will be equal to the predicted tendon excursions of earlier studies[34,89] only when more than 300 g of tension is applied to the repair site.[61] A component of active motion has been recommended for true tendon excursion for repairs at the A_3 and A_4 levels because of poor excursions in these regions with passive motion.[57]

The protocols for flexor zones I and II combine standard splinting and passive motion protocols with a component of active motion in tendons repaired with conventional sutures. Internal tendon forces transmitted to the FDP in the position of SAM with drag calculated are estimated to be 82 g, and 1210 g to the FDS.[46] These forces allow for a safety margin when compared to the tensile strength of the modified Kessler technique with an epitenon 2280 g at week 0 (1140 g 1 week postrepair). The FDS repaired with a mattress suture should not tolerate the forces imposed by the SAM position, however, clinically this repair has not been a problem using this technique. The Tajima technique provides tensile strength for the FDS in a safer range.[15] In the full fist position

*References 8, 32, 36, 41, 43, 114.

†References 12, 20, 73, 90, 103, 107, 120, 128.

internal tendon forces rise dramatically and exceed the tensile strength of conventional repairs (see Table 43-2).

The technique described in the SAM protocol, which uses specific joint angles (wrist extension 20°, MP flexion 80°, PIP 75° flexion, and DIP flexion 40°) and a measured external load of 15 to 20 g, allows the application of force to be reliable and repeatable. This may explain why so few ruptures occurred with clinical application to tendons repaired with standard technique. The modified Kessler technique with an epitendinal suture may have some advantage with this limited active program in that, with less suture and possibly less edema, less WOF will be required. Programs that rely on the patients' judgment only to reproduce certain forces will definitely require a stronger suture technique.

In zone II the greatest improvement in IP motion was at the DIP joint where the SAM group averaged 48° and the passive group averaged 29°. Improvements in PIP motion were less impressive. The greatest advantage of the active program over the passive program may be with independent FDP glide and DIP joint flexion. This observation has also been reported by Silverskiöld and May in a recent study on combined passive and active motion in tendons repaired with the epitendinal cross-stitch.[109] They noted no improvement in PIP flexion (1°) with their new method, but an increase from 50° to 63° with DIP flexion. Another interesting correlation of this work and that of Silverskiöld and May[109] is that they concluded that motion beyond 75° for the PIP joint was not necessary in the early stages of the active motion program.

The limited zone I protocol[39] has been changed with the SAM program to provide active tension to the FDP in zone I. The active hold for injury at this level probably better ensures a true proximal migration of the FDP at the A₄ pulley level where excursion is small[57] and a tendency to develop adhesion is great. Both techniques limit distal migration of the FDP by limiting the last 40° to 45° of DIP extension during the first 3 postoperative weeks. Theoretically, this prevents gap formation in an area where excursion is small, and rests the tendon proximal to its normal resting position during the healing phase.[39] The rationale for this protocol has been defined in detail.[39]

Within the described parameters for joint angle and external load, active tension was tolerated by the tensile strength provided by a modified Kessler technique and an epitendinal suture in these cases treated by only one therapist. FDP gliding and DIP motion benefitted the most from the addition of active tension to the passive regimen. An experienced therapist may be a critical variable. The application of light active tension does have to be altered to some degree dependent on tissue stiffness or resistance encountered with each individual case.

Extensor zones III and IV

Technique of rehabilitation. A protocol for immediate active SAM for the repaired central slip injury (zones III, IV)

has been defined[45] and supported clinically.[40] Controlled active motion is initiated in zones III and IV, 24 to 48 hours postoperatively with this regimen: Except during exercise, the PIP and DIP joints of the involved digit are immobilized in a volar static thermoplastic splint. One inch transpore plastic tape is applied directly over the PIP and DIP joints to ensure that both joints rest at 0° (Fig. 43-7, *A*). Two exercise splints are used by the patient during exercise sessions to control stress application and excursion of the repaired central slip and zone IV extensor tendon. Template splint 1 (Fig. 43-7, *B*) for PIP joint motion is a volar static splint with a 30° PIP joint flexion angle and a 20° to 25° flexion angle for the DIP joint. Template splint 2 (Fig. 43-7, *D*) for DIP flexion is a volar static extension splint for the proximal and middle phalanges with the PIP joint at 0° and the DIP joint free.

The patients are instructed to remove the immobilization splint (see Fig. 43-7, *A*) every waking hour for an empirical 20 repetitions for PIP and DIP exercise. The wrist is positioned at 30° of flexion, the MP joint at 0° to slight flexion. The patients are instructed to manually support the proximal phalanx in template splint 1, which allows the PIP to flex to 30° and unrestrained DIP to 20° to 25°. The patients actively flex (see Fig. 43-7, *B*) and extend (see Fig. 43-7, *C*) the PIP through this 30° range with 20 repetitions. The patients are instructed that each exercise should be performed slowly and sustained briefly in a fully extended position. Template splint 2 is then applied with manual pressure to stabilize the PIP joint at 0° of extension. If the lateral bands were not repaired, the distal joint is fully flexed and extended to 0° (Fig. 43-7, *E*). If the lateral bands were repaired, the distal joint is flexed only 30° to 35° with active extension emphasized (Fig. 43-7, *F*).

The patients are instructed in a technique of *minimal active tension*[45,46,102] (the minimal amount of force required to overcome the elastic resistance of the antagonistic muscle-tendon unit) with the active extension component. The active phase must be carried out in the predescribed joint angles with repetitions performed slowly and frequently.[40,45,46]

The patients are cautioned that the IP joints must be held at absolute 0° of extension within the digital immobilization splint to prevent extensor lag. If no lag develops after 2 weeks of controlled motion in the above-described parameters, then template splint 1 is altered to allow 40° at the PIP joint during the third postoperative week and 50° during the fourth postoperative week.

The wrist, MP joint of the affected digit, and other digital joints are free to move through a normal range of motion during the healing phase while only the IP joints of the affected digit are splinted (Fig. 43-7, *G* and *H*). Controlled mobilization and intermittent splinting at 4 weeks provide protection for the healing tendon as PIP joint flexion is gradually increased.[42] Digital edema is controlled with a

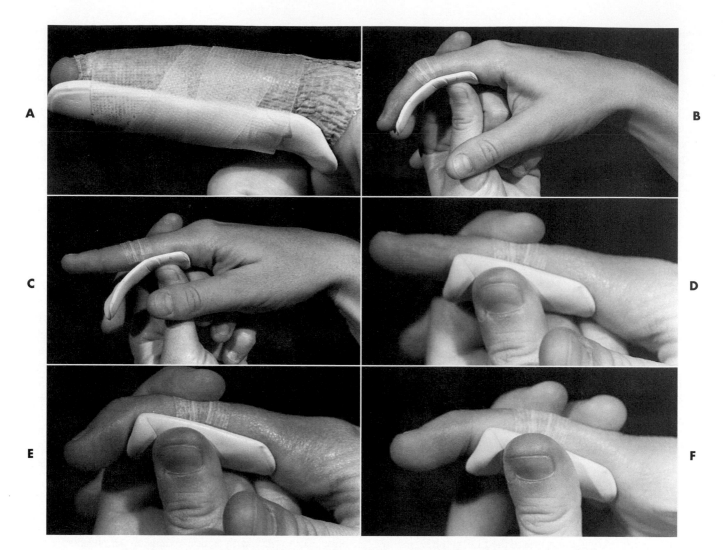

Fig. 43-7. A, The repaired central slip is immobilized in a volar static digital thermoplastic splint, which positions the proximal interphalangeal (PIP) and distal interphalangeal (DIP) joints at absolute 0°. Dorsal pressure is applied over both joints with one inch transpore tape, securely positioning the interphalangeal (IP) joints in extension. **B,** The exercise template splint allows 30° at the PIP joint and 20 to 25° at the DIP joint, preventing the patient from attenuating the repair by allowing only the precalculated excursion of the zone III and IV tendon. **C,** The position of active exercise for the repaired central slip is wrist flexion 30°, MP extension 0°, and active flexion and extension of the PIP joint through the 30° range. The proximal phalanx of the injured digit is held against the splint by the contralateral hand. **D,** The exercise template splint for DIP flexion immobilizes only the PIP joint. The DIP joint is free, allowing isolated distal joint motion to create gliding of the lateral bands. **E,** The DIP joint is fully flexed if the lateral bands are not repaired to create excursion of the lateral bands. The PIP is manually stabilized at 0° during this exercise. **F,** If the lateral bands are repaired, the DIP is flexed only to 30° to 35°.

single layer of Coban wrap for the first 4 weeks, and the usual antiedema measures are utilized.

Clinical experience. The results of 64 digits with open injury and repair of the zone III extensor tendon in 55 patients have been reported[40] and are summarized in Tables 43-6 and 43-7. The patients were divided into two groups depending on postoperative management technique. Sur-

gical management was not controlled and complex injury was not excluded. The patients in group I (30 patients) were treated with 3 to 6 weeks (mean 33 days) of immobilization before any PIP motion was initiated. The patients in group II were treated with the SAM protocol initiated between 2 and 11 days postoperatively (mean 5 days). Group I patients treated during the first 2 of the

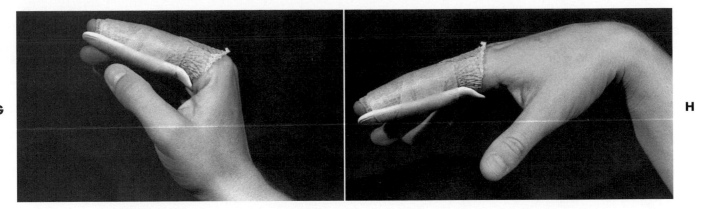

Fig. 43-7, cont'd. G, The position of wrist extension encourages flexion at the metacarpophalangeal (MP) joint through a natural tenodesis action. The sagittal bands will glide distally as the MP joint flexes decreasing tension on the central slip. The repair is protected with the digital extension splint. **H,** The position of wrist flexion will encourage digital extension through tenodesis action. Any increased tension in the extensor system as the muscle tendon unit lengthens appears to be physiologic and compatible with combined central slip repair and digital extension splinting. (From Evans RB: Early active short arc motion for the repaired central slip, *J Hand Surg* 1994; 19A:993.)

Table 43-6. Final results and statistical analysis zone III

Results	Group I (Immobilization)	Group II (SAM)	Statistical Significance *t* Test	Statistical Significance Chi Sq.
Number digits	38	26		
Mean age	39.9	42.2	>0.5 NS	
% Male sex	86.8%	80.8%		>0.5 NS
% Complex injury	76.3%	76.9%		>0.5 NS
Mean day motion initiated	32.9	4.59	<0.001 S	
Mean day injury to discharge	76.07	51.38	<0.001 S	
PIP extension lag on 1st motion day	13°	3°	<0.01 S	
PIP extension lag on discharge day	8.13°	2.96°	<0.01 S	
PIP motion at 6 weeks	44°	88°	<0.001 S	
PIP motion at discharge	72°	88°	<0.01 S	
TAM (PIP and DIP) at discharge	110.7°	131.5°	<0.01 S	
DIP motion at discharge	37.63°	45°	<0.01 S	

From Evans RB: Early active short arc motion for the repaired central slip, *J Hand Surg* 1994; 19A:994.

PIP, Proximal interphalangeal; *TAM,* total active motion; *DIP,* distal interphalangeal; *S,* statistically significant; *NS,* not statistically significant.

7 years reviewed were evaluated retrospectively. All other patients treated during the last 5 years were evaluated prospectively (some group I, all group II).

The two groups were further subdivided into two categories depending on the severity of the injury. *Simple injury* was defined as extensor tendon laceration and repair with or without lateral band repair. *Complex injury* was defined as tendon laceration with associated injury to cartilage, ligament, bone, or distal joint. Patients were excluded only for insufficient follow-up or associated flexor tendon injury. Demographics and results for each digit have been defined and reported in detail.[43]

The results of each digit repair were calculated as a percent of normal utilizing the formula[116] cited previously that excludes MP joint motion. The results of this study should be considered in light of the high percentage of complex injuries in both groups (76% of group I and 77% of

Table 43-7. Classification of results zone III (Strickland-Glogovac formula)

	Group I (Immobilization)	Group II (SAM)
Excellent: 85% to 100%, ≥150°	5 (13%)	5 (19%)
Good: 70% to 84%, 125° to 149°	11 (29%)	12 (46%)
Fair: 50% to 69%, 90° to 124°	12 (32%)	7 (27%)
Poor: 0% to 49%, >90°	10 (26%)	2 (8%)
	38 digits	26 digits

From Evans RB: Early active short arc motion for the repaired central slip, *J Hand Surg* 1994; 19A:994.

group II). By all criteria, evaluated patients in the SAM group demonstrated significantly better results at discharge compared to patients treated with 3 to 6 weeks of immobilization. No patient in the SAM group developed extensor lag or boutonniere deformity. Extensor lag averaged 3° for the early motion group versus 8° for the immobilized group.

Discussion. Early controlled motion for the zone III extensor tendon injury has been described, but most reports are for simple tendon injury, and most protocols have problems with the position of splint immobilization, timing of the application of stress, or parameters for PIP joint motion.[1,62]

The exercise parameters outlined in the SAM protocol are based on a detailed study of extensor tendon anatomy at the zone III and IV levels, and mathematic modeling of extensor tendon excursions and internal tendon forces.[45]

The effects of joint positional changes and the dynamic anatomy of the surrounding tissues to extensor tendon gliding and work requirement have been studied[45] and will only be reviewed briefly here. The exercise position of modest wrist flexion reduces the work requirement of the EDC by reducing the resistance of the digital extrinsic flexors[46,102] and through the action of the interossei muscles, which help extend the digits when the wrist is flexed.[28] As the wrist extends, the MP joints will flex because of the viscoelasticity of the flexors. The sagittal bands glide distally with MP flexion, actually reducing tension on the central slip.[137] Movement of the phalanges can be independent of wrist position through the action of the interossei.[123] The exercise position of MP extension causes the sagittal bands to glide proximally.[137] The attachment of the dorsal hood with the MP extended is slack and allows distal transmission of power to the EDC.[110] Thus the position of MP extension facilitates EDC function, yet minimizes its work requirement because in this position the lumbricals assist IP extension both directly through their action on the PIP joint and indirectly by neutralizing the resistance of the FDP.[80,81] The interossei assist in PIP extension by transmitting force through the lateral bands.[126]

The SAM protocol creates approximately 4 mm of extensor tendon excursion through zones III and IV with 0° to 30° of flexion (calculated by radians)[16,45] (Fig. 43-8). Internal tendon forces in the exercise position of 20° wrist flexion, MP at 0° of extension, and active extension from 30° flexion to 0° extension are calculated to be approximately 300 g (200 g less than the lowest tensile strength measured for extensor tendon repairs gapping at 2 mm[93]). The prescribed distal joint motion addresses the problem of lateral band adherence.

This early controlled motion in zones III and IV not only improves intrinsic healing, but also prevents tendon to bone adhesion along the broad tendon-bone interface in zone IV. The immobilized repair in zone III may attenuate or gap with late mobilization programs because its proximal segment is

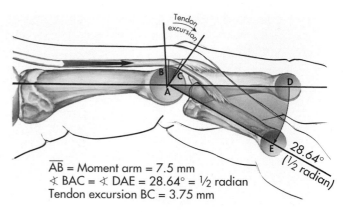

$\overline{AB}$ = Moment arm = 7.5 mm
∢ BAC = ∢ DAE = 28.64° = ½ radian
Tendon excursion BC = 3.75 mm

Fig. 43-8. Excursion of the central slip (zone III) as calculated by radians. $\overline{AB}$ = the moment arm of the central slip. Angle BAC = ½ radian, or 28.64°. If the proximal interphalangeal (PIP) joint is moved through ½ radian, the central slip excursion will equal ½ the moment arm of the long finger central slip. Brand has calculated the mean moment arm for the extensor tendon of the long finger PIP joint to be 7.5 mm. (From Evans RB, Thompson DE: An analysis of factors that support early active short arc motion of the repaired central slip, *J Hand Ther* 1992; 5:193.)

adherent and nongliding (Fig. 43-9). Extensor lag at the PIP level was found to be less in tendons treated with SAM (mean 3°) than those treated with immobilization (mean 8°). The PIP must be splinted at absolute 0° in the protective splint except during exercise to prevent extensor lag.

The SAM technique for zones III and IV has proven itself to be safe, simple, effective, comfortable, and inexpensive. Central slip injuries treated with the SAM protocol are improved in all regards compared with those treated with immobilization.

Extensor zones V, VI, VII, TIV, TV

The techniques for early passive motion have been applied to extensor tendon injuries in zones V, VI, VII, TIV, and TV for the past decade.* The addition of an active component to supplement passive protocols has recently been described,[43] and a large series of cases comparing the results of treatment by immobilization, early passive motion, and combined passive and active motion have been reported[43] (Table 43-8).

The passive component of the combined passive and active protocol has been described.[44] Ideally, therapy is initiated 24 to 48 hours postoperative. Controlled stress is applied to the extrinsic zones V, VI, VII, TIV, and TV tendons by allowing the tendons to glide the predicted 5 mm within a forearm-based dynamic extension splint.

The forearm-based splint positions the wrist between 30° and 40° of extension. Dynamic traction rests all digital joints at 0° (Fig. 43-10, *A*). An interlocking palmar blocking splint permits the predetermined angular changes at the MP level (30° for the index and long digits, 40° for the ring and small digits) (Fig. 43-10, *B*). A high profile moving spring steel

*References 1, 19, 24, 37, 38, 44, 46, 48, 62.

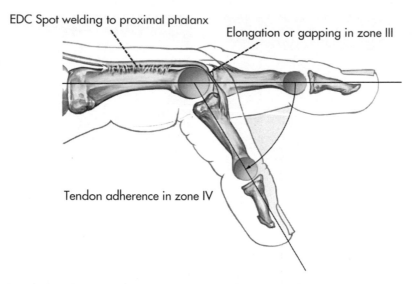

EDC Spot welding to proximal phalanx

Elongation or gapping in zone III

Tendon adherence in zone IV

Fig. 43-9. This schematic drawing illustrates the problem of tendon to bone adhesions following injury to the dorsal aspect of the proximal phalanx and proximal interphalangeal joint. The broad tendon-bone interface in zone IV and their intimate relationship result in functional gliding problems following injury at this level. Repair in zone III may gap or attenuate with late mobilization programs because of elevated tension at the repair site resulting from an adherent, nongliding tendon in zone IV. (From Evans RB, Thompson DE: An analysis of factors that support early active short arc motion of the repaired central slip, *J Hand Ther* 1992; 5:193.)

Table 43-8. Summary of extensor tendon results zones V, VI, VII, TIV, TV

Zones V, VI	Group I (Immobilization)	Group II (EPM)	Group III (EPM + SAM)
Number of patients	14	84	18
Number of tendons	24	151	31
Percent complex	80%	67%	44%
TAM*	189	235	248
MP extensor lag	25	10	0
Zone VII			
Number patients	4	8	2
Number tendons	16	25	7
Percent complex	100%	100%	100%
TAM*	199	242	240
MP extensor lag	25	12	3
Zones TIV, TV			
Number patients	6	8	3
Number tendons	6	8	3
Percent complex	50%	63%	33%
TAM†	120	116	121

From Evans RB: Immediate active short arc motion following extensor tendon repair, *Hand Clinics* 1995; 11(3):508.

*TAM = MP + PIP + DIP − extensor lag.

†TAM = CMC = MP + IP − extensor lag.

EPM, Early passive motion; *TAM,* total active motion; *MP,* metacarpophalangeal.

outrigger is utilized to reduce the forces required for flexion.[14]

The patient is instructed to actively flex the digits at the MP joint until the fingers touch the volar block, and then to relax the digits allowing the outriggers to return the digits to full extension. If the patient has difficulty flexing the fingers at the MP level or if the PIP joints do not rest at 0° of extension within the traction slings, then a volar static digital extension splint can be slipped inside each finger sling to ensure that motion takes place at the MP joint. The patient is also instructed to place the sling under the proximal phalanx during exercise sessions and to manually hyperextend the proximal phalanx while actively moving the digit through at least 70° to 80° of motion at the PIP level. These exercises for the MP and PIP joints should be repeated about 20 times each waking hour.

The repaired EPL in zones TIV and TV is splinted with a dorsal forearm-based splint that positions the wrist between 30° and 40° of extension, carpometacarpal (CMC) joint at neutral, and MP joint at 0°. The IP joint is held at 0° in dynamic traction (Fig. 43-11, *A*). An interlocking volar component is cut away at the IP level to allow 60° of IP flexion allowing the extensor pollicis longus (EPL) the predicted 5 mm of passive excursion at the level of Lister's tubercle during the exercise phase of treatment. The patient is instructed to actively flex the IP joint and to allow the traction to passively return the joint to its resting position (Fig. 43-11, *B*).

The patient is seen in therapy for wound care, splint adjustments, controlled passive motion for the digital and thumb joints, controlled active place and hold exercises, and

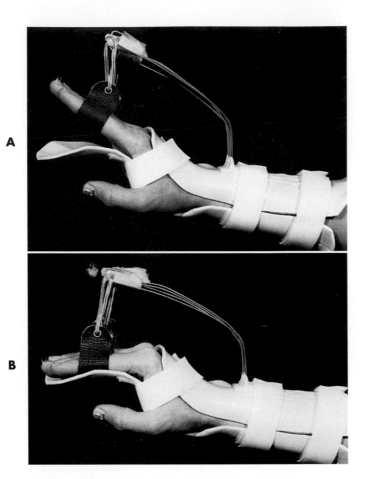

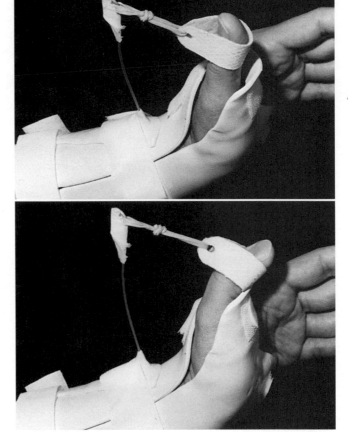

Fig. 43-10. A, A dorsal forearm-based dynamic extension splint immobilizes the wrist at 45° extension and rests all finger joints at 0°. A volar block permits only the predetermined metacarpophalangeal joint flexion, allowing slightly more flexion for the ulnar digits to achieve the necessary tendon excursion (From Evans RB, Burkhalter WE: A study of the dynamic anatomy of extensor tendons and implications for treatment, *J Hand Surg* 1986; 11A:776.) **B,** The digits are actively flexed to the volar block to create approximately 5-mm excursion for the extensor tendons. While the splint is designed to allow the dynamic traction to return the digits to an extended position passively, most patients inadvertently move the digits actively within this splint.

Fig. 43-11. A, The repaired extensor pollicis longus in zones IV and V is splinted with the wrist extended, carpometacarpal joint in neutral position, metacarpophalangeal joint at 0°, and interphalangeal joint resting at 0° in the dynamic traction. **B,** The distal joint is actively flexed about 60° to effect 5 mm of passive glide of the extensor pollicis longus. The dynamic traction returns the distal phalanx to a resting position of 0°. (From Evans RB, Burkhalter WE: A study of the dynamic anatomy of extensor tendons and implications for treatment, *J Hand Surg* 1986; 11A:777.)

wrist tenodesis exercises.[30] Under a therapist's supervision the hand is removed from the splint, washed and massaged in a protected position, and moved through controlled ranges of motion. The digital IP joints are moved individually through at least 70% to 80% passive range of motion, while the wrist and MP joints are manually held in extension. With the wrist and IP joints held in extension, the MP joints are passively moved at least to 30° for the index and long fingers and to 40° for the ring and small fingers. With all digital joints held at 0° the wrist is passively moved to 20° of flexion when the repair level is in zones V and VI, and to 10° of extension when the repair is in zone VII. The wrist is then moved passively to full extension while the MP joints are

simultaneously moved to 40° flexion and the IP joints are manually held in extension.

The passive thumb exercise performed by the patient in the dynamic splint is supplemented in therapy with supervised passive exercise to the wrist, CMC, MP, and IP joints. The IP joint is moved from 0° to 60° while all proximal joints are held in maximum extension; the MP joint is moved from 0° to 30° while all other joints are manually held in extension; and the CMC joint is moved from 20° to 50° palmar abduction and from neutral to full radial abduction while all other joints are supported in extension. Wrist tenodesis exercises position the wrist at 0° while the thumb kinetic chain is held in maximum extension followed by full passive extension of the wrist while the thumb is allowed to simultaneously relax into moderate flexion.

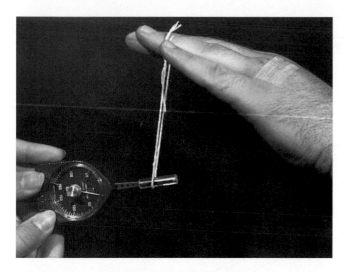

Fig. 43-12. The active hold exercise for the repaired extensor tendon in zones V, VI, and VII is performed with the wrist flexed at about 20° while the digital joints are positioned at 0°. The patient can be instructed in the minimal hold technique by demonstrating allowable external load with the Haldex pinch meter. (From Evans RB, Thompson DE: The application of force to the healing tendon, *J Hand Ther* 1993; 6[4]:276.)

Immediate active short arc motion (SAM). Passive motion is supplemented with an active exercise component in therapy by the therapist who ensures that only minimal active tension is applied to the repair sites. The SAM active exercise component is preceded by slow, repetitious passive motions in the previously described parameters until passive torque[18] is estimated to be <200 to 300 g of force. The therapist then places the wrist in 20° of flexion, and with all digits held by the therapist at 0° of extension the patient is asked to actively hold this position with minimal tension. The MP joints are moved actively from 30° of flexion to 0° extension for approximately 20 repetitions with the wrist in this position of moderate flexion. These two exercises under therapist supervision comprise the active exercise supplement to the passive program.

The small calibrated Haldex pinch meter (<150 g) can be used to demonstrate to the patient how gentle the forces of active extension must be and also to provide the inexperienced therapist with a repeatable and reliable technique for applying force to the tendon repair site in a range compatible with the tensile strength of the repair[46] (Fig. 43-12). The weight of the digit in the joint positions described is the only external load that should be applied with the extensor system.

To provide minimal active tension to the repaired EPL, the wrist is placed in 20° of flexion while the CMC, MP, and IP joints are held in extension by the therapist. The patient is then asked to gently hold this position actively with minimal tension. This active component supplements the passive exercise and wrist tenodesis for the EPL described previously.

Clinical experience. Clinical results are summarized in Table 43-8. These data were compiled from extensor tendon injury treated in the senior author's clinic from 1979 to 1994,[38,43,44] with the exception of 84 tendons in 44 patients that were treated by participants in a multicenter study.[38]

Digital tendons in group III (combined early passive motion and SAM) demonstrated modest improvement compared with tendons treated with passive motion only (group II) (13° in zones V and VI and 2° in zone VII), but significant improvement compared with tendons treated by immobilization (group I) (59° in zones V and VI and 41° in zone VII). Results for the EPL treated with all three techniques were similar in regard to range of motion, but treatment time was decreased by an average of 3 weeks for the 2 early motion groups compared with the immobilization group.

Digital extensor tendons in these zones tolerate the passive and minimal active motion described in the protocols for groups II and III as well as the modified wrist tenodesis exercise. Repaired extensor tendons treated with the combined active and passive protocols demonstrate improved TAM, decreased extensor lag, and decreased treatment time compared with similar injuries treated with immobilization. Thumb extensor tendons also tolerate early motion, but in these cases, demonstrated improvement only in regard to rehabilitation time over treatment by immobilization. Only three extensor tendons have ruptured, and in all cases they occurred in patients who removed their splints for activity during the first 3 weeks of healing.

Discussion.   *Tendon excursion* as it relates to joint motion for zones V, VI, and VII has been studied by literature review, Brand's radian theory, and intraoperative measurement.[44] In the pilot study of early passive motion,[44] the desired passive excursion to minimize extrinsic adhesion at a repair site in these zones was thought to be 5 mm based on the work of Duran[34] and Gelberman.[50] Transposing desired tendon excursion into joint range of motion has been described[44] and can be applied to clinical situations simply by moving the MP joints through approximately ½ radian (30°) for the index and long digits and a little more (40°) for the ring and small digits (Fig. 43-13, *A* and *B*). Burkhalter confirmed the relationship between tendon excursion and these MP joint motions intraoperatively.

Others report good results with greater excursions for the extensor tendons[19]; however, our clinical results indicate that SAM is sufficient to obtain good functional results. Greater excursions that will increase the internal tendon tension at a repair site should probably be reserved for stronger tendon repair techniques designed for active motion protocols.

EPL excursion cannot be calculated by radians because of the multiple moments of adduction and external rotation at the CMC level and because alterations in thumb position alter the moment arms at each joint.[16,63] Intraoperative

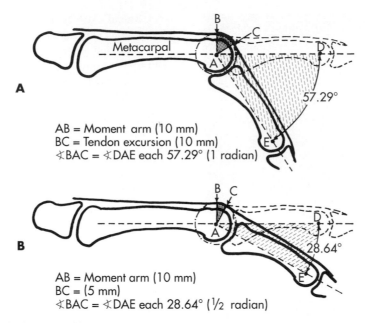

Fig. 43-13. A, If the head of the metacarpal is considered in terms of a circle, the moment arm of the extensor tendon is equal to the radius of that circle. If metacarpophalangeal joint motion equals 57.29°, or 1 radian, tendon excursion is equal to the moment arm or AB = BC. If the moment arm equals 10 mm, angular change of 57.29° affects 10 mm of extensor tendon excursion. (From Evans RB, Burkhalter WE: A study of the dynamic anatomy of extensor tendons and implications for treatment, *J Hand Surg* 1986; 11A: 776.) **B,** Angular change of 0.5 radians or 28.3° affects the 5 mm or extensor tendon excursion recommended for the early passive motion program.

measurements determined that 60° of IP flexion will glide the EPL distally 5 mm at the level of Lister's tubercle if the wrist is neutral and the CMC and MP joints are at 0° of extension.[44]

Internal tendon forces with the SAM protocol in these zones as they relate to various joint angles and applied external loads have been defined.[46] A biomechanical analysis of extensor tendon forces is presented in a series of mathematical models that negate resistance from the antagonistic muscle-tendon group, and any other drag, and then apply a known external force. The results of this mathematical study estimate that with the wrist positioned at approximately 20° of flexion (a position which reduces the resistance of the antagonistic flexors) and with only the weight of the finger as an external load, that active motion at the MP joint from 30° of flexion to 0° of extension will transmit approximately 300 g of internal tendon tension to repairs in zones V, VI, and VII. However, as the wrist is extended, these forces rise dramatically to approximately 1200 g of force, as the extensors have to overcome the viscoelastic resistance from increased tension in the flexor system.[46] The position of 20° of wrist flexion for the active hold component is compatible with the tensile strength[93] most commonly used in repair techniques for extensor tendons.

The wrist tenodesis exercise[30] is an important part of the SAM protocol and may help to ensure that the predicted excursion is indeed occurring at the repair sites in these zones. Wrist position significantly alters tendon excursions

and internal tendon tensions.[46,91,102] In a cadaver study of extensor tendon excursion it has been demonstrated that if the wrist is extended more than 21°, the extensor tendons glide with little or no tension in zones V and VI throughout full simulated grip to full passive digital extension.[91] These measurements made in cadaver hands may not apply in vivo.

We observe clinically and it has been demonstrated by electromyographic analysis[92] that with the MP joints splinted at 0° of extension that the EDC tendons are active within the confines of dynamic splints used with passive protocols. It is likely that extensor tendons treated with passive protocols already are moving actively even without the active hold components. This may explain the similarity in results between the tendons treated with passive only protocols and the combined passive and active protocols.

It is important to rest all digital joints at 0° within the dynamic splints. This position will prevent extensor lag and also ensure that some active tension is transmitted to the EDC. Splinting the MP at 20° of flexion keeps the EDC quiescent.[92] The high profile spring steel outrigger is preferred by the senior author because flexion forces are reduced by using an outrigger with a larger moment arm[14] and a moving outrigger as opposed to a static outrigger.

SUMMARY

The shift from passive only to combined passive and active rehabilitation protocols following digital tendon repair is a part of researchers' efforts to improve functional results by ensuring that some true proximal migration of a tendon repair site is taking place with the controlled early motion exercises in the early healing phases. Force application with active motion protocols must be less than the tensile strength of the repair with adjustments made for increased internal tension from drag and decreased tensile strength associated with early tendon softening. It is especially critical with standard repair techniques that external load and joint positions are precise during the active exercise components to ensure that the internal tendon forces noted in this chapter are reproduced with an element of precision.

REFERENCES

1. Allieu Y, Ascencio G, Rouzaud JC: Protected passive mobilization after suturing the extensor tendons of the hand: a survey of 120 cases. In Hunter JM, Schneider LH, Mackin EJ, eds: *Tendon surgery in the hand,* St. Louis, 1987, Mosby.
2. Amiel D, Gelberman R, Harwood F, Siegel D: Fibronectin in healing flexor tendons subjected to immobilization or early controlled passive motion, *Matrix II* 184-189, 1991.
3. An K-N, Berglund L, Uchiyama S, Coert JH: Measurement of friction between pulley and flexor tendon, *Biomechanical Scientific Instrumentation* 1993; 29:1-7.
4. Aoki M, Manske PR, Pruitt DL, Larson BJ: Tendon repair using flexor tendon splints: an experimental study, *J Hand Surg* 1994; 19A(6): 984-991.
5. Aoki M, Manske PR, Pruitt DL, Larson BJ: Work of flexion after tendon repair with various suture methods, *J Hand Surg* 1995; 20B(3):310-313.
6. Aoki M, Pruitt DL, Kubota H, Manske PR: Effect of suture knots on tensile strength of repaired canine flexor tendons, *J Hand Surg* 1995; 20B(1):72-75.
7. Arbuckle JD, McGrouther DA: Measurement of the arc of digital flexion and joint movement ranges, *J Hand Surg* 1995; 20B(6):836-840.
8. Bainbridge LC, Robertson C, Gillies D, Elliot D: A comparison of postoperative mobilization of flexor tendon repairs with "passive flexion–active extension" and "controlled active motion" techniques, *J Hand Surg* 1994; 19B:512-521.
9. Barmakian JT, Lin H, Green SM, et al: Comparison of a suture technique with the modified Kessler method: resistance to gap formation, *J Hand Surg* 1994; 19A:777-781.
10. Becker H: Primary repair of flexor tendons without mobilization: preliminary report, *Hand* 1978; 10:37-47.
11. Becker H, Davidoff M: Eliminating the gap in flexor tendon surgery: a new method of suture, *Hand* 1977; 9(3):306-311.
12. Becker H, Orak F, Duponselle E: Early active motion following a bevelled technique of flexor tendon repair: report on fifty cases, *J Hand Surg* 1979; 4:454-460.
13. Bhatia D, Tanner KE, Bonfield W, Citron ND: Factors affecting the strength of flexor tendon repair, *J Hand Surg* 1992; 17B(5):550-553.
14. Boozer JA, Sanson MS, Soutas-Little RW, et al: Comparison of the biomechanical motions and forces in high-profile versus low-profile dynamic splinting, *J Hand Ther* 1994; 7:171-182.
15. Boulas HJ, Strickland JW: Strength and functional recovery following repair of flexor digitorum superficialis in zone 2, *J Hand Surg* 1993; 18B:22-25.
16. Brand PW, Hollister A, eds: *Clinical mechanics of the hand,* ed 2, St Louis, 1993, Mosby.
17. Brand PW, Thompson DE: Mechanical resistance. In Brand PW, Hollister A, eds: *Clinical mechanics of the hand,* ed 2, St Louis, 1993, Mosby.
18. Breger-Lee D, Bell-Krotoski J, Brandsma JW: Torque range of motion in the hand clinic, *J Hand Ther* 1990; 3:14-19.
19. Browne EZ, Ribik CA: Early dynamic splinting for extensor tendon injuries, *J Hand Surg* 1989; 14A:72-76.
20. Brunelli G, Vigasio A, Brunelli F: Slip-knot flexor tendon suture in zone II allowing immediate mobilization, *Hand* 1983; 15:352-358.
21. Bunker TD, Potter B, Barton NJ: Continuous passive motion following flexor tendon repair, *J Hand Surg* 1989; 14B:406-411.
22. Burge PD, Brown NM: Elastic band mobilization after flexor tendon repair: splint design and risk of flexion contracture, *J Hand Surg* 1990; 15B:443-448.
23. Cannon NM, Strickland JW: Therapy following flexor tendon surgery, *Hand Clin* 1985; 1:147-165.
24. Chow JA, Dovelle S, Thomes LJ, et al: Postoperative management of repair of extensor tendons of the hand—dynamic splinting versus static splinting, *Orthop Trans* 1987; 11(2):258-259.
25. Chow J, Thomes LJ, Dovelle S, et al: A combined regimen of controlled motion following flexor tendon repair in "no man's land," *Plast Reconstr Surg* 1987; 79:447-453.
26. Chow SP, Stephens MM, Ngai YC, et al: A splint for controlled active motion after flexor tendon repair, *J Hand Surg* 1990; 15A:645-651.
27. Cieslik K, Pieniazek M, Kaozmarczyk D, et al: Early mechanical strength in sutures of the finger flexor tendons, *Handchir Mikrochir Plast Chir* 1986; 18:347-360.
28. Close JR, Kidd CC: The functions of the muscles of the thumb, the index, and the long finger, *J Bone Joint Surg* 1969; 51A:1601-1620.
29. Coert JH, Uchiyama S, Amadio PC, et al: Flexor tendon-pulley interaction after tendon repair: a biomechanical study, *J Hand Surg* 1995; 20B(5):573-577.
30. Cooney WP, Lin GT, An K-N: Improved tendon excursion following flexor tendon repair, *J Hand Ther* 1989; 2:102-106.
31. Craver JM, Madden JW, Penwik EE: The effect of sutures, immobilization, and tenolysis on healing tendons: a method for measuring work of digital flexion in a chicken foot, *Surg* 1964; 64:437-441.
32. Cullen K, Tolhurst P, Lang D, Page R: Flexor tendon repair in zone II followed by controlled active motion, *J Hand Surg* 1989; 14B:392-395.
33. Dennerlein JT, Mote CD, Diao E, et al: A new in vivo finger tendon force transducer, *Bio-5C International Mechanical Engineering Congress and Exposition,* ASME, San Francisco, Nov 12–17, 1995.
34. Duran RJ, Houser RG: Controlled passive motion following flexor tendon repair in zones 2 and 3. In *AAOS symposium on tendon surgery in the hand,* St Louis, 1975, Mosby.
35. Edinburg M, Widgerow A, Biddulph S: Early post-operative mobilization of flexor tendon injuries using a modification of the Kleinert technique, *J Hand Surg* 1987; 12A:34-38.
36. Elliot D, Moiemen NS, Flemming AFS, et al: The rupture rate of acute flexor tendon repairs mobilized by the controlled active regimen, *J Hand Surg* 1994; 19B(5):607-612.
37. Evans RB: Therapeutic management of extensor tendon injuries, *Hand Clin* 1986; 2:157-169.
38. Evans RB: Clinical application of controlled stress to the healing extensor tendon: a review of 112 cases, *Phys Ther* 1989; 68(12): 1041-1049.
39. Evans RB: A study of the zone I flexor tendon injury and implications for treatment, *J Hand Ther* 1990; 3:133-148.
40. Evans RB: Early active short arc motion for the repaired central slip, *J Hand Surg* 1994; 19A:991-997.
41. Evans RB: Immediate active short arc motion for the repaired zone I and II flexor tendon, *J Hand Surg* (submitted for publication).
42. Evans RB: An update on extensor tendon management. In Hunter JM, Mackin EJ, Callahan AD, eds: *Rehabilitation of the hand: surgery and therapy,* ed 4, St Louis, 1995, Mosby.
43. Evans RB: Immediate active short arc motion for the repaired extensor tendon, *Hand Clin* 1995; 11(3):483-512.

44. Evans RB, Burkhalter WE: A study of the dynamic anatomy of extensor tendons and implications for treatment, *J Hand Surg* 1986; 11A:774-779.

45. Evans RB, Thompson DE: An analysis of factors that support early active short arc motion of the repaired central slip, *J Hand Ther* 1992; 5:187-201.

46. Evans RB, Thompson DE: The application of force to the healing tendon, *J Hand Ther* 1993; 6(4):266-284.

47. Freehan LM, Beauchene JG: Early tensile properties of healing flexor tendons: early controlled passive motion versus postoperative immobilization, *J Hand Surg* 1990; 15A:63-68.

48. Frère G, Moutet F, Sarrorius C, et al: Controlled postoperative mobilization of sutured extensor tendons of the long fingers, *Ann Chir Main* 1984; 141-144.

49. Gault DT: A review of repaired flexor tendons, *J Hand Surg* 1987; 12B:321-325.

50. Gelberman RH, Botte MJ, Spiegelman JJ, et al: The excursion and deformation of repaired flexor tendons treated with protected early motion, *J Hand Surg* 1986; 11A:106-110.

51. Gelberman RH, Nunley JA, Osterman AL, et al: Influence of the protected passive mobilization interval in flexor tendon healing, *Clin Orthop* 1991; 264:189-196.

52. Gelberman RH, Steinberg D, Amiel D, et al: Fibroblast chemotaxis after tendon repair, *J Hand Surg* 1991; 16A:686-693.

53. Gelberman RH, VandeBerg JS, Manske PR, Akeson WH: The early stages of flexor tendon healing: a morphologic study of the first fourteen days, *J Hand Surg* 1985; 10A:766-784.

54. Gratton P: Early active mobilization after flexor tendon repairs, *J Hand Ther* 1993; 6:285-289.

55. Greenwald D, Shumway S, Allen C, Mass D: Dynamic analysis of profundus tendon function, *J Hand Surg* 1994; 19A:626-635.

56. Haddad RJ, Kester MA, McCluskey GM, et al: Comparative mechanical analysis of a looped suture tendon repair, *J Hand Surg* 1988; 13A:709-713.

57. Hagberg L, Selvik G: Tendon excursion and dehiscence during early controlled mobilization after flexor tendon repair in zone II: an x-ray stereophotogrammetric analysis, *J Hand Surg* 1991; 16A:669-680.

58. Harmer TW: Tendon suture, *Boston Med Surg J* 1917; 177(23):808-810.

59. Hitchcock TF, Light TR, Bunch WH, et al: The effect of immediate contrained digital motion on the strength of flexor tendon repairs in chickens, *J Hand Surg* 1987; 12A:590-595.

60. Horibe S, Woo SL-Y, Spiegelman JJ, et al: Excursion of the human flexor digitorum profundus tendon, *Trans 35th Ann Mtg Orthop Res Soc* 1989; 14:252.

61. Horii E, Lin GT, Cooney WP, et al: Comparative flexor tendon excursions after passive mobilization: an in vitro study, *J Hand Surg* 1992; 17A:559-566.

62. Hung LK, Chan A, Chang J: Early controlled active mobilization with dynamic splintage for treatment of extensor tendon injuries, *J Hand Surg* 1990; 15A:251-257.

63. Kapandji IA: Biomechanics of the thumb. In Tubiana R, ed: *The hand,* Philadelphia, 1985, Saunders.

64. Karlander LE, Berggren M, Larsson M, et al: Improved results in zone 2 flexor tendon injuries with a modified technique of immediate controlled motion, *J Hand Surg* 1993; 18B:26-30.

65. Kessler I, Allissim F: Primary repair without immobilization of the flexor tendon division within the digital sheath, *Acta Orthop Scand* 1969; 40:587-601.

66. Kessler I: The "grasping" technique for tendon repair, *Hand* 1973; 5(3):253-255.

67. Ketchum LD, Martin NL, Kappel DA: Experimental evaluation of factors affecting the strength of tendon repairs, *Plast Reconstr Surg* 1977; 59(5):708-719.

68. Ketchum L, Thompson D, Pocock G, Wallingford D: A clinical study of the forces generated by the intrinsic muscles of the index finger and the extrinsic flexor and extensor muscles of the hand, *J Hand Surg* 1978; 3:571-578.

69. Kleinert HE, Kutz JE, Cohen MJ, et al: Primary repair of zone 2 flexor tendon lacerations. In *AAOS symposium on hand tendon surgery,* St Louis, 1975, Mosby.

70. Kleinert HE, Schepel S, Gill T: Flexor tendon injuries, *Surg Clin North Am* 1981; 61(2):267-286.

71. Lahey FH: A tendon suture which permits immediate motion, *Boston Med Surg J* 1923; 188(22):851-852.

72. Lane JM, Black J, Bora FW: Gliding function following flexor-tendon injury, *J Bone Joint Surg* 1976; 58A(7):985-990.

73. Lee H: Double loop locking suture: a technique of tendon repair for early active mobilization, part I: evolution of technique and experimental study, *J Hand Surg* 1990; 15A(6):945-952.

74. Lee H: Double loop locking suture: a technique of tendon repair for early active mobilization, part II: clinical experience, *J Hand Surg* 1990; 15A(6):953-958.

75. Lexer E: Verwethung der Freien, Sehnentransplantation, *Arch Klin Chir* 1912; 98:818.

76. Lin GT, An K-N, Amadio PC, Cooney WP: Biomechanical studies of running suture for flexor tendon repair in dogs, *J Hand Surg* 1988; 13A:553-558.

77. Lindsay WK, Thompson HG, Walker FG: Digital flexor tendons: an experimental study: the significance of gap occurring at the line of suture, *Br J Plast Surg* 1960; 13:1-9.

78. Lister GD, Kleinert HE, Kutz JE: Primary flexor tendon repair followed by immediate controlled mobilization, *J Hand Surg* 1977; 2(6):441-445.

79. Llorens WL: An experimental analysis of finger joint stiffness, Baton Rouge, Louisiana State University, 1986 (MSME thesis).

80. Long CH: Intrinsic-extrinsic muscle control of the finger electromyographic studies, *J Bone Joint Surg* 1970; 52A:853-867.

81. Long CH: Electromyographic studies of hand function. In Tubiana R, ed: *The hand,* vol I, Philadelphia, 1981, Saunders.

82. Manske P: Flexor tendon healing, *J Hand Surg* 1988; 13B:237-245.

83. Martin BF: The tendons of the flexor digitorum profundus, *J Anat* 1958; 92:602-608.

84. Mashadi ZB, Amis AA: Strength of the suture in the epitenon and within the tendon fibers: development of stronger peripheral suture technique, *J Hand Surg* 1992; 17B(2):171-175.

85. Mashadi ZB, Amis AA: The effect of locking loops on the strength of tendon repair, *J Hand Surg* 1991; 16B:35-39.

86. Mason ML, Allen HS: The rate of healing of tendons: an experimental study of tensile strength, *Ann Surg* 1941; 113:424-459.

87. Matthews JP: Early mobilization after tendon repair, *J Hand Surg* 1989; 14B(4):363-367.

88. May E, Silverskiöld K, Sollerman C: Controlled mobilization after flexor tendon repair in zone II: a prospective comparison of three methods, *J Hand Surg* 1992; 17A:942-952.

89. McGrouther DA, Ahmed MR: Flexor tendon excursion in "no man's land," *Hand* 1981; 13:129-141.

90. Messina A: The double armed suture: tendon repair with immediate mobilization of the fingers, *J Hand Surg* 1992; 17A:137-142.

91. Minamikawa Y, Peimer CA, Yamaguchi T, et al: Wrist position and extensor tendon amplitude following repair, *J Hand Surg* 1992; 17A:268-271.

92. Newport ML, Shukla A: Electrophysiologic basis of dynamic extensor splinting, *J Hand Surg* 1992; 17A:272-277.

93. Newport ML, Williams MS: Biomechanical characteristics of extensor tendon suture techniques, *J Hand Surg* 1992; 17A:117-123.

94. Papandrea R, Seitz WH, Shapiro P, Borden B: Biomechanical and clinical evaluation of the epitenon-first technique of flexor tendon repair, *J Hand Surg* 1995; 20A:261-266.

95. Pruitt DL, Manske PR, Fink B: Cyclic stress analysis of flexor tendon repair, *J Hand Surg* 1991; 16A:701-707.

96. Rank BK, Wakefield AR, Hueston JT: *The Surgery of repair as applied to hand injuries,* ed 4, Edinburgh, 1973, Churchill Livingstone.

97. Robertson GA, Al-Qattan MM: A biomechanical analysis of a new interlock suture for flexor tendon repair, *J Hand Surg* 1992; 17B(1):92-93.

98. Rothkopf DM, Webb S, Szabo RM, et al: An experimental model for the study of canine flexor tendon adhesions, *J Hand Surg* 1991; 16A:694-700.

99. Saldana MI, Chow JA, Gerbino P, et al: Further experience in rehabilitation of zone II flexor tendon repair with dynamic traction splinting, *Plast Reconstr Surg* 1991; 87:543-546.

100. Sanders WE: Advantages of "epitenon-first" suture placement technique in flexor tendon repair, *Clin Orthop* 1992; 280:198-199.

101. Savage R: In vitro studies of a new method of flexor tendon repair, *J Hand Surg* 1985; 10B(2):135-141.

102. Savage R: The influence of wrist position on the minimum force required for active movements of the interphalangeal joints, *J Hand Surg* 1988; 13B:262-268.

103. Savage R, Ristano G: Flexor tendon repair using a "six strand" method of repair and early active mobilization, *J Hand Surg* 1989; 14B:396-399.

104. Schink W, Gersbach B: Eine eperimentelle Studie uber die festigkeit genahter sehnen bei verschiedenen Nahtmethoden langen, *Arch Klin Chir* 1961; 297:191-235.

105. Schuind F, Garcia Elias M, Cooney WP, An K-N: Flexor tendon forces: in vivo measurements, *J Hand Surg* 1992; 17A:291-298.

106. Seradge H: Elongation of the repair configuration following flexor tendon repair, *J Hand Surg* 1983; 8:182-185.

107. Silfverskiöld KL, Andersson CH: Two new methods of tendon repair: an in vitro evaluation of tensile strength and gap formation, *J Hand Surg* 1993; 18A(1):58-65.

108. Silverskiöld K, May EJ, Tornvall AH: Gap formation during controlled motion after flexor tendon repair in zone II: a prospective clinical study, *J Hand Surg* 1992; 17A:593.

109. Silverskiöld KL, May EJ: Flexor tendon repair in zone II with a new suture technique and an early mobilization program combining passive and active flexion, *J Hand Surg* 1994; 19A:53-60.

110. Simmons BP, De La Caffiniere JY: Physiology of flexion of the fingers. In Tubiana R, ed: *The hand,* vol I, Philadelphia, 1981, Saunders.

111. Singer M, Maloon S: Flexor tendon injuries: the results of primary repair, *J Hand Surg* 1988; 13B:269-272.

112. Slattery PG: The modified Kleinert splint in zone II flexor tendon injuries, *J Hand Surg* 1988; 13B:273-376.

113. Slattery RG, McGrouther DA: The modified Kleinert controlled mobilization splint following flexor tendon repair, *J Hand Surg* 1984; 9B(2):217-218.

114. Small J, Brennen M, Colville J: Early active mobilization following flexor tendon repair in zone II, *J Hand Surg* 1989; 14B:383-391.

115. Stewart K, Van Strien G: Therapists' management of flexor tendon injury. In Hunter JM, Schneider LH, Mackin EJ, Callahan A, eds: *Rehabilitation of the hand,* ed 4, St Louis, 1995, Mosby.

116. Strickland JW, Glogovac SV: Digital function following flexor tendon repair in zone 2: a comparison study of immobilization and controlled passive motion, *J Hand Surg* 1980; 5:537-543.

117. Strickland JW: Flexor tendon surgery: part I: primary flexor tendon repair, *J Hand Surg* 1989; 14B(3):261-272 (review article).

118. Strickland JW: Biologic rationale, clinical application, and results of early motion following flexor tendon repair, *J Hand Ther* 1989; 2(2):71-83.

119. Strickland JW: Flexor tendon injuries: I. foundations of treatment, *J Am Acad Orthop Surg* 1995; 3:44-54.

120. Strickland JW: Flexor tendon injuries: II. operative treatment, *J Am Acad Orthop Surg* 1995; 3:55-62.

121. Takai S, Woo SL, Horibe S, et al: The effects of frequency and duration of controlled passive mobilization on tendon healing, *J Orthop Res* 1991; 9(5):705-713.

122. Trail 9A, Powell ES, Noble J: The mechanical strength of various suture techniques, *J Hand Surg* 1992; 17B:87-91.

123. Tubiana R: Architecture and functions of the hand. In Tubiana R, ed: *The hand,* vol 1, Philadelphia, 1981, Saunders.

124. Uchiyama S, Coert JH, Berglund L, et al: A method for measurement of frictional between tendon and pulley, *J Orthop Res* 1995; 13:83-89.

125. Urbaniak JR, Cahill JD, Mortenson RA: Tendon suturing methods: analysis of tensile strengths. In *AAOS symposium on tendon surgery in the hand,* St Louis, 1975, Mosby.

126. Valentine P: The interossei and the lumbricals. In Tubiana R, ed: *The hand,* vol 1, Philadelphia, 1981, Saunders.

127. Wade PJF, Muir IFK, Hutcheon LL: Primary flexor tendon repair: the mechanical limitations of the modified Kessler technique, *J Hand Surg* 1986; 11B:71-76.

128. Wade PJ, Wetherell RG, Amis AA: Flexor tendon repair: significant gain in strength from the Halsted peripheral suture technique, *J Hand Surg* 1989; 14B:232-235.

129. Wagner WF, Carroll C, Strickland JW, et al: A biomechanical comparison of techniques of flexor tendon repair, *J Hand Surg* 1994; 19A:979-983.

130. Wainwright SA, Biggs WD, Currey JD, Gosline JM: Mechanical design in organisms, Princeton, 1976, Princeton University Press.

131. Walbeehm ET, McGrouther DA: An anatomical study of the mechanical interactions of flexor digitorum superficialis and profundus and the flexor tendon sheath in zone 2, *J Hand Surg* 1995; 20B(3):269-280.

132. Wehbé MA, Hunter JM: Flexor tendon gliding in the hand: I. in vivo excursions, *J Hand Surg* 1985; 10A:570-575.

133. Wehbé MA, Hunter JM: Flexor tendon gliding in the hand: II. differential gliding, *J Hand Surg* 1985; 10A:575-579.

134. Werntz JR, Chesher SP, Breiderbach WC, et al: A new dynamic splint for postoperative treatment of flexor tendon injury, *J Hand Surg* 1989; 14A:559-566.

135. Williams RJN, Amis AA: A new type of flexor tendon repair: biomechanical evaluation by cyclic loading, ultimate strength and assessment of pulley friction in vitro, *J Hand Surg* 1995; 20B(5): 578-583.

136. Wray RC, Weeks PM: Experimental comparison of techniques of tendon repair, *J Hand Surg* 1980; 5:144-148.

137. Zancolli EA: *Structural and dynamic bases of hand surgery,* ed 2, Philadelphia, 1979, Lippincott.

SUGGESTED READING

O'Dwyer FG, Quinton DN: Early mobilization of acute middle slip injuries, *J Hand Surg* 1990; 15B:404-406.

Peterson WW, Manske PR, Bollinger BA, et al: Effect of pulley excision on flexor tendon biomechanics, *J Orthop Res* 1986b; 4(1):96-101 (reference to work of flexion).

Peterson WW, Manske PR, Dunlap J, et al: Effect of various methods of restoring flexor sheath integrity on the formation of adhesions after tendon injury, *J Hand Surg* 15A(2):48-56 (reference to work of flexion).

Peterson WW, Manske PR, Kain CC, Lesker PA: Effect of flexor sheath integrity on tendon gliding: a biomechanical and histological study, *J Orthop Res* 1986a; 4(4):458-465 (reference to work of flexion).

Thomes LJ, Thomes BJ: Early mobilization method for surgically repaired zone III extensor tendons, *J Hand Ther* 1995; 8(3):195-198 (support for early controlled motion extensor zone III).

Walsh MT, Muntzer E, Patel J, Sitler MR: Early controlled motion with dynamic splinting for zones III and IV extensor lacerations, *J Hand Ther* 1994; 7:232-236 (support for immediate short arc motion for extensor zones III and IV).

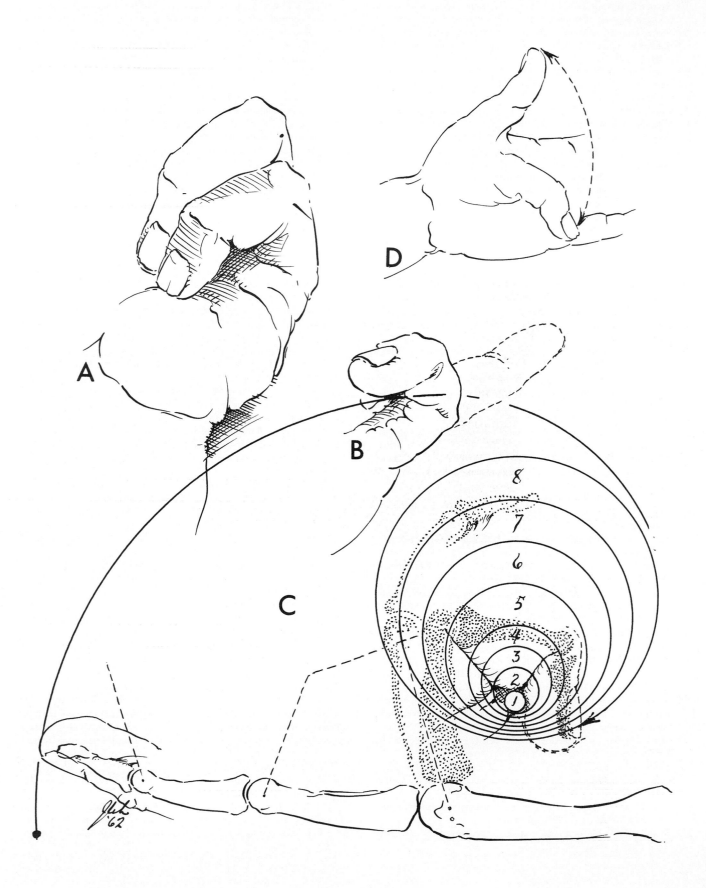

A

B

C

D

1
2
3
4
5
6
7
8

Part X

TENDON GRAFTS

A successful tendon graft permits near full extension of the finger (to 180°) and is capable of flexing the interphalangeal (IP) joints through a range that permits relatively small diameters to be grasped. An index of success is the diameter of the smallest rod effectively encircled by the flexed phalanges and palm *(C)*. The useful functional segment of the normal extension-flexion are restored should be the criterion for flexor tendon evaluation. Fixation in acute flexion of the IP joints following tendon repair *(A* and *B)* renders the digit useless.

At the proximal interphalangeal (PIP) joint some restraint of extension is desirable in preventing a recurvatum deformity, and ease of flexion through the singular profundus tendon graft should act primarily on the PIP joint rather than on the distal one to produce a coordinated and efficient flexion arc.

D, Extension-flexion arc of the thumb. Stability in good position is the special characteristic of the thumb. Interphalangeal and metacarpophalangeal extension and flexion show great individual variation. The grafted thumb must be compared with its mate for evaluation. The range of movement will be modified by wrist position, especially when the repair has been made proximal to the radiocarpal joint. (From Converse JM: *Reconstructive plastic surgery: principles in correction, reconstruction and transplanation,* vol. iv, Philadelphia, 1964, Saunders.)

Chapter 44

TENDON GRAFTING
A historical perspective

Raoul Tubiana

The first tendon graft was attempted at the end of the nineteenth century. The exact date is difficult to pinpoint because of the confusion surrounding the term *tendon transplant,* which should be used only to describe a tendon graft, although it was used inaccurately to signify a tendon transfer. In 1882 Heuck, a German surgeon, repaired an extensor pollicis longus (EPL) using a tendon graft.[12] In 1886 at the Surgical Society of Paris, Peyrot reported a case of "transplantation in man of the tendon of a dog" to replace the flexor tendons of a middle finger "which had been destroyed"; this resulted in "good healing with partial functional recovery."[33] In 1887 at a meeting of the same society, Monod reported a case in which a 5-cm tendon graft taken from the Achilles tendon of a rabbit was successfully used to repair the EPL.[30] In 1888 Robson took a tendon from an injured digit to fashion an extensor graft on the same hand.[37]

The beginning of the twentieth century saw extensive clinical and experimental work being done, especially in Germany, by Lange,[19] Kirschner,[17] Rehn,[36] and more particularly by Biesalski[1] from Berlin. Biesalski reconsidered the problem of adhesions and the action of tension on sutures, and his work had a profound influence on his contemporaries. In 1912 Lexer from Iena published the results of the first series of 10 autografts of flexor tendons.[21] However, it was in the United States that tendon surgery had its greatest advances.

In 1911 Lewis and Davis made an experimental study of direct tendon and fascial transplant.[20] Mayer, who had worked in Lange's department in Munich, published a number of works, including three articles[26-28] on "The physiological method of tendon transplantation." In these articles he described the anatomy and physiology of the peritendinous structures and mentioned the necessity for a precise surgical technique, which he called the "physiological method." He also stressed the importance of ensuring the correct tension of the transfer and the necessity for preserving the gliding planes. He also recommended that the surgeon should personally supervise the postoperative care and resumption of movements.

While the clinical applications of Mayer's work were directed more toward the foot and the ankle joint, Bunnell in San Francisco turned his interest more toward surgery of the hand. Between the time of his first article on tendon repair in the fingers, published in 1918,[4] and his masterly book, *Surgery of the hand,* (first edition, 1944),[6] he had formulated the principles that now form the basis of tendon surgery.

At that time, primary suturing of flexor tendons was almost always doomed to failure in the digital canal. Although the tendon healing was usually satisfactory, adhesions were so extensive that tendon mobility was nil. In the face of such consistently poor results following primary suturing in what he called "no man's land," in 1922[5] Bunnell gave this advice: "Close the skin, wait for the wound to heal, then perform a secondary repair as follows: excise the two flexors and graft the profundus tendon alone from the lumbrical to the digital extremity."

This teaching was held as a dogma by generations of surgeons (Boyes, Pulvertaft, Graham, Littler, Tubiana) for the treatment of lesions within "no man's land."*

*References 2, 3, 11, 22, 35, 39, 40.

Tendon grafting is an ingenious attempt at solving some of the biologic problems of tendon repair. Not only can a tendon graft compensate for a loss of substance, but it also offers the advantage that the sutures are tension-free and can be placed in an optimal position, away from the fibrous pulleys. In practice, most grafts are autogenous.

ALLOGRAFTS (HOMOLOGOUS) AND XENOGRAFTS (HETEROLOGOUS)

The possibility of using preserved grafting material has been considered for a long time. This would allow the creation of tendon banks and obviate the need for autogenous grafts.

For many years, Iselin[15] has advocated the use of acellular grafts preserved in a mercurial solution of Cialit, (1 g of Cialit powder in 5 L of sterile water). These grafts are easy to handle and are immunologically more inert than fresh grafts containing live cells. Seiffert and Schmidt[38] have followed the life cycle of these grafts by radioactive labeling techniques (Cproline) and have shown that the collagen is gradually replaced and that the allograft is repopulated in 6 or 8 weeks.

In a series of experiments in dogs in which homologous freeze-dried grafts were transplanted into the digital sheaths, Potenza showed that the graft is well tolerated and its repopulation by the recipient's cells is not accompanied by adhesion formation in the sheath.[34] As Potenza pointed out, the term *dead graft* is too often applied to allografts and heterografts, for although the cells themselves disappear, extracellular collagen remains. An important question is whether this collagen is denatured in the course of transplantation.[9]

COMPOSITE TISSUE TENDON ALLOGRAFTS

Peacock has carried out a series of fascinating experiments on homologous transplantation of the whole flexor tendinous apparatus of the digits with a view to applying his methods to humans.[32] His basic premise is that adult tendons and their sheaths are devoid of cells capable of synthesizing collagen. If the tendon sheath could be taken intact with its contents, the scarring would proceed between the recipient's bed and the outside of the sheath and the tendons. Animal experiments confirm this view and show that immunologic reactions are of little significance. This method has been used successfully in humans by several surgeons.[13,32] Chacha[8] has used composite autogenous grafts taken from the flexor apparatus of the toes (second toe), first in the monkey and then in humans, with interesting functional results.

RECONSTRUCTING THE FIBROUS TENDON SHEATH

Restoring or reconstructing the flexor tendon sheath after tendon repair has been an important step forward. The attitude toward the flexor sheaths has changed considerably over the years. For a long time the tendency was to resect as much of the sheaths as possible and to preserve only narrow pulleys. The reasoning was that the sheaths formed a barrier against vascularization of the graft and that there was a risk of the grafts becoming adherent to a fixed structure. Since the studies of Peacock, Potenza, Lundborg, Matthews, Doyle and Blythe, Manske, and many others,[10,23-25,33,34] the mechanical and nutritional actions of the digital flexor sheath are better understood. The most important pulleys must be reconstructed around the graft. In some cases to prevent adhesions, it seems preferable to reconstruct the pulleys around a tendon implant.

RECONSTRUCTING THE PSEUDOTENDON SHEATH

In 1959 Carroll and Bassett[7] used silicone rods to induce pseudosheath formation. Since 1960, Hunter[14] has progressively developed a two-stage procedure using a silicone rod for preliminary preparation of a pseudosheath. The basic concept of this technique is that when a pseudosynovial sheath is formed in response to a biologically inert implant, the cells adapt so that they can effectively accept the tendon graft. Hunter's technique is now widely used and will be discussed later.

PEDICLE TENDON GRAFT

In 1965 Paneva-Holevich[31] from Sofia reported a new technique for secondary reconstruction of flexor tendon injuries in zone II. The operation involves use of the superficial flexor of the same finger as a predicle graft after suturing it at an earlier operation to the flexor profundus at the lumbrical muscle level.

Later, this procedure was combined with the Hunter two-stage technique.[16] In the first stage, both flexors are cut at the level of the lumbrical muscle and their proximal stumps are sutured to each other. A pseudosheath is prepared in the digit by temporary placement of a silicone rubber implant. Two to three months later, the end of the pedicle graft is temporarily sutured to the silicone rubber implant, pulled through the digital canal, and fixed to the distal phalanx. This technique is used in "unfavorable" cases.

The proper time to *begin motion* following a tendon graft has created enormous controversy. For a long time, a 3-week period of immobilization was the rule after a tendon graft. Now a technique of early passive mobilization is used after two-stage tendon grafting. A one-stage graft requires greater care for fear of tendon rupture.

CONCLUSION

During the last century, tendon grafting has been the subject of numerous studies that have given rise to a variety of different techniques. This ingenious method is still evolving and seems to be indicated mostly for secondary tendon repairs. Progress in the technique of primary tendon suture[18,41] has considerably reduced the indications for primary tendon grafting.

SUMMARY

The first attempt of tendon grafts started a century ago in Western Europe.* Extensive clinical and experimental work has been done in the United States by Mayer[26-28] and by Bunnell[4] who formulated the principles that form the basis of flexor tendon surgery in "no man's land" in 1922. A tendon graft offers the advantage that the sutures are tension-free and can be placed in an optimal location.

Progress in the technique of primary repair of flexor tendons[18,41] has considerably reduced the indications of primary tendon grafting. Secondary tendon grafting has benefited from numerous studies and new procedures trying to avoid the adhesions that occur when a tendon is grafted onto an injured bed:

- Composite tissue tendon allografts[32]
- Inert gliding implants that produce a pseudosynovial sheath[14]
- Pedicle tendon grafts[31]

REFERENCES

1. Biesalski K: Über Sehnenscheidenauswechslung, *Deutsche Med Wochnschr* 1910; 36:1615-1618.
2. Boyes JH: Flexor tendon grafts in the fingers and thumb: an evaluation of end results, *J Bone Joint Surg* 1950; 32A:489.
3. Boyes JH, Stark HH: Flexor tendon grafts in the finger and thumb: a study of factors influencing results in 1000 cases, *J Bone Joint Surg* 1971; 53A:1332.
4. Bunnell S: Repair of tendons in the fingers and description of two new instruments, *Surg Gynecol Obstet* 1918; 26:103.
5. Bunnell S: Repair of tendons in the fingers, *Surg Gynecol Obstet* 1922; 35:88-97.
6. Bunnell S: *Surgery of the hand*, Philadelphia, 1944, Lippincott.
7. Carroll RE, Bassett AL: Formation of tendon sheath by silicone rod implants, *J Bone Joint Surg* 1963; 45A:884-885.
8. Chacha P: Free autologous composite tendon grafts for division of both flexor tendons within the digital theca of the hand. In Tubiana R, ed: *The hand*, vol 2, Philadelphia, 1988, Saunders.
9. Flynn JE, Graham JH: Healing following tendon suture and tendon transplants, *Surg Gynecol Obstet* 1962; 115:467-472.
10. Doyle JR, Blythe WF: The finger flexor tendon sheath and pulleys: anatomy and reconstruction. In *AAOS symposium on tendon surgery in the hand*, St Louis, 1975, Mosby.
11. Graham WC: Flexor tendon grafts to the finger and thumb, *J Bone Joint Surg* 1947; 29:553-559.
12. Heuck G: Ein Beitrag zur Sehnenplastik, *Zentralbl Chir* 1881; 9:289-292.
13. Hueston JT, Hubble B, Rigg BR: Homografts of the digital flexor tendon system, *Aust N Zeal J Surg* 1967; 36:269.
14. Hunter JM: Artificial tendons: early development and application, *Am J Surg* 1965; 109:325.
15. Iselin F: Preliminary observations on the use of chemically stored tendinous allografts in hand surgery, In *AAOS symposium on tendon surgery in the hand*, St Louis, 1975, Mosby.

16. Kessler F: Use of pedicled tendon transfer with silicone rod in complicated secondary flexor tendon repairs, *Plast Reconstr Surg* 1972; 49:439-443.
17. Kirschner M: Über freie Sehnen und Fascientransplantation, *Beitr Klin Chir* 1909; 65:472-503.
18. Kleinert HE, Kutz JE, Atasoy E, et al: Primary repair of flexor tendons, *Orthop Clin North Am* 1973; 4:865.
19. Lange F: Über periostale Sehnenverpflanzungen bei Lahmungen, *Münchener Med Wochnschr* 1900; 47:486-490.
20. Lewis D, Davis CB: Experimental direct transplantation of tendon and fascia, *JAMA* 1911; 57:540-546.
21. Lexer E: Die Verwertung der freien sehnentransplantation, *Langenbecks Arch Klin Chir* 1912; 98:818-852.
22. Littler JW: Free tendon grafts in secondary flexor tendon repair, *Am J Surg* 1947; 74:315.
23. Lundborg G, Myrhage PD, Rydevik B: The vascularization of human flexor tendons within the digital synovial sheath region: structural and functional aspects, *J Hand Surg* 1977; 2(6):417-427.
24. Manske PR, Whiteside LA, Lesker PA: Nutrient pathways to flexor tendons using hydrogen washout technique, *J Hand Surg* 1978; 3(1):32-36.
25. Matthews P, Richards H: The repair potential of digital flexor tendons, *J Bone Joint Surg* 1974; 56B:618.
26. Mayer L: The physiological method of tendon transplantations. I. historical: anatomy and physiology of tendons, *Surg Gynecol Obstet* 1916; 22:182.
27. Mayer L: The physiological method of tendon transplantations. II. operative techniques, *Surg Gynecol Obstet* 1916; 22:198.
28. Mayer L: The physiological method of tendon transplantations. III. experimental and clinical experiences, *Surg Gynecol Obstet* 1916; 22:472.
29. Mayer L: Reconstruction of digital tendon sheaths, *J Bone Joint Surg* 1936; 18:607-616.
30. Monod C: Plaies des tendons: greffe tendineuse, *Bull Mem Soc Chir Paris* 1887; 13:297-299.
31. Paneva-Holevich E: Two stage tenoplasty in injury of the flexor tendon of the hand, *J Bone Joint Surg* 1969; 5A:21-32.
32. Peacock EE, Madden JW: Human composite tissue tendon allografts, *Ann Chir* 1967; 166:624.
33. Peyrot JJ: Transplantation chez l'homme d'un tendon emprunté à un chien. Guérison avec rétablissement partiel de la fonction, *Bull Mem Soc Chir Paris* 1886; 12:356-361.
34. Potenza AD: The healing of autogenous tendon grafts within the flexor digital sheath in dogs, *J Bone Joint Surg* 1964; 46A:1462-1484.
35. Pulvertaft RG: Tendon grafts for flexor tendon injury in the fingers and thumb, *J Bone Joint Surg* 1956; 38B:175.
36. Rehn E: Die homoplastische Sehnentransplantation in Tierexperiment, *Beitr Klin Chir* 1910; 68:417-447.
37. Robson AWH: A case of tendon grafting, *Trans Clin Soc London* 1889; 22:289.
38. Seiffert K, Schmidt KP: Preserved tendon grafts in hand surgery, *Trans Fifth Internat Congr Plast Surg*, London, 1971, Butterworths.
39. Tubiana R: Greffes des tendons fléchisseurs des doigts et du pouce. Technique et résultats, *Rev Chir Orthop* 1960; 46:191-214.
40. Tubiana R: Incisions and technique in tendon grafting, *Am J Surg* 1965; 109(3):339-345.
41. Verdan C: Half a century of flexor tendon surgery, *J Bone Joint Surg* 1972; 54A:472.

*References 1, 12, 21, 30, 33, 37.

Chapter 45

ISOLATED FLEXOR DIGITORUM PROFUNDUS INJURY

Treatment by tendon grafting

Lawrence H. Schneider

Disruption of the function of the flexor digitorum profundus (FDP) by laceration or closed rupture but with an intact flexor digitorum superficialis (FDS) calls for a direct repair for patients with a recent injury (within 3 to 4 weeks) if wound conditions allow. When seen later, this injury creates a difficult judgment problem for the surgeon. It is unusual that direct repair can be performed after 3 to 4 weeks have elapsed unless the short vinculum to the FDP has remained intact and has kept the tendon well out in the finger.[18,21] This may not be known until surgical exploration. In a closed rupture the tendon may have been avulsed with a piece of its distal phalangeal bony insertion, so an x-ray examination may be of value in determining the location of its proximal end.

When more than 3 to 4 weeks have elapsed and the FDS is fully functional, one must consider carefully before offering the patient a free tendon graft to restore distal joint function.[21] Most of the useful arc of motion of the finger has been maintained[11] when the FDS is fully functional, but there is considerable risk to this function if, while passing the tendon graft through or around the superficialis decussation, damage is done to this complex area that results in adhesion formation and an overall decrease in function. In cases where, in addition to the FDP injury, the FDS is not fully functional because of partial injury of this tendon with resultant adhesion formation or because of adhesions of the FDS instigated by the tearing through of the ruptured FDP,

there is a good indication for surgical exploration with evaluation under local sedative anesthesia.[8] If tenolysis of the injured FDS can restore 90° of active motion at the proximal interphalangeal (PIP) joint through the function of the lysed FDS, one might elect just to fuse or tenodese the distal interphalangeal (DIP) joint as agreed with the patient, or if a graft is planned, do stage 1 of a staged tendon reconstruction. I would not do a standard one-stage tendon graft at the time of FDS lysis.

In fingers with a fully functional FDS, the patient is at risk to lose function if an FDP graft fails. Because of these considerable risks to FDS function, many surgeons have advised a conservative approach in these cases.* Despite the difficulties and not inconsiderable risks, others have shown, with varying degrees of enthusiasm, satisfactory results with tendon grafts placed through an intact FDS in selected patients.† One of the reasons for the discrepancy in these papers can be attributed to variations in the evaluation techniques used by the different authors. This concerns not only the method of grouping the results, but also is as basic as the technique used in measuring the degrees of motion attained at the involved finger joints. It is stressed here that the end results must be measured in the first position if they are to be regarded as valid as well as comparable to other

---

*References 2, 6, 10, 11, 13, 14, 16, 26.
†References 1, 3, 4, 9, 12, 15, 22, 23, 25, 27.

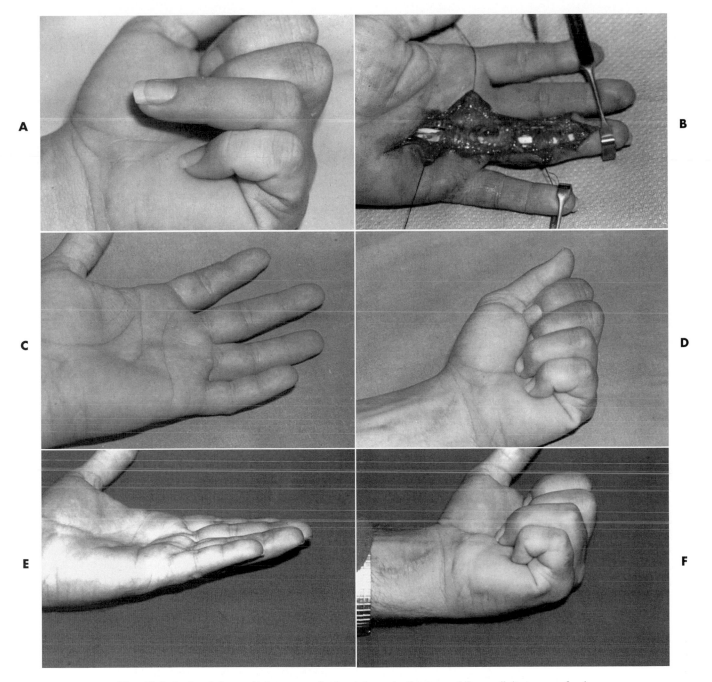

Fig. 45-1. Isolated flexor digitorum profundus injury. **A,** Rupture of flexor digitorum profundus tendon in ring finger 16 months before surgery. **B,** A scarred bed and contracted pulleys indicated the placement of a tendon implant. **C, D, E, F,** Range of motion 6 months after stage 2 tendon graft.

series.[17] Many authors do not state their methods of measurement, whereas others patently measure the range of motion attained by the distal joint using a blocked position of the more proximal joints, thereby giving an inaccurate estimation of the movement returned to the joint.[19]

It has also been stated that tendon grafting, even when it fails to provide active distal joint motion, acts to stabilize the distal joint, which is true, but if that is the only result, this

is a rather risky technique for such a limited goal, an objective that could also be attained by distal joint fusion.

In fingers that are not particularly soft or supple, but show good FDS function, it may be justified to offer no treatment, particularly when the distal joint is not hyperextensible. If the distal joint is unstable, fusion, tenodesis, using the FDP stump is offered. At times I have combined a tenolysis of the adherent FDS with a fusion of the DIP joint in an effort to improve function without using a tendon graft. This salvage has been referred to as the "superficialis finger."[20] At the same time I might excise the proximal portion of the FDP if it is coiled into the palm and causing a troublesome mass at that location. If at the time of tenolysis of the intact but adherent FDS, a graft for distal joint function has been elected, the staged technique would be used.[7,24,28]

In patients who have met strict criteria, I have used a single-stage tendon graft on 25 occasions in almost 30 years. These patients were young, had supple joints with minimal scarring, and at least one neurovascular bundle intact. Occupational need has been given as an indication for this surgery, but I hesitate to emphasize this criterion in the decision as most occupations can be performed well with a stable DIP joint. It should be noted that when the FDS is completely normal in function there is less indication for a grafting procedure than in the finger with a poorly functioning FDS. This is in contradistinction to the writing of other authors.[22] The grafting procedure is also more often indicated in the ring and little fingers, where power grasp demands greater and stronger flexion, than in the index and long fingers, where loss of FDP function will be missed less in precision activities.

TECHNIQUE

The technique is similar to that used in grafting for loss of both flexors.[18,21] An intact functioning FDS is never sacrificed at the time of grafting although a nonfunctioning or injured FDS may have to be removed. Harrison[5] has advocated removal of one tail of the FDS to allow room for the passage of the graft, but I have only found the need to do this on one occasion. Under *no* conditions is it ever justifiable to remove an intact, fully functioning FDS tendon. Great care is exercised to create as little damage to the FDS decussation and insertion as possible. The palmaris longus is the usual donor tendon, but a thin graft such as the plantaris is useful. The graft is usually passed through the decussation of the FDS, but it may be passed around the FDS if necessary. As much of the uninjured flexor retinaculum in the finger is preserved as is possible. The distal juncture technique used is that described by Bunnell, and the Pulvertaft interweave is used at the proximal juncture in the palm.[19,21]

Postoperatively, I use immediate mobilization with a rubber band attached to the nail and allow active extension and passive rubber-band flexion on the day after surgery. At 10 days to 2 weeks, gentle active motion is begun at the PIP joint. Most of the early postoperative activities are directed to the preservation of FDS function so that, at the worst, the patient would not lose that function.

On occasion the procedure has been done in two stages,[18,21] placing a tendon implant as the first stage, particularly if there has been some element of injury to the FDS or the flexor tendon bed or pulley system. Despite at least one negative report,[24] the use of the staged tendon graft has been gratifying here, but should be restricted to those fingers with a poor bed (Fig. 45-1).

RESULTS

All involved must realize that there are considerable risks when a tendon graft is to be placed in a finger that has a normal FDS. Of the 25 one-stage tendon grafts placed in almost 30 years, none have been made worse, but 14 patients were subjected to tenolysis to obtain distal joint function. An additional four patients probably would have benefitted from tenolysis, but never underwent the secondary procedure. Early motion with attention to the recovery of FDS function in the early postoperative program is critical in preventing a negative result. These tenolyses were performed 6 or more months after the tendon graft operation. At the present time all patients selected for tendon grafting are advised of the possibility of a tenolysis being needed as a secondary procedure.

SUMMARY

FDP tendon grafting through the intact FDS is a procedure that is not frequently indicated because of the considerable risk to the overall function of the finger. With appropriate conditions the procedure has returned excellent distal joint function, but a secondary tenolysis was required in the majority of patients. Some patients may benefit from the procedure being done in stages with a temporary silicone rubber tendon placed at the first stage.

REFERENCES

1. Bora FW: Profundus tendon grafting with unimpaired sublimis function in children, *Clin Orthop* 1970; 71:118.
2. Carroll RE, Match RM: Avulsion of the profundus tendon insertion, *J Trauma* 1970; 10:1109.
3. Chang WHJ, Thoms OJ, White WL: Avulsion injury of the long flexor tendons, *Plast Reconstr Surg* 1972; 50:260.
4. Goldner JL, Coonrad RW: Tendon grafting of the flexor profundus in the presence of a completely or partially intact flexor sublimis, *J Bone Joint Surg* 1969; 51A:527.
5. Harrison S: Repair of digital flexor tendon injuries in the hand, *J Plast Surg* 1961; 14B:211.
6. Honner R: The late management of isolated lesion of the flexor digitorum profundus tendon, *Hand* 1975; 7:171.
7. Honner R: Treatment of isolated flexor digitorum profundus injuries. In Hunter JM, Schneider LH, Mackin EJ, eds: *Tendon surgery in the hand,* St Louis, 1987, Mosby.
8. Hunter JM, Schneider LH, Dumont J, Erickson JC: A dynamic approach to problems of hand function using local anesthesia supplemented by intravenous fentanyl-droperidol, *Clin Orthop* 1974; 104:112.
9. Jaffe S, Weckesser E: Profundus tendon grafting with the sublimis intact, *J Bone Joint Surg* 1967; 49A:1298.
10. Leddy JP, Packer JP: Avulsion of the profundus insertion in athletes, *J Hand Surg* 1977; 2:66.
11. Littler JW: The physiology and dynamic function of the hand, *Surg Clin North Am* 1960; 40:259.
12. McClinton MA, Curtis RM, Wilgus S: One hundred tendon grafts for isolated flexor digitorum profundus injuries, *J Hand Surg* 1982; 7: 224.

13. Nalebuff EA: The intact sublimis. In Verdan C, ed: *Tendon surgery of the hand,* Edinburgh, 1979, Churchill Livingstone.

14. Nichols HM: The dilemma of the intact superficialis tendon, *Hand* 1975; 7:85.

15. Pulvertaft RG: The treatment of profundus division by free tendon graft, *J Bone Joint Surg* 1960; 42A:1363.

16. Reid DAC: The isolated flexor digitorum profundus lesion, *Hand* 1969; 1:115.

17. Schneider LH: Re-one hundred tendon grafts for isolated flexor digitorum profundus injuries, *J Hand Surg* 1983; 8:225 (letter to the editor).

18. Schneider LH: *Flexor tendon injuries,* Boston, 1985, Little, Brown.

19. Schneider LH: Treatment of isolated flexor digitorum profundus injuries by tendon grafting. In Hunter JM, Schneider LH, Mackin EJ, eds: *Tendon surgery in the hand,* St Louis, 1987, Mosby.

20. Schneider LH, Hunter JM, Fietti VG: The flexor superficialis finger: a salvage procedure. In Hunter JM, Schneider LH, Mackin EJ, eds: *Tendon surgery in the hand,* St Louis, 1987, Mosby.

21. Schneider LH, Hunter JM: Flexor tendons—late reconstruction. In Green DP, ed: *Operative hand surgery,* ed 3, New York, 1993, Churchill Livingstone.

22. Stark HH, Zemel NP, Boyes JH, Ashworth CR: Flexor tendon graft through intact superficialis tendon, *J Hand Surg* 1977; 2:456.

23. Strandell G: Tendon grafts in injuries of the flexor tendons in the fingers and thumb: end results in a consecutive series of 74 cases, *Acta Chir Scand* 1956; 111:124.

24. Sullivan DJ: Disappointing outcomes in staged flexor tendon grafting for isolated profundus loss, *J Hand Surg* 1986; 11B:231-233.

25. Versaci AD: Secondary tendon grafting for isolated flexor digitorum profundus injury, *Plast Reconstr Surg* 1970; 46:57.

26. Wakefield AR: The management of flexor tendon injuries, *Surg Clin North Am* 1960; 40:267.

27. Wexler MR, Lie K: Tendon grafts for isolated injuries of the flexor digitorum profundus tendon, *Isr J Med Sci* 1974; 10:1448.

28. Wilson RL, Carter MS, Holdeman VA, Lovett WL: Flexor profundus injuries treated with delayed two-stage grafting, *J Hand Surg* 1980; 5:74.

Chapter 46

TENDON GRAFTING TO THE SYNOVIAL SPACES OF THE HAND

A biologic basis for the selection of the donor tendon

John Gray Seiler III
Richard H. Gelberman

Autogenous flexor tendon grafting using donor tendons taken from extrasynovial donor sites to replace injured flexor tendons has resulted in a significant incidence of poor digital function.[1,6,7,13] Until recently most researchers have focused on the soft tissue problems within the injured digit as being the primary factors that affect outcome. Little information has been available regarding the various mechanisms of donor tendon incorporation in the specialized environment of the digital synovial sheath.

Because of recent reports that suggest that the structural differences between intrasynovial donor tendons may indicate different metabolic requirements, we postulated that these two types of dense regular connective tissue may have different fates when grafted into the synovial space for the purpose of reconstructing digital flexion.[10,12]

This chapter summarizes our findings on the biologic outcome of the two most common types of regular dense connective tissue that may be used to reconstruct digital flexion. We attempt to identify the biologically optimal source of autogenous tissue for tendon grafting and to gain insight into the other potential causes of digital stiffness following tendon grafting.

DEVELOPMENT OF THE MODEL

Because of the similarity of its flexor apparatus, a survival canine model for single-stage tendon grafting was developed.[8] All tendon grafts were done using the peroneus longus tendon as the extrasynovial donor tendon and the flexor digitorum longus (FDL) as the intrasynovial donor tendon. The peroneus longus tendon was chosen because of its paratenon covering and the similarity of its caliber to the flexor digitorum profundus (FDP) tendon. The hind paw FDL was chosen as the intrasynovial donor tendon because of its homology to the FDP tendon of the forepaw. After inducing general endotracheal anesthesia, a midlateral incision was made on the second and fifth digits of the forepaw exposing the flexor apparatus. The FDL tendon was divided distally through a 1-cm incision in the synovial sheath and the tendon retracted proximal to the mesotenon reflection. This tendon segment was excised and replaced with the FDL tendon or the peroneus longus tendon. The distal repair was done by placing a modified grasping suture of 3-0 nylon in the tendon graft and passing it out to the dorsum of the distal phalanx through drill holes. The suture was secured over a padded dorsal button. Proximally, the repair was done using an end–to–side Pulvertaft weave secured with 4-0 braided dacron suture. Postoperatively all

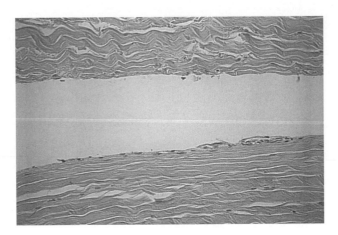

Fig. 46-1. A longitudinal section of an intrasynovial tendon graft *(bottom)* healing without the formation of surface adhesions. The gliding surface of the tendon has been preserved.

animals were immobilized in a polyurethane shoulder spica cast and underwent a program of controlled passive motion.

Using this model, experiments were designed to assess morphologic characteristics during tendon graft incorporation, the revascularization of the graft, the cellular viability within the graft, DNA content and synthesis, collagen synthesis, and the biomechanical function of the two types of tendon grafts.[2-5,9-11]

METHODS OF EVALUATION

One hundred fifty-six tendon grafts were evaluated at regular intervals from 10 days to 6 weeks following tendon grafting. The morphologic changes in the epitenon and endotenon were studied with light and transmission electron microscopy. The neovascularization of free tendon grafts was evaluated by microangiography, and the survival characteristics of tendon graft fibroblasts were studied with intravital staining and confocal microscopy. Biochemical studies were done to characterize the changes in tendon graft cellularity and to determine alterations in the extracellular matrix for the two types of donor tendons. The structural properties of the healing grafts were evaluated with a new device designed to measure proximal interphalangeal (PIP) joint angular rotation, linear tendon excursion, and the tensile strength of the repair site.

Morphology

To study the general methods of tendon graft incorporation and to focus on the morphologic changes that occur on the gliding surface of the tendon graft, we evaluated tendon grafts with light and transmission electron microscopy.[5,9]

The study of specimens showed striking differences between intrasynovial and extrasynovial tendon grafts at all time intervals. The incorporation of intrasynovial tendon grafts was accomplished with preservation of the grafts'

Fig. 46-2. By 6 weeks, dense adhesions encased extrasynovial tendon grafts.

gliding surface and with minimal apparent change in the internal architecture of the graft (Fig. 46-1). Electron microscopic examination of these specimens confirmed the findings of the light microscopy by demonstrating internal fibroblasts that appeared to be viable. In contrast, the incorporation of extrasynovial tendon grafts was characterized by early internal tendon fibroblast necrosis and by the early obliteration of the gliding tendon surface from peripherally ingrown adhesions. By 6 weeks extrasynovial tendon grafts appeared to have undergone substantial internal remodeling and were hypercellular compared with control tendon specimens. During the 6 postoperative weeks the peritendinous adhesions thickened and increased in number effectively encasing the tendon graft in a number of specimens (Fig. 46-2).

Neovascularization

To correlate the histologic findings with the neovascularization of the tendon grafts, we used a modified Spalteholz method and studied the sources, pattern, and extent of new blood vessel ingrowth for both types of tendon grafts during the first 6 postoperative weeks.[4]

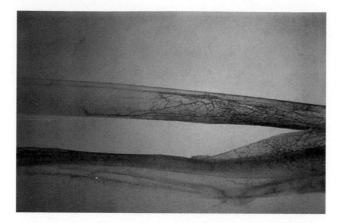

Fig. 46-3. A longitudinal view of an intrasynovial tendon graft demonstrating intrinsic neovascularization of the tendon graft.

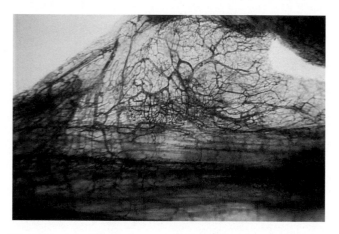

Fig. 46-4. A longitudinal section of an extrasynovial tendon graft at 3 weeks with surface adhesions welding the sheath to the tendon graft *(bottom)*.

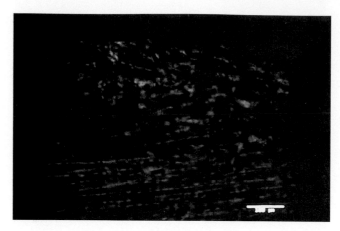

Fig. 46-5. Throughout the 6 weeks of study the intrasynovial tendon grafts were characterized by a preponderance of green-staining viable cells within the tendon graft.

The neovascularization of intrasynovial donor tendons were characterized by an intrinsic process of vascular buds growing into the tendon graft largely through the site of the proximal repair (Fig. 46-3). In contrast, extrasynovial tendon grafts were vascularized through an extrinsic process of new vessel formation extending randomly from the digital sheath to the surface of the tendon graft (Fig. 46-4). These new vessels increased in both size and number during the 6 weeks of study. Oblique radicals arborized from the surface of the tendon into the internal collagen bundles providing new vascular supply to the tendon interior.

DNA content and DNA synthesis

To give additional insight into the cellularity and cellular turnover of intrasynovial and extrasynovial tendon grafts, DNA content and DNA synthesis were measured using the methods of Bonting and Jones and of Abrahamsson.[3] Again suggesting early tendon fibroblast survival, the intrasynovial tendon grafts showed only modest increases in DNA content and synthesis during the 6-week period of study. In contrast,

extrasynovial tendon grafts showed massive increase in DNA content and an increase in DNA synthesis to over 6 times that of control specimens. The findings for the extrasynovial tendon grafts were consistent with the early densely cellular peritendinous adhesion formation and late tendon graft hypercellularity seen following graft repopulation on morphologic study with light microscopy.

Cellular survival

To evaluate variations in cellular survival, tendon grafts were stained with vital dyes and examined using confocal microscopy.[3] Intravital staining of the tendon grafts was done using calcein-AM and ethidium bromide, two chemical probes known to measure recognized parameters of cell viability and cell death. With this method, live cells stain bright green and nonviable cells appear red.

Confocal microscopy showed that the cells of intrasynovial tendon grafts were nearly uniformly viable throughout the period of study (Fig. 46-5). At 6 weeks only occasional nonviable cells were seen, consistent with a slower tendon remodeling. In contrast, extrasynovial tendon grafts underwent nearly complete early cell death, which was followed by massive cellular repopulation by 6 weeks (Figs. 46-6, 46-7, and 46-8).

Collagen production

The cellular expression of type I procollagen messenger ribonucleic acid (mRNA) and levels of reducible collagen crosslinks of intrasynovial and extrasynovial donor grafts were assessed to determine if structural evidence of increased survival translated into fundamental metabolic differences at the cellular level.[2]

After harvest of the tendon graft specimens, paraffin sections were prepared from the central portions of intrasynovial and extrasynovial grafts. Following in situ hybridization, autoradiography, and staining of sections, the levels

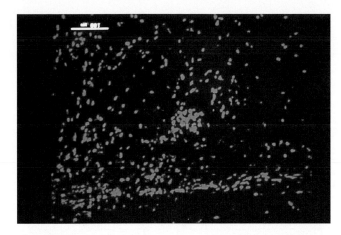

Fig. 46-6. At 10 days extrasynovial tendon grafts showed nearly complete necrosis, demonstrated by the red-staining necrotic cells.

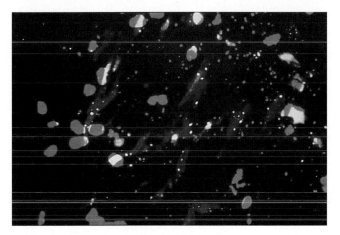

Fig. 46-7. By 3 weeks extrasynovial tendon grafts showed significant cellular repopulation demonstrated by the presence of both red (nonviable) and green (viable) cells.

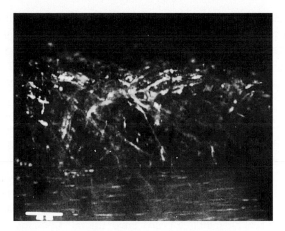

Fig. 46-8. By 6 weeks extrasynovial tendon grafts were hypercellular compared to control specimens, indicating complete cellular repopulation of the graft.

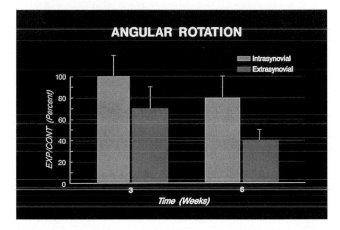

Fig. 46-9. Graph showing the values for angular rotation of the proximal interphalangeal joint for intrasynovial and extrasynovial tendon grafts (*exp,* experimental; *cont,* control).

of procollagen mRNA were assessed by microscopic examination.

The two types of tendon grafts exhibited different levels of pro-α1 (I) collagen mRNA expression at all study intervals. Intrasynovial tendon grafts displayed no areas of increased type I mRNA at 2, 4, and 6 weeks. The extrasynovial tendon grafts displayed increased surface levels of type I procollagen mRNA at 2 and 4 weeks, which decreased by 6 weeks to background levels. The high levels of procollagen mRNA exhibited by the extrasynovial grafts suggest increased collagen synthetic activity indicative of a cellular response to injury, whereas preservation of the low levels of expression in the intrasynovial grafts may signify minimal tissue requirements for satisfactory tendon repair when grafted to the synovial space.

Biomechanics

To evaluate the functional performance of the two types of tendon grafts a biomechanical assessment was done at 3 and 6 weeks following tendon grafting.[9] The linear excur-

sion (gliding function) of the tendon grafts within the sheaths was evaluated with a device designed to measure angular rotation of the PIP with a 1.5 N load applied to the proximal tendon end. The strength of the distal repair site was determined by uniaxial tensile testing to failure on an Instron testing machine. Specially designed clamps were used to secure the phalanx and to grasp the proximal tendon end. To obtain tissue equilibrium, clamped specimens were immersed in a 37° C, 0.9% saline bath for 15 minutes before testing. After a 0.5 N preload was applied to the tendons, the specimens were loaded at a crosshead speed of 20 mm/min until failure occurred.

The results of biomechanical testing showed consistent functional differences between the two tendon types. Intrasynovial tendon grafts demonstrated significantly greater angular rotation of the PIP joint than did extrasynovial tendon grafts ($p < 0.5$) (Fig. 46-9). The values for angular rotation of the intrasynovial tendon grafts were not significantly different when comparing the 3-week and the

6-week values, indicating the gliding surface of the tendon was functioning well. In contrast, the early loss of angular rotation seen with extrasynovial tendon grafts correlates well with the previous morphologic study indicating early obliteration of the gliding surface, which restricts normal tendon excursion and PIP joint rotation.

DISCUSSION

Traditionally the choice of the donor tendon used for flexor tendon grafting has been based on the accessibility, expendability, and availability of extrasynovial tendons such as the palmaris longus. Complications have not been infrequent and the poor outcomes reported in the literature have been attributed to associated digital problems such as digital and flexor apparatus scarring, associated fracture, or associated nerve injury. Although these factors certainly play a role in the ultimate function of the digit, it is possible that the selection of the donor tendon also has a role in affecting tendon graft incorporation and ultimately digital function.

Weber and colleagues were among the first to report the findings of a detailed morphologic study of intrasynovial digital flexor tendons.[12] They observed pores within the tendon surface, which were connected to intratendinous canaliculi, and postulated that this canal system facilitated synovial fluid diffusion and tendon nutrition in an area of the tendon known to be hypovascular. Other light microscopic studies directly comparing tendon morphologies have concluded that most tendons (extrasynovial tendons) are covered with an areolar, vascular paratenon.[10,11] Some specialized tendons, such as the digital flexor tendons (intrasynovial tendons), are characterized by an absence of paratenon and have a covering layer of flattened fibroblasts and hyaluronic acid that forms the gliding surface layer that is critical to efficient digital flexion. Although there are obvious morphologic differences between tendons with a paratenon covering (extrasynovial tendons) and those without such a covering (intrasynovial tendons), the potential for incorporation within the digital sheath for these two types of tendons has not been systematically examined in a clinically relevant animal model until recently.[11,12]

The striking findings of the experiment characterizing the morphologic tendon changes during graft incorporation suggest that the two tendon types have different metabolic requirements and that the incorporation of dense regular connective tissue when grafted to the synovial space is donor tissue specific (Fig. 46-10).[9] Intrasynovial donor tendons have the capability to incorporate without the formation of dense peritendinous adhesions and with the preservation of the gliding surface that is critical to tendon function.

The findings of the morphologic study were confirmed by the experiments examining DNA content, DNA synthesis, and cellular survival with vital microscopy.[2,3] These studies also suggested that intrasynovial and extrasynovial donor tendons were characterized by different methods of soft

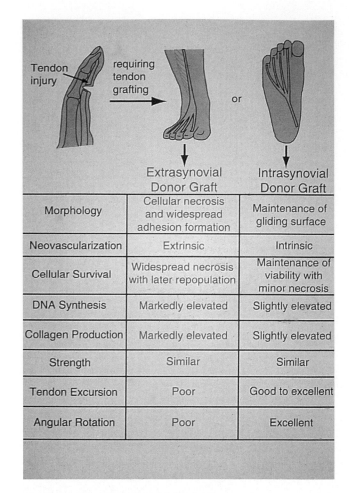

	Extrasynovial Donor Graft	Intrasynovial Donor Graft
Morphology	Cellular necrosis and widespread adhesion formation	Maintenance of gliding surface
Neovascularization	Extrinsic	Intrinsic
Cellular Survival	Widespread necrosis with later repopulation	Maintenance of viability with minor necrosis
DNA Synthesis	Markedly elevated	Slightly elevated
Collagen Production	Markedly elevated	Slightly elevated
Strength	Similar	Similar
Tendon Excursion	Poor	Good to excellent
Angular Rotation	Poor	Excellent

Fig. 46-10. Summary table of the findings.

tissue incorporation. For extrasynovial donor tendons the large increases in DNA synthesis and DNA content, at all intervals studied, reflected the early and thorough cellular substitution that was also seen on vital microscopy. In contrast, intrasynovial donor tendons were able to, in large part, survive the grafting process to the synovial space. While these studies cannot confirm the specific cellular mechanism for the improved survival of intrasynovial tendons, it seems likely that it is related to the metabolic requirements of the intrasynovial donor tendons and the specialized structural features of these tendons, which facilitate synovial fluid nutrition.

Most importantly, our studies indicate that the improved survivability associated with preservation of the gliding surface for intrasynovial donor tendons results in improved functional performance.[9,11] Biomechanical testing of the intrasynovial tendon graft specimens showed significantly improved angular rotation of the PIP joint, indicating that in the experimental setting improved outcome could be expected by using tendon grafts of this type.

Although a number of factors impact digital function following tendon grafting, it now seems likely that the selection of the donor tendon may also have a role in outcome. In contrast to the traditional selected extrasynovial palmaris longus tendon, intrasynovial tendon grafts appear specially adapted to survive and repair in the specialized environment of the digital synovial sheath. These tissue-specific effects explain, in part, the variable results reported in clinical trials examining traditional methods of digital flexor tendon grafting. Incorporation of intrasynovial tendons can experimentally be accomplished with preservation of the gliding surface, slow intratendinous neovascularization, slightly increased cellularity, and improved angular rotation of the PIP joint.[2-5,9,11] The results of these experimental studies will need to be confirmed in anatomic and clinical trials of digital flexor tendon grafting that specifically examine the variable of the donor tendon.[11]

REFERENCES

1. Amadio PC, Wood MB, Cooney WP, Bogard SD: Staged flexor tendon reconstruction in the fingers and hand, *J Hand Surg* 1988; 13A:559-562.
2. Amiel D, Harwood FL, Gelberman RH, et al: Intrasynovial and extrasynovial autogenous tendon grafts: an experimental study of mRNA procollagen expression in dogs, *J Orthop Res* (in press).
3. Ark JW, Gelberman RH, Abrahamsson SO, et al: Cellular survival and proliferation in autogenous flexor tendon grafts, *J Hand Surg* 1994; 19:249-258.
4. Gelberman RH, Chu CR, Williams CS, et al: Angiogenesis in healing autogenous flexor tendon grafts, *J Bone Joint Surg* 1992; 74A:1207-1216.
5. Gelberman RH, Seiler JG, Rosenberg AE, et al: Intercalary flexor tendon grafts: a morphological study of intrasynovial and extrasynovial donor tendons, *Scand J Plast Reconstr Hand Surg* 1992; 26(3):257-264.
6. Hunter JM, Salisbury RE: Flexor tendon reconstruction in severely damaged hands: a two stage procedure using a silicone dacron reinforced gliding prosthesis prior to tendon grafting, *J Bone Joint Surg* 1971; 53A:829-858.
7. LaSalle WB, Strickland JW: An evaluation of the two-stage flexor tendon reconstruction technique, *J Hand Surg* 1983; 8A:263-267.
8. Noguchi M, Seiler JG, Chan SS, et al: Tensile properties of intrasynovial and extrasynovial flexor tendon autografts, *J Orthop Res* (submitted for publication).
9. Seiler JG, Gelberman RH, Williams CS, et al: Autogenous flexor tendon grafts: a biomechanical and morphological study in dogs, *J Bone Joint Surg* 1993; 75A:1004-1013.
10. Seiler JG, Chu CR, Abrahamsson SO, Gelberman RH: The fate of autogenous flexor tendon grafts, *Iowa J Orthop* 1993; 13:56-62.
11. Seiler JG, Simpson L, Reddy A, et al: The flexor digitorum longus: an anatomical study of its use as a donor tendon for tendon grafting, *J Hand Surg* (in press).
12. Weber ER: Optimizing tendon repairs within the digital sheath. In Tubiana R, ed: *The hand,* vol 3, Philadelphia, 1988, Saunders.
13. Wehbé MA, Hunter JM, Schneider LH, Goodwyn BL: Two-stage flexor tendon reconstruction: ten year experience, *J Bone Joint Surg* 1986; 68A, 742-763.

Chapter 47

FLEXOR TENDON GRAFTS IN THE FINGERS AND THUMB

An evaluation of end results*

Joseph H. Boyes

Reconstruction of the flexor tendon mechanism in digits is most difficult in the area lying between the distal crease of the palm and the middle flexion creases of the fingers. In this critical zone, so aptly called "no-man's land" by Bunnell, both flexor tendons pass through the fibrous tunnels or pulleys: Any scarring from injury, infection, or previous surgery impairs the gliding motion of the tendon and restricts the flexion of the digits. In order to flex the interphalangeal (IP) joints of the finger completely, the deep flexor tendon must make an excursion of three fourths of an inch in the proximal segment of the finger and one and three-eighths inches in the palm.[1] If this excursion is limited, the tip of the finger fails to touch the distal crease of the palm. The measurement of this distance, *the lack of flexion to the distal crease,* thus becomes an easily recorded and readily understood index of the results of flexor tendon action in the fingers. In the thumb, the long flexor tendon acts primarily on the IP joint. Flexion here is best measured in degrees of the arc that the tip of the thumb makes from a line parallel to the proximal phalanx. Its percentage of motion is determined by comparison with the range of passive motion in the same joint.

This study is limited to cases involving damage to flexor tendons in the "critical" zone,[1] because reconstruction in this area offers the most rigid test of operative technique. A total of 138 grafts were used in 118 patients. Twenty-

three of these were in the thumb, 43 in the index finger, 29 in the long finger, 13 in the ring finger, and 30 in the little finger. Multiple tendon reconstructions were done in 11 patients: the thumb and index finger together twice; the thumb and long finger once; the index finger and long finger five times; the index finger and ring finger once; the index finger, long finger, and ring finger once; and all four fingers once. The end results are known in all but 13 cases. Therefore the final figures are based upon a study of 104 flexor tendon grafts in the fingers and 21 flexor tendon grafts in the thumb.

The basic technique used throughout this study was that described by Bunnell, namely, a full-length tendon graft extending from the lumbricalis origin in the palm to the terminal phalanx of the digit; the distal attachment was tendon-to-bone, the proximal suture being in the palm, inserted according to the Bunnell technique. Pulleys were reconstructed at the metacarpal heads by free graft when necessary, and the pulley mechanisms in the fingers were restored by suture of the deeper tissues. To provide material for the graft, either the proximal portion of the sublimis tendon from the involved digit was used, or the palmaris longus tendon from the forearm. In a few instances it was necessary to take the long extensor tendons of the toes. In the majority of cases digital nerve damage accompanied the tendon injury; whenever possible, this was repaired at the time of the tendon operation.

An evaluation of the end results of flexor tendon reconstruction must take into consideration the preoperative condition of the hand. Three major factors influence the

*Read at the Annual Meeting of The American Academy of Orthopaedic Surgeons, New York, N.Y., February 15, 1950. (From *J Bone Joint Surg* 1950; 32A[3]:489-499.)

410

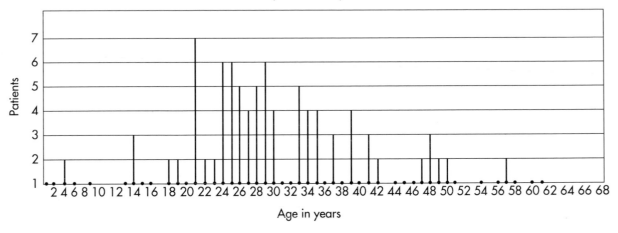

Fig. 47-1. Age affects the end results of flexor tendon grafting in the fingers only in the very young, where there is lack of cooperation in the after-care.

results: scar tissue, stiff joints, and trophic changes from nerve damage. The reconstruction of more than one digit at the same time usually impairs the result, and there are other factors that cannot be foretold, such as the individual's reaction to trauma and the patient's willingness to work and exercise for a better result, in spite of some discomfort. Fig. 47-1 shows the age groups involved in this study, and indicates that age in itself apparently does not influence the end results, except in the very young, where there is lack of cooperation in the after-care.

CLASSIFICATION OF CASES

In this study all cases were classified preoperatively into one of five groups, based upon the condition seen when the patient was first examined. In a few cases, preliminary operation was done to improve the function of the joint or to remove excessive or deforming scars. In many instances a period of slow, gradual, elastic traction was used to mobilize the joints before tendon reconstruction was attempted. The criteria used in classifying cases were as follows:

Good. This was the ideal group, with minimal scarring in the skin and soft tissue, good supple joints, no ligamentous or capsular contractures, and no major trophic changes from nerve damage. The loss of function of one or both of the digital nerves was not considered detrimental, and such cases were classed in this group unless trophic changes were severe.

Cicatrix. In this group were included cases in which there was scarring from the injury or from ill-advised midline incisions, or in which deep cicatrix followed infection from attempted primary repair. The contractures resulted from deep scar tissue rather than from joint stiffness. In a few instances a preliminary Z-plasty

was done or a pedicle flap was applied to repair the soft tissue damage before tendon reconstruction was carried out.

Joint damage. Cases were classed in this group when the range of passive motion of an IP joint was restricted. A period of slow, gradual, elastic traction was carried out, and as much easy, free, passive motion as possible was obtained before the tendon was reconstructed.

Nerve damage. This was a small group, limited to those cases in which damage to the major nerve trunks caused trophic changes in the fingers and resulted in smooth, shiny skin and secondary stiffness of the joints. In some instances the major nerve damage was repaired, and the tendon was reconstructed after regeneration had taken place.

Multiple damage. Where tendon damage was not confined to one digit, an attempt was made to reconstruct all the damaged tendons at one operation. Many of these cases were complicated by other factors, such as cicatrix and joint stiffness. These were combined into one group.

The number and proportions of the 104 tendon grafts in the fingers in each classification are shown in Fig. 47-2, *A*.

RESULTS

The results of tendon grafts in the fingers are best presented graphically, the percentage of cases (shown on the vertical line) being plotted against the distance by which the pulp of the finger failed to reach the distal crease of the palm (shown on the horizontal axis). Fig. 47-2, *B* shows the ideal result which would occur if flexion were sufficient in all cases so that the tip of the finger could touch the distal crease of the palm. In the succeeding charts, improvement may be noted as the curve representing results approaches this theoretically perfect picture.

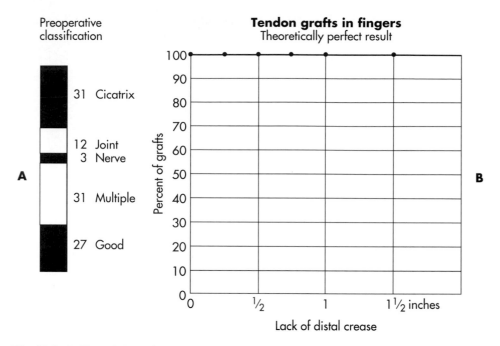

Fig. 47-2. A, The relative proportion of cases having factors which influence the results of flexor tendon grafting in the fingers, as seen in this series of 104 consecutive cases. B, Showing the ideal result which would occur if in all cases in a series, flexion of the finger to the distal crease of the palm were possible after tendon grafting.

Fig. 47-3 shows the results in all 104 cases of tendon grafts in the fingers, and the effect of the preoperative condition upon the end result. Whereas in 10% of cases in the "good" classification flexion was sufficient so that the pulp of the finger touched the distal crease of the palm, in not a single case in the other classifications was flexion possible to this complete degree. In the "cicatrix" group, the best result was flexion to one-half inch from the distal palmar crease, whereas in the group classified as "good," 35% had flexion to that degree and all patients had flexion to within one and one-half inches of the distal crease. In the "cicatrix" group, only 40% had flexion to within one and one-half inches of the distal crease in the palm; in the "multiple" group, 59% and in the "joint" group, 60%. The results in the "joint" cases approximate those in the "good" cases, because elastic traction and mobilization were carried out before tendon reconstruction was done. However, in these patients the same tendency for stiffness of the joints followed the operation as well as the injury and, therefore, the end results are not so good as in the ideal group.

Fig. 47-4 shows the effect on the end result of four variations in technique. In the first group, silk was used both at the suture line in the palm and at the distal insertion into the phalanx.

In the second group, silk was again used in the palm, but a Bunnell type of pullout wire suture of stainless steel, passed through a drill hole in the terminal phalanx and tied to a button over the nail, was used at the insertion of the graft into the terminal phalanx. This wire was removed after three

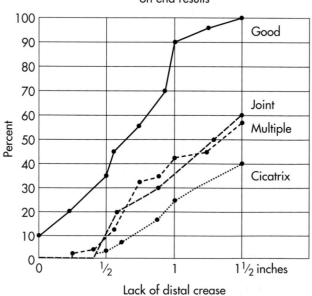

Fig. 47-3. Illustrating the effect of preoperative factors on the end results. Whereas almost 90% of cases in the "good" group had flexion to within one inch of the distal crease, less than half of those having stiff joints and only one quarter of the "cicatrix" group had such a good degree of flexion.

Influence of technique on end results

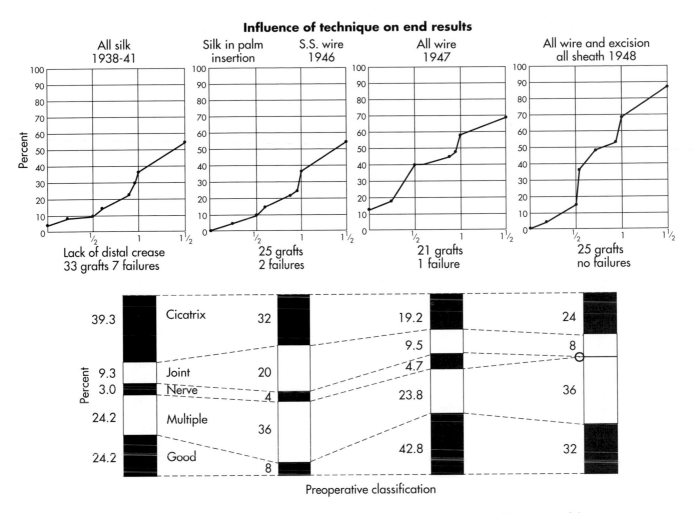

Fig. 47-4. Regardless of all other factors, the progressive increase in steepness of the curves of the four graphs indicates improvement in results due to the one variable—technique. The large number of failures in the period from 1938 to 1941 were caused by complications from the buried silk sutures; this difficulty had been overcome in the 1948 series. The lower bars illustrate in percentage the preoperative factors present in the various groups. (See Fig. 47-5 for the effect of technique on comparable classes.)

weeks. It can be seen from Fig. 47-4 that there was relatively little difference in the end results. However, the classification in the lower portion of the chart shows that only 8% of the cases in this group were "good" as compared with 24.2% in the group in which only silk sutures were used. The greatest difference, however, is seen in the number of failures. There were seven failures in the silk series, all due to infection occurring around the silk, whereas there were only two failures in the second group, neither of which was due to complications at the insertion of the graft.

In the third group, stainless-steel wire was used throughout, both at the insertion and as a buried suture in the palm. Here the end results were better, with flexion to the distal crease in the palm in 13% and only one failure. The percentage of "good" cases was slightly higher here than in any other group, although hardly enough to account for the marked improvement in results.

In the last series, not only was stainless-steel wire used throughout, but a deliberate excision of all remaining sheath tissue was done in the fingers, and in most instances the pulley in the middle segment was excised. Its action was restored by suturing the deep fascia with nonabsorbable cotton sutures. In this series there were no failures and, in spite of the smaller percentage of "good" cases, the end results were better. Although none of the fingers had complete flexion to the distal crease in the palm, 7% flexed to within one and one-half inches. The curve can now be seen to rise more steeply and thus is approaching the ideal shown in Fig. 47-2, *A*.

Fig. 47-5 illustrates more clearly the effect of these changes in technique. A comparison is made of results in two series of cases in which the only variable factor was a change in technique, the 1938 series consisting entirely of silk sutures and the 1948 series entirely of wire with excision of

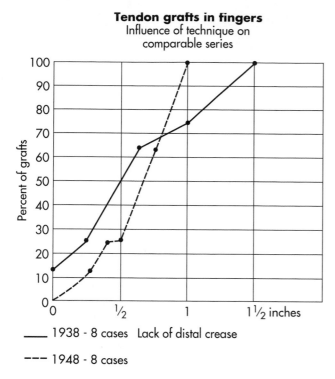

Tendon grafts in fingers
Influence of technique on
comparable series

_____ 1938 - 8 cases   Lack of distal crease

- - - 1948 - 8 cases

Fig. 47-5. The results of flexor tendon grafting in the fingers in two series of similar cases are shown. In 1938, silk sutures were used entirely; in 1948, wire was used in all. All cases were selected from the "good" classification. Flexion was possible to within one and one-half inches of the distal crease when silk was used, but in only 73% was flexion possible to within one inch. Use of wire in a similar group resulted in all cases in flexion to within one inch, and in 25% in flexion to within one-half inch of the distal crease of the palm.

the sheath. Each series comprised eight "good" cases; thus 12.5% on the vertical line represents one case. In the 1938 series, one case had flexion to the distal crease and all had flexion to within one and one-half inches. In 1948, one case had flexion to within one-quarter inch of the distal crease and all had flexion to within 1 inch.

INFLUENCE OF SOURCE OF GRAFT

Tendons to be used as grafts are better if of small diameter, so that they can be easily nourished by the surrounding tissues, which are often scarred from injury; the tendons should have a smooth, gliding surface. The palmaris longus tendon is ideal. However, it is absent in about 10% of patients and is often too short. The proximal portion of the sublimis tendon of the involved digit is next best. This, however, lacks the true paratenon layer, which makes up the gliding surface of the palmaris longus, and is sometimes of greater diameter than is desired. Comparison of results (Fig. 47-6) shows that a greater number of those fingers in which the palmaris was used can flex to touch the palm. Recent experience indicates that a deliberate block removal of the true paratenon layer with the palmaris longus produces even better results, especially when much scarring is present. It

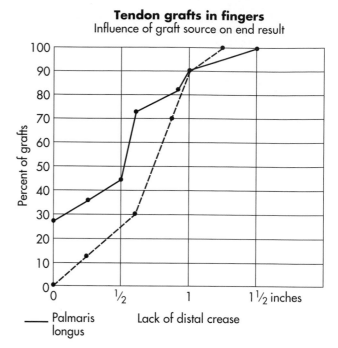

Tendon grafts in fingers
Influence of graft source on end result

_____ Palmaris   Lack of distal crease
        longus

- - - Sublimis

Fig. 47-6. In the cases classified as "good," with similar technique, the palmaris longus tendon gives better results as a graft than the sublimis of the same digit. This finding is most noticeable in this series in the high percentage of cases with flexion to less than one-half inch from the distal crease of the palm.

has not been felt necessary to make a new sheath by the preliminary insertion of celloidin, plastic or stainless-steel ribbons, or tubes.

COMPLICATIONS AND FAILURES

Of the 104 grafts in the fingers, there were 10 instances in which the IP joints failed to flex to any appreciable degree following operation. These cases were classified as failures. Seven of these occurred in the series in which only silk sutures were used; in each instance there was a severe foreign body reaction with drainage, requiring removal of the suture material. In three patients the complication occurred at the proximal suture line in the palm. One case involved all four fingers, accounting for four of the failures. In the second series, where silk sutures were used in the palm and pullout wire sutures at the insertion, there were only two failures, both due to complications in the palm. One failure occurred in the third series and none in the last series.

Ten secondary operations were performed—four in the first series, and three each in the second and third series. These operations were done after several months, in order to remove excess scar, free the tendons, or, in a few instances, to insert paratenon-like gliding tissues.

Minor flexion contracture, limiting extension of the digit at the middle joint, is not disabling. In 27 instances (26%)

Tendon grafts in the thumb
End results in good cases

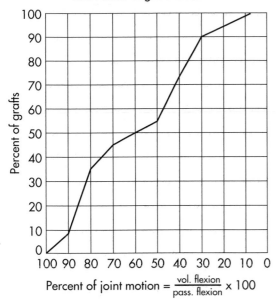

Percent of joint motion = $\frac{\text{vol. flexion}}{\text{pass. flexion}} \times 100$

Fig. 47-7. Results of flexor tendon grafting in the thumb, in a series of 21 cases treated by varying techniques. Better results were obtained by a long graft, extending from the terminal phalanx to the musculotendinous junction of the forearm, than by a proximal suture line placed in the thenar eminence.

there were flexion contractures of 5° or more; in only 5 of these (4.8%) was the limitation more than 30°.

TENDON GRAFTS IN THE THUMB

The end results are known in 21 of 23 cases in which flexor tendon grafts were used in the thumb. Function was recorded by measuring in degrees the voluntary flexion of the IP joint. This figure was used as a numerator, the passive flexion of the joint being taken as a denominator. The fraction was then reduced to a percentage. The cases classified as "cicatrix," "joint," "trophic," and "multiple"

are too few to be shown graphically, but the same general effect of preoperative condition on the end results was noted as in the series in the fingers. The results for the 11 cases in the "good" group are shown graphically in Fig. 47-7. As all injuries were in the thumb itself, the grafts were inserted into the distal phalanx and the proximal suture line was usually placed in the thenar eminence. In two cases a longer graft was used, and the proximal suture line was placed at the musculotendinous junction in the forearm. The results in these two cases were the best in the series, one attaining flexion of 95% of normal and the other 80%. Utilization of a long graft to avoid a suture line in the palm should be done wherever possible.[2]

CONCLUSIONS

A study of the end results in a series of flexor tendon grafts in the fingers and thumb, inserted because of damage to the tendons in the "critical" zone, shows that the influencing factors, in order of importance, are cicatrix from injury or infection, stiffened joints, trophic changes, and damage to more than one digit. Improvement in results has followed the use of Bunnell-type stainless-steel wire sutures in place of silk, combined with meticulous excision of scar and thickened sheath tissue. The use of the palmaris longus tendon as a graft has given better results than use of other tendons. In the thumb, a graft from the musculotendinous origin to the insertion is preferred. It has been shown that, under ideal conditions, the results of digital flexor tendon grafts are as follows: In 25% of the cases flexion is complete, so that the pulp of the finger reaches the distal crease of the palm; in 50%, the pulp reaches to within one-half inch of the distal crease of the palm.

REFERENCES

1. Boyes JH: Immediate vs. delayed repair of the digital flexor tendons, *Ann Western Med Surg* 1947; 1:145-152.
2. Bunnell S: *Surgery of the hand*, ed 2, Philadelphia, 1948, Lippincott.

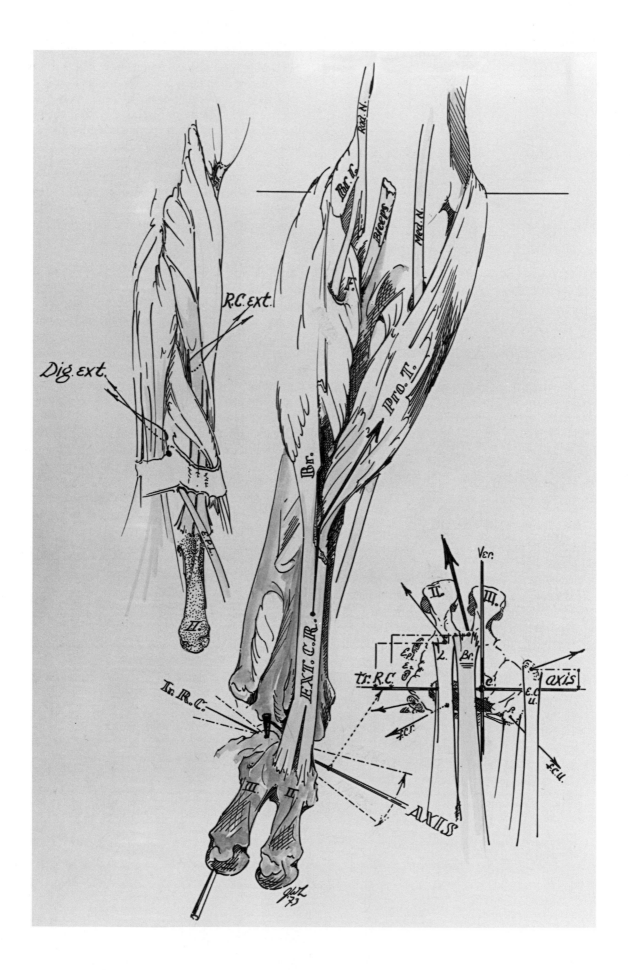

Part XI

TENDON TRANSFERS

Dynamic wrist stabilization is fundamental to hand function. (From Converse JM: *Reconstructive plastic surgery: principles in correction, reconstruction and transplantation,* ed 2, vol vi, Philadelphia, 1977, Saunders.)

Chapter 48

ASPECTS OF FLEXOR TENDON FUNCTION

Paul W. Brand

Hand surgeons and therapists have a practical interest in the functions of flexor tendons in two major groups of conditions: when tendons are injured and when the function of flexor tendons is disturbed by paralysis and other problems that affect flexor tendon function from outside the tendon. This chapter addresses aspects of the function of uninjured flexor tendons that have had their biomechanics modified by other factors affecting the balance of the hand.

All flexor tendons have in common the fact that they cross many joints, and none of them has the ability to change the distribution of tension and, therefore, of torque between the various joints that they cross. Each flexor muscle has control of the tension it can produce, but that tension is the same along the whole length of its tendon. This results in *flexor torque,* also called *flexor moment,* at every joint that the tendon crosses, differing only in proportion to the moment arm at each joint.

Consider first the way in which external load affects the flexor torque at each joint and then the way in which static structures within the hand may affect and may be affected by the torque at each joint. Then consider the role of surgery and conservative therapy in attempts to restore balance to the sequence of flexion of the joints of the hand.

Fig. 48-1 shows a diagram of a finger in which the only flexor tendon is the flexor digitorum profundus (FDP). I have marked the flexor torque at each joint, assuming that there is a tension of just 2 kg of force (kgF) in the tendon. It is convenient to remember the following sequence of flexor tendon moment arms for the joints of the middle finger of an average hand. The moment arm at the metacarpophalangeal (MP) joint is about 1 cm, the proxi-

mal interphalangeal (PIP) joint is 0.75 cm, and the distal interphalangeal (DIP) joint is 0.5 cm. This sequence is proportional to the tapering thickness of the digit and, thus, probably also to the stiffness or resistance because of normal soft tissue around the joint that needs to be folded or stretched as the joint moves.

Thus, in a newly paralysed hand, a single remaining active profundus muscle and tendon can flex the whole digit in a smooth curve that appears normal. Long[3] has shown that such unopposed flexion in a normal hand is usually carried out by the profundus muscle alone, with the superficialis muscle and tendon just going along for the ride, having little or no active contraction at all.

Things are very different when the hand is at work and there is an opposing external load, especially when the load is on the distal segment of the finger (Fig. 48-2). A distal external load exercises an extensor thrust at every joint, causing an extensor torque directly opposing torque from flexor tendon tension. However, this opposing torque is not in proportion to the thickness of the digit, it is in proportion to the length of the digit between the point of application of the load and the axis of the affected joint.

In Fig. 48-3, a distal external force of 2 kg is seen to result in an extensor torque of 4 kg/cm at the distal joint, which is 2 cm proximal to the load, and of 21 kg/cm at the MP joint, 10.5 cm down the finger. As soon as the finger senses the effect of the external thrust at the DIP joint, the profundus muscle increases its tension to 8 kg, so that with its 0.5-cm moment arm, it may create a matching torque of 4 kg/cm at the distal joint. With the distal joint in balance, the tendon tension is much too weak to control the PIP joint where 8 kg of tension at a 0.75-cm moment arm gives only 6 kg/cm

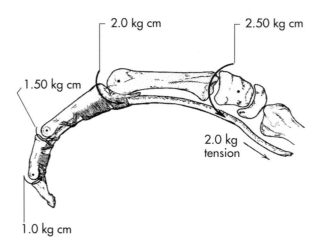

Fig. 48-1. Finger with only a profundus tendon exerting 2 kg of tension, resulting in flexor torque at each joint in proportion to the moment arm at that joint.

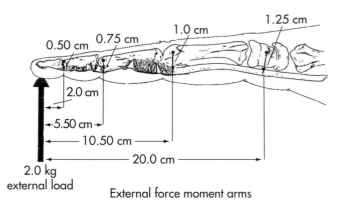

External force moment arms

Fig. 48-2. The same finger being subjected to an external force at its tip, which results in extensor torque at each joint in proportion to the moment arm of the force at the axis of each joint.

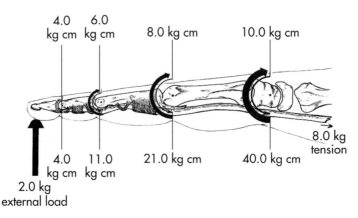

Fig. 48-3. Finger as in Fig. 48-2, with 2 kg of external extensor force at the tip. The profundus is now exerting 8 kg of tension to balance the DIP joint at the 0.5-cm moment arm (= 4 kg/cm of torque) against the opposing external force of 2 kg at a 2-cm moment arm (= 4 kg/cm torque). At this tension of the profundus, no balance is possible without additional muscles at any of the more proximal joints, which are forced into extension by much higher torque from the larger moment arms for the external force.

torque to match the extensor torque of 12 kg/cm, resulting from 2 kg at 6 cm. To prevent hyperextension at the proximal joints, the profundus increases its tension, which now becomes too high at the DIP joint, resulting in hyperflexion there. This sequence of events is most commonly observed in the thumb, where it is called Froment's sign. Those of us who have done long-term follow-up studies on fingers that have been deprived of their flexor superficialis tendons for transfer elsewhere have all seen the late development of sharp flexion of the DIP joint, sometimes followed by hyperextension of the PIP joint, resulting in an ugly "swan-neck" deformity in many such deprived fingers (Fig. 48-4).

These deformities are so biomechanically predictable, especially in slender, highly mobile fingers, that I find it hard to understand why the old Stiles-Bunnell[1,2] operation and the relatively new Lasso operation of Zancolli[4,5] are still so widely practiced. Both these operations leave the PIP joint without its own independent flexor tendon and are only justifiable in fingers that have so much stiffness, preoperatively limiting extension at the PIP joint, that full correction appears unlikely, and overcorrection still more unlikely.

If, for any reason, transfer of a superficialis tendon seems indicated, I recommend follow-up examinations after several months. If an early flexion deformity of the DIP joint is seen, the patient should be informed that this is a progressive condition and may become quite ugly. The surgeon should recommend a tenodesis of half the thickness of the profundus tendon near the base of the middle phalanx, at a tension that holds the DIP joint at an acceptable and functional position. This operation turns the profundus tendon functionally into a superficialis tendon with a tenodesis extension for the DIP joint. It is

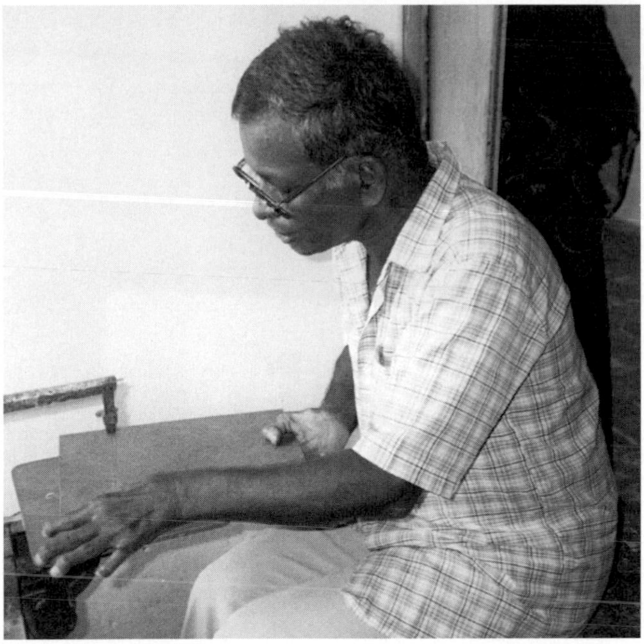

Fig. 48-4. Recent unposed photograph sent to me from India, of a man I operated on 45 years ago, using sublimis transfers for claw hands, with an excellent result at that time. Note that he now has swan-neck deformities of his fingers.

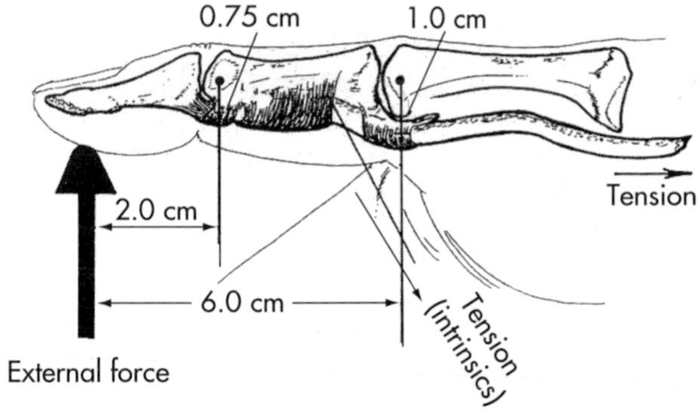

Fig. 48-5. Normal thumb with flexor pollicis longus exerting enough tension at the interphalangeal joint to balance the extensor torque produced by the external force at its tip. The same external force will create three times as much extensor torque at the metacarpophalangeal joint. The additional flexor torque that is needed to balance this joint is provided by the intrinsic muscles, adductor policis and flexor policis brevis.

better to have a PIP joint under good control and a DIP joint stabilized in good position, than a swan-neck deformity.

The condition in which a single isolated long flexor tendon remains as the only flexor in a digit is more common in the thumb, where the flexor pollicis longus (FPL) may be left as the only flexor after ulnar palsy (Fig. 48-5). Here a flexed terminal joint with a hyperextended MP joint is a well-recognized problem (Figs. 48-6 and 48-7). In the thumb, however, if a joint is to be fixed it is usually better to arthrodese the MP joint than the interphalangeal (IP) joint, because the end of the thumb needs to be free to adapt its posture to the surface of the digit it is opposing in pinch. Once the MP joint is either arthrodesed or given an independent flexor, the previously flexed IP joint comes under control, so long as its passive range of motion has been restored.

Now, moving proxially to look at the biomechanics of the third joint from the tip of a digit, (the MP joint of the fingers and the carpometacarpal [CMC] joint of the thumb) we come across some interesting contrasts. In all digits, paralysis of the intrinsic muscles deprives these basic joints of their prime flexors. The result in the fingers and in the thumb are quite different from each other. In the fingers the palmar plates become gradually stretched under the relatively unopposed pull of the extensors, together with the extensor torque of external loads using long moment arms. The MP joints become hyperextended, and the IP joints become clawed.

Most hand surgeons now respond by adding a transferred muscle-tendon graft or transfer to restore independent active MP flexion. There are still a few who use the biomechanical trick of capsuloplasty, both to form a passive block to MP hyperextension and to advance the pulley of the flexor sheath so that the long flexors are allowed to bowstring across the joint and increase their moment arm there. The result is supposed to allow MP flexion to begin ahead of IP flexion, thus correcting clawing of the digits and promoting the normal sequence of finger flexion.

There are two biomechanical errors in this procedure. The first is that in any kind of bow, bowstringing occurs only when the bow is bent. Thus, when the finger is straight, the long flexor tendons still lie on the skeletal plane, with no increase of moment arm. Thus the distal joints still flex ahead of the MP joint, especially when there is a distal load. Only after the finger has begun to bend does tendon bowstringing give any mechanical advantage at the MP joint by the pulley advancement. At that late stage of grasp, torque is most needed distally and can be spared proximally.

The second error is the assumption that a tightened palmar plate will stay tight in the presence of unbalanced tendon tensions for month after month and year after year. I once visited the late Dr. Borsani in Rosario, Argentina (a dedicated surgeon who had performed many hundreds of these operations on leprosy patients). We reviewed some of his patients, and he smiled wryly as we noted recurrent MP hyperextension in many of the cases. He said, "Those were done in the days I tried to be neat and meticulous, like a real hand surgeon. I soon learned that I had to make a mess in front of the MP joint if I wanted to avoid recurrence. Now I scratch the bone and the capsule and everything I can see except the tendon itself. In that way I make a lot of scar, and that holds up better than the palmar plate by itself." The problem is that the palmar plate is less than 1 cm from the

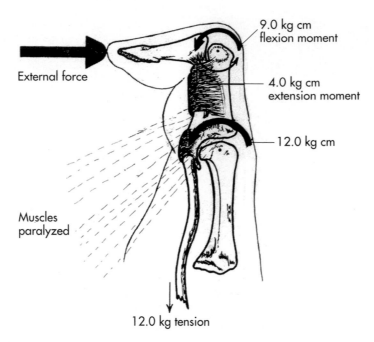

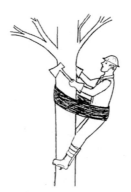

External force

Muscles
paralyzed

9.0 kg cm
flexion moment

4.0 kg cm
extension moment

12.0 kg cm

12.0 kg tension

Fig. 48-6. Thumb with ulnar nerve paralysis has only the flexor pollicis longus (FPL) to flex the distal interphalangeal (DIP) and the metacarpophalangeal (MP) joints. To prevent hyperextension from the extensor torque at the MP joint, the FPL increases its tension, thereby providing excessive torque at the DIP joint, which goes into acute flexion. This results in the disability known as Froment's sign.

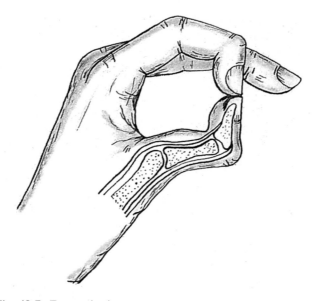

Fig. 48-7. Froment's sign.

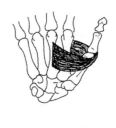

Fig. 48-8. A lumberjack climbing a tree has two choices about how to support himself while he works. (1) He may use muscles—his arms. (2) He may use a passive sling around his hips and around the tree trunk. He may now lean back in the sling (passive fascia), leaving his hands free to work. The thumb metacarpal, to prevent itself from falling away from the palm in hyperextension at the carpometacarpal joint, usually uses muscles. If these intrinsic muscles are paralyzed, it uses a passive sling (thumb web) as the lumberjack does.

axis of the joint, so it has only a small moment arm and is subjected to high tension whenever the extensor tendons or a distal load force the finger back. Little by little the palmar plate becomes lengthened by this high tension.

At the base of the thumb the situation is different. It is similar in that in the absence of the intrinsic muscles, the joint has very weak flexion torque. The FPL has less than 1.5 cm moment arm for flexion at the CMC joint, no more than it has at the MP joint. Yet it is subject to extensor torque from external force at the tip of the thumb, which has a leverage or moment arm of 10 cm. There is no contest. It should become hyperextended. Yet most surgeons, including myself, have been content in such cases to do a tendon transfer only to restore abduction and opposition to the thumb at the CMC joint and do nothing to support the base of the thumb against the huge extensor torque at the CMC joint every time the thumb takes part in pinch. Our results were not bad, either.

I have to confess that only in the past few years have I stopped to wonder how the balance of the base of the thumb is maintained in pinch when all the prime flexors of the joint are missing and the flexor pollicis longus alone resists hyperextension, with a severely reduced moment arm.

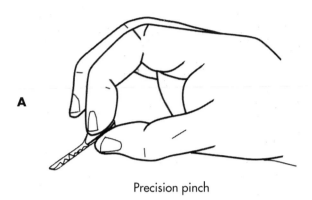

Precision pinch

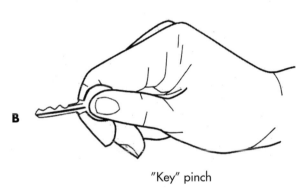

"Key" pinch

Fig. 48-9. A, Precision pinch, or "tip pinch" contrast with **B,** "key pinch." A normal hand can choose which one to use. A hand with severe muscle paralysis may be limited to one or the other as the pinch of choice. The choice may have to be made before surgery enhances one or the other.

The answer, of course, is that the joint is held and stabilized by the passive fascia and skin of the thumb web. And why does that dermofascial sling not *stretch* and lengthen under the strain as the palmar plate does in the finger MP joints? Simply because it gives its support a long way from the joint axis. It exerts its effective passive torque through a moment arm of between 3 and 4 cm. Thus it is not subjected to a significant tensile force and rarely becomes stretched.

The metacarpal of the thumb swings around a cone, the center of which is along the third metacarpal. In a normal hand, the fascia of the web is rarely subjected to stretch because its position is maintained by the active adductor and flexor pollicis brevis muscles that originate along that line. However, when those muscles are paralyzed, it is not the FPL that takes over from them but the passive fascia of the web.

This diagram of a lumberjack up a tree (Fig. 48-8) demonstrates how a passive sling, supporting the man's thighs and buttocks (his metacarpal) gives him freedom to move his distal segments without worrying about the danger of hyperextending his whole body away from the tree.

Finally I want to demonstrate how profoundly different the biomechanics of the flexor tendon of the thumb are in what we call "tip pinch" or "precision pinch" from "key pinch," (Fig. 48-9) when we study them at the CMC joint of the thumb.

Fig. 48-10, *A* is a picture of my hand, pinching in the tip-pinch fashion. The pencil will not move, and my thumb scarcely moves either (Fig. 48-10, *B*). Almost *all* the movement of tip pinch is *finger movement.* Contrast this with the key pinch. Again the pencil does not move (Fig. 48-11, *A*). Notice that all the movement is *thumb motion* (Fig. 48-11, *B*), and the fingers remain still, like the anvil to a hammer.

Where there is a shortage of available muscles for transfer, one may have to choose one type of pinch or the other, because their biomechanics are so different from each other. If one has good confidence in the control of the fingers,

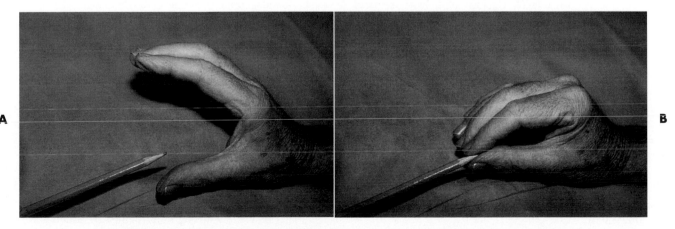

Fig. 48-10. A, My hand poised to pinch a pencil point, using tip pinch. **B,** Tip pinch accomplished. Note that all the active movement is finger motion. The thumb need not move.

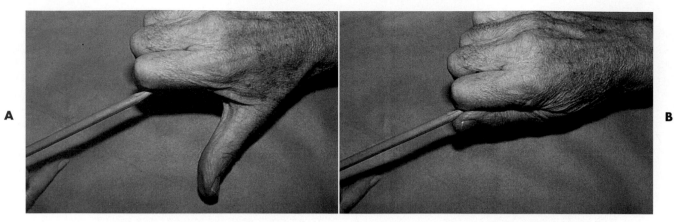

Fig. 48-11. A, My hand poised to pinch a pencil point, using key pinch. **B,** Key pinch accomplished. Note that all the movement is thumb motion. Fingers remain semiflexed and need not move.

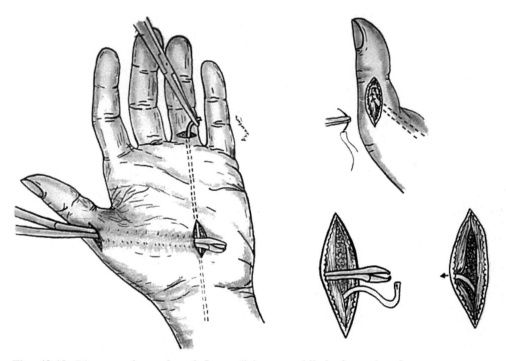

Fig. 48-12. Diagram of transfer of flexor digitorum sublimis from ring finger, to serve as adductor-flexor for the MP joint of the thumb and to reinforce flexion of the carpometacarpal (CMC) joint as well. Note that the tendon is retrieved through palmar fascia and is then tunnelled to the thumb, superficial to the palmar fascia, to ensure that the tendon will not slip proximally and lose its moment arm for the CMC joint.

especially at the MP joints, then it is usually best to aim for a tip pinch, because it places no demands on the long flexor tendon at the CMC joint of the thumb. The thumb metacarpal may lie sleeping in its dermofascial cradle of the thumb web and leave all the work to the fingers. If, however there is residual stiffness or paralysis in the fingers, and if the patient seems happy with the key pinch, then the surgeon has to make drastic alterations in the biomechanics of the FPL if that pinch is to work.

The thumb web is of no use in key pinch. It may limit the spread of the open extended thumb, but it folds up and

becomes loose as the thumb closes in key pinch. In the absence of other supporting muscles, the action of the FPL will flex the DIP joint. Because key pinch is normally done with an extended IP joint, it may be best to arthrodese this joint in extension. This will leave the FPL to flex the MP joint. This, however, will be useless if flexion of the CMC is so weak that the thumb metacarpal is pushed into extension at every pinch.

This is where a strong muscle must be added across the palm, along the line of the transverse fibers of the adductor pollicis. Such a muscle may be arranged to have a 1.5-cm

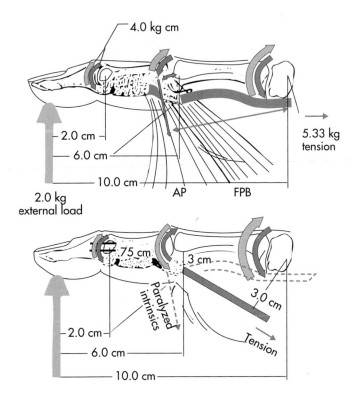

Fig. 48-13. In tetraplegia, where there may be no muscles available for transfer, the distal interphalangeal joint must be arthrodesed and a single long flexor tendon (perhaps the flexor pollicis longus) may serve to flex the metacarpophalangeal (MP) and carpometacarpal (CMC) joints. At the MP joint it will have a 1.5-cm moment arm, and may then leave the thumb and cross the palm, behind all tendons, and be routed into the forearm, around the hook of the hamate and passed through Guyon's canal on its way either to an active forearm muscle or to a tenodesis across the wrist. Such a pathway will ensure an effective moment arm at the CMC joint.

moment arm at the MP joint, and will then have about 3 cm at the CMC joint (Fig. 48-12).

If, as in tetraplegia, there are no muscles to spare, then the FPL tendon itself must be rerouted to enter the palm from around the hook of the hamate bone (Fig. 48-13) and approach the thumb behind the flexor tendons to the fingers, being attached to the proximal phalanx about 1.5 cm distal to the axis of the MP joint, as is the adductor pollicis. In such a position the tendon will have about a 3-cm moment arm to the CMC joint and will be able to give a strong key pinch without the assistance of any fascial support from the web.

REFERENCES

1. Bunnell S: Surgery of the intrinsic muscles of the hand other than those producing opposition of the thumb, *J Bone Joint Surg* 1942; 1:24.
2. Bunnell S: *Surgery of the hand,* New York, 1948, Lippincott.
3. Long C, Conrad PW, Hall EA, Furler SL: Intrinsic-extrinsic muscle control of the hand in power grip and precision handling, *J Bone Joint Surg* 1970; 52A(5):853-867.
4. Zancolli EA: Claw-hand caused by paralysis of the intrinsic muscles: a simple surgical procedure for its correction, *J Bone Joint Surg* 1957; 39A:1076.
5. Zancolli EA: *Structural and dynamic bases of hand surgery,* ed 2, Philadelphia, 1979, Lippincott.

Chapter 49

TENDON TRANSFERS IN RHEUMATOID ARTHRITIS

Yves Allieu
Michel Chammas

Tendon transfers in patients who have rheumatoid arthritis are indicated if there are deformities of the wrist or fingers and tendon ruptures. Compression neuropathies rarely lead to paralysis, and they require palliative procedures such as tendon transfers.

TENDON TRANSFERS FOR DEFORMITIES IN THE RHEUMATOID HAND
Wrist deformities

Tendon transfers to restore wrist balance are part of dorsal wrist surgery,[2,10,16] also called *conservative surgery.* The procedures included are dorsal synovectomy, extensor tenosynovectomy[15] and extensor tendon reconstruction (if necessary), and resection of the ulnar head and stabilization-realignment of the wrist. In dorsal synovectomy, the posterior interosseus nerve is also resected to complete the pain relief effect of the synovectomy.

Stabilization-realignment of the wrist is carried out by soft tissue release and tendon transfers. The principal procedures are outlined here.

In extensor carpi ulnaris (ECU) realignment, the ECU is repositioned dorsally and fixed by part of a reticular ligament anteriorly transposed under the extensor tendon of the wrist and fingers. This repositioning tends to correct the supination of the carpus and the posterior luxation of the distal radioulnar joint.

Transfer of the extensor carpi radialis longus (ECRL) to the ECU (Fig. 49-1) is advocated to correct excessive radiometacarpal shift. The ECRL is detached from the base of the second metacarpal and transferred subcutaneously to

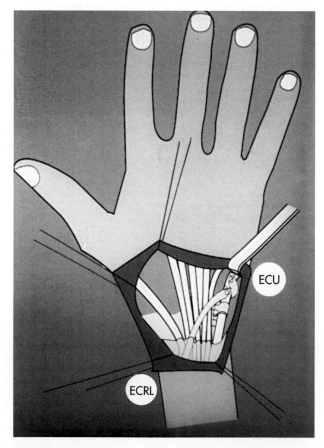

Fig. 49-1. Stabilization and realignment of the wrist by soft tissue procedures, specifically extensor carpi ulnaris (ECU) realignment and extensor carpi radialis longus (ECRL) transfer on the ECU joint.

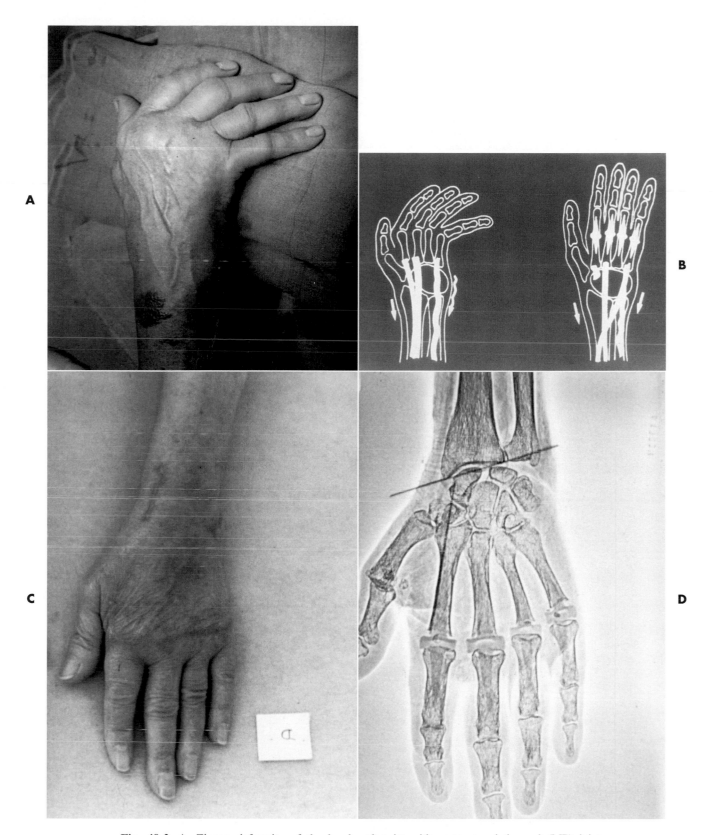

Fig. 49-2. A, Zigzag deformity of the hand and wrist with metacarpophalangeal (MP) joint destruction. **B,** MP joint arthroplasty by Swanson implants and transfer of the extensor carpi radialis longus joint on the extensor carpi ulnaris joint. **C,** Postoperative result. **D,** Postoperative radiograph. The MP joints are realigned. Note the absence of an osteoarticular lesion of the wrist.

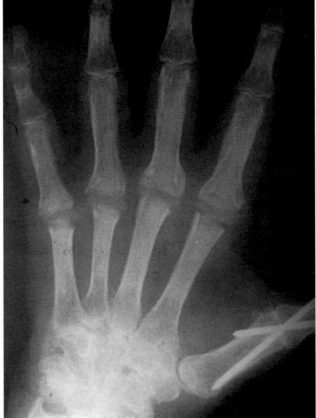

Fig. 49-3. A, Extensor indicis proprius (EIP) transfer to the base of the first phalanx after having passed it under the first interosseous muscle to place it in a dorsal position. **B,** Preoperative radiograph. **C,** Postoperative radiograph of metacarpophalangeal (MP) arthroplasties using Swanson implants with tendinous realignment and EIP transfer.

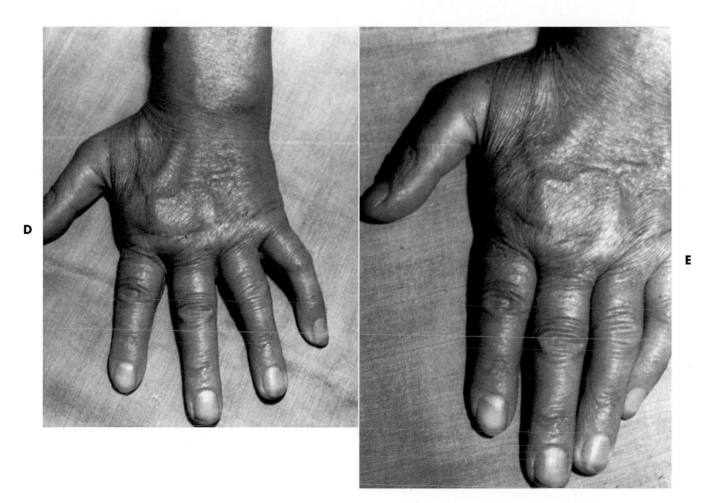

Fig. 49-3, cont'd.   D and **E,** Clinical results after arthroplasties using Swanson implant on the MP joints' realignment of extensor tendons, and EIP transfer.

the ECU on the ulnar side of the carpus. This transfer tends to correct the radial deviation of the carpus and to maintain the ECU in a dorsal position.

Rheumatoid arthritis is a progressive disease and, in time, realignment of the wrist using soft tissue transfers becomes insufficient.[1,11,20] Tendon transfers are credited with good results for a limited period of time.[4,6,7] We only use this method when there is an existing radial deviation of the carpus associated with an ulnar deviation of the metacarpophalangeal (MP) joint (zigzag deformity) without affecting any osteoarticular structure (Larsen grade 0 or 1)[12] (Fig. 49-2).

For instability or partial destruction of the carpus, dorsal wrist surgery is now supplemented by partial wrist arthrodesis or, particularly, radiolunate arthrodesis, according to Chamay.[5]

Ulnar deviation of the fingers

The extensor indicis proprius (EIP) is transferred to the base of the first phalanx after having passed under the first dorsal interosseus muscle to place it in a dorsal position. This

avoids the negative action of having the first dorsal interosseus muscle displaced toward the palm, which leads to palmar subluxation of the MP joint. Thus the role of abductor of the first dorsal interosseus muscle is restored[3] (Fig. 49-3, *A*).

This transfer is more often associated with MP joint arthroplasties using Swanson implants (Fig. 49-3). These implants are the only way to correct the palmar subluxation associated with ulnar deviation.

Transfer of the EIP does not affect isolated extension of the index finger.[25] Correction of ulnar deviation of the MP joints must only be carried out after correction of the radial deviation of the carpus. Persistence of this wrist deformity risks the recurrence of ulnar deviation and secondary rupture of the implants (Fig. 49-4).

TENDON TRANSFERS FOR TENDON RUPTURES

Essentially, tendon transfers are indicated for extensor tendon ruptures. In rheumatoid arthritis, rupture of a flexor tendon usually requires palliative procedures other than tendon transfers.[13,22-24]

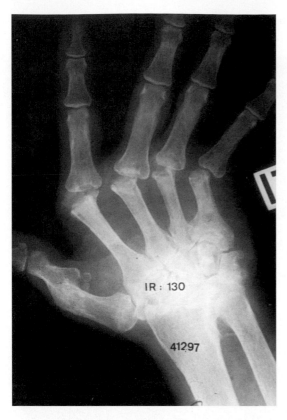

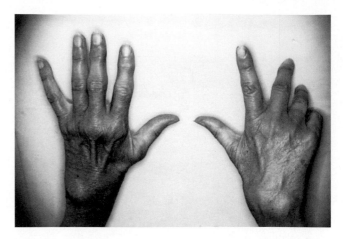

Fig. 49-6. Extensor tendon rupture of the three ulnar fingers of the right hand. Note the subluxation of the ulnar head.

Fig. 49-4. Recurrence of the ulnar deviation of the fingers with fracture of the implants postoperatively. The radial deviation of the wrist had not been previously corrected.

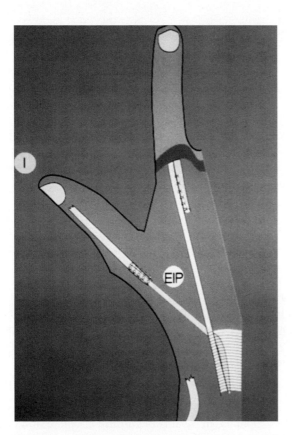

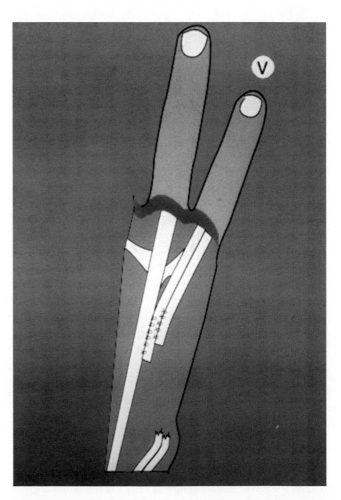

Fig. 49-5. Reconstruction of an extensor pollicis longus rupture by transfer of the extensor indicis proprius (EIP).

Fig. 49-7. Single extensor tendon rupture treated by side-by-side transfer to the adjacent tendon.

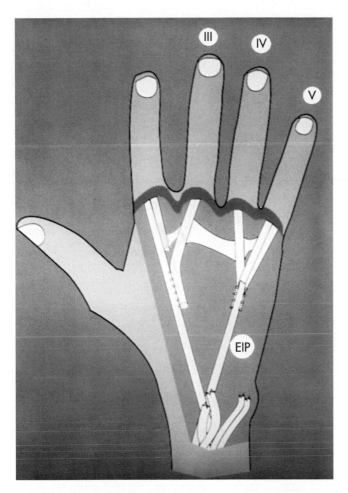

Fig. 49-8. Triple tendon rupture treated by side-to-side transfer in combination with extensor indicis proprius (EIP) transfer.

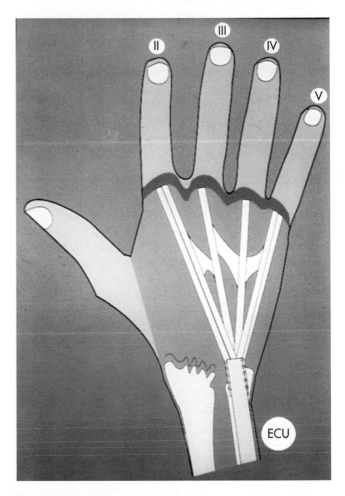

Fig. 49-9. Multiple extensor tendon ruptures treated by extensor carpi ulnaris (ECU) transfer.

Extensor pollicis longus ruptures

Extensor pollicis longus (EPL) ruptures occur near Lister's tubercle and are commonly observed in rheumatoid arthritis, although overshadowed by the articular affliction of the thumb interphalangeal (IP) and MP joints.[8] Such ruptures are often well tolerated, with variable loss of function. Usually the patient maintains the ability to extend the IP joint but cannot extend the thumb with the palm resting on a flat surface.[18]

To restore EPL function, we prefer to use the EIP transfer (Fig. 49-5).[21] The EIP tendon has an excursion similar to that of the EPL tendon. Therefore the patient does not lose independent extension of the index finger as a result of this transfer.[26]

In rheumatoid arthritis the EIP tendon is an important motor transfer that can be preserved for future purposes. Other available motor tendons are the extensor pollicis brevis (EPB)[9] and the ECRL. We have never used the ECRL tendon for this transfer. In three cases where the condition of the MP joint necessitated an arthrodesis, an EPB tendon was used. We do not necessarily think that this method is the best, despite its simplicity, because there is destabilization of the thumb MP joint, which, in rheumatoid arthritis, tends to pull itself into flexion.

Rarely, rupture of the EPL tendon is repaired using a free interposition tendon graft of the palmaris longus, and sometimes an arthrodesis of the IP joint of the thumb can be performed.

Extensor tendon ruptures of the four ulnar fingers

One must differentiate between tendon ruptures and the inability to extend the finger, which is a consequence of compression of the posterior interosseus nerve.[14,17] This lesion results from synovitis of the elbow. It is not common, but it is important to be aware of it in the differential diagnosis of extensor tendon lesions. More commonly, tendon extensor rupture must be differentiated from MP joint dislocation with flexed and ulnar deviation of the fingers or ulnar displacement of the extensor tendon between the metacarpal heads.

Extensor tendon ruptures of the fingers usually occur on the ulnar side of the wrist, secondary to attrition over a damaged subluxed ulnar head (Fig. 49-6). The little finger is affected more often. The extent of functional loss depends on whether or not both the extensor digiti minimi (EDM) and the extensor digitorum communis (EDC) tendons are ruptured. Commonly, after rupture of the extensor tendon of the little finger, the ring finger extensor also ruptures. Thus the usual progression of extensor tendon ruptures is in a radial direction, finally affecting the index finger.

In combination with ulnar head resection and dorsal tenosynovectomy, several types of tendon transfers are used, depending on the type and extent of the tendon rupture.

Single extensor tendon rupture. For single tendon rupture, our procedure of choice consists of suturing the distal tendon stump to an adjacent intact tendon under adequate tension (Fig. 49-7).

Multiple extensor tendon ruptures. Double extensor tendon ruptures are not infrequent and affect the ring and little fingers. The etiology is typically the Vaughan-Jackson lesion. We use side-to-side transfer between the distal stumps of the ruptured tendons and adjacent tendon. However, a supplementary extensor tendon (EIP) transfer is indicated if it is possible when the distal tendon stump of the little finger is too short.

Triple tendon ruptures include lesions of the two extensor tendons of the little finger and the EDC of the ring finger. We prefer to use transfer of the distal stump of the extensor tendons of the fourth finger to the adjacent (third digit) tendon (Fig. 49-8). Then the EIP tendon is transferred to the combined distal stumps of the EDM and the EDC of the little finger.

When rupture of four or more extensor tendons occurs, side-to-side transfer cannot be performed. No excellent functional result can be expected, especially if the MP joint is subluxed and deviated. Because of the risk of swan-neck deformity, we usually do not use the flexor digitorum sublimis as a motor transfer in rheumatoid arthritis.[19] Depending on the extent of extensor tendon rupture, we choose between EIP, EPL, EPB, ECRL, and ECU transfers. Despite its weakness, the ECU tendon is useful (Fig. 49-9). The surgical technique is simple, and the dorsal position transfer stabilizes the ulnar stump.

With multiple ruptures of the extensors, the subluxed palmar MP joint necessitates arthroplasties more often using Swanson implants. When these are associated with transfers, the fingers are maintained in extension and allow the use of the hand. The quality of the functional result depends essentially on the active range of motion of the proximal interphalangeal and distal interphalangeal joints of the fingers. Postoperatively, we use a dynamic splint to immobilize the wrist in extension and allow active flexion but provide passive extension of the fingers (Fig. 49-10).

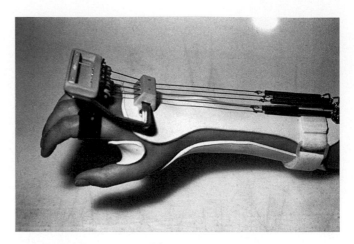

Fig. 49-10. Dynamic splint after extensor tendon repair.

Wrist extensor tendon rupture. Rupture of the wrist extensor tendon is usually observed in combination with all extensor tendon ruptures of the fingers and requires wrist arthrodesis.

REFERENCES

1. Allieu Y, Lussiez B, Asencio G: The long term results of synovectomy of the rheumatoid wrist: a report of sixty cases, *Rev Chir Orthop* 1989; 3(2):188-194.
2. Allieu Y, Brahin B: La chirurgie du "poignet dorsal" dans la polyarthrite rhumatoïde. Synovectomies et réaxation du carpe, *Ann Chir* 1977; 31:279-289.
3. Allieu Y, Dimeglio A, Pech J: Les arthroplasties des metacarpophalangiennes avec implants de Swanson dans la main rhumatismale. Evaluation critique des résultats, *Ann Chir* 1974; 28(10):873-882.
4. Boyce T, Youm Y, Sprague BL, et al: Clinical and experimental studies of the effect of extensor carpi radialis longus transfer in the rheumatoid hand, *J Hand Surg* 1978; 3:390-394.
5. Chamay A, Della Santa D, Vilaseca A: L'arthrodèse radio-lunaire, facteur de stabilité du poignet rhumatoïde, *Ann Chir Main* 1983; (2):5-17.
6. Clayton ML, Ferlic DC: Tendon transfer for radial rotation of the wrist in rheumatoid arthritis, *Clin Orthop* 1974; 100:176-185.
7. Goldner JL: Tendon transfers in rheumatoid arthritis, *Orthop Clin North Am* 1974; 5:425-444.
8. Harris R: Spontaneous rupture of the tendon of extensor pollicis longus as a complication of rheumatoid arthritis, *Ann Rheum Dis* 1951; 10:298-306.
9. Harrison SH, Swannell AJ, Ansell BM: Repair of extensor pollicis longus using extensor pollicis brevis in rheumatoid arthritis, *Ann Rheum Dis* 1972; 31:490-492.
10. Kessler I, Vainio K: Posterior (dorsal) synovectomy for rheumatoid involvement of the hand and wrist. A follow-up study of sixty-six procedures, *J Bone Joint Surg* 1966; 48A:1085-1094.
11. Kulick RG, De Fiore JC, Straub LR, Ranawat CS: Long-term result of dorsal stabilization in the rheumatoid wrist, *J Hand Surg* 1981; 3:272-280.
12. Larsen A, Dale K, Eek M, Pahle J: Radiographic evaluation of rheumatoid arthritis by standard references films, *J Hand Surg* 1983; 5:667-669.
13. Laine VAI, Vainio KJ: Spontaneous ruptures of tendons in rheumatoid arthritis, *Acta Orthop Scand* 1955; 24:250-257.
14. Marmor L, Lawrence JF, Dubois EL: Posterior interosseous nerve palsy due to rheumatoid arthritis, *J Bone Joint Surg* 1967; 49A:381-383.

15. Millender LH, Nalebuff EA: Preventive surgery—tenosynovectomy and synovectomy, *Orthop Clin North Am* 1975; 6:765-792.

16. Millender LH, Nalebuff EA, Albin R, et al: Dorsal tenosynovectomy and tendon transfer in the rheumatoid hand, *J Bone Joint Surg* 1974; 56A:601-610.

17. Millender LH, Nalebuff EA, Holdsworth DE: Posterior interosseous nerve syndrome secondary to rheumatoid synovitis, *J Bone Joint Surg* 1973; 55A:753-757.

18. Nalebuff EA: Surgical treatment of tendon rupture in the rheumatoid hand, *Surg Clin North Am* 1969; 49:811-822.

19. Nalebuff EA, Patel MR: Flexor digitorum sublimus transfer for multiple extensor tendon ruptures in rheumatoid arthritis, *Plast Reconstr Surg* 1973; 51:530-533.

20. Ramaya G, Thirupathi RG, Ferlic DC, Clayton ML: Dorsal wrist synovectomy in rheumatoid arthritis—a long term study, *J Hand Surg* 1983; 8:848-856.

21. Schneider LH, Rosenstein RG: Restoration of extensor pollicis longus function by tendon transfer, *Plast Reconstr Surg* 1983; 71:533-537.

22. Straub LR, Wilson EH: Spontaneous rupture of extensor tendons in the hand associated with rheumatoid arthritis, *J Bone Joint Surg* 1956; 38A:1208-1217.

23. Straub R, Wilson EH: Spontaneous rupture of extensor tendons in the hand associated with rheumatoid arthritis, *J Bone Joint Surg* 1956; 38A:1208.

24. Vaughan-Jackson OJ: Attrition ruptures of tendons in the rheumatoid hand, *J Bone Joint Surg* 1958; 40A:1431.

25. Wadstein T: Spontaneous rupture of the long extensor tendon of the extensor pollicis longus. Transplantation of the extensor indicis proprius, *Acta Orthop Scan* 1946; 16:194-202.

26. Weiland AJ, Naiman J: Independent index extension after extensor indicis proprius transfer, *J Hand Surg* 1985; 10A:427.

Chapter 50

EXTENSOR TENDON RUPTURES IN RHEUMATOID HANDS

Sung Tack Kwon
Lawrence H. Schneider

Vaughan-Jackson brought attention to attrition ruptures of extensor tendons in rheumatoid arthritis in 1948.[30,31] Since those reports many authors have studied the application of reconstructive surgery after this devastating event.* This problem can be detrimental to the function of the hand in these patients who, in addition to hand problems, often have multiple other areas of involvement by their disease.

Typically, patients with extensor tendon rupture will present with a history of recent loss of ability to fully extend one or more fingers. There may be a history of recent flareup of their disease with dorsal wrist tenosynovitis being an obvious predecessor to the rupture. Almost all of our cases had considerable dorsal tenosynovitis, wrist synovitis, and distal radioulnar joint damage. Especially frequent in these extensor tendon ruptures is the involvement of the distal radioulnar joint by the arthritic process, a finding well documented by the original work of Vaughan-Jackson.[30]

There are several etiologic mechanisms for rupture of extensor tendons in rheumatoid arthritis. The first, already alluded to, is caused by attrition of the tendons at the distal ulna, which is often subluxed dorsally and can with bone erosion take on a knifelike distal end. The distal ulna just under the tendons will ultimately sever these tendons.[6]

A second mechanism involves direct invasion of the involved tendons by the diseased tenosynovium or pannus.[6,28]

A third mode presumes circulatory deprivation of the tendons by the surrounding tenosynovium, which competes with the tendon for its blood supply.[7,23]

The diagnosis is usually obvious when a patient presents with inability to actively extend one or more fingers at the metacarpophalangeal (MP) joints. Other conditions have to be ruled out when first examining these patients. These include tendon subluxation into the ulnar gutters on the sides of the MP heads as a possible etiology.[29] Another relatively rare cause is posterior interosseous nerve paralysis secondary to elbow joint synovitis, which is well documented in the literature.†

Treatment for extensor tendon ruptures is a relatively urgent problem, because the tendency for progression exists with additional ruptures from the ulnar to radial aspect of the hand occurring as time passes. As a general rule, surgical exploration reveals more tendons injured than are diagnosed in the preoperative examination. The surgeon should be prepared to find more tendons involved than predicted preoperatively and be suitably prepared with various reconstructive possibilities.

CLINICAL EXPERIENCE

The experience of the senior author with this problem in the rheumatoid hand includes 45 operations for cases of extensor tendon ruptures in 37 patients in a 15-year period. A total of 127 tendons were ruptured in these hands.

---

*References 2, 8, 13, 14, 16, 19-22, 25, 29, 32.

†References 4, 9, 12, 15, 17, 26.

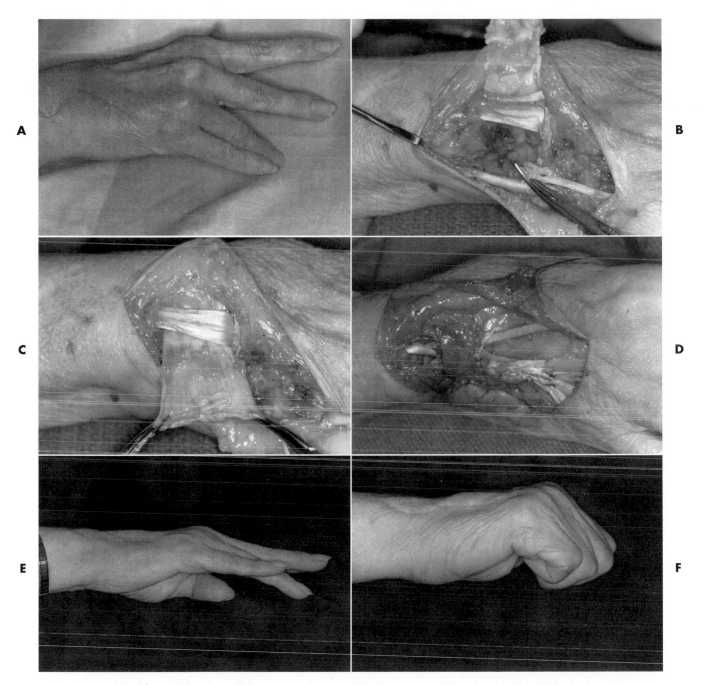

Fig. 50-1. A 52-year-old patient with rupture of extensors to ring and little fingers. **A,** Loss of active extension at the ring and little finger MP joints. **B,** The retinaculum has been reflexed radially. The ulnar head has been excised. The clamp is on the distal tendon segment of the ruptured EDC 4 and 5. **C,** The retinaculum is placed beneath the intact extensors. **D,** The EIP is transferred to the distal stumps of the EDC 4 and 5 and the EDM. **E** and **F,** Extension and flexion restored at 6 months.

These patients all had documented rheumatoid arthritis and were between 24 and 84 years old, with an average age of 55 years. Most of the patients were in the 5th through 7th decade. Ruptures occurred as early as 1.5 years after the diagnosis of rheumatoid arthritis; one patient ruptured her tendons 34 years after onset of the disease. The mean time between onset of disease and diagnosis of rupture was 12.3 years. Local steroid injections preceded rupture in 14 hands. Although many patients had intervals of systemic steroid intake during the course of their illness, there was no correlation between the use of these medications, regardless of the route of administration and extensor tendon rupture. The ruptures were more common on the ulnar side of the hand progressing to the radial side with the little finger most frequently involved.

TREATMENT

Although tendon grafting has been successfully reported,[2] this technique was not used in these patients. In our opinion the graft would be expected to have a lesser prognosis in the poor beds provided and the need for two junctures would also increase the risk for failure.

Direct repair is not usually feasible because of the nature of the condition, which often occurs with loss of tendon substance because of the attritional nature in most of these cases. It was possible in only one case with rupture of the extensor digiti minimi (EDM) and extensor digitorum communis (EDC) localized at the MP joint level in a solitary little finger rupture.[5]

The usual treatment is by tendon transfer,[13,14,16,19-22,32] and the treatment carried out in the remaining 46 operations was either a transfer of the distal end of the ruptured tendon to an adjacent intact tendon in an end-to-side juncture or by tendon transfer of an available motor, usually the extensor indicis proprius (EIP) or flexor digitorum superficialis (FDS) to the distal end of the ruptured extensor tendon. End-to-side transfer was employed in 8 cases, and tendon transfer end-to-end was the most common procedure either alone (33 cases) or in combination with end-to-side attachment (2 cases). The EIP was used most frequently for tendon transfer (25 cases). For the hands with multiple ruptures and those in which repeat surgery was performed, where the extensor indicis proprius or other extensors were no longer available or themselves ruptured, an FDS (seven cases) was used as the motor tendon. The extensor pollicis brevis (EPB) and the extensor carpi radialis longus (ECRL) were each used in one case.

Ancillary procedures

In many hands, associated procedures included excision of distal ulna (22 cases)[10,31] and dorsal tenosynovectomy.*

*References 1, 3, 10, 11, 18, 24, 28.

Current procedure

Given our experience it is the treatment policy at this time to proceed as follows in these cases.

When only the fifth finger extensors (EDM and EDC-5) are involved, we transfer the distal stump of the EDM, side-to-side, to the intact extensor of EDC-4.

When extension is lost at both the fourth and fifth fingers, the EIP is transferred to the distal stumps of the ring and little extensors (Fig. 50-1).

Rupture of extensors of long, ring, and little fingers are treated by transfer of the EIP to ring and little fingers with the distal stump of the long finger sutured end-to-side to the intact extensor of the index EDC.

When all the finger extensors are ruptured, it is necessary to bring in another source of motor power and we use the FDS of the long or ring fingers, or both (Fig. 50-2).

RESULTS

The follow-up of these cases averaged more than 3 years, ranging from 2 months to 12 years. Thirty-three hands of 45 had extension lags of less than 15°. Ten hands had a lag between 15 and 30°. Two cases lagged more than 30°. Four of the hands had ongoing rupture more radial to the originally treated ruptures and needed further surgery. There was one infection that was treated without loss of the tendon transfer. Flexion loss was not a major problem, with only three hands suffering some loss of flexion.

DISCUSSION

Rheumatoid arthritis is a systemic disease that greatly affects the lives of its victims. Our patients had more than two major joint problems of varying severity when their ruptures occurred. The hand problems themselves are often of secondary concern and many of our patients are referred too late, when earlier treatment may have been simpler. Most of them had severe wrist problems, which may have benefitted from earlier tenosynovectomy with ulnar head resection. That procedure might have averted the ultimate rupture.†

Clinically, synovitis precedes the dorsal subluxation and damage to the ulnar head. Tendons weakened by synovitis might become very susceptible to attrition and eventually rupture. Once rupture occurs, tendon transfer is the best option and is considered a standard treatment modality at this time.‡ Prevention would be a better approach, but as stated earlier, these are patients with widespread and complex problems. Attention to medical management is important. From the surgical viewpoint, the tendon reconstruction, tenosynovectomy or wrist synovectomy (with or without resection of ulnar head) was done simultaneously

†References 3, 10, 11, 18, 24, 28.
‡References 8, 13, 14, 16, 27, 32.

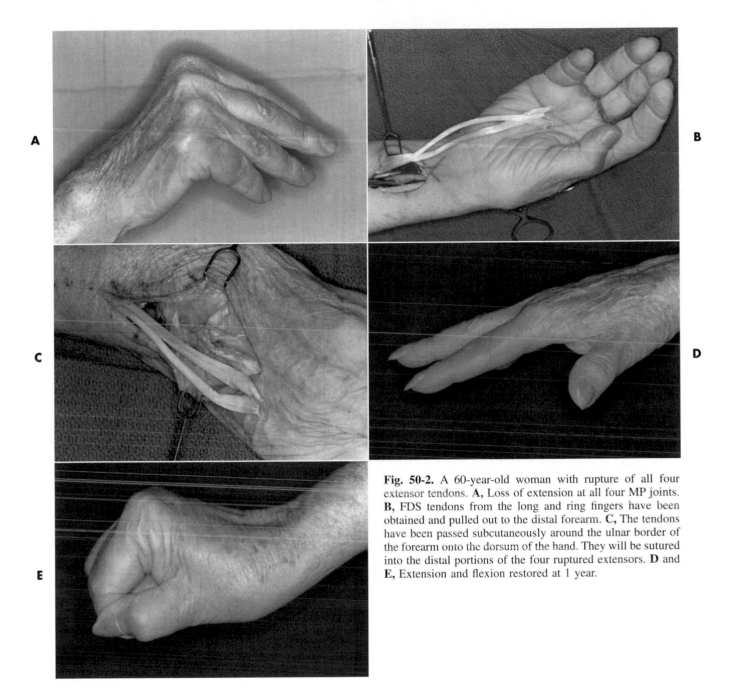

Fig. 50-2. A 60-year-old woman with rupture of all four extensor tendons. **A,** Loss of extension at all four MP joints. **B,** FDS tendons from the long and ring fingers have been obtained and pulled out to the distal forearm. **C,** The tendons have been passed subcutaneously around the ulnar border of the forearm onto the dorsum of the hand. They will be sutured into the distal portions of the four ruptured extensors. **D and E,** Extension and flexion restored at 1 year.

to try to prevent further ruptures. Four patients in this series did have additional rupture in the same hand, which required further surgery. In several patients, long-term hand function did deteriorate, as would be expected in this ongoing pernicious condition.

REFERENCES

1. Aernathy PJ, Dennyson WG: Decompression of the extensor tendons at the wrist in rheumatoid arthritis, *J Bone Joint Surg* 1979; 61B:64-68.
2. Bora FW, Osterman AL, Thomas VJ, et al: The treatment of ruptures of multiple extensor tendons at wrist level by a free tendon graft in the rheumatoid patient, *J Hand Surg* 1987; 12A:1038-1040.
3. Brown FE, Brown M-L: Long-term results after tenosynovectomy to treat the rheumatoid hand, *J Hand Surg* 1988; 13A:704-708.
4. Chang LW, Gowans JDC, Granger CV, Millender LH: Entrapment neuropathy of the posterior interosseous nerves: a complication of rheumatoid arthritis, *Arthritis Rheum* 1972; 15:350-352.
5. Clayton ML, Thirupathi RG, Ferlic DC, et al: Extensor tendon rupture over the metacarpal heads, *Hand* 1983; 15:149-150.
6. Ehrich GE, Peterson LT, Sokoloff L, et al: Pathogenesis of rupture of extensor tendons at the wrist in rheumatoid arthritis, *Arthritis Rheum* 1959; 2:332-346.
7. Engkvist O, Lundborg G: Rupture of the extensor pollicis longus tendon with fracture of the lower end of the radius, *Hand* 1979; 11:76-86.

8. Goldner JL: Tendon transfer in rheumatoid arthritis, *Orthop Clin North Am* 1974; 5:425-444.

9. Goodfellow JW, Mowat A: Posterior interosseous nerve palsy in rheumatoid arthritis, *J Bone Joint Surg* 1988; 70B:468-471.

10. Ishikawa H, Hanyu T, Tajima T: Rheumatoid wrists treated with synovectomy of the extensor tendons and the wrist joint combined with a Darrach procedure, *J Hand Surg* 1992; 17A:1109-1117.

11. Kessler I, Vainio K: Posterior (dorsal) synovectomy for rheumatoid involvement of the hand and wrist, *J Bone Joint Surg* 1966; 48A:1085-1094.

12. Leffert RD, Dorfman HD: Antecubital cyst in rheumatoid arthritis, *J Bone Joint Surg* 1972; 54A:1555-1557.

13. Leslie BM: Rheumatoid extensor tendon ruptures, *Hand Clin* 1989; 5:191-202.

14. Mannerfelt LG: Tendon transfers in surgery of the rheumatoid hand, *Hand Clin* 1988; 4:309-316.

15. Marmor L, Lawrence JF, Dubois EL: Posterior interosseous nerve palsy due to rheumatoid arthritis, *J Bone Joint Surg* 1967; 49A:381-383.

16. Millender LH, Nalebuff EA, Albin R, et al: Dorsal tenosynovectomy and tendon transfer in the rheumatoid hand, *J Bone Joint Surg* 1974; 56A:601-610.

17. Millender LH, Nalebuff EA, Holdsworth DE: Posterior interosseous nerve syndrome secondary to rheumatoid synovitis, *J Bone Joint Surg* 1973; 55A:753-757.

18. Millender LH, Nalebuff EA: Preventive surgery tenosynovectomy and synovectomy, *Orthop Clin* 1975; 6:765-792.

19. Miller-Breslow A, Millender LH, Feldon PG: Treatment considerations in the complicated rheumatoid hand, *Hand Clin* 1989; 5:279-289.

20. Moore JR, Weiland AJ, Valdata L: Tendon ruptures in the rheumatoid hand: analysis of treatment and functional results in 60 patients, *J Hand Surg* 1987; 12A:9-14.

21. Nalebuff EA: Surgical treatment of tendon rupture in the rheumatoid hand, *Surg Clin North Am* 1969; 49:811-822.

22. Nalebuff EA, Patel MR: Flexor digitorum sublimus transfer for the multiple extensor tendon ruptures in rheumatoid arthritis, *Plast Reconstr Surg* 1973; 52:530-533.

23. Neurath MF, Stofft E: Ultrastructural causes of ruptures of hand tendons in patients with rheumatoid arthritis: a transmission and scanning electron microscopic study, *Scand J Plast Reconstr Surg* 1993; 27:59-65.

24. Nicolle FV, Holt PJL, Calna JS: Prophylactic synovectomy of joints of the rheumatoid hand, *Ann Rheum Dis* 1971; 30:476-480.

25. Ohshio I, Ogino T, Minami H, et al: Extensor tendon rupture due to osteoarthritis of the distal radioulnar joint, *J Hand Surg* 1991; 16B:450-453.

26. Roth AI, Stulberg BN, Fleegler EJ, et al: Elbow arthrography in the evaluation of posterior interosseous nerve compression in rheumatoid arthritis, *J Hand Surg* 1986; 11B:120-122.

27. Schneider LH, Rosenstein RG: Restoration of extensor pollicis longus function by tendon transfer, *Plast Reconstr Surg* 1982; 71:533-537.

28. Thirupathi RG, Ferilic DC, Clayton ML: Dorsal wrist synovectomy in rheumatoid arthritis: a long-term study, *J Hand Surg* 1983; 8:848-856.

29. Vaccaro AR, Kupcha P, Schneider LH: The operative repair chronic nontraumatic extensor tendon subluxations in the hand, *Hand Clin* 1995; 11:431-440.

30. Vaughan-Jackson OJ: Rupture of extensor tendons by attrition at the inferior radioulnar joint: report of 2 cases, *J Bone Joint Surg* 1948; 30B:528-530.

31. Vaughan-Jackson OJ: Rheumatoid hand deformities considered in the light of tendon imbalance I, *J Bone Joint Surg* 1962; 44B:764-775.

32. Williamson SC, Paul F: Extensor tendon ruptures in rheumatoid arthritis, *Hand Clin* 1995; 11:449-459.

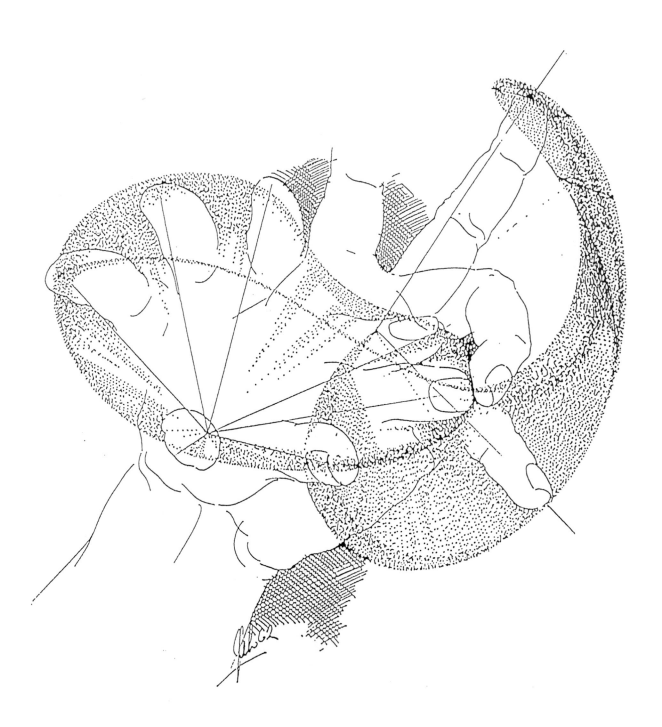

Part XII

TENOLYSIS

This sketch indicates the ellipsoidal range of the thumb and the equiangular pathway of the fingers. (From Converse JM: *Reconstructive plastic surgery: principles in correction, reconstruction and transplantation,* vol. iv, Philadelphia, 1964, Saunders.)

Chapter 51

FLEXOR TENOLYSIS
A *personal experience*

James W. Strickland

Although the biologic basis and clinical efficacy of tenolysis has been questioned by some authors,[3,5,14,16] I have found that when carried out properly, the procedure is a worthwhile effort at restoring or improving digital function.[4] Tenolysis should always be considered as a potential, final salvage procedure following tendon repair, grafting, or staged reconstruction, and patients should be forewarned that a certain percentage of those procedures results in tendon adherence sufficient to require lysis.[2,3] The procedure must be approached as a major surgical effort with great consideration for patient selection, operative technique, and postoperative management. It is perhaps the most demanding of all flexor tendon operations, demanding attention to detail and strong teamwork on the part of the patient, physician, and therapist.[12]

In this chapter I present the preoperative, operative, and postoperative considerations for flexor tenolysis, as well as my technique and personal results achieved from the procedure. The important contributions of others to this procedure are documented, and differing opinions are discussed.[26]

PREOPERATIVE MANAGEMENT

Tenolysis may be indicated following flexor tendon repair or grafting whenever the passive range of digital joint flexion significantly exceeds the patient's ability to actively flex the same joints. The decision to perform the procedure should be based on serial joint measurements that indicate there has been no appreciable improvement in active flexion after several months, despite a good therapy program and the conscientious efforts of the patient.[21-23,27,29]

The prerequisites for tenolysis as outlined by Fetrow,[9] Hunter et al.,[10] Schneider and Hunter,[18] and Schneider and Mackin[19,20] should be closely adhered to. All fractures should be healed, and wounds should have reached tissue equilibrium with soft, pliable skin and subcutaneous tissues, and minimal reaction around scars. In addition, joint contractures must have been overcome and a normal or near-normal passive range of digital motion achieved. Satisfactory sensation and muscle strength must also be present, and the patient must be carefully informed as to the objectives, techniques, postoperative course, and pitfalls of the procedure. Many patients will be content with considerably less than normal active digital motion, whereas others who have returned a fairly good digital range may be desirous of near-normal function and, in most circumstances, should be offered the operation. When he or she elects to undergo tenolysis, the patient must understand that if the findings at surgery preclude the possibility of returning a satisfactory functional flexor system, it may be necessary to proceed with the implantation of a silicone rod as the first stage of a staged flexor tendon reconstruction sequence.

The proper timing for tenolysis following a tendon injury, repair, or graft is somewhat controversial. Wray et al.[30] concluded from an experiment on chicken tendons that waiting 12 weeks appeared to be optimum for the procedure in that this time period did not weaken the tendon and resulted in an increased blood supply. Fetrow[9] and Pulvertaft[13] have both recommended waiting 3 months following a primary tendon repair and 6 months following a flexor tendon graft before tenolysis is performed. Rank et al.[16] have advocated waiting 6 to 9 months after tendon repair whether by sutures or a graft. Weeks and Wray[28] have shown that 86% of the total active motion attainable 1 year following tendon grafting in a favorable recipient bed and 90% of the total action motion attainable 1 year following a two-stage silicone rubber rod–flexor tendon graft procedure was present at 22 weeks. This indicates that 5 to 6 months following tendon grafting would be an appropriate time for tenolysis for those patients in whom serial examinations revealed no significant improvement. My policy is to consider tenolysis for those patients in whom serial examinations revealed no significant improvement in 3 months or more after a repair or graft, provided the previously mentioned criteria for the procedure have been fulfilled and there has been no improvement in active motion in the previous 4 to 8 weeks.

SURGICAL MANAGEMENT

The use of local anesthesia supplemented by intravenous analgesia and tranquilizing drugs has become the accepted technique for most tenolysis procedures. With the patient awake and the forearm musculature functional, the patient is able to actively demonstrate the completeness of flexor lysis by flexing the involved digit during surgery. The use of a sterile pediatric tourniquet applied to the midforearm is an effective method of dealing with the problems of tourniquet pain and muscle paralysis. The patient is slightly sedated before entering the operating room and, at that time, a local anesthetic may be administered 15 to 30 minutes before the beginning of the surgical preparation and inflation of tourniquet. This allows the drug to have maximal effect and to have been absorbed by the soft tissues before the beginning of surgery, so that the anesthetic fluid will not impede the direct visualization of the delicate hand structures and the ability to carry out a meticulous surgical extrication of the involved tendons. I prefer to use bupivacaine, 0.5% (Marcaine), because of its long duration (10 to 14 hours), which will tend to minimize the immediate postoperative discomfort. I prefer to infiltrate the anesthetic fluid directly into the skin and subcutaneous tissues at the base of the finger and into the distal palm. Administration of the anesthetic should include a transmetacarpal block to the involved digit, and if extensive palmar dissection is anticipated or more than one finger is to undergo tenolysis, I may elect to use a wrist block. The only disadvantage of a wrist block is that it paralyzes the intrinsic muscles and may compromise the patient's ability to demonstrate normal digital kinetics following tenolysis. It is, however, very effective at permitting full function of the extrinsic flexor system and is an excellent alternative to direct palmar injection in certain instances. An anesthesiologist provides supplementary analgesia or sedation so that the patient's comfort is assured throughout the dissection necessary to free the flexor tendons.

Although the benefits of local anesthesia[17] in allowing the patient to actively demonstrate the restored performance of the flexor system are known, it must be remembered that tourniquet ischemia results in muscle paralysis in approximately 30 minutes and, although active function returns after the tourniquet has been released, this delay is a surgical inconvenience. In addition, tourniquet discomfort may sometimes limit the patient's ability to tolerate its use for more than 20 to 40 minutes, depending on the effectiveness of supplementary analgesia. An excellent method of dealing with the problem of muscle paralysis and tourniquet pain had been the use of a sterile pediatric pneumatic tourniquet, which can be placed around the mid forearm and secondarily inflated, following which the upper arm tourniquet is deflated. Homeostasis is preserved, the discomfort from the forearm tourniquet is usually minimal, and function of the extrinsic forearm flexors can usually be restored following their revascularization. When the dressing is applied, the proximal tourniquet can be reinflated and the pediatric tourniquet removed.

With the patient in the supine position, the arm is abducted onto a standard hand table and a pneumatic tourniquet is applied to the upper arm. After a routine 6 to 10 minutes of preparation of the hand, wrist, and forearm, draping is carried out using the following technique. The table is first draped with at least one layer of a water impervious material following which two surgical towels are used to block drape the arm so that it can be lifted and moved during the procedure without compromising sterility. Both towels are folded longitudinally and the bottom towel is placed beneath the arm while it is still elevated after prepping. The edges of the lower towel are directed toward the hand and are positioned so that they are well inside of the prepped area. The arm is then lowered onto the hand surgical table and a second folded towel is laid across the arm directly above the open edges of the bottom towel, but with the folded edge directed toward the hand. The corners of the top layer of the bottom towel are then brought around the arm so that they cross each other, and a towel clip is used to secure the two towel edges together. Additional clips are employed to fasten both the folded edges of the top towel and the corners of the remaining layer of the bottom towel to the table. An additional sterile sheet is then brought across the patient and over an ether screen, so that its folded edge can be secured to the block drape and to the table. This technique allows the arm to be lifted and repositioned or rotated without jeopardizing the sterile field.

Thorough tenolysis requires wide surgical exposure, and the exact incisions employed depend on the wounds resulting from the original injury and subsequent operative efforts. My preference for the tenolysis procedure is a midlateral incision as described by Rank and Wakefield[16] in which the neurovascular bundles are left in a dorsal position. I believe that this approach results in the least amount of scar formation directly over the flexor tendons and creates less wound tension with the initiation of early digital motion following lysis. In the lateral digits, the incision can be carried down the border of the hand to the level of the distal palmar crease and then turned across the palm.

Continuous exposure of the flexor tendon sheath is provided in this manner, and there is no need to cross over the neurovascular bundles, as would be required in the midlateral technique in which the neurovascular bundles are reflected with the palmar flap. Oblique digital-palmar extensions of midlateral incisions permit wide exposure of the flexor system to the long and ring fingers. As the dissection proceeds, every attempt should be made to preserve as much of the pulley system as possible. If a great deal of scar tissue exists within the digit, it will be very difficult to define the neurovascular structures and it is often preferable to reflect the skin flaps off of the lateral portions of the digit in a subcutaneous manner. Extending the dissection in the midline of the digit permits exposure of the flexor tendon system with little likelihood of violating the digital nerves and arteries. From a biomechanical point of view, it is particularly important to retain the A_2 and A_4 annular pulleys[8] to minimize moment arm alterations between the flexor tendons and the digital joints and to negate the requirement for additional tendon amplitude to produce full digital flexion. If the pulley system has been damaged by injury or previous surgery, the forces acting on the remaining pulleys will be much greater during active digital flexion, and the likelihood of secondary pulley rupture is increased. It may be necessary to excise badly scarred sections of the flexor sheath, but careful protection of existing uninjured components usually results in the preservation of an adequate system.

All limiting adhesions are meticulously divided, and care is taken to define the borders of the flexor tendons. When possible, I individualize the profundus and superficialis tendons, and the judicious use of small knife blades and elevators may help in this effort to extricate the flexor systems from their scarred beds on the floor of the fibro-osseous canal and underneath the pulleys. When indicated, small pediatric urethral dilators can be used to widen the annular pulleys slightly and allow for smoother gliding of the lysed tendons.

When the procedure is carried out under local anesthetic,[18] it is possible to periodically ask the patient to flex the involved digit and, in doing so, determine the adequacy of the lysis. Occasionally, this active motion on the part of the patient will rupture a few remaining adhesions and permit full excursion of the lysed tendon. At approximately 30 minutes, tourniquet paralysis of the flexor musculature may preclude the patient's ability to actively flex and, at this point, dissection is continued without patient participation. When an active demonstration is again desirable, I apply and inflate a sterile pediatric tourniquet on the midforearm following which the upper arm tourniquet can be released. After several minutes, the patient will regain extrinsic flexor muscle tendon activity and the proximal tourniquet discomfort will also be resolved.

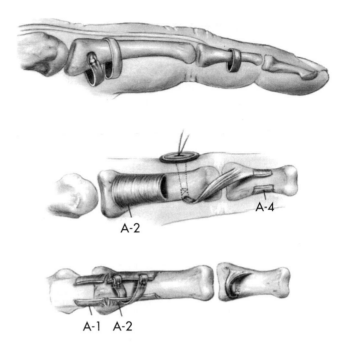

Fig. 51-1. Techniques of pulley reconstruction. Reconstruction using flexor tendon grafts passed circumferentially around proximal and middle phalanges *(top)*. Tendon graft passes under extensor tendon at proximal phalangeal levels and over it at middle phalangeal level. Tendon junction is rotated away from palmar surface of digit to provide a smooth, gliding surface. Use of slip of flexor digitorum superficialis (FDS) for middle digital pulley reconstruction *(middle)*. Tendon woven through remnant of annular flexor tendon sheath over proximal phalanx and use of slip of FDS stump to create a new middle phalangeal pulley *(bottom)*. (Modified from Doyle JR, Blythe W: The finger flexor tendon sheath and pulleys: anatomy and reconstruction. In *AAOS symposium on tendon surgery in the hand,* St Louis, 1975, Mosby.)

Surgical dissection is continued throughout the digit and palm until the adequacy of the release is demonstrated by active patient flexion or by a gentle proximal traction check in the palm. If necessary, the tourniquet can be released at this point and revascularization of the flexor muscles will return the patient's ability to actively participate. If the patient can fully flex the digit within the passive limits and if an adequate pulley system has been preserved, the procedure is deemed successful and wound closure and dressing application may ensue. If, however, annular pulleys are absent, attenuated, or inadequate, I believe it is appropriate to carry out immediate pulley reconstruction.

Although some surgeons believe that reconstructing pulleys at the time of tenolysis is contradictory and precludes an effective postoperative therapy regimen, I believe that the reconstructed pulleys can be adequately protected during the postoperative rehabilitation and do not hesitate to include annular pulley reconstruction (Fig. 51-1). I prefer to reconstruct pulleys at the proximal and mid portion of the proximal phalanx and mid portion of the middle phalanx to provide tendon restraint similar to that normally supplied by the A_2 and A_4 pulleys. I believe this is best accomplished by creating circumferential pulleys using the method of Bunnell, which has proven to be an effective method of restoring digital mechanics in the pulley-deficient finger. A curved cardiovascular ligature carrier is passed around the phalanx beneath the extensor mechanism at the level of the proximal phalanx and over it at the middle phalangeal level. Sutures placed through the graft are attached to the tip of the carrier and drawn around the phalanx. The tendon follows the suture into position and the second or third pass may be used to add additional width to the pulley and better distribute the forces of the tendon during strong flexion. The graft ends are woven tightly over the tendon and stitched with 3-0 braided suture. The junction site is then rotated away from the palmar portion of the digit so that a smooth interface is created between the tendon and the new pulley. When it is necessary to initiate immediate postoperative digital motion, reconstructed pulleys may be protected by the use of circumferential taping and later by the use of an orthoplast ring.

Capsulectomy may occasionally be combined with flexor tenolysis and the procedure usually involves a release of the palmar scar or tightened check-rein extensions of the palmar plate at the level of the proximal interphalangeal (PIP) joint to restore digital extension at that level. It should be emphasized, however, that every effort should be made to achieve full passive digital joint motion before surgery, because the concomitant lysis of tendons and joint release complicate the postoperative program and almost inevitably compromise the final result.

Although I previously believed that the local administration of triamcinolone was effective[7,11,31] in modifying the recurrence of tendon adhesions following tenolysis, I now doubt that there is any meaningful difference in results with or without the use of intraoperative steroids. However, for extremely difficult cases in patients who have shown a propensity for rapid and aggressive reformation of scar tissue or when some repeat lysis procedures are being carried out, several milliliters of triamcinolone may be locally administered. Although wound healing has not been a problem following the installation of cortisone preparations, the infection rate may be somewhat higher and tendon rupture may be an increased possibility.

The quality of flexor tendon or tendons at the time of surgery may give rise to serious concern as to whether the tendon will remain intact during the rigors of the obligatory postoperative therapy program. While the integrity of the tendon may often appear tenuous and create strong concern for its survival, I have rarely opted to excise the tendon and initiate a staged reconstruction procedure. I have, in several instances, combined the procedures by placing a Hunter tendon implant beneath the lysed tendon from the base of the distal phalanx to either the palm or distal forearm. It is hoped that this rod will serve as both a gliding base for the tendon and a potential stage I reconstruction if the tendon should

rupture. As of this writing, I have not had to proceed with a staged reconstruction and several badly scarred digits have performed well with this compromise technique. Although the procedure is certainly not recommended for general use, it may on occasion be a helpful method following difficult tenolysis in which tendon quality is judged to be marginal.

At the conclusion of the procedure, when maximum active digital motion compatible with the passive limits of the digital joints has been achieved, the wound is carefully repaired using 5-0 prolene. The tubing from scalp vein set may be left in the digit if it appears there will be substantial postoperative bleeding, and the needle component can be placed in a vacuum collecting tube as a drain, which is incorporated in the bandage. A compressive dressing is employed, and it is my preference to splint the involved digit in flexion with the thought that this position is the most appropriate from which to begin the postoperative mobilization program. Patients usually have much less difficulty bringing the finger from a flexed to an extended attitude, and extension should produce obligatory movement of the lysed tendon over a short distance, whereas passive flexion does not necessarily ensure any gliding.

POSTOPERATIVE MANAGEMENT

Before initiating a postoperative therapy program following flexor tenolysis, the hand therapist must carefully consider many factors pertaining to the specific clinical situation presented by the patient. The surgeon and therapist should have direct communication regarding the patient's history, previous surgery, and preoperative status; the condition of the tendon; and the status of the pulley system. Some understanding of the patient's motivation and of pain tolerance also add immeasurably to the preparation for a given therapy program. In addition, an effort should be made to identify patients who have a tendency to develop excessive edema, those who have diminished vascularity resulting from previous injury or surgery, and those who have previously been infected. This information is useful in establishing realistic goals and in implementing a treatment program that can best achieve such goals.

The surgical finding of a poor quality tendon or the need to reconstruct pulleys also requires special postoperative techniques designed to minimize the stress placed on the tendons or pulleys, or both. A strong tendon that appears near-normal in a minimally scarred bed with an adequate pulley system would be a candidate for a more aggressive postoperative mobilization program. Some aspects of the postoperative therapy are dictated by the appearance of the involved digit and hand at the time of removal of the surgical dressing. Excessive swelling, bleeding, infection, wound breaking, or inordinate pain may all have a prejudicial effect on the initial efforts to gain motion.

The rapid formation of new adhesions can be at least partly avoided by early tendon movement and immediate motion compatible with wound healing is desirable. I believe that it is extremely important to initiate digital motion within 12 hours following a flexor tenolysis procedure. It is equally important that the surgeon or a confident and experienced hand therapist personally supervise the initial active and passive motion program and that the patient's progress be monitored very closely thereafter. The performance of the digit in the first several days following tenolysis is critical, and it is rare to see a substantial improvement in range of motion that is actively achieved during that first week.

When I am concerned about the quality of the lysed tendons, I ask our therapist to employ a technique that we originally designated as the "frayed tendon program." This protocol involves the passive manipulation of the fingers into full flexion followed by efforts by the patient to actively maintain the flexion. The rationale for the regimen is simply that the tendon excursion required to hold the passively produced flexed position of the digit should be exactly the same as that required to actively bring the digit from extension to flexion. The major difference, of course, is that the tensile loading of the lysed flexor tendon is markedly less when a passive assist is used to flex the digit, particularly when the finger is somewhat swollen and stiffened by the recent surgery. The desired tendon excursion is achieved with much less effort by the patient and less stress on the tendon. Although we are without statistical verification, it is our impression that there is less discomfort associated with therapy, that it is easier for the patient to maintain the excursion of the lysed tendon, and that the rupture rate has been diminished by this approach. The frayed tendon program has now become the standard postoperative regimen for almost all my patients who have undergone flexor tenolysis.

During the initial postoperative visit, and after the goals and methods of therapy have been discussed with the patient, the bulky compressive dressing is removed and a lighter dressing is applied that is compatible with the control of edema. When necessary, areas of pulley reconstruction are identified and protected by circumferential taping or the use of a thermoplastic ring.[6] This protection is continued for 10 to 12 weeks and has resulted in very few ruptures. Finger socks or Coban wraps are generally applied to control digital edema. In addition to reducing swelling, these small dressings are aesthetically acceptable to the patient and tend to obviate the limitation of motion, pain, and bleeding that can sometimes hamper the early mobilization of the digit that has just undergone extensive surgery.

The initial exercise program consists of active and passive exercises designed to take the involved digit through the full range of motion that was passively present preoperatively. This session is usually not terminated until the patient can actively achieve essentially the same flexion that was demonstrated at surgery. The patient is instructed to exercise with the wrist in various positions and to place equal emphasis on both extension and flexion. These exercises maximize the required excursion of the lysed flexor tendons. At the conclusion of the first effort at postoperative mobilization, the patient is instructed to continue the exercise program for 10 to 15 minutes each waking hour. The ability to carry out self-therapy is carefully monitored. Postoperative splinting varies, depending on the tendency toward joint stiffening in a given digit and the difficulty that the patient may have initiating motion from either a flexed or an extended position. The majority of posttenolysis digits are managed by extension splinting between exercise sessions to place the digits at rest and diminish the tendency for PIP joint flexion contracture. When passive extension is easily achieved, it may be better to splint the digit in a flexed attitude between motion efforts. Other methods that have proved to be helpful in enhancing tendon excursion subsequent to flexor tenolysis include the following[6]:

1. Wrist and metacarpophalangeal (MP) flexion block splinting in full extension in an effort to isolate the long flexors
2. Blocking exercises to maximize the effect of profundus and superficialis function at the PIP and distal interphalangeal (DIP) joints, respectively
3. Scar massage, particularly at wrist level, to separate skin and subcutaneous tissues from the underlying tendons

During the course of the postoperative effort to maintain the excursion and digital performance that was achieved in surgery, it may be necessary to employ several adjunctive modalities to assist the patient. The use of transcutaneous nerve stimulators (TENS) units have been shown to be valuable in reducing postoperative pain, and electrical stimulation may be of considerable value when the muscle of the tenolysed tendon is weakened and requires augmentation to produce full tendon excursion. The use of muscle stimulation is compatible with the passive flexion–active maintenance program that I have described. For patients who tend to protectively counteract their own efforts to flex their fingers by simultaneously using antagonistic extensor muscle contraction, the use of biofeedback indicators may be of value. Other adjunctive equipment such as continuous passive motion (CPM) machines may also be beneficial to the postoperative therapy effort, but must be combined with active flexion efforts on the part of the patient. If digital joints begin to soften, the use of dynamic extension or flexion splinting may be helpful depending on the specific needs of the individual patient. As already mentioned, circumferential taping or the use of orthoplast rings may be required to protect the reconstructed pulleys after the procedure.

Above all, the clinical course of the patient must be carefully monitored. Every effort must be made to maintain the gains achieved at surgery, and serial measurements must be frequently assessed to be sure that the patient is progressing appropriately. Failure to proceed aggressively following this procedure may result in either a rapid or gradual readherence of the lysed tendons and a loss of the gains achieved at surgery.

COMPLICATIONS

Despite the surgical demonstration of complete lysis of one or more flexor tendons, an occasional patient is unable to achieve or maintain adequate digital flexion in the immediate postoperative course. In those instances, it is important for the surgeon and therapist to identify the problem and devote every effort to gaining maximum excursion of the tendon before it readheres. Regardless of these efforts, there are patients who simply fail to demonstrate the expected result. I have sometimes elected to return the patient to surgery and have usually been able to salvage good function by placing gentle, sustained, proximal traction on the involved tendon at the distal forearm level. It appears that some patients have a propensity for a rather rapid readherence of their lysed tendons and that a return to the operating room within 1 or 2 weeks while the restricting adhesions are still immature offers a chance for a simple mechanical rupture of the peritendinous restraints without the need for a formal reopening of the entire operative site. This is a *salvage procedure for selected patients* in whom the posttenolysis result has been inconsistent with the operative findings and the demonstrable performance of the digit during surgery. There have been a few instances of partial wound separation following this procedure given the fact that the motion program may place considerable stress on the surgical wound, especially if the digit is swollen. Such wounds may expose the underlying tendon and the risks of infection or tendon necrosis creates considerable concern. I believe that this complication should be approached by rapid return to the operating room and repair of the involved wound with enhanced efforts made to protect it when the therapy motion program resumes.

The most devastating postoperative complication is probably the rupture of the lysed tendon, and despite the most conscientious efforts on the part of the surgeon, patient, and therapist, this complication occasionally occurs. If a rupture does occur, it must be addressed immediately and the surgeon's options include to do nothing, to allow the wound to heal and return at a later date to begin a staged flexor tendon reconstruction by implanting a silicone rod in the involved digit, or to return to the operating room to repair the ruptured tendon. I usually prefer to return the patient promptly to the operating room, when the soft tissues of the digit permit, for an effort at surgical repair of the ruptured tendon. Immobilization of the wrist and digit for 3 to 4 weeks to permit healing and, in all likelihood, readherence will occur. An additional surgical lysis can then be carried out, and, somewhat surprisingly, it will frequently return function that is comparable with or better than that which could be expected from a staged reconstruction sequence.

The length of the therapy program varies depending on the individual performance of the involved digits in each patient. Some patients easily regain excellent motion with little tendency toward digital stiffening in between exercise efforts. If these patients are reliable, there is little need to prolong the formal therapy program, and a home exercise protocol will suffice. Others may have a much more reactive soft tissue response to surgery and their course will be complicated by swelling, recurring stiffness, and even a tendency to develop contractures. For these patients, the therapy is more intense and longer in duration. Edema control, dynamic splinting, and the use of adjunctive modalities such as a CPM machine or some type of electrical muscle stimulation is required. At times, a short course of oral steroids may be of value in diminishing this untoward biologic response. Usually, therapy can be discontinued by 6 weeks posttenolysis; however, I advise patients not to carry out any strong grasping or heavy lifting for up to 3 months following the procedure. This will avoid the uncommon but catastrophic late tendon rupture.

SUMMARY

The results of thorough tenolysis of the flexor tendons in the palm and digits in selected patients can be gratifying.[22,25] Preoperative requirements include a well-motivated patient with a supple digit and an established wide discrepancy between active and passive ranges of digital motion. Careful preservation of reconstruction of annular pulleys and the demonstration of the adequacy of the lysis at the time of surgery are extremely important.

Every effort must be made to achieve active digital motion compatible with passive motion as quickly as possible after tenolysis. In some instances, however, the patient fails to achieve the expected result, and it is important to monitor these patients very closely. Serial measurements of the performance of a given digit should provide useful information as to whether the patient will be able to maintain the tendon and joint motion that was surgically achieved. It has been my impression that when there is good isolated function of the flexor digitorum superficialis and flexor digitorum profundus that is gradually improving, it is usually possible to regain full active flexion compatible with passive limitations within 2 weeks.

The postoperative maintenance of the tendon excursion and joint motion following flexor tenolysis is a difficult and challenging responsibility. Therapists must be mindful of all the factors that affect the patient's preoperative course, including the initial injury, previous surgery, the preoperative status of the involved digit, and the findings at surgery. A well-designed treatment program can then be implemented, following careful consultation between the surgeon and therapist. A close rapport between therapist and patient is also essential. Special efforts may be required to modify pain, control edema, preserve passive motion, eliminate antagonistic muscle activity, protect pulleys, and, above all, maintain tendon excursion.

When this surgical-therapy program proceeds without complication, the improvement in digital flexion should be consistent, often with restoration of near-normal function. At the time of this writing, incidences of tendon rupture, infection, or delayed wound healing have been few.

REFERENCES

1. Reference deleted in proofs.
2. Boyes JH: The great flexor tendon controversy. In Cramer LM, Chase RA, eds: *Symposium on the hand,* vol 3, St Louis, 1971, Mosby.
3. Brooks DM: Problems of restoration of tendon movements after repair and grafts, *Proc R Soc Med* 1970; 63:67.
4. Bruner JM: The zigzag volar digital incision for flexor tendon surgery, *Plast Reconstr Surg* 1967; 40:571.
5. Bunnell S: *Surgery of the hand,* ed 2, Philadelphia, 1967, Lippincott.
6. Cannon NM, Strickland JW: Therapy following flexor tendon surgery, *Hand Clin* 1987; 1(1):147.
7. Carstam N: The effects of cortisone on the formation of tendon adhesions and on tendon healing: an experimental investigation in the rabbit, *Acta Chir Scand* 1953; 182(suppl):1.
8. Doyle JR, Blythe W: The finger flexor tendon sheath and pulleys: anatomy and reconstruction. In *AAOS symposium on tendon surgery in the hand,* St Louis, 1975, Mosby.
9. Fetrow KW: Tenolysis in the hand and wrist, *J Bone Joint Surg* 1967; 49A:667.
10. Hunter JM, Seinsheimer F, Mackin EJ: Tenolysis: pain control and rehabilitation. In Strickland JW, Steichen JB eds: *Difficult problems in hand surgery,* St Louis, 1982, Mosby.
11. Reference deleted in proofs.
12. James JIP: The value of tenolysis, *Hand* 1969; 1:118.
13. Ketchum LD: The effects of triamcinolone on tendon healing and function, *Plast Reconstr Surg* 1971; 47:471.
14. Peacock EE, Van Winckle W: *Surgery and biology of wound repair,* Philadelphia, 1970, Saunders.
15. Pulvertaft RG: Experience in flexor tendon grafting in the hand, *J Bone Joint Surg* 1959; 41B:629 (abstract).
16. Rank BK, Wakefield AR, Hueston JJ: *Surgery of repair as applied to hand injuries,* ed 4, Baltimore, 1973, Williams & Wilkins.
17. Schneider LH, Hunter JM: Flexor tenolysis. In *AAOS symposium on tendon surgery in the hand,* St Louis, 1975, Mosby.
18. Schneider LH, Hunter JM: Flexor tendon—late reconstruction. In Green DP, ed: *Operative hand surgery,* New York, 1982, Churchill Livingstone.
19. Schneider LH, Mackin EJ: Tenolysis. In Hunter JM, Schneider LH, Mackin EJ, Bell JA, eds: *Rehabilitation of the hand,* St Louis, 1978, Mosby.
20. Schneider LH, Mackin EJ: Tenolysis: dynamic approach to surgery and therapy. In Hunter JM, Schneider LH, Mackin EJ, Callahan AD, eds: *Rehabilitation of the hand,* ed 2, St Louis, 1984, Mosby.
21. Strickland JW: Flexor tenolysis: a personal experience. In Hunter JM, Schneider LH, Mackin EJ, eds: *Tendon surgery in the hand,* St Louis, 1987, Mosby.
22. Strickland JW: Flexor tenolysis, *Hand Clin* 1985; 1(1):121-132.
23. Strickland JW: Functional recovery after flexor tendon severance in the finger: the state of the art. In Strickland JW, Steichen JB, eds: *Difficult problems in hand surgery,* St Louis, 1982, Mosby.
24. Strickland JW: Management of acute flexor tendon injuries, *Orthop Clin North Am* 1983; 14:827.
25. Strickland JW: Results of flexor tendon surgery in zone II, *Hand Clin* 1985; 1(1):167.
26. Verdan CE: *Tendon surgery of the hand,* Edinburgh, 1979, Churchill Livingstone.
27. Verdan CE, Crawford GP, Martini-Benkeddache Y: The valuable role of tenolysis in the digits. In Cramer LM, Chase RA, eds: *Symposium on the hand,* vol 3, St Louis, 1971, Mosby.
28. Weeks PM, Wray RC: The rate and extent of functional recovery after flexor tendon grafting, with and without silicone rod, *J Hand Surg* 1976; 1:174.
29. Whitaker J, Strickland JW, Ellis RG: *The role of tenolysis in the palm and digit,* J Hand Surg 1977; 2:462.
30. Wray RC, Moucharafieh B, Weeks PM: Experimental study of the optimal time for tenolysis, *Plast Reconstr Surg* 1978; 61:184.
31. Wrenn RL, Goldner JL, Markee JL: An experimental study of the effect of cortisone on the healing process and tensile strength of tendons, *J Bone Joint Surg* 1954; 36A:588.

Chapter 52

DIGITAL FLEXOR TENDON TENOLYSIS

Improvement by maintained flexion in postoperative regimen

Guy Foucher
Giorgio Padjardi

Adhesions of flexor tendons is a normal response to tendon injury. Tenolysis is the procedure that frees all adhesions and maintains gliding of the flexor apparatus.

All types of injuries could be followed by attachment of the mobile tendons to fixed structures. Two etiologies deserve to be isolated as giving very limited adhesion and subsequently not involving a real tenolysis, but a much more limited procedure. They are partial lesion of the flexor tendon with hypertrophic callus and blockage (different from triggering, another complication) and fixation of the profundus tendon to an amputation stump, giving a quadriga syndrome described by Verdan.[19] Other etiologies can be separated according to the presence or absence of a direct lesion of the flexor tendon. As demonstrated by Peacock, edema is rich in proteins providing a real biologic "glue." When edema is present, a soft tissue crush injury or a phalangeal fracture, followed by immobilization, could be complicated by tendon adhesion. First phalanx fractures are particularly prone to this complication, but direct injury or "catching" of the flexor tendon at the fracture or healing site have to be ruled out. A good lateral x-ray examination is always mandatory.

Infection of the flexor sheath can cause extensive adhesions when treated late, at a point when tenolysis is not technically possible.

But the major etiology of direct lesions of the flexor tendon remains. Even in the tight space of no man's land,

tendon adhesion is not now considered a normal consequence of the extrinsic healing process, but rather a complication secondary to tendon injury either caused by the type of injury (crush) or to surgical technique. Meticulous suturing of divided flexor tendons, followed by early mobilization, encourages intrinsic healing and reduces the incidence of adhesions. However, the range of mobility of the tendon suture in semiactive (Kleinert[12]), passive (Duran[5]), or combined postoperative regimen, remains largely unpredictable. Adhesions occurred in 22% of patients in our series of primary tendon suture with the Tsuge technique, followed by semiactive mobilization.[2] The occurrence was more relevant in immobilized tendons with crush and complex injuries.

Scarce experimental studies have proved that recurrence of adhesions could happen in a few hours,[13] giving relevance to the postoperative regimen based on early mobilization. We developed an original postoperative regimen in 1978,[8] and have consequently reported the results[10] in the digital canal (zones 1 and 2).

CLINICAL EXAMINATION

Careful examination is mandatory before deciding on a tenolysis. General examination of the patient needs to consider age, associated vascular disease, psychologic status, and motivations. Time off from work could be anticipated according to the job (and leisure activities). In strenuous manual occupations, 4 months leave may be necessary to avoid tendon rupture, and the patient must know this in advance.

A hand examination must include assessment of tissue equilibrium, quality and extension of scar tissue, arterial supply of the finger, bone stability, sensibility, functional use (or exclusion) of the finger, limitation of passive motion, and range of active flexion (with or without flexor bowstringing). An x-ray image is taken in cases of previous finger or joint fracture. In the absence of any active motion, palpation may reveal a gap or coiling of the flexor tendon in the palm, and in our experience magnetic resonance imaging has been useful in ruling out a tendon rupture and allowing preoperative discussion of the possibility of a two-stage tendon graft.

Indications and contraindications

Indication of flexor tenolysis is contemplated in a compliant healthy patient, with a well-vascularized finger with bone stability, when the passive range of motion (PROM) largely exceeds the active range of motion (AROM).

Definite contraindications are uncompliant or psychiatric patients, injuries that are too old (when the flexor motor is atrophic or fibrotic), or excluded fingers (e.g., bypassed index finger).

Other problems are only temporary contraindications: patients who are too young, nonunion of bones, recent infection, heavy palmar scar, stiff finger in extension with associated extensor adhesion. In such cases, a previous surgical step is often mandatory with bone grafting, skin flap replacement, extensor tenolysis, or intrinsic release. We avoid combining these procedures with flexor tenolysis to ensure that postoperative edema remains limited and nothing interferes with the regimen of active motion. We avoided collateral nerve grafting for the same reason, until vein tube grafting became available, which can be performed at the same time.

TIMING OF THE PROCEDURE

Timing of the procedure is important. Many limited tendon adhesions can be managed by a combined program of active rehabilitation and splinting to improve PROM and AROM. This trial period, even if not fully successful in active gain, improves PROM and provides a timely approach of the patient's psychologic status, compliance, motivation, and pain threshold. In a previous study,[9] we have tried to assess the minimum duration of the splinting period. We have demonstrated that if the PROM has not sufficiently improved after 12 weeks in a well-fitting splint, only surgery will lead to further improvement.

Otherwise, we apply the criteria of tissue equilibrium as proposed by Fetrow,[6] Hunter et al.,[11] and Verdan et al.[19] These criteria are healed fractures, absence of joint contracture, and good muscle strength.

The optimal timing of tenolysis has been extensively discussed in the literature. After fracture, the delay may be shorter and after infection of the tendon sheath it may be longer. Following flexor tendon suture Fetrow[6] recommended 3 months, and Rank et al.[14] 6 to 9 months. Whitaker waited 7.2 months,[21] and the delay was 5.2 months in our series (excluding 3 cases in which the delay was more than 2 years). Experimentally, the ideal delay in performing tenolysis after tendon suture has been studied by Wray et al.[22] Their study revealed that chickens demonstrate good tensile strength and increased vascularization when the tenolysis is performed at 12 weeks.

The patient needs to understand the procedure and subsequent rehabilitation and should realize that there may have to be a change of plans during the operation, including a tendon graft, tenodesis, or arthrodesis. Information should also be given about complications, including skin breaks, infection, rupture, and recurrent adhesions.

TECHNIQUE

We have performed all procedures under regional anaesthesia on an outpatient basis. We abandoned local anaesthesia,[11,15,16] and the technique of selective sensory blocks[7] intended to allow preoperative checking of AROM, except in late tenolysis where we have doubts about a muscle's performance.

Like Schneider and Hunter,[15] we favor the Bruner incision[4] for its direct approach, but we agree that the angles of the flaps are at risk when previous incisions are crossed. Strickland[16] prefers the midlateral incision leaving the neurovascular bundle with the finger. A separate incision in the palm or forearm is frequently used to check flexion after the procedure.

We proceed from the unaffected to the affected area, freeing both flexors as a block, trying to save as many pulleys as possible.[11] For this purpose, we use multiple transverse incisions in the pulleys, maneuvering gently with a spatula to develop a plane of cleavage. Discrete bands of adhesions are formally incised with a blade. Only then are the two tendons separated from each other. Having verified the continuity of the flexor digitorum profundus (FDP), we are prepared to remove the less well-preserved slip of flexor digitorum superficialis (FDS). A thread loop passed around the tendons can be helpful for pulling out adhesion through incisions in the pulley (Lister, 1993, personal communication).

The procedure is considered complete when traction through the proximal incision produces good muscle excursion proximally, and free and full flexion of the digit distally. Trimming the tendon is frequently necessary to achieve this goal at the site of a previous suture, and all foreign material must be removed.

Additional procedures

Sometimes additional procedures are required. Some, such as pulley reconstruction, arthrolysis, tendon length-

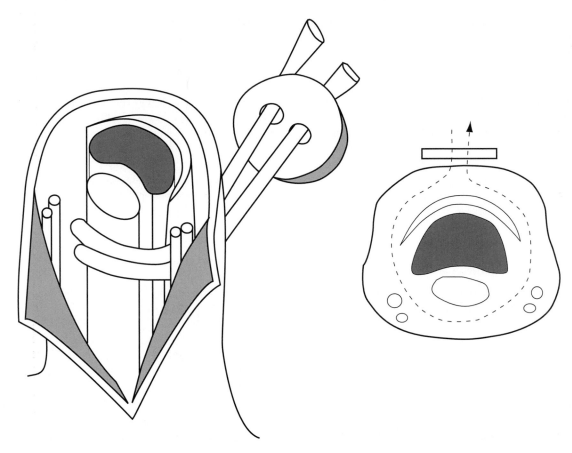

Fig. 52-1. Technique of strong pulley reconstruction used to allow early motion after tenolysis. (From Foucher G, Lenoble E, Youssef K-Ven, Sannut D: A post-operative regime after digital flexor tenolysis: a series of 72 patients, J Hand Surg 1993; 18B:35-40.)

ening, and silicone underlay, concern the operation itself.

Pulley reconstruction. Many procedures are available for pulley reconstruction. But the basic requirement, when an active program of motion is contemplated, is whether a pulley is easy to protect or strong enough. If the A$_1$ pulley can be protected by immobilizing the metacarpophalangeal (MP) joints in extension, it is best to do so as we have been disappointed by any external ring protection (at least in the early postoperative period). This is why in 1980 we developed a modification of Bunnell[3] technique, consisting of a double encirclement of tendon graft around skeleton and extensor tendon.[8,10] The two ends of the graft are exteriorized and anchored on a button. Because this reconstruction is narrow, it must be sited close to the axis of rotation of the joint (Fig. 52-1).

Check-rein release. Check-rein release is considered only in cases with extensor deficit after complete flexor liberation. The technique has been extensively described by Watson et al.[20]

Silicone underlay. Silicone underlay is rarely used, and is restricted to covering bone after spur resection or after extensive periosteum loss.[1]

Last steps of the procedure

Mainly in case of pulley reconstruction, a further check of the PROM by means of wrist tenodesis effect is performed. This involves full passive extension of the wrist, allowing finger flexion in cascade, and flexion of the wrist allowing the finger to passively extend.

The three ultimately important steps are meticulous hemostasis, maximal proximal migration of the flexor tendon and, to minimize pain, insertion of one or two percutaneous catheters at the wrist level close to the nerve trunks supplying the tenolysed digits. Long-acting local anesthetics are then injected to provide postoperative pain relief.

The distal skin incision is closed first and the finger flexed by traction on the tendon through the proximal incision that is still open. The fingers are immobilized in slight flexion in a bulky boxing glove bandage, encouraging the tendon to adhere initially in flexion. Excessive interphalangeal (IP) joint flexion is avoided to prevent skin ischemia.[8,10]

POSTOPERATIVE MANAGEMENT

Forty hours after surgery, a small amount of local anesthetic is injected through the catheter(s) before the first dressing change. The patient is asked to extend the digits actively. If this is difficult or extension is incomplete, the surgeon passively extends the digits by gentle traction while maintaining the wrist and MP joints in flexion. It is common to feel crepitus as adhesions are broken. Active extension and flexion is repeated five or six times, ending with active flexion, and the hand is then placed in a splint maintaining some metacarpal and phalangeal flexion. This splint is worn continuously for 3 weeks, but during waking hours the patient removes it, each hour, to perform three or four full extension-flexion exercises. To facilitate extension, an extension spring is used by the patient each morning and following each session of active motion (for a period of 5 minutes or longer in case of preoperative deficit of extension). Compliance with the instructions is supervised the following day (at this stage the catheter is usually removed) and if good, a visit is scheduled each week.

No activity requiring force is permitted for 6 weeks, but if necessary, from the third week, extension is gradually increased in a night splint.

SERIES

The details of our series of 78 digits treated have been reported previously[10]; only general results and relevant factors are mentioned here. Cases of replantation or toe transfers were excluded. Forty-nine patients (68%) were referred after initial management elsewhere. Some known complications had occurred: three cases of impaired skin healing, two infections, and six supposed ruptures. In our department, all of the 23 flexor tendon injuries were sutured using Tsuge's method.[18] Postoperatively, 9 were mobilized using Kleinert's method,[12] 2 were mobilized passively,[5] and 12 were immobilized. Excluding the three tenolyses performed after a delay of more than 2 years, the average interval between injury and treatment was 5.2 months. Pulley reconstruction, according to the technique previously cited, was done in 10 cases, and a volar proximal interphalangeal (PIP) arthrolysis was necessary in 24 cases.

After a mean follow-up of 21.5 months, ranging from 16 to 28 months, assessment was done by measuring each individual joint with a goniometer and comparing the findings with the preoperative measurement. These figures were then expressed according to Swanson's system[17] to assess functional improvement. Statistical analysis has been unifactorial and multifactorial (Lotus 1-2-3 and Fischer tables) taking improvement in total active movement as an index of outcome and a number of other factors including age, profession, affected fingers, preoperative range of motion, preoperative and postoperative complications, and specific surgical technique. Time off from work averaged 3.4 months.

COMPLICATIONS

Complications are listed in Table 52-1. Two tendons (2.5%) ruptured. Out of the nine thumbs tenolysed in zone

Table 52-1. Complications

	Number of Cases (%)
Delayed healing	2
Flexor tendon exposed	2 (1 cross finger, 1 rupture)
Flexor tendon rupture	2 (2.5%)
Reflex sympathetic dystrophy	2*
Infection	none
Unimproved	4 (5%)
Aggravated	9 (11.5%)

From Foucher G, Lenoble E, Youssef K-Ven, Sannut D: A post-operative regimen after digital flexor tenolysis: a series of 72 patients, *J Hand Surg* 1993; 18B:35-40.
*Diagnosis was confirmed by three-phase bone scan; in both cases this was a localized form.

2, two cases (22%) were unimproved. In the fingers, two cases (3%) were unimproved, and nine cases (13%) were made worse, with total AROM deteriorating from 148.6° to 123.2°. These bad results may be explained by the poor initial condition of the tendons (in two fingers FDP was absent), by associated procedures (five cases of PIP joint stiffness requiring arthrolysis), and by postoperative complications (two cases of delayed healing, including one exposed tendon followed by rupture and another independent rupture).

RESULTS IN IMPROVED CASES

Seven thumbs (78%) improved. Total AROM increased from 65° to 115° following tenolysis (Table 52-2). Swanson's[17] assessment accords equal functional importance to the IP and the MP joints in the thumb. The improvement in function is the result of improvement in the IP joint.

Fifty-eight fingers (84%) improved. Average preoperative total AROM went from 134.7° to a postoperative average of 202.9° (Table 52-3). Using Swanson's assessment, the functional deficit averaged 41.4%, improving to a deficit of 19.8% postoperatively. Virtually, the entire functional deficit is at the level of the IP joint.

Most of the variables examined had no correlation with the degree of improvement in total active movement. However, the improvement is inversely proportional to the AROM at the IP joint at presentation—the poorer the presenting IP joint ranges, the greater the improvement will be.

DISCUSSION

If complications are excluded, this series of tenolyses has achieved an increased AROM from 135° to 203° in the fingers and from 65° to 115° in the thumbs. Using Swanson's method of evaluation, the functional impairment for the thumb in this series decreased from 12% to 1.9% (10.1%) and for the fingers from 41.4% to 19.8% (21.6%). Four cases (5%) were unimproved, and 9 (11.5%) were made worse by the procedure (with an average total active movement loss of 25.4°). The total failure rate was 17%, which means that 83%

Table 52-2. Comparison of preoperative and postoperative joint mobility in the thumb with regard to the seven patients improved by tenolysis

AROM	Preoperative		Postoperative	
	Average	Standard	Average	Standard
MP	53.5°	15.7°	60°	0°
IP	11.4°	9.8°	64.1°	11.7°
Degrees	65°	15.3°	115°	24.9°
Percent	12%	12.6%	1.9%	1.2%

From Foucher G, Lenoble E, Youssef K-Ven, Sannut D: A post-operative regimen after digital flexor tenolysis: a series of 72 patients, *J Hand Surg* 1993; 18B:35-40.
AROM, Active range of motion; *MP,* metacarpophalangeal; *IP,* interphalangeal.

Table 52-3. Comparison of preoperative and postoperative total active movement for long digits in those patients improved by tenolysis

AROM	Preoperative		Postoperative	
	Average	Standard Deviation	Average	Standard Deviation
MP	87.1°	10.7°	87.3°	8.8°
PIP	36.8°	26.2°	73.7°	20.9°
DIP	17.6°	22°	53.3°	23.8°
IP	47.6°	35.8°	115.6°	44.9°
Degrees	134.7°	39.1°	202.9°	46.4°
Percent	41.4%	17.4%	19.8%	14%

From Foucher G, Lenoble E, Youssef K-Ven, Sannut D: A post-operative regimen after digital flexor tenolysis: a series of 72 patients, *J Hand Surg* 1993; 18B:35-40.
AROM, Active range of motion; *MP,* metacarpophalangeal; *PIP,* proximal interphalangeal; *DIP,* distal interphalangeal; *IP,* interphalangeal.

of fingers were improved. This is close to the results reported by the literature (Table 52-4), but with a lower rate of rupture. Only two tendons (2.5%) ruptured, which can be explained by the protection of the splinting in flexion, which avoids incidental use of the hand. In our series, rupture occurred early (first and second week) and we have not observed very late rupture such as the one mentioned by Whitaker 2 months after the operation.[21] The policy of immobilizing the fingers initially in flexion has several advantages. Gliding of the flexor tendon decreases rapidly after the operation, as demonstrated by Lane et al.[13] and collageneous adhesions form within hours. The patient may be unable to break these adhesions due to persistent pain and muscle weakness. This can be performed gently by the surgeon at the first dressing change and later on by an extension spring applied early in the morning. However, this position could increase the risk of skin necrosis and lack of PIP extension. There were two cases of wound breakdown

Table 52-4. Published series

	Improved Finger (%)	Rate of Rupture (%)
Whitaker[21]	79	9
Verdan[19]	74	6.3
Schneider[15]	72	5.5
Foucher[10]	83.4	2.5

From Foucher G, Lenoble E, Youssef K-Ven, Sannut D: A post-operative regimen after digital flexor tenolysis: a series of 72 patients, *J Hand Surg* 1993; 18B:35-40.

apparently due to the excessively flexed position adopted early in our series using a Bruner incision. There was no such complication in the last 52 consecutive cases. Rather, preoperative extension deficit has constantly improved in all cases thanks to extension splinting.

Tenolysis is an acceptable major procedure for digital flexor tendon adhesions. In 83% of cases it provided an improvement in the active range of motion averaging 68° for the fingers and 50° for the thumbs. According to Swanson et al.,[17] this corresponds to an improvement in function of 10.1% for the thumbs and 21.6% for the fingers.

REFERENCES

1. Ashworth CR, Blatt G, Chuinard RG, Stark HH: Silicone-rubber interposition arthroplasty of the carpometacarpal joint of the thumb, *J Hand Surg* 1977; 2(5):345-357.
2. Berard V, Lantieri L, Ebelin M, Foucher G: Resultats de la réparation tendineuse des fléchisseurs selon la technique de Tsuge. A propos de 95 doigts, *Ann Chir Main* 1995; 16:69-73.
3. Bunnell S: *Surgery of the hand,* Philadelphia, 1944, Lippincott.
4. Bruner JM: The zig-zag volar digital incision for flexor-tendon surgery, *Plast Reconstr Surg* 1967; 40(6):571-574.
5. Duran RJ, Houser RG: Controlled passive motion following flexor tendon repair in zones 2 and 3, *AAOS symposium on tendon surgery in the hand,* St Louis, 1975, Mosby.
6. Fetrow KO: Tenolysis in the hand and wrist, *J Bone Joint Surg* 1967; 49A(4):667-685.
7. Foucher G, Haberer JP, Farny J, et al: Interêt des blocs nerveux sélectifs sensitifs en chirurgie de la main, *Ann Chir* 1978; 32(9):615-618.
8. Foucher G, Marin Braun F: Technique originale de mobilisation après ténolyse des tendons fléchisseurs en zone 2, *Ann Chir Main* 1989a; 8(3):252-253.
9. Foucher G, Greant PH, Ehrler S, et al: Le rôle de l'orthèse dans les raideurs de la main, *Chirurgie* 1989b; 115:100-105.
10. Foucher G, Lenoble E, Ben-Youssef K, Sammut D: A post-operative regime after digital flexor tenolysis: a series of 72 cases, *J Hand Surg* 1993; 18B:35-40.
11. Hunter JM, Seinsheimer F, Mackin EJ: Tenolysis: pain control and rehabilitation, In Strickland JW, Steichen JB, eds: *Difficult problems in hand surgery,* St Louis, 1982, Mosby.
12. Kleinert HE, Kutz JE, Cohen MJ: Primary repair of zone 2 flexor tendon lacerations, *AAOS symposium on tendon surgery in the hand,* St Louis, 1975, Mosby.
13. Lane JM, Black J, Bora FW: Gliding function following flexor tendon injury: a biomechanical study of rat tendon function, *J Bone Joint Surg* 1976; 58A(7):985-990.
14. Rank BK, Wakefield AR, Hueston JT: *Surgery of repair as applied to hand injuries,* ed 4, Edinburgh, 1973, Churchill Livingstone.
15. Schneider LH, Hunter JM: Flexor tenolysis. In *AAOS symposium on tendon surgery in the hand,* St Louis, 1975, Mosby.

16. Strickland JW: Flexor tenolysis, *Hand Clin* 1985; 1(1):121-132.

17. Swanson AB, Göran-Hagert C, Swanson G de G: Evaluation of impairment in the upper extremity, *J Hand Surg* 1987; 12A:5(2):896-926.

18. Tsuge K, Ikuta Y, Matsuishi Y: Repair of flexor tendons by intratendinous tendon suture, *J Hand Surg* 1977; 2(6):436-440.

19. Verdan CE, Crawford GP, Martini-Benkeddach Y: The valuable role of tenolysis in the digits, In Cramer LM, Chase RA, eds: *Symposium on the hand,* vol 3, St Louis, 1971, Mosby.

20. Watson HK, Light TR, Johnson TR: Check-rein resection for flexion contracture of the middle joint, *J Hand Surg* 1979; 4(1):67-71.

21. Whitaker JH, Strickland JW, Ellis RK: The role of flexor tenolysis in the palm and digit, *J Hand Surg* 1977; 2(6):462-470.

22. Wray RC, Moucharafieth B, Weeks PM: Experimental study of the optimal time for tenolysis, *Plast Reconstr Surg* 1978; 61(2):184-189.

Chapter 53

COMPLEX TENOLYSIS OF THE HAND
Guidelines for treatment

Antonio Landi
Antonio Saracino
Giuseppe Caserta
Marco Esposito

Early active mobilization of all primary repairs of flexor and extensor tendons is gaining growing consensus[8,15] independently from the level of repair. In 1992 we sent out a detailed questionnaire probing surgeons' criteria for treating acute tendon lesions. For the majority of surgeons (Table 53-1) repair of the extensor tendons of the fingers in no man's land was considered of equal difficulty as those of the flexor tendons, although for different reasons. The trend toward early active mobilization after primary repair of the flexor and extensor tendons has been confirmed.[8,12,15] As a consequence of current surgical and rehabilitative techniques, the incidence of secondary tenolysis after tenorrhaphy has decreased to 2% of the operated cases. This finding reflects the widespread use of immediate passive gliding techniques during rehabilitation and early controlled active mobilization.

However, in contrast to the decrease in the incidence of tenolysis, the incidence of tendon rupture has increased slightly in the various centers.

As we approach the turn of the century, the global results of simple tenorrhaphy of both the flexors and extensors appear improved across all continents because of the use of new suture materials, techniques, and rehabilitation methods. Tendon tenolysis is consistently performed via standardized methods and leads to reproducible results. In this chapter we examine the problem of complex lesions and thus exclude isolated tendon sequelae. We attempt to identify criteria for clinical evaluation within the pooled complex tenolysis group and the priority for the various surgical steps. The need for tenolysis of both the extensor and flexor apparatus is discussed on the basis of the clinical experience acquired from 1978 to 1994 at the Orthopedic Clinic of the University of Modena. In this chapter, we describe the technical aspects of complex tenolysis and the possible clinical outcomes following surgery.

GENERAL CONSIDERATIONS

Tenolysis is considered complex when surgery aims not merely to release the tendon, but is associated with preliminary or ancillary interventions on the skin or contiguous anatomic structures (joints, tendons, pulleys), without which tenolysis per se would not produce significant functional improvements. We may thus define a complex tenolysis as occurring when interventions are requested on at least one other functionally correlated structure or neighboring anatomic tissue. The possible associations can be very varied, and are listed in the box on p. 457.

Tenolysis is a delicate surgical procedure, and its success strictly depends on a concerted effort among the patient, surgeon, and hand therapist. The patient must be instructed on how to be dedicated to guided rehabilitation.

Table 53-1. List of world-wide experts interviewed on tendons repair

Europe

Italy	G. Brunelli, L. Cugola, A. Landi, P. Raimondi
Switzerland	U. Buchler, D. Della Santa, D.W. Egloff, V. Meyer, A. Narakas
France	Y. Allieu, J. Baudet, R. Gomis, J.C. Rouzaud
Germany	U. Lanz, C. Wulle
Sweden	A. Ejeskär, G. Lundborg, A.K. Nachemson, K. Silfverskiöld
Finland	M. Vastamaki, S. Vilkki
Spain	F. Fonseca, G. Julve, A. Lluch
UK	N. Burton, J. Colville, M.C. Grouther, J.K. Stanley
Bulgaria	I. Matev

Asia

China	Da-De Pan, S.L. Huang, T.Y. Shen, J.K. Zhu
Singapore	R.W. Pho
Hong Kong	S.P. Chow, P.C. Leung
Japan	H. Saito, T. Satoshi, T. Tajima, S. Tamai, K. Tsuge, Y. Watanabe

Australia | B. Connoly, R. Hamilton, W. Morrison, M.A. Tonkin |

North America

USA	P. Amadio, G. Blatt, F. Bora, W.E. Bulkhalter, C. Hamlin, V. Hentz, M. Jabaley, J. Jupiter, H. Kleinert, P. Manske, J. Pribaz, R. Schenck, L. Schneider, B. Strauch

Africa

South Africa	S.L. Biddulph

Classification of complex tenolysis of the hand

- Tenolyses that are preceeded by other reconstructive procedures on skin, bones, nerves, and vessels
- Tenolyses dealing with tendons alone or of structures functionally related to tendon function
  - Tenolysis of flexor tendons with reconstruction of the pulleys
  - Tenolysis of the tendon grafts
  - Tenolysis of both extensor and flexor tendons
- Tenolysis associated with simultaneous joint release
  - Tenoarthrolysis of the dorsal apparatus (TADA)
  - Total anterior tenoarthrolysis (TATA)
- Tenolysis on a scarred environment that requires the following
  - Interposition of inert material (silicon sheet or rods)
  - Simultaneous reconstruction of a vascularized gliding tissue

---

Moreover, what will be done during the operation and what outcome can be expected must be explained in simple terms.

Tendon rupture following tenolysis must be advanced as a possible complication, and if this is foreseeable, an accurate prophylaxis by limiting rehabilitation to place-holding exercises must be selected.

The surgeon together with the therapist must make a detailed preoperative evaluation and verify the realistic possibilities of the patient taking part in a rehabilitation program as an outpatient.

Active patient collaboration is imperative for both flexor and extensor tenolysis. Accordingly, local anesthetic techniques that allow the patient to appreciate the results obtained immediately at the end of the surgical procedure are preferred.

A static splint is a crucial aid, depending on whether tenoarthrolysis of the dorsal apparatus (wrist extended, metacarpophalangeal [MP] joint and interphalangeal [IP] joint flexed), or tenolysis of the flexors (wrist in neutral position, MP joint flexed 10°, IP joint extended) have been performed, and its use must be limited to sleeping hours. With simultaneous tenolysis of the extensors and flexors, the two types of splints can be alternated. Any drains must be removed early (within 24 hours) to obviate microbial colonization of the wound, which can lead to serious complications such as septic arthritis and chronic synovitis of the new sheath, especially in complex tenolyses.

Postoperative edema of the released tendon might lead to friction at the level of the pulleys, especially on the flexor apparatus. This conflict is often audible and should not worry the patient; it should be treated by curtailing rehabilitation for a short period. Once the surgical scar has healed, frequent massage, the use of ultrasound, and standard techniques for reducing edema are helpful.

Active grip exercises differ substantially depending on whether tenolysis has been performed on an intact or sutured tendon or on a tendon graft. In the latter, active grip exercises should be postponed for at least 3 weeks. However, late tendon rupture remains a risk,[2] and it is strictly related to rehabilitation errors.

The thin or narrow pulleys that are at risk should be protected with artificial external pulleys. Even after complex tenolysis, patients can return to work activities on average 3 to 4 months after surgery, because tenolysis generally represents the final surgical act in the context of a complex lesion. The same precautions must be maintained for the joint's range of motion (ROM) if arthrolysis of the MP or IP joint has been carried out.

Thus, we will analyse the following conditions:

1. Dorsal tenoarthrolysis of the extensor apparatus and in particular after extensor tendon suture and grafts
2. Complex tenolysis of the flexor apparatus in zone 2
3. Tenolysis of both extensor and flexor tendons

In case of complex lesions where tenolysis is indicated, we follow the general principle that all interventions requiring immobilization of the limb, such as secondary nerve grafts, bone transplants, tendon transfers, etc., must, if possible, be grouped together, and releasing interventions, such as arthrolysis and tenolysis, should represent the final surgical step. Moreover, when stiffness results from adhesions of both the extensor and flexor apparatus, we perform dorsal tenolysis or tenoarthrolysis before flexor tenolysis. In complex tenolysis, initial evaluation is essentially based on active and passive ROM,[13,10] and the final outcomes have been correlated with the data on the functional ROM of the joints of the hand for various types of grip.[14] We mainly base final evaluation on the gain in active ROM[13] and a global clinical judgment of the patient.

TENOARTHROLYSIS OF THE DORSAL APPARATUS

Tenoarthrolysis of the dorsal apparatus (TADA) becomes necessary when adhesions and joint stiffness occur as sequelae of infection, inflammatory reactions (Fig. 53-1), closed trauma, and tenorrhaphy of the extensors at the dorsum of the hand and fingers. In complex trauma of the

hands, it is often difficult to ascertain whether joint rigidity is secondary to tenodesis, and once that resolves, joint excursion should return to normal on its own, or if it is primary and related to the outcome of intraarticular disorders such as hematoma or capsular-ligamentous lesions.

The effects of tenodesis are basically evaluated by clinical maneuvers[5,13] by sequentially placing the joints in a position of biomechanical advantage starting from the wrist. In this way, we can almost always identify the point of greatest fixation of the extensor apparatus. However, if fixation is located at or near a single joint, it became impossible to clinically identify the intraarticular or extraarticular etiology of stiffness.[6]

The patient's medical history can help us define the site and initial pathology. If stiffness follows tenorrhaphy of the extensor apparatus, tenolysis must begin at the site of the suture. In agreement with Creighton,[9] we found that in the majority of cases TADA became necessary after open fractures of the IP joint and closed, plurifragmented fractures

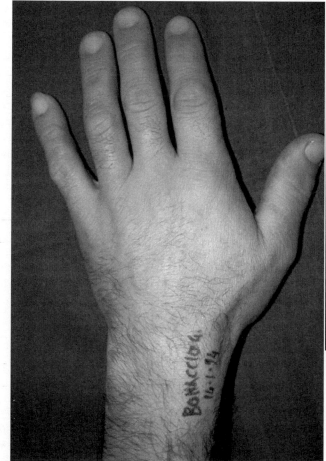

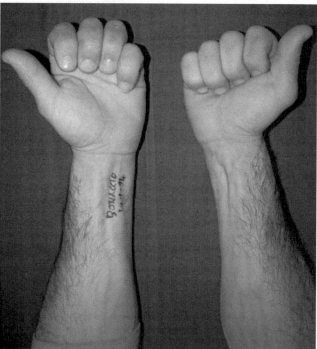

Fig. 53-1. *Case 1, Table 53-2.* Abnormal fibrous reaction following a sting from a viper fish (*Trachinus draco*). **A** and **B**, Range of motion before the operation.

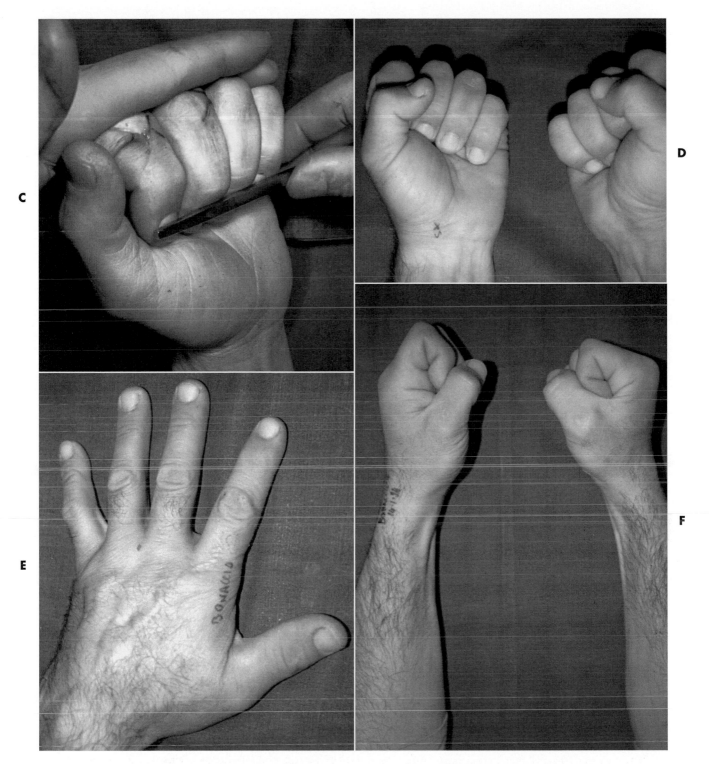

Fig. 53-1, cont'd. C, TADA was performed through a Y-shaped incision. A dense scar that was 1-cm thick had to be cut through before approaching the extensor mechanism. The tip of the spike was found during the operation; no granulomatous reaction was described at histology. **D, E,** and **F,** Excellent clinic result at 3 years follow-up, but the intraoperative gain of excursion was not maintained completely.

Table 53-2. TADA after closed trauma or inflammatory reaction

Sex, Age	Etiology	Operation		Gain in Joint Mobility				Follow-up (years)	Final Outcome
Male, 33	Reaction to a venomous fish sting	EDC tenolysis MP arthrolysis	MP	2nd 35°	3rd 35°	4th 41°	5th 30°	3	Excellent
Male, 36	Carpal metacarpal sprain	Ext. tenolysis 2nd to 5th MP arthrolysis	MP	2nd 72°	3rd 80°	4th 80°	5th 80°	4	Excellent
Male, 36	Fractured 4th metacarpal	Ext. tenolysis 4th finger MP arthrolysis	MP	4th 60°				1	Good
Male, 54	Crush injury, fractured wrist and metacarpal	Ext. tenolysis 3rd finger MP arthrolysis	MP	3rd 25°				2	Satisfactory
Male, 31	Fractured P_1 of 3rd and 4th	Ext. tenolysis 3rd, 4th, 5th MP + 4th and 5th PIP arthrolysis	MP PIP	3rd −5° 5°	4th 10° 7°	5th n.r. n.r.		10 months	Satisfactory
Male, 29	Crush injury P_1 2nd and 3rd sublux MP 4th, fracture subluxation MP 5th	Ext. tenolysis 3rd arthrolysis PIP 3°	MP PIP DIP	3rd 13° 5° 25°				2	Poor
Male, 21	Fractured 3rd-4th metacarpal	Ext. tenolysis 5th MP arthrolysis	MP PIP DIP	5th 84° 74° 90°				1	Good

EDC, Extensor digitorum communis; MP, metacarpophalangeal; ext., extensors; PIP, proximal interphalangeal; DIP, distal interphalangeal; flex., flexion; n.r., not reported.

Table 53-3. TADA in outcomes of tenorraphy of extensor tendons

Age, Sex	Etiology	TADA		Gain in range of motion				Follow-up (years)	Final Outcome
Male,* 23	Section Ext. 2nd finger	Ext. tenolysis + arthrolysis PIP 2nd	PIP DIP	2nd 60° 45°				1	Good
Male,* 38	Section Ext. at PIP 2nd finger	Ext. tenolysis arthrolysis PIP 2nd	PIP DIP	2nd 45° 45°				2	Good
Male, 29	Section EDC	Ext. tenolysis 4th MP arthrolysis Interposition of Silastic	MP	2nd 6°	3rd 24°	4th 27°	5th 10°	2	Satisfactory
Male, 29	Cut lesions with section of the EDC at wrist	Tenolysis ELP, EDC, extensors of the wrist Arthrolysis of wrist		Wrist 16° 1st ray: normal range				1	Good

*Interconnected rigidity of PIP and DIP. In the final evaluation, the improvement of excursion of DIP was taken into account.
PIP, Proximal interphalangeal; DIP, distal interphalangeal; MP, metacarpophalangeal; ext., extensors; EDC, extensor digitorum communis; EPL, extensor pollicis longus.

of the first phalanx (P1) and metacarpal bones rather than after primary extensor tendons suture (Tables 53-2 and 53-3).

Case series

Our experience with tenolysis of the extensor apparatus encompasses 24 patients, for a total of 45 fingers and 62 operations. We divided the operations into the following 5 groups:

1. Dorsal tenoarthrolysis after closed trauma: 7 patients, with 17 operations on 20 fingers (Table 53-2)
2. Dorsal tenoarthrolysis as outcomes of tenorrhaphy of the extensor apparatus: 4 patients with operations on 6 fingers and the wrist, for a total of 7 interventions (Table 53-3)
3. Dorsal tenoarthrolysis as outcomes of tendon grafts: 3 patients for 3 single fingers, for a total of 4 interventions (Table 53-4)

Table 53-4. TADA after extensor tendon grafting

Age, Sex	Etiology	Operation	Gain in Range of Motion		Follow-up (years)	Final Outcome
Male, 20	Section ext. primary tenolysis grafting 4th finger	Tenolysis graft + arthrolysis PIP 4th	PIP	4th 90°	2.5	Good
Male, 17	Fractured P_1 4th and 5th les. ext. and flex, 4th and 5th	Tenolysis graft ext. + flex., arthrolysis PIP 4th	PIP	4th 45°	2	Satisfactory
Male, 54	Crush injury to right hand	Tenolysis graft ext. 2nd		2nd	3	Good
		Opening 1st web perichondral graft to head 2nd	MP	62°		
		metacarpal arthrolysis MP-PIP 2nd	PIP	56°		

PIP, Proximal interphalangeal; *MP*, metacarpophalangeal; *ext.,* extensors; *les.,* lesion; *flex.,* flexors.

Table 53-5. TADA and tenolysis of flexors

Age, Sex	Etiology	Operation	Gain in Range of Motion				Follow-up (years)	Final Outcome
Male,* 7	Amputation 4th finger left hand	TAD 4th + arthrolysis PIP Tenolysis flex. 4th-5th	MP PIP	4th 92° 42°	5th 86° 110°		7	Good
Male,* 18	Crush injury, disartic; 2nd fractured 4th metacarpal	TAD 3° arthrolysis MP and PIP tenolysis flex. 3rd	MP PIP DIP	3° 55° 35° 50°			5	Good
Male, 22	Amputation of 3rd, 4th, and 5th fingers of right hand	Tenolysis extensor 4th-5th arthrolysis MP Tenolysis flex. 2nd	MP PIP DIP	2nd 0° 110° 40°	4th 64° 40° 30°	5th 60° 60° 10°	7	2° excellent 3°-4°-5° Good
Male, 17	Fractured P_1 4th and 5th les. ext. and flex. 4th and 5th	Tenolysis graft ext. + flex. arthrolysis PIP 4th	PIP	4th 45°			2	Satisfactory
Male, 54	Fractured 3rd metacarpal and P_1 4th, trapezium-capitate, sect. flex. and ext. 3rd and 4th	EDC tenolysis MP and 4th PIP arthrolysis flex. tenolysis 4th, 2nd, 3rd	MP PIP DIP	2nd 30° 68° 48°	3rd 53° 42° 21°	4th 70° 38° 26°	1.5	2nd good 3rd good 4th satisfactory

*Indicates where microvascular procedures have been carried out.

TADA, Tenoarthrolysis-dorsal apparatus; *PIP,* proximal interphalangeal; *DIP,* distal interphalangeal; *MP,* metacarpophalangeal; *flex.,* flexors; *les.,* lesion; *ext.,* extensors.

4. Dorsal tenoarthrolysis and tenolysis of the flexor apparatus: 5 patients, for a total of 16 interventions on 7 fingers (Table 53-5)

5. Dorsal tenoarthrolysis as outcomes of reimplantations: 8 patients, 16 fingers operated on, for a total of 18 interventions. This group includes 2 subjects who had an associated tenolysis of the flexor apparatus (Table 53-6).

Surgical technique

Tenoarthrolysis of the dorsal apparatus can be accomplished via two modalities, depending on whether tenolysis is required following tenorrhaphy and tendon graft of the extensor apparatus or a closed trauma of the fingers and hand. In the former, tenolysis extends in both directions from the site of anatomic fixation, and it involves more drastic surgical choices, because at the proximal interphalangeal (PIP) joint the central band must be isolated from the lateral bands, and at the MP joint, the extensor hood must almost always be sacrificed. The saggital bands are usually the only retinacular structures that are preserved.[42] Conversely, in closed lesions, the extensor hood might be retained (Fig. 53-2).

The tendon cannot always be freed easily from the periosteal plane, and we have found a 15 blade to be the best surgical tool. If active flexion of the finger is possible at this point, the extrinsic type of stiffness has been completely resolved. However, extrinsic stiffness is often associated with an intrinsic stiffness of the MP and PIP joints.[3] In this case, one proceeds with a dorsal capsulotomy at the MP joint (the capsule after edema or hematoma becomes particularly thick, up to 1 or 2 mm). By a vertical approach between the extensor hood and the sagittal band,[20] the collateral ligaments are released partially bilaterally, or even totally at the PIP joint, without negative repercussions on joint stability.[11] The retrocondylar recess is then released using a curved rougine.[20]

Table 53-6. Tenolysis after reimplantation

Sex, Age	Level of Reimplant	TADA	Tenolysis Flexors	Gain in Range of Motion					Follow-up (years)	Final Outcome
Male, 26	2nd, 3rd, 4th, 5th right hand	—	2nd		2nd				3	Poor
				PIP	20°					
Male, 1.3	3rd, 4th left hand	—	4th, 5th	n.r.					2	Good
Male, 19	2nd, 3rd left hand	—	2nd, 3rd		2nd	3rd			6	Good
				PIP	40°	68°				
				DIP	60°	65°				
Male,* 22	3rd, 4th, 5th right hand	4th-5th + arthrolysis MP	2nd		4th	6th			7	2° excellent 3°-4°-5° Good
				MP	64°	60°				
				PIP	40°	60°				
				DIP	30°	10°				
Male,* 7	4th left hand	4th + arthrolysis PIP	4th, 5th		4th				7	Good
				MP	92°					
				PIP	42°					
Male, 61	Left arm	Arthrolysis MP 2nd, 3rd, 4th, 5th	—		2nd	3rd	4th	5th	5	Satisfactory
				MP	65°	60°	48°	55°		
Male, 16	Left thumb	—	—	n.r.					3	Good
Male, 22	2nd, 3rd	—	2nd, 3rd	n.r.					2	Poor

*Cases where tenolysis has been performed both on flexor and extensor tendons.
MP, Metacarpophalangeal; *PIP,* proximal interphalangeal; *DIP,* distal interphalangeal; *n.r.,* not reported.

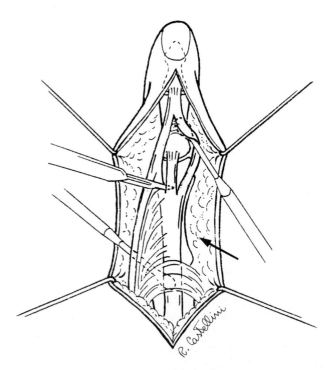

Fig. 53-2. *Top,* the scalpel shows the space between the lateral and central band which needs to be created in order to perform a TADA. *Bottom,* a curved rougine is used to free the oblique and transverse fibers of the extensor mechanism, which are preserved on the left side. On the right (*arrow*), the scarred retinacular system has been removed, and only the sagittal band has been maintained.

If the joint then bends up to 90° but opens as a book, this means that arthrolysis was incomplete, as the residual rigidity is linked to shortening of the collateral ligaments or obliteration of the retrocondylar space. TADA at the level of the MP joint is also compatible with some types of joint resurfacing procedures, but we feel that only one side of the joint (generally the metacarpal head) should be restored and a free perichondral transplant used for this purpose. Under these conditions, the motility obtained in the three cases operated on was always within a useful range[13] (Fig. 53-3).

TADA was satisfactory (see Table 53-2) providing that an accurate postoperative rehabilitation followed (Fig. 53-4).

The results remain acceptable even for TADA after repair of the tendon apparatus by tendon graft (see Table 53-4, Fig. 53-5), if sufficient time (at least 3 to 6 months) has passed from the tendon grafting procedure and all points of fixation have been released (Figs. 53-2 and 53-6).

The traditional pessimism toward tenolysis of the extensor apparatus[5] should be reevaluated in light of available techniques of hand rehabilitation. The tendency of adhesions to recur can be prevented by using, where adhesions are limited, a small silicone bar[35] sutured to the volar aspect to the extensor tendon. This seems to offer advantages over the use of silicone sheets, which, even in our series, have not provided significant improvements. In case of an extensively scarred bed, vascularized tendon grafts might be considered

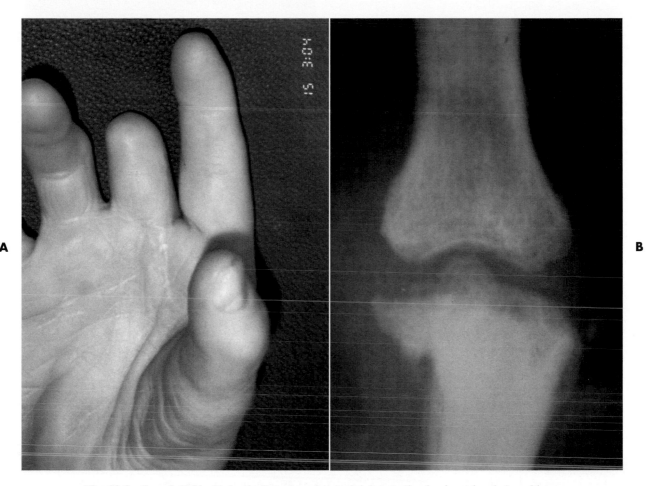

Fig. 53-3. *Case 3, Table 53-4.* **A,** Sequelae of a crush injury to the dominant hand. A multistage program was established for this patient. At this point, a tendon graft for extensor pollicis longus and the index finger in addition to a first web release and EPDV to APB had already been performed. Therefore all immobilizing procedures had been ultimated at this stage. **B,** Corresponding x-ray image of the MP joint of the index ankylosed in the neutral position. *Continued.*

from the beginning, or living gliding tissue planned as a secondary procedure.[27]

Results

The patients were given a clinical follow-up examination after an average of 2.8 years (range 10 months to 7 years). To evaluate the results, we took as end points both the values of active mobility, and thus the gain in ROM,[13] and the patients' subjective judgment of improvement. We achieved the following outcomes:

- 12 patients with excellent results (19.35%): MP active flexion > 80°, PIP > 100° and no extension deficit
- 20 patients with good results (32.25%): MP active flexion > 70°, PIP > 90° and extension deficit < 30°
- 14 patients with satisfactory results (22.5%): MP active flexion > 50°, PIP > 60° and extension deficit < 30°
- 4 patients with poor outcomes (6.5%): MP active flexion > 50°; PIP < 60° and extension deficit > 30°

COMPLEX TENOLYSIS OF THE FLEXOR TENDONS IN ZONE 2

At our institution from January 1970 to May 1990, we performed 144 tenolyses of the flexors in zone 2; these are reported in Table 53-7 and subdivided on the basis of their etiology. In this section, we limit our discussion to complex tenolyses, namely, only those of the flexor superficialis, flexor grafts secondary to iatrogenic causes, and total anterior tenoarthrolysis (TATA).

A simple tenolysis might become complex when early complications arise. Tourniquet lesions following tenolysis are rare, but they interfere with the functional outcome, because early active mobilization by the patient is no longer possible.[22,23] Retenolysis after tenolysis (Fig. 53-7) is tied to an incorrect evaluation at surgery of the real gliding capacities of the flexor tendons. Reexploration, which must be immediate, can reveal echimotic and edematous tendons and, at this point, it becomes mandatory

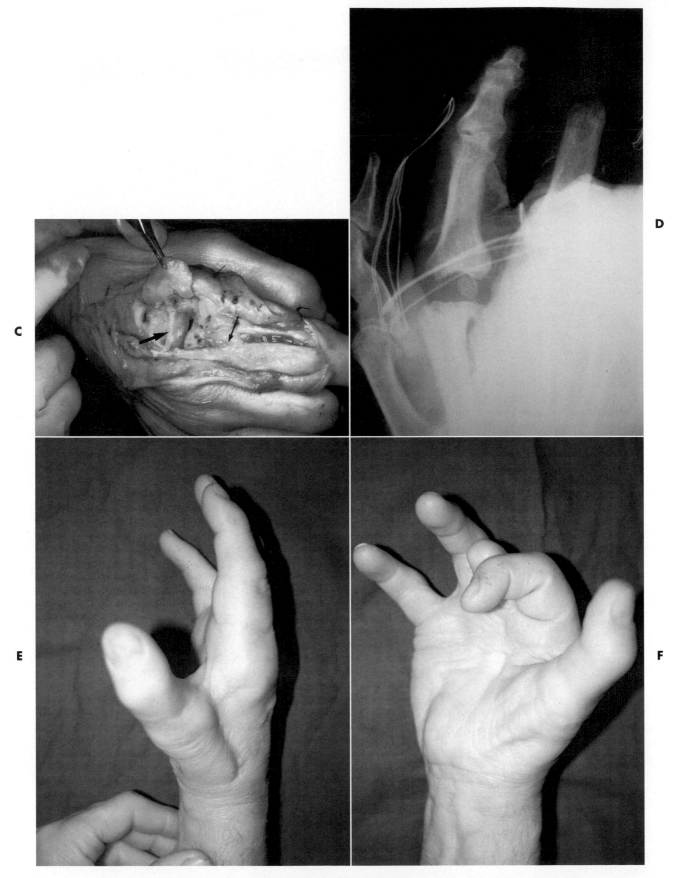

Fig. 53-3, cont'd. C and **D,** A TADA of the index finger has been carried out and both MP and IP joints fully released. At the MP joint, perichondrial graft for the metacarpal head (*heavy arrow*) and tenolysis of the extensor tendon graft (*thin arrow*) have been accomplished. **E** and **F,** The patient was finally able to resume his part-time activity as a lumberjack.

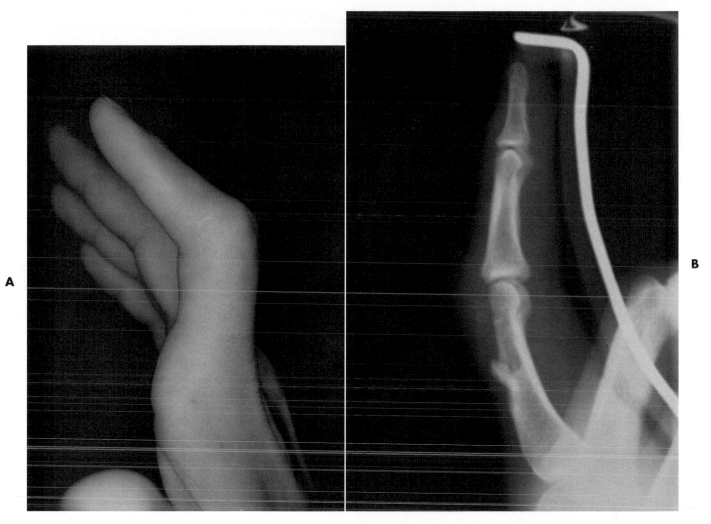

Fig. 53-4. *Case 2, Table 53-3.* **A,** Circular saw injury in a cardiac surgeon. The extensor tendon had been repaired elsewhere. A flexion contracture of PIP joint with complete stiffness of the DIP joint represents the real handicap for this patient. **B,** Corresponding x-ray image that shows the tangential resection by the saw of roughly one fourth of the dorsal aspect of P2. *Continued.*

to sacrifice crucial pulleys (Fig. 53-7, *C*) to obtain sufficient tendon gliding.

Biologic considerations

Survival and function of the flexor tendons in zone 2 are strictly dependent on vascularization and synovial fluid. Tenolysis represents a serious biologic insult that for the first 48 hours compromises both metabolic supplies of the tendons.[19]

In an in vivo experimental model reproducing hypovascular tendon stress,[19] tenolysis causes central necrosis of the tendon with processes of remodelling stemming from undifferentiated cells of the epitenon, which present glucose-6-phosphate dehydrogenase (G6PD) activity that is absent in adult tenocytes. However, in the first 48 hours, vascular congestion of the epitenon (see Fig. 53-7, *C*) represents the first phase of a series of events that leads either to successful

tenolysis or to tendon rupture. In this delicate phase, the only protection until the tendon sheath reforms (as soon as 24 hours after tenolysis in the rabbit), seems to be provided by the residual intrinsic circulation of the tendon. This constitutes the basis of the generally accepted axiom[25,26,33,40] that tenolysis must be performed at least 3 months after tenorrhaphy and 6 months after tendon grafting.

General surgical indications

Tenolysis of the flexor tendons is technically difficult,[33,37,40] undoubtedly more than tenorrhaphy, a fact that must be clear to both the patient and surgeon. The requisites for a simple tenolysis are adequate sensation in the fingers, good passive joint motion,[40] and full recovery from any associated lesions. Swollen or rigid fingers must thus be submitted to an intense cycle of specific reeducation before surgery. If the outcome after rehabilitation is poor and the

Text continued on p. 470.

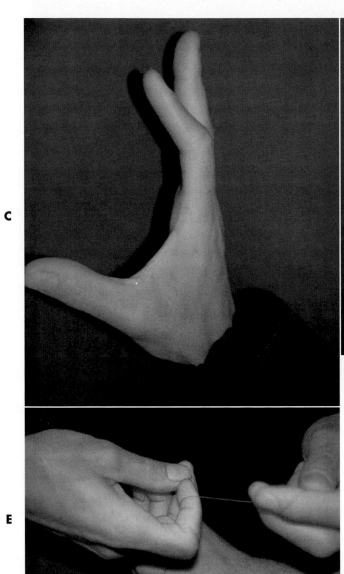

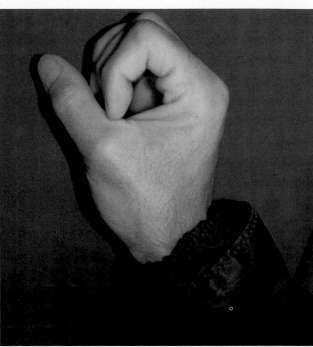

Fig. 53-4, cont'd. C, D, and **E,** Clinical follow-up after TADA was performed. The overall gain at PIP and DIP joints was 90° of active excursion. The patient gained his original ability to execute surgical knots and returned to his original job.

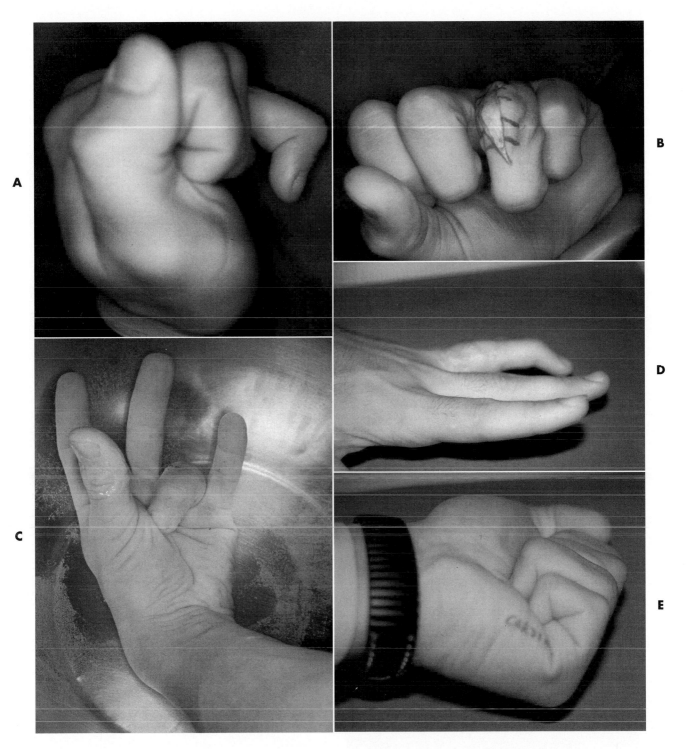

Fig. 53-5. *Case 1, Table 53-4.* **A,** A lesion with tendon loss of the extensor apparatus of the left ring finger was reconstructed with a palmaris longus (PL) tendon graft in an emergency operation; the patient ended up with an ankylosed PIP joint in the neutral position. **B,** A TADA had been carried out. **C,** Active exercises are performed in antiseptic solution 24 hours after the operation. **D** and **E,** The final outcome was favorable.

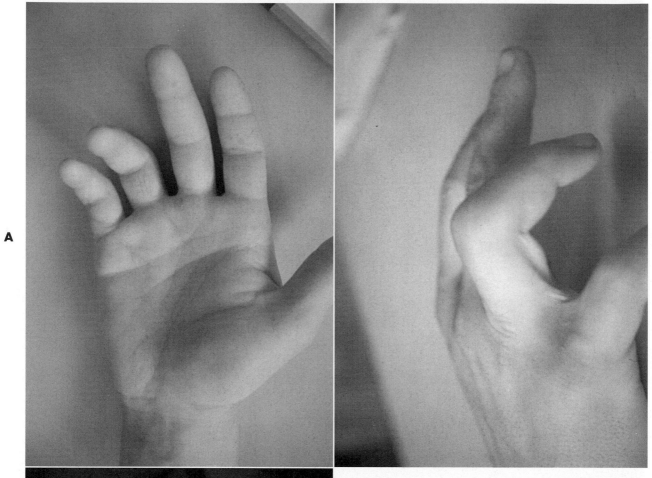

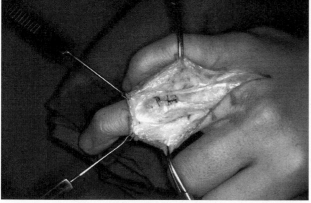

Fig. 53-6. *Case 2, Table 53-4 and Case 4, Table 53-5.* Sequelae of multifragmented fractures at the first phalanx of right ring and little finger. **A,** Flexor and extensor tendon tenolysis was carried out simultaneously on the ring finger. The flexor apparatus was found extensively entrapped at the level of intraarticular fracture at the PIP joint of the little finger so that no reconstructive procedures were attempted for this ray. Flexor tenolysis of the ring finger provided an excellent result but the extensor mechanism ruptured early at the level of the PIP joint. **B,** A tendon graft to the extensor mechanism was carried out but led to a stiff PIP joint in neutral position. **C and D,** A TADA was subsequently performed.

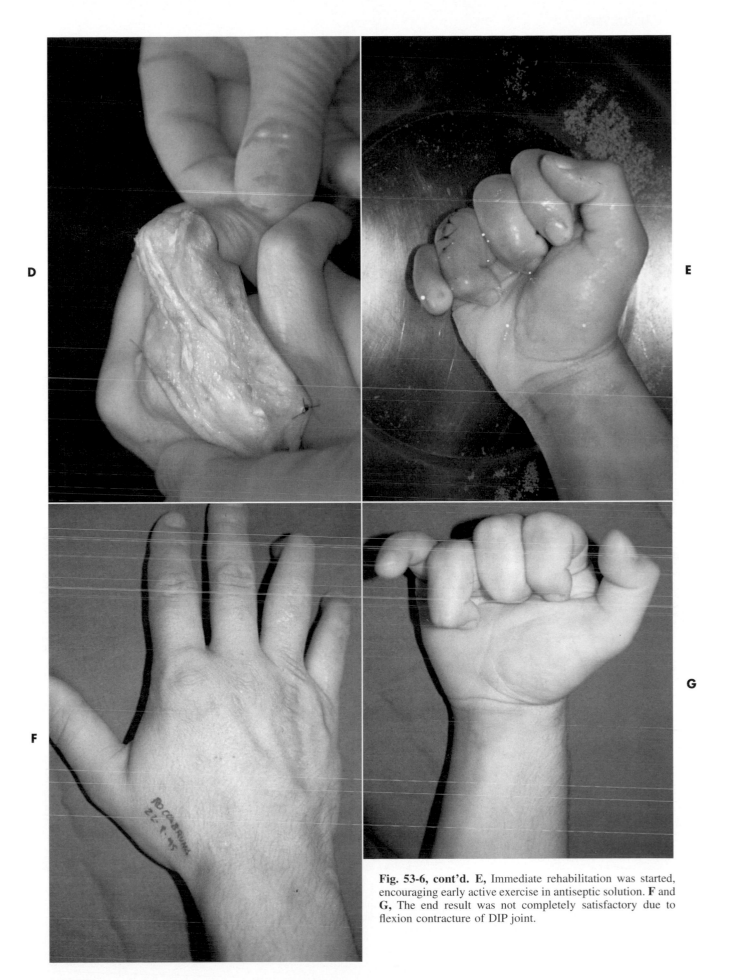

Fig. 53-6, cont'd. E, Immediate rehabilitation was started, encouraging early active exercise in antiseptic solution. **F** and **G,** The end result was not completely satisfactory due to flexion contracture of DIP joint.

PIP joint remains stiff in the neutral position, tenolysis of the flexors should be preceded by dorsal tenoarthrolysis (see Tables 53-5 and 53-7).

Anesthesiologic considerations

The success of tenolysis is also connected to active collaboration by the patient, which begins at the time of surgery. Except for Tsuge,[38] who routinely uses generalanesthesia or brachial plexus block, the majority of authors[21,33,37,40] advocate neuroleptoanalgesic techniques. After sedation, local anesthesia is induced, which, when associated with administration of benzodiazepines, fentanyl, and droperidol, provide a good tolerance to surgery and allow active patient collaboration. One limit of this method is that sedation is difficult to regulate; indeed, collaboration falls off at the end of surgery when it is needed most. Because the entire first part of the operation is performed under the strict requirement of the tourniquet, which produces motor paralysis after 20 minutes, patient cooperation becomes technically impossible at this stage. A valid alternative is the use of a specific benzodiazepine antagonist, which allows the immediate reversal of the

Table 53-7. Case series tenolysis of flexors in zone 2 (1970-1990)

Open Lesions		Closed Lesions	
Simple skin lesions	15	Crush injuries of the fingers	8
Outcome of tenorrhaphy	79	Fracture and subluxaton	11
Outcome of tendon graft	5	Burns	1
Outcome of compound fractures without tenorraphy	4		
Outcome of joint dislocation	2		
Postoperative adhesions (Dupuytren + trigger finger)	2		
Postinfective adhesions	2		
Complex lesions, reimplant revascularizations	15		
Total of cases	124		20

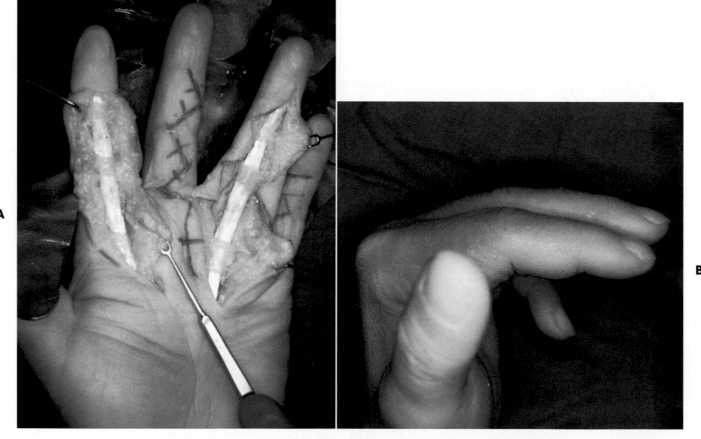

Fig. 53-7. A 56-year-old worker who in September, 1988 accidentally injured the flexor superficialis tendons of the 2nd, 3rd, and 5th fingers of the left hand with a paper cutter. The injury was treated with simple skin sutures. Active flexion of PIPJ before surgery. **A,** May, 1989: tenolysis of the deep flexors of the 2nd, 3rd, and 4th fingers. **B,** Tenolysis failed in the postoperative period.

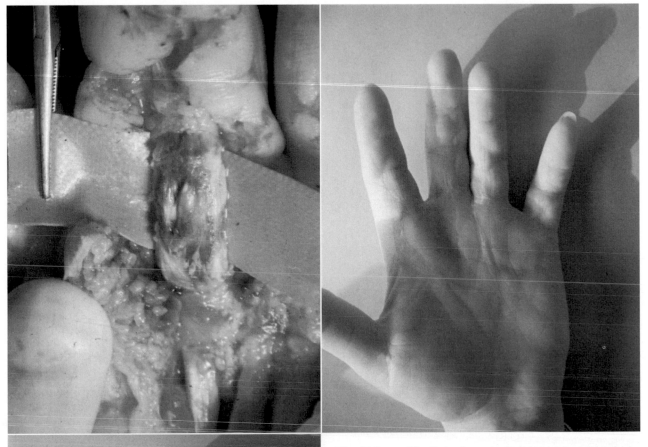

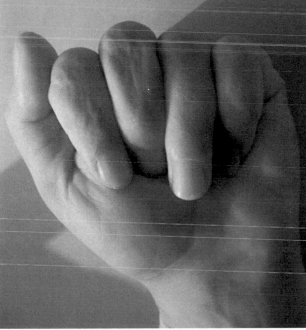

Fig. 53-7, cont'd. C, At the seventh day, revision of tenolysis: flexors and the surrounding soft tissue appear remarkably edematous, thus limiting tendon gliding. The A₁ pulley is sectioned and myotomy of the lumbrical muscle performed. Tenolysis was extended to the palm, where the sectioned and retracted superficial flexors appeared to be stuck to the deep flexors. **D** and **E,** Clinical follow-up after 1 year. (From Aulo Gaggi Editore Bologna, *GIOT* 1994; 20[3]:347-358.)

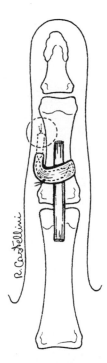

Fig. 53-8. Reconstruction of a pulley utilizing one band of the flexor superficialis, which is fixed to the stump of the flexor sheath and fixed to the dorsal skin by a pull-out suture. (From Aulo Gaggi Editore Bologna, *GIOT* 1994; 20[3]:347-358.)

sedative effect without collateral symptoms.[21,39] The combination of local anesthesia, anesthetic ointment at the level of the tourniquet, and benzodiazepines and associated antagonists seems today to be a very promising anesthesiologic approach.[21]

Surgical technique

1. Skin incisions are often compulsory in operations secondary to tenorrhaphy or tendon grafting. Nonetheless, under these circumstances, it is usually possible to make them similar to the zigzag incision of Bruner. In outcomes of closed trauma, we agree with Strickland[37] on the use of a mediolateral incision, which offers the twofold advantage of low wound tension during mobilization and low recurrence of adhesions. Tenolysis must be performed on both the superficialis and deep flexor tendons.[40] Often the space available is no longer sufficient for both, and in this case the superficialis is sacrificed. One should also consider that the superficialis might have been removed during the first operation or sutured to the distal stump of the deep flexor.

2. The number and quality of the pulleys represent the absolute essential for success of tenolysis. According to Schneider,[33] the absence of pulleys is an indication to proceed to a tendon graft, even though we feel that some crucial pulleys constructed *ex novo* may be sufficient to limit oneself to tenolysis. Considering the

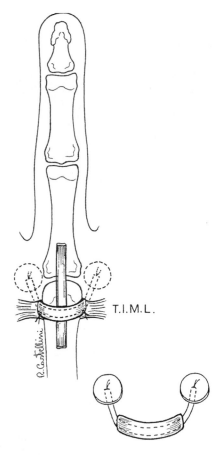

Fig. 53-9. Reconstruction of A_1 pulley by a free PL tendon graft. The new pulley has a double fixation at the level of the intermetacarpal ligament and of the dorsal skin through a pullout suture. The strength of the new pulley is considered adequate to allow early motion. (From Aulo Gaggi Editore Bologna, *GIOT* 1994; 20[3]:347-358.)

residual pulleys, the most important are located at the PIP joint,[16] namely, at the distal part of A_2 and A_3 pulleys, and the proximal part of A_4. The cruciform pulleys can in part replace the annular pulleys in preventing the bowstringing effect of the tendon. The A_5 will usually be sacrificed, so that a three-pulley system (A_1, A_2, and A_3), as we usually adopt, is sufficient from a biomechanical standpoint. According to Strickland, with a good A_1 pulley, a single pulley that replaces the A_2 may suffice. Following tenolysis, the pulley must present biomechanical prerequisites of resistance, and this holds true for both residual and reconstructed pulleys.

Subcutaneous rupture of an inadequate pulley represents an acute event associated with an immediate bowstring effect and limitation of the flexion obtained at surgery. In uncertain cases, the pulley at risk should be protected during rehabilitation with an external pulley made of velcro or felt.[25]

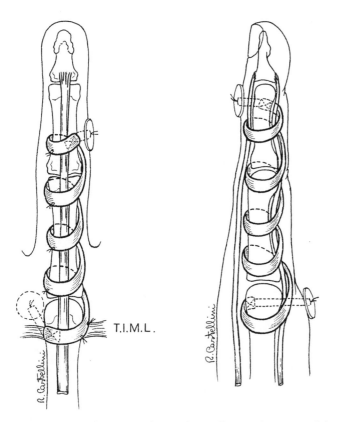

T.I.M.L.

Fig. 53-10. The circumferential running pulley can be very useful when the original pulley system is too weak. The pulley is double-fixed proximally at the transverse intermetacarpal (TIM) ligament and to the dorsal skin. It is then passed beneath the extensor tendon at P_1 and above it at P_2. Distal fixation is secured through a pull-out suture. This arrangement allows immediate active flexion exercises. (From Aulo Gaggi Editore Bologna, *GIOT* 1994; 20[3]:347-358.)

A biomechanical study by Windstrom et al.[41] indicates that the pulleys with the greatest resistance used during tenolysis are those constructed with one and a half loops of palmaris tendon wrapped around itself, whereas the weakest pulley is that constructed with a tendon graft passed through the residues of A_2 and A_4, as proposed by Weilby. During tenolysis, we resort to pulleys derived from the superficialis flexor tendon, as suggested by Bunnel, and fixed there by means of a pullout passed through the tendon (Fig. 53-8). A free tendon graft (Fig. 53-9), which can be woven around the remains of the digital sheath (Figs. 53-10 and 53-11), represents an alternative means of pulley reconstruction after tenolysis.

Special technical aspects

The technical difficulties of tenolysis are linked to the necessity of preserving the pulleys, especially at the periarticular sites, where the convex condylar plane covered by the volar plate does not always allow easy access to the surgical instruments. In order not to weaken the pulley, the

hook-shaped arthroscopic blades, the minimeniscus, and the right and left semicurved blades[34] can be very useful, as well as a small curved mosquito and a curved rougine (Fig. 53-12).

In this phase, active patient cooperation has the double advantage of contributing to breaking the remaining adhesions and to allowing the patient to view the fingers that are now free, fostering a responsible active role in postoperative rehabilitation.

Intraoperative evaluation

Faced with a tendon whose diameters are reduced by more than 30%, rupture becomes a significant risk.[16] However, the intrinsic qualities, more than the size of the residual tendon, are important criteria. A clean continuity of tendon tissue offers a greater guarantee than a continuity consisting of scar tissue alone. According to Verdan et al.,[40] the finger submitted to tenolysis should, in the end, touch the Kanavel crease, or more realistically, we feel it should actively repeat the passive preoperative excursion. It is indispensable to verify the full excursion of the tendon by exploiting the patient's active flexion capacity. Indeed, flexors apparently freed up to the palm are often blocked at the base of the hand by residual stumps of the superficialis flexor tendons (see Fig. 53-7). During general anesthesia or brachial plexus block, a direct verification of this parameter is obtained by a counterincision at the level of the wrist and passive traction on the tendon.[37]

Complications

Tendon rupture is the most frequent and feared complication. Out of 136 grafts, Pulvertaft[29] reported this complication in 6% of his series. This untoward effect can be minimized by an accurate intraoperative evaluation and protected rehabilitation. Indeed, ruptures after 2 to 3 weeks are related to an excessively vigorous rehabilitation program.[2]

Early recurrence of adhesions can be prevented by accurate planning of the surgical incision and an appropriate rehabilitation program.

Peculiar aspects

Tenolysis of the superficialis tendon alone

In some circumstances a finger with only the superficialis flexor tendon must be opted for if anchylosis or arthrodesis of the DIP joint is present. This choice can be freely made when, for example, only the superficialis tendon has been sutured during the primary operation. The alternative to a finger with only a superficialis tendon is a two-stage tenoplasty. In both circumstances, however, especially for the radial finger, the superficialis finger can be functionally adequate as long as the pulley system (A_1, the distal portion of A_2, and the proximal portion of A_4) is efficient.

When simultaneous reconstruction of the pulleys is required, we tend to protect them by adopting pullout sutures (see Fig. 53-10).

Fig. 53-11. A 19-year-old male with primary tendon suture of the flexor tendon at the level of the distal palmar crease. He subsequently underwent two interventions of flexor tendon tenolysis. **A,** The A$_1$ and A$_2$ pulleys were removed, and bowstringing of the flexor tendon became apparent. **B** and **C,** At exploration, the deep flexor tendon appeared to have good structural continuity. Reconstruction with a circumferential running pulley was selected (see Fig. 53-10). Because the myostatic contracture the profundus flexor was lengthened at the myotendinous junction.

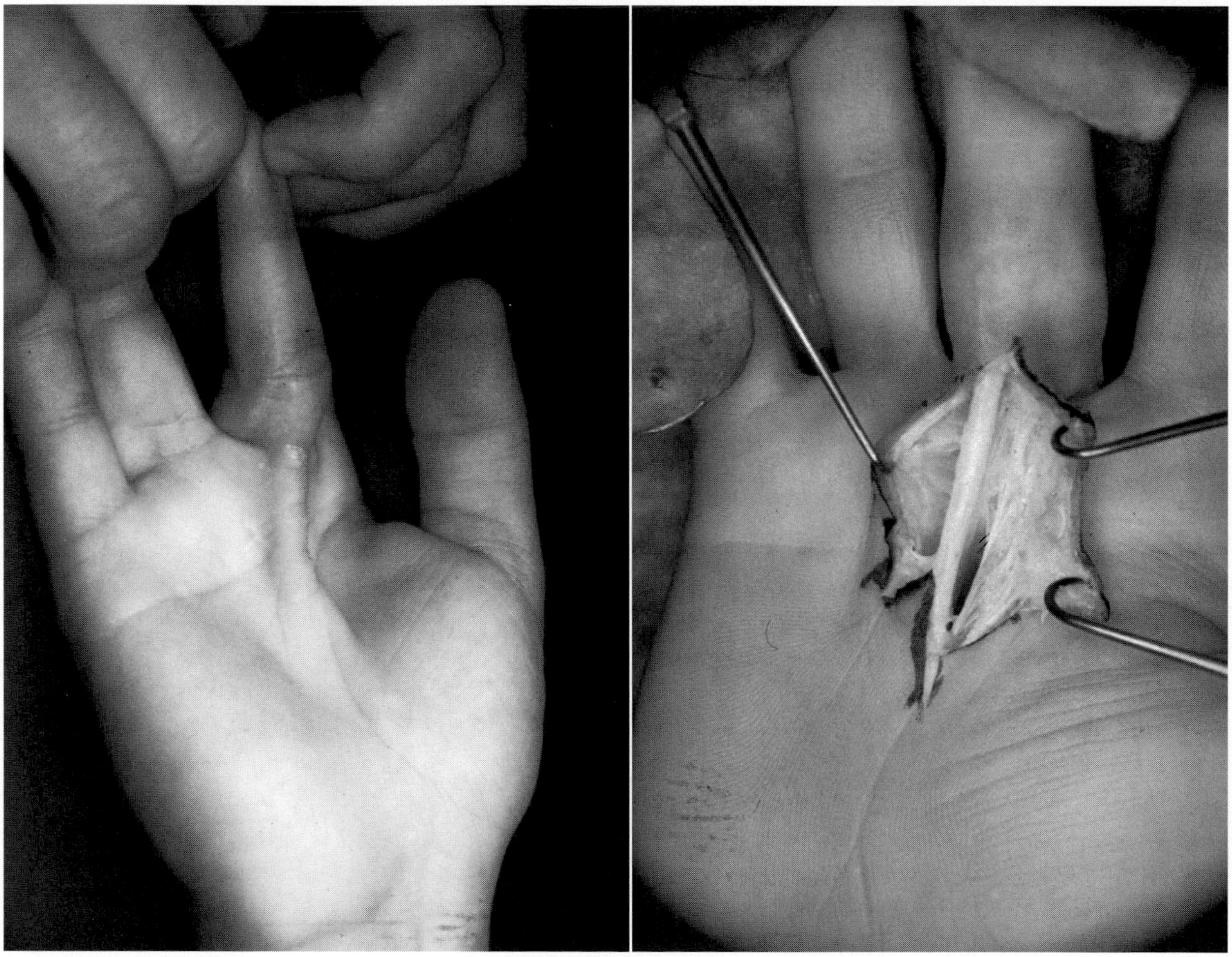

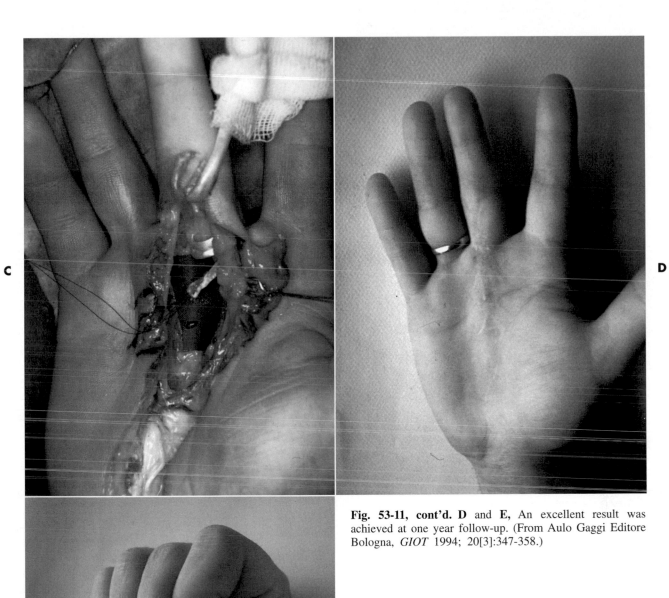

Fig. 53-11, cont'd. D and **E,** An excellent result was achieved at one year follow-up. (From Aulo Gaggi Editore Bologna, *GIOT* 1994; 20[3]:347-358.)

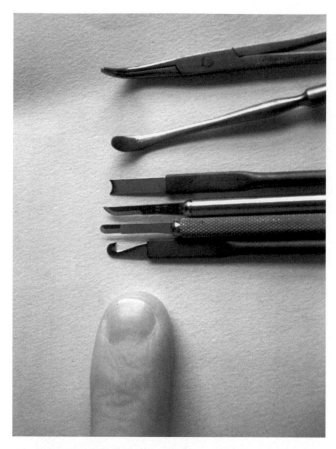

Fig. 53-12. Surgical instruments for tenolysis or pulley release. (From Aulo Gaggi Editore Bologna, *GIOT* 1994; 20[3]:347-358.)

Tenolysis after tendon grafts. The percentages of tenolysis after tendon grafts reflects the time span of the respective case series, passing from 47% in the series by Strickland,[37] and 27% in that by Chamay et al.,[7] to 16% in Amadio et al.[1] This significant decrease may be tied to a more widespread use of passive early mobilization (Fig. 53-13).

Swan-neck deformity. The swan-neck deformity is a possible complication of a tendon graft. It must be prevented and the most appropriate way during the first phase is by bridging the superficialis tendon over the PIP joint so as to maintain flexion at 10° to 20°. Unfortunately, once a swan-neck deformity has been established and tenolysis is required due to objective lack of gliding of the tendon graft, we believe that it should be delayed until the swan-neck deformity has resolved. If a swan-neck deformity has already become rigid at the PIP joint, a dorsal release should be performed first.

Flexor tendons missing the A_1 and A_2 pulleys

This condition must be distinguished from the intrinsic plus hand described by Zancolli,[42] where the intrinsic plus posture of the MP joint reflects a defensive mechanism produced by the patient to protect a painful palm, fre-

quently related to a neuroma. The deformity that we describe also presents a flexion deformity of the MP joint, but it is more obviously associated with bowstringing of the flexor apparatus. This condition may be secondary to excessive release of a trigger finger or to tenolysis where neither A_1 nor A_2 pulleys were reconstructed. It is invalidating because it might ultimately lead to a stiff swan-neck deformity. Moreover, myostatic contracture of the flexor apparatus might ensue. In simple cases the deformity can be corrected by means of tenolysis and reconstruction of the A_1 pulley. In complex cases, where the key pulleys are not available, we suggest the following surgical steps: (1) tenolysis of the flexor apparatus, (2) reconstruction of a running system of pulleys (see Fig. 53-10), and (3) lengthening of the flexor at the myotendinous junction.

This surgical strategy usually yields good functional results.

Total anterior tenoarthrolysis

Skin and flexion contracture often coexist at the PIP joint in cases of sequelae of multiple interventions to the flexor tendon in zone 2 or sequelae of surgical treatment of Dupuytren's syndrome. Under these circumstances, the surgeon is faced with a drastic choice. The options for treating the "hook deformity" range from an additional tenolysis of the flexor and release of the volar plate at the PIP and DIP joints, to arthrodesis in a more extended position of one of the two IP joints (with shortening of the finger), to amputation of the digit in the case of a severe deformity. As an alternative, Saffar introduced in 1978 the total anterior tenoarthrolysis (TATA),[30] later described by the same author in 1983[31] and by Quenod.[28]

The surgical technique includes the following surgical procedures: access through the lateral surface (Fig. 53-14), always choosing the side of a previous incision, and extension from the middle of the proximal phalanx to the tip of the distal phalanx (Fig. 53-15). After incising the subcutaneous tissue and isolating neurovascular bundle, the periostium is dissected with a straight rougine or scalpel from the diaphasis of the first two phalanges.

The volar fibers of the collateral ligament are incised, removing the volar plate that becomes continuous with the previously detached periosteum (see Fig. 53-15).

This surgical procedure is performed both at the PIP and DIP joints so that all elements of the volar surface of the two phalanges are detached from the bone. Sectioning of the collateral ligaments proceeds from volar to dorsal, sparing the most dorsal fibers.

At times, part of the collateral ligaments of the DIP joint must also be sectioned (see Fig. 53-15). If we attempt to extend the finger and extension is possible at the expense of flexion of the DIP, the flexor digitorum profundus (FDP) must be sectioned, leaving the tendon attached to the surrounding tissues (see Fig. 53-15).

When the pulp skin is isolated, the finger can finally be extended. The degree of gliding is proportional to the

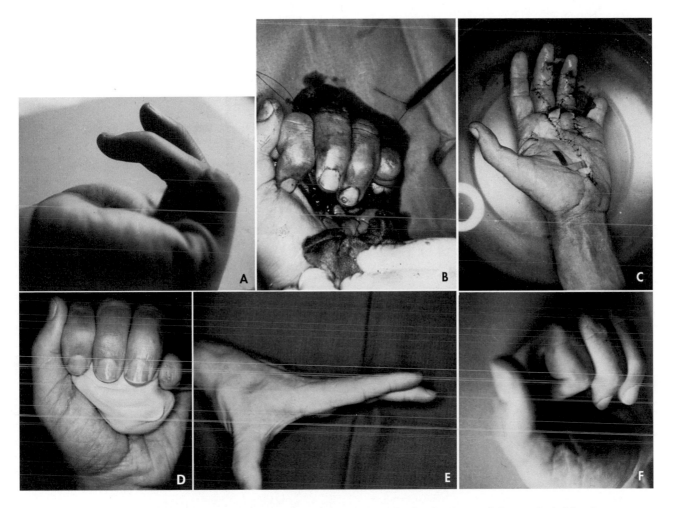

Fig. 53-13. In September 1987, a 42-year-old male, sustained a circular saw injury to the left hand with primary suture of flexor tendons of the third and fourth fingers. **A,** In September 1988, two-stage tendon reconstruction of the flexor tendons of the third and fourth fingers was performed. Active flexion was incomplete with normal passive excursion. **B,** Tenolysis was then performed under local anesthesia with active collaboration from the patient. **C,** Postoperative rehabilitation started after 24 hours, by means of active exercises performed in an antiseptic solution until the wound healed. **D,** Active grip exercises with play-dough can be started 3 to 4 weeks after tenolysis. **E** and **F,** Clinical follow-up 2 years after tenolysis. Active extension and flexion of the fingers has returned to within normal ranges. (From Aulo Gaggi Editore Bologna, *GIOT* 1994; 20[3]:347-358.)

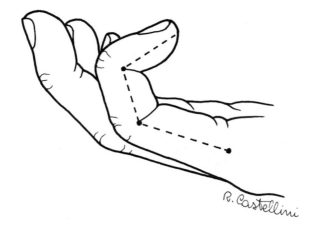

Fig. 53-14. TATA: access through the lateral surface.

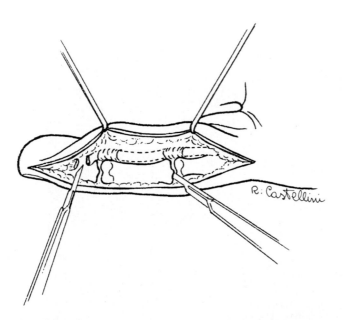

Fig. 53-15. TATA: The proximal scalpel at the proximal interphalangeal joint indicates the release of the volar plate and accessory collateral ligaments. The scalpel at the distal interphalangeal joint indicates the volar release of the joint and tenotomy of distal insertion of FP performed to complete the release if needed.

severity of the hook deformity. Moreover, the condition of the articular cartilage of the PIP and DIP joints must be verified.

It is not always necessary to obtain a complete extension of the digit. If a small area of skin remains uncovered, it can be left to heal by secondary intention.

When gliding of the pulp tissue is limited, the consequent skin loss might be covered in different ways by incising the digitopalmar fold (Fig. 53-16), by fusing the DIP joint but, under those circumstances, the FDP should not be detached because this would decrease the blood supply to the distal phalanx.[32]

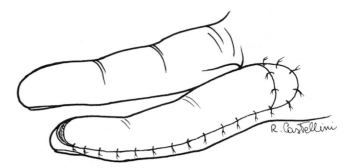

Fig. 53-16. The consequent skin loss might be covered in different ways by advancing the volar skin.

TENOLYSIS OF THE EXTENSORS AND TENOLYSIS OF THE FLEXOR TENDONS

A TADA in association with flexor tendon tenolysis is usually a delayed intervention. Crush injuries, outcomes of lesions from chemical or physical agents, and especially the sequelae of revascularization and reimplantation are the most frequent causes that require associated tenolyses. In double tenolyses of the digits, when dealing with a closed trauma, TADA is almost always performed first but might also be performed simultaneously.[13]

In outcomes of reimplantation (see Table 53-6) or complex trauma (see Table 53-5) the two tenolyses are performed separately after a sufficient time has passed for the fingers and hand to regain their full passive range of motion (PROM), and the surgical scar has softened.

In any case, contraindications for associated tenolysis are reflex sympathetic dystrophy and reimplantations followed by vascular complications, where survival of the segments has been achieved at the expense of atrophy of subcutaneous tissues and elasticity and mobility of the skin, which appears thin and adherent.

We have performed double tenolyses after fracture of the phalanges and after complex trauma and reimplantation to the hand (see Tables 53-5 and 53-6).

Tenolysis after fracture of the metacarpals or phalanges

To our knowledge, this topic has only been treated in depth by Strickland.[4] The second phalanx together with the metacarpal bones are the most frequent site of adhesions. Spiroid fractures, in particular, might eventually violate the floor of the flexor sheath and interfere with tendon gliding (see Table 53-2). The fractures, especially if comminute, must be immobilized until definitive consolidation, and tenolysis must be performed afterward. Alternatively, one might try to prevent tendon adhesions by using external fixation, which allows immediate mobilization. Often, the outcomes will involve stiffness in extension of the PIP joint. It is best to perform tenolysis of the extensor mechanism first to regain PROM of this joint. In this phase,

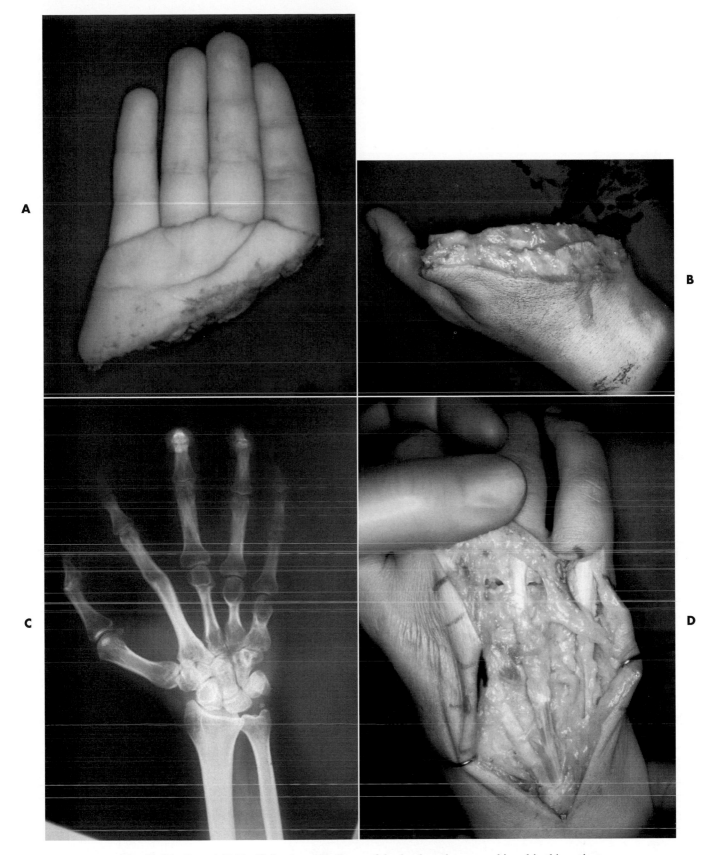

Fig. 53-17. *Case 4, Table 53-6.* **A** and **B,** Successful reimplantation was achieved in this patient following amputation by a circular saw. **C,** The MP joint of the index finger was first fused as a result of a transarticular amputation. The other metacarpal bones have been shortened. **D,** TADA of little and ring fingers was carried out and was promptly followed by tenolysis of the flexor tendon of the index finger. *Continued.*

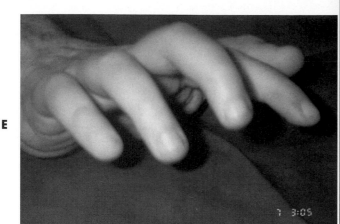

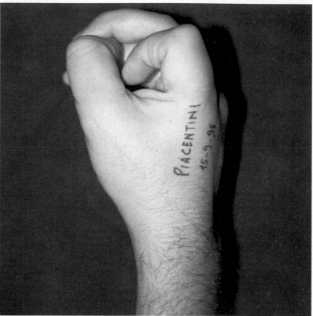

Fig. 53-17, cont'd. E and **F,** Overall, the outcome was satisfactory.

normal PROM is rarely obtained for two reasons: adhesions on the volar side of the flexor tendon and obliteration of the retrocondylar space. Tenolysis through a volar approach will follow the dorsal intervention, generally allowing active joint motion of the finger to be restored. A similar guideline has permitted Strickland to obtain significant improvements in 20 out of 27 cases of associated tendon-skeletal lesions, with a mean increase of active motility of 67.7°. A TADA followed by flexor tenolysis has led to improved functional results in our case series (see Table 53-5).

Tenolysis after reimplantation

Contrary to the findings of Meyer and Buck-Gramcko (quoted by Jupiter[17]), our results[18,24] and those of Jupiter[17] on tenolysis following reimplantation are relatively favorable. The technique does not differ greatly from tenolysis after simple tenorrhaphy. TADA (Fig. 53-17) always anticipates tenolysis of the flexor apparatus. However, it is advisable, before the operation, to obtain a Doppler investigation on the patency of the sutured vessels. Moreover, the original surgical notes must be carefully consulted, any available drawings examined, and particular attention paid to arterial transpositions. To avoid damaging the sutured digital arteries, after reimplantation we perform a more central mini-Bruner incision, which gives a direct approach to the flexor tendon.

Jupiter performed flexor tenolysis in 22 patients (13% reimplants), of which 13 were in zone 2. In five fingers the tendon was obviously ischemic, and a tendon graft was carried out immediately. Simultaneous tenolysis of both tendons was performed in two subjects, and the tendon ruptured in the postoperative period in another two subjects, but the complications did not correlate with the number of arteries sutured. According to Jupiter[17] the functional results of tenolysis do not differ from those after simple tenorrhaphy. Our experience in 8 subjects (see Table 53-6) has been that tenolysis of the flexors in this type of lesion remarkably improves the ROM of the fingers. The best results with tenolysis are achieved on outcomes of cleancut lesions (Fig. 53-18). In avulsions and crush injuries, where long venous grafts are used, extensive devascularization of the sheath does not promote good results of tenorrhaphy and tenolysis (see Table 53-6).[36]

Tenolysis after complex trauma of the hand

The strategies described in the previous paragraphs apply here as well. The dorsal approach is followed by tenolysis of the flexors, which is often associated with a release of the first web and arthrolysis of the trapezium-metacarpal (TM) joint.[24] In this field, an interconnected stiffness will usually form and it is often underevaluated; it is clinically expressed by flexion contracture of the MP joint and extension contracture of the IP joint of the thumb.[24] If the surgical or rehabilitation plan is performed according to staged criteria, the results of double tenolyses even in complex trauma of the hand will achieve useful ranges of motion (see Table 53-5 and Fig. 53-19).

CONCLUSIONS

We define tenolysis as complex when surgery to the tendon is performed in conjunction with interventions on functionally correlated anatomic tissues or structures.

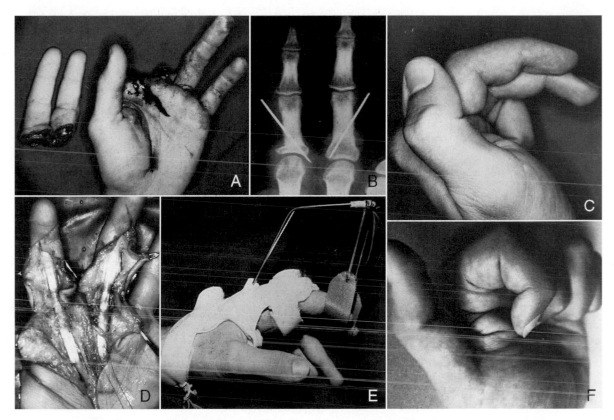

Fig. 53-18. *Case 3, Table 53-6.* **A,** Amputation of the second and third finger of the left hand by a paper cutter. **B,** Reimplantation of the fingers was performed via the following phases: osteosynthesis with K wires, tenorrhaphy of the flexor according to the Tsuge technique and of the extensors, radial and ulnar digital arteriorrhaphy of the second finger, and radial digital arteriorrhaphy of the third finger. Three dorsal veins for each finger and neurorrhaphy of the common sensory digital nerve were carried out. **C,** Clinical follow-up shows limitation of active flexion of the second and third fingers. **D,** At operation, tenolysis of the flexors of the index and middle finger was satisfactory, as an efficient three-pulley system could be preserved. **E,** Dynamic splint for extension of the PIP joint was utilized to prevent flexion contracture. **F,** Good clinical result at 6-year follow-up examination. (From Aulo Gaggi Editore Bologna, *GIOT* 1994; 20[3]:347-358.)

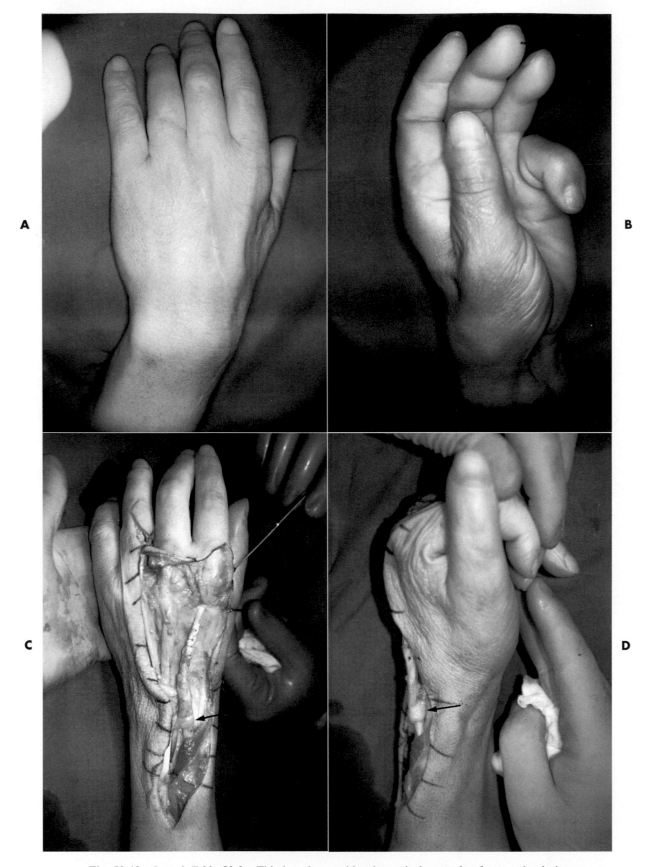

Fig. 53-19. *Case 6, Table 53-2.* This is to be considered a typical example of a complex lesion caused by a circular saw. The clinical status when the patient was referred to our center is shown in **A** and **B.** A multiple-staged program was outlined. In the static phase, multiple nerve grafts to the sensory common digital nerves of the median nerve were undertaken as this had been cut distal to its motor branch. **C,** Subsequently, a TADA was performed when sensation had returned in the median nerve distribution. The extensor indicus proprius was lengthened because of its tightness, and pulley reconstruction *(arrow)* was carried out at the distal forearm. **D** and **E,** Good passive range of motion was achieved at the MP joint level, and passive exercises were started immediately. *Continued.*

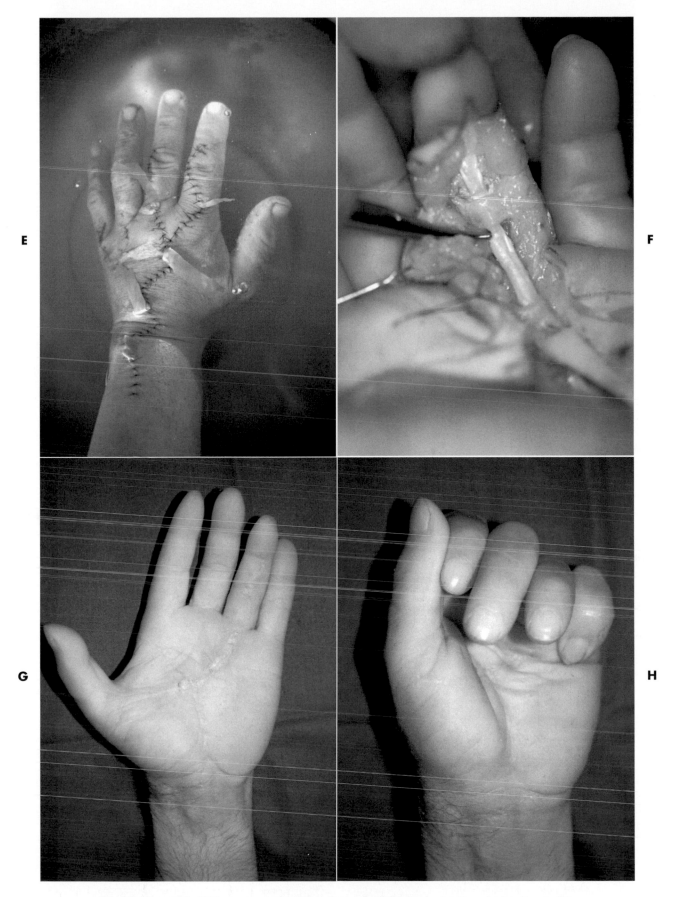

E

F

G

H

Fig. 53-19, cont'd. F, Flexor tenolysis of the index and middle fingers (at the wrist level) and of the ring finger in no man's land were the next surgical steps. **G** and **H,** The end result was satisfactory.

In this chapter we described the following conditions that are to be considered difficult tenolyses: dorsal tenoarthrolysis (TADA), complex tenolyses of the flexors in zone 2(defining the various subgroups), and associated tenolyses of the flexor and extensor tendons.

Our goal was to verify whether it is possible, when initially faced with a difficult hand, to intervene favorably on the outcome and predict a functional prognosis.

The prerequisites to successful intervention are tied to the patient's capacity and willingness to undergo successive surgical interventions. This implies that the health care system (public and private) must be able to provide the patient with the opportunity for multistage surgical interventions, with the understanding that these will markedly change the outcome of a lesion of the hand, which was initially classified as complex. Public and private insurance conditions permitting, the patient must then be sufficiently motivated to undergo the reconstructive procedure, which including rehabilitation programs, generally exceeds a period of 1 year.

The patient must be clearly informed on all the steps of the various operations. We have, when dealing with complex lesions of the hand, grouped all the immobilizing procedures (bone grafts, arthrodesis, tendon transfers) in the first phase. Only as the final step are the releasing interventions (tenoarthrolysis dorsal-apparatus [TADA], TATA, and combined tenolysis of the flexor-extensors) performed, once a good static function has been obtained.

The review of the present case series points out that this multistage surgical approach, when applicable, and also because of the contribution of complex tenolyses, provides a significant improvement in the outcome of complex lesions of the hand.[12]

REFERENCES

1. Amadio PC, Wood MB, Cooney WP, Bogard ST: Staged flexor tendon reconstruction in the fingers and hand, *J Hand Surg* 1988; 13A:559-562.
2. Buck-Gramcko D, Dietrich FE, Gogge S: Ewertungskriterien bei Nachuntersuchungen von Beugesehnewieder herstellungenen, *Handchirurgie* 1976; 8:65-69.
3. Bufalini C, Angeloni R, Innocenti M, Nigi M: Le rigidità delle metacarpo-falangee ed interfalangee della mano, *GIOT* 1995; 23(suppl)3:211-215.
4. Burrows WB, Hartwig RH, Kleinman WB, Strickland JW: The role of tenolyses after phalangeal fractures. In Strickland JW, ed: *Difficult problems in hand surgery,* St Louis, 1982, Mosby.
5. Burton RI: Extensor tendons—late reconstruction. In Green DP, ed: *Operative hand surgery,* New York, 1988, Churchill Livingstone.
6. Carreri G, Di Leo P, Santucci A, Barbarella R: Le rigidità articolari post-traumatiche e post-chirurgiche: definizione, classificazione, eziopatogenesi, *GIOT* 1995; 21(suppl)3:59-69.
7. Chamay A, Verdan C, Simonetta C: The two stage graft: a salvage operation for the flexor apparatus. A clinical study of 28 cases. In Verdan C, ed: *Tendon surgery of the hand,* Edinburgh, 1979, Churchill Livingstone.
8. Colville J: Tenorrafia dei tendini flessori con mobilizzazione immediata. In Landi A, ed: *Atti 2, Corso Italiano Permanente di Ortesi e Riabilitazione dell'Arto Superiore: "Patologia dei tendini della mano dall'infanzia all;età adulta,"* 177-182. Modena 4-6, Dicembre 1991, (in Italian).
9. Creighton JJ Jr, Steichen B: Complications in phalangeal and metacarpal fracture management: results of extensor tenolysis, *Hand Clin* 1994; 10(1):111-116.
10. De La Caffinière JY: Raideur post-traumatic des doigts longs, *Rev Chir Ort* 1981; 67:515-570.
11. Diao E, Eaton RG: Total collateral ligament excision for contractures of the proximal interphalangeal joint, *J Hand Surg* 1993; 18A: 395-402.
12. Foucher G, Lenoble E, Benyoussef K, et al: A post-operative regime after digital flexor tenolysis, *J Hand Surg* 1993; 18B:35-40.
13. Guelmi K, Sokolow C, Mitz V, Lemerle JP: Teno-arthrolyse dorsale de l∞tetphalangienne proximale. A propos de dix-neuf cas, *Ann Chir Main* 1992; 11(4):307-313.
14. Hume CM, Hellman H, McKellop H, Brumfield RH Jr: Functional range of motion of the joints of the hand, *J Hand Surg* 1990; 15A:240-243.
15. Hung LK, Chan A, Chang J, et al: Early controlled active mobilization with dynamic splintage for treatment of extensor tendon injures, *J Hand Surg* 1990; 15A:251-257.
16. Hunter JM, Cook JF, Ochiai N, et al: The pulley system, *J Hand Surg* 1980; 5:283-286.
17. Jupiter JB, Pess GM, Bour CC: Results of flexor tendon tenolysis after reimplantation in the hand, *J Hand Surg* 1989; 14A:35-44.
18. Landi A, Cugola L, Luchetti R, et al: I reimpianti pluridigitali di mano, *GIOT* 1985; 11:53-63.
19. Landi A: Oxidative metabolism in rabbit intrasynovial flexor tendons III changes in enzyme activity of hypovascular tendon after physical activity, *J Hand Surg Res* 1980; 29:287-292.
20. Landi A, Pederzini L, Soragni O, Luchetti R: La mètacarpo-phalangienne bloquée: facteurs etiologique et traitement, *Ann Chir Main* 1988; 7(3):232-237.
21. Landi A, Cavana R, Caserta G, et al: Il punto sulla tenolisi dei tendini flessori nella zona 2, *GIOT* 1994; 20(3):347-358.
22. Landi A, Luchetti R, Schoenhuber R: Peripheral nerve injuries. In Leung PC, ed: *Microsurgery in orthopaedic practice,* Singapore 1995, World Scientific.
23. Landi A, Saracino A, Pinelli M, et al: The tourniquet paralysis in microsurgery, *Ann Acad Med Singapore* 1995; 28(suppl): 89-93.
24. Landi A, Caserta G, Saracino A, Facchini MC: Le rigidità del 1° raggio, *GIOT* 1995; 21(suppl)3:205-210.
25. Mackin EJ: Benefits of early tendon gliding after tenolysis. In *Difficult problems in hand surgery,* St Louis, 1982, Mosby.
26. McCarty JA, Lesker PA, Peterson WW, Manske PR: Continuous passive motion as an adjunct for tenolysis, *J Hand Surg* 1986; 11B: 88-90.
27. Morrison WA, Cleland H: Vascularized flexor tendon grafts, *Ann Acad Med Singapore* 1995; 28(suppl):26-31.
28. Pittet-Cuenod B, Della Santa D, Chamay A: Total anterior teno-arthrolysis to treat inveterate flexion contraction of the fingers: a series of 16 patients, *Ann Plast Surg* 1991; 26:358-364.
29. Pulvertaft RG: Tendon grafting for the isolated injury of flexor digitorum profundus, *Bull H J D Ort Inst* 1984; 44:424-434.
30. Saffar PH, Rengeval JP: La teno-arthrolyse totale anterieure. Technique de traitement des doigts en crochet, *Ann Chir Main* 1978; 32(9):579-582.
31. Saffar PH: Teno-arthrolyse totale anterieure a propos d'une serie de 72 cas, *Ann Chir Main* 1983; 2(4):345-350.
32. Saffar Ph: La tèno-arthroliyse totale anterieure. In Tubiana R, ed: *Traitè de chirurgie de la main,* vol 3, Paris, 1986, Masson.
33. Schneider LH: Flexor tenolyses. In Strickland JW, ed: *Difficult problems in hand surgery,* St Louis, 1982, Mosby.
34. Schreiber DR: Arthroscopic blades in flexor tenolysis of the hand, *J Hand Surg* 1986; 11A:144-145.

35. Skoff HD: Extensor tenolysis: a modern version of an old approach, *Plast Reconstr Surg,* 1994; 93:1056-1061.

36. Steichen JB: Management of flexor tendon injury associated with digital replantation or revascularization. In Hunter J, Mackin E, eds: *Tendon surgery of the hand,* St Louis, 1987, Mosby.

37. Strickland JW, ed: Flexor tenolysis: a personal experience. In *Difficult problems in hand surgery,* St Louis, 1982, Mosby.

38. Tsuge K, ed: *Atlante di chirurgia della mano,* New York, 1988, McGraw-Hill.

39. Uhl RL: Salvage of extensor tendon function with tenolysis and joint release, *Hand Clin* 1995; 11(3):461-470.

40. Verdan CE, Crawford GP, Martini-Benkeddache Y: The valuable role of tenolysis in the digits. In *AAOS symposium on the hand,* St Louis, 1971, Mosby.

41. Windstrom CJ, Doyle JR, Manske PR, et al: A mechanical study of six digital pulley reconstruction techniques: comparative breaking strength and mechanical effectiveness, *Communication 44th Congr Am Soc Surg Hand,* Seattle, Sept 1989.

42. Zancolli E, ed: Structural and dynamic bases of hand surgery, ed 2, Philadelphia, 1979, Lippincott.

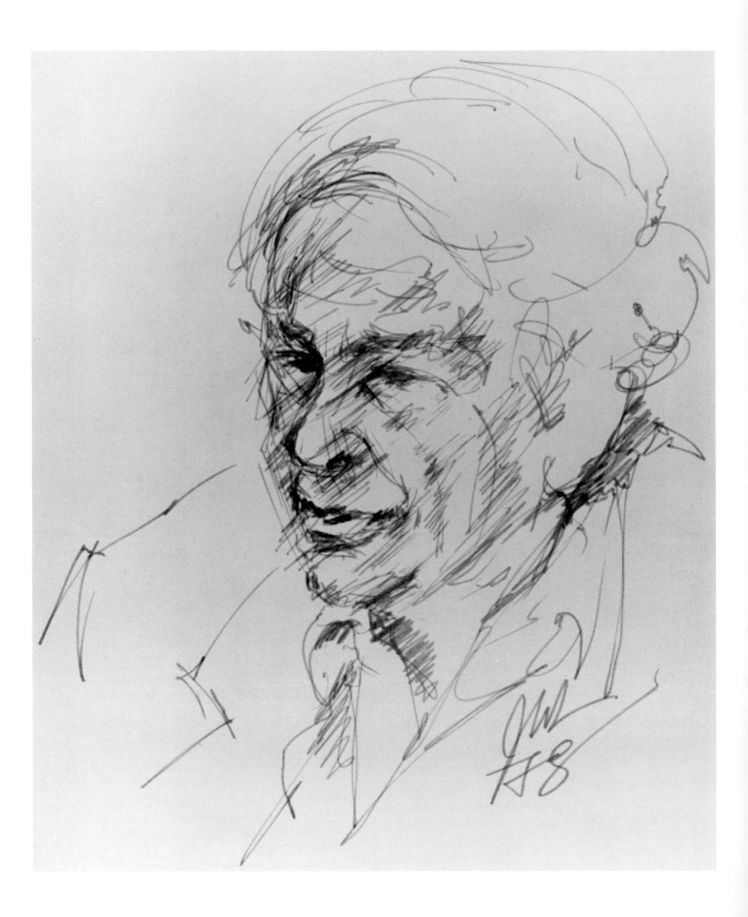

Part XIII

FLEXOR TENDON RECONSTRUCTION

Sketch of James M. Hunter, M.D., by J. William Littler, M.D.

Chapter 54

HISTOLOGY AND ULTRASTRUCTURE OF THE NORMAL TENOSYNOVIUM AND PSEUDOSHEATH IN CHICKENS AND HUMANS

Antal Salamon
Vilmos Biró
László Vámhidy
Károly Trombitás
László Józsa

The healing of the injured, especially the severely injured, flexor tendon in zone 2 is a very complicated process depending on biologic, functional, and clinical factors. Hunter[7] has described a two-stage procedure for the reconstruction of scarred tendon in this zone using a silicone rubber implant to develop a new tendon sheath. This method has been proposed by other authors as well. During the last 20 years a lot of experimental and clinical data were published, but nowadays different opinions exist in the judgment of the repair process. The origin of the ingrowing cells, the nutrition of the tendon graft, and the capacity of the new collagen synthesis are uncertain.

In recent work the following questions were investigated using light microscopic, scanning electron microscopic, and transmission electron microscopic investigations:

1. What is the structure of the parietal and visceral layers of the normal tenosynovium and the pseudosheath?
2. Where are the synovial cells and what is the morphology and function of these cells?

3. What is the mechanism of tendon healing within the pseudosheath?

MATERIAL AND METHODS

Young adult chickens were used as experimental animals because of the anatomic similarity between their digits and those of humans. Fresh human cadaver digits, amputated fingers, and little pieces of the tendon sheath of injured patients were studied. A total of 45 chickens and 18 human materials were used. Ten chickens and 6 humans served as controls. All the animals that suffered postoperative infection or an operative failure were excluded from the recent study. The experimental model was similar to human flexor tendon injuries, including scar formation and the two-stage reconstruction. All chickens were anesthetized with ketamine and local nerve block was given to the digital nerves using 1% lidocaine. First the flexor digitorum profundus (FDP) tendon of the long toe of the chicken foot was injured at the level of the insertion of the flexor digitorum superficialis (FDS). After 4 weeks the

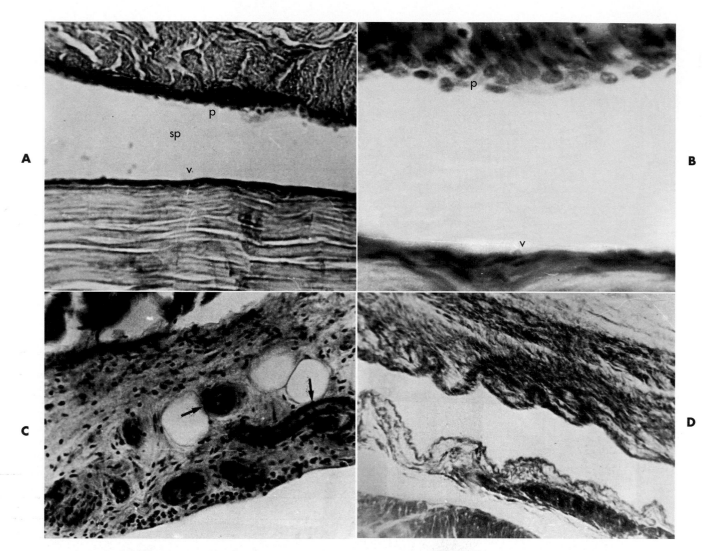

Fig. 54-1. A, Longitudinal section of normal chicken synovium showing the visceral (*V*) and parietal (*P*) sheath of the synovial space (*SP*), H.E. stain (×25). **B,** Chicken tenosynovium at higher magnification. The visceral *(V)* and parietal *(P)* lining cells are visible, hematoxylin-eosin stain (×160). **C,** Human parietal tendon sheath showing synovial cells, loose connective tissue, capillaries *(arrows),* and collagen fibers, hematoxylin-eosin stain (×40). **D,** Human tenosynovium stained with Krutsay trichrome (×40).

long toe was explored using a zigzag incision, and the scarred tissues were removed together with the remaining FDP stumps from the territory of the tendon sheath. At 2 weeks a plaster cast fixation was applied. Six weeks after the silicone rubber implantation, the silicone rubber implant was replaced with a tendon graft taken from the other foot using only a small proximal and distal incision. A plaster cast fixation was applied immobilizing the metatarsophalangeal (MTP) and interphalangeal (IP) joints in flexed position for 2 weeks. Normal activity was allowed for the animals after the cast was removed. Specimens were obtained from the normal tendon sheath and from the

pseudosheath 6 weeks after silicone implantation and 4 weeks after replacing the silicone implant by autogenous tendon graft. For light microscopy, paraffin sections were stained with haematoxylin-eosin and with Krutsay trichrome.

For scanning electron microscopy, samples were fixed in 2.5% glutaraldehyde at pH 7.4, were dehydrated in grading alcohol, and dried in a critical point dryer apparatus. The specimens were coated with gold and examined in a TESLA BS 300 scanning electron microscope. For transmission electron microscopy, tissue was fixed in 4% glutaraldehyde and 2% osmium tetroxide, embedded

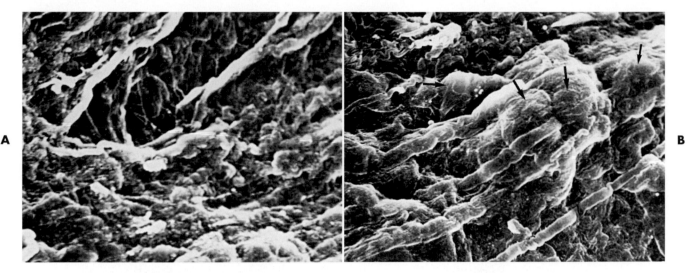

Fig. 54-2. Surface structure of normal chicken tenosynovium (SEM). **A,** Surface architecture of the parietal layer showing folds, fine fibrillar network (×300). **B,** Protrusions of synovial cells *(arrows)* covered with fibrils. Parietal tenosynovium (×1000).

in Durcupan ACM and examined with a JEM 100 B type electron microscope.

RESULTS
Group I: Light microscopic and ultrastructural morphology of normal chicken and human tendon tendon-sheath unit

Light microscopy. In the longitudinal sections of the normal chicken tendon tendon-sheath unit, the synovial cells of the visceral part form one layer and the lining cells of the parietal sheath are generally in two layers. The cells have ovoid nuclei. The parietal membrane shows rich vascularization in loose connective tissue. The outer layer of the tendon sheath consists of dense collagen bundles (Fig. 54-1, A and B). The histology of the human flexor tendon tendon-sheath unit is similar to the structure described previously (Fig. 54-1, C and D).

Scanning electron microscopy. The architecture of the surface of the chicken visceral tenosynovium shows slight, parallel folds. The surface is covered with fibrils and vesicular particles (Fig. 54-2).

Transmission electron microscopy. Two types of synovial cells are observable in the chicken and human tenosynovium (Fig. 54-3). The type A cells are present at different levels of the synovium. These phagocytic cells have many vacuoles, vesicles, lysosomes, filopodia, a prominent Golgi complex, but only little endoplasmic reticulum is visible. The type B cells have distinct endoplasmic reticulum, wide cisternae, namely, the ultrastructural features of a secretory cell. There are intermediary cells between types A and B, as well (Figs. 54-4, 54-5, and 54-6).

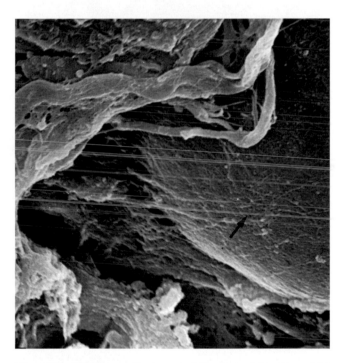

Fig. 54-3. Chicken parietal synovium. Synovial cell at high magnification *(arrow)*. Fibrils and vesicular particles attached to the cellular surface (×6000).

Group II: The structure of the newly formed synovium (pseudosheath) 6 weeks after silastic rod implantation

Light microscopy. The newly formed sheath appeared thicker than normal and varying in different places. The

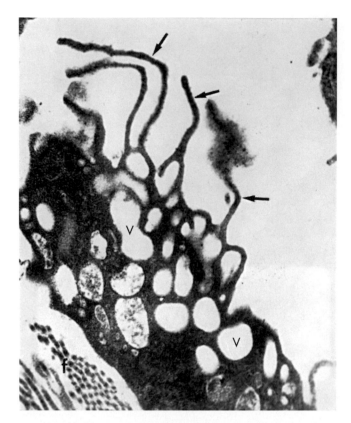

Fig. 54-4. Normal chicken tenosynovium (TEM). Cytoplasmic part of a type A cell with many filopodia *(arrows)*, vacuoles *(V)*, collagen fibrils *(F)* (×8000).

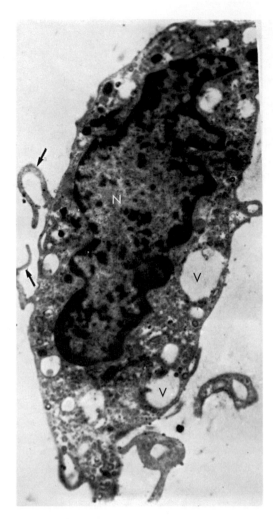

Fig. 54-6. Normal human tenosynovium. Type A lining cell shows scanty endoplasmic reticulum, vacuoles *(V)*, filopodia *(arrows)*, nucleus *(N)* (×5000).

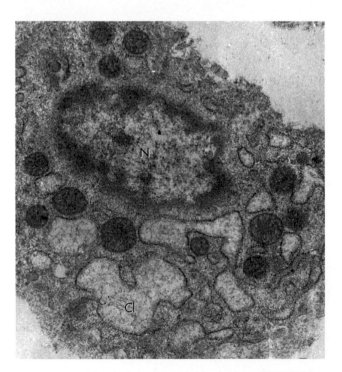

Fig. 54-5. Type B cell with profuse rough endoplasmic reticulum: wide cisternae *(CI)*, mitochondria *(M)* in the chicken parietal synovium, nucleus *(N)* (×13,000).

synovial cells of the chicken parietal sheath were arranged in two or three different layers in the longitudinal sections supported by vascular connective tissue (Fig. 54-7).

Scanning electron microscopy. The surface of the parietal pseudosynovium is similar to the normal chicken tenosynovium. Uneven surface is visible. The fold and lining cells are generally in a longitudinal direction (Fig. 54-8).

Transmission electron microscopy. Human pseudosheath was investigated, finding a similar ultrastructure to the normal chicken and human tenosynovium. Ultrastructure of type A cells possesses characteristics of phagocytic capacity (vacuoles, filopodia, lysosomes, little endoplasmic reticulum). The type B cells have ultrastructural features of a secretory cell showing extensively developed endoplasmic reticulum, wide cisternae, prominent Golgi complex (Figs. 54-9, 54-10, and 54-11).

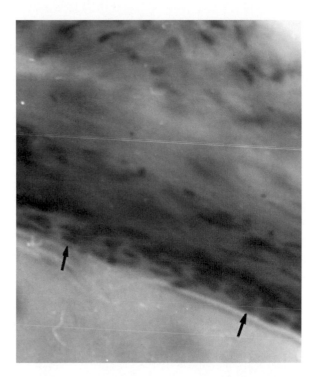

Fig. 54-7. Longitudinal section of chicken pseudosheath. Lining cells *(arrows)* and underlying connective tissue, hematoxylin-eosin stain (×160).

Group III: The structure of the pseudosheath 6 weeks after replacing the silicone rubber implant by autologous tendon graft

Light microscopy. The histology of the newly formed parietal and visceral sheath is similar to that of the normal flexor tendon sheath. The synovial cells of the parietal synovium are in two or three layers, and the surrounding tissue contains more bundles (Fig. 54-12).

Scanning electron microscopy. On the surface of the newly formed visceral sheath, flat lining cells are covered with fine fibers and vesicles. The structure of the parietal sheath is uneven. The synovial cells and fibril network is similar to the normal parietal sheath (Figs. 54-13 and 54-14).

DISCUSSION

The structure of the synovial layer is controversial in the literature. Some authors did not find a continuous cellular lining of the normal synovial sheath or of the pseudosheath, observing only an irregular amorphous layer.[3-5,11] Others have observed a regular tenosynovial surface, using scanning and transmission electron microscopy.[2,8,13,15,16] According to the scanning electron microscopic observations the cellular protrusions of the lining cells of the vincula and parietal sheath are covered with

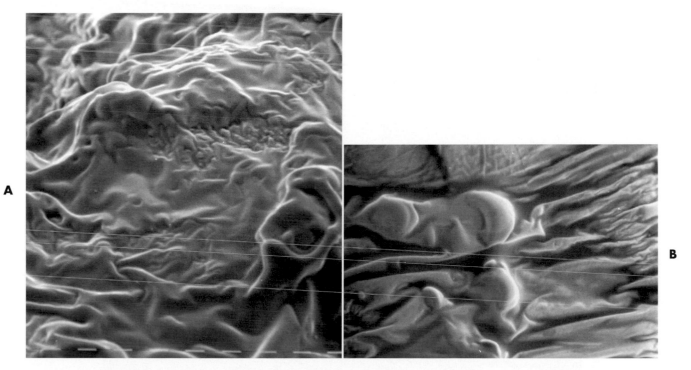

Fig. 54-8. A, Chicken pseudosynovium. SEM demonstrates the surface structure of the pseudosheath after removal of silicone rubber implant (×300). **B,** Surface folds and lining cell protrusions at higher magnification (×1000).

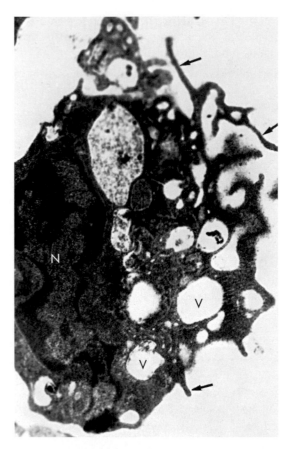

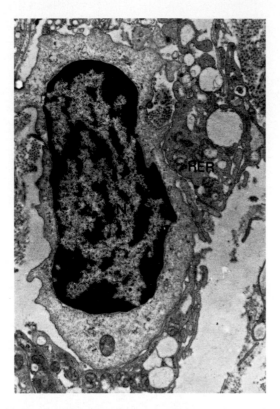

Fig. 54-9. Type A synovial cell in human pseudosheath showing nucleus *(N)*, vacuoles *(V)*, filopodia *(arrows)*, little rough endoplasmic reticulum (×8000).

Fig. 54-10. Type B cell in the human pseudosynovium nucleus *(N)*. Well-developed rough endoplasmic reticulum (RER), wide cisternae and mitochonria are visible (×12,000).

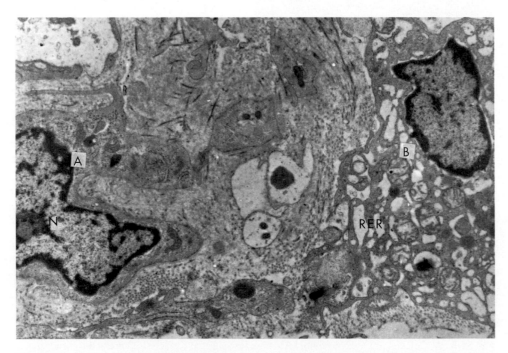

Fig. 54-11. Human tenosynovium. Type A cell *(A)* characterized by little endoplasmic reticulum. Type B cell *(B)* shows an abundant endoplasmic reticulum *(RER)* nucleus *(N)* (×6000).

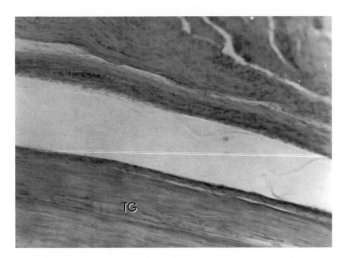

Fig. 54-12. Newly formed chicken pseudosheath. *TG:* tendon graft. Hematoxylin-eosin stain (×25).

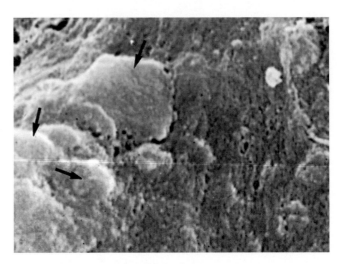

Fig. 54-13. Scanning electron micrograph demonstrates flat lining cells *(arrows)*, fibrils, and vesicles on the visceral pseudosynovium (×3000).

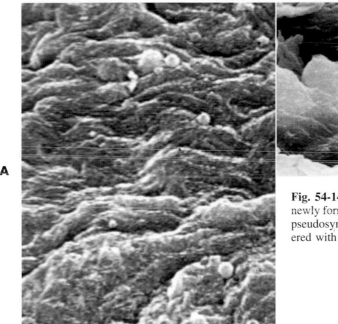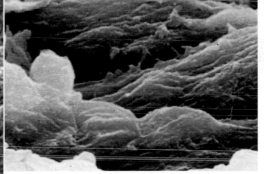

Fig. 54-14. A, Surface folds and visicles on the newly formed parietal synovium (×30). **B,** Parietal pseudosynovium. Protrusions of lining cells covered with fibrillar network (×3000).

fibrils and vesicular particles, the synovial cells of the visceral surface are flat, enmeshed with filamentous fibrils. The structure described above has a similar buildup in both the normal and in the pseudosheath. The same regular architecture was found both in the chicken and human sheath.

The ultrastructure and function of the synovial cells were studied first in the joint synovial membrane. Two types of synovial cells have been recognized by transmission electron microscopy. Type A cells have phagocytic capacity with features of absorptive macrophagic cells. Type B cells have

the ultrastructural characteristics of secretory cells producing probably protein and hyaluronic acid.[1,6,10,14] According to Yehia and Duncan[16] and Eiken et al.,[3] plasma dialysate, containing protein, flows from the surrounding vascular tissue between the synovial cells to the joint space, to which is added mucin, secreted by the type B cells to lubricate and nourish the joint cartilage. The same situation can be found in the tendon sheath. Similar data have been found only by Schmidt and Mackay[13] concerning the tendon sheath. These authors described the type A and type B cells in the normal human tenosynovium. We have also found two

Biologic factors

Biochemical factors ↓	*Biomechanical factors* ↓	*Functional factors* ↓
I. Exudation Infiltration ↓	Silicone rubber implant Pseudosheath ↓	State of rest Movement Active Passive ↓
II. Proliferation Granulation tissue Neovascular- ization Fibroblasts Collagen synthesis ↓	Tendon graft Short Long Tensile strength Original collagen frame New collagen	↓
III. Repair Synovial membrane Collagen re- modeling ↓	↓	↓

Development of a gliding surface
Reconstruction of the smooth surface of the tendon graft
Repairing of the continuity of collagen fibers

types of synovial cells, and we have described the ultrastructural characteristics both in normal and pseudosheath in chicken and in human cases. The regular ultrastructure of the synovial membrane guarantees the nutritional supply and provides a gliding surface after tendon transplantation, not only under normal conditions, but under reconstruction as well. The fact that a very important area for future research is the synovial fluid formed in the tendon sheath was declared by Lundborg in 1978.[9] The components of the synovia could probably prevent adhesion formation around the tendon. The normal and the newly formed synovial membranes are well vascularized. The undistributed microcirculation and the adequate production of synovial fluid make the tendon or graft nutrition possible. Under such circumstances, first of all the epitenon cells proliferate and migrate into the suture zone and into the deeper part of the tendon graft synthesizing new collagen. The results of our experiments proved that the reorganization of the tendon graft takes place in this way undergoing a gradual reorganization.[12] There is a possibility for intrinsic repair of the tendon graft under ideal conditions during the two-stage procedure, according to the data from the literature and our experiments. The synovial fluid has probably important components to lubricate the newly formed sheath preventing adhesion formation. The neurovascular supply and the

remodeling of collagen and early function are other important factors as well (see the box on the left). This chapter deals mainly with the morphology and the function of the lining cells.

In some cases it is difficult to achieve the ideal healing conditions in clinical practice. Further investigations are necessary for the better understanding of the biologic healing process altogether with its adaptation to the clinical practice. These efforts can result in the improvement of the final outcome after tendon reconstruction.

CONCLUSIONS

1. The normal visceral and parietal flexor tendon sheath contain regular layers of synovial cells. At 6 weeks the pseudosheath has a similar appearance to the normal sheath.
2. The morphology and probably the function of type A and B synovial cells are also similar in the newly formed sheath.
3. Under ideal conditions the nutritional supply of the tendon graft is very important for the proliferation of the epitenon cells during the repairing process. According to our observation, the tendon graft undergoes gradual reorganization.

SUMMARY

The histology and ultrastructure of the intact flexor tendon sheath and the pseudosheath of the chicken foot and the human hand were studied. A regular visceral and parietal layer was found both in the normal sheath and in the pseudosynovium using light microscopy and scanning electron microscopy. The surface of the normal synovium shows folds and cellular protrusions covered with fibrils and vesicles. The architecture of the pseudosynovial surface is similar after silicone rubber implant. Two types of synovial lining cells were observed using transmission electron microscopy. The ultrastructural features and the possible function of these cells are discussed. Type A cells have phagocytic characteristics, type B cells possess secretory capacity. These findings were similar concerning the normal tendon sheath and pseudosynovium both in chickens and humans. Hypothetically, the described regular structure of the newly formed tenosynovium should guarantee the nutritional supply and the gliding of the transplanted tendon under ideal conditions. The elaborate healing process and the influencing factors of the tendon healing are emphasized.

REFERENCES

1. Barland P, Novikoff A, Hamerman D: Electron microscopy of the human synovial membrane, *J Cell Biology* 1962; 14:207.
2. Cohen MJ, Kaplan L: Histology and ultrastructure of the human flexor tendon sheath, *J Hand Surg* 1987; 12A:25.
3. Eiken O, Lundborg G, Rank F: The role of the digital synovial sheath in tendon grafting, *Scand J Plast Reconstr Surg* 1975; 9:182.

4. Eskeland G, Eskeland T, Hovig T, Teigland T: The ultrastructure of normal digital flexor tendon sheath and of the tissue formed around silicone and polyethylene implants in man, *J Bone Joint Surg* 1977; 59B:206.

5. Farkas LG, McCain WG, Sweeney P, Wilson W: An experiment of the changes following silastic rod preparation of a new tendon sheath and subsequent tendon grafting, *J Bone Joint Surg* 1973; 55A:1149.

6. Ghadially FN, Roy S: Ultrastructure of rabbit synovial membrane, *Am Rheum Dis* 1966; 25:318.

7. Hunter JM, Salisbury R: Flexor tendon reconstruction in severely damaged hands, *J Bone Joint Surg* 1971; 53A:829.

8. Inoue H, Takasugi H, Akahori O: Surface study of tenosynovium in hens and humans by electron microscopy, *Hand* 1976; 8:222.

9. Lundborg G, Rank F: Experimental intrinsic healing of flexor tendons based upon synovial nutrition, *J Hand Surg* 1978; 3:21.

10. Moller Graabeck P: Characteristics of the two types of synoviocytes in rat synovial membrane, *Lab Invest* 1984; 50:690.

11. Potenza AD: Tendon healing within the flexor tendon sheath in the dog: an experimental study, *J Bone Joint Surg* 1962; 44A:49.

12. Salamon A, Hamori J, Deak G, Mayer F: Submicroscopic investigation of autogenous tendon grafts, *Acta Morph Ac Sci Hung* 1970; 18:23.

13. Schmidt D, McKay B: Ultrastructure of human tendon sheath and synovium: implications for tumor histogenesis, *Ultrastructural Pathology* 1982; 3:489.

14. Schumacher HR: Ultrastructure of the synovial membrane, *Ann Clin Lab Sci* 1975; 5:489.

15. Takashi M: Micro-constructive studies of human digital flexor tendon and tendon sheath: observations by scanning electron microscope and light microscope, *J Jap Orthop Ass* 1981; 56:133.

16. Takasugi H, Inoue H, Akahori O: Scanning electron microscopy of repaired tendon and pseudosheath, *Hand* 1976; 8:228.

Chapter 55

FLEXOR-TENDON RECONSTRUCTION IN SEVERELY DAMAGED HANDS

A two-stage procedure using a silicone-Dacron reinforced gliding prosthesis prior to tendon grafting*

James M. Hunter
Roger E. Salisbury

In 1965, one of us (J.M.H.) presented evidence that a new tendon bed and sheath would form in response to a gliding tendon prosthesis and that a free tendon graft could be inserted in the new sheath and remain function functional.[26,27] He reviewed the literature and reported his results in 29 clinical cases of severe tendon damage in which several types of silicone-dacron reinforced tendon prostheses were used both in the reconstruction of flexor and extensor tendons and for opponens transfers. From this review of the literature, it was concluded that research aimed at overcoming the damaging effects of scar tissue on tendon grafting had developed in three principal directions: (1) the use of devices or implants to prevent or block out scar tissue formation†; (2) the placement of rigid, semirigid, or flexible implants in damaged connective-tissue beds to enhance pseudosheath formation prior to tendon grafting;‡ and (3) the use of artificial tendon substitutes to bridge tendon gaps.§

*Reprinted from *The Journal of Bone and Joint Surgery* 53A(5):829-858, July 1971. Copyrighted 1971 by *The Journal of Bone and Joint Surgery, Inc.*
†References 3, 4, 19-21, 24, 25, 31, 38, 48.
‡References 1, 5, 13, 14, 18, 23, 36-38, 45.
§References 2, 17, 22, 24, 30, 32, 43, 44.

It was also noted in 1965 that Mayer and Ransohoff, in 1936,[36] building on the earlier work of Biesalski, in 1910,[6] had introduced the pseudosheath concept when they used celloidin tubes as implants in scarred tendon beds and that Milgram[37] had continued this work in 1945 using stainless-steel implants. Neither method gained acceptance, however, because the rigid materials caused stiffness of the fingers during the period of implantation. In 1958, Carroll and Bassett[14] showed that a flexible silicone-rubber rod could be safely implanted in scarred tendon beds in the hands.

These findings stimulated one of us (J.M.H.) to study pseudosheath formation in response to implants in the laboratory.[28] Mesothelial cells were found aligned on the surface of the implant as early as 5 days and by 3 weeks a well-developed bursa had formed. The type of implant (stiff, rigid, or flexible) did not affect pseudosheath formation provided no joint motion was involved. Studies with several types of dacron-reinforced silicone gliding tendon prostheses in dogs showed a more advanced sheath formed when there was gliding and fluid resembling synovial fluid was found to be lubricating the prosthesis. When the prosthesis was removed and replaced by a tendon graft, the sheath

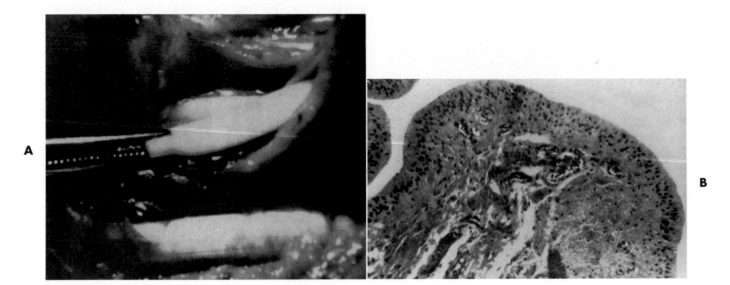

Fig. 55-1. A, Proximal end of prosthesis (in hemostat) and sheath 4 months after stage I. Opening of sheath can be seen to the right. **B,** Biopsy specimen of sheath shown in **A.** Note well-formed synovial membrane and absence of inflammatory cells (hematoxylin-eosin, × 40).

seemed to afford nourishment and a gliding surface for the central one-third of the graft. On all occasions, the tendons remained viable both grossly and histologically. Since the presentation of these laboratory findings, our progressively improving clinical results in the salvage of fingers with severe tendon injuries has led us to believe that a reliable tendon prosthesis inserted as one stage in tendon reconstruction is the additional step needed to improve the results of flexor-tendon reconstructive surgery.

The method has been applied in more than 150 tendon reconstructions of various types. It is the purpose of this report to describe the presently used two-stage technique for flexor-tendon reconstruction in hands in which the conditions are less than optimum and to report the results in 74 of 86 consecutive cases in which this method has been employed.

Until 1965, tendon prostheses made of silicone rubber extruded over polyester sutures and tapes were employed. These implants were used in badly damaged fingers and were sutured to the distal phalanx and to the appropriate superficialis or profundus tendon in the distal part of the forearm. Although tendon function was sometimes achieved and was maintained as long as 5 years in one thumb,[28] in many fingers the anastomosis gave way, compromising the results of the tendon grafting, which was done as a second-stage free tendon graft about 4 months after the insertion of the prosthesis or sooner if there were certain complications. In several cases in which the proximal suture line of the prosthesis gave way, regular passive motion of the finger maintained gliding of the prosthesis and kept the joints supple so that when the tendon graft was performed at the second stage, the sheath was found to be well formed with no evidence of synovitis

(Fig. 55-1, *B*). In view of this finding and the need to develop a more reliable method, the use of an active tendon prosthesis was abandoned at least temporarily. Since that time, a passive gliding prosthesis has been used that is secured to the distal phalanx while its proximal end is left free to glide in the palm or forearm as the finger is passively flexed and extended.

THE PROSTHESIS

With the cooperation of the Holter Company, the Philadelphia College of Textiles and Science, and the Orthopaedic Research Laboratories at Jefferson Medical College, a new prosthesis, now commercially available as the Hunter tendon, was developed to serve this passive function. This new design is ovoid in cross-section so as to glide well and to produce a sheath of proper contour for the tendon graft, which is inserted at the second stage. The details of fabrication are most important. The central dacron core is woven especially (1) to resist tearing out of the stainless-steel or dacron sutures used for fixation of the prosthesis at the time of implantation and (2) to provide the requisite stiffness to ensure push-pull excursion of the implant and sufficient durability to withstand repeated bending and straightening caused by passive finger motion. The proper type of medical grade silicone must be used and molded under high pressure in highly polished stainless-steel molds. The vulcanizing and curing of the silicone must also be carried out in a meticulous fashion.

When properly fabricated the prosthesis has the necessary combination of firmness and flexibility, as well as the smooth glistening surface required to ensure ease of insertion and free passive gliding of the implant throughout the finger,

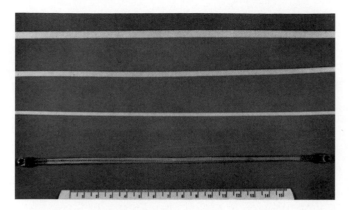

Fig. 55-2. Passive prostheses as they are currently produced. From top down: large, medium, and small. At the bottom is an experimental active prosthesis with polished metal rings for tendon-loop anastomosis (see text).

palm, and forearm. A smooth surface free of any type of contaminant[5] is essential to minimize foreign-body reaction and to stimulate the formation of a smooth sheath capable of lubricating and nourishing a tendon graft.

The currently available prostheses are 23 cm long and 3 widths are available (Fig. 55-2): small (3 mm), medium (4 mm), and large (5 mm). At the time of insertion, the implant may be cut to proper length. Based on our experience to date, a larger implant is needed. This will soon be available and the three-millimeter implant currently designated *small* will be provided only on special request. The regularly available implants will then be: *large,* 6 mm wide and 23 cm long; *medium,* 5 mm wide and 23 cm long; and *small,* 4 mm wide and 23 cm long.

The tape used in the prosthesis is woven 70-denier dacron yarn (Type 55) textured by the Fluflow process. The tensile strength of the tapes and of the prostheses was determined using a Thwing-Albert electrotensiometer and a slow strain rate of 30.5 cm/min. The breaking strength of the large and medium tapes was 13.6 to 18.1 kg and of the small tape, 9.1 kg. After completion of the silicone coating, the breaking strength was increased by 2.3 to 3.2 kg.

The breaking strengths of the sutured ends of the prostheses were also determined using a Dillon tensiometer and a strain rate of 50.8 cm/min. No. 4 monofilament or multifilament stainless-steel wire on atraumatic needles was used and a double figure-of-eight suture was placed in the end of the prosthesis under test. When tested, the sutures broke at about 4.1 kg, or at 25% of the breaking strength of the prosthesis. When No. 0 monofilament wire was used, the tendons tore at 50% of the tensile strength of the prosthesis.

Randomly selected tendon prostheses, removed 3 to 6 months after implantation, showed no significant change in breaking strength compared with the new tendons. Currently, new yarns and cables, made of stainless steel, titanium, and a combination of tantalum and platinum, are being tested in the hope that, with proper design and fabrication of the yarn and end devices, an active tendon prosthesis can be developed that may be used for extended periods before a second-stage procedure for tendon grafting is required.

The present report concerns our experience to date using the original active and the presently employed passive prostheses in hands with significant damage to the tendon gliding mechanism. It is believed that inclusion of both types of prosthesis is justified. Because the active prostheses provided only limited function and were used guardedly prior to tendon grafting, they were essentially the same as the passive grafts insofar as their mechanical effects on the surrounding tissues were concerned. The passive prosthesis with no proximal anastomosis has been the most reliable method and is now used in the majority of cases.

TECHNIQUE

Patients selected for the two-stage tendon reconstruction to be described are put on a program of physical therapy under the supervision of our hand therapist. The program is designed to mobilize stiff joints and to improve the condition of the soft tissues as much as possible before the first stage.

Stage I

The damaged flexor tendons and their scarred sheath are exposed. In the finger, this is done through a midlateral incision or the zigzag incision of Bruner.[11] In the palm, exposure is accomplished through a transverse incision or through a proximal continuation of Bruner's zigzag incision. In the forearm, an ulnarly curved volar incision (Fig. 55-3, *A*) is made to expose the proximal portions of the flexor tendons and their musculotendinous junctions. A stump of the profundus tendon, one centimeter in length, is left attached to the distal phalanx. Scarred tendons, sheath, and retinaculum are then excised. If the excision is stopped in the palm at the lumbrical level, the contracted and scarred lumbrical muscle is excised (Fig. 55-4). Contracted or scarred lumbricals should always be excised.[29] This is done to prevent the paradoxical motion of the lumbrical, which is seen after some tendon grafts.[39] This motion causes the finger to extend rather than flex as the patient attempts to flex the finger completely.

Undamaged portions of the flexor fibro-osseous retinaculum, which are not contracted, are retained. Any portion of the retinaculum that can be dilated instrumentally with a hemostat is also preserved. The rest is excised. The retinacular pulley system (Figs. 55-5 and 55-6) should be preserved or reconstructed proximal to the axis of motion of each joint, otherwise normal gliding of the tendon will not be restored. Four pulleys are preferred: one proximal to each of the three finger joints and one at the base of the proximal phalanx.

The implant to be inserted must have been prepared by the prescribed method.[5] After sterilization, the prosthesis is kept

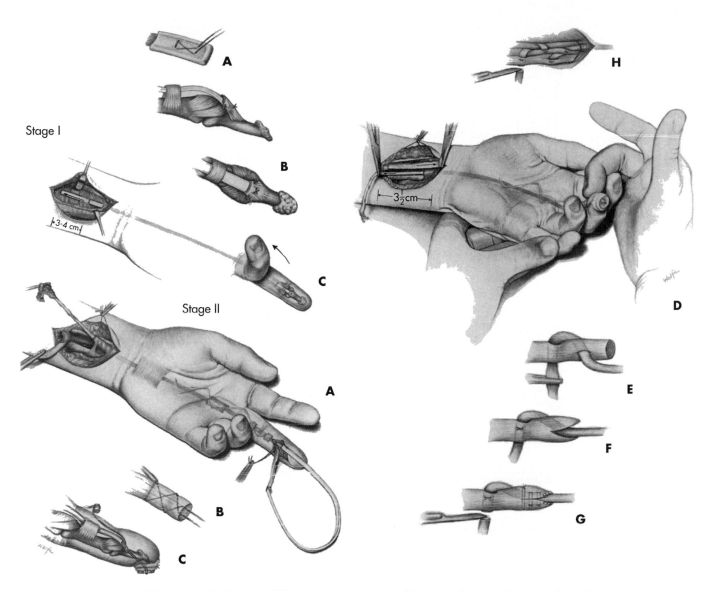

Fig. 55-3. A and **B,** Passive gliding program, using the Hunter tendon prosthesis. *A:* Stage I. Placement of tendon prosthesis. After excision of scar and formation of pulleys. *A.* Figure-of-eight suture in distal end of the prosthesis. *B.* Distal end of prosthesis sutured to stump of profundus tendon and adjacent fibrous tissue on distal phalanx. *C.* Prosthesis in place showing free gliding and excursion of its proximal end during passive finger flexion. Stage II. Removal of prosthesis and insertion of tendon graft. *A.* Graft has been sutured to proximal end of the prosthesis and then pulled distally through the new tendon bed. Note mesentery-like attachment of new sheath visible in the forearm. *B.* Distal anastomosis. Bunnell pullout suture in distal end of tendon graft. *C.* Distal anastomosis. Complete Bunnel suture with button over fingernail. Reinforcing sutures are usually placed through the stump of the profundus tendon. *D.* Proximal anastomosis. Measuring excursion of tendon graft and selecting motor. If the procedure is done under local anesthesia (see text) the true amplitude of active muscle contraction can be measured. *E.* Proximal anastomosis. Graft is threaded through tendon motor muscle two or three times for added strength. *F.* Proximal anastomosis. Stump is fish-mouthed after the method of Pulvertaft, the tension is adjusted, and one suture is inserted as shown. Further adjustment of the tension can be accomplished simply by removing and shortening or lengthening as need be. *G.* Proximal anastomosis. After appropriate tension has been selected the anastomosis is completed. *H.* Proximal anastomosis. Technique when graft is anastomosed to common profundus tendon (see text).

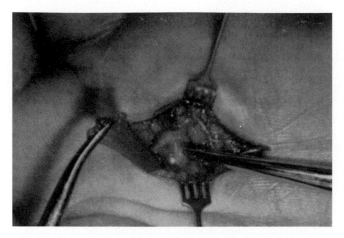

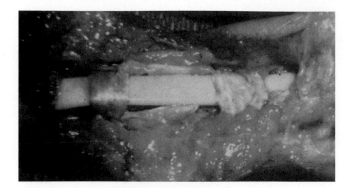

Fig. 55-6. Both pulleys, the one on the left proximal to the distal interphalangeal joint and the one on the right proximal to the interphalangeal joint, have been made with free tendon grafts sutured to the remnants of the old retinaculum, which is visible between pulleys and dorsal to the prosthesis. When the retinaculum cannot be dilated sufficiently to prevent binding of the prosthesis, new pulleys must be fashioned.

Fig. 55-4. Excision of the scarred lumbrical muscle through an oblique palmar incision. The tip of the dissecting scissors is on the proximal stump of the severed profundus tendon. Because the profundus will be used as the motor in stage II, it is left in situ at this time. The tendon is adherent in the palm; hence some function of the profundus is maintained as the wrist is flexed and extended. In addition, by leaving the tenosynovium in the proximal part of the palm and wrist undisturbed during stage I, scarring as the result of insertion of the prosthesis is minimized.

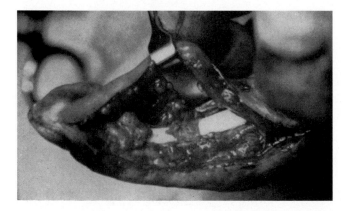

Fig. 55-5. A large prosthesis in place after excision of the scarred tendons through a midlateral incision. The retinaculum has been preserved and dilated sufficiently to accept the prosthesis. The distal end of the prosthesis has been sutured beneath the stump of the profundus tendon.

flat in a lint-free receptacle. When handled at operation, gloves should be freshly moistened with Ringer's solution before contact with the implant, or sponges wet with Ringer's solution should be used to hold the device. A large tendon prosthesis (5 mm) is preferred. It is first placed on sponges moistened with Ringer's solution on the volar aspect of the forearm, and then a tendon passer, with a diameter slightly larger than that of the prosthesis, is passed proximally from the palm through the carpal tunnel into the forearm. The distal end of the prosthesis is secured to this and pulled into the palm, whence it can be pushed through the retinaculum and pulleys to the distal end of the finger—a process facilitated by moistening the pros-

thesis with Ringer's solution. An alternative method is to insert the prosthesis in a proximal direction by seeking a free plane in the carpal canal by blunt instrumentation. The superficialis and profundus tendons may be transected either proximal or distal to the carpal canal. If proximal, the tendon is sutured to the fascia beneath the flexion crease of the wrist. The purpose of this suture is (1) to prevent the muscle (a potential motor for the free tendon graft to be inserted during stage II) from shortening, (2) to provide for some isometric function of the muscle during the interval between stages I and II, and (3) to facilitate identification of the muscle during stage II and hence to reduce the amount of dissection required.

The distal end of the prosthesis is sutured beneath the stump of the profundus tendon after resecting all but the most distally attached fibers of the tendon (see Fig. 55-3, A). A figure-of-eight suture of No. 32 or 34 monofilament stainless-steel wire on an atraumatic taper-cut needle is used. In addition, medial and lateral sutures of No. 35 multifilament wire are usually put through the tendon, prosthesis, and fibroperiosteum for further fixation. Any excess of profundus tendon is resected. Traction is then applied on the proximal end of the prosthesis in the forearm, to be sure that the attachment of the prosthesis is distal to the distal interphalangeal joint and its volar plate and that there is no binding of the tendon during flexion (Fig. 55-7) and extension. The prosthesis is also observed during passive flexion and extension of the finger (see Fig. 55-3, A) to make sure that it glides freely with no binding or buckling distal to some part of the pulley system that is too tight. If any portion of the system is tight, it must be removed and replaced with a new pulley constructed from a free tendon graft (see Fig. 55-6).

The proximal end of the prosthesis should also be observed during passive flexion and extension to make sure

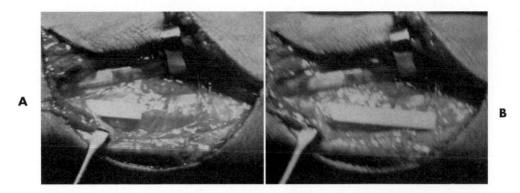

Fig. 55-7. Proximal end of prosthesis has been cut off to appropriate length. Fingers extended (**A**) and flexed (**B**). Note passive gliding of prosthesis, which should be of sufficient length to cause the new sheath to form as far proximal as the musculotendinous junction of the flexor muscles in the forearm.

that it glides properly (see Fig. 55-7, *A* and *B*). Preferably, this end of the prosthesis should be in the forearm so that the newly formed sheath will extend to the region of the musculotendinous junction of the motor muscle (see Fig. 55-3, *A* and *C*). The prosthesis may be placed superficial or deep to the antebrachial fascia or deep in one of the intermuscular planes. The track for the prosthesis can be fashioned by separating connective tissues and tendon mesenteries with the moistened gloved finger. The track must permit free passive gliding of the prosthesis during passive flexion and extension of the finger. If such a track cannot be established by spreading and adjusting of the tissues, the prosthesis should be shortened so that, when the finger is fully extended, the proximal end of the prosthesis lies just proximal to the flexion crease at the wrist.

When multiple prostheses are threaded through the carpal canal, the superficialis tendons are generally removed from the canal. To date, we have not observed a carpal tunnel syndrome in association with one or more prostheses traversing the canal.

Finally, before the wound is closed, traction should again be applied to the prosthesis and the amount of active finger motion determined and recorded (Fig. 55-8). If this maneuver does not produce full flexion it may be necessary to modify the pulley system. This is a most important point and is a unique feature of this technique, because use of the prosthesis permits preservation or reconstruction of the four-pulley system with direct observation of its function at operation and, in addition, ensures the development of gliding surfaces before the tendon graft is inserted.

Following skin closure, a standard postoperative hand dressing is applied, with the wrist and metacarpophalangeal (MP) joints in moderate flexion (40° to 50°) and the interphalangeal (IP) joints in slight flexion (20° to 30°). In this position the new sheath will be formed proximally and free excursion of the prosthesis distally will be possible when passive motion is begun at 3 weeks. Where there were

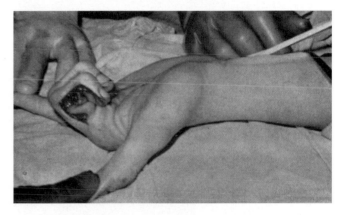

Fig. 55-8. Finger flexion produced by traction on the prosthesis during stage I. This maneuver permits a prediction of the future range of active motion, which in these grade 5 fingers was flexion to a pulp-to-crease distance of 0.6 cm. Any visible bowstringing of the prosthesis with resultant loss of flexion should be corrected by appropriately placed free-tendon-graft pulleys. After this maneuver the distal anastomosis should be inspected to be sure it is sound.

joint contractures prior to insertion of the prosthesis, intermittent dynamic splinting may be required to prevent recurrence of the contracture. This periodic elastic traction on the fingers, while the wrist and MP joints are maintained in position by splinting, may be started during the first postoperative week. Gentle passive motion of all joints is started gradually during the second to the fourth week. Regular passive stretching, under the supervision of the hand therapist, is begun in the fifth week and the patient is taught at this time to flex the finger whenever possible, using an adjacent finger hooked over the damaged one. Usually, by the sixth week, there is a functional range of passive motion. During this time the hand should be examined regularly for evidence of synovitis in the new sheath. If this has not developed within the first 6 weeks, it is not likely to occur and the patient may resume normal activities, including going back to work, until the patient is ready for the second stage.

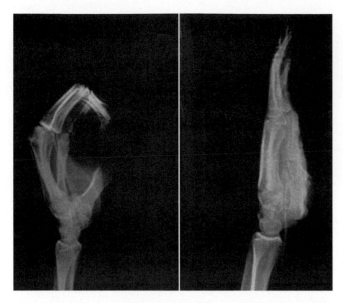

Fig. 55-9. Roentgenograms made between stages I and II. Patient is using adjacent normal fingers to flex the two digits in which prostheses have been inserted. Note excursion of proximal ends of the prostheses with no buckling. Compare with Fig. 55-10.

A small amount of barium sulphate is incorporated in the prosthesis so that its function can be checked roentgenographically at 6 weeks and again just before insertion of the tendon graft (Fig. 55-9). Anteroposterior and lateral roentgenograms of the hand and distal one half of the forearm are made with the fingers and wrist in full extension and full flexion. These roentgenograms will demonstrate how much the proximal end of the prosthesis moves with respect to the distal end of the radius. If there is a full range of motion of the wrist and all finger joints, an excursion of 5 to 7 cm is not unusual. These roentgenograms will also show any evidence of buckling. Slight or intermittent buckling may cause no difficulty. However, if there is appreciable buckling (Fig. 55-10), synovitis is likely to occur and the patient should be followed carefully. If synovitis develops, the finger should be immobilized promptly and if the synovitis persists, the second-stage procedure should be done sooner before chronic fibrosis develops.

Stage II

The interval between stage I and stage II should be 2 to 6 months, or long enough to permit maturation of the tendon bed to the point where it can nourish and lubricate the gliding tendon graft. In fingers in which fixed flexion contractures of many months' duration are mobilized for the first time at the

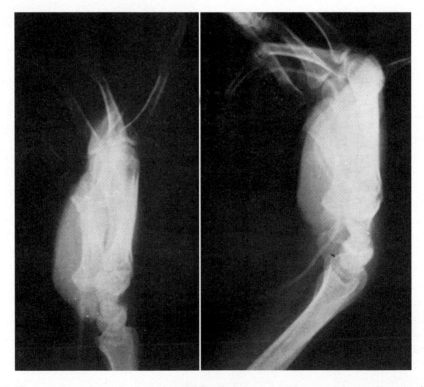

Fig. 55-10. Buckling of prosthesis at the middle phalanx caused by too tight a pulley proximal to this level and by poor placement of the proximal part of the prosthesis in the tissues of the forearm. With the finger extended (*left*) the prosthesis is virtually straight. During flexion, however, the prosthesis buckles distal to the proximal interphalangeal joint and the proximal end of the implant in the forearm abuts against the antebrachial fascia.

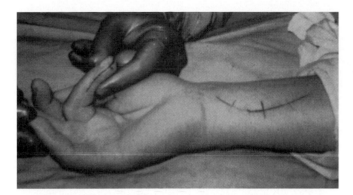

Fig. 55-11. Incision used for stage II.

stage I procedure, stage II should be delayed until maximum softening of the tissues and mobilization of the stiff joints have been achieved. Each case must be individualized and the decision to do the second-stage procedure must be made by the surgeon on the basis of the findings in the hand.

When stage II is begun, the limits of extension and flexion of the finger must first be accurately measured and recorded. A short midlateral or Bruner zigzag incision is then made to locate the distal end of the prosthesis where it is attached to the distal phalanx (Fig. 55-11). This attachment is left intact and a second ulnarly curved volar incision is made in the forearm through the original stage I incision to expose the proximal end of the prosthesis and the musculotendinous junction of the superficialis or profundus tendon, whichever is to be used as a motor for the tendon graft.

With the prosthesis still in place, the excursion of the proximal end of the prosthesis, as the finger is moved from full extension to full flexion, should also be measured as an additional check on the amount of excursion that the motor muscle must have to provide full finger motion (see Fig. 55-3, *B* and *D*).

A long tendon graft is then obtained from one leg—the plantaris preferably—but if this is missing, a long toe extensor tendon may be used. If a toe extensor must be employed, the graft is obtained using a modified Brand tendon stripper and two or more incisions, so that the portion of the tendon proximal to the retinaculum is obtained. Any attached fat or muscle is removed and one end of the graft is sutured to the proximal end of the prosthesis with a catgut or polyester suture (Fig. 55-12). Leaving the distal end of the prosthesis attached to the distal phalanx, the rest of the prosthesis, with the attached tendon graft, is pulled distally, thereby threading the graft through the new sheath (see Fig. 55-3 *A, Stage II, A*). The prosthesis is then removed and discarded. Free motion of the graft in the sheath can now be confirmed by grasping each end of the graft with a hemostat and pulling it proximally and distally.

The tendon graft is first secured to the distal phalanx using a Bunnell button pullout wire suture, with the button on the fingernail and medial and lateral reinforcing sutures through

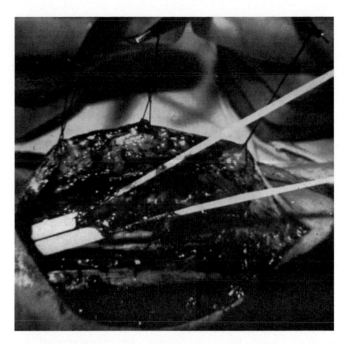

Fig. 55-12. Stage II. Proximal incision at the level of the musculotendinous junction. Long free-tendon grafts have been sutured to the proximal ends of the two prostheses preparatory to threading the grafts into the newly formed sheaths by pulling the prostheses distally.

the profundus tendon stump (see Fig. 55-3, *A, Stage II, B* and *C*). Traction is now applied to the proximal end of the graft and the predicted range of active flexion, measured as the distance of the finger pulp from the distal palmar crease, is determined. After this maneuver, the attachment of the graft to the distal phalanx is inspected, to check on the security of the fixation.

The condition of the tissues at the site of the proximal anastomosis is critical. Atraumatic technique should be used during the dissection. Scar tissue and thickened antebrachial fascia are excised to minimize motion-restricting adhesions. When the firm fascia is carefully dissected away from the newly formed tendon sheath, the sheath is found to be soft, with loose mesentery-like attachments to the surrounding tissues (see Figs. 55-1, *A* and *B*, 55-3-A, *Stage II, A*). If the sheath is thickened or scarred as the result of synovitis, it is resected far enough distally so that there will be no scar in the region of the tendon suture. If the anastomosis is small in diameter, the sheath may be placed around it. This is not always possible, however, because of the bulk of the graft-tendon junction. In this event the sheath is either dissected away completely so that there is no contact between the anastomosis and the sheath, or the sheath may be left open so that one side of the anastomosis glides on the sheath.

In most patients in the series reported here, the proximal anastomosis was in the forearm. For the index finger when either the superficialis or the profundus muscle was available as a motor, the graft was anastomosed to the proximal segment of the motor tendon according to the method of Pulvertaft (see Fig. 55-3, *B, E, F,* and *G*). For the long, ring, and little fingers, on the other hand, the graft was woven through oblique stab incisions in the common profundus tendon securing the different tendons together as one tendon unit (see Fig. 55-3, *B* and *H*). In a few instances in which the palm was not involved, a palmaris longus graft was used and the proximal end of the graft was sutured to the profundus tendon at the origin of the lumbrical muscle. If the proximal anastomosis is done in the palm, the superficialis or profundus of the injured finger or the superficialis of an adjacent finger may be used as the motor. If the forearm is the site of the anastomosis, the same three options are available.

It is essential to adjust the length of the graft accurately. The excursion of the prosthesis during flexion and extension has already been determined. The excursion of the tendon graft should now be checked by pulling on the graft, starting with the finger in full extension (see Fig. 55-3, *B* and *D*). Having determined the excursion necessary to produce a full range of flexion, the excursions of the available motors are then determined and the one is selected that has the requisite excursion. Obviously, if the motor lacks sufficient excursion, active motion will not be complete, even if the anastomosis is exact and the tendon graft glides perfectly.

The tension of the graft is adjusted so that, with the wrist in neutral, the involved finger rests in slightly more flexion than that of the adjacent fingers. When the anastomosis has been completed, the tension is checked with the wrist in both flexion and extension to assess the tenodesis effect and to make sure that the tension of the graft is correct. Currently, all uncomplicated stage II procedures are done under local anesthesia, supplemented with Innovar and releasing the tourniquet intermittently to assess active function. After the distal anastomosis is completed and the distal wound is closed, the graft is sutured tentatively to the motor tendon; and, after the tourniquet has been deflated for ten to fifteen minutes, the patient is asked to flex and extend the finger. If the predicted amount of active flexion is not achieved, the tension of the graft is readjusted or a motor with more excursion is selected. When the patient can accomplish the predicted amount of flexion or the best possible function has been achieved, the anastomosis is completed and the wound is closed and dressed.

This procedure eliminates the guess work in establishing optimum tension in the graft and the results to date have been very encouraging. Removal of the tendon graft from the leg under this type of anesthesia has not caused difficulty. The technique previously described is employed using local anesthesia in the skin and subcutaneous tissues combined with Innovar and a leg tourniquet. If a tendon stripper is used, the patients have some, but not excessive, discomfort as the tendon is being stripped. No patient has complained that the procedure was unduly uncomfortable.

When the proximal anastomosis is made (see Fig. 55-3, *B, E* through *H*), great care is taken to preserve the sheath and peritenon. First the peritenon is gently pushed proximally until the musculotendinous junction is exposed; then, after completion of the anastomosis, the peritenon is pulled distally and sutured to the proximal end of the newly formed sheath or to the surrounding tissues as far distally as possible. The wound is irrigated with sterile saline solution and then closed, and the final dressing is applied, with a plaster splint to maintain the wrist and MP joints in moderate flexion and the IP joints in slight flexion.

Early protected active flexion of the grafted finger is encouraged, while a padded dorsal splint prevents sudden forceful extension. Each patient is instructed at the first postoperative dressing, usually after 5 to 7 days, to splint the MP joints while the proximal and distal IP joints are actively flexed and extended. If necessary, intermittent splinting is continued during the fourth week while the pullout suture and button are still in place. In the fifth week the pullout wire is removed and light passive stretching exercises may be started if necessary. Some vigorous patients with full excursion of the graft may require intermittent splinting during the fourth week to protect the proximal anastomosis from excessive stress. If stubborn contractures were present prior to tendon grafting, a supervised program of passive stretching and splinting may be required after the fifth week. Patients should achieve a full range of active motion during the sixth to the twelfth week. Intensive training in active exercises personally supervised by the operating surgeon during this period are essential.

MATERIAL

Between December 1960 and July 1970, 86 old flexor-tendon injuries were treated by the two-stage technique and were followed from 6 months to 8 years. Five patients were lost to follow-up before 1962, and seven had their second-stage procedure done too recently for the result to be evaluated. The remaining 74 cases included 69 flexor-tendon reconstructions in the fingers and 5 in the thumb.

For purposes of evaluation, the patients' status at their initial examination was graded according to the following classification, modified from the one proposed by Boyes.[8,9]

Grade 1 (good): Good soft tissues, supple joints, and no significant scarring. (No grade 1 patients were included in this series, since in all of these conventional tendon grafts can be used.)

Grade 2 (scar): Deep cicatrix, resulting from injury or previous surgery, as well as mild soft-tissue contractures which, in a few instances, were severe enough to require preliminary plastic procedures.

Grade 3 (joint): Limitation of passive joint motion, usually in the proximal interphalangeal (PIP) joint, sufficient to require mobilization by traction and dynamic splinting. (In this series, all grade 3 patients had scarring of the tendon bed. Those with extensive scarring were classed grade 5.)

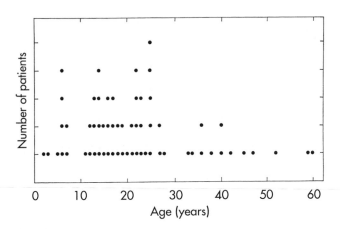

Fig. 55-13. Age distribution of the 63 patients with flexor tendon injuries of the fingers.

Grade 4 (nerve): Nerve damage with associated trophic changes in addition to scarring of the tendon bed and joint stiffness. (There were no grade 4 patients in this series; but, in future studies, patients with injuries to both digital nerves in one finger will be included.)

Grade 5 (multiple): Soft-tissue scarring or joint changes in more than one digit, or a combination of injuries in a single digit of such character that grades 2, 3, and 4 did not apply, and, in addition, involvement of the palm in many cases.

The result in each patient was correlated with the preoperative grade.

Thumbs

There were 5 patients, 3 male and 2 female, 14 to 27 years old, with thumb injuries—two in grade 2 and three in grade 5. Two injuries were the result of trauma alone; and three, the result of trauma and previous unsuccessful surgery. In all five thumbs, the scarring of the flexor-tendon bed and contractures contraindicated simple flexor-tendon grafting. Intensive physiotherapy and stretching splints were used preoperatively in each patient. The flexor-tendon mechanism was completely resected at the first stage and a large tendon prosthesis was inserted for 4 months or more.

At the second stage, in two thumbs, because the amplitude of the flexor pollicis longus (FPL) was poor, the superficialis tendon of the ring finger was transferred into the new sheath.

In the other three, a plantaris tendon graft was used, with the FPL serving as motor.

Fingers

There were 63 patients, 51 male and 12 female, with 69 finger injuries. Their ages ranged from 2 to 60 years (Fig. 55-13). All had old injuries, with one exception: a 26-year-old pharmacist who had severe lacerations of the volar surface of both index fingers. One finger was treated by primary repair and subsequent tenolysis. The other was treated by a two-stage procedure with a short prosthesis inserted initially and a subsequent tendon graft. The finger treated by the two-stage procedure had the better result (its tip flexing to within a distance of 1.3 cm from the distal palmar crease), despite the fact that it had the more severe injury.

Preoperatively the 69 fingers were graded as follows: 12 in grade 2, 13 in grade 3, and 44 in grade 5. Thirty-five of these fingers had had previous tendon surgery and were classified as follows: 4 in grade 2, 8 in grade 3, and 23 in grade 5. Thirty-four had not had previous surgery and were classified: 8 in grade 2, 5 in grade 3, and 21 in grade 5.

RESULTS
Thumbs

The results in the five thumbs were evaluated using the method described by Boyes, in which active flexion of the IP joint is expressed as the percentage of available passive motion in this joint. The results in all five thumbs in this series were in the ninetieth percentile.

Fingers

The results in the 69 fingers, according to pretreatment grade and final function (distance between finger pulp and distal palmar crease at maximum active flexion), are summarized in Table 55-1. As can be seen in this table, complete flexion was restored in 17 (25%) and the pulp-to-crease distance was 1.3 cm or less in 35 (57%), 2.5 cm or less in 45 (80%), and 3.2 cm or less in 49 (85%). Ten (15%) were rated as failures (pulp-to-crease distance more than 3.8 cm).

It is surprising that the grade 3 (joint) fingers had the highest incidence of success—4 of 13 regaining complete flexion. During the first-stage procedure in these fingers, the greatest correction of the joint contractures occurred when the scarred tendon, sheath, and peritendinous tissue spanning the volar aspect of the finger joints were resected. In some instances, at the PIP joint, it was necessary to release the proximal and lateral attachments of the volar plate on the proximal phalanx.

If this procedure resulted in some tendency for the joint to hyperextend, it was fixed in 10° of flexion by a small Kirschner wire across the joint. The wire was removed 3 weeks later, but hyperextension was prevented by splinting for 2 weeks more while flexion was permitted. In our experience, if some of the contracted tissue on the sides of the joint is preserved, recurvatum does not occur. Fixation of the joint with a Kirschner wire is, therefore, seldom necessary.

After the first-stage procedure, all IP joint contractures were reduced to 30° or less in each individual joint, or to a combined total of 40° or less for all of the joints of each finger.

Table 55-1. Results of finger flexor-tendon reconstruction according to preoperative grade distance of pulp from distal palmar crease at maximum active flexion

Preoperative Grades	Results (cm)							More or Failed	Totals
	0	0.6	1.3	1.9	2.5	3.2	3.8		
2 Scar	2	2	3	2	1	0	0	2	12
3 Joint	4	3	1	0	3	0	0	2	13
5 Multiple	11	3	6	6	8	4	0	6	44
Totals	17	8	10	8	12	4	0	10	69

Table 55-2. Results of finger flexor-tendon reconstruction in terms of the difference between the passive pulp-to-palmar crease distance before stage II and the active pulp-to-crease distance after stage II

Preoperative Grades	Results (cm)							More or Failed	Totals
	0	0.6	1.3	1.9	2.5	3.2	3.8		
2 Scar	5 (42%)	4	2	0	0	0	0	1	12
3 Joint	7 (54%)	2	1	0	2	0	1	1	13
5 Multiple	14 (30%)	8	11	1	4	0	0	6	44
Totals	26	14	14	1	6	0	1	8	69

Table 55-3. Results of finger flexor-tendon reconstruction according to preoperative grade in 35 patients who had previous tendon surgery: distance of pulp from distal palmar crease at maximum active flexion

Preoperative Grades	Results (cm)							More	Totals
	0	0.6	1.3	1.9	2.5	3.2	3.8		
2 Scar	1	1	1	1	0	0	0	0	4
3 Joint	3	1	1	0	0	0	0	3	8
5 Multiple	7	2	3	3	5	0	0	3	23
Totals	11	4	5	4	5	0	0	6	35

Of the 44 grade 5 fingers (the ones that traditionally have the worst results), 11 (25%) regained full flexion, while the pulp-to-crease distance was 1.3 cm or less in 20 (45%) and 2.5 cm or less in 34 (75%).

In order to evaluate the tendon function and eliminate the other factors influencing finger function, such as joint contractures, the results were also evaluated by subtracting the postoperative active pulp-to-crease distance from the passive pulp-to-crease distance as determined prior to the second-stage procedure (Table 55-2). By this method of evaluation, the percentages of fingers in which active flexion was equivalent to passive flexion were: 42% in the grade 2 fingers, 54% in the grade 3 fingers, and 30% in the grade 5 fingers.

The results in the 35 fingers in which previous tendon surgery had failed are given in Table 55-3. The results in such cases are notoriously poor because there is scarring, not only at the site of injury, but also at the site of proximal anastomosis in the palm. The results in this group of 35 fingers were virtually the same as in the overall group of 69 fingers.

Analysis of failures

The result was rated as a failure if the active pulp-to-crease distance was 3.8 cm or more, of if the difference between the passive and the active pulp-to-crease distance was more than 3.8 cm. There were 10 failures. In eight of them, the difference between the active and passive pulp-to-crease distance exceeded 3.8 cm.

As can be seen from Table 55-4, the failures occured in grade 2 and grade 5 fingers (five of each) and were caused by rupture of the prosthesis or tendon anastomosis in three

Table 55-4. Failures

Case	Age of Patient (yr)	Year of Surgery	Type of Prosthesis	Finger	Cause of Failure	Preoperative Grade	Final Result
1	48	1962	Active	Long	Previous infection; after stage I, anastomosis ruptured; prosthesis eroded through scar at proximal flexion crease	5+ Skin scars	Prosthesis removed; acceptable result after arthrodesis of proximal interphalangeal joint
2	32	1962	Active	Long	Previous infection; recurrent infection after stage I	5	Prosthesis removed; acceptable result after skin grafts and arthrodesis of proximal interphalangeal joint
3	28	1964	Active	Ring and little	Synovitis after stage I; soiled materials; tendon-graft adhesions after stage II in both digits	5	Acceptable functional result for heavy work despite contractures
4	38	1967	Passive	Long and ring	Poor circulation; poor tendon sheath; adhesions of tendon graft in long finger after stage II	5	Good range of passive motion; adjacent fingers used to flex digit
5	36	1968	Passive	Long	Rupture of proximal anastomosis due to forceful manipulation by surgeon after stage II	2	Acceptable result after distal interphalangeal arthrodesis and sublimis tendon transfer from adjacent finger
6	60	1968	Passive	Little	Stage I after infection; previous infection; prosthesis removed	2	Good range of passive motion; adjacent finger used to flex digit
7	14	1968	Passive	Ring and little	Poor circulation; synovitis stage I; dense adhesions of tendon graft in little finger after stage II; graft removed	5	Full range of passive motion; adjacent finger used to flex digit; two-stage procedure could be repeated
8	4	1969	Passive	Long	After stage I superficial infection in palmar incision, then spread along sheath of prosthesis	2	Stage I redone one year later followed by stage II; active pulp-to-crease distance 0.6 cm
9	15	1969	Passive	Long	Rupture of proximal anastomosis after stage II; poor patient control	2	Full range of passive motion; two-stage procedure could be redone
10	4	1970	Passive	Long	Synovitis after stage I; poor patient control	2	Prosthesis removed; full range of passive motion; two-stage procedure could be redone

cases, infection in three, synovitis in two, and diffuse adhesions in two, apparently the result of poor circulation in the digit.

COMPLICATIONS

The complications related to the stage I and stage II operations were analyzed separately. Those related to use of an active tendon prosthesis were reviewed in 1965[26] and will not be discussed here.

Stage I

Eleven patients had synovitis characterized by the following (singly or in combination): pain in the finger tip, swelling along the volar surface of the finger, and swelling and erythema at the site of the incision in the forearm. In most patients, there was swelling just proximal to the crease of the distal joint, sometimes associated with palpable fluid within the sheath. In some of the earlier cases, this complication was caused by soiling of the prosthesis (see Table 55-4, Case 3). After the technique was perfected, synovitis occurred either when there was excessive motion of the prosthesis too soon after stage I (see Table 55-4, Cases 1 and 10) or when there was mechanical obstruction to the gliding of the prosthesis during finger flexion, as seen on roentgenograms (see Fig. 55-10). As reported in 1965, rupture of one of the anastomoses of an active prosthesis was also a cause of synovitis.

Of the 11 cases of synovitis in this series, 5 were associated with buckling of the prosthesis caused by scarring and tightness of the pulleys in the tendon bed or an obstruction preventing proximal movement of the proximal end of the prosthesis during finger flexion, the result of a fascial block; 2 in children, 2 and 3 years old, associated with overuse; 2, with contaminants on the prosthesis resulting from the fabrication of homemade end loops for use in an active prosthesis; and 2 with rupture of an active prosthesis.

If the synovitis did not respond to 5 to 7 days of immobilization followed by the gradual resumption of activity, the stage II procedure was performed earlier and the thickened synovium was excised in the region of the proximal anastomosis. In four patients, immobilization controlled the synovitis without other modification in treatment. In six, stage II was performed sooner, and in one, the prosthesis had to be removed. In the case in which removal was required, the patient was a 4-year-old boy whose synovitis appeared to have been primarily the result of excessive use. Because control of this young child was inadequate, it was elected to remove the prosthesis and to defer redoing stage I until he was older. In the meantime he flexed the finger passively using an adjacent finger.

There were three wound infections, all in patients who had had previous surgery. Two of them had also had previous infections. All infections healed promptly after removal of

the prosthesis and irrigation of the sheath (see Table 55-4, Cases 2, 6, and 8).

Stage II

Six patients had adhesions that limited tendon function to a significant degree. In three, synovitis had developed after the stage I procedure. In the other three, the injury was grade 5 (multiple digits) and, prior to stage I, the circulation in the digit, in which adhesions developed, had been noted to be poor. Given these circumstances, special precautions are necessary to make the operation as atraumatic as possible and to supervise the postoperative program very closely, to gain maximum strength and excursion of the forearm muscles.

Restrictive adhesions may form around the proximal anastomosis particularly when there has been previous trauma to this area with subsequent scarring. The functional significance of adhesions about the proximal end of the tendon graft cannot be overemphasized. These adhesions, of course, are part of the normal healing reaction, but at times they may be the only adhesions preventing good function. Under these circumstances the adhesions can best be released under direct vision.

The procedure is usually performed three months after stage II using local anesthesia, Innovar analgesia, and a tourniquet. Since tourniquet ischemia rather consistently produces paralysis of the extrinsic muscles after 25 minutes and of the intrinsic muscles after 30 minutes, the tourniquet should be released at 25-minute intervals so that active function of the finger flexors can be tested. Thus during the first 25 minutes, active function can be tested with the tourniquet inflated. It then must be deflated and reinflated as need be to test function.

By this means it is possible to visualize the problem while the patient actively flexes and extends his or her fingers. The region of the proximal anastomosis should be explored first, with attention directed initially to the junction of the new tendon sheath and the tendon graft; next, to the proximal anastomosis; and, last, to the tendon graft within the new sheath. Only adhesions that actually restrict motion should be lysed.

Tenolysis was carried out in five patients in this series. Three of them were failures (see Table 55-4, Cases 3, 4, and 7). In the other two, there was significant improvement. After tenolysis, active flexion, measured as the pulp-to-palmar crease distance, was 1.3 cm less than passive flexion (the potential flexion possible in the digit). In both of these patients there were adhesions about the proximal anastomosis but there was free gliding of the graft within the sheath distally in the finger. The results were eventually rated *good* (pulp-to-palmar crease distance, 1.3 cm).

The three failures after tenolysis occurred in patients who had two-digit reconstructions (see Table 55-4, Cases 3, 4, and 7). The failures were in both digits in Case 3 and in one digit in Cases 4 and 7. In these fingers the adhesions extended along the full length of the graft. The circulation in these fingers had been poor initially, a circumstance that suggests that the sheath, formed about the prosthesis, may have had poor nutritional function and hence had failed to nourish the tendon graft adequately.

In Case 3 there also appeared to be some soiling of both prostheses (in the ring and little finger) related to homemade loops at their proximal ends. Acute synovitis developed after the stage I procedure, which could not be controlled by splinting. At stage II the large amount of scar formation found in relation to the proximal loops suggested some sort of foreign-body reaction in addition to uncontrolled syno- vitis. When the tenolysis was performed, a large amount of scar had reformed proximally and each graft was adherent throughout the sheath. These findings suggested that the grafts had become fixed proximally shortly after stage II with the result that no gliding had occurred.

In Cases 4 and 7, only one of the two grafts in each hand was a failure. In Case 4, the reconstructions in the long and ring fingers were performed 10 years after injury and the motor muscle for the long finger failed to function adequately, but the finger remained supple. The patient could flex it using the index finger and the adjacent ring finger in which good function had been restored by the graft.

In Case 7, grafts were placed in the ring and little fingers. An excellent result was achieved in the ring finger, but the proximal anastomosis of the graft in the little finger became adherent because of synovitis. The patient could flex the little finger passively with the ring finger. In both Cases 4 and 7, the patients did not want further treatment, but the two-stage procedure could have been repeated.

Two failures were due to separation of the proximal anastomosis (see Table 55-4, Cases 5 and 9). In Case 5, a short graft could not be repaired until 4 weeks after separation. At exploration the graft could not be resutured in a good bed; hence, an adjacent superficialis tendon was transferred into the old sheath in the palm and the DIP joint was arthrodesed with a satisfactory functional result. In Case 9, a boy 15 years old, the proximal anastomosis separated 10 days after removal of the cast while the patient was performing gymnastics against advice. His parents refused further surgery.

In a third patient not listed as a failure, separation of a technically poor proximal anastomosis occurred after the patient had gained gliding motion very early. At reanasto- mosis 8 weeks after stage II, the proximal 3.8 cm of the graft was visualized and no adhesions were seen (Fig. 55-14). This finding is believed to be consistent with our concept that when early free gliding of the tendon graft has occurred the portions of the graft away from the sites of anastomosis are nourished by fluid within the sheath and not by blood vessels entering through adhesions. The final result in this patient was rated *good.*

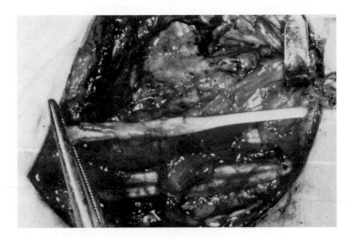

Fig. 55-14. Rupture of proximal anastomosis, 8 weeks after stage II, and 3 weeks after rupture occurred. Tension is being applied to the proximal end of the tendon graft, flexing the finger and pulling 3.8 cm of the graft out of the sheath. Adhesions were present at the site of the anastomosis but not within the sheath. This graft had functioned for 2 weeks prior to rupture, suggesting that if the grafts have begun to glide in the new sheath, they do not become adherent within the sheath.

The following case reports of successful reconstructions are cited to illustrate more graphically the results that can be obtained with this procedure in a variety of circum- stances.

CASE REPORTS

Case 11. M.D., a left-handed female cafeteria worker, had sustained a severe laceration of the left palm on a broken bottle. Primary skin closure was performed, followed 1 month later by tenorrhaphies in the palm. Six months later, the patient was referred for treatment of her persistent numbness and lack of flexion of the left long, ring, and little fingers.

Four neurorrhaphies were performed and the scarred superfi- cialis tendons of the long and ring fingers were excised. Five months later, after the patient had received intensive physical therapy and had acceptable sensation and active flexion of the long and ring fingers but not in the little finger, a stage I procedure was performed on the little finger. This included excision of dense scar that extended from the base of the finger proximally for the full extent of the tendon bed in the palm. The tissues in the finger were atrophic, an appearance consistent with what would be expected after absence of function for one year. A medium prosthesis was inserted from the distal phalanx to the forearm and the finger pulleys were preserved or reconstructed. The potential range of motion was then from full extension to full flexion and the finger was assigned grade 2, because the defect was primarily scarring of the bed.

The postoperative course was uneventful and, 5 months later, a stage II procedure was performed. A long toe-extensor tendon was used as the graft. In the forearm, the common tendon of the profundus muscle of the ring and little finger was used as the motor.

Two months later, the pulp of the little finger could be actively flexed to within 0.6 cm of the palmar crease, and 1 month later, flexion was complete.

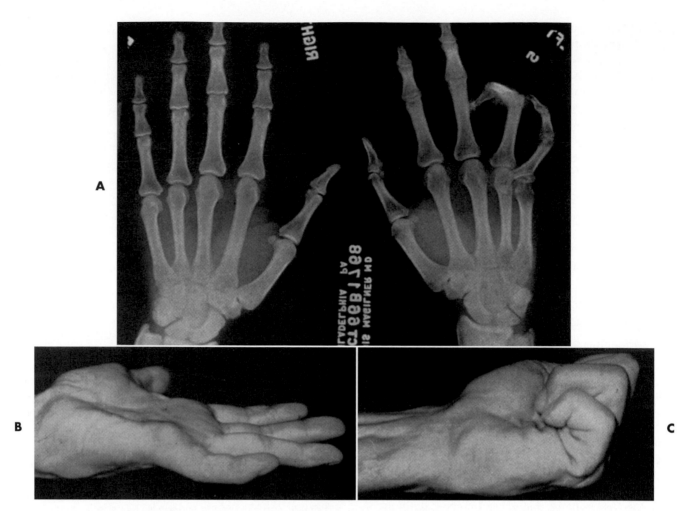

Fig. 55-15. Case 12. R.R., a 21-year-old man with residual deformity and contractures of the ring and little fingers caused by a conveyor-belt injury. **A,** Preoperative roentgenogram showing flexion contractures of both fingers and malunion of a fracture at the base of the proximal phalanx of the little finger that was classified grade 5. **B** and **C,** Extension and flexion 20 months after osteotomy of the proximal phalanx of the little finger and 16 months after stage I and 1 year after stage II procedures on the ring and little fingers. Two prostheses extending into the forearm were inserted at stage I and two long plantaris grafts were inserted at stage II with the profundus muscle of these two fingers as the motors.

The good result in this patient is believed to be significant because this finger was of the type in which a conventional graft is often attempted with a poor result. Typically the tissues are soft and the joints are mobile but there is extensive scarring in the palm (in this patient in the finger also at the site of the deep glass laceration).

The excellent result obtained in this little finger suggests that this procedure has a place in the treatment of borderline injuries that do not belong in the salvage category, yet often do not do well after conventional tendon grafts.

Case 12. R.R., a right-handed man, 21 years old, received a crushing injury in a conveyor belt, which caused fractures and flexor-tendon lacerations of the left ring and little fingers at the level

of the MP joints (Fig. 55-15, *A* through *C*). After initial treatment, he was left with a hyperextension deformity in the proximal phalanx of the little finger and no flexion of either the ring or little finger.

A corrective osteotomy was performed first, to eliminate the deformity of the little-finger proximal phalanx. Four months later, a stage I procedure was performed on both the ring and little fingers, resecting the scarred profundus tendons at the level of the lumbrical origin at the base of the palm and the superficialis tendon proximal to the transverse carpal ligament of the wrist, thereby leaving enough room in the carpal tunnel for the subsequent placement of two large prostheses. Contractures of both proximal and distal IP joints were released while the essential pulleys were preserved. Two large prostheses were then inserted, one in each finger, extending from the distal phalanx into the forearm. Both fingers were

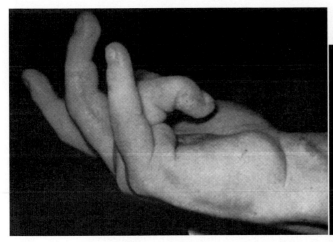
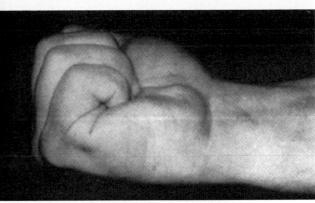

Fig. 55-16. Case 13. R.K., a 21-year-old man, who, 3 years before treatment, had sustained a crushing injury of the right ring finger. The preoperative findings were: a fixed 25° hyperextension deformity of the proximal interphalangeal (PIP) joint and partial loss of sensation in this finger. Treatment included (1) intensive preoperative physiotherapy; (2) a stage I procedure that included scar excision, reconstruction of pulleys, proximal displacement of the volar plate of the PIP joint to correct the hyperextension deformity, and insertion of a long prosthesis extending into the forearm; and (3) a stage II procedure performed at 2½ months because of synovitis caused by buckling of the prosthesis. The superficialis tendon of the adjacent long finger was transferred into the new sheath because the injury was 3 years old and an effective motor for a free graft was not available. It was also feared that the patient might not cooperate completely and that, therefore, a tendon transfer might give a better result. **A,** Independent flexion of the ring finger, 8 weeks after stage II. **B,** Flexion of all fingers 8 weeks after stage II.

rated grade 5 because both scar and joint problems were present. Both fingers were thought to have potential flexion sufficient to bring the pulp to the distal palmar crease. Postoperatively, stretching splints were used as well as physiotherapy. The patient returned to work at 8 weeks.

Four months after the stage I procedure, two long plantaris tendon grafts were inserted from the distal phalanx to the common tendon of the profundus of the ring and little finger at a point just distal to the musculotendinous junction. The profundus sheath in the forearm was folded around the anastomosis. The postoperative course was uneventful and the patient returned to work 3 months after operation. At 1 year, both fingers could be flexed so that their pulps came to within 1.3 cm of the distal palmar crease (see Fig. 55-15, *B* and *C*).

Case 13. R.K., a right-handed male electrician, 21 years old, 3 years before he was first evaluated had sustained a deep crushing laceration on the volar aspect of the right ring finger with severance of both flexor tendons and injury to the volar plate of the PIP joint. The initial pertinent findings were disuse atrophy of the finger, IP joint stiffness, and a 25° hyperextension deformity of the PIP joint.

An intensive program of physiotherapy prior to stage I restored flexibility so that, with passive flexion, the finger pulp came to within 0.6 cm of the distal palmar crease.

Stage I was performed using a Bruner zigzag volar incision. After the scarred tendon remnants had been removed, approximately two thirds of both the middle and the proximal phalanges were exposed as bare bone. Four pulleys were reconstructed from the scarred retinaculum. The hyperextension deformity was corrected by shifting the proximal attachment of the volar plate

proximally and suturing it in place. Grade 5 was assigned to the finger because of the scarring, joint damage, some loss of sensation, and the delayed reconstruction. A medium prosthesis was inserted, which extended from the distal phalanx to the level of the musculotendinous junction of the muscles of the forearm. Although not noticed at the time, the pulley proximal to the DIP joint was too tight and there was a tendency for the prosthesis to buckle distal to the PIP joint.

Despite close postoperative supervision, synovitis developed and the stage II procedure was done at 2½ months to prevent further fibrosis of the new sheath. At that time passive flexion would bring the pulp to within 1.3 cm of the distal palmar crease. Because the finger had not functioned for 3 years and there was some doubt as to the patient's motivation, it was decided to transfer the superficialis of the long finger to the new sheath rather than to use a graft. The palmar fascia and the thickened sheath in the palm proximal to the retinaculum were resected, but the sheath in the forearm, which was also thickened because of synovitis, was left undisturbed. The transferred tendon was threaded through the palmar retinaculum of the ring finger and through the new sheath to the distal phalanx after first irrigating the inflamed sheath with sterile saline.

Postoperatively, the potential flexion of the ring finger was achieved actively by the fifth week. By means of splinting, a flexion contracture of the DIP joint was partially corrected at the eighth week, at which time the finger pulp could be flexed to the distal palmar crease (Fig. 55-16, *A* and *B*). Because a graft was not used and there was no proximal anastomosis, earlier and more vigorous active motion was possible in this patient. Although the superficialis transfer worked well in this patient, our experience with this type of transfer has not been uniform, particularly when the superficialis

Fig. 55-17. Case 14. J.R., a 33-year-old man with a functionless right hand because of an old rattlesnake bite and steak knife lacerations of the left long, ring, and little fingers with resultant severance of both flexor tendons in the ring and little fingers and of the profundus tendon in the long finger. The little finger was not treated and the profundus tendon was advanced in the long finger. The ring finger was treated by the two-stage procedure using a long, plantaris tendon graft anastomosed to the superficialis of the long finger in the forearm. **A,** Eight months after stage II, independent flexion of the ring finger. **B,** Combined flexion at this time.

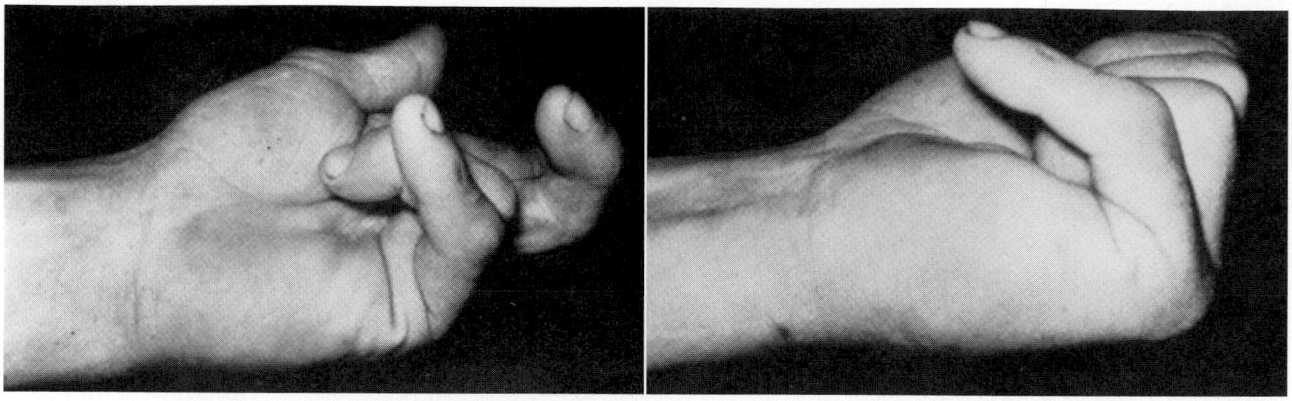

tendon was transferred in the forearm through the new sheath to the finger. The poor function under these circumstances may have been due to the discrepancy between the size of the newly formed sheath and that of the superficialis tendon.

Case 14. J.R., a 33-year-old bulldozer operator, had sustained steak knife lacerations of his long, ring, and little fingers of his left, dominant hand 1 month prior to evaluation. Primary treatment had been wound closure. Examination revealed that both flexor tendons had been divided in the long, ring, and little fingers. The right hand was almost functionless as the result of a rattlesnake bite eighteen years before.

Because this man's livelihood depended on this hand, it was elected simply to advance the profundus tendon of the long finger, to do a two-stage reconstruction of the ring finger, and not to treat the little finger initially. At stage I, on the ring finger, both tendons were found to be severed at the level of the PIP joint with dense cicatrix extending from the proximal one third of the proximal phalanx to the distal one third of the middle phalanx. The scarred tendons and their sheaths were resected as far proximal as the lumbrical origin, preserving and reconstructing pulleys as need be. A large (5 mm) prosthesis was then inserted from the forearm through the palm and finger to the distal phalanx. The proximal end of the prosthesis was placed deep to the superficialis tendons at the level of the musculotendinous junctions. The ring finger was rated grade 2. The superficialis tendon of the long finger was advanced at the time of the stage I procedure on the ring finger. Some scarring of the bed of this tendon was noted.

At the stage 2 procedure 4 months later, a plantaris tendon graft was inserted from the distal phalanx of the ring finger to the musculotendinous junction of the flexor digitorum superficialis (FDS) of the long finger. Eight months later, the patient could flex the ring finger pulp to within 1.3 cm of the crease independently, and all the way to the crease when all fingers were flexed simultaneously (Fig. 55-17, A and B). Function of the ring finger was considerably better than that of the long finger, and the patient

then wished to have the contractures of the long finger released and long and little finger treated by the two-stage procedure used in the ring finger.

DISCUSSION

The two-stage procedure for tendon reconstruction using a gliding silicone Dacron-reinforced prosthesis has important advantages. A new tendon bed and anatomic pulley system, with gliding surfaces, is established prior to the insertion of the graft. At the first stage, it is possible to do multiple procedures, such as digital neurorrhaphy, osteotomy, and capsulotomy,[15,16] in addition to resection of scar, construction of the pulley system, and insertion of the prosthesis, without fear of jeopardizing function. By careful preoperative planning it is therefore possible to reduce the number of operations necessary to reconstruct a severely damaged hand. It should be emphasized, however, that fingers that are stiff, as the result of severe injury or repeated unsuccessful operations, cannot be benefitted by this procedure. Restoration of a tendon sheath and a gliding tendon will not mobilize a stiff finger.

The indications for this procedure are not yet completely defined. It is, we believe, the procedure of choice for tendon grafting when the tendon gliding system of the fingers and hand has been damaged and is less than optimum. We believe, also, that all patients who are to have flexor-tendon grafting are potential candidates for this procedure, because only at operation can the extent of damage to the tendon bed be determined.

When there has been extensive damage to the palm, the two-stage procedure, with a long graft and the proximal anastomosis in the forearm, has great advantages and is the procedure of choice. When this is done, the proximal anastomosis may be placed beneath the profundus peritenon,

Table 55-5. Comparison of results in this series with those of Boyes in hands graded 2, 3, and 5*: preoperative grade versus distance of fingertip pulp from distal palmar crease

	Grades	0	1.3	2.5	3.8	Number of Cases
Hunter and Salisbury 1970	2 Scar	16†	57	85	85	12
	3 Joint	31	62	85	85	13
	5 Multiple	25	45	79	79	44
	Total Cases					69
Boyes 1955	2 Scar	8	24	49	82	79
	3 Joint	12	30	64	82	33
	5 Multiple	2	6	45	—	64
	Total Cases					176

*No grade I fingers included in this series.
†Figures are in percentages, which are cumulative.

within the superficialis peritenon, or within the newly formed sheath, thereby reducing the formation of restrictive adhesions.

Although we have received enthusiastic verbal reports from surgeons who have used silicone implants for the treatment of acute tendon injuries, we suggest that until a precise plan of treatment has been worked out and tested, and statistically valid results are known, that use of this procedure for acute injuries is not justifiable because more dissection is required and the risk of infection is increased.

However, the results in this study lead us to believe that primary tendon suture in no man's land should perhaps be reconsidered.[47] The experienced hand surgeon can now do this procedure with reasonable assurance that if it fails, the two-stage tendon graft described in this chapter can be done with the probability that an acceptable result can be obtained.

The evidence from our clinical experience suggests that the sheath that forms about the gliding tendon prosthesis after the stage I procedure can provide the nutritional requirements of a free tendon graft with minimum or no adhesions. When the gliding prosthesis is removed, the sheath that has formed around it apparently has both the physiologic and the anatomic characteristics necessary to nourish a tendon graft that has started gliding in the early postoperative period. The new sheath is a closed sac which will confine either the fluid associated with mechanical synovitis caused by buckling of the prosthesis or the pus accompanying an infection.

It is difficult to compare the results of tendon repair reported by different authors[33,34,46] because criteria for selection and methods of grading the preoperative status of the hands have varied. However, if these differences are kept in mind, a meaningful comparison of the results reported here with those of Boyes, White, and Pulvertaft seems possible.

The results in the thumb were reported as a percentage— the active flexion divided by the passive flexion. Boyes[8]

reported on 21 cases, 11 of which were in the good categories preoperatively. Ten percent of his patients achieved 90% motion. Most of them were treated with short grafts with the proximal suture line in the thenar eminence. The two best results in his series were obtained when the proximal anastomosis was placed at the musculotendinous junction in the forearm.

Pulvertaft reported on 42 cases in which there were all grades of involvement preoperatively. All of his patients were treated with tendon grafts and 30% of them achieved 90% motion in their thumbs.

In our five thumbs, all graded in the poor categories preoperatively and all treated by the two-stage method, 90% motion was achieved.

The fingers reported on by Boyes and by us were selected and graded preoperatively in essentially the same manner. The results in these two series are compared in Table 55-5, eliminating Boyes' cases, which were classified *good*. The incidence of fingers that postoperatively could flex sufficiently to bring the pulp to within 2.5 cm or less of the distal palmar crease is strikingly higher in our series. Although our series is considerably smaller, the comparison, nonetheless, strongly suggests that the procedure described here can produce results better than those attained by conventional methods in less than optimum cases.

White classified his cases as *good* and *less than good* preoperatively, and reported that of the 48 patients with less than good fingers, 35% could flex the pulp of the involved finger postoperatively to within 2.5 cm of the distal palmar crease. Of our 69 patients, all with a less than good rating preoperatively, 80% could flex their finger to within 2.5 cm or less of the distal palmar crease at follow-up. These results represent a considerable improvement over those reported by White.

Pulvertaft grouped all of his tendon grafts together and reported that 70% of his 90 patients achieved pulp-to-crease flexion of 2.5 cm or less. Again our results compare very favorably.

Finally, it is worth noting that, in their *good* cases, 2.5-cm pulp-to-crease flexion was achieved in 84% by Boyes (grade I) and in 79% by White. The percentages in these *good* cases are essentially the same as the percentages in our cases, all of which were less than good.

Although the results with the passive prosthesis have been distinctly encouraging, it would seem that a reliable active prosthesis would have advantages under certain circumstances. From our limited experience it would appear that an active tendon prosthesis results in better organization of the tissues in the region of the proximal anastomosis so that at the stage II procedure there is a good connective tissue mesentery that can be preserved when the graft is inserted. As a result, there is an earlier return of function after grafting. In addition, with an active prosthesis the muscle, which is to be the motor for the graft, continues to function, fewer adhesions form, and functional training after grafting is simplified.

In elderly patients or in patients in whom the condition of the local tissues would make it unlikely that a tendon graft could function, an active prosthesis may help to gain some useful function. In younger patients, the ones who have most of the flexor-tendon injuries, the aim of therapy is, of course, eventually to provide a permanent viable tendon by the insertion of a tendon graft. However, even in these patients a reliable active tendon prosthesis would have advantages. Thus a working person could return to work for a limited period with active function of the finger while the new sheath is forming.

In the development of an active prosthesis the major problem will be the proximal attachment of the prosthesis to the tendon or musculotendinous junction of the motor muscle. An active prosthesis will only be practical if a durable attachment at this level can be developed. Various types of anastomoses have been investigated. The best long-term results, for as long as 5 years, were achieved with free Mersalene sutures to bone distally and to tendon proximally; the best short-term results, for as long as ten months, were achieved with loop-to-loop anastomoses distally to tendon and proximally to tendon. Continuing research with metal fabrics and metal end devices suggests that these are the basic directions for our research in the development of active artificial tendons in the future.

The prosthesis, as it is now produced, should be used primarily as a passive gliding device with no proximal attachment. However, in carefully selected and closely supervised patients, the prosthesis may be made active by suturing its proximal end to the proximal tendon stump or musculotendinous junction of the motor muscles in the palm or forearms.

SUMMARY

Our experience with a dacron-reinforced silicone tendon prosthesis in the reconstruction of flexor tendons of the hand, first reported in 1965, is brought up to date. Currently the prosthesis is usually used as a passive gliding device which is attached only to the distal phalanx. This implant, inserted as the first stage of a two-stage procedure in conjunction with excision of scar and the reconstruction of a proper pulley system, has been demonstrated to stimulate the formation of a sheath, which provides a durable gliding surface and a nutritional mechanism for a tendon graft that begins to glide early.

The indications for this procedure, as well as the preoperative, operative, and postoperative management, are described. The results in 5 thumbs and 69 fingers, all with less than good conditions for tendon grafting (Boyes' grades 2, 3, and 5), after follow-ups ranging from 6 months to 8 years, are presented. The complications are also described. The results are compared with those in previously reported comparable cases.

The distinctly better results obtained in our series lead us to conclude that the two-stage procedure described is the one of choice for properly selected old injuries where the conditions are less than optimum for tendon grafting.

REFERENCES

1. Anzel SH, Lipscomb PR, Grindlay JH: Construction of artificial tendon sheaths in dogs, *Am J Surg* 1961; 101:355-356.
2. Arkin AM, Siffert RS: The use of wire in tenoplasty and tenorrhaphy, *Am J Surg* 1953; 85:795-797.
3. Ashley FL, Polak T, Stone RS, Marmor L: Healing of tendons in silicone rubber sheaths, *Bull Dow-Corning* 1962; 4:3.
4. Ashley FL, Stone RS, Alonso-Artieda M, et al: Experimental and clinical studies on the application of monomolecular cellulose filter tubes to create artificial tendon sheaths in digits, *Plast Reconstr Surg* 1959; 23:526-534.
5. Bassett CA, Campbell JB: Keeping silastic sterile, *Bull Dow-Corning* 1960; 2:1.
6. Biesalski K: Ueber Sehnenscheidenauswechslung, *Deutsche Med Wochnschr* 1910; 36:1615-1618.
7. Biesalski K, Mayer L: *Die physiologische Sehnenverpflanzung*, Berlin 1916, Springer.
8. Boyes JH: Flexor tendon grafts in the fingers and thumb: an evaluation of end results, *J Bone Joint Surg* 1950; 32A:489-499.
9. Boyes JH: Evaluation of results of digital flexor tendon grafts, *Am J Surg* 1955, 89:1116-1119.
10. Brand P: Principles of free tendon grafting, including a new method of tendon suture, *J Bone Joint Surg* 1959; 41B:208.
11. Bruner JM: The zigzag volar-digital incision for flexor-tendon surgery, *Plast Reconstr Surg* 1967; 40:571-574.
12. Bunnell S: *Bunnell's surgery of the hand*. Revised by Boyes JH, ed 4, Philadelphia, 1964, Lippincott.
13. Bunnell S, ed: *Hand surgery in World War II*, p. 49. Medical Department of the United States Army. Washington, Office of the Surgeon General, Department of the Army, 1955.
14. Carroll RE, Bassett AL: Formation of tendon sheath by silicone-rod implants, Proceedings—American Society for Surgery of the Hand, *J Bone Joint Surg* 1963; 45A:884-885.
15. Curtis RM: Joints of the hand. In Flynn JE: *Hand Surgery*, Baltimore, 1966, Williams & Wilkins.
16. Curtis RM: Capsulectomy of the interphalangeal joints of the fingers, *J Bone Joint Surg* 1954; 36A:1219-1232.
17. Cushman P: Personal communication.

18. Davis L, Aries LJ: An experimental study upon the prevention of adhesions about repaired nerves and tendons, *Surgery* 1937; 2:877-888.
19. Goenicdtian SA: A new method of canalization tendon sutures with vein grafts, *Arch Surg* 1949; 26:181.
20. Gonzalez RI: Experimental tendon repair within the flexor tunnels: use of polyethylene tubes for improvement of functional results in the dog, *Surgery* 1949; 26:181-198.
21. Gonzalez RI: Experimental use of teflon in tendon surgery, *Plast Reconstr Surg* 1958; 23:535-539.
22. Grau HR: The artificial tendon: an experimental study, *Plast Reconstr Surg* 1958; 22:562-566.
23. Hanisch CM, Kleiger B: Experimental production of tendon sheaths: a preliminary report on the implantation of a flexible plastic in the tissues of rabbits and guinea pigs, *Bull Hosp Joint Dis* 1948;9:22-31.
24. Henze CW, Mayer L: An experimental study of silk-tendon plastics with particular reference to the prevention of post-operative adhesions, *Surg Gynec Obstet* 1914; 19:10-24.
25. Hochstrasser AE, Broadbent TR, Woolf R: Sheath replacement in tendon repair: experimental study with Ivalon, *Rocky Mountain Med J* 1960; 57:30-33.
26. Hunter JM: Artificial tendons: early development and application, *Am J Surg* 1965; 109:325-338.
27. Hunter JM: Artificial tendons–their early development and application. In Proceedings of the American Society for Surgery of the Hand, *J Bone Joint Surg* 1965; 47A:631-632.
28. Hunter JM, Salem AW, Steindel CR, Salisbury RE: The use of gliding artificial tendon implants to form new tendon beds. In Proceedings of the American Society for Surgery of the Hand, *J Bone Joint Surg* 1969; 51A:790.
29. Hunter JM, Salisbury RE: Use of gliding artificial implants to produce tendon sheaths. Techniques and results in children, *Plast Reconstr Surg* 1970; 45:564-572.
30. Iwauchi S, Shoji N, Abe I: Experience with artificial tendon-grafting in the hand. In Proceedings of the Fourth Annual Meeting of the Japanese Society for Surgery of the Hand, *J Bone Joint Surg* 1961; 43A:152.
31. Koth DR, Sewell WH: Freeze-dried arteries used as tendon sheaths, *Surg Gynec Obstet* 1955; 101:615-620.
32. Lange Fritz: Ueber periostale Sehnenverpflanzungen bei Lähmungen, *Münchener Med Wochnschr* 1900; 47:486-490.
33. Littler JW: Free tendon grafts in secondary flexor tendon repair, *Am J Surg* 1947; 74:315-321.
34. Littler JW: Principles of reconstructive surgery of the hand. In *Reconstructive plastic surgery* by Converse JM, vol 4, pp. 1612-1674. Philadelphia, 1964, Saunders.
35. Mayer L: The physiological method of Tendon Transplantation, *Surg Gynec Obstet* 1916; 22:182-197.
36. Mayer L, Ransohoff N: Reconstruction of the digital tendon sheath. A contribution to the physiological method of repair of damaged finger tendons, *J Bone Joint Surg* 1936; 18:607-616.
37. Milgram JE: Transplantation of tendons through performed gliding channels, *Bull Hosp Joint Dis* 1960; 21:250-295.
38. Nichols HM: Discussion of tendon repair. With clinical and experimental data on the use of gelatin sponge, *Ann Surg* 1949; 129:223-234.
39. Parks A: The "lumbrical plus" finger, *J Bone Joint Surg* 1971; 53(B):236-239.
40. Potenza AD: Tendon healing within the flexor digital sheath in the dog. An experimental study, *J Bone Joint Surg* 1962; 44A:49-64.
41. Pulvertaft RG: Experiences in flexor tendon grafting in the hand, *J Bone Joint Surg* 1959; 41B:629-630.
42. Pulvertaft RG: Tendon grafts for flexor tendon injuries in the fingers and thumb. A study of technique and results, *J Bone Joint Surg* 1956; 38B:175-194.
43. Sakata Y: Experimental study on the combined use of arterial tissues with nylon thread in artificial tendon formation, *J Japan Orthop Assn* 1962; 36:1021.
44. Sarkin TL: The plastic replacement of severed flexor tendons of the fingers, *British J Surg* 1956; 44:232-240.
45. Thatcher H vH: Use of stainless steel rods to canalize flexor tendon sheaths, *Southern Med J* 1939; 32:13-18.
46. Tubiana R: Greffes des tendons fléchisseurs des doigts et du pouce. Technique et résultats, *Rev Chir Orthop* 1960; 46:191-214.
47. Verdan CE: Primary and secondary repair of flexor and extensor tendon injuries. In *Hand Surgery,* by Flynn JE, pp. 220-275. Baltimore, 1966, Williams & Wilkins.
48. Wheeldon T: The use of cellophane as a permanent tendon sheath, *J Bone Joint Surg* 1939; 21:393-396.
49. White WL: Secondary restoration of finger flexion by digital tendon grafts. An evaluation of seventy-six cases, *Am J Surg* 1956; 91:662-668.

Chapter 56

STAGED TENDON RECONSTRUCTION
History and current perspective

Lawrence H. Schneider

The placement of a silicone rubber tendon implant as a preparatory stage to induce the formation of a bed favorable for tendon grafting at a second stage, as described by Hunter in 1971, is now a well-established procedure in the treatment of the severely damaged flexor system.

This operation was designed for patients with flexor tendon injuries in whom reconstruction by the usual tendon grafting techniques had a low probability of success. The reasons for this are numerous and include the severity of the original trauma (i.e., crushing injuries associated with underlying fracture or overlying skin damage). The procedure is indicated in cases of excessive scarring of the tendon bed secondary to the patient's particular healing response or secondary to failed prior surgery as well as complications of healed infection. Other indications include significant loss of the retinacular pulley system caused by the original injury or prior surgery. Joints that are restricted by contractures not responsive to therapy measures are also poor prognostic factors in flexor tendon surgery, and they can serve as an indication for this procedure.

Patients with all or some of the problems described above, in whom conventional tendon grafting is not likely to offer a reasonable chance of success, are offered the staged tendon reconstruction procedure in an attempt to salvage finger function. Most of these candidates were found to have had failures of prior surgery, particularly where primary repair had failed.

HISTORICAL REVIEW

In 1965 Hunter[28] first published his personal experience with a tendon implant and in 1971, with Salisbury,[31] he presented more than 10 years' experience with this technique, in which severely damaged flexor tendons were excised and the system rebuilt around a silicone-Dacron reinforced implant. A Dacron woven tape was added within the rubber to give body to the implant, to enhance its gliding in the passive motion program, and to supply better hold for the distal sutures. The implant, attached only at its distal end, was left free at its proximal end in the distal part of the forearm. During wound healing, a passive exercise program was used to mobilize the finger before the second stage. In response to the implant, a smooth, well-organized pseudosheath was formed, ideally creating order in a previously chaotic tendon bed. The proximal end of the implant was placed in the distal forearm, because many of the patients had severe scarring that involved the palm in addition to zone II. This gave the surgeon the option to create the proximal juncture above the wrist, bypassing the scarred palm and using an area relatively favorable for tendon juncture.[29]

At the second stage (performed 3 months later) the implant was replaced with a long tendon graft, an operation carried out with as little disturbance as possible to the newly formed sheath. The second stage was, therefore, a tendon graft carried out in a manner greatly simplified by the tendon implant. This work was partially based on earlier studies of artificial tendons and silicone tendon implants by Bassett and Caroll.[6]

Many authors have subsequently written of their experiences in tendon salvage using the staged technique in which the silicone rubber implant is placed at the first stage.*

During the development period there was considerable interest concerning the response of the tissues to the silicone rubber implant. The exact nature and the physiologic activity of the pseudosheath formed in response to a flexible rubber implant was debated in the literature.[31,56] Before an inert, yet flexible material was available, there were many attempts to solve this problem. Rigid implants, such as bands of stainless steel, tantalum, and Vitallium, were placed in an effort to attain a smooth-gliding bed before tendon graft or transplantation.[50] Milgram described the formation of a smooth bursalike sac clinging to the implant contour with a liquid that was similar to synovial fluid on the implant surface. Microscopically, the sheath was lined by flat "mesothelial cells," surrounded by a fibrovascular supportive layer. This wall became thicker and more fibrous with time. A rigid implant would not allow passive motion during the important sheath-building stage and, therefore, could not create a favorable situation when used in the fingers. The availability of medical-grade silicone rubber improved the possibilities for this reconstructive approach.

The structure and function of the silicone-induced sheath has been studied in many laboratories.† Hunter's group, working in the 1960s, published studies on the sheath formed when silicone implants were placed in the paravertebral soft tissues of dogs[34] and found an orderly pattern of cellular organization on the surface of the implant. A parallel study was designed to evaluate the response to an actively gliding implant in the extensor system of the dog.[35] Evidence was obtained that the system could function as a physiologic sheath that would support a long tendon graft by fluid nutrition and with time by the formation of vascular, yet mobile, adhesions. Conway, Smith, and Elliott[15] and Urbaniak and colleagues[72] confirmed these observations. Urbaniak's experiments were carried out in the flexor system and actually demonstrated revascularization of the dog tendon by infratendinous vessels in the sheath.

Electron microscopic studies of the silicone-rubber-induced sheaths in chickens by Salisbury and colleagues[59] and Talasugi, Inoue, and Akahoti[71] showed that the pseudosheath closely resembled normal synovium in reference to architecture and biologic properties.

The final word on the exact nature of the sheath created in response to a low reactive flexible implant used in a passive gliding program, in humans, is not completely elucidated. Some of the varying observations may be a result of species differences and conditions of the experiments. The presence of a soft, pliable, translucent

sheath, seen with frequency in clinical cases and associated with an uncomplicated Stage 1, encourages surgeons in the clinical use of this technique to salvage severely damaged flexor systems.[33]

RECONSTRUCTION OF THE PULLEY SYSTEM

Probably the most useful application of the staged flexor tendon reconstruction technique is in cases in which there is need to reconstruct the flexor pulley system. Successful reconstruction of the flexor tendon system within the finger is not only dependent on the treatment of the tendon itself, but must also involve the important structural aspects of the supportive retinacular system. The pulley system plays an important role in controlling the effect of a given flexor tendon excursion on the motion at the joints in the finger.[17,27,46] In the ideal, uninjured situation the pulley system serves to prevent bowstringing of the tendon across the volar aspect of the joint in flexion. This provides for the most efficient use of the flexor tendon excursion, thereby allowing maximum range of motion of the digital joints. Bunnell[8] taught us that pulley loss results in the tendon taking the shortest distance between the next two adjacent pulleys (i.e., bowstringing). If significant, the bowstringing results in a decreased range of joint motion as well as a flexion deformity at the involved joint. Tendon adhesions and increased risk of rupture of the remaining pulleys, caused by stress, also become a possibility.

A reconstructed pulley, therefore, should be not only of optimal location but also of the proper diameter and strong enough to resist breakdown or attenuation. It must hold the tendon as close to the underlying bone as possible without restricting gliding. The relative importance of the individual pulleys has been studied by Doyle and Blythe,[16-18] Hunter and colleagues,[30] and others‡ who confirmed the work of Barton,[5] who stated in 1969 that at least two pulleys (A_2 and A_4) need to be retained or reconstructed, including one over the middle phalanx (A_4). I believe that two pulleys may not be enough; in general, a system of three or even four pulleys should be reconstructed for optimal efficiency. Practically speaking, because reconstruction may interfere with volar plate or collateral ligament function, pulleys should be reconstructed just distal to the metacarpophalangeal and proximal interphalangeal joints at the bases of the proximal and middle phalanges as a minimum requirement. In the clinical situation, it is often necessary to settle for less than optimal conditions when reconstructing the pulley system.

When considering the literature on flexor tendon grafting, it is interesting to find that some authors concerned themselves with the problems related to pulley disruption,[4,8,39,44,74] while others completely ignored this aspect of flexor tendon reconstruction.

In a staged reconstruction, even an injured pulley may be acceptable over the implant if the pulley is reparable by

*References 1-3, 11, 13, 14, 22-24, 26, 34, 38, 41, 42, 52, 57, 58, 61-64, 73, 75-77.
†References 10, 20, 21, 25, 31, 48, 51.

‡References 7, 19, 43, 44, 54, 60, 68, 70.

suture. Damaged pulleys, if strong, are also useful as they will not adhere to the implant as they would to a tendon graft. For this reason, all pulley material is saved at stage 1 if possible. If a pulley is constricted, an attempt is made to dilate the tissue available to accept the implant. If the original pulley material is unsalvageable or absent, reconstruction must be carried out.

Methods of pulley reconstruction

The tail of the superficialis can be used as a pulley if it is long enough.[66] It can be left attached at its insertion and the free end sutured over the implant to the contralateral side either to periosteum or the rim of the original pulley, or sutured via small drill holes to bone. This is done with nonabsorbable Dacron, which is used in all pulley reconstructions. This will make an excellent pulley in the A_3 area.

When doing staged tendon reconstruction, there is generally sufficient tendon material available to construct free tendon graft pulleys. Various techniques have been advocated for the fixation of this material. As pointed out by Kleinert and Bennett,[39] there is often a remnant of the destroyed pulley left to which one can suture this free graft material. They interwove the pulley material in the rim itself; if the rim is adequate, we use this technique. The material should be thin and the remnant strong enough to hold the pulley graft.

Another technique uses tendon graft encircling the phalanx[9,40,53,66] superficial to the extensor apparatus in the middle phalanx and deep to the extensor mechanism in the area of the proximal phalanx. It is desirable to support the flexor system with a long pulley at the important A_2 area; thus, if possible, the phalanx is encircled two or three times in the proximal phalangeal area, creating a pulley 10 mm long. This encircling technique is the preferred technique today when critical pulleys are needed at the A_2 level. Lister[45] has described good results with a technique in which a segment of the extensor retinaculum from the dorsum of the wrist is passed around the phalanx for pulley reconstruction. Another technique that uses the volar plate in reconstruction of the pulleys has been published.[37] Recent articles have suggested that this "belt-loop" technique is nearly as strong as a normal annular band,[44] but did not provide as normal joint motion as reconstruction of the A_2 and A_4 pulleys.[43]

The reconstructed pulley must be strong[49] and should be vigorously tested under direct visualization at the operating table. The forces generated against the pulley in flexion are considerable.

Artificial materials have been used in the reconstruction of pulleys. These materials include knitted Dacron arterial graft,[78] silicone rubber sheeting,[4] xenograft materials,[12] polytetraflouroethylene (PTFE),[36] and woven nylon and fascia lata.[19,55] The plentiful availability at operation of tendon remnants to be used as pulley grafts is such that I have not needed these materials.

COMPLICATIONS OF STAGED TENDON RECONSTRUCTION

Synovitis in the sheath forming in response to the implant was formerly recognized in about 15% to 20% of post-stage 1 patients.[62] It is noted now that this complication has been reduced to 8% in an evaluation of cases done in 1986.[76] This problem is characterized by increased heat, crepitus, and obvious swelling with fluid in the sheath and will be associated with a thickened, less pliable sheath at stage 2. This serious complication is often, but not necessarily always, followed by a less successful end result after stage 2. Cultures for bacteria in the fluid found within these sheaths have consistently shown no growth.[65] Foreign materials, such as talc, on the implant surface are reduced by minimizing handling of the implant and careful cleansing of the surgeon's gloves. Sterile packaging of the implant has reduced this potential source of problem, and breaking the actual implant out of the package as late as possible in the procedure has further shortened the implant's exposure time.

When synovitis is recognized, the patient's exercise program should be decreased, with return to resting splints except for limited periods of passive range of motion exercises. An earlier stage 2 may be advisable if the problem is not controllable.

Postoperative infection following stage 1 is a disastrous complication, as in any implant procedure. When confronted with infection in the sheath, I have tried antibiotic irrigations using small-bore catheters and, on at least one occasion, have salvaged the sheath. In general, however, established infection calls for removal of the implant, with a healing period of 3 to 6 months, and, if feasible, replacement with a new implant.

COMPLICATIONS AFTER STAGE 2

Breakdown at the proximal or distal juncture of the graft has been seen in staged tendon reconstruction as with any tendon graft.[65] Good surgical technique should make this a rare complication, and the application of a closely supervised postoperative hand therapy program is also advisable. When rupture of a graft juncture is recognized early, the procedure can often be salvaged by early reoperation. The patient usually can localize the juncture that has pulled free, and exploration may allow reattachment. This complication occurs more commonly at the distal juncture, and if the tendon cannot be advanced to the original insertion, the end of the graft can be inserted into the middle phalanx creating a superficialis finger.[67]

A proximal level juncture disruption is usually represented by a slippage of the graft interweave in the distal forearm. Exploration of the distal forearm wound will often allow reattachment and salvage.

Pulley breakdown is another failure point seen and is confirmed by reduction in regained range of motion, with bowstringing of the tendon graft. Blocking support of the flexor tendon using the patient's other hand, a wood block, or an external ring will help maintain tendon gliding while consideration for secondary pulley reconstruction is undertaken. Use of the encircling method for pulley reconstruction at A_2 has virtually eliminated this problem.

Late flexion deformity is seen mostly in poorer cases and may be related to a poor nutritional status in the finger or by a particular patient's collagen formation. This deformity is rarely seen in a patient with a good range of movement early after stage 2. This problem is aggravated by inadequate pulley structure and bowstringing. In addition to complete release of joints at stage 1 and the construction of stronger pulleys, a prolonged retentive splinting program (up to 1 year), along with gentle stretching in the postoperative period is advocated.

Most of the problems described previously are now rare after the performance of the staged flexor reconstruction. Unfortunately, the most common problem that remains after this procedure is the inability to restore full gliding function, that is, the ongoing formation of adhesions, which can occur and reduce gliding function of the tendon.

SUMMARY

This procedure is demanding and needs the postoperative attention of a skilled hand therapist. The contribution of the therapist to the success of staged tendon reconstruction in my patients cannot be overestimated.[47,69]

With the improvement in techniques for early direct repair of the injured flexor tendon, there is much less need for secondary tendon reconstruction at this time. However, when confronted with the need for this procedure, the surgeon should stick closely to the indications and treatment protocols. This still is the only operation that offers hope of salvage in severely injured flexor systems.

REFERENCES

1. Allieu Y, Asencio G, Bahri H, et al: Two-step reconstruction of the flexor tendons (Hunter's technique) in the treatment of fingers "en crochet," *Ann Chir Main* 1983; 2:341-344.
2. Amadio PC, Wood MB, Cooney WP, Bogard SD: Staged flexor tendon reconstruction in the fingers and hand, *J Hand Surg* 1988; 13A:5559-5562.
3. Bader KF, Curtin JW: A successful silicone tendon prosthesis, *Arch Surg* 1968; 97:406-411.
4. Bader KF, Sethi G, Curtin JW: Silicone pulleys and underlays in tendon surgery, *Plast Reconstr Surg* 1968; 41:157-164.
5. Barton NJ: Experimental study of optimal location of flexor tendon pulleys, *Plast Reconstr Surg* 1969; 43:125-129.
6. Bassett CAL, Carroll RE: Formation of tendon sheaths by silicone rod implants. In Proceedings of the American Society for Surgery of the Hand, *J Bone Joint Surg* 1963; 45A:884.
7. Brand PW, Cranor KC, Ellis JC: Tendon and pulleys at the metacarpophalangeal joint of a finger, *J Bone Joint Surg* 1975; 57A:779-784.
8. Bunnell S: Repair of tendons in the fingers and description of two new instruments, *Surg Gynecol Obstet* 1918; 26:103-110.
9. Bunnell S: *Surgery of the hand,* Philadelphia, 1944, Lippincott.
10. Chamay A, Gabbiani G: Digital contracture deformity after implantation of a silicone prosthesis: Light and electron microscopic study, *J Hand Surg* 1978; 3:266-270.
11. Chamay A, Verdan C, Simonetta C: The two-stage graft: a salvage operation for the flexor apparatus. In Verdan C, ed: *Tendon surgery of the hand,* Edinburgh, 1979, Churchill Livingstone.
12. Cheng JCY, Hsu SYC, Chong YW, Leung PC: Use of bioprosthetic tendon in digital pulley reconstruction–an experimental study, *J Hand Surg* 1986; 11B:225-230.
13. Chong JK, Cramer LM, Culf N: Combined two-stage tenoplasty with silicone rods for multiple flexor tendon injuries in "no man's land," *J Trauma* 1972; 12:104-121.
14. Chuinard RG, Dabezies EJ, Mathews RE: Two-stage superficialis reconstruction in severely damaged fingers, *J Hand Surg* 1980; 5:135-143.
15. Conway H, Smith JW, Elliott MP: Studies on the revascularization of tendons grafted by the silicone rod technique, *Plast Reconstr Surg* 1970; 46:582-587.
16. Doyle JR: Anatomy of the flexor tendon sheath and pulley system, *J Hand Surg* 1988; 13A:473-484.
17. Doyle JR, Blythe WF: The finger flexor tendon sheath and pulleys: anatomy and reconstruction. In *AAOS symposium on tendon surgery in the hand,* St Louis, 1975, Mosby.
18. Doyle JR, Blythe WF: Anatomy of the flexor tendon sheath and pulleys of the tendon sheath and pulleys of the thumb, *J Hand Surg* 1977; 2:149-151.
19. Dunlap J, McCarthy JA, Manske PR: Flexor tendon pulley reconstruction—a histological and ultrastructural study in non-human primates, *J Hand Surg* 1989; 14B:273-277.
20. Eskeland G, Eskeland T, Hovig T, Teigland J: The ultrastructure of normal digital flexor tendon sheath and of the tissue formed around silicone and polyethylene implants in man, *J Bone Joint Surg* 1977; 59B:206-212.
21. Farkas LG, McCain WG, Sweeney P, et al: An experimental study of the changes following silastic rod preparation of a new tendon sheath and subsequent tendon grafting, *J Bone Joint Surg* 1973; 55A:1149-1158.
22. Gaisford JC, Hanna DC, Richardson GS: Tendon grafting: a suggested technique, *Plast Reconstr Surg* 1966; 38:302-308.
23. Grau HR: The artificial tendon: an experimental study, *Plast Reconstr Surg* 1958; 22:562-566.
24. Helal B: The use of silicone rubber spacers in flexor tendon surgery, *Hand* 1973; 5:85-90.
25. Hernandez-Jauregui P, Esperanza GC, Gonzalex-Angulo A: Morphology of the connective tissue grown in response to implanted silicone rubber: a light and electron microscopic study, *Surgery* 1974; 75:631-637.
26. Honnor R, Meares A: A review of 100 flexor tendon reconstructions with prosthesis, *Hand* 1977; 9:226-231.
27. Hoving EW, Hillen B: Functional anatomy of the vagina fibrosa of the flexors of the fingers, *J Hand Surg* 1989; 14B:99-101.
28. Hunter JM: Artificial tendons: early development and application, *Am J Surg* 1965; 109:325-338.
29. Hunter JM: Staged flexor tendon reconstruction, *J Hand Surg* 1983; 8:789-793.
30. Hunter JM, Cook JF: The pulley system: rationale for reconstruction. In Strickland JW, Steichen JB, eds: *Difficult problems in hand surgery,* St Louis, 1982, Mosby.
31. Hunter JM, Salisbury RE: Flexor tendon reconstruction in severely damaged hands: a two-stage procedure using a silicone dacron reinforced gliding prosthesis prior to tendon grafting, *J Bone Joint Surg* 1971; 53A:829-858.
32. Hunter JM, Jaeger SH, Matsui T, Miyaji N: The pseudosynovial sheath—its characteristics in a primate model, *J Hand Surg* 1983; 8:461-470.

33. Hunter JM, Singer DI, Jaeger SH, Mackin EJ: Active tendon implants in flexor tendon reconstruction, *J Hand Surg* 1988; 13:849-59.

34. Hunter JM, Steindel C, Salisbury R, Hughes D: Study of early sheath development using static nongliding implants, *J Biomed Mater Res* 1974; 5:155.

35. Hunter JM, Subin D, Minkow F, Konikoff J: Sheath formation in response to limited active gliding implants (animals), *J Biomed Mater Res* 1974; 5:155.

36. Kain CC, Manske PR, Reinsel TE, et al: Reconstruction of the digital pulley in the monkey using biologic and nonbiologic materials, *J Orthop Res* 1988; 6:871-877.

37. Karev A: The "belt loop" technique for the reconstruction of pulleys in the first stage of flexor tendon grafting, *J Hand Surg* 1984; 9A:923-924.

38. Kessler FB: Use of a pedicled tendon transfer with a silicone rod in complicated secondary flexor tendon repairs, *Plast Reconstr Surg* 1972; 49:439-443.

39. Kleinert HE, Bennett JB: Digital pulley reconstruction employing the always present rim of the previous pulley, *J Hand Surg* 1978; 3:297-298.

40. Kleinert H, Schepel S, Gill T: Flexor tendon injuries, *Surg Clin North Am* 1981; 61:267-286.

41. La Salle WB, Strickland JW: An evaluation of the two-stage flexor tendon reconstruction technique, *J Hand Surg* 1983; 8:263-267.

42. Leonard AG, Dickie WR: Observations on the use of silicone rubber spacers in tendon graft surgery, *Hand* 1976; 8:66-68.

43. Lin G-T, Amadio PC, An K-N, et al: Biomechanical analysis of finger flexor pulley reconstructions, *J Hand Surg* 1989; 14B:278-282.

44. Lin G-T, Cooney WP, Amadio PC, An K-N: Mechanical properties of human pulleys, *J Hand Surg* 1990; 15B:429-434.

45. Lister GD: Reconstruction of pulleys employing extensor retinaculum, *J Hand Surg* 1979; 4:461-464.

46. Littler JW: The digital flexor-extensor system. In Converse JM, ed: *Reconstructive plastic surgery,* ed 2, Philadelphia, 1977, Saunders.

47. Mackin EJ: Therapist's management of staged flexor tendon reconstruction. In Hunter JM, Schneider LH, Mackin EJ, Callahan A, eds: *Rehabilitation of the hand,* St Louis, 1984, Mosby.

48. Mahoney J, Farkas LG, Lindsay WK: Silastic rod pseudosheaths and tendon graft healing, *Plast Reconstr Surg* 1980; 66:746-750.

49. Manske PR, Lesker PA: Strength of human pulleys, *Hand* 1977; 9:147-152.

50. Milgram JE: Transplantation of tendons through performed gliding channels, *Bull Hosp Joint Dis* 1960; 21:250-295.

51. Neuman Z, Ben-Hur N, Tritsch IE: Induction of tendon sheath formation by the implantation of silicone tubes in rabbits, *J Plast Surg* 1966; 19B:313-316.

52. Nicolle FV: A silastic tendon prosthesis as an adjunct to flexor tendon grafting: an experimental and clinical evaluation, *Br J Plast Surg* 1969; 22:224-236.

53. Okutsu I, Ninimiya S, Hiraki S, et al: Three-loop technique for A₂ pulley reconstruction, *J Hand Surg* 1987; 12A:790-794.

54. Peterson WW, Manske PR, Bollinger BA, et al: Effect of pulley excision on flexor tendon biomechanics, *J Orthop Res* 1986; 4:96-101.

55. Peterson WW, Manske PR, Lasker PA, Kain CC, Schaefer RK: Development of a synthetic replacement for the flexor tendon pulleys—an experimental study, *J Hand Surg* 1986; 11A:403-409.

56. Rayner CRW: The origin and nature of pseudosynovium appearing around silastic rods, an experimental study, *Hand* 1976; 8:101-109.

57. Rowland SA: Palmar fingertip use of silicone rubber followed by free tendon graft. In *AAOS symposium on tendon surgery in the hand,* St Louis, 1975, Mosby.

58. Sakellarides HT: Severe injuries of the flexor tendons in no man's land and with excess scarring and flexion contracture, *Orthop Rev* 1977; 6:51.

59. Salisbury RE, Levine NS, McKeel DW, Pruitt BA, Wade CWR: Tendon sheath reconstruction with artificial implants: a study of ultrastructure. In *AAOS symposium on flexor tendon surgery in the hand,* St Louis, 1975, Mosby.

60. Savage R: The mechanical effect of partial resection of the digital fibrous flexor sheath, *J Hand Surg* 1990; 15B:435-442.

61. Schmitz PW, Stromberg WB: Two-stage flexor tendon reconstruction in the hand, *Clin Orthop Rel Res* 1978; 131:185-190.

62. Schneider LH: Staged flexor tendon reconstruction using the method of Hunter, *Clin Orthop Rel Res* 1983; 171:164-171.

63. Schneider LH: *Flexor tendon injuries,* Boston, 1985, Little, Brown.

64. Schneider LH: Staged tendon reconstruction, *Hand Clin North Am* 1985; 1:109-120.

65. Schneider LH: Complications in tendon injury and surgery, *Hand Clin North Am* 1986; 2:361-371.

66. Schneider LH, Hunter JM: Flexor tendons—late reconstruction. In Green DP, ed: *Operative hand surgery,* New York, 1982, Churchill Livingstone.

67. Schneider LH, Hunter JM, Fietti VG: The flexor superficialis finger: a salvage procedure. In Hunter JM, Schneider LH, Mackin EJ, eds: *Flexor tendon surgery in the hand,* St Louis, 1986, Mosby.

68. Solonen KA, Hoyer P: Positioning of the pulley mechanism when reconstructing deep flexor tendons of the fingers, *Acta Orthop Scand* 1967; 38:321-328.

69. Stanley BG: Flexor tendon injuries: late solution, therapist's management, *Hand Clin North Am* 1986; 2:139-147.

70. Strauch B, de Moura W: Digital flexor tendon sheath: an anatomic study, *J Hand Surg* 1985; 10A:785-789.

71. Takasugi H, Inoue H, Akahori O: Scanning electron microscopy of repaired tendon and pseudosheath, *Hand* 1976; 8:228-234.

72. Urbaniak JR, Bright DS, Gill LN, Goldner JL: Vascularization and the gliding mechanism of free flexor tendon grafts inserted by the silicone rod method, *J Bone Joint Surg* 1984; 56A:473-482.

73. Van Der Meulen JC: Silastic spacers in tendon grafting, *J Plast Surg* 1971; 24B:166-173.

74. Watson AB: Some remarks on the repair of flexor tendons in the hand, with particular reference to the technique of free grafting, *J Surg* 1955; 43B:35-42.

75. Weeks PM, Wray RC: Rate and extent of functional recovery after flexor tendon grafting with and without silicone rod preparation, *J Hand Surg* 1976; 1:174-180.

76. Wehbé MA, Hunter JM, Schneider LH, Goodwyn BL: Two-stage of flexor-tendon reconstruction, *J Bone Joint Surg* 1986; 68A:752-763.

77. Weinstein SL, Sprague BL, Flatt AE: Evaluation of the two-staged flexor tendon reconstruction in severely damaged digits, *J Bone Joint Surg* 1976; 58A:786-791.

78. Wray CR, Weeks PM: Reconstruction of digital pulleys, *Plast Reconstr Surg* 1974; 53:534-536.

Chapter 57

RECONSTRUCTION OF FLEXOR TENDON FUNCTION AND STRENGTH

The Hunter active tendon sublimis finger method

James M. Hunter
Evelyn J. Mackin
Patricia M. Byron
Scott H. Jaeger

The use of a Hunter-designed Dacron-reinforced silastic molded tendon implant* to convert an unfavorable tendon bed into one that is much less inclined to adhesions after tendon grafting has proved to be a consistently reliable method of salvaging scarred tendon systems.[8-13,15,17,18] The scarred bed and adhered tendon is resected at stage I and replaced with a gliding tendon implant that will restore a new tendon bed. Pulley systems are reconstructed as uninjured pulley retinaculam are preserved. Capsular joint contractures are released. Stage II involves surgical removal of the tendon implant and insertion of a tendon graft at a later time when normal gliding biomechanics and a fluid nutrition system have been established. The system, using passive or active tendons, can function for indefinite periods. The new biologic sheath that forms around the tendon surface during the period of gliding that follows stage I surgery becomes biologically stable and develops a synovial fluid system by 6 weeks that supports gliding indefinitely. The synovial fluid nutrition system developed during stage I aids the hand therapy recovery by maximizing postoperative digital motion by a biologic softening of the ligamentous connective tissue of the fingers.

Flexor tendon surgery, in general, has the objective for restoring active motion in both the proximal interphalangeal (PIP) and distal interphalangeal (DIP) joints. However, despite advancement in surgical and therapy techniques, the failure rate or poor results following primary flexor tendon repair are in the 30% range.[28] Patients who have sustained flexor tendon injuries often require cost-ineffective multiple salvage procedures because of failed primary repair and failed tenolysis. Therefore restoring the ideal one-tendon, three-joint system may require a realistic change in plan for the maximum benefit of the patient with manual work requirements. In these patients, basic function and strength take precedence and the more reliable metacarpophalangeal (MP) joint, PIP joint "sublimis (superficialis) finger" is recommended.

---

*Phoenix Biomedical, Valley Forge, PA.

Note: Only Hunter tendon implants are reinforced by textile engineered high tenacity polyester tapes or cords to produce stability during passive and active gliding and hence reliability. Other silicone rods may buckle and migrate in soft tissue or frequently show distal loosening causing sheath synovitis.

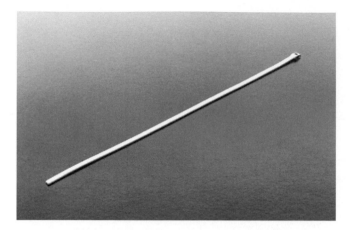

Fig. 57-1. MARK I active tendon implant (Phoenix Biomedical).

The clinical experiences of Burkhalter[4] and Hunter working separately showed that a sublimis finger active tendon method fulfilled the reconstructive need for the working hand. Applying the MARK I (Fig. 57-1) active tendon implant method could return these patients with flexor tendon injury back to early work by producing early MP and PIP function. The distal metal plate of the tendon implant is attached to the middle phalanx. Arthrodesis in a functional position or tenodesis is performed on the distal joint and A_1 and A_2 pulleys are reconstructed as needed. The proximal loop of the tendon implant is attached to the sublimis muscle tendon in the forearm to produce an efficient one-tendon, two-joint flexor system.[14-21]

HISTORY OF SUBLIMIS FINGER

The concept of the sublimis finger was initially described by Osborne from Liverpool, England, as the "redemption operation."[24,25] The operation was performed on patients who had a failing flexor tendon retinaculum that resulted in a bowed flexor tendon graft. The patients had useful finger flexion, but the extension loss of usually 40° to 60° at the PIP and DIP joints was not accceptable. The surgery included a tenotomy and recession of the tendon graft at the distal phalanx, and then reinsertion of the shortened tendon to the proximal one third of the middle phalanx. Some years later, Pulvertaft[25] introduced the senior author to the procedure as a means of salvage for the digit affected by adhesions and a bowed tendon graft. The loss of distal joint function becomes a good compromise if the MP joint and especially the PIP joint can be expected to produce a good arc of flexion. Although the sublimis finger procedure was initially described by Osborne as a salvage procedure, the senior author has used the MARK II and MARK III active tendons in sublimus finger reconstruction successfully for the past decade.[12,14,21]

Littler[22,23] demonstrated that 85% of the arc of motion can be achieved with full MP and PIP flexion (Fig. 57-2).

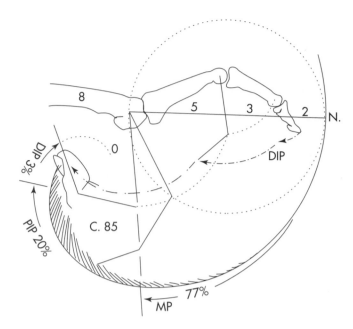

Fig. 57-2. *Grasp or encompassment.* This composite figure drawn by Dr. J. William Littler shows the following: *(A)* A finger skeleton in the intrinsic minus posture (i.e., intrinsic muscle paralysis). The metacarpophalangeal (MP) joint is hyperextended and the interphalangeal (IP) joints rest in varying degrees of flexion. *(B)* The phalangeal skeletal lengths which correspond to the Fibonacci ratio of $1/1.618$. *(C)* A dotted circle that represents the axis of proximal interphalangeal (PIP) rotation as the center of the digit. *(D)* The shaded flexion/extension spiral arc of the fingertip in a normal finger; its normal equiangular pathway is illustrated by the linked, straight black lines. The relative areas provided by individual joint flexion are: MP = 77% flexion by intrinsic muscles or "intrinsic" flexion; PIP = 20% flexion by extrinsic flexors; and DIP = 3% "extrinsic" flexion. The 77% of the total encompassment provided by MP flexion is the placement arc. The 23% of total encompassment area provided by IP flexion is the vitally important final encompassment. The PIP joint contributes 85% of this final encompassment. *(E)* The clawed hand pathway, which is illustrated by the dots and dashes (.–.—), is provided only by such MP flexion that is possible. *(F)* The O beneath the metacarpal head is the polar axis of the normal flexion/extension spiral pathway. (*MP,* metacarpophalangeal; *PIP,* proximal interphalangeal; *DIP,* distal interphalangeal.) (From Littler JW, Thompson JS: Surgical and functional anatomy. In Bowers WH, ed: *The interphalangeal joints,* New York, 1987, Churchill Livingstone.)

Adjustable grasp is based on the MP flexion curve executing the equiangular spiral. When an object is grasped, 77% of the total encompassment is provided by MP joint flexion; the remaining 23% is supplied by flexion of the interphalangeal (IP) joints. In this vitally important encompassment the PIP joint provides 85% of the closing motion. Curtis[5] named the joint the epicenter of hand surgery. The axis of the PIP joint lies exactly at the mathematical center of the four-bone chain of a finger; it is the anatomic and functional locus of finger function.[5,6]

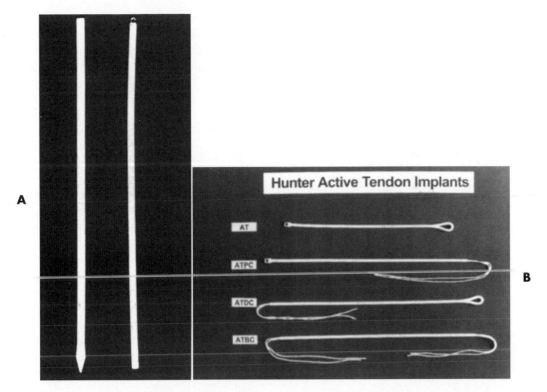

Fig. 57-3. A, MARK I passive, gliding tendon implants reinforced by textile inguinal Dacron •• with high–pressure-molded silicone covers.* **B,** Active gliding tendon implants. *AT,* MARK II fixed-length implants with plate distally and loop proximally. *ATPC,* MARK III adjustable-length implant with plate distally and porous cords proximally. *ATDC,* adjustable-length implant with porous cords distally and loop proximally. *ATBC,* adjustable-length implant with porous cords both distally and proximally. (From Hunter JM, Taras JS, Mackin EJ, et al: Staged flexor tendon reconstruction using passive and active tendon implants. In Hunter JM, Mackin EJ, Callahan AD, eds: *Rehabilitation of the hand: surgery and therapy,* ed 4, St Louis, 1995, Mosby.)

INDICATIONS FOR THE SUBLIMIS FINGER USING THE ACTIVE AND PASSIVE TENDON METHODS

The need for basic strength and basic function is addressed in the following section. Indications for the sublimis finger active tendon procedure are as follows:
1. Extensor lag of the DIP joint caused by extensor tendon rupture or attenuation
2. Joint contracture or DIP arthritis
3. A_4 pulley failure with bowing of a flexor tendon graft
4. Two or more annular pulleys requiring reconstruction
5. DIP joint volar skin failure (i.e., slough, scarring)
6. Multiple digit injuries
7. Multiple prior failed procedures on the flexor tendon system
8. Digit is graded 4 to 5 on the Boyes scale

Indications for a sublimis finger passive tendon implant over the sublimis active tendon follow. (Some of the patients may qualify for the active tendon with the exposed porous cord.)
1. Places where metal plate and screw are too bulky
   a. Children

b. Fifth finger reconstruction because of digit size
   c. PIP implant arthroplasty as the cord is compatible with the stem of the Swanson implant
2. Multiple reconstructions in the hand (i.e., replantation)
3. Poor patient compliance

IMPLANT DESIGN: DESIGNED FOR THE YEAR 2000

The experimental and clinical experience that has accumulated over the past 35 years is reflected in two basic types of Hunter tendon implants: passive and active (Fig. 57-3). The active tendon or tendon prosthesis was the design concept from the beginning of artificial tendon research.[8,9] Many clinical and laboratory hours later, there evolved a basic tendon graft replacement for our time—1990 to 2000—the sublimis finger active tendon replacement. It is versatile, strong, and capable of restoring basic flexor sublimis tendon function.

The Hunter Dacron-reinforced passive tendon implant can be used in salvage surgery to prepare for stage II tendon grafting. The Hunter active tendon implant, designed and engineered to replace the human tendon, is a temporary

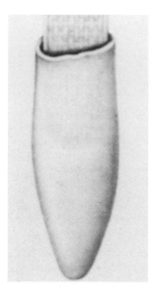

Fig. 57-4. MARK I implant. Silicone rubber has been cut away to show Dacron woven tape added to give body to implant. (From Hunter JM, Singer DI, Mackin EJ: Staged flexor tendon reconstruction using passive and active tendon implants. In Hunter JM, Schneider, LH, Mackin EJ, Callahan AD, eds: *Rehabilitation of the hand: surgery and therapy,* ed 3, St Louis, 1990, Mosby.)

tendon implant that can produce tendon function for extended periods (years) before replacement with a second implant or a tendon graft.

All Hunter tendon implants have special cores of woven Dacron that is pressure-molded into a radiopaque silicone rubber (Fig. 57-4). Passive implants are sometimes called rods (i.e., passive rods, Hunter rods); all rods used by Hunter or Hunter and Schneider are reinforced by a high-tech Dacron tape to produce stability for gliding and a secure method of attachment to tendon or bone. The surface has a smooth finish, and the cross-sectional design is ovoid to optimize development of the pseudosheath.

Passive flexor tendon implants

The accepted implant design for difficult cases of flexor tendon reconstruction is the Hunter passive tendon implant with or without a screw-fixation terminal device. This reinforced Hunter passive tendon implant is designed to be firm and flexible, with the distal end securely fixed, and covered by the flexor digitorum sublimis (FDS) tendon stump. This secure distal fixation reinforced by a secure A_2 and A_1 pulley system offers the surgeon assurance of push-pull, flexion and extension, and gliding of the tendon in the finger, palm, and forearm. Soft unreinforced silicone rods (Swanson-Hunter type) do not have these characteristics and therefore the Swanson-Hunter implant is no longer recommended in flexor tendon reconstruction. The Dacron-reinforced passive tendon implant without a metal plate is held in place by securing it under the sublimis tendon stump with a 4-0 monofilament wire or a 3-0 ethibond suture woven through its distal end: care is taken

to place the suture through the central Dacron core. This distal juncture is also reinforced with lateral sutures of ethibond 3-0. The implant is available in the following sizes: 3 mm × 23 cm, 4 mm × 23 cm, 5 mm × 25 cm, and 6 mm × 25 cm. These implants can be shortened by sharp cut at the proximal end.

The passive tendon implant is used in young patients when flexion or extension of the distal joint has been compromised. The 3-mm size can be used in children who have an open epiphyseal plate. A new active tendon designed for children will be available in a smaller implant using two 1-mm porous cords for bone and tendon attachment. The distal end is sutured either to the stump of the sublimis tendon or to the bone. Again, in the passive tendon implant, the ethibond sutures (4-0 for children) must be placed through the Dacron core of the tendon.

A second type of passive tendon implant differs from the first in its distal juncture. Its distal end has a stainless steel plate that attaches to the middle phalanx by a screw. This attachment provides secure fixation to bone and eliminates any possibility of proximal migration of the implant and sheath synovitis. The A_0 mini-fragment using the 2-mm screw is recommended. The thread cutter, however, is not used with the plate fixation system. After a two-cortex 1.5-mm hole is drilled, the 2-mm screw must self-tap to thumb pressure. Select the ideal screw length to penetrate both cortices of the middle phalanx. When secure, test the excursion of the tendon by pulling the proximal end of the tendon. Florascan for security of location and position of the plate and screw is helpful but not necessary. The screw should be long enough to engage the dorsal cortex of the phalanx but not pass more than 2 mm beyond it, because this may result in pain dorsally. The screw plate fixation in sublimis finger reconstruction is easy and efficient. The Hunter passive tendon implant is available in diameters of 3, 4, 5, or 6 mm and lengths of either 23 or 25 cm. The plate and screw technique is not recommended for children because of the large size.

Active tendon implants—stage I

Stage II tendon grafting using a passive tendon implant was traditionally performed 3 to 4 months after stage I. Attached distally to bone of the middle phalanx and proximally to the motor tendon in the forearm at stage I, the Hunter active tendon creates an interface between the implant and tendon in the forearm so that the proximal juncture matures while the new sheath is forming. By the time stage II surgery is to be performed, which could be 4 months or years after stage I, the finger is in much better condition and the patient's morale and motivation have substantially improved.

The active tendon implant may have its greatest value in workers who are permitted to return to their occupations for extended periods of time during stage I while a new sheath and muscle tendon juncture is forming throughout the

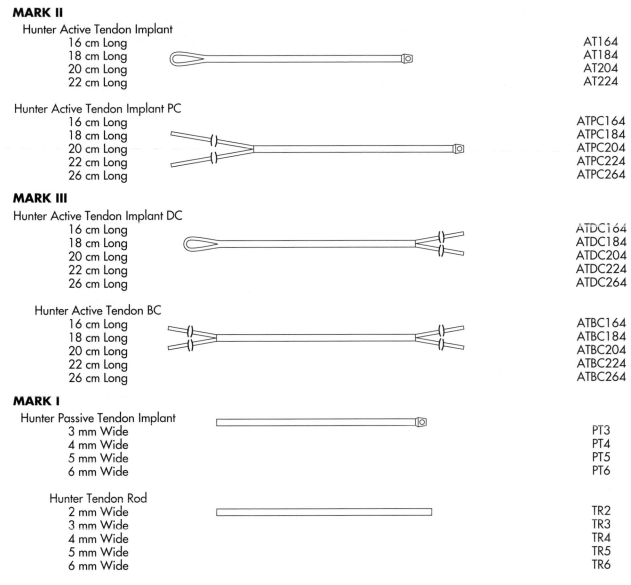

MARK II

Hunter Active Tendon Implant
- 16 cm Long AT164
- 18 cm Long AT184
- 20 cm Long AT204
- 22 cm Long AT224

Hunter Active Tendon Implant PC
- 16 cm Long ATPC164
- 18 cm Long ATPC184
- 20 cm Long ATPC204
- 22 cm Long ATPC224
- 26 cm Long ATPC264

MARK III

Hunter Active Tendon Implant DC
- 16 cm Long ATDC164
- 18 cm Long ATDC184
- 20 cm Long ATDC204
- 22 cm Long ATDC224
- 26 cm Long ATDC264

Hunter Active Tendon BC
- 16 cm Long ATBC164
- 18 cm Long ATBC184
- 20 cm Long ATBC204
- 22 cm Long ATBC224
- 26 cm Long ATBC264

MARK I

Hunter Passive Tendon Implant
- 3 mm Wide PT3
- 4 mm Wide PT4
- 5 mm Wide PT5
- 6 mm Wide PT6

Hunter Tendon Rod
- 2 mm Wide TR2
- 3 mm Wide TR3
- 4 mm Wide TR4
- 5 mm Wide TR5
- 6 mm Wide TR6

Fig. 57-5. Hunter Tendon Implants. (Phoenix Biomedical Corp. P.O. Box 80390, Valley Forge, PA 19484. Phone: [800-462-2563].)

middle phalanx of the finger, palm, and sublimis muscle of the forearm.

Hunter active tendon implants (available, researched and developed by the historic Holter Co., and manufactured and distributed by Phoenix Biomedical, Fig. 57-5) are constructed of two 2-mm helical porous cords of high-tenacity polyester fibers that are presssure-molded into a shaft of radiopaque silicone rubber. The two cords are 66,000 polyester fibers each, totaling 132,000 high-tenacity Dacron fibers in each tendon. Beiler, the textile engineer, created this tubular twill design for the first aerospace suit.[10] It was possible to convert the special design to our ligament research program for use in the hand and upper extremity for non–weight-bearing joint reconstruction. The high tenacity porous tendon is compatible with medical-grade silicone rubber as well as with human tendon and bone. The dacron

fibers are woven in a never-ending helix that because of minimal shear effect there is ingrowth of fibroblastic cells and eventual collagen support of the implant cord (Fig. 57-6).

There are currently four types of active tendon implants (active tendon [AT] implant, ATPC, ATDC, ATBC), and they are distinguishable by their proximal and distal junctures (see Fig. 57-5).

1. The AT implant, fixed in length, has a plate for distal fixation and has a preformed reinforced silicone loop at its proximal end; it has an overall diameter of 4 mm and comes in lengths of 16, 18, 20 and 22 cm. This implant is especially recommended for sublimis finger and thumb flexor tendon reconstruction. The proximal silicone loop allows a simple attachment of the sublimis motor tendon to the prosthesis or the flexor

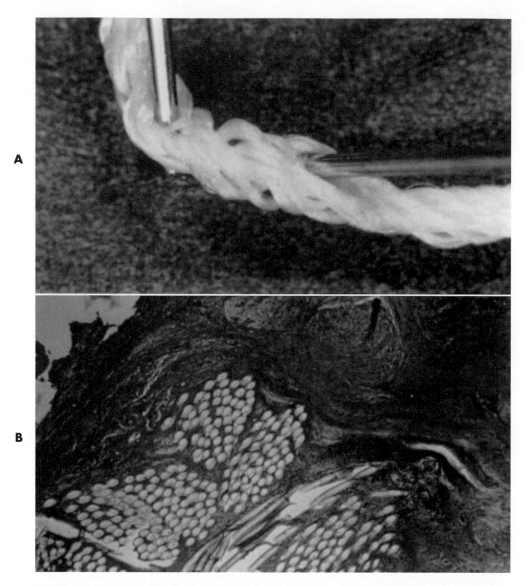

Fig. 57-6. A, The MARK III Dacron fibers are woven similar to the collagen helix. **B,** A magnified view reveals the helical configuration of the polyester weave with ingrowth of the collagen providing biologic fixation. (From Hunter JM, Taras JS, Mackin EJ, et al: Staged flexor tendon reconstruction using passive and active tendon implants. In Hunter JM, Mackin EJ, Callahan AD, eds: *Rehabilitation of the hand: surgery and therapy,* ed 4, St Louis, 1995, Mosby.)

pollicis longus (FPL) of the thumb in the forearm passed through the loop. The patient's sublimis tendon is then fixed to the tendon loop using the Pulvertaft interweave. The distal plate allows secure fixation to the middle phalanx with a screw or wire. The tensile strength of the juncture between the plate and the implant shaft has been rated at more than 100 pounds. The three implants are not adjustable in length and are most effective in the early trauma flexor tendon defect where early active motion and return to function is advised. The implant is sometimes called the MARK II tendon.

2. The ATPC implant has a plate for distal fixation and porous cords for intertendon weave proximally. This implant is recommended as an alternative proximal juncture rather than the loop to loop.

3. The ATDC implant has porous cords for distal fixation and a preformed silicone loop proximally. The two free distal porous cords can be placed through drill holes in the bone. This implant is recommended for flexor and extensor tendon reconstruction in situations where plate and screw fixation are not indicated.

4. The ATBC implant has porous cords for both proximal and distal fixation. This implant is indicated in the

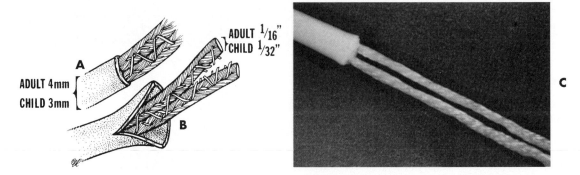

Fig. 57-7. A, Shortening of the MARK III implant. The silicone is divided sharply, then peeled back to reveal the polyester cords. **B,** The cords are then separated by dividing those stitches that keep the cords held together. **C,** The total width is 4 mm for the adult implant and 3 mm for the child's implant. (From Hunter JM, Taras JS, Mackin EJ, et al: Staged flexor tendon reconstruction using passive and active tendon implants. In Hunter JM, Mackin EJ, Callahan AD, eds: *Rehabilitation of the hand: surgery and therapy,* ed 4, St Louis, 1995, Mosby.)

complex flexor and extensor tendon reconstruction where long tendon grafts at stage II would be needed but are not available. This system is at times the only choice, for example, in the case of severe burns, infection that has destroyed the tendons and nerves, and mutilating trauma where tendons have been destroyed.

These adjustable-length implants allow for implant shortening by pulling the silicone away from the two porous cords and hand separating the woven polyester cords (Fig. 57-7). Care must be taken not to damage the fine polyester weave when peeling away the silicone.[18] This special technique must be applied before the tendon is in place for a distal attachment. The proximal forearm weave attachment requires that the distal attachment be completed so the exact measurements for tendon tension and length can be determined.

Active tendon implants are used as temporary tendon prostheses for months or years. The delay to stage II is the surgeon's choice, based on the needs of the patient. During the stage I period with the active tendon all the benefits of the active tendon functions are achieved. The new gliding tendon bed is prepared for a stage II tendon graft while the patient has useful hand function. Importantly, the functioning anatomic muscle tendon bed in the forearm is prepared dynamically for the ideal stage II tendon graft. The proximal motor juncture in the forearm is easily identified in stage II. The fibrous sheath motor tendon unit is kept intact as the active tendon is removed. The graft is woven through the healed tendon complex. The tension is set and the graft is secured by the Pulvertaft technique. All Phoenix-Hunter tendon implants are ready for immediate use—sterile, lint free, double packaged. The Hunter tendons as packaged are not for reuse. When placed on the surgical field the following precautions are suggested:

1. Place tendon in clean pan in normal saline or antibiotic solution, such as bacitracin (50,000 U/L normal saline solution) or polymyxin B (500,000 U/L of normal saline solution).
2. Handle the implants with saline-moistened gloves.
3. Place tendon on fluid-soaked sponge.
4. Irrigate the tendon during the procedure.
5. Antibiotic irrigation solutions prepared in the operating room are recommended.

PREOPERATIVE STAGE I

Before surgical reconstruction, a hand therapy program prepares the patient's hand for surgery. Joint contractures are corrected, soft tissue is softened, and range of motion (ROM) is maximized. The passive potential for active ROM is recorded. Sensibility evaluation is important, as an insensate finger may not be a candidate for two-stage tendon reconstruction.[18] The hand and wrist should be evaluated for median nerve entrapment syndromes and the upper extremity should be studied anatomically to rule out a neurologic thoracic outlet syndrome.

In special instances of flexor and extensor tendon reconstruction, the surgeon needs to perform an active functional assessment of the tendons and joints after tenolysis and joint release. The extent of the extensor hood gliding and PIP motion may show a sublimis finger reconstruction to be the better procedure even in the first stages of reconstruction.

ANESTHESIA

If expert anesthesia support is available, the operation can be started with local and pain sedation for active motion assessment of the hand. At times, with a good patient and anesthesia compliance, an entire procedure can be done with multiple tourniquet releases and the benefit of a display by the patient of the final active ROM. This is a great benefit to the post stage I hand therapy program as the actual predicted ROM can be recorded at surgery for postoperative goal attainment.[7]

STAGE I—ACTIVE TENDON SURGICAL TECHNIQUE

As with most orthopedic implants, a 48- to 72-hour course of antibiotic prophylaxis is suggested before surgery.

At stage I, the damaged flexor tendon system is explored. The volar zigzag incision, popularized by Bruner, spares the deep vascular connections to the tendon bed while completely exposing the bed. The incision begins at the tip of the finger for the FDS finger reconstruction and enters the palm proximally. It must reach the distal aspect of the transverse carpal ligament in order to facilitate tenolysis and subsequent passage of the tendon implant. The skin flaps should be of full thickness with the corners lying over the neurovascular bundles. The digital neurovascular bundles must be identified and protected. After the entire canal has been exposed, an isolated curvilinear incision is made proximal to the wrist crease, usually on the ulnar aspect of the forearm. The ulnar artery, ulnar nerve, and median nerve are identified and protected.

The plane between the profundi and sublimis tendons in the forearm is identified and enlarged with blunt finger dissection. In the finger, by making transverse window incisions in the flexor tendon sheath between A_1 and A_2 pulleys and the mid A_2 and distal A_2 pulley levels, the scarred and adherent flexor tendons are gradually removed in segments. The palmar segment of tendon is excised at the lumbrical level while preserving uninjured portions of the sheath retinaculum. At the levels of the three cruciate pulleys, the proper digital arteries impart four transverse arteries that supply the synovial bed and the vincular system. If possible, these arterial branches are spared. A portion (approximately 2 cm) of the sublimis tendon attachment to the middle phalanx is preserved for later coverage of the plate and screw or porous Dacron cord of the tendon implant. The length remaining should not pass the PIP joint. PIP joint release and capsulectomy is often necessary to optimize PIP passive and active motion.

If the palm is uninjured, the lumbrical muscle and profundus tendon with surrounding mesotenon are carefully preserved as an occasional alternative location for stage II graft attachment. A scarred or shortened lumbrical muscle is resected to prevent the problem of a lumbrical-plus finger. The active tendon implant is inserted from the palm distal through remaining pulleys and flexor tendon sheath using a no-touch technique. Pass a grasping or hooking instrument from the forearm to the palm and palm the proximal end to the forearm. Moistening the device with Ringer's solution will facilitate this process. Severe PIP contractures with skin loss may be salvaged by shifting skin flaps proximally in the finger and skin grafting the distal defects over a DIP joint arthrodesis.

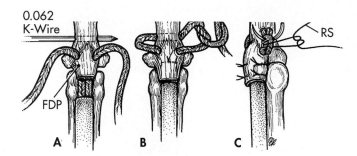

Fig. 57-8. MARK III distal implant fixation—porous cord technique. **A,** With a free needle, the porous cords are passed through the flexor digitorum profundis stump. Next, a 0.062-inch K-wire is used to drill through the distal phalanx parallel to the joint line. **B,** One of the cords is passed through the drill hole and tied to the other with a square knot. **C,** The square knot is reinforced with 3-0 nonabsorbable sutures using a tapercut needle. The flexor digitorum superficialis stump is secured over the active tendon. (From Hunter JM, Taras JS, Mackin EJ, et al: Staged flexor tendon reconstruction using passive and active tendon implants. In Hunter JM, Mackin EJ, Callahan AD, eds: *Rehabilitation of the hand: surgery and therapy,* ed 4, St Louis, 1995, Mosby.)

Four types of active tendons are available to enhance flexibility of reconstruction.

AT fixed length. Single-unit tendon referred to as the MARK II Active Tendon with metal plate distal and reinforced loop proximal. Pass a wet umbilical tape through the metal plate screw hole and pass the tape through A_1 and A_2 pulleys. Irrigate the wound using instrument. While pulling on the tape, walk the end plate to the middle phalanx of the finger. Instrument the proximal loop into the forearm for its FDS tendon juncture.

ATPC. A metal plate distal, two porous cords silicone-covered tendon shaft, and free porous cords proximal. This is an adjustable-length tendon. The proximal end to be adjusted in the forearm method: After clearing the tendon bed, pull the two porous cords distal to proximal through pulleys A_2 and A_1 to proximal in the forearm. After the plate is fixed to the middle phalanx, the proximal end is shortened by stripping the rubber to length, separating the two cords, and suturing the cords to the FDS tendon by Pulvertaft-type tendon weave in the distal one third of the forearm.

ATDC. A loop proximal and two porous cords distal method: Pass the two cords from the palm distally through the A_1 and A_2 pulley to the middle phalanx. Pass loop of tendon from palm to forearm. Pass Alice forceps through loop and hold. Length will be adjusted distally and the free end passed through bone drill hole (Fig. 57-8). The cord system through bone works well in the fifth finger, and in all fingers in combination with the Swanson PIP joint stem implant arthroplasty and in children while preserving the epiphyseal plate.

ATBC. Porous cords distal and proximal. It is recommended that the distal fixation be completed first. The proximal attachment should follow as it sets the muscle-tendon tension in the operation. This particular implant is used in opponents-plasty of the thumb.

Pulley reconstruction

The precise biomechanical design of the flexor tendon pulley system permits lubricated gliding of tendons while transmitting the power of the forearm musculature to the bones and joints of the fingers. Unless the flexor sheath and pulley system can be restored at stage I surgery, the functional arc of motion cannot be acceptable despite good postoperative therapy. Pulleys that are absent or appear weak at stage I require reconstruction.

Discarded tendon material from an injured finger may be used for pulley reconstruction. The palmaris longus tendon or plantaris tendon may also be used. We prefer to wrap the tendon material around the proximal phalanx extraperiosteally but under the extensor apparatus; it is wrapped three times around the phalanx and sutured to itself and to the rim of the fibro-osseous canal. A small dorsal incision through skin and tendon aids tendon passage maneuver (Fig. 57-9). This is performed over a trial implant to prevent making the pulley too tight. The pulley should be as broad as possible but not too close to the joints, and the implant used should fill the tendon bed but not bind on glide testing.[18] An advantage of the sublimis finger is that only A_1 and A_2 pulleys need to be intact for functional flexion at the MP and PIP joints. If A_3 pulley is intact at the PIP joint, it is left in place for passage of the tendon implant.

Distal fixation: metal plate FDS method

At stage I, the distal end of the active tendon is carried to the base of the middle phalanx and fixed in place by plate screw fixation (Fig. 57-10) or by passing the porous cords through a transverse drill hole. The DIP joint is either arthrodesed or tenodesed to a fixed angle of flexion.[17] The distal metal plate component must be secured to bone in a way that will provide a strong, durable, and immediate juncture. The following steps are performed:

1. As one bears in mind that the ideal position of the distal end plate is with the metal points in the proximal one third of the middle phalanx, the point where the screw should enter the bone is visualized or measured and marked on the bone.
2. The plate is centered over the mark. The dorsum of the patient's finger is placed on a firm part of the operative table, a bone impacter is positioned against the plate, and the impacter is struck firmly; this drives the four sharp spikes into the bone so that the plate is secure and evenly aligned.
3. A 1.5-mm drill bit is passed through both cortices of the bone at an angle $15°$ dorsal to the joint line and a lateral x-ray image is taken. The drill should miss the

joint and be located in the central portion of the cortical bone.
4. A 2-mm cancellous screw is turned through a 1.5-mm drill hole. *No thread cutter is used.* With the joint held securely, the proper screw length is chosen. The distal end is secured by carefully turning the self-cutting screw through both cortices of bone to thumb tightness. The screw should appear dorsally with less than 2 mm protruding. The fit should feel firm throughout and final fixation should be secure. If the final screw turns are loose, the system may not stand cyclic force; therefore, the screw should be reinserted more distally in the middle phalanx in bone or fixed with twisted wires.
5. The preserved stump of the sublimis tendon is drawn over the distal component and sutured laterally at the level of the middle phalanx to provide a soft-tissue buffer that prevents irritation of the overlying skin.
6. The tourniquet is released, the wounds are irrigated, hemostasis is obtained, and the distal incision is closed.

Note: the distal component is designed to allow fixation by twisted wires through the bone or by screw. If the bone has been fractured or is osteoporotic, wiring is preferred. In addition, wire fixation using two drill holes is preferred if the bone is deformed during the preparation for screw insertion. The distal component must be held securely to bone to prevent movement and wire fracture. Fixation must be strong enough to prevent the plate from lifting off the phalanx (Fig. 57-11).

Distal fixation: porous cords, the FDS method

The long-term results of fixation by porous cords are not yet available; however, there are data indicating that porous cord material is biocompatible and maintains its strength beyond 2 years of cyclic motion.[19] Porous cord is not recommended in acute trauma or tissue areas that might be susceptible to infection.

The porous polyester cords are passed through drill holes in the middle phalanx, a process that may be facilitated by a Swanson tendon passer. The cords are then tied with a square knot, and the knot is reinforced with 3-0 nonabsorbable suture. It is important that a tapercut (R-Ethicon, Inc.) needle be used for this reinforcing stitch, because a cutting needle will damage the fine polyester fiber. The knot should be pressed to the side away from contact or grip.

Distal fixation with the helical porous cords is particularly useful for salvage when a PIP joint arthroplasty with intramedullary stems is necessary in sublimis finger reconstruction (Fig. 57-12).

The use of the open porous cords has other advantages. They pass through the pulleys more easily than does the metal plate. They are useful for smaller fingers and in young people, where the metal plate may be too large.[18]

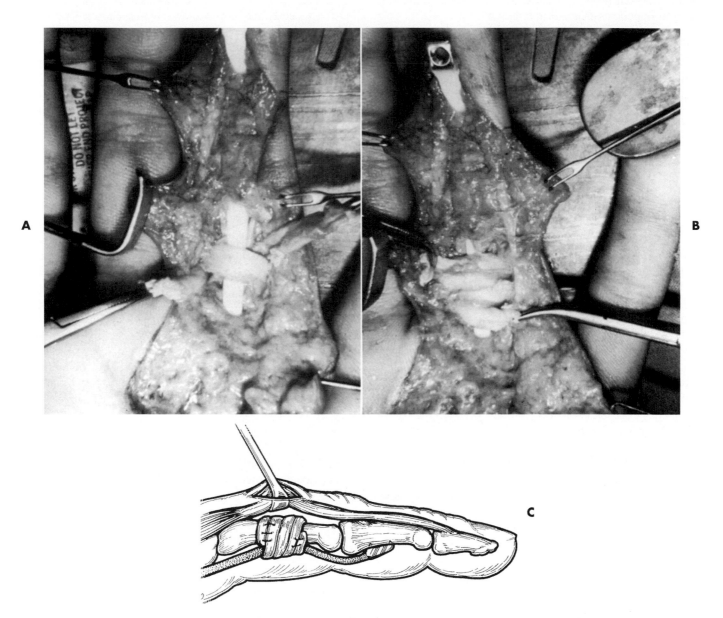

Fig. 57-9. A, Sublimis remnant is wrapped under the extensor apparatus and over the implant to reconstruct the A₂ pulley. **B,** After tendon is wrapped around twice, it is sewn to itself and the rim of the fibro-osseous canal. Pulley should be as wide as possible without blocking motion itself. **C,** Diagram of pulley reconstruction in a superficialis finger. A retractor is placed into a split, which is made centrally in the extensor hood. This is performed via a dorsal skin incision to retract the extensor hood to allow for passage of the tendon graft. Four loops are used to reconstruct the A₂ pulley. (From Hunter JM, Taras JS, Mackin EJ, et al: Staged flexor tendon reconstruction using passive and active tendon implants. In Hunter JM, Mackin EJ, Callahan AD, eds: *Rehabilitation of the hand: surgery and therapy,* ed 4, St Louis, 1995, Mosby.)

The proximal juncture is completed by the loop method or porous cord weave method.

Arthrodesis of the DIP joint is performed before establishing the tendon juncture to avoid excessive manipulation of the tendon-to-bone attachment.[14] Arthrodesis is achieved using a cup-and-cone technique with the Kirschner wire fixation through a dorsal approach. Tenodesis of the DIP joint may be considered instead of arthrodesis, but failure of the tenodesis causing instability of the DIP joint has been a more frequent problem in the senior author's experience than pseudoarthrosis. He prefers arthrodesis of the DIP joint in 20° of palmar flexion.

Proximal juncture: loop method

The motor tendon must be long enough to pass through the proximal loop and return proximally for at least two 90° (Pulvertaft) passes through the tendon (Fig 57-13). Desired excursion of the motor tendon wrist neutral is 3 cm for the FDS. If the patient can be aroused from anesthesia, an accurate assessment of the muscle amplitude is possible. Otherwise, the traditional technique of flexing the wrist to secure a cascade of balance in the fingers is effective. We prefer that the operated finger be placed in slightly greater flexion compared with that in the normal cascade of the uninjured digits.[18]

The selected proximal tendon is passed through the implant loop and then through a small longitudinal split in the tendon (Fig. 57-14). One suture is placed through the tendon for temporary fixation. The implant surface is moistened, and tension is tested by flexing and extending the wrist. The finger should lie in extension during wrist flexion and show a position of balance with the adjacent fingers on wrist extension. If the balance is acceptable, a second suture is placed and the tendon is turned 90° through one or two additional longitudinal splits in the tendon. Tendon balance is then retested to be certain there has been no loss of tension.

Proximal juncture: porous cord weave method

The silicone rubber is peeled away from the polyester cords, as previously described, to obtain the appropriate-length implant. With a free needle or fine point passing hemostat, the helical porous cords are then woven into the

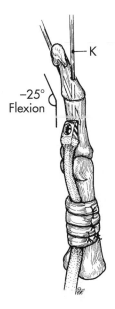

Fig. 57-10. MARK II or III. In the construction of a superficialis finger, the distal end of the active tendon is fixed to the base of the middle phalanx. In this patient, the A₂ pulley has been reconstructed, and the distal interphalangeal joint has been fused in 25° of flexion. (From Hunter JM, Taras JS, Mackin EJ, et al: Staged flexor tendon reconstruction using passive and active tendon implants. In Hunter JM, Mackin EJ, Callahan AD, eds: *Rehabilitation of the hand: surgery and therapy,* ed 4, St Louis, 1995, Mosby.)

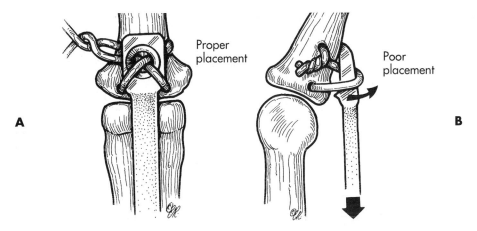

Fig. 57-11. A, Distal implant fixation—wire technique. The wire is passed in a figure-of-eight fashion through drill holes to secure the plate. The wire should pass over the proximal portion of the plate to prevent it from lifting up during active finger flexion. **B,** As the distal interphalangeal joint is actively flexed, the force of the tendon tends to elevate the proximal aspect of the plate. It is extremely important to secure the proximal portion of the plate with the wire.

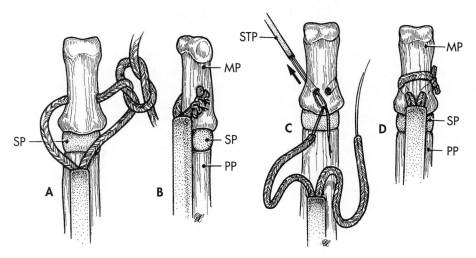

Fig. 57-12. MARK III distal implant fixation—porous cord technique using the Swanson proximal interphalangeal (PIP) implant. **A,** The porous cords are passed through the previously made drill hole in the middle phalanx and tied with a square knot. **B,** The square knot is reinforced with 3-0 nonabsorbable sutures. The stump of the superficialis tendon can then be sutured down over the implant (not shown). **C,** Alternatively, the porous cords are passed through two previously made drill holes in the middle phalanx. **D,** One cord is then passed over the volar surface of the middle phalanx, the cords are tied with a square knot, and the knot is reinforced (*STP,* Swanson tendon passer; *SP,* Swanson PIP implant; *MP,* middle phalanx; *PP,* proximal phalanx). (From Hunter JM, Taras JS, Mackin EJ, et al: Staged flexor tendon reconstruction using passive and active tendon implants. In Hunter JM, Mackin EJ, Callahan AD, eds: *Rehabilitation of the hand: surgery and therapy,* ed 4, St Louis, 1995, Mosby.)

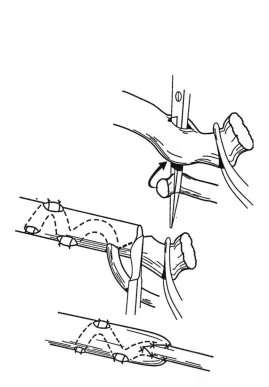

Fig. 57-13. Pulvertaft type of weave of motor tendon graft juncture. Care must be taken to assure passage of the sutures through the donor and recipient tendons to avoid complication of the proximal anastomosis rupture. (From Hunter JM, Taras JS, Mackin EJ, et al: Staged flexor tendon reconstruction using passive and active tendon implants. In Hunter JM, Mackin EJ, Callahan AD, eds: *Rehabilitation of the hand: surgery and therapy,* ed 4, St Louis, 1995, Mosby.)

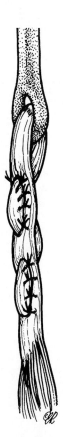

Fig. 57-14. Proximal implant fixation—loop technique. The tendon is passed through the porous cord silicone loop and sutured to itself. Several weaves are made for firm fixation. Tension is checked after the first weave. (From Hunter JM, Taras JS, Mackin EJ, et al: Staged flexor tendon reconstruction using passive and active tendon implants. In Hunter JM, Mackin EJ, Callahan AD, eds: *Rehabilitation of the hand: surgery and therapy,* ed 4, St Louis, 1995, Mosby.)

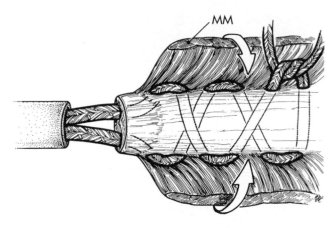

Fig. 57-15. Proximal MARK III implant fixation—porous cord technique. Each of the cords is woven through the proximal tendon in crisscross fashion. Each cord pass should be fixed with a nonabsorbable suture after the muscle has been stripped off the musculotendinous junction. The cords are then tied with a square knot, and the knot is reinforced. The muscle is repaired over the cords with fine absorbable sutures (*mm,* muscle). (From: Staged flexor tendon reconstruction using passive and active tendon implants. In Hunter JM, Mackin EJ, Callahan AD, eds: *Rehabilitation of the hand: surgery and therapy,* ed 4, St Louis, 1995, Mosby.)

lateral borders of the tendon and fixed with nonabsorbable 3-0 or 4-0 sutures at points of exit (Fig. 57-15).

After the first two sutures, tendon balance is tested, as previously described, and readjusted if necessary. After three or four passes, the cords can be tied securely with a square knot, reinforced with 3-0 nonabsorbable suture, and the ends cut with approximately 2000° F electrocautery. Only TAPERCUT needles should be used during all reinforcement procedures, because cutting needles will seriously damage the delicate polyester weave. The final balance of the fingers is checked again. When satisfactory tendon tension has been achieved, the proximal juncture is tucked beneath the muscle folds and the muscle is gently closed.

If the proximal juncture fails during stage I and x-ray film demonstrates that full passive gliding remains, stage II surgery can be delayed, providing there are no signs of synovitis.[14] Splint rest with daily controlled gliding is recommended followed by early stage II tendon grafting.

POSTOPERATIVE STAGE I

Postoperatively, the patient's hand is kept in a protective dorsal splint with the wrist in 30° of flexion, the MP joints in approximately 70° of flexion, and the PIP joints in extension (Fig 57-16).

Postoperative goals are to increase functional movement, to restore good gliding biomechanics, and to maintain a fluid nutrition system that can nourish the gliding tendon implant as well as the subsequent stage II tendon graft.

Therapy begins the first postoperative day with a passive hold exercise. To perform the passive hold exercise, the

patient must relax the forearm muscles of the involved extremity. The patient gently presses the fingers into flexion with the uninvolved hand and then is asked to maintain the position actively with a gentle muscle contraction. The rationale for the passive hold is that it takes less force to maintain the position of an already flexed finger than to actively pull the finger into flexion from an extended position. The benefits of tendon excursion with place-hold exercises are the same as those derived from active flexion. We ask the patient to perform this exercise in full flexion and at two ranges of partial flexion (i.e., slight flexion, mid flexion, and full flexion). Three repetitions at each range are performed three to four times a day. Place-hold protocols are discussed in Chapter 40.

In addition, gentle passive flexion of the IP joints is performed several times a day within the dorsal splint. If the patient begins to glide the tendon very early and excellent tendon pull-through is demonstrated, we slow them at 2 weeks by applying elastic-band traction. The patient still can do the passive hold exercise, but the elastic band traction program adds protection for the healing tendon juncture.

If pulleys were reconstructed at stage I surgery, the postoperative program must take them into account.

If the patient does not have full active IP joint extension, a contracture-control program must be initiated during the first postoperative week. A PIP joint passive extension splint is fitted within the dorsal splint (Fig. 57-17). This insert splint includes a counterforce applied over the reconstructed pulley to prevent its attenuation as the contracted joint is gently pulled into extension.

Light grip strengthening may begin with a foam squeeze after the *fourth postoperative week.* The passive hold exercise is continued. Overzealous use of the digit soon after surgery is to be avoided because this may result in synovitis. This complication generally responds to rest and splinting.

At *6 weeks,* the protective dorsal splint may be removed and a wristlet and elastic band traction applied; these permit wrist extension to neutral and full extension of the MP and IP joints. An active patient may need a dorsal splint for an additional 2 weeks. By *8 weeks,* patients usually are permitted full activities with restrictions on full-power grip until 12 weeks. During *weeks 8 to 12,* the goal is improvement of strength and endurance through beginning of putty exercise and light sustained grip activities (woodworking), progressing to the weight well and resistance exercise. A return-to-work program is initiated. At *12 to 14 weeks,* the patient, depending on job description, can return to work using the gliding tendon implant. Lifting should be limited to 100 pounds bilaterally and 50 pounds unilaterally. Young men in jobs requiring forceful active use of their hand average at least 1 year with full power before stage II replacement. Patients with easier demand occupations may go many years before stage II.

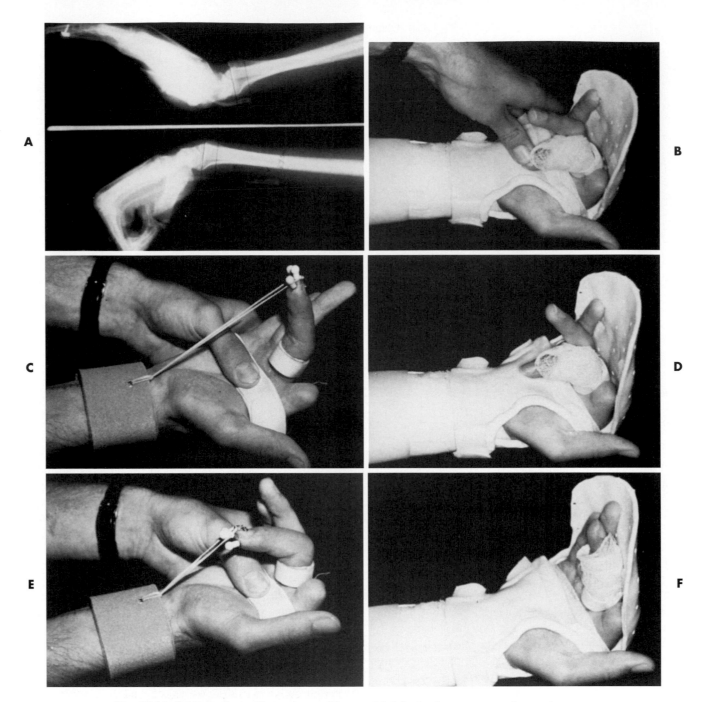

Fig. 57-16. Sublimis finger. The patient, a 23-year-old right-dominant surveyor, incurred a severe injury to his right hand with a log splitter. The index finger was shattered and unsalvageable. The long finger was amputated and replanted. Vascularity was reestablished to the long finger, but the tendons were badly damaged and not repaired primarily. Subsequently the patient underwent a tendon graft procedure 8 months after injury. A swan-neck deformity developed, and the patient underwent a secondary revision 8 months later. Approximately 2 years after the injury the patient was seen at the Philadelphia Hand Center. He had good neurovascular function in the finger but lacked active flexion. He had maintained good passive range of motion, which made the finger salvageable for flexor tendon reconstruction using the active tendon implant and sublimis finger method. The flexor tendon graft was excised. A volar plate advancement tenodesis was performed to prevent hyperextension of the proximal interphalangeal (PIP) joint. **A,** The active tendon implant was fixed to the base of the middle phalanx. A_1 and A_2 pulleys were reconstructed. **B,** The distal interphalangeal joint was arthrodesed. Note excursion. A dorsal protective splint was applied at surgery. Therapy begins the first postoperative day with a passive hold exercise. Reconstructed A_1 and A_2 pulleys are protected with pulley rings. **C** and **D,** Wristlet and elastic-band traction were applied *6 weeks* after surgery. Direct digital pressure from the uninvolved hand adds support to the reconstructed A_1 pulley during the early training program. **E,** During *weeks 8 to 12* the goal is improvement of strength and endurance. A return-to-work program is initiated. At *12 to 14 weeks* the patient, depending on his job description, can return to work using his functioning gliding tendon implant. **F, G,** and **H,** Stage II: Passive hold exercise.

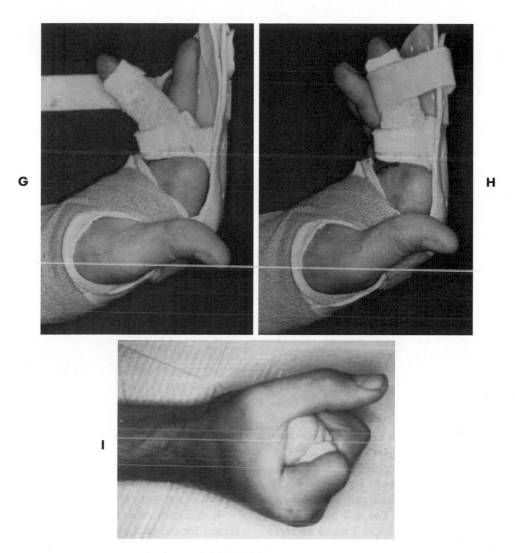

Fig. 57-16, cont'd. I and **J,** Passive extension of PIP joint. Felt wedge places the proximal phalanx in more flexion. With the felt wedge in place, the Velcro strap gently pulls the PIP joint into −20° of extension. Passive extension splint delayed in this patient because of volar plate reconstruction. Postoperative therapy stage II is similar to stage I, but because very early pain-free gliding generally occurs, protective splinting may be extended. (**A** and **C** through **J** from Hunter JM, Taras JS, Mackin EJ, et al: Staged flexor tendon reconstruction using passive and active tendon implants. In Hunter JM, Mackin EJ, Callahan AD, eds: *Rehabilitation of the hand: surgery and therapy,* ed 4, St Louis, 1995, Mosby.)

POSTOPERATIVE CARE OF RECONSTRUCTED PULLEYS

Reconstructed pulleys in the presence of an active tendon implant must be protected actively with digital pressure and passively with a pulley ring so that the active muscle force transmitted through the implant does not stretch the pulley reconstruction. Protection during the first postoperative days may be provided by a Velcro and felt pulley ring (Fig. 57-18). When postoperative edema decreases, the soft pulley ring can be replaced with a thermoplastic pulley ring and eventually a metal ring in some cases. Pulley reconstruction is as sensitive as tendon repair and should be protected for 6 months. The A_1 pulley leads and protects the A_2 pulley by reducing the angular power drive at the proximal edge of the construction. Firm pressure on the A_1 pulley during rehabilitation training is important. A thermoplastic palmar support may be fabricated to protect the A_1 pulley, however, it is difficult to obtain firm support. Additional support should be applied by pressure from a finger from the opposite hand during active flexion.[18] Even with the use of pulley supports, the reconstructed pulley is susceptible to elongation because it does not near collagen maturity for 4 to 6 months postoperatively (Fig. 57-19).[2]

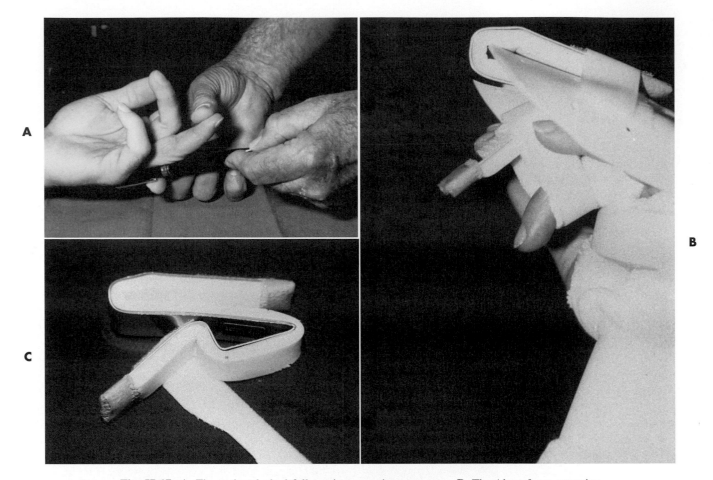

Fig. 57-17. A, The patient lacked full passive extension at surgery. **B,** The Alumafoam extension splint was fabricated to correct the contracture. It was applied 1½ weeks postoperatively. The initial wearing schedule was ½ hour, four times per day with gentle tension. The finger responded well to treatment. Had the finger not responded, wearing time could have been increased to include night use with only maintenance tension. **C,** The proximal interphalangeal extension insert.

STAGE II—TENDON GRAFTING SURGICAL TECHNIQUE

The immature mesothelial sheath is formed around the tendon implant by 4 weeks and becomes mature by 4 months. A minimum of 4 to 6 months is required between stage I and stage II so that the patient can derive the full benefit of the tendon implant, especially the biologic softening of digital connective tissues. Patients who have returned to work and a normal lifestyle will benefit by waiting longer than 1 year before stage II tendon grafting. As time passes with the tendon implant in the digit, the motor unit becomes stronger, ROM is maximized, and soft tissue becomes more pliable, thus making the digit better prepared for stage II tendon grafting.

Stage II involves the surgical removal of the active tendon implant and insertion of a tendon graft through the new pseudosheath. The patient's assistance in setting the tension of the graft in stage II is helpful if the patient can be temporarily awakened for an active trial. Local anesthesia

with intravenous sedation is preferred, but routine general anesthesia can be selected as required. The patient under fentanyldro-peridol (Innovar) and local anesthesia is able to produce muscle contraction on command bringing the finger actively into extension and returning it actively into flexion.[7]

After the distal juncture has been exposed, it is left intact and the proximal juncture is exposed. An ulnarly curved volar incision through the previous stage I incision in the forearm exposes the proximal end of the device. The tendon implant is grasped with an instrument (rubber-shod forceps) and the sheath and the site of the juncture are carefully examined.

Portions of soft sheath may be retained at the surgeon's discretion. If synovitis* has been present, the thickened

---

*This synovitis implies mechanical failure from a loosened distal juncture of the implant. (So-called *silicone synovitis* has never been observed in staged tendon implant surgery in the senior author's thirty years of experience.)

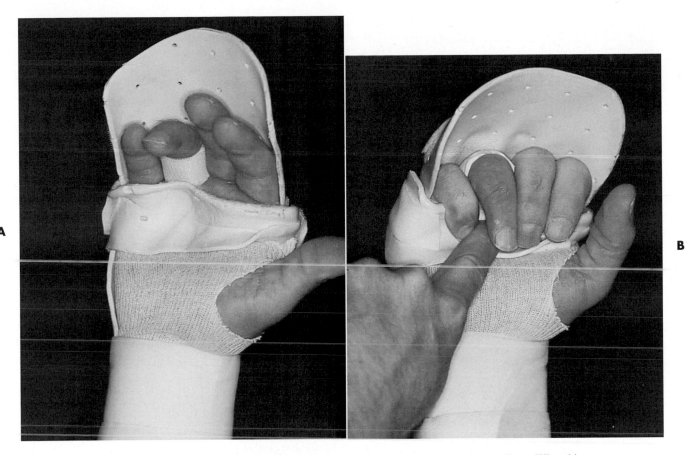

Fig. 57-18. DH had previously undergone pulley reconstruction at A_1 and A_2 pulleys. When his active tendon implant was placed, the previously reconstructed pulleys, weakened during an earlier tenolysis, were reinforced with Dacron. Postoperatively, they required protection. In the early stage, this was accomplished with Velcro and orthopedic felt ring placed at the A_2 level **(A)**. A wide palmar strap was placed to protect A_1. It is padded with orthopedic felt that is contoured to maintain the palmar arch. **B**, Additionally, the patient applied pressure over the reconstructed A_1 pulley with his uninvolved hand during active extension and during place-hold exercises.

sheath must be completely removed from the proximal juncture site to the wrist flexion crease. The active potential ROM of the finger and the excursion necessary to produce it are determined by laying the hand and finger flat on the table and firmly pulling the implant proximally. The surgeon should note the following:

1. The implant excursion needed to produce a ROM from maximum extension to maximum flexion,
2. The distance between the finger pulp and the distal palmar crease (DPC), and
3. Joints with restricted motion

The palmaris tendon is preferred, however, if it is absent, the plantaris tendon and toe extensor tendons may be used. The tendon graft is sutured to the proximal end of the tendon implant and pulled through the new tendon bed. The tendon implant is detached from the middle phalanx and discarded. A Bunnell-type weave is placed through the distal end of the

graft with monofilament stainless steel or nonabsorbable suture. A separate pullout wire is no longer used.[12] Care is taken to protect the remaining or reconstructed pulleys, especially the A_2 pulley. Two drill holes are made through the middle phalanx under the sublimis stump remnant and enlarged with a curette. A Keith needle is drilled at the base of the middle phalanx and exits dorsally, angulating distally. The suture is then pulled through the middle phalanx by threading it through the Keith needle. As the Keith needle is advanced through the middle phalanx, one must watch the graft being pulled into the drill holes on the volar side of the finger. This tendon-to-bone juncture is most important and will prevent any distal ruptures of the graft when healed. A nice technique is to tie the suture directly over the middle phalanx dorsally through a small dorsal incision. This prevents complications related to the dorsal button technique.

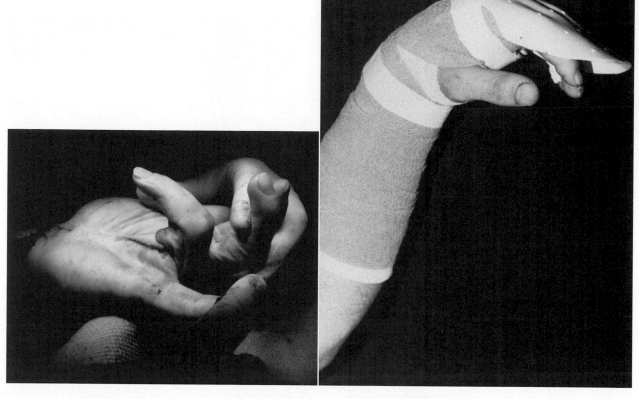

Fig. 57-19. DH is a 36-year-old, right-dominant male who sustained an injury to his right hand about 13 years before presentation at the Philadelphia Hand Center. He had undergone 10 surgeries since the injury, three over the year before his initial evaluation at the center, including a tendon graft, pulley reconstruction, and finally a tenolysis, which ended in rupture. He had also had difficulty with healing of the incision on the proximal phalanx. The remainder of the hand was intact. **A,** As the active tendon implant was placed in the digit, but before closure, the patient's active potential was demonstrated. **B,** Postoperatively, the patient was placed in a dorsal protective splint with wrist at 30°, metacarpophalangeals at 70°, and interphalangeals able to extend to 0°.

The final phase of stage II surgery is the completion of the proximal juncture. The sublimis muscle power may be used to an advantage when grafting to the middle phalanx to create a sublimis finger. After the motor is selected and the graft is passed through the motor tendon, the tension of the graft is set and fixed with a braided nonabsorbable suture. The attitude of the finger with the wrist in neutral should be one of slightly more flexion than the adjacent digit. At this point the patient's compliance can be enhanced under leptoanalgesia, alleviating the guesswork in setting the tension of the graft. The patient is asked to flex and extend the involved fingers, and the tension of the graft is adjusted accordingly. The selected tendon motor must supply sufficient excursion if a good result is to be achieved. When the tension is correct, the graft is further woven through the motor tendon and sutured into place using the technique described by Pulvertaft (see Fig. 57-13).[26,27]

The Pulvertaft end-weave technique is preferred for single-tendon junctures (i.e., the profundus of the index finger, the flexor pollicis longus, or the sublimis). The multiple end-weave is preferred for a juncture with the profundus of the long, ring, or little finger. It is extremely important to be certain that the suture passes through the graft and into the motor tendon to prevent subsequent slipping of the proximal juncture. One also must be sure that the pseudosheath does not impede excursion of the tendon graft juncture; if necessary, more of the proximal sheath should be excised to permit full extension.[18]

After repeated manipulation of the finger, the digit should remain in slightly more flexion than normal. The juncture is completed by a second interweave and suture fixation, and the wound is closed.[18]

POSTOPERATIVE STAGE II THERAPY

Postoperatively, the patient's hand is kept in the protective dorsal splint applied at surgery with the wrist in 30° of flexion, the MP joints in approximately 70° of flexion, and the IP joints in full extension. Early mobilization with

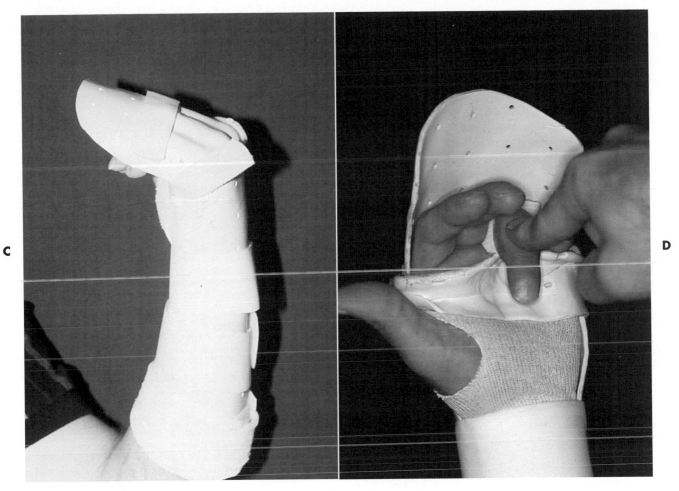

Fig. 57-19, cont'd. C, At 3 weeks, the wrist was extended to neutral in the dorsal protective splint. **D,** Velcro pulley protection applied postoperatively was replaced with a thermoplastic splint to provide additional support. It was still reinforced at A_1 with pressure from the uninvolved hand during active extension and place-hold exercises.

elastic-band traction begins the first postoperative day. The patient actively extends the finger and then reciprocally relaxes it, permitting the elastic band to flex the digit. Ten repetitions of this exercise are performed every working hour. Gentle passive motion is performed; 10 repetitions are performed several times a day, with care given to avoiding extensor tendon attenuation by overstretching. Attention continues to be devoted to controlling the development of contractures. Postoperative therapy is similar to that after stage I. However, because very early pain-free gliding generally occurs, protective splinting may be extended beyond the usual 6-week period if necessary to protect against excessive force on the tendon junctures. Initiation of the wristlet at 6 weeks after surgery may be delayed until 8 weeks, and active exercise at 8 weeks delayed until 10 weeks. Timetables always should be adjusted according to the patient's progress.

CONCLUSION

Sublimis finger flexor tendon reconstruction offers the surgeon another option when dealing with a scarred tendon bed and the failed biomechanics of a flexor tendon system.

Tenodesis or arthrodesis of the distal joint combined with stage I fixation of the active tendon implant and a subsequent stage II tendon graft to the middle phalanx establishes a simplified one-tendon, two-joint flexor tendon system. Restoration of motion at the PIP joint with sacrifice of motion at the DIP joint is based on the concept that the PIP joint makes the greatest contribution to hand function in the salvage finger.

Postoperative therapy care for a sublimis finger offers a quicker, more reliable recovery than for the FDP three-joint reconstruction. Because fewer pulleys require repair, there are fewer potential areas for the flexor tendon to bowstring away from the phalanx. The preservation of pulley repairs enhances the ability of the tendon graft at stage II to maintain an effective moment arm at the MP and PIP joints: The maintenance of the moment arms facilitates maximal flexion of the digit.[1,3,14]

Because fewer pulleys are needed for force transmission, tendon drag and potential stage II adhesions are minimized. Less excursion is required for the finger to flex to the palm. With decreased excursion demand there is also a decrease in the amount of tension required from the muscle to enable flexion. Because less tension is needed for PIP flexion, earlier active flexion is less stressful to tendon junctures, again optimizing postoperative function.[1] Fixation of the distal joint at stage I surgery eliminates the need to manage a recurrent DIP flexion contracture or elongated terminal position of the extensor tendon.

The two-stage tendon graft procedure using a Hunter tendon implant has proven to be a consistently reliable method of salvaging a scarred tendon system. Complex injuries in zone II and failed tendon grafting procedures may require a compromise of the goal of restoring an FDP two-tendon, three-joint flexor tendon system. When the MP joint has full ROM, and PIP joint motion can be restored, useful digital motion can be achieved with a one-tendon, two-joint flexor system; therefore, a reasonable alternative in flexor tendon reconstruction is the sublimis finger.

SUMMARY

The principles and fine details of staged flexor tendon reconstruction using passive and active tendon implants, secondary tendon grafting, and postoperative management are described here and in the literature.[8-18] The principles of the redemption operation, Osborne/Pulvertaft, can be applied to two-stage flexor tendon and a sublimis finger reconstruction when conditions warrant a salvage procedure and a sublimis finger reconstruction. The Dacron-reinforced passive tendon implant is a standard for staged flexor tendon reconstruction. In many cases, however, an active tendon implant is preferred. This chapter highlights the indications, technique, and postoperative therapy of tendon reconstruction by using the Hunter Active Tendon to create a functioning sublimis finger.

REFERENCES

1. Blackmore SM, Hunter JM, Kobus RJ: Superficialis finger reconstruction: a new look at a last resort procedure. In Mackin EJ, Callahan AD, eds: *Hand clinics: frontiers in hand rehabilitation,* vol 7, no 3, Philadelphia, 1991, Saunders.
2. Brand PW, Thompson DE, Micks JE: The biomechanics of the interphalangeal joints. In Bowers WH, ed: *The interphalangeal joints,* New York, 1987, Churchill Livingstone.
3. Brand PW: *Clinical mechanics of the hand,* St Louis, 1985, Mosby.
4. Burkhalter WE: Personal communication.
5. Curtis RM: Capsulectomy of the interphalangeal joints of the fingers, *J Bone Joint Surg* 1954; 36A:1219-1232.
6. Flatt AE: *Anatomy and kinesiology: the care of the arthritic hand,* ed 5, St Louis, 1995, Quality Medical Publishing, Inc.
7. Erickson JC III, Hunter JM, Schneider LH: *Neuroleptanalgesia and local anaesthesia for a dynamic approach to surgery of the hand.* Videotape narrative description and scientific exhibit for American Association of Surgeons. Philadelphia, April 11-14, 1976.
8. Hunter JM: Artificial tendons: early development and application, *Am J Surg* 1965; 109:325.
9. Hunter JM: Staged flexor tendon reconstruction, *Hand Surg* 1983; 8:789.
10. Hunter JM: Active tendon prosthesis—techniques and clinical experiences. In Hunter JM, Schneider LH, Mackin EJ, eds: *Tendon surgery in the hand,* St Louis, 1984, Mosby.
11. Hunter JM. Staged tendon reconstruction: technique and rationale. In Hunter JM, Schneider LH, Mackin EJ, eds: *Tendon surgery in the hand,* St Louis, 1987, Mosby.
12. Hunter JM: Artificial tendons: early development and application. In Hunter JM, Schneider LH, Mackin EJ, eds: *Tendon surgery in the hand,* St Louis, 1987, Mosby.
13. Hunter JM, Jaeger SH, Matsui T, Miyaji N: The pseudosynovial sheath—its characteristics in a primate model, *J Hand Surg* 1983; 8(4):461-470.
14. Hunter JM, Blackmore S, Callahan AD: Flexor tendon salvage and functional redemption using Hunter tendon implant and superficialis finger operation, *J Hand Ther* 1989; 2(2):259-266.
15. Hunter JM, Salisbury R: Flexor tendon reconstruction in severely damaged hands: a two stage procedure using a silicone-Dacron reinforced gliding prosthesis prior to tendon grafting, *J Bone Joint Surg* 1971; 53A(5):829.
16. Hunter JM, Schneider LH, Fietti VG: Reconstruction of the sublimis finger, *Orthop Trans* 1979; 3:321.
17. Hunter JM, Singer DI, Mackin EJ: Staged flexor tendon reconstruction using passive and active tendon implants. In Hunter JM, Schneider LH, Mackin EJ, Callahan AD, eds: *Rehabilitation of the hand: surgery and therapy,* St Louis, 1990, Mosby.
18. Hunter JM, Taras JS, Mackin EJ, et al: Staged flexor tendon reconstruction using passive and active tendon implants. In Hunter JM, Mackin EJ, Callahan AD, eds: *Rehabilitation of the hand: surgery and therapy,* St Louis, 1995, Mosby.
19. Hunter JM, Sattel AB, Belkin J, Masada K: Collateral ligament reconstruction of the metacarpophalangeal and proximal interphalangeal joints porous Dacron tendon. In Mackin EJ, Callahan AD, eds: *Hand clinics: frontiers in hand rehabilitation,* 1991; 7(3):557-568.
20. Kirkpatrick WH, Kobus RJ: The superficialis finger procedure. *Orthopaedic Specialists,* Philadelphia, 1993, Saunders.
21. Kobus RJ, Kirkpatrick WH: The superficialis finger: an alternative in flexor tendon surgery. In Hunter JM, Mackin EJ, Callahan AD, eds: *Rehabilitation of the hand: surgery and therapy.* St Louis, 1995, Mosby.
22. Littler JW: The physiological and dynamic function of the hand, *Surg Clin North Am* 1960; 40(2):259-266.
23. Littler JW, Thompson JS: Surgical and functional anatomy. In Bowers WH, ed: *The interphalangeal joints,* New York, 1987, Churchill-Livingstone.
24. Osborne G: Redemption operations for flexor tendon injuries. In Stack HG, Bolton H, eds: *Proceedings of the Second Hand Club,* London, 1975, British Society for Surgery of the Hand.
25. Osborne G: The sublimis tendon replacement technique in tendon injuries. Proceedings of the British Orthopaedic Association, *J Joint Bone Surg* 1960; 42B:647.
26. Pulvertaft RG: Experiences in flexor tendon grafting in the hand, *J Bone Joint Surg* 1959; 41B:629.
27. Pulvertaft RG: Tendon grafts for flexor tendon injuries in the fingers and thumb—a study of technique and results, *J Bone Joint Surg* 1956; 38B:175.
28. Strickland JW. Results of flexor tendon surgery in zone II, *Hand Clin* 1985; 1:16.

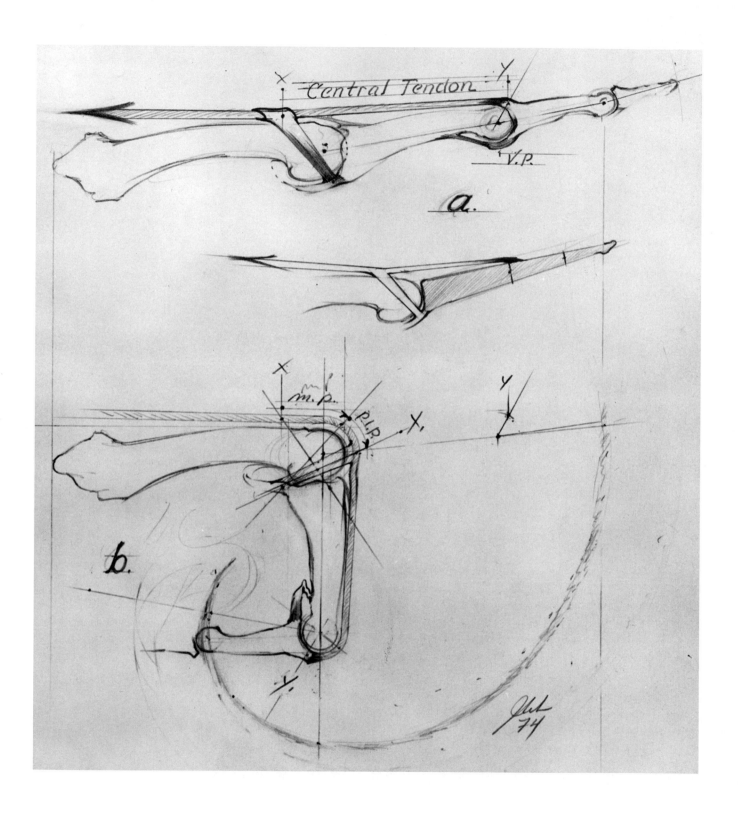

Part XIV

EXTENSOR TENDONS

Basic format of the extrinsic extensor system on the MP-unit, showing primary insertion on the dorsal base of the middle phalanx and the control restraints of both the PIP volar plate and the sagittal bands at the MP level; the finger in full extension and in full flexion.

Chapter 58

ANATOMY OF THE EXTENSOR TENDON SYSTEM OF THE FINGERS

Raoul Tubiana

The extensor apparatus of the fingers is formed by extrinsic muscles, by intrinsic muscles, and by fixed fibrous structures.

EXTRINSIC EXTENSORS

The extensor digitorum communis (EDC) and the two extensor proprius tendons pass under the dorsal retinaculum on the back of the wrist before diverting toward the fingers (Fig. 58-1). The extensor indicis and extensor digiti minimi (EDM) have independent muscles that allow independent function. Their tendons run on the ulnar side of the EDC tendon. On the dorsum of the hand the extensor communis tendons are interconnected by the juncturae tendinum. These bands assist extension of adjacent connected fingers. Interruption of an extensor tendon proximally may be masked by the effect of these bands[18] (Fig. 58-2). The extensor communis tendon to the little finger may be absent and is replaced by an oblique junctura from the ring finger.[12]

The shape of the extensor tendons changes at the level of the metacarpophalangeal (MP) joints. They become thin and flat. Halfway down the proximal phalanx of each finger, the broad flat extensor tendon splits into three parts: an extensor central band and two extensor lateral bands.

The extensor communis has four sites of insertion (Fig. 58-3):

1. The most proximal on each side of the MP joint by the sagittal bands fixed to the volar plate. They contribute to the stability of the tendon on the dorsum of the MP joint.
2. An inconstant insertion into the base of the proximal phalanx, stretched when the proximal interphalangeal (PIP) joint is extended, and relaxed when the PIP is flexed.
3. The most important insertion is that of the central tendon into the base of the middle phalanx. It extends the middle phalanx, except when the MP joint is in hyperextension, and contributes to extension of the proximal phalanx by pushing its head dorsally when the proximal phalanx is flexed. It also contributes to the extension of the distal phalanx.
4. Insertion of the terminal extensor tendon into the distal phalanx.

The multiple insertions at all the levels of the digital osseous chain distribute the action of the extrinsic tendons to the three phalanges. However, they cannot ensure the complete extension of the finger. Isolated contraction of the EDC, under normal physiologic conditions, extends mainly the proximal phalanx (Fig. 58-4 and 58-5). The two distal phalanges remain flexed in a clawlike position. To act on the distal phalanges, the EDC tendons must lose their anchorage to the proximal phalanx (Fig. 58-6), or the antagonist action of the long flexors must be suppressed (Fig. 58-7). These are abnormal experimental or pathologic conditions. Landsmeer showed that to control in all positions two joints in a polyarticular chain of bones, such as the fingers, at least three muscles are necessary.[14] The proximal phalanx, which is a typical intercalated bone, is controlled by three muscular systems: two extrinsic muscles (flexor and extensor) and one diagonal intrinsic muscle. For the middle phalanx the third diagonal component is not a muscle but the oblique retinacular ligament (Fig. 58-8). Each phalanx has a wide

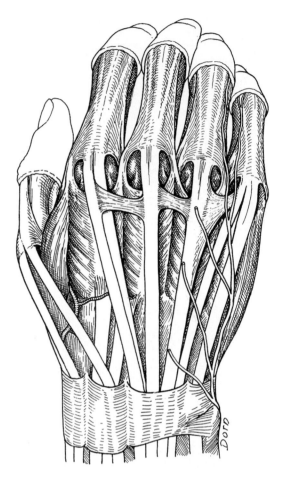

Fig. 58-1. Extensor tendons on the dorsal aspect of the wrist and hand.

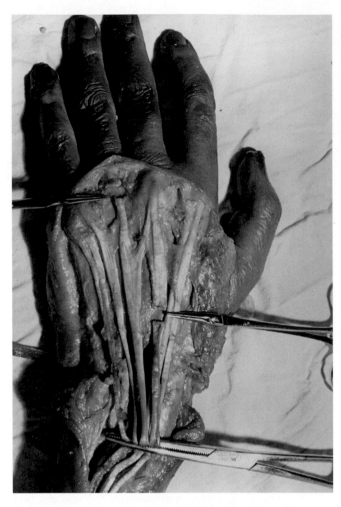

Fig. 58-2. Traction on the extensor digitorum tendons. Extension of the long finger is possible in spite of the division of its extensor tendon proximal to the juncturae tendinum.

range of movement in flexion and extension. Flexion is ensured by the exceptionally large excursion of the long flexors; that of the long extensors is much less. Their action has to be relayed by the intrinsic muscles: the interossei and lumbrical muscles.

INTRINSIC MUSCLES

The intrinsic muscular system consists of the interossei and lumbrical muscles.

Interossei muscles

In the sixteenth century, Fallopio from Padova established the action of the interossei as extensors of the distal phalanges.[6] Winslow was more precise when he found that the interossei and lumbricals act as flexor of the proximal phalanx and extensor of the two distal ones.[27] Albinus described the interossei, according to their origins, into palmar-adductors and dorsal-abductors of the fingers.[1] This classification was accepted for almost 200 years. All these authors considered these muscles to be weak auxilliaries of the long flexors and extensors of the digits.

Duchenne demonstrated that the intrinsic muscles were indispensable to ensure the freedom of movement of each phalanx.[4] However, he thought that the intrinsic muscles were the only extensors of the IP joints. Testut states that extension of the IP joints can be performed by the long extensor.[25] Fowler further clarified the interplay between extrinsic and intrinsic muscles.[7]

The usual anatomic descriptions distinguish four dorsal and three palmar interossei (Fig. 58-9). The dorsal interossei have a double origin from the two metacarpals that bound the space. For Landsmeer[13] and for Eyler and Markee[5] they are made up of two distinct muscles: the deep[13] or dorsal[5] component, which is inserted mostly on the lateral tubercle on the base of the proximal phalanx, and the superficial or ventral component, which inserts chiefly into the extensor aponeurosis.

The palmar interossei originate on only one metacarpal, on the face of the metacarpal facing the axis of the hand. Most anatomists describe three palmar interossei situated in the palmar aspect of the second, third, and fourth in-

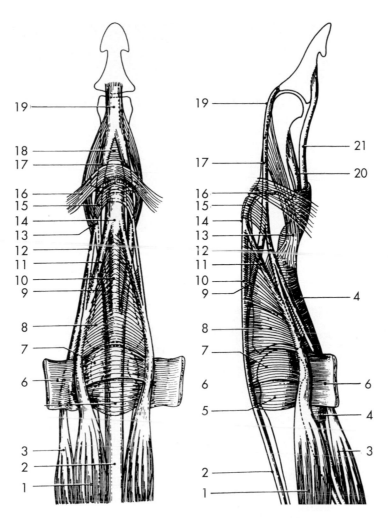

Fig. 58-3. Extensor apparatus of the fingers: frontal and lateral views. *1,* Interosseous muscle; *2,* extensor digitorum communis tendon; *3,* lumbrical muscle; *4,* flexor tendons fibrous sheath; *5,* sagittal band; *6,* intermetacarpal ligament; *7,* transverse fibers of the interosseous hood; *8,* oblique fibers of the hood; *9,* lateral band of extensor tendon; *10,* central or middle band of extensor tendon; *11,* central or middle band of interosseous tendon; *12,* lateral band of interoseous tendon; *13,* oblique retinacular ligament; *14,* middle or central extensor tendon; *15,* spiral fibers of extensor apparatus; *16,* transverse retinacular ligament; *17,* lateral extensor tendon; *18,* triangular ligament (or lamina); *19,* terminal extensor tendon. At the dorsal aponeurosis level the term *tendon* is used for the distal portion of the tendons formed by the junction of *bands* arising from the extrinsic and intrinsic muscles. (From Tubiana R: Extensor apparatus of the fingers. In Hunter JM, Schneider LH, Mackin EJ, eds: *Tendon surgery in the hand,* St Louis, 1987, Mosby.)

terosseous spaces. They have an essentially aponeurotic insertion on the ulnar side of the index and on the radial side of the ring and little fingers. The osseous insertion on the base of the proximal phalanx is inconstant and accessory.

There are, within the first space, some muscle fibers that arise from the ulnar side of the first metacarpal and become inserted on the extensor aponeurosis of the thumb. Some anatomists regard these fibers as a palmar interosseous muscle,[19] others as part of the flexor pollicis brevis (FPB).

In fact, each interosseous muscle is composed of a number of muscular bundles of different lengths that have their origins on the lateral or palmar surfaces of the

metacarpal shafts. The relative importance of the components differs in the various interspaces. The muscular bundles have a relatively independent nerve supply, arising from the deep branch of the ulnar nerve. They continue as tendinous slips that cross the MP joint on the dorsal aspect of the deep intermetacarpal ligament, and insert distally at different levels in the fingers. These anatomic peculiarities allow for several classifications, according to their origins or according to their distal insertion: deep or superficial for Salisbury,[20] proximal or distal for Stack.[22]

1. The deep insertions are into the lateral tubercles on the base of the proximal phalanx and into the capsule of the MP joint.

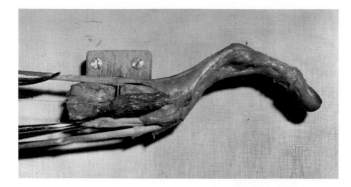

Fig. 58-4. Traction on extensor digitorum communis tendon extends mainly the proximal phalanx. (From Tubiana R: Extensor apparatus of the fingers. In Hunter JM, Schneider LH, Mackin EJ, eds: *Tendon surgery in the hand,* St Louis, 1987, Mosby.)

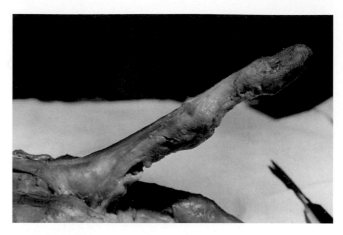

Fig. 58-7. The flexor tendons are divided. Traction on the extensor digitorum communis extends all the digital joints.

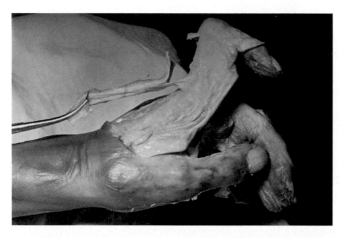

Fig. 58-5. Traction on the extensor communis tendon after division of the tendon over the proximal phalanx. The proximal insertions of the tendon hyperextend the proximal phalanx. The proximal interphalangeal joint is completely flexed; this joint was only partly flexed in Fig. 58-14.

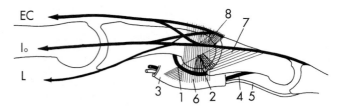

Fig. 58-8. Diagrammatic lateral view of the extensor apparatus at the proximal interphalangeal joint level (*IO,* interosseous; *L,* lumbrical). *1,* Volar plate; *2,* collateral ligament; *3,* fibrous flexor tendon sheath; *4,* flexor superficialis tendon; *5,* flexor profundus tendon; *6,* transverse retinacular ligament; *7,* oblique retinacular ligament; *8,* spiral fibers.

2. The superficial insertions occur at three separate levels in the finger (Fig. 58-10):
   a. A first group of muscle bundles runs into the transverse fibers surrounding the posterior aspect of the MP joint and into the base of the proximal phalanx and forms the interosseous hood.
   b. A second group runs more distally over the dorsal aspect of the proximal phalanx. The oblique fibers blend with the central band of the extensor tendon and form the central extensor tendon, which inserts into the base of the middle phalanx.
   c. A third group of distal fibers runs into the lateral band of the extensor tendon and forms the lateral extensor tendon.
   d. The two lateral extensor tendons cross the PIP joint at the junction of its dorsal and lateral surfaces and then join together to form the terminal extensor tendon inserted onto the base of the distal phalanx.

This is the general arrangement. There are different patterns in the insertions of the interossei and lumbrical muscles for each finger and even for each side of the finger allowing greater functional individuality.

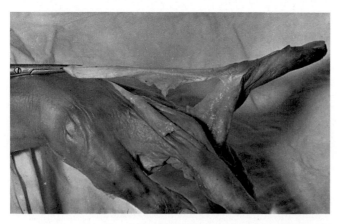

Fig. 58-6. The proximal insertions of the extensor digitorum communis (EDC) are divided. Traction on the EDC puts the interphalangeal joints into complete extension.

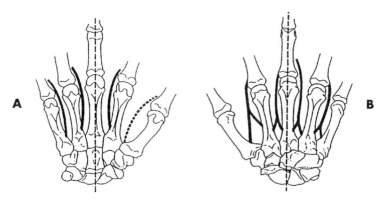

Fig. 58-9. **A,** Diagram of the palmar interossei muscles, which approximate the fingers. The palmar interosseous of the first interspace (in dotted lines) is not described by all anatomists. **B,** Diagram of the dorsal interossei muscles, which open out the fingers. They have a double origin from the two metacarpals that bound the space.

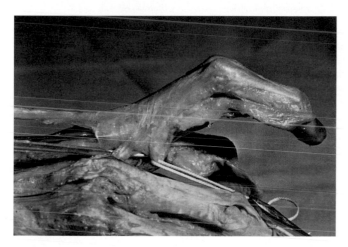

Fig. 58-10. Lateral side of the left ring finger. At the level of the metacarpophalangeal joint: the sagittal band, the tendon of the lumbrical muscle (pulled forward by a stitch), the interglenoid (or intermetacarpal) ligament, and on its dorsal aspect, the interossei muscles tendon with their transverse and oblique fibers forming the interosseous hood. At the level of the proximal interphalangeal joint: the central extensor tendon, the lateral extensor tendons, the spiral fibers, the oblique retinacular ligament. At the level of the distal interphalangeal joint, the two lateral extensor tendons join each other to form the terminal extensor tendon.

The index and the little fingers, because of their peripheral location, have specialized intrinsic muscles. The index has the first dorsal interosseous, whose distal insertion is entirely interosseous. The radial aponeurotic wing is formed almost entirely by the first lumbrical. On the little finger, the tendinous wing on the ulnar side is formed by the abductor digiti minimi (ADM).

Lumbrical muscles

The lumbricals are four small fasciculi that arise from the tendons of the flexor profundus in the palm. Each passes to the radial side of the corresponding finger, superficial to the transverse intermetacarpal ligament and

terminates on the lateral extensor tendons. The angle of approach to the dorsal aponeurosis is greater than that of the interossei.

ACTIONS OF THE INTRINSIC MUSCLES
Interossei Muscles

The introssei muscles produce lateral movements of fingers not only through their insertions on the lateral aspect of the base of the proximal phalanges but also through their more distal aponeurotic expansion. The dorsal interossei abduct the fingers, the palmar interossei adduct then. If they are paralyzed, slight lateral movement persists, because of the proximal convergence of extensor communis tendons.

The interossei muscles also play an essential role in flexion-extension movements of the three phalanges. Schematically, they flex the proximal phalanx and extend the two distal phalanges, but this extension is only possible when the MP joint is in extension. The position of the MP joint determines the application of forces of the interossei (Fig. 58-11).

The interossei also contribute to the extension of the distal phalanx. Viewed from the dorsal aspect, Stack has noted that the extensor apparatus can be seen to form a diamond figure.[22] The tendons of the interossei are attached to the lateral angles of the diamond. As they pull on these angles, the diamond becomes broader and shorter (Fig. 58-12).

Lumbrical muscles

The lumbricals are longer than the interossei, giving them a greater contractile potential, though their volume is much less than that of the palmar interossei. Unlike the interosseous muscles, the lumbrical muscles are able to extend the two distal phalanges whether the MP joint is in extension or flexion (Fig. 58-13).

The integrity of the lumbricals at the level of the index and long fingers, in cases of isolated paralysis of the ulnar nerve, is sufficient to prevent development of the claw deformity. However, this deformity is latently present even

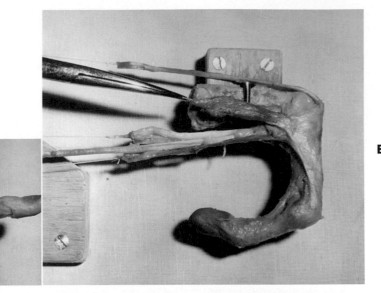

Fig. 58-11. A, When the metacarpophalangeal (MP) joint is extended, traction on the interosseous muscle extends the two distal phalanges. **B,** When the MP joint is flexed, the interosseous hood slides distal to the joint. Traction on the interosseous flexes the proximal phalanx and cannot extend the distal phalanges. (From Tubiana R: Extensor apparatus of the fingers. In Hunter JM, Schneider LH, Mackin EJ, eds: *Tendon surgery in the hand,* St Louis, 1987, Mosby.)

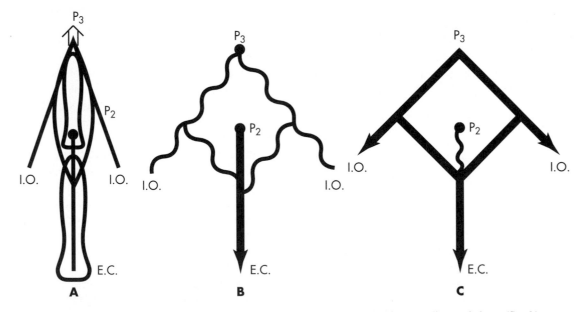

Fig. 58-12. Extension of the distal phalanx. The extensor apparatus forms a diamond shape (Stack) to the angles of which are attached the intrinsic muscles. **A,** Extensor apparatus at rest. **B,** Traction on the central extensor tendon contributes to the extension of the distal phalanx. **C,** When the intrinsic muscles contract, they widen the shape of the diamond, which is shortened. The central extensor tendon inserted on the middle phalanx is relaxed and the force of the common extensor is then completely transmitted to the distal phalanx (*EC,* extensor communis; *IO,* interosseous muscle; *P2,* middle phalanx; *P3,* distal phalanx). (From Tubiana R: Extensor apparatus of the fingers. In Hunter JM, Schneider LH, Mackin EJ, eds: *Tendon surgery in the hand,* St Louis, 1987, Mosby.)

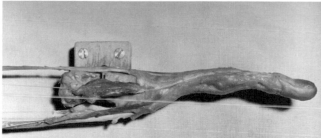
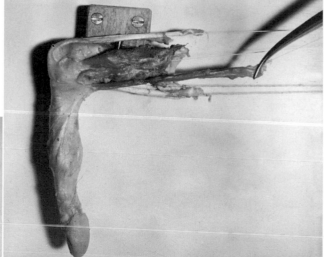

Fig. 58-13. Action of the lumbrical muscles. **A,** When the metacarpophalangeal (MP) joint is extended, traction on the lumbrical muscle extends the two distal phalanges. **B,** When the MP joint is flexed, traction on the lumbrical muscle also extends the distal phalanges. (From Tubiana R: Extensor apparatus of the fingers. In Hunter JM, Schneider LH, Mackin EJ, eds: *Tendon surgery in the hand,* St Louis, 1987, Mosby.)

though it is not exhibited. During a strong grip between the thumb, index, and long fingers, the MP joint has a tendency to hyperextend while the IP joints are hyperflexed—hyperflexion sign of Mannerfelt.[16] This latent deformation is evident when the patient is asked to flex the index and long finger MP joints while maintaining the IP joints in extension (lumbrical plus position). Slight pressure on the volar aspect of the proximal phalanx causes immediate flexion of the PIP joint. These patients are hindered in their ability to grasp small objects with precision and strength, although movements of the index and long fingers made without effort appear normal.

However, the lumbricals appear primarily to be IP extensors, following which (and only then) they could possibly act as MP flexors.[2] The action of these small slender muscles between the flexor profundus tendons and the extensor apparatus is subtle: They participate in extension of the distal phalanges by pulling distally on the flexor digitorum profundus (FDP) tendon when this muscle is at rest. As has been shown by Long,[15] this permits a reduction of the viscoelastic resistance of the flexor profundus and indirectly facilitates the action of the common extensor on the distal phalanges. Contraction of the lumbrical muscles, whose relatively free play is little impaired by attachments to the dorsal hood, also contributes directly to the extension of the distal phalanges, regardless of the position of the MP joint, whether the proximal phalanx is extended or flexed.

By contrast, the interossei muscles have a decreasing extensor effect at the IP joints as flexion of the MP joint increases. This explains why, despite their feebleness, lumbrical muscles can form an active diagonal system between the flexors and extensors at the proximal part of the finger.

Thus these muscles, which have the same innervation as the corresponding flexor profundus, play a coordinating role between the extensor and flexor systems. Rabischong[17] demonstrated the richness of the sensory receptors at their level; thus these small, weak muscles are true proprioceptive organs.

FIXED FIBROUS STRUCTURES OF THE EXTENSOR APONEUROSIS

The expansions of the extensor tendons and of the intrinsic muscles on the dorsal aspect of the finger form a veritable fibrous plexus, the extensor aponeurosis, activated at various levels by the tendinous slips of the extensor communis, the interossei, the lumbricals, and anchored by fixed fibrous structures (Fig. 58-14).

The triangular laminae is comprised of the transverse fibers arising from the medial borders of the lateral extensor tendons at the level of the middle phalanx. They form a fine triangular membrane at the apex at which the two tendons unite.

The spiral fibers curl from the lateral extensor tendons to the central tendon over the PIP joint. These fibers were described by Hauck in 1923.[11] Their action has been recently defined by Gaul[8] and by Van Zwieten.[28]

The transverse retinacular ligament is nontendinous. The fibers form a thin fibrous lamella on the lateral and dorsal surfaces of the extensor apparatus to which they adhere on either side of the PIP joint. They are attached to the skin and subcutaneous layers.

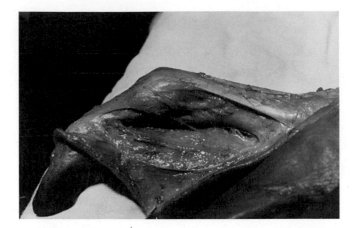

Fig. 58-14. The extensor aponeurosis.

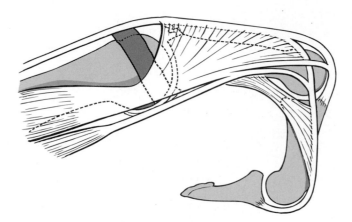

Fig. 58-15. Lateral gliding. As the proximal interphalangeal joint flexes, the lateral extensor tendons move volarly over each side of the joint.

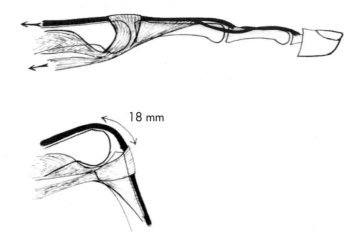

Fig. 58-16. Distal gliding. The sagittal band and the interosseous hood are displaced distally during flexion of the metacarpophalangeal joint.

The oblique retinacular ligament was identified by Weitbrecht[26] and has been described by Landsmeer.[13] This fibrous bundle extends on either side of the PIP joint and has no muscular connection.[21] These ligaments, which cross the axis of rotation of the PIP joint diagonally, are placed under tension by extension of PIP joint or by flexion of the DIP joint and act as an active tenodesis to initiate extension of the distal IP joint. This mechanical action of the oblique retinacular ligament that we tested with Valentin on cadavers[24] has been challenged by Harris and Rutledge,[9,10] because the structure and extent are variable from one finger to another in the same hand and even from one side to the other of a particular finger. If the functional value of these ligaments is probably variable and limited in normal fingers, their role becomes evident under pathologic circumstances; when thickened and contracted, they contribute to fixation of a boutonnière deformity. The same applies to the transverse retinacular ligament.

Gliding movement

Because of the nonelastic structure of the extensor aponeurosis, the lengthening, which must occur when the fingers are flexed, is achieved by gliding movement in two directions, laterally and distally.

Lateral gliding

As the PIP joint flexes, the lateral extensor tendons move volarly over each side of the joint. This lateral gliding (Fig. 58-15) is controlled by the lateral transverse structures. It is the spiral fibers that normally play the essential role in the control of coordination between the lateral tendons by virtue of their obliqueness and their combined attachment to the lateral and the central extensor tendons.

Distal gliding

The extensor apparatus glides distally in complete flexion of the MP and PIP joints between 18 and 24 mm according to the finger.

The distal gliding (Fig. 58-16) is especially important at the level of the MP joints. It is made possible and later checked by the peculiarities of the proximal insertions of the long extensor. The sagittal bands, attached into the volar plates of the MP joints, are directed obliquely forward and distally when the joint is extended. Their dorsal attachments are then proximal to the joint; in full flexion they cover the joint. The central extensor tendon is attached to the base of the proximal phalanx by means of a long, thin inconstant insertion, which is relaxed during flexion of the IP joints and is taut during extension. The interosseous hood is displaced distally during flexion. The hood covers the metacarpal head in extension but slides distal to the joint in flexion.

This gliding has important physiologic results:
1. In complete flexion of the MP and PIP joints, the extensor communis tendon fails, from this position, to control the extension of the distal phalanx. If the index and the little fingers are in complete extension and the

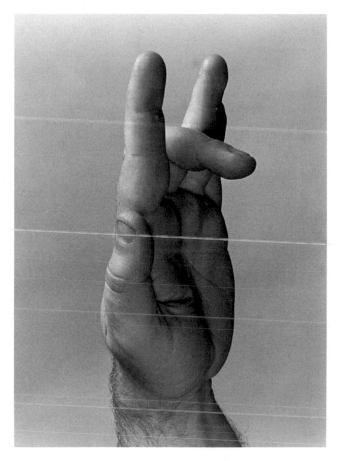

Fig. 58-17. The floating distal phalanx. When the long finger is flexed with the other fingers extended, the extensor apparatus has lost its action on the distal phalanx and the flexor profundus is neutralized by the phenomenon of quadrige. The distal phalanx floats.

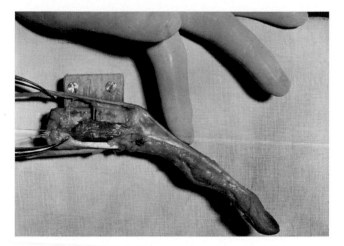

Fig. 58-18. The ulnar claw hand is corrected by stabilization in slight flexion of the metacarpophalangeal joint.

ring or middle fingers in flexion, the flexor profundus is also neutralized by the phenomenon of quadrige of Verdan and the distal phalanx is floating (Fig. 58-17).

2. The position of the MP joint determines the application of the forces of the interossei. In flexion of the MP joint, the interosseous hood slides distal to the joint, the contraction of the interossei tightens the hood against the dorsum of the proximal phalanx and increases the flexion (see Fig. 58-11).

3. In extension of the MP joint, the contraction of the interossei is transmitted via the central and lateral bands of the interosseous tendons and contributes to the extension of the distal phalanges.

Although the actions of the interossei are dependent on the position of the MP joint, they are independent of wrist movement.

Each one of the two systems, the long extensors and the intrinsics, can extend the interphalangeal articulations, provided that the MP joint cannot be put into hyperextension. The stabilization of the MP joint is normally due to the action of the intrinsics. Should they be paralyzed, the long

extensors act unopposed at the level of their proximal insertions and hyperextend the MP joint. Holding the MP joints in slight flexion, as described by Bouvier,[3] allows extension of the distal phalanges (Fig. 58-18). Various surgical procedures can prevent hyperextension of the MP joints (tendon transfers, tenodesis, capsulodesis)[29] so that the long extensors will be allowed to extend the distal phalanges.

SUMMARY

The extensor tendon system has four sites of insertion, the most proximal at the level of the interglenoid ligament or deep intermetacarpal ligament provided on each side of the metacarpophalangeal articulation by the sagittal bands, and the most distal at the level of the base of the distal phalanx. The most important insertion is that of the central tendon into the base of the middle phalanx, the insertion of the base of the proximal phalanx being inconstant. These multiple insertions at all the levels of the digital osseous chain distribute the action of the extrinsic extensor tendons to the three phalanges. However, they cannot ensure complete extension of the finger. The long extensors, whose range of movement is inferior to the range of the flexors, exhaust their action at the level of their proximal insertions, acting solely on the proximal phalanx. Nature has provided supplementary muscles, the intrinsic muscles, to relay the action of the long extensors and ensure the autonomy in extension of the two distal phalanges. The expansions of the extensor tendons and of the intrinsic muscles on the dorsal aspect of the finger form a veritable fibrous plexus, the extensor aponeurosis. This is activated at various levels by the tendons of the long extensors, the palmar and dorsal interosseous muscles, and the lumbricals and also anchored by fixed fibrous structures, such as the oblique retinacular ligaments, which act like a tenodesis. Because of the nonelastic structure of the extensor aponeurosis, the lengthening that must occur when the fingers are flexed is achieved by a gliding movement in two directions: laterally and distally.

CONCLUSION

The complex arrangement of the extensor system of the fingers allows muscles that have only a small excursion to act at each phalangeal level with a large amplitude of extension. This subtle mechanism is fragile and any lesion at one level of the digital kinetic chain may alter the balance of the whole finger.

REFERENCES

1. Albinus BS: *Historia musculorum hominis,* Leiden, 1724.
2. Backhouse KM: Functional anatomy of the hand, *Physiotherapy* 1968; 54:114-117.
3. Bouvier: Note sur un cas de paralysie de la main, *Bul Acad Med* 1851; 27:125.
4. Duchenne GB: *Physiologie des mouvements,* Paris, 1867, JB Baillière.
5. Eyler DL, Markee JE: The anatomy of the intrinsic musculature of the fingers, *J Bone Joint Surg* 1954; 36A:1.
6. Fallopio: *Observaciones anatomicae,* 1561.
7. Fowler SB: Extensor apparatus of the digits, Proceedings of the British Ortho Assoc, *J Bone Joint Surg* 1949; 31B:477.
8. Gaul SJ: *The ratio of motion of the interphalangeal joints* (unpublished report), 1971.
9. Harris C, Rutledge GL: The functional anatomy of the extensor mechanism of the finger, *J Bone Joint Surg* 1972; 54A:713-726.
10. Harris CE: Intrinsic balance of the extensor system. In Hunter JM, Schneider LH, Mackin EJ, eds: *Tendon surgery in the hand,* St Louis, 1987, Mosby.
11. Hauck G: Die Ruptur der Dorsalaponeurose am ersten Interphalangeal-gelenk; zugleich ein Beitrag zur Anotomie und Physiologie der Dorsalaponeurose, *Arch Klin Chirugie* 1923; 123:197-232.
12. Kaplan EB: *Functional and surgical anatomy of the hand,* ed 2, Philadelphia, 1965, Lippincott.
13. Landsmeer JMC: The anatomy of the dorsal aponeurosis of the human finger and its functional significance, *Anat Rec* 1949; 104:35.
14. Landsmeer JMC: The coordination of finger joint motion, *J Bone Joint Surg* 1963; 45A:1654-1662.
15. Long C, Brown ME: Electromyographic kinesiology of the hand: muscles moving the long finger, *J Bone Joint Surg* 1964; 46A:1683-1706.
16. Mannerfelt L: Studies on the hand in ulnar nerve paralysis: a clinical experimental investigation in normal and anomalous innervation, *Acta Orthop Scand* 1966; (suppl 87).
17. Rabischong P: Innervation proprioceptive des muscles lombricaux de la main chex l'homme, *Rev Chir Orthop,* 1963; 25:927.
18. Rosenthal EA: The extensor tendons. In Hunter JM, Schneider LH, Mackin EJ, Callahan AD, eds: *Rehabilitation of the hand,* ed 3, St Louis, 1990, Mosby.
19. Rouvière H: *Anatomie humaine,* Paris, 1943, Doulin.
20. Salisbury RC: The interosseous muscles of the hand, *J Anat* 1936; 71:395.
21. Shrewsbury MM, Johnson RK: A systematic study of the oblique retinacular ligament of the human finger: its structure and function, *J Hand Surg* 1977; 2:194.
22. Stack GH: Muscle function in the fingers, *J Bone Joint Surg* 1962; 44B:899-909.
23. Testut L: *Traité d'anatomice humaine,* Paris, 1896, Doulin.
24. Tubiana R: Extensor apparatus of the fingers, In Hunter JM, Schneider LH, Mackin EJ, eds: *Tendon surgery in the hand,* St Louis, 1987, Mosby.
25. Tubiana R, Valentin P: Anatomy of the extensor apparatus and the physiology of the extension of the fingers, *Surg Clin North Am* 1964; 44:897-906, 907-918.
26. Weitbrecht J: Syndesmologia sive historia ligamentorum corporis humani, quam secundum observationes anotomicas concinnavit, et figuris and objecta recentia adumbratis illustravit, *Academy of Sciences,* Petropoli, 1742.
27. Winslow JB: Exposition anatomique de la structure du corps humain, ed 2, Amsterdam, 1742.
28. Van Zwieten KJ: The extensor assembly of the finger in man and non-human primates, *Thesis,* 1980, Leiden.
29. Zancolli E: *Structural and dynamic bases of hand surgery,* ed 2, Philadelphia, 1979, Lippincott.

Chapter 59

DYNAMICS OF THE EXTENSOR SYSTEM*

Erik A. Rosenthal

The anatomic attributes of the extensor tendons are largely responsible for their functional dynamics. Composite tendon excursions, anatomic interconnections, variable moment arms, an integrated retinacular fiber system, and inflexible dependency on skeletal integrity are features that define the extensor tendon system. These attributes maintain tendon stability, integrate mobility between articulated segments, and synchronize function.

The extensor tendons that diverge distal to the extensor retinaculum display composite excursions that include longitudinal as well as transverse vectors. The juncturae tendinum link the extensor digitorum tendons and transfer forces that provide stability. The central tendon and intrinsic tendons exchange fibers about the proximal interphalangeal (PIP) joint that have dual insertions on the middle and distal phalanges; these coordinate balanced extension of the interphalangeal (IP) joints. Wrist extensor tendons acquire variable moment arms for extension, radial, and ulnar deviation that respond to forearm rotation. The lateral bands about the PIP joint level are variably effective for IP joint extension as their moments reflect PIP joint flexion and extension. Extensor tendons are modulated by a retinacular fiber system that includes the extensor retinaculum about the wrist, the sagittal bands about metacarpophalangeal (MP) joints, and transverse fibers about the PIP joint that comprise the transverse retinacular and triangular ligaments. Tension balance in the extensor tendons is exquisitely responsive to alterations in the

skeleton, particularly in the digits: Attachments at the MP, PIP, and distal interphalangeal (DIP) joints deprive the extensor tendons of the ability to self-adjust when the skeleton is angulated or foreshortened.

THE WRIST (ZONE 7)

The extensor retinaculum and contiguous fibro-osseous septa are dorsal pulleys that maintain the stations of the extensor tendons over the distal radius and ulna. The retinaculum restrains bowing during wrist extension; the septa resist displacement with radial and ulnar wrist deviation. The deep fascia distal to the extensor retinaculum exerts restraint against dorsal bowing similar to the extensor retinaculum. In the absence of the retinaculum, the dorsal fascia is the sole determinant of the distal moment of the finger extensors as the wrist extends (Fig. 59-1).

Steindler's force vector diagram, published in 1950, portrayed the direction and magnitude of extensor tendon forces relative to the axis of wrist motion.[5,14] The extensor carpi radialis longus (ECRL) has a larger moment for radial deviation but a smaller moment for wrist extension than the extensor carpi radialis brevis (ECRB). The extensor digitorum communis (EDC) has a large extension moment but a relatively small ulnar deviation moment. The extensor carpi ulnaris (ECU), the most powerful of the wrist extensor muscles, has a strong moment for ulnar deviation, but its moments are influenced by the position of forearm rotation (Fig. 59-2).

Extensor carpi radialis longus and brevis

The moment arms of the ECRL and ECRB for wrist extension and radial deviation change as the wrist moves

*The original presentation of *Dynamics of the extensor system* was dedicated to Carol W. Stoddard, OTR/L, CHT of Springfield, MA, for 20 years of leadership in developing quality hand therapy for western Massachusetts.

557

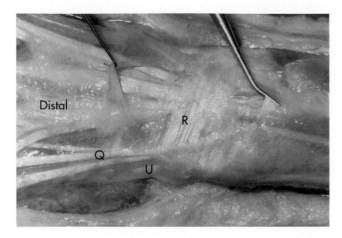

Fig. 59-1. Extensor retinaculum. The extensor retinaculum and the deep dorsal fascia of the forearm and hand function as pulleys that restrain dorsal bowing of the extensor tendons. They enhance the efficiency of extensor muscle contraction and tendon excursion. Septa beneath the extensor retinaculum fix the stations of the extensor tendons that determine their moments for extension, radial, and ulnar deviation (*R,* extensor retinaculum; *U,* extensor carpi ulnaris; *Q,* extensor digiti quinti tendons).

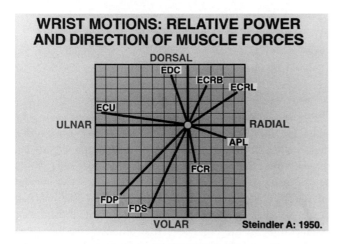

Fig. 59-2. Steindler depicted the relative power of muscles by the length of the directional moment arms. Current convention defines a muscle's relative capacity for producing tension as its *tension fraction* and is proportional to the cross-sectional area of a muscle. The ECU has a larger *tension fraction* than either the ECRL or ECRB.[6] (Adapted from Steindler A: Postgraduate lectures, vol 1, Springfield, IL, 1950, Charles C. Thomas.)

from radial extension to ulnar flexion. The ECRB has a larger moment arm than the ECRL for extension in all positions; the moment arms of both tendons decrease as the wrist ulnar deviates and flexes until the wrist is in ulnar flexion when their moment arms are smallest (Fig. 59-3). The moment arms of both tendons for radial deviation also vary with wrist position. They increase slightly as the wrist ulnar deviates. The ECRL, the more radial tendon, has a proportionally larger moment arm for radial deviation through the entire excursion (Fig. 59-4).

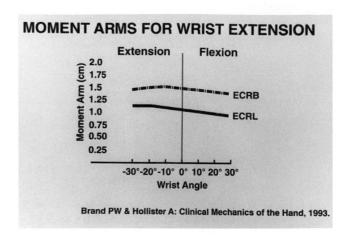

Fig. 59-3. The ECRB has a larger moment arm than the ECRL for wrist extension in all positions between radial extension and ulnar flexion. The moment arms of both tendons decrease as the wrist ulnar deviates and flexes. Their moment arms are smallest in ulnar flexion. (Adapted from Brand PW, Hollister A: *Clinical mechanics of the hand,* ed 2, St Louis, 1993, Mosby.)

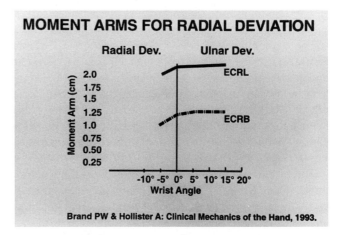

Fig. 59-4. The moment arms of both ECRL and ECRB for radial wrist deviation vary with wrist position. They increase slightly as the wrist ulnar deviates. The more radial ECRL maintains a larger moment through the entire excursion range. (Adapted from Brand PW, Hollister A: *Clinical mechanics of the hand,* ed 2, St Louis, 1993, Mosby.)

Dorsal convex anatomic pulley

The wrist extensor tendons are at a functional disadvantage for initiating wrist extension as their moment arms are progressively reduced during ulnar flexion. The dorsal proximal pole of the flexed scaphoid with the dorsal convexities of the lunate and distal radius depict a dorsal convex anatomic pulley that facilitates the initiation of wrist extension from the ulnar-flexed position. The distal radius and lunate lift the EDC; the distal radius and scaphoid lift the ECRL and ECRB. These contours enlarge the moments for wrist extension and facilitate the initiation of wrist extension[1] (Fig. 59-5).

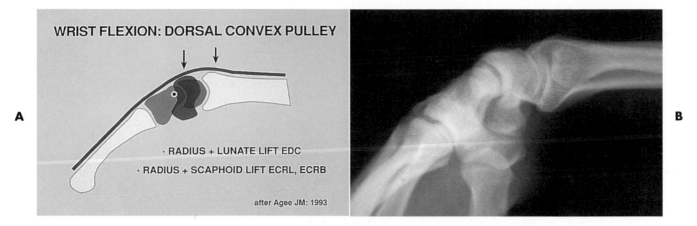

Fig. 59-5. Dorsal anatomic pulley. **A,** Schematic drawing illustrates the configuration of the dorsal anatomical pulley that enlarges the moments of the extensor digitorum communis, extensor carpi radialis longus and brevis when the wrist is in ulnar flexion. Arrow is moment arm for wrist extension (see Color Plate 6). **B,** Comparable lateral x-ray film.

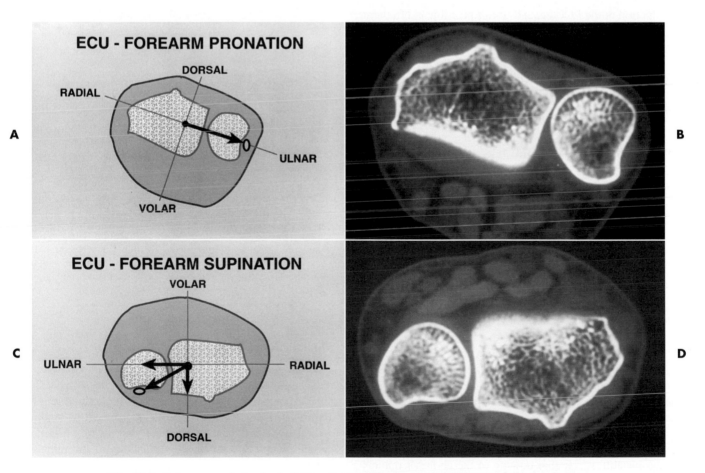

Fig. 59-6. Extensor carpi ulnaris. **A,** Schematic drawing of transaxial CT through distal radioulnar joint in forearm pronation. The extensor carpi ulnaris (ECU) has a significant moment for ulnar deviation but no significant moment for wrist extension. **B,** Comparable transaxial CT scan in pronation. **C,** Schematic drawing of transaxial CT through distal radioulnar joint in forearm supination. The ECU has a decreased moment for ulnar deviation but has acquired a significant moment for wrist extension relative to pronation. **D,** Comparable transaxial CT scan in supination.

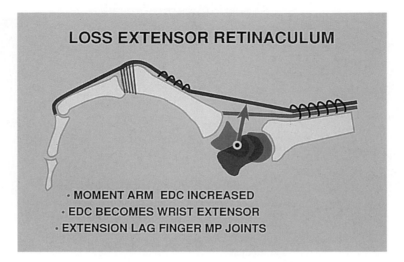

Fig. 59-7. Loss of extensor retinaculum. Schematic drawing depicting biomechanical changes associated with loss of the extensor retinaculum (see Color Plate 7).

Extensor carpi ulnaris

Function of the ECU depends on its position and forearm rotation. In forearm pronation the ECU has a large moment for ulnar deviation but no significant moment for wrist extension. When the forearm supinates, the ECU acquires a larger dorsal extension moment with a reduced moment for ulnar wrist deviation. The variable function of the ECU reflects variable moments at the wrist that depend on forearm rotation (Fig. 59-6).

Loss of extensor retinaculum

The extensor retinaculum is critical for normal function of the EDC and wrist extensor tendons. There is normally slight dorsal bowing of the ECRL and ECRB at the wrist during extension. Progression of this bowing is arrested by the tendon insertions at the bases of the second and third metacarpals. The EDC tendons, however, are not anchored to the metacarpals and bow dorsally when the extensor retinaculum is removed; their dorsal moments increase. The effective point of application of extensor forces moves distally on the metacarpals to the level of retained fascia where further bowing is restrained. The EDC then acts to extend the metacarpals and is effectively a wrist extensor. Normal excursion is dissipated in wrist extension, there is insufficient compensatory excursion for finger extension, and an extension lag of the finger MP joints is observed clinically (Fig. 59-7).

Excessive fasciotomy distal to the extensor retinaculum during surgery for deQuervain's disease may introduce tendon instability.[16] Radial bowing of the abductor pollicis longus and extensor pollicis brevis (EPB) tendons can produce exaggerated extension of the first metacarpal with an extension lag at the thumb MP joint, a deformity that is analogous to the extension lag of the finger MP joints associated with loss of the extensor retinaculum.[11]

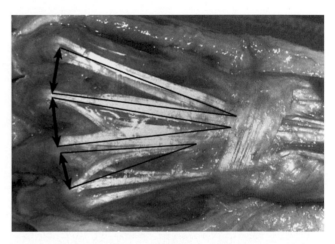

Fig. 59-8. Composite extensor tendon excursions. The extensor tendons diverge distal to the extensor retinaculum. Their composite excursions include longitudinal and transverse vectors. These excursions are influenced by the juncturae tendinum and distal attachments to the sagittal bands over the metacarpophalangeal joints.

ZONE 6
Dynamic force redistribution

The digital extensor tendons diverge distal to the extensor retinaculum relative to the axis of the third metacarpal. They display composite excursions that contain both longitudinal and transverse vectors (Fig. 59-8). The juncturae tendinum diverge distally from the EDC tendon of the ring finger, and variably connect with the EDC tendons to the remaining fingers.[15]

Agee and Guidera[2] conceived of a redistribution of dynamic forces about the dorsum of the hand by tensions transmitted by the EDC tendons through the juncturae tendinum that are secondarily transmitted to the sagittal bands on the radial and ulnar borders of the hand. They

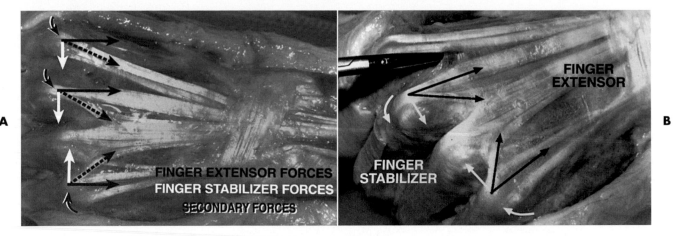

Fig. 59-9. Tension forces through extensor digitorum communis and junctural tendinum. Primary forces transmitted through the extensor digitorum tendons and juncturae tendinum result in *longitudinal extensor forces* that extend the metacarpophalangeal joints and transverse *finger stabilizer forces* that compress the metacarpals. Secondary forces are transmitted through the radial sagittal bands of the index and long fingers and ulnar sagittal bands of the small finger. **A,** Dorsum of the hand illustrating disposition of these forces. Forces through index communis tendon and juncturae tendinum from ring communis tendon are primary. **B,** Force distributions about the ulnar fingers.

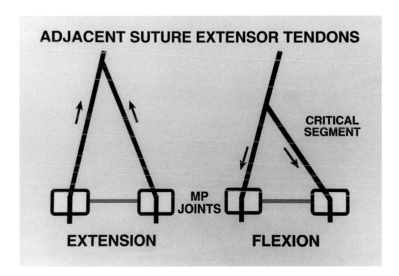

Fig. 59-10. Adjacent suture of ruptured extensor digitorum communis tendon. The critical length is the segment between the metacarpophalangeal (MP) joint of the ruptured tendon and the suture junction with the intact adjacent tendon. Tension should be adjusted with the MP joint in flexion to ensure that this segment is sufficiently long to permit flexion. A short segment will tether adjacent fingers and restrict flexion.

proposed that tension in the EDC tendon of the index finger results in two forces: a longitudinal *finger extensor force* that extends the MP joint and a smaller, ulnar-directed *finger stabilizer force* transmitted through the radial sagittal bands about the index MP joint. Similarly, forces transmitted by the EDC tendon of the ring finger through the juncturae tendinum to the EDC tendons of the long and small fingers create longitudinally directed *finger extensor forces* and transverse *finger stabilizer forces* through the radial sagittal bands of the long finger and ulnar sagittal bands of the small finger. These forces dynamically stabilize the hand. They compress the metacarpal heads centrally and oppose the tendency of the metacarpals to splay during grip[2] (Fig. 59-9).

Adjacent tendon suture

The divergent tendon pathways and composite excursions acquire clinical significance when a ruptured extensor tendon is reconstructed by adjacent suture to an intact tendon. The junction angle between the sutured tendon and intact tendon is smallest with their MP joints in extension.

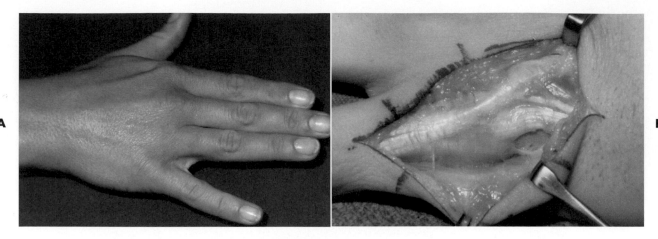

Fig. 59-11. Wartenberg's sign. **A,** Clinical appearance caused by unopposed action of abductor digiti quinti and extensor digiti in low ulnar nerve palsy with loss of third palmar interosseous muscle without claw deformity. **B,** The anatomic basis for the deformity. Extensor digiti quinti inserts with the abductor digitis quinti into the lateral tubercle of the proximal phalanx in association with an oblique juncturae tendinum from the ring finger communis tendon.

This angle increases with flexion; it is greatest when both MP joints are fully flexed. The critical length segment is between the MP joint of the ruptured tendon and the suture junction when the MP joints of both fingers are fully flexed. If this distance is shorter than that required by the functional excursions, a proximal tether will prevent flexion and interfere with normal function of these adjacent fingers (Fig. 59-10).

Wartenberg's sign

The extensor digiti quinti (EDQ) has a common insertion, with the abductor digiti quinti (ADQ) tendon, into the lateral tubercle of the base of the proximal phalanx of the small finger. Some patients with a low ulnar palsy with inherent stability of the MP joints do not develop a claw deformity but may acquire an abduction deformity of the small finger (Wartenberg's sign) because of paralysis of the third palmar interosseous muscle. Their abducted small finger is associated with an oblique junctura from the ring finger, a weak biomechanical link that leaves the EDQ relatively unopposed. Palsied patients without this deformity reportedly have a transversely oriented junctura, a biomechanically forceful link that opposes the deformity[4] (Fig. 59-11).

THE MP JOINTS (ZONE 5)

There is a linear relationship between extensor tendon excursion and MP joint angle.[3] The position of the EDC tendons over the finger MP joints is controlled by the sagittal bands. Ulnar displacement of the extensor tendon is more likely in the middle finger where the attachment of the tendon to the underlying sagittal bands is tenuous compared with the other fingers. The forces required to stabilize the extensor tendon at the level of the MP joint decrease normally during the initial 60° of flexion and then increase

slightly. If the tendon is displaced, however, there is a linear acceleration in the amount of force necessary to stabilize the tendon with progressive flexion. Propagation of an imbalance is fostered by the imbalance itself. Attenuation of radial sagittal bands with ulnar displacement of the extensor tendon establishes a situation that demands considerably more force to counteract the deformity than is required to sustain equilibrium in the normal state without deformity[8] (Fig. 59-12).

PROXIMAL PHALANX AND PIP JOINT (ZONES 3 AND 4)
Lateral band shift

Lateral band shift adjusts tensions between the intrinsic and extrinsic tendons, compensates for the different radius of the PIP and DIP joints, and permits balanced extension of the IP joints. Extension of the IP joints is partly interdependent because of the double insertions of the intrinsic and extrinsic tendons on the base of the middle and distal phalanges.[13] If lateral band shift were blocked by scar from trauma or surgical tenodesis, IP extension would then become totally interdependent. The extensor moment arms of the PIP and DIP joints have been estimated at 0.75 cm and 0.50 cm, respectively; the PIP joint is approximately one-third larger.[7] Joint motion, for a given tendon excursion, is proportional to the radius of the joint. If lateral band shift is blocked, 60° PIP joint extension would accompany 80° extension at the DIP joint, with awkward functional implications (Fig. 59-13). Normally, however, the PIP joint has approximately 110° of motion, and the DIP joint has approximately 60° of motion. It is the lateral band shift that permits this adjustment and balances forces between the larger PIP and smaller DIP joints.

Normal shift of the lateral bands is influenced by numerous factors. These include the trapezoidal slope of the

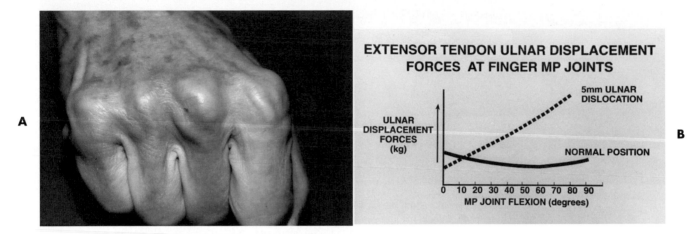

Fig. 59-12. Stability of the extensor tendon by the sagittal bands over the finger metacarpophalangeal (MP) joint. **A,** Clinical appearance of ulnar subluxation of the extensor digitorum communis tendon. **B,** Ulnar displacement forces normally decrease slightly through the initial 60° of flexion. There is a linear acceleration of ulnar displacement forces by the ulnar displaced extensor tendon as the MP joint flexes.

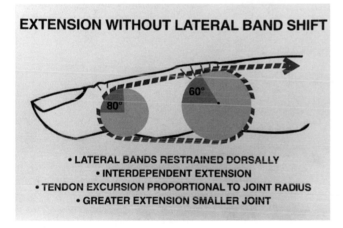

Fig. 59-13. Interdependent extension of interphalangeal (IP) joints. Dorsal scarring or surgical tenodesis of the lateral bands creates interdependent extension of the IP joints that is proportional to the radius of each joint for a given tendon excursion.

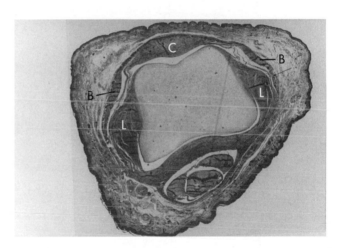

Fig. 59-14. Trapezoid configuration of the proximal phalanx. The lateral slopes of the proximal phalanx are raised by the bulges of the collateral ligaments. This configuration facilitates ascent and resists descent of the lateral bands during extension and flexion of the interphalangeal joints (*B,* Lateral band; *L,* collateral ligament; *C,* central tendon).

PIP joint, the retinacular ligaments, interconnections between the intrinsic and extrinsic tendons, a crisscross fabric arrangement of the extensor mechanism about the proximal phalanx, and variable moment arms about the PIP joint.

Trapezoidal proximal phalanx. The head of the proximal phalanx depicts a trapezoid on cross-section; the broader palmar surface slopes dorsally.[9] The bulk of the collateral ligament within the sulcus on each side alters the slope and surface contour and influences displacement of the lateral band. This physical configuration modulates descent and facilitates ascent of the lateral bands during flexion and extension of the PIP joint, respectively (Fig. 59-14).

Retinacular ligaments. The retinacular system about the PIP joint consists of transversely oriented, contiguous fibers that originate from the flexor fibro-osseous sheath and

encircle the finger dorsally. Fibers palmar to the lateral bands, the transverse retinacular ligaments, regulate lateral band ascent during PIP joint extension. Fibers dorsal to the lateral bands, the distal fibers of which comprise the triangular ligament, restrict descent of the lateral bands during flexion (Fig. 59-15).

Crisscross extensor fibers. Schultz described a two-layered fabric arrangement consisting of superficial extrinsic and deep intrinsic fibers that comprise the extensor tendons about the proximal phalanx. The fiber layers move, one on the other, as the finger flexes and extends. The delicate panoply of fibers intersect at approximately 30° in extension. The fabric unfolds as the lateral bands shift palmar during flexion and the angle between the extrinsic and intrinsic

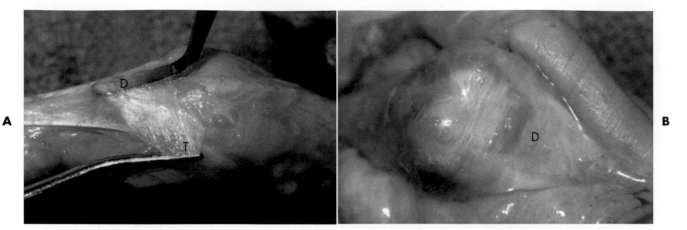

Fig. 59-15. Retinacular ligaments about the proximal interphalangeal joints. **A,** Fibers palmar to the lateral bands, the transverse retinacular ligaments, are contiguous with dorsal fibers. Palmar fibers restrict ascent and dorsal fibers restrict descent of the lateral bands during IP extension and flexion, respectively. **B,** Distal, dorsal fibers comprise the triangular ligament (*T,* Transverse retinacular ligament; *D,* triangular ligament).

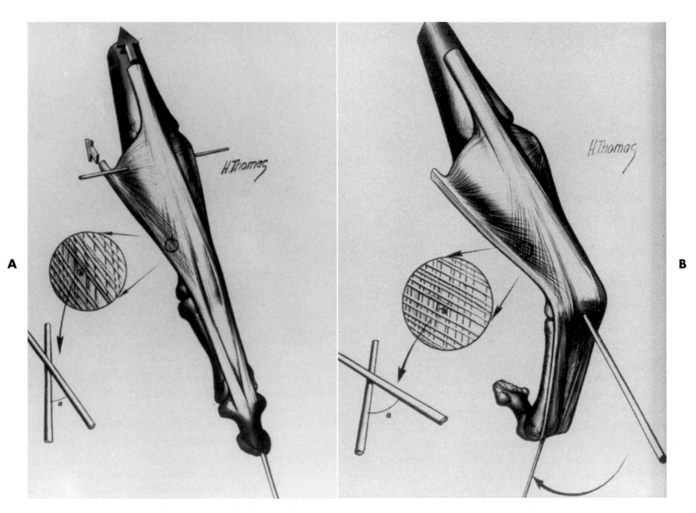

Fig. 59-16. Fabric arrangement of the extensor mechanism about the proximal phalanx. The delicate fibers of the extrinsic and intrinsic tendons form a layered fabric about the proximal phalanx. This geometric arrangement may influence lateral band migration. **A,** In extension the angle between the superficial extrinsic and deeper intrinsic fibers approximates 30°. **B,** In flexion the angle between the fibers approaches 50°. (*A* and *B* from: Schultz RJ, Furlong J II, Storace A: Detailed anatomy of the extensor mechanism at the proximal aspect of the finger, *J Hand Surg* 1981; 6A:498.)

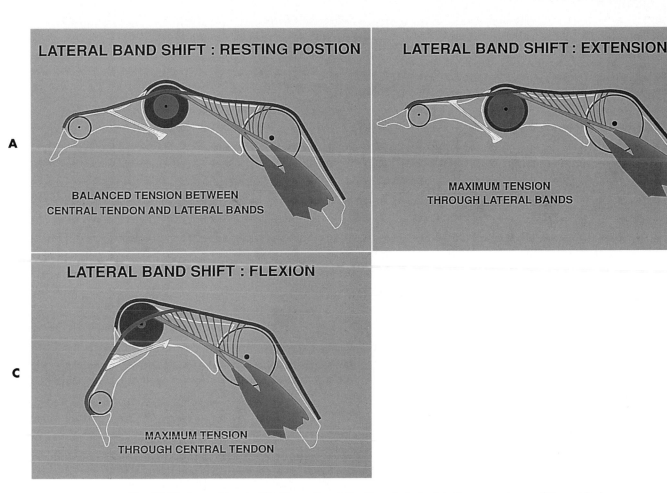

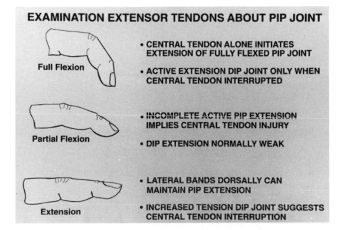

Fig. 59-17. Lateral band shift. The radius of the blue circle depicts the moment arm of the extrinsic central tendon for extension of the proximal interphalangeal (PIP) joint. The radius of the green circle depicts the moment arm of the lateral band for extension of the PIP joint. **A,** There is balanced tension between the central tendon and lateral bands in the resting position. **B,** Tension through the lateral bands increases with interphalangeal (IP) extension as their moments enlarge. Tension and the moment for extension of both IP joints is greatest in full extension. **C,** The moments of the lateral bands decrease during flexion as the moment for extension by the central tendon increases. Only the central tendon can initiate extension of the fully flexed PIP joint normally (see Color Plates 8, 9, and 10.)

Fig. 59-18. Clinical examination of extensor tendons about the proximal interphalangeal joint. Facets of the examination apply the biomechanical attributes illustrated in Fig. 59-17.

fibers increases to 50°. The delicate individuality of this fiber system is a marvel of anatomic design. This action of the crisscross fiber pattern, by altering the geometric arrangement between extrinsic and intrinsic extensor tendon fibers, may regulate displacement of the lateral bands[12] (Fig. 59-16).

Variable moment arms. In the resting position there is balanced tension between the central tendon and the lateral bands that maintain relative positioning of the PIP and DIP joints. A balance exists between extrinsic and intrinsic tendons. There is an increase in tension through the lateral bands as they shift dorsally during extension. The moment for PIP extension increases and, concurrently, the potential for DIP extension also increases. In the extended position, there is maximum tension through the lateral bands. As the finger flexes, the moment for lateral band extension of the PIP joint decreases while the moment of the central tendon for extension of the PIP joint increases progressively. In flexion there is maximum tension through the central tendon. Only the central tendon can initiate extension of the flexed PIP joint; the central tendon weakly influences DIP extension in this position. The lateral bands are incapable of initiating extension of the flexed PIP joint and have little control of DIP extension in this position (Fig. 59-17).

CLINICAL APPLICATION

These anatomic and biomechanical observations can be applied in the clinical setting. When an injured PIP joint is examined to ascertain the status of the central tendon or the lateral bands, the digit should be examined in three positions: full flexion, partial flexion, and extension. In full PIP joint flexion, the central tendon alone can initiate PIP joint extension. The lateral bands are lax, have no potential for PIP joint extension, and are loosely connected to the DIP joint, which permits distal joint flexion. Active DIP joint extension only occurs in this position when the central tendon has been interrupted and the entire extensor mechanism has shifted proximally, transferring tension to the DIP joint. With the finger in partial flexion, there is weak or incomplete DIP extension unless the central tendon has been interrupted. Distal joint extension normally is weak with the finger in partial flexion. In full extension, the lateral bands are dorsal and can maintain extension. Even a single lateral band can maintain extension if it is positioned dorsally. Increased extension tension at the DIP joint—relative to adjacent fingers—with the PIP joint in extension suggests that the central tendon has been injured and the extensor tendons have displaced proximally[10,11] (Fig. 59-18).

REFERENCES

1. Agee JM: Mechanics of tendons that cross the wrist. In Brand PW, Hollister A, eds: *Clinical mechanics of the hand,* ed 2, St Louis, 1993, Mosby.

2. Agee JM, Guidera M: The functional significance of the juncturae tendinum in dynamic stabilization of the metacarpophalangeal joints of the fingers, *J Hand Surg* 1980; 5:288.

3. An KN, Ueba Y, Chao EY, et al: Tendon excursion and moment arm of index finger muscles, *J Biomechanics* 1983; 16:419.

4. Blacker GJ, Lister GD, Kleinert HE: The abducted little finger in low ulnar palsy, *J Hand Surg* 1976; 1:190-196.

5. Boyes JH: *Bunnell's surgery of the hand,* ed 4, Philadelphia, 1964, Lippincott.

6. Brand PW, Beach RB, Thompson DE: Relative tension and potential excursion of muscles in the forearm and hand, *J Hand Surg* 1981; 6:209-219.

7. Brand PW, Hollister A: *Clinical mechanics of the hand,* ed 2, St Louis, 1993, Mosby.

8. Kettlekemp DB, Flatt AE, Moulds R: Traumatic dislocation of the long finger extensor tendon: a clinical, anatomical and biomechanical study, *J Bone Joint Surg* 1971; 53A:229-240.

9. Landsmeer JMF: *Atlas of anatomy of the hand,* London, 1976, Churchill Livingstone, p. 191.

10. Riordan DC: Discussion. In Dobyns JH, Chase RA, Amadio PC, eds: *Year book of hand surgery,* Chicago, 1988, Year Book Medical publishers, p. 68.

11. Rosenthal EA: The extensor tendons: anatomy and management. In Hunter JM, Mackin EJ, Callahan AD, eds: *Rehabilitation of the hand: surgery and therapy,* ed 4, vol I, St Louis, 1996, Mosby.

12. Schulz RJ, Furlong J II, Storace A: Detailed anatomy of the extensor mechanism at the proximal aspect of the finger, *J Hand Surg* 1981; 6:493.

13. Smith RJ: Balance and kinetics of the fingers under normal and pathological conditions, *Clin Orthop Rel Res* 1974; 104:92.

14. Steindler A: *Post graduate lectures,* vol 1, Springfield, IL, 1950, Thomas.

15. Wehbé MA: Junctura anatomy, *J Hand Surg* 1992; 17A:1124.

16. White GM, Weiland AJ: Symptomatic palmar tendon subluxation after surgical release for deQuervain's disease: a case report, *J Hand Surg* 1984; 9A:704.

Chapter 60

TREATMENT OF ACUTE EXTENSOR TENDON INJURIES

Robert Lee Wilson
Frank Fleming

Injuries to the extensor tendons of the fingers and the thumb occur more frequently than to the flexors. The extensors have a superficial location and a minimal amount of soft tissue protection. However, these features predispose the dorsal tendons to involvement following lacerations as well as crush and abrasion injuries. Extensor tendon trauma may be associated with skin and soft tissue loss and can occur after open fractures and burns. Unless the patient has received prompt and appropriate treatment, injuries to the extensor mechanism can result in lost motion, lengthy morbidity, and weakness.

The anatomy and physiology of the extensor apparatus has been discussed in a previous chapter. Important articles that have expanded our knowledge of extensor tendon anatomy and function should be known to all treating these problems.[9,25,38-40,46,54] A few points pertaining to tendon injuries will be mentioned. The juncturae tendinum are intertendinous connections that run distally from the ring finger common extensor tendon to the middle and little finger tendons. There are several anomalies of the juncturae described in the literature,[43] a knowledge of which is important in the reconstruction and repair of extensor tendon injuries. If the extensor digitorum communis tendon to the little finger is absent, the extensor digiti quinti proprius receives a junctura from the ring finger.[37] Division of a common extensor tendon proximal to a junctura may allow full extension of the finger and can mask the seriousness of the injury.[48] Similarly, partial injuries to the extensor mechanism at any level may not become apparent initially, but at a later stage a deformity will manifest itself. In the intervening period the interconnections of the extrinsic and intrinsic systems may partially, but incompletely, compensate for these injuries.

Extension of the interphalangeal (IP) joints is carried out by the efforts of both the extrinsic and intrinsic tendons. All of the intrinsics pass volar to the axis of the metacarpophalangeal (MP) joint, dorsal to the axis of the IP joints, and interconnect with the extrinsic extensor tendons. The intrinsics include the four lumbricals and seven interossei. The lumbrical muscles originate from the profundus tendons in the palm and progress on the palmar aspect of the deep transverse metacarpal ligament to insert into the dorsal aponeurosis on the radial side of each finger. The principal function of the lumbricals is IP joint extension. With lumbrical relaxation, the profundus advances proximally allowing IP joint flexion. Should the profundus tendon be lacerated in the finger, the lumbrical retracts along with the proximal profundus. With profundus muscle contraction, the lumbrical transmits force to the dorsal apparatus causing extension of the IP joints rather than flexion. This paradoxical action has been described as a lumbrical-plus finger[30] and is representative of the imbalances that can occur in the tendon system.

The important factors when managing extensor tendon injuries are the anatomic characteristics of the area, the correct position of immobilization, and postinjury remobilization. Because the nature of extensor tendon anatomy varies throughout the hand, it is necessary to classify tendon trauma[17] as occurring in various zones (Fig. 60-1). Numbers have been assigned beginning distally with the odd numbers overlying each of the joints and the even numbers overlying the intermediate segments. The subsequent descriptions

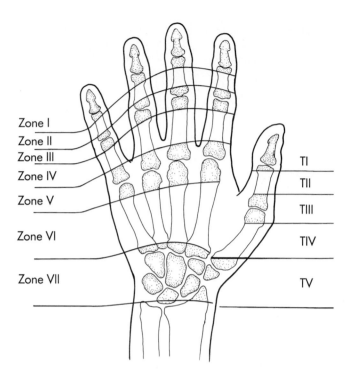

Fig. 60-1. Classification of extensor tendon injury by zones. (From Wilson RL: Management of acute extensor tendon injuries. In Hunter JM, Schneider LH, Mackin EJ, eds: *Tendon surgery in the hand,* St Louis, 1987, Mosby; with permission.)

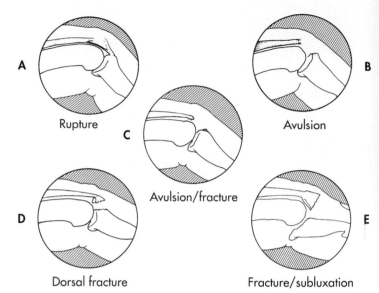

Fig. 60-2. Mallet injuries. **A,** Attenuation of rupture. **B,** Avulsion. **C,** Avulsion fracture. **D,** Dorsal fracture. **E,** Fracture/subluxation. (From Wilson RL: Management of acute extensor tendon injuries. In Hunter JM, Schneider LH, Mackin EJ, eds: *Tendon surgery in the hand,* St Louis, 1987, Mosby; with permission.)

will use these zones to discuss patterns of injury, repair techniques, and rehabilitation. Postoperative treatment can be simplified by treating tendon injuries occurring between the joints in a manner similar to those at the next most distal level.[51] For instance, an extensor tendon divided over the middle phalanx (zone II) will be managed postinjury in the same fashion as one injured at the distal interphalangeal joint (DIP) (zone I).

ZONE I—DIP JOINT

Disruption of the terminal extensor tendon at the distal joint of the finger can produce a flexion deformity at the DIP joint. This familiar lesion is known by several synonyms, including mallet finger, dropped tip finger, and baseball finger (Fig. 60-2). Mallet deformities may be classified as closed, open, those associated with fractures, or as pathologic.[52] Closed mallet injuries are the most common and are produced by sudden acute forceful flexion of the DIP joint while the proximal interphalangeal (PIP) joint is held in active extension. This may occur in a variety of sports or occupational activities. Disruption of the tendon can also occur after trivial trauma such as flicking a cigarette ash or tucking in bed sheets, and it may be explained by the relative avascularity in the distal aspect of the extensor tendon mechanism.[49] The sex and age incidence of mallet finger vary somewhat, depending on the population. However, generally speaking, in males it usually occurs in the younger

ages (11 to 40 years) and in females the incidence is usually in the older age groups (41 to 60 years).[1,34]

The tendon rupture in closed mallet injuries can occur within its substance or be avulsed from the distal insertion. The resulting deformity can vary from a few degrees of extension lag to a 75° drop. With partial or incomplete tears, the initial minimal loss of extension may become progressively worse with further trauma or active distal joint flexion. Although the finger deformity occurs immediately in some cases, the drop may be delayed by hours or days.

In closed mallet finger deformities, occasionally the tendon is avulsed with a small bone fragment from the distal phalanx. The piece of bone attached to the tendon will retract and may serve as a marker to determine the distance that the tendon has retracted. A mallet finger injury may be associated with a swan-neck deformity. This is most notable in individuals that have laxity at the middle joint level. PIP joint hyperextension is produced as the extension forces from the extrinsic and intrinsic tendons concentrate their power at the PIP joint.

The treatment of choice for closed injuries is continuous immobilization of the DIP joint in extension for 4 to 6 weeks, followed by 2 additional weeks of night splinting. There are a number of splinting regimens and materials described for this treatment. Regardless of which method is chosen, it must be remembered that, with as little as 15° of hyperextension, blanching of the skin over the DIP joint occurs and prolonged splinting in this position may result in tissue ischemia.

The most common method used in the immobilization of mallet injuries involves splinting of the DIP joint in extension. This may be done using an aluminum splint with foam padding, either on the dorsal or volar aspect of the middle and distal phalanx or using prefabricated plastic splints. Whether the PIP joint as well as the distal joint is to be included in the splint has been a matter of controversy. Bunnell recommended immobilizing the PIP joint in flexion, while extending the DIP joint to allow for advancement of the lateral bands and approximation of the torn extensor tendon at the DIP joint. Most authors have not found it necessary to immobilize the PIP joint in the treatment of mallet finger. McFarland and Hampole[21] reviewed 50 cases of mallet finger treated by immobilizing only the DIP joint in extension and had an 80% rate of excellent to good results. This treatment method may be successful, even if the patient presents up to 6 months following the injury. It is believed that splinting the DIP joint in extension, even at this late date, promotes scar contracture about the ruptured tendon, resulting in correction of the deformity.

The method of involving both the PIP and DIP joints in a plaster splint may be useful in certain cases when the patient is unreliable or unable to consistently apply the removable splint correctly. Of concern, however, is the potential for a PIP joint flexion contracture, which may prove difficult to correct.

Another option for closed injuries is K-wire fixation of the distal joint to provide internal immobilization. This was described by Cassels and Strange in 1957,[5] who placed their K-wire in a longitudinal fashion. This method was modified by Tubiana[47] in which he recommended oblique placement of the transarticular K-wire to avoid fibrous scarring of the pulp. Placing the K-wire in an oblique fashion also permits removal of the K-wire at its proximal aspect as it exits the cortex of the middle phalanx and allows the distal aspect of the K-wire to remain at the distal edge of the cortex of the distal phalanx, thus minimizing irritation. This method of treatment is usually reserved for surgeons and dentists. Potential complications include pin-track infections, osteomyelitis, and pin breakage.

Operative repair of closed mallet injuries has been described. The operative complication rate is over 50%,[45] and the results are no better than closed management, therefore, making surgical treatment of closed injuries a rarely indicated procedure. The only routine reason for opening acute closed deformities is an associated major articular fracture, which is discussed later.

Another management option is no treatment at all. In some cases, the mallet deformity causes no functional problem to the patient and, in fact, depending on the patient's occupation, the possible loss of full DIP joint flexion after the prolonged period of extension splinting could result in decreased function.[3]

Open mallet deformities are an indication for surgical treatment. If there is a cuff of distal tendon present, the tendon ends may be approximated alone or the injury may be treated by suturing the skin and tendon together as a single unit. If gross contamination exists, the wound should be left open and the tendon problem treated by splinting alone.

Open injuries may be produced by abrasion with loss of skin and tendon. Treatment of these injuries may involve skin grafting, tendon grafting, or local skin flaps over a tendon graft.[16] The fourth option in such cases may involve DIP joint fusion.

A bone fragment may be avulsed along with the terminal extensor tendon. Larger fragments, involving between 20% to 50% of the dorsal articular surface, need to be carefully evaluated. These can often be adequately treated closed with a splinting program.[50] A lateral x-ray film of the digit, with the splint in place, will confirm the position of the fracture fragment relative to the remaining distal phalanx and the joint. Open reduction of the fracture is technically exacting and often frustrating. This is perhaps only indicated when a large fragment is displaced more than 2 mm in association with a significant flexion deformity or volar subluxation of the distal phalanx.[26]

In children, mallet deformities are frequently associated with transepiphysial fractures. The treatment of these injuries involves closed reduction with splinting for 3 to 4 weeks.

Mallet deformities are frequently seen in patients with rheumatoid arthritis. This may be due to synovitis at the DIP joint producing attenuation of the extensor mechanism or as a part of the swan-neck deformity. The causes of a swan-neck deformity in a rheumatoid patient are multiple and treatment is decided after first assessing the causes.[53]

A review of the results following treatment of mallet deformities shows that 75% of the patients will have an extensor lag of 15° or less. Although reconstruction procedures are recognized for the management of more severe deformities, the best advice for the mild extensor lag is acceptance.[47]

ZONE II—MIDDLE PHALANX

Injuries to the extensor mechanism in this area are usually caused by lacerations or crushing trauma. Partial lacerations involving less than 50% of the tendon can be treated with skin closure, splinting, and active motion after 7 to 10 days. Even with greater involvement of the extensor apparatus, if the oblique retinacular ligament has been preserved, there will be no lag at the distal joint when attempting to extend both IP joints. Complete lacerations of the extensor tendon mechanism in zone II should be treated with operative tendon repair, followed by the same splinting and remobilization regimen as zone I injuries. However, extensor tendon loss in zone II presents an additional problem: If the tendon is approximated end to end, this will result in

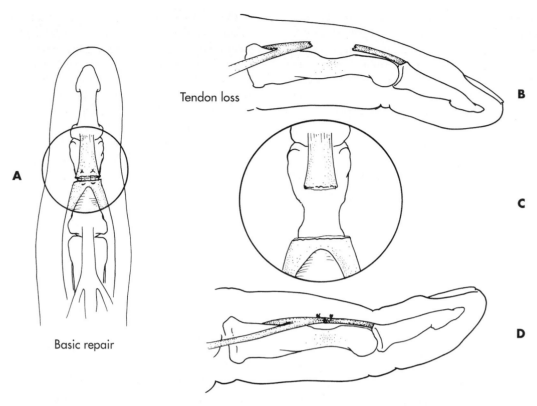

Tendon loss

Basic repair

Fig. 60-3. In zone II, an incised extensor tendon is repaired end-to-end with sutures, **A,** with extensor tendon loss from a laceration, **B** and **C,** approximation of the tendon will limit joint flexion, **D.** (From Wilson RL: Management of acute extensor tendon injuries. In Hunter JM, Schneider LH, Mackin EJ, eds: *Tendon surgery in the hand,* St Louis, 1987, Mosby; with permission.)

hyperextension of the DIP joint, which will never flex sufficiently afterward (Fig. 60-3). Treatment options include a flexor tendon graft or a proximally based tendon flap to bridge the area of tendon loss,[41] or a distal joint fusion.

ZONE III

An open or closed injury to the extensor mechanism at the PIP joint can result in the boutonnière deformity. Division, avulsion, or attenuation of the central slip is followed by a tearing of the dorsal extensor apparatus. The head of the proximal phalanx then buttonholes through the dorsal defect. This allows the lateral bands to shift volar to the PIP joint axis. The extensor forces are then focused entirely on the DIP joint, resulting in hyperextension at this level. Untreated, the retinacular ligaments become contracted, resulting in fixation of the displaced lateral bands in a volar position. The boutonnière deformity may not appear immediately, because all of the components may not be injured completely or to the same degree.[22] In fact, it may develop slowly over 10 to 21 days. The usual scenario develops after sudden forceful PIP joint flexion or blunt trauma producing a hemarthrosis and resulting in central slip laxity. Diagnostic clues to a central slip injury include a 15° to 20° extensor lag at the PIP joint, with the wrist and MP joints fully flexed, or weak extension versus resistance. If the patient maintains full PIP

and DIP joint extension, this indicates that at least one lateral band is functioning. If the patient can slowly extend the PIP joint from 90° of flexion against resistance, this means that the central slip is intact.[12] Boutonnière injuries are notoriously difficult to treat. The factors associated with the worst prognosis (a fixed PIP contracture, age greater than 45 years, associated fracture or prior surgery) should be recognized.[44] All open injuries, even partial division of the central tendon or lateral bands, require repair and immobilization. Boutonnière deformities are most commonly secondary to closed, blunt trauma, associated with acute forceful flexion at the PIP joint that produces avulsion or rupture of the central extensor tendon slip from its middle phalanx. Closed boutonnière injuries that present with an extension lag of 45° or less at the PIP joint should initially be treated closed, with the PIP joint maintained in full extension for 4 to 5 weeks. During this time, the distal joint is actively moved to prevent lateral band adherence.[51] A variety of splints have been devised to achieve PIP joint extension, including plaster cylinder casts, metal or plastic splints, and dynamic splints.

Indications for operative intervention in closed injuries include individuals with a significant extensor lag, an avulsion fracture of the middle phalanx base, and some volar PIP dislocations. The patient with an extensor lag greater than 60°, associated with an injury of significant force, will probably have complete disruption of the entire extensor mechanism at the PIP joint. This injury is not amenable to conservative treatment. Another indication for exploration of an acute, closed boutonnière injury, is when the PIP joint cannot be fully extended passively or remains dislocated volarly. Surgical exploration will usually reveal displacement of a lateral band volar to a proximal phalanx condyle and central slip avulsion. Surgical repair of the injured tendons and supporting structures is the appropriate treatment.

Another indication for operative treatment after closed injuries is when the central slip has been avulsed with a bone fragment, which remains displaced from its insertion at the dorsum of the middle phalanx. In this case, the surgical treatment entails excision of the small fragment and reattachment of the central slip. The repair is protected with a transarticular wire and continuous splinting of the PIP joint in full extension, with active flexion of the distal joint.[20] Depending on whether the size of the fracture is sufficient, the fragment may be reattached to the middle phalanx.

Besides damage to the central slip and lateral bands at this level, collateral ligament and volar plate injuries may be seen with anterior or volar dislocations of the PIP joint. Because of the extensive soft tissue trauma seen with these injuries, Spinner and Choi[42] have recommended gradual remobilization of the PIP joint after 3 weeks of rest in extension to minimize joint stiffness. Open treatment of these injuries may not be necessary if closed reduction is achieved. However, interposition of tissue (lateral band, collateral ligament) will render the joint irreducible and open reduction with tissue retraction and repair is required.[53]

Lacerations at the middle joint level are likely to involve the PIP joint space, and treatment must be directed to preventing infection with adequate cleansing and aeration of the joint. The central slip and the lateral bands should be repaired primarily, and the repair protected with a transarticular wire for 4 to 6 weeks. Again, as in closed injuries, the distal joint is actively flexed to maintain motion of the lateral bands. Saldana has described dynamic splinting for these injuries and demonstrated a significantly shorter rehabilitation period.[35]

Loss of tendon substance at the PIP joint level is usually associated with loss of soft tissue coverage. Reconstruction of the tendon may be accomplished using a retrograde extensor flap,[41] a lateral band repair as described by Aiche,[2] or a free tendon graft.[51] The repair should be protected with a transarticular wire. Soft tissue coverage may then be accomplished using a cross-finger or distant flap. After the wire is removed, remobilization of the PIP joint and extensor tendon is begun. Initially, emphasis should be placed on PIP joint extension. The patient is advised to first relax the involved finger and then to actively extend the middle joint. A volar splint is worn for protection until active flexion exercises are begun at 6 weeks. If an extension lag occurs at any time, the finger is splinted in extension for another 2

weeks or longer. A patient over 50 years of age or those who have formed a dense immobile scar should have the immobilization time shortened by 1 to 2 weeks.

McCue[23] has described a condition having an appearance similar to a boutonnière deformity but having different causation, such as a pseudo boutonnière deformity. Rather than an injury to the extensor mechanism, a pseudo boutonnière deformity is caused by PIP joint hyperextension with an injury to the volar plate's proximal attachment and the collateral ligaments. Examination of these patients will reveal a PIP flexion contracture and slight residual hyperextension at the distal joint. When the PIP joint is passively extended to its maximum, complete active and passive DIP flexion is still present. In contrast, when an injury to the extensor mechanism happens and the same test is performed, neither active nor passive DIP flexion can occur. There may be radiologic evidence of calcification near the volar plate's proximal attachment. Treatment to correct this problem, if necessary, involves a volar PIP joint capsulotomy.

ZONE IV—PROXIMAL PHALANX

Most tendon injuries in zone IV over the proximal phalanx are partial, but can affect the extensor mechanism's tendon balance (Fig. 60-4). Isolated lateral band injuries should be repaired, then remobilized with protective splinting. For complete division of the extensor apparatus in zone IV, treatment consists of operative repair, followed by immobilization for 4 to 5 weeks. The postinjury exercise program for zone IV injuries is the same as that for zone III injuries. Care must be taken not to stretch out the healing tendon, because a permanent extension lag might occur. Two problems can arise after dorsal injuries in the fingers. The first is the formation of an exostosis following closed blunt or deep open injuries over the proximal phalanx. Bone enlargement increases tension on the extensor mechanism, eventually assuming the shape of a turret. Patients demonstrate pain with motion and decreased finger flexion. Treatment of a turret exostosis can be directed at the bone, with removal of the lesion. However, symptoms may also be relieved by a tendon release alone.[51] A second problem following dorsal digital injury is extensor adherence over the proximal phalanx. This may occur after an open fracture, and in turn may prevent full digital flexion. Littler has reported that a partial resection of the extensor mechanism over the proximal phalanx with separation of the intrinsics from the extrinsic system may allow increased finger motion. He has shown that only one lateral band is needed to extend the PIP joint.[19] Large central extensor tendon defects may be bridged with a tendon graft.

Conventional extensor tendon rehabilitation following injuries in this zone consists of splinting in full extension for a period of 4 to 5 weeks postinjury. Remobilization is started in the fifth postoperative week, beginning with gentle extension and rest periods in extension. During the sixth week, active flexion is encouraged, as well as continuation

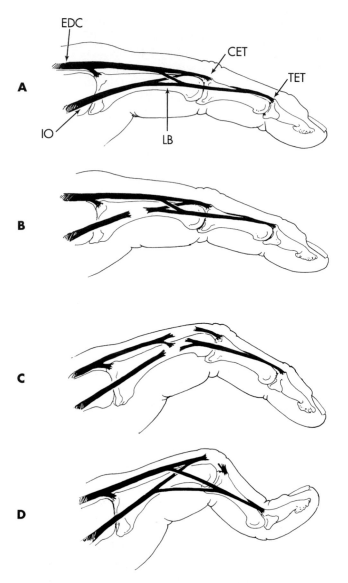

Fig. 60-4. Extensor tendon injuries in zones III and IV. **A,** Normal anatomy; extensor digitorum communis *(EDC),* central extensor tendon *(CET),* interosseous tendon *(IO),* lateral band *(LB),* terminal extensor tendon *(TET).* **B,** Isolated lateral band injury. **C,** Complete division extensor mechanism. **D,** Central tendon injury with boutonniere deformity.

of extension splinting. After 8 weeks, use of a splint is discontinued and therapy is directed at achieving full flexion in the injured digit. During the seventh and eighth weeks postoperatively, if an extension lag develops, the digit is then splinted for 2 additional weeks.

Recently, there has been increased interest in immediate postoperative motion for the rehabilitation of extensor tendon repairs. The electrophysiologic basis for dynamic splinting, after flexor tendon repair, may be extrapolated to dynamic splinting after extensor tendon repair.[28] Evans and Thompson have described the short arc of motion (SAM) program.[15] An additional set of parameters was established regarding range of motion during postoperative rehabilita-

tion. This allows for sufficient tendon excursion without compromising the repair and improved range of motion both initially and at the end of the treatment program.

ZONE V—MP JOINT

Injuries to the extensor mechanism at the MP joint are often open injuries. These are technically easy to repair because proximal tendon retraction is prevented by the sagittal bands and juncturae. The wrist should be immobilized in at least 45° of extension to take tension off of the repair[8,24] and the MP joint rested in 15° to 20° of flexion. After 3½ to 4 weeks, the digit and tendon are rapidly remobilized. A secondary tenolysis at this level is rarely required. Other injuries to the extensor mechanism at this level can be caused by human bite wounds and a high index of suspicion should be present when examining lacerations in this area. If a human bite is suspected, the wound should be extended, the joint debrided and left open.

Lacerations to the extensor hood or sagittal bands at this level should be repaired to prevent subluxation of the extensor tendon in a radial or ulnar direction. Displacement of the extensor tendon from its central location may be associated with an extensor lag. Closed sagittal band injuries may also occur spontaneously or secondary to blunt trauma.[18] Rupture of the sagittal fibers usually occurs on the radial side of the middle finger. The extensor tendon is thus displaced in an ulnar direction as is the digit. This results in a loss of full MP joint extension and possible PIP joint hyperextension. Untreated, an intrinsic contracture can occur. Management of this spontaneous dislocation includes splinting in extension for 4 weeks, if treatment is initiated early, followed by a gentle remobilization program.[33] If unsuccessful, surgical treatment usually includes repair of the torn sagittal band, with reinforcement using the junctura or a slip of the extensor tendon routed around a lateral band or the radial collateral ligament. Chronic cases will require release of the ulnar sagittal band and centralization of the extensor using a strong segment of tendon. A rare injury to the extensor mechanism over the MP joint has been described as boxer's knuckle.[31] This occurs with direct blows to the MP joint area, resulting in injury not only to the sagittal bands of the extensor tendon mechanism at this level, but also to the underlying articular capsule. These tears of the joint capsule may cause prolonged pain and the treatment is surgical repair (Fig. 60-5). Crush injuries in this area may also affect extension of the digits by causing interosseous-lumbrical adhesions known as the saddle deformity.[6]

ZONE VI—DORSUM OF THE HAND

Extensor injuries over the dorsum of the hand occur less frequently, but are often associated with multiple tissue involvement, including fractures and major soft tissue injuries. The tendon at this level is substantial enough to accept strong sutures and withstand an early dynamic splinting program. Complex injuries require prolonged

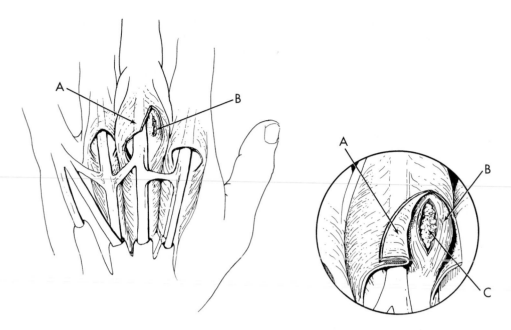

Fig. 60-5. Boxer's knuckle. **A,** Saggital band tear. **B,** Rupture of the joint capsule. **C,** Hypertrophic synovitis filling the gap between the retracted capsular edges.

Table 60-1. EDC excursion

	Total excursion (mm)	Excursion (mm)/10°
Distal interphalangeal	4	0.65
Proximal interphalangeal	7	0.75
Metacarpal phalangeal	16	1.38
Wrist	23	1.85

From Elliot D, McGrouther DA: The excursions of the long extensor tendons of the hand, *J Hand Surg* 1986; 11B:77-80.

rehabilitation, and this can result in extensor lag from tendon adherence to bone.[7] Joint contractures and stiffness of the noninjured digits are also recognized complications. To prevent these problems, Evans and Burkhalter[14] have described early motion protocols for injuries at this level involving dynamic extension splints. They report full extension in over 90% of their patients and no tendon ruptures. It is believed that 5 mm of tendon excursion are sufficient to prevent adherence of the repaired extensor tendons, and this can be correlated with range of motion at the various joints as outlined by Elliot[10] (Table 60-1). Injuries limited to one or more extensor tendons can be safely treated with immobilization for four weeks followed by a standard rehabilitation program. However, complex injuries should be promptly remobilized as mentioned above and further described in Chapter 43. Patients with complex injuries requiring soft tissue coverage may have better results if tendon reconstruction is performed emergently with free tissue transfer.[36] Multiple tendon loss at this level may not lead to significant dysfunction, however, even if reconstruction is not performed.[32]

ZONES VII, VIII, AND IX—WRIST, DISTAL AND PROXIMAL FOREARM

Correct identification of extensor tendons that have been divided at the wrist and forearm level can prove difficult. Furthermore, before repair can be accomplished, extensive dissection may be required to locate the retracted proximal tendons ends. At the wrist level (zone VII), the tendons are repaired using a strong core suture. Should the tendon repair be situated within the area of the extensor retinaculum, only a small portion of this band should be resected. The possibility of repair site impingement should be checked by passive motion of the wrist and fingers and a portion of the divided retinaculum reapproximated if necessary to prevent bowstringing. The wrist is traditionally immobilized in 30° to 40° extension, with the MP joints held in neutral or slight flexion and the PIPs in full extension for 3 to 4 weeks. Remobilization is initiated with further protection for 2 to 3 weeks. Resistance and dynamic splinting is begun at 7 to 8 weeks.

The most common tendon rupture in zone VII involves the extensor pollicis longus (EPL). This usually occurs following a minimally displaced distal radial fracture secondary to devascularization of the tendon.[13] The tendon ends frequently demonstrate sufficient degeneration to prevent an end-to-end repair. Reconstructive possibilities include an extensor indicis proprius transfer and an intercalary graft.

Lacerations over the forearm may traumatize tendons as well as nerves (superficial radial and lateral antebrachial cutaneous) in the area. With more proximal forearm injuries, longitudinal extension of the wound is necessary. What might appear as trivial trauma may actually involve multiple extensor tendon divisions, and exposure is required. For injuries in zones VIII and IX, proximal muscle retraction should be expected and dissection will be required to identify the fibrous muscle septa, which can be realigned to its distal portion with a 3-0 or 4-0 nonabsorbable suture. The exposed muscle ends should be reapproximated with figure-of-eight absorbable sutures. After the repair, the wrist is splinted in 30° to 40° of extension with the MPs at neutral for 10 to 15 days. Thereafter, increasing MP joint flexion is allowed with continuous immobilization for 4 weeks and protection for another 2 weeks.

With multiple tendon injuries at the forearm level, repair of all of the divided structures is recommended, but may not be possible. When this situation occurs, the priority should be to repair independent wrist and thumb extensor tendons and create mass extension of the digits. Divided wrist extensor tendons must be protected for 6 weeks as attenuation or rupture of the repair will diminish use of the hand by producing a weak grasp. Injuries at the musculotendinous junction will require reapproximation with strong sutures and postoperative immobilization of the wrist in 40° extension and slight MP joint flexion (15°).

Injuries near the elbow can be classified as in zone IX. These are often produced by a penetrating wound to the proximal forearm. The major difficulty is distinguishing division of the muscle-tendon tissue from transection of the posterior interosseous nerve. Injury to both tendons and nerve may occur. It is essential that the nerve be visualized and repaired if divided. The muscle bellies are repaired with figure-of-eight sutures. Postoperative care is the same as in zone VIII, but above-elbow immobilization is required if the muscles are injured close to the epicondyle.

EXTENSOR TENDON REHABILITATION—ZONES V, VI, AND VII

Conventional postoperative treatment for tendon injuries in these zones has involved immobilization for 3 to 4 weeks, with the wrist in 30° to 40° extension, the MP joints in neutral or in slight flexion, and the IPs in full extension. A further 2 to 3 weeks of protective splinting is also used. Resisted extension and dynamic splinting is then instituted at 7 to 8 weeks.

As previously stated, dynamic splinting and early remobilization have been shown to be beneficial and safe.[4] The caliber of the extensor tendons in zones V, VI, and VII allows for stronger tendon repairs. These areas, therefore, are better suited to dynamic splinting protocols than the more distal zones. Dynamic splinting is instituted 3 days postoperatively and supported by elastic traction to an outrigger. The details of treatment are described in Chapter 43.

THUMB

Treatment of extensor tendon injuries of the thumb has many similarities to management of finger injuries with exceptions as noted. Closed zone I injuries are treated by splinting in extension for 6 weeks. Open tendon division in zone I is managed with a surgical repair and a similar splinting program. Injuries in zone II are usually open injuries, which will require tendon suture and splinting the IP joint in the extended position. In zone III, at the MP joint, the EDL and EPB tendons are often injured along with the joint capsule. All are reapproximated and repaired. Postinjury, the thumb is immobilized for 3 to 4 weeks in extension at the IP and MP joints, as well as the wrist. In zone IV, after tendon repair, the wrist is splinted in 40° of extension and the MP joint in complete extension for 3 to 4 weeks. At the base of the thumb, in zone V, the EPB abductor pollicis longus, as well as the radial nerve, are usually injured. The nerve is repaired if easy reapproximation is possible. If not, the nerve is resected so that the ends will fall into a nontraumatized area. The retinaculum should be resected over the repair site and the thumb should be rested in abduction as well as extension. The wrist is also immobilized in 40° extension for 4 weeks, with protective splinting for 2 more weeks.

CONCLUSION

Because the end results following repairs of extensor tendon injuries are conventionally considered to be satisfactory, the initial care is often relegated to individuals with limited exposure to hand surgery,[11] and rehabilitation often consists of insufficient splinting and unprotected remobilization. A recent study has clarified a number of these misconceptions.[27] More than half of their patients who sustained extensor tendon trauma had associated injuries, such as a fracture, joint trauma, or flexor tendon damage. Good or excellent results, which can be defined as an extension lag of 10° or less and a loss of flexion of 20° or less, occurred in 64% of those patients that did not have any associated injuries and in less than half of the patients that had associated injuries, as mentioned previously. Less motion occurred after injuries more distally in the hand than those over the dorsum of the hand and wrist. The overall total active motion was 83% of normal, and the biggest problem following extensor injury and repair was loss of finger flexion. The question raised is why does this occur? Does the act of tendon repair create tendon shortening or do adhesions form between the extensor tendons and the adjacent tissues? A recent cadaver study with sequential extensor shortening from 1 to 8 mm in zone IV concluded that the proximal dorsal hood fibers were capable of rotating distally to compensate for tendon reduction. The implication of this study is that the tendons can accommodate to the tendon loss or the bunching that may occur with repair and that adhesions are the most likely cause of lost digital flexion.[29]

The connection between the zone of injury and end result is important. It has been observed previously, that injuries over the dorsum of the hand have far superior results to those occurring in the digits. Extensor tendon injuries in the zones III and IV have the worst results. Careful evaluation of both the extension lag and loss of active flexion has been recently assessed, and the flexion loss was greater than the extensor lag. The conclusion is that rehabilitation programs need to be monitored and adjusted to restore better flexion. Careful attention should be directed toward understanding the relationship between the zone of injury, associated trauma, technique of repair, and postoperative management.

REFERENCES

1. Abouna JM, Brown H: The treatment of mallet finger, the results in a series of 148 consecutive cases and a review of the literature, *Br J Surg* 1968; 55:653-667.
2. Aiche A, Barsky AJ, Weiner DL: Prevention of boutonniere deformity, *Plast Reconstr Surg* 1979; 46:164-167.
3. Blair WF, Steyers CM: Extensor tendon injuries, *Orthop Clin North Am* 1992; 31:141-148.
4. Brown EZ Jr, Ribik CA: Early dynamic splinting for extensor tendon injuries, *J Hand Surg* 1989; 14A:72-76.
5. Casscells SW, Strange TB: Intramedullary wire fixation of mallet finger, *J Bone Joint Surg* 1957; 39A:521-526.
6. Chicarilli ZN, Watson HK, Linberg R, Sasaki G: Saddle deformity: post traumatic interosseous-lumbrical adhesions, *J Hand Surg* 1986; 11A:210-218.
7. Creighton JJ, Steichen JB: Complications in phalangeal and metacarpal fracture management: results of extensor tenolysis, *Hand Clin* 1994; 10:111-116.
8. Dagum AB, Mahoney JL: Effect of wrist position on extensor mechanism after disruption separation, *J Hand Surg* 1994; 19A:584-589.
9. El-Gammal TA, Steyers CM, Blair WF, Maynard JA: Anatomy of the oblique retinacular ligament of the index finger, *J Hand Surg* 1993; 18A:717-721.
10. Elliot D, McGrouther DA: The excursions of the long extensor tendons of the hand, *J Hand Surg* 1986; 11B:77-80.
11. Elliott RA Jr: Injuries to the extensor mechanisms of the hand, *Orthop Clin North Am* 1970; 1:335-354.
12. Elson RA: Rupture of the central slip of the extensor hood of the finger: a test for early diagnosis, *J Bone Joint Surg* 1986; 68B(2):229-231.
13. Engkvist O, Lundborg G: Rupture of the extensor pollicis longus tendon after fracture of the lower end of the radius: a clinical and microangiographic study, *Hand* 1979; 11:76-86.
14. Evans RB, Burkhalter WE: A study of the dynamic anatomy of extensor tendons and implications for treatment, *J Hand Surg* 1986; 11A:774-779.
15. Evans RB, Thompson DE: An analysis of factors that support early active short arc motion of the repaired central slip, *J Hand Ther* 1992; 5:187-201.
16. Foucher G, Debry R, Merle M, Dury M: Treatment of dorsal tissue defects of the proximal interphalangeal joint of the fingers, *Ann Chir Plast Esthet* 1986; 31(2):129-136.
17. Kleinert HE, Verdan C: Report of the committee on tendon injuries, *J Hand Surg* 1983; 8:794-798.
18. Koniuch MP, Peimer CA, VanGorder T, Moncada A: Closed crushed injury of the metacarpophalangeal joint, *J Hand Surg* 1987; 12A:5 (part 1).
19. Littler JW: The finger extensor mechanism, *Surg Clin North Am* 1967; 47:415-432.
20. Lovett WL, McCalla MA: Management and rehabilitation of extensor tendon injuries, *Orthop Clin North Am* 1983; 14:811-826.
21. McFarlane RM, Hampole MK: Treatment of extensor tendon injuries of the hand, *Can J Surg* 1973; 16:366.
22. Matev I: The boutonnière deformity, *Hand* 1969; 1:90-95.
23. McCue FC, Honner R, Gieck JH, et al: A pseudoboutonniere deformity, *Hand* 1975; 7:166-170.
24. Minamikawa WA, Peimer CA, Yamaguchi T, et al: Wrist position and extensor tendon amplitude following repair, *J Hand Surg* 1992; 17A:268-271.
25. Moore JR, Weiland AJ, Valdata L: Independent index extension after extensor indicis proprius transfer, *J Hand Surg* 1987; 12A:232-236.
26. Niechajev IA: Conservative and operative treatment of mallet finger, *Plast Reconstr Surg* 1985; 76:582-585.
27. Newport ML, Blair WF, Steyers CM Jr: Long-term results of extensor tendon repair, *J Hand Surg* 1990; 15A:961-966.
28. Newport ML, Skukla A: Electrophysiologic basis of dynamic extensor splinting, *J Hand Surg* 1992; 17A:272-277.
29. Newport ML, Pollack GR, Williams CB: Biomechanical characteristics of suture technique in extensor zone IV, *J Hand Surg* 1995; 20A:650-656.
30. Parkes A: The lumbrical plus finger, *Hand* 1970; 2:164-165.
31. Posner MA, Ambrose L: Boxer's knuckle—dorsal capsule rupture of the metacarpophalangeal joint of the finger, *J Hand Surg* 1989; 14A(2):229-236 (part 1).
32. Quaba AA, Elliot D, Sommerlad BC: Long-term hand function without long finger extensors: a clinical study, *J Hand Surg* 1988; 13B:66-71.
33. Rayan GM, Murray D: Classification and treatment of closed sagittal band injuries, *J Hand Surg* 1994; 19A:590-594.
34. Robb WAT: The results of treatment of mallet finger, *J Bone Joint Surg* 1959; 41B:546-549.
35. Saldana MJ, Choban S, Westerbeck P, Schacherer TG: Results of acute zone three extensor tendon injuries treated with dynamic extension splinting, *J Hand Surg* 16A(6):1991.
36. Scheker LR, et al: Primary extensor tendon reconstruction in dorsal hand defects requiring free flaps, *J Hand Surg* 1993; 18B:568-575.
37. Schenck RR: Variations of the extensor tendons of the fingers: surgical significance, *J Bone Joint Surg* 1964; 46A:103-110.
38. Schultz R, Furlong J II, Storace A: Detailed anatomy of the extensor mechanism at the proximal aspect of the finger, *J Hand Surg* 1981; 6:493-498.
39. Smith RJ: Non-ischemic contractures of the intrinsic muscles of the hand, *J Bone Joint Surg* 1971; 53A:1313-1331.
40. Smith RJ: Balance and kinetics of the finger under normal and pathological conditions, *Clin Orthop* 1974; 104:92-111.
41. Snow JW: Use of a retrograde tendon flap in repairing a severed extensor tendon in the PIP joint area, *Plast Reconstr Surg* 1973; 51:555-558.
42. Spinner M, Choi BY: Anterior dislocation of the proximal interphalangeal joint, a cause of rupture of the central slip of the extensor mechanism, *J Bone Joint Surg* 1970; 52A:1329.
43. Steichen JB, Petersen DP: Juncture tendinum between extensor digitorum communis and extensor pollicis longus, *J Hand Surg* 1984; 9A:674-676.
44. Steichen JB, Strickland JW, Call WH, Powell SG: Results of surgical treatment of chronic boutonniere deformity, *Difficult problems in hand surgery,* St Louis, 1982, Mosby.
45. Stern PJ, Kastrup JJ: Complications and prognosis of treatment of mallet finger, *J Hand Surg* 1988; 13A:329-334.
46. Taleisnik J, Gelberman RH, Miller BW, Szabo RM: The extensor retinaculum at the wrist, *J Hand Surg* 1984; 9A:495-501.
47. Tubiana R: Surgical repair of the extensor apparatus of the fingers, *Surg Clin North Am* 1968; 48:1015.

48. Von Schroeder HP: The functional significance of the long extensors and juncturae, *J Hand Surg* 1990; 15A:595-602.

49. Warren RA, Kay NRM, Norris SH: The microvascular anatomy of the distal digital extensor tendon, *J Hand Surg* 1988; 13B(2):161-163.

50. Wehbé MA, Schneider LH: Mallet fractures, *J Bone Joint Surg* 1984; 66A:658-669.

51. Wilson RL: Management of acute extensor tendon injuries. In Hunter JM, Schneider LH, Mackin EV, eds: *Tendon surgery in the hand,* St Louis, 1987, Mosby.

52. Wilson RL: Mallet finger in panel discussion: extensor tendons. In Hunter JM, Schneider LH, Mackin EV, eds: *Tendon surgery in the hand,* St Louis, 1987, Mosby.

53. Wilson RL, Liechty BN: Complications following small joint injuries, *Hand Clin* 1986; 2:329-345.

54. Woodburn KR, McGrouther DA: Tendon excursions of the interossei and superficial hypothenar muscles: an anatomical study, *J Hand Surg* 1988; 13B(4):415-420.

Chapter 61

CLINICAL APPLICATION OF EARLY MOTION TO EXTENSOR TENDON REPAIR

Randall W. Culp

Extensor tendon injuries can be associated with as much compromise of hand function as injuries to the flexor tendon counterpart.[1-3] Yet only recently has similar vigor been applied to their rehabilitative protocols.[1-5,7] Traditionally, extensor tendon lacerations were treated with operative repair and static splinting.[6,9,10] Problems associated with this protocol include adhesion formation, extensor lag, joint stiffness, and loss of flexion.[12] Several factors have been implicated to explain observed results. Extensor tendons tend to be flat and difficult to suture, they have less excursion than flexor tendons, the surrounding tissue is thin, and they can often be associated with disruption of the underlying bone. To improve outcome, newer rehabilitative programs have been forwarded.[1-5,7] Based on the widespread acceptance of the benefits of early controlled motion after flexor tendon repair, protocols following similar principles on the extensor side have been suggested and form the basis of this chapter.

ZONES OF INJURY

The committee on tendon injuries for the International Federation of the Society for Surgery of the Hand has determined zones of injury referable to the extrinsic extensor tendons for the fingers and thumb (Fig. 61-1). Guidelines for surgical repair and postoperative rehabilitation are dependent on the zone of injury. Because the preponderance of recent research in early controlled motion has been described after injuries in zones V to VII, this chapter focuses on that area.

LITERATURE REVIEW

Most recent studies have based their splint designs and rehabilitation protocols on the biomechanics and anatomy of the extensor system. For example, Evans and Burkhalter[4] have demonstrated that to create 5 mm of extensor digitorum communis (EDC) tendon glide in zones V to VII, metacarpophalangeal (MP) joint flexion required would be index 28.3°, long 27.5°, ring 40.9°, and small 38.3°. In their dynamic extensor tendon protocol, the wrist is placed in 45° of extension to relieve tension on the repair site. The metacarpophalangeal (MP) and interphalangeal (IP) joints are supported to 0° with elastic traction slings. A palmar block limiting MP flexion in the arc of motion mentioned above was used. Exercises allowing active flexion but passive extension were done 10 times per hour.

Several recent studies have verified the efficacy of dynamic extension splinting after injury. Brown[2] studied 52 well-motivated patients who began dynamic extension splinting 3 days after injury. Therapy was designed to achieve 70° of MP flexion, 90° proximal interphalangeal (PIP) flexion, and 50° of distal interphalangeal (DIP) flexion. Dynamic splinting was discontinued after 5 weeks, but static splinting was used for another month. Full extension was achieved in 77 of 82 digits. There were no ruptures.

Chow[3] conducted a comparative study between two centers; one group was treated postoperatively with static splinting, the other with dynamic splinting. Faster recovery and return to work, better functional results, and avoidance

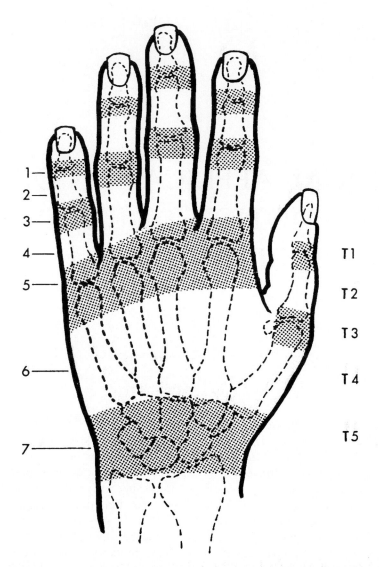

Fig. 61-1. Zones of injury referable to the extrinsic extensor tendons for the fingers and thumb.

of secondary procedures was noted in the dynamic extension splint protocol.

Finally, Hung[5] in a prospective study, reported on 38 patients with 48 digit injuries after extensor tendon repair and dynamic extension splinting. He noted that injuries distal to the MP joint had poorer results than those proximal. There were again no ruptures.

CURRENT PROTOCOL ZONES V TO VII

Based on the literature review, our current protocol with dynamic extension splinting is as follows.

A custom-made dynamic extension outrigger is fabricated with thermoplastic material, the wrist at 45° of extension. An outrigger with a rubber band is attached to a broad finger strap at the level of the PIP joint. The rubber band is adjusted so that the MP joint of the required finger is held in full extension. If the EDC is lacerated, all digits are included. If

the extensor indicis proprius or extensor digiti quinti are involved, only the affected digit need be treated. Full motion at the MP and PIP joint are allowed based on a study by Minamikawa[11] that demonstrated no tension after extensor tendon repairs with full flexion of the digits when the wrist is in 45° of extension. Patients are instructed to actively flex 10 times per hour. Patients are often fitted with a static extension splint at night.

At the end of the 5-week program, the splint is discarded and active exercises are performed. Emphasis on finger flexion is made at this time. At 7 weeks, resistance and dynamic flexion splints are used as necessary.

CONCLUSION

Dynamic splinting has been demonstrated to be a useful adjunct in the treatment of both simple and complex extensor tendon injuries in zones V to VII. It is most successful in cooperative patients who have a skilled hand therapist. Traditional postoperative immobilization still may be used in children or uncooperative patients.

REFERENCES

1. Allieu Y, Asencio G, Rouzaud J-C: Protective passive mobilization after suturing of the extensor tendons of the hand. In Tubiana R, ed: *The hand,* vol 3, Philadelphia, 1988, Saunders.
2. Browne EI, Ribik CA: Early dynamic splinting for extensor tendon injuries, *J Hand Surg* 1989; 14A:72.
3. Chow JA, Doouelle S, Thomas J, et al: A comparison of results of extensor tendon repair followed by early controlled mobilization versus static immobilization, *J Hand Surg* 1989; 14B:18.
4. Evans RB, Burkhalter WE: A study of the dynamic anatomy of extensor tendons and implications for treatment, *J Hand Surg* 1986; 11A:774.
5. Hung LK, Chan A, Chang J, et al: Early controlled mobilization with dynamic splinting for treatment of extensor tendon injuries, *J Hand Surg* 1990; 15A:251.
6. Kelly AP: Primary tendon repairs: a study of 789 consecutive tendon severences, *J Bone Joint Surg* 1959; 41A:581.
7. Kerr CD, Burczak JR: Dynamic traction after extensor tendon repair in zone 6, 7 and 8: a retrospective study, *J Hand Surg* 1989; 14B:21.
8. Lovett WC, McCalla MA: Management and rehabilitation of extensor tendon injuries, *Orthop Clin North Am* 1983; 14:811.
9. Mason ML, Allen HS: The rate of healing of tendons: an experimental study of tensile strength, *Ann Surg* 1941; 113:424.
10. Miller H: Repair of severed tendons of the hand and wrist, *Surg Gynecol Obstet* 1942; 75:693.
11. Minamikawa Y, Peimer CA, Yamaquchi T, et al: Wrist position and extensor tendon amplitude following repair, *J Hand Surg* 1992; 17A:268.
12. Newport ML, Blair WF, Steyers CM. Long-term results of extensor tendon repair, *J Hand Surg* 1990; 15A:961.

Chapter 62

BOUTONNIÈRE DEFORMITY TREATMENT
Immediate and delayed

François Iselin

Three situations should be considered in boutonnière deformity treatment: (1) fresh lacerations and ruptures, (2) old but correctible boutonnière deformities, and (3) fixed boutonnière deformities.

FRESH LACERATIONS OR RUPTURES OF THE EXTENSOR TENDON IN ZONE III

Whenever possible, conservative treatment by a dorsal extension splint is preferred because there will be no retraction of the central slip (Fig. 62-1). Spontaneous healing with normal length should be expected within 5 weeks, and if the distal phalanx has been free to move, no retraction of the retinacular ligaments should occur.

If the wound is deep and large, we do an exact repair of the joint capsule and of the central slip by a crisscross nonabsorbable suture and immobilize the proximal interphalangeal (PIP) joint in extension with an oblique Kirschner-wire[2] (Fig. 62-2, A and B). The wire should be removed as soon as an extension splint can be placed safely over the dorsal skin, about the third week (Fig. 62-2, C). This splint should be maintained until the fifth week while progressive, protected active flexion is encouraged; then the splint can be worn intermittently until week 12. (It can be replaced by a Capener type splint.) During the whole immobilization period, it is extremely important that the distal phalanx should be kept completely free and the patient instructed to move constantly to maintain a functional retinacular system.

If the extensor apparatus is still anatomically recognizable in its three elements, it will be possible to identify a central slip and to shorten it by a resection that should not exceed 2 mm[1] (Fig. 62-3, A). An end-to-end suture (Fig. 62-3, B) is then made with a single loop of nonabsorbable material. This suture should allow full passive PIP joint flexion without rupture. Then the PIP joint is pinned in full extension with an oblique Kirschner-wire for 3 weeks (see Fig. 62-3, B). The lateral bands should not be sutured, but merely released from any surrounding fibrous scar tissue.

When the extensor apparatus is totally fibrotic, the forces should be rebalanced in the extensor mechanism by the operation described by Littler and Eaton in 1967.[5] By a short, dorsal median skin incision, the lateral elements are separated between the dorsal aspect and the retinacular elements by a V-shaped tendon incision from the dorsal aspect of the middle phalanx.

When the retinacular system is totally contracted, the corresponding distal interphalangeal (DIP) joint hyperextension should be corrected by a careful and progressive lengthening[3] of the distal extensor system, which, if overdone, would cause a mallet deformity.[6]

THREE STIFF BOUTONNIÈRE DEFORMITIES

The situation is a fixed deformity in flexion of the PIP joint and in hyperextension of the DIP joint. All attempts, even prolonged, at correction by splinting or therapy have failed.

Anatomically, the lateral bands are fibrotic and fixed volarly to the PIP joint, the triangular ligament has disappeared or is fibrotic and unable to bring back dorsally

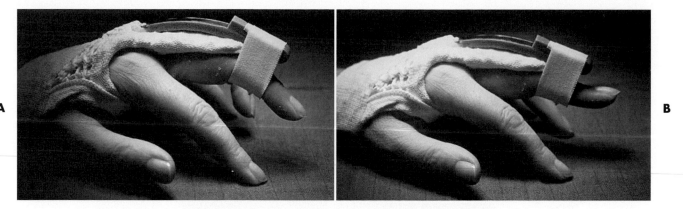

Fig. 62-1. Late postoperative splint. **A,** Distal phalanx in flexion. **B,** Distal phalanx in extension.

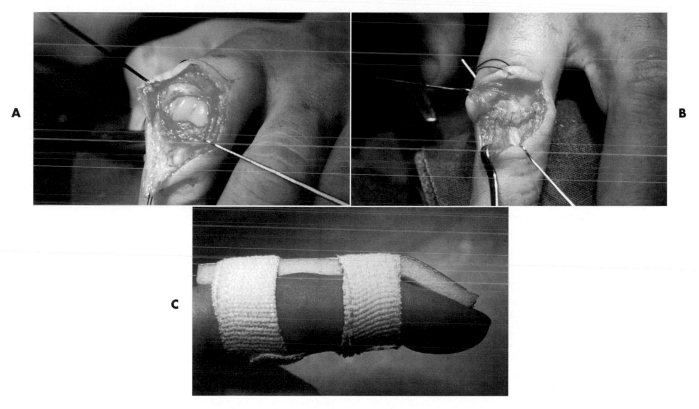

Fig. 62-2. A, Fresh wound in zone III. **B,** Repair by suture, K-wire fixation. **C,** Early postoperative splint.

the lateral elements. The retinacular system is contracted, hyperextending the DIP joint. The dorsal elements are beyond recognition.

We have noticed that long-term joint stiffness leads to alteration of the joint cartilages, even if they were not initially involved. Finally, a fixed boutonnière deformity is a combined lesion of tendon and joint.

It is impossible for a normal PIP joint to move with a damaged extensor system in zone III. It is also obvious that a damaged joint will have no function even with a normal extensor tendon. But a damaged joint, if still mobile, can be moved in flexion by an intact flexor system and can be "recalled" in extension by some elastic, even if fibrotic, extensor system.

Therefore we state the following "equation": *A damaged extensor tendon should correspond to a simplified PIP joint*[4] (Fig. 62-4).

The simplest joint is a resected joint, and the interposition of a silastic Swanson's implant will give stability, alignment, and joint encapsulation.

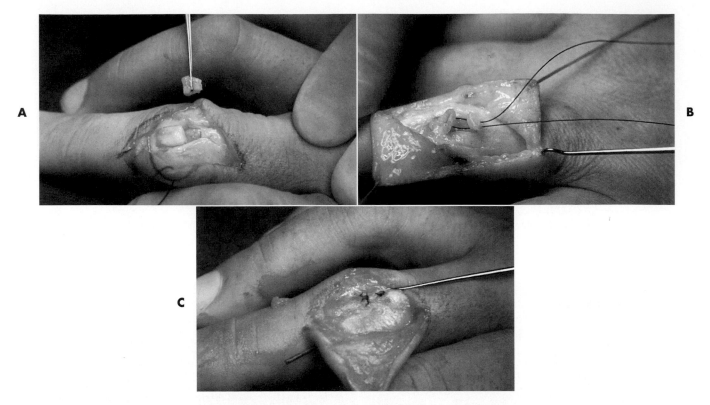

Fig. 62-3. Secondary repair. **A,** Resection of 2 mm of central slip. **B,** End-to-end suture. **C,** K-wire temporary fixation.

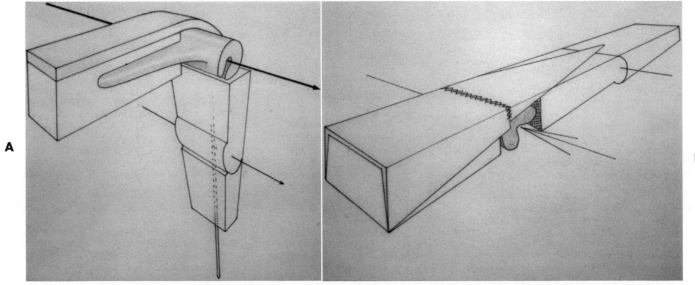

Fig. 62-4. A and **B,** "A damaged extensor tendon should correspond to a simplified PIP joint."

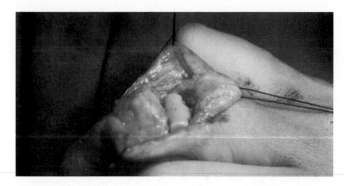

Fig. 62-5. Intraoperative view with sizer of PIP joint arthroplasty for a stiff boutonnière deformity.

A resection arthroplasty with a silastic implant is, therefore, the preferred solution to fixed boutonnière deformities (Fig. 62-5).

CONCLUSION

Between 1979 and 1988 I treated 40 fixed boutonnière deformities in 26 patients, aged 14 to 40 (mean 26), with a follow-up from 2 to 15 years. The preoperative, stiff, average extension lag was 57°.

The postoperative, average, *active* range of motion is 23° to 58°.

This improvement is mainly toward extension as the chief complaint was a stiff flexion deformity. It appears that the flexion improvement is slight, but it corresponds to active motion. Six are now stiff in extension, which is considered an improvement by the patients. Thirty-six digits of 40 have satisfactory cosmetic correction; 38 are stable and pain free, except during adverse weather conditions.

Only 2 had to be secondarily amputated, and 24 of 26 patients are satisfied, although only 15 have actual joint mobility.

Fourteen of 26 patients had previously sustained at least 2 surgical attempts at correction.

Finally, the difficulties and the poor results in fixed boutonnière deformities should be compared with the better results of early repair.

REFERENCES

1. Burton RI: Extensor tendons—late reconstruction. In Green DP, ed: *Operative hand surgery,* New York, 1982, Churchill Livingstone.
2. Curtis RM, Reid RL, Provost UM: A staged technique for the repair of traumatic boutonnière deformity, *J Hand Surg* 1983; 8(2):167-171.
3. Dolphin JA: The extensor tenotomy for chronic boutonniere deformity, *J Bone Joint Surg* 1965; 47A:161-164.
4. Iselin F, Pradet G: Traitement des lésions anciennes des extenseurs en boutonnières invétérées par résection arthroplastique avec implant, *Ann Chir Main* 1987; I:11-17.
5. Littler JW, Eaton RG: Redistribution of forces in correction of boutonnière deformity, *J Bone Joint Surg* 1967; 49A:1267-1274.
6. Tubiana R: Les déformations en boutonnière, *Traité de chirurgie de la main,* vol 3, Paris, 1986, Masson

Chapter 63

REHABILITATION FOR SWAN-NECK DEFORMITIES OF THE LONG DIGITS OCCURRING WITH RHEUMATOID ARTHRITIS

Jean-Claude Rouzaud
Yves Allieu

The Swan-neck deformity (Fig. 63-1) creates the most inconvenience for hand function. In the severest cases, grasp becomes impossible. The constraint that a swan-neck deformity produces is much more important in terms of function than that caused by a boutonnière deformity. It is an intrinsic plus deformity, with the proximal interphalangeal (PIP) joint in hyperextension and the distal interphalangeal (DIP) joint in flexion.[8]

ETIOLOGY

Origin is multifactorial. Swan-neck deformity may be secondary to *extrinsic causes* (Fig. 63-2), such as a carpal collapse, a palmar dislocation, a mallet finger, or tendinous imbalance; or to *intrinsic causes* (Fig. 63-3), for example, PIP joint synovitis with dorsal adhesions of the extensor system or articular forces destroying in volar plate, with or without flexor digitorun sublimis (FDS) rupture.

STAGES OF SWAN-NECK DEFORMITY

The following stages can be seen as swan-neck deformity develops:
1. Free PIP joint in every range of motion: reducible deformity
2. Fully or partially stiff PIP joint: fixed or reducible deformity
3. Destroyed PIP joint

TREATMENT

Whether the swan-neck deformity is reducible (Fig. 63-4) or fixed (Fig. 63-5) considerably modifies the therapeutic approach. In some cases PIP joint flexion is maintained, but, when the deformity is fixed, it is impossible to carry out global flexion of the digits. To determine which type is

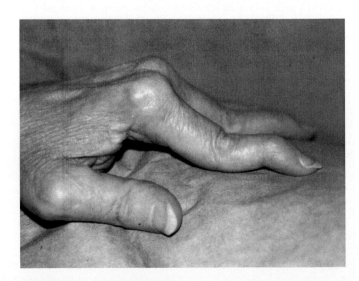

Fig. 63-1. Swan-neck deformity.

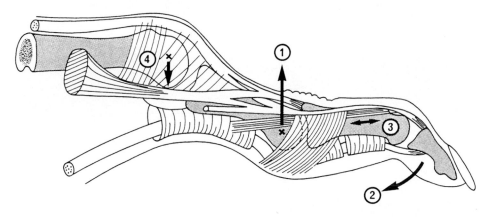

Fig. 63-2. *1,* Dorsal displacement of the traction axis of the extensor system. *2,* Flexion of P3. *3,* Retraction of the oblique retinacular ligament. *4,* Displacement of the traction forces of the intrinsics when there is an existing anterior MP subluxation.

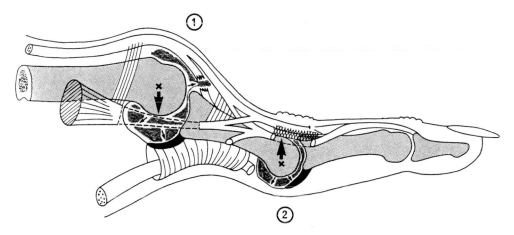

Fig. 63-3. *1,* Metacarpophalangeal causes. *2,* Proximal interphalangeal causes.

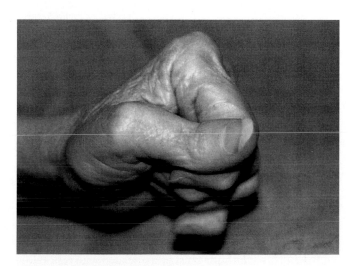

Fig. 63-4. Reducible swan-neck deformity.

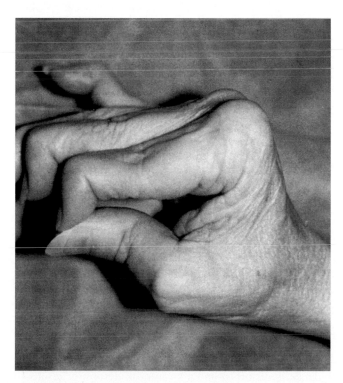

Fig. 63-5. Irreducible swan-neck deformity.

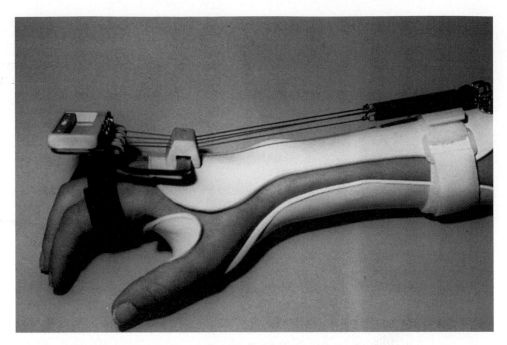

Fig. 63-6. Dynamic extension splinting.

present, a reduction test of the metacarpophalangeal (MP) joint must be carried out. Palmar luxation of the MP joint causes loss of intrinsic muscle balance, which provokes a swan-neck deformity. Reducing the MP joint restores muscle balance and corrects the deformity at the PIP joint level. In fixed swan-neck deformity, where the joint is in a nonfunctional position and cannot be reduced, making any hand function impossible, surgery is the only treatment option.[1,13]

General principles

Treatment of swan-neck deformity rests on two principles:
1. A simple surgical procedure is used for the rheumatoid arthritis.
2. A limited PIP joint extension is used to obtain balanced PIP joint flexion contracture at 30°.

Goals

The aim of the treatment is to restore stable pinch of the second and third digits. Arthrodesis is often proposed at this level. Use of this procedure assumes a free or mobile MP joint after an arthroplasty, as with a Swanson implant. Grasp is obtained using the fourth or fifth digit, so a PIP joint arthroplasty could be used.

Treatment focusing on causative factors

Carpal collapse is responsible for reducing the length of the longitudinal arch, as shown by Shapiro.[10] Muscle balance is disturbed and a swan-neck deformity results by reciprocity.

Metacarpophalangeal joint subluxation carries extrinsic tension at the level of the PIP joint. A Swanson implant in the MP joint prevents any secondary PIP joint deformity. A dynamic extension splint using gauged springs (Fig. 63-6) produces tendinous balance and realignment of the digits.

PIP joint synovitis suppresses the intrinsic cause of the disease. With respect to the extensor system, tenolysis, at the dorsal side of the PIP joint, produces a ventral repositioning of the lateral bands.

A *DIP joint lesion,* specifically an *isolated mallet finger,* can degenerate into a secondary swan-neck deformity. Arthrodesis in 0° of extension restores tendinous balance. The spiral oblique retinacular ligament[6-7,14] surgical procedure may be a solution, but it is difficult and must only be used in special cases of rheumatoid arthritis. DIP joint arthrodesis presents another solution for this condition.

Treatment at the PIP level

Free PIP joint. Treatment consists of tenodesis by FDS band, as described by Swanson[12] (modified by Bosse). The dorsal tenodesis uses an extensor lateral band. The goal is to limit PIP joint dorsal extension.

Stiffened PIP joint. Dorsal tenoarthrolysis, which liberates the extensor system, allows the two lateral bands to take up a ventral position.

Destroyed PIP joint. PIP joint arthrodesis focusing on the second and third rays in functional position or the Swanson arthoplasty on the fourth and fifth rays' PIP joint may be used. However, Swanson arthroplasty on a PIP joint with rheumatoid arthritis must be associated with restoration of tendinous balance to avoid recurrence of the deformity.

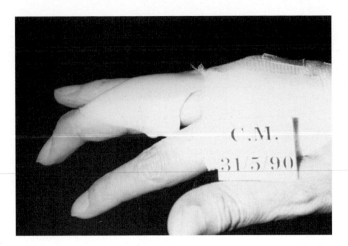

Fig. 63-7. Orthotic device that reduces metacarpophalangeal joint subluxation.

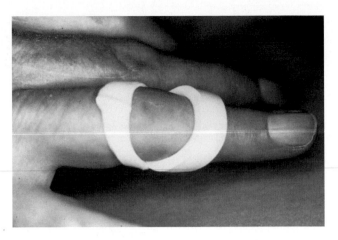

Fig. 63-8. Restrictive splint.

REHABILITATION[2-4]

Prevention

Orthotics that reduce MP joint subluxation (Fig. 63-7) correct the muscle imbalance at the MP joint level. Restrictive splints that limit PIP joint extension (Fig. 63-8) along with a strap maintaining the PIP joint in flexion can prevent settlement of the PIP extension.[5]

Postoperative measures

Tenodesis effect. Tenodesis may be used with an FDS or extensor apparatus band. Active mobilization in flexion is used beginning at the third week postoperatively. In both cases a temporary pin fixes the PIP joint at −30° extension. A dorsal protective splint is required until the sixth week postoperatively.

PIP joint dorsal tenoarthrolysis. Immediate active and passive mobilization begins on the fourth day postoperatively. A dorsal protective splint is used at 30° of PIP joint flexion for 3 weeks.

Dorsal tenoarthrolysis associated with tenodesis. Protection is continued for 3 weeks postoperatively, then active mobilization in flexion is begun.

PIP joint arthroplasty by Swanson implant. This technique is rarely indicated for patients with rheumatoid arthritis. It is only for the fourth and fifth rays to help restore grasp.[9-15]

Protocol

We use the Swanson protocol. A dorsal static orthotic device is set up on the PIP joint at −30° of extension. We never use dynamic extension orthotic devices because the extensor system here is the strongest and must not be assisted. Flexion training has priority. Dorsal static orthotics ensure the alignment and avoid any lateral deviation in the PIP joint.[12,13]

Timing. A static orthotic device is used during the first 3 weeks and may be worn until the sixth week. As of the third

week, active PIP joint flexion begins. At the sixth week, active extension is fixed at −30°. An active static splint may be needed until the sixth month.

CASE SUMMARIES

Following the principles outlined in this chapter, we have performed the following procedures:

- In 45% of cases, tenodesis, using all types of techniques
- In 28% of cases, dorsal tenoarthrolysis
- In 19% of cases, arthrodesis
- In 8% of cases, Swanson arthroplasty

CONCLUSION

The treatment of the long digit deformities must not be considered as an isolated therapy, but must be included in a global program of rheumatoid arthritis management. The proximodistal strategy must be respected, and the rehabilitation technique must include some ergonomic education. Finally, rheumatoid arthritis is a systemic disease, and one must take into account the different accessories and technical aides the patient can use, such as walking sticks for lower limb lesions, which may suggest an alternative surgical indication or rehabilitation program.

REFERENCES

1. Allieu Y: Déformations de la main rhumatoide et leurs traitements, *Documenta Geigy*, 1985; 1:73-86.
2. Allieu Y: Principles généraux de rééducation postopératoires de la main rhumatoide. Traitement chirurgical de la polyarthrite rhumatoide. *Acquisitions rhumatologiques,* Paris, 1986, Masson.
3. Allieu Y, Laurent J, Dotte P: Rééducation et main rhumatoide opérée. *Actualités Réed Réadapt Fonct,* Paris, 1976, Masson.
4. Allieu Y, Mailhé D, Asencio G, et al: La readaptation chirurgicale globale dans les sequelles de l'arthrite chronique juvenile a l'age adulte. Acquisitions rhumatologiques, Paris, 1984, Masson.
5. Delprat J, De Godebout J, Mansat M, Allieu Y: *Rééducation post op des arthroplasties par implants dans la main rhumatoide.* Traitement chirurgical de la PR, Paris, 1986, Masson.

6. Kleinman WB, Petersen DP: Oblique retinacular ligament reconstruction for chronic mallet finger deformity, *J Hand Surg* 1984; 9A:399-404.

7. Littler JW: Commentary on a new method of treatment of mallet finger by Weinberg H, et al: *Plast Reconstr Surg* 1976; 58:499-500.

8. Mackin EJ: Post operative management of wrist implant, *Cycle d'enseignement de pathologie et de chirurgie de la main,* Allieu, Montpellier, 1984.

9. Nalebuff EA, Millender LH: surgical treatment of the swan-neck deformity in rheumatoid arthritis, *Orthop Clin North Am* 1975; 6:733-752.

10. Shapiro JS, Heijna W, Nasatir S, Ray RD: The relationship of wrist motion to ulnar phalangeal drift in the rheumatoid patient, *Hand* 1971; 3:68-75.

11. Simon L, Houlez G: Ergothérapie et main rhumatoide, *Actualités de Réed et Réadap Fonct,* Paris, 1976, Masson.

12. Swanson AB: Pathogenesis and pathomechanics of rheumatoid déformities in hand and wrist, *Orthop Clin North Am* 1973; 4:1039-1056.

13. Swanson AB: Postoperative rehabilitation programs in flexible implant. In Hunter JM, ed: *Tendon Surgery in the Hand,* ed 2, St. Louis, 1984, Mosby.

14. Thompson JS, Littler JW, Upton J: The spiral oblique retinacular ligament (SORL), *J Hand Surg* 1978; 3:482-487.

15. Tubiana R, Achach PC: La place de la chirurgie dans le traitement de la main rhumatoide, *GEM la main rhumatoide,* Paris, 1969, Expansion Scientifique.

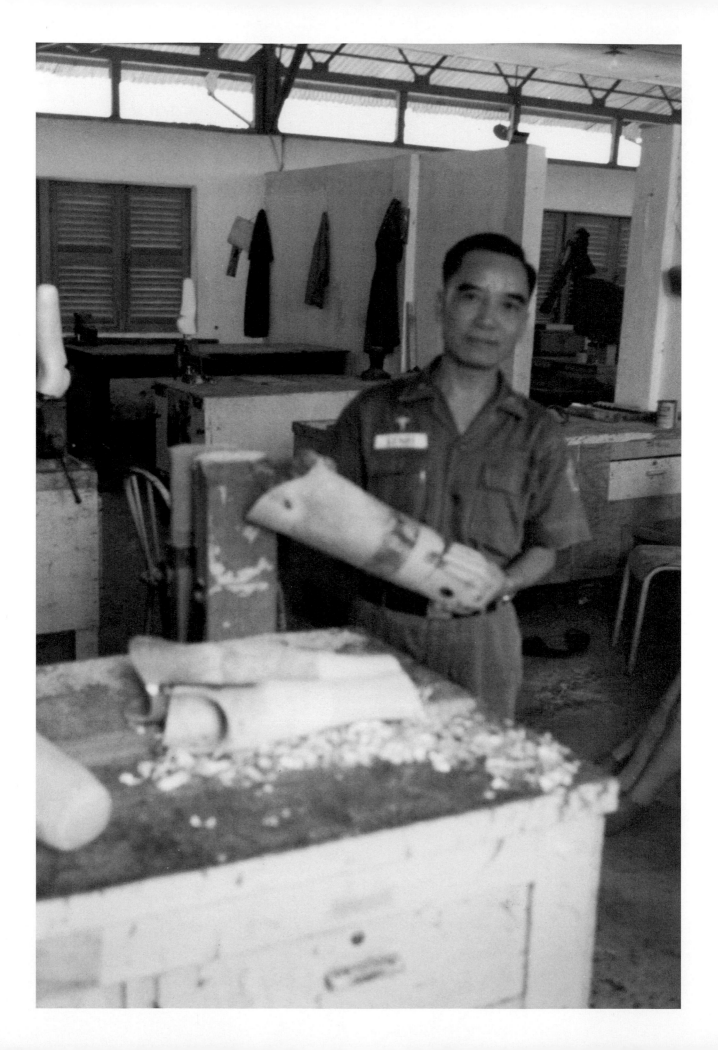

Part XV

PEDIATRIC TENDON INJURIES

Great credit must be given Major Linh for getting a fine prosthetic department under way at Cong Hoa. His men now turn out 100 leg prostheses per month. Delightful lunch with Maj. Linh in the old French air officers club. More casualties at Cong Hoa, as many as 60 per day. (Notes by J. William Littler, from his "A Surgical Diary: Vietnam 1969.")

Chapter 64

FLEXOR TENDON INJURIES AND REPAIR IN CHILDREN

A. Lee Osterman
Nader Paksima

Although the treatment of flexor tendon injuries in children is in many ways similar to that in the adult, there are some special considerations unique to the pediatric population. There is the obvious difference in the size of the tendons. The smaller, more delicate tendon is harder to suture and to work with. The donor tendons, the plantaris and the palmaris longus, are often too thin to be of use. Controversy exists as to the type of repair, the material to be used, the period and type of immobilization, the rehabilitation, the use of tendon grafts, and primary versus delayed repair.

Growth retardation has been reported in the digit with a flexor tendon laceration. Cunningham et al.[5] reported on four cases in which flexor tendon lacerations were not repaired, with subsequent growth retardation. They postulated that the growth disturbance was related to an absence of the mechanical force of flexion. This causes dedifferentiation of cartilage with retardation of the bone growth. Gaisford and Fleegler[7] have shown that growth retardation can also occur in repaired flexor tendons in the chicken model and the growth disturbance in unrepaired tendons was more pronounced. Also working on the chicken model, Nishijima et al.[16,17] have shown that longitudinal growth disturbance can occur in the digit with a repaired flexor tendon, and tendon growth occurred along the whole tendon.

ANATOMY

Although the anatomy in children is similar to adults, it is important to review the embryology and the blood supply.

Embryology

The upper limb bud is visible by the beginning of the fourth week of intrauterine life. The outline of the hand becomes visible at 37 days as a flattened paddle-like structure. The apical ectodermal ridge directs growth distally differentiating into five fingers, with the mesoderm condensing to form the metacarpals. The hand initially has a tridactyl architecture similar to birds, the thumb and little finger at first being only proximal buds. The flexor tendons form from the mesoderm during the sixth week of gestation. The majority of differentiation is completed by the eighth week.[14]

Blood supply

The blood supply to the tendon is segmental. In the musculotendinous portion, vessel groups composed of one artery and two veins pass through the mesotenon and split into T-shaped branches. In the nonsynovial tendon, the tendon vasculature is longitudinally oriented with two channels in the profundus and three, one artery and two veins, in the superficialis. These vessels are fed and drained by the vincula. The vincula are condensations of the mesotenon, which are the main source of blood supply to the tendon.[19] In the palm, the tendon has abundant secondary blood supply. Healing in this region, zones III and IV, is quite rapid.[6] In the synovial tendon, within the fibro-osseous tunnel, the vincula again lie on the dorsal surface of the tendon. Here the mesotenon forms vincula that act as mesenteric bands; fanning out at their attachments, they wrinkle and stretch with the movements of the tendons. The shorter vincula are referred to as *vincula brevus* and the longer as *vincula longus*. In the child the distance between the vincula is shorter; therefore, the blood supply is richer, which may lead to more rapid healing with less adhesions.[6]

The tendons also derive nutrition from the synovial fluid lubrication. Completely avascular segments of flexor tendon have been shown to heal by diffusion through the synovial fluid.[11,13,15]

Tendon and bone

Pulley development and location is constant through the postnatal period with gross characteristics resembling that of the adult.

The epiphysis of the distal, middle, and proximal phalanx have a broad range of appearance and ossification. In general the range of appearance is between 5 months to 2 years, with fusion being completed between 14 to 21 years.[14] It should be noted that the extensor tendon attaches to the epiphysis in both the proximal interphalangeal (PIP) and distal interphalangeal (DIP) joints, while the flexor tendon attaches to the metaphysis.

DIAGNOSIS

Diagnosis can be difficult in the child who is not old enough to cooperate fully with the examination. One helpful tool is to observe the normal resting cascade of the digits. A finger lying in extension is clinical evidence of a loss of flexor tendon tone. It should be noted that an intact profundus tendon can deceive the examiner by flexing across both joints. Another method to test the integrity of the tendon is to place the digit in the appropriate position and ask the child to hold that position. The tenodesis effect, that is, observing the motion of the digits as the wrist is repeatedly flexed and extended, has also proven valuable. Another clinical tool is to put pressure on the distal forearm at the myotendinous junction of the flexor tendons. This causes contraction and movement of the corresponding joint if the tendon is intact.

A high index of suspicion must be maintained for associated digital nerve lacerations. The sensory examination may be unreliable and surgical exploration may be warranted. In our experience 52% of flexor tendon lacerations required digital nerve repair, and this compares with other reported series.

During examination of the injured child, especially in the case of chronic unrepaired tendon laceration, the physician must be alerted to the phenomenon of *trapping*. Here the child compensates for the loss of motion in one of the digits and uses the adjacent finger to seemingly move the tendon-deficit finger.

Two cases have been reported in which the superficialis and profundus were completely cut, and the patient still had full flexion at the PIP joint.[20] This was made possible by the action of an intact short vincula. We stress the need for examining the strength of contraction to avoid misdiagnosis (see the box above).

> **KEYS TO THE DIAGNOSIS OF FLEXOR TENDON INJURY IN CHILDREN**
> 1. Suspicion
> 2. Loss of normal resting cascade
> 3. Squeeze test
> 4. Tenodysis effect
> 5. Active motion examination
> 6. Watch out for vicarious motions and trappings

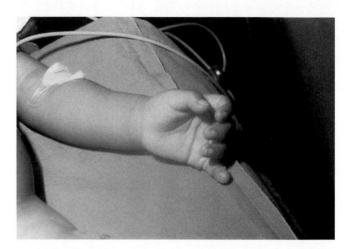

Fig. 64-1. A 5-year-old child with simple laceration at the base of the small finger. Note the resting posture of the right fifth finger. Surgery confirmed laceration of both the profundus and sublimis tendon in zone II, and they were repaired.

Flexor tendon injuries in children are most commonly caused by sharp laceration, over 50% of the time from broken glass.[8,9,21,25] Up to 25% of the injuries are initially missed.

REPAIR BY ZONE
Zone I: profundus only

Acute. As mentioned previously, the diagnosis of isolated profundus injury is often missed, because the patient can still move the interphalangeal (IP) joint and it is often assumed by the patient or the parents that the distal tip motion will return after the swelling decreases. Because swelling is often present at the PIP joint, it often leaves the examiner the false impression that the major injury is present at the PIP joint rather than at the profundus. Inability to actively flex the DIP joint on fist making should alert the physician to the possibility of profundus avulsion or laceration (Fig. 64-1).

Early direct repair of the profundus tendon has given excellent results. Direct repair can often be carried out up to 4 weeks postinjury, but best results are seen when repaired within 1 week. In a recent paper, O'Connell et al.[18] reported on 10 isolated profundus lacerations treated with direct primary repair, all with excellent results. Wakefield, in 1964,[26] reported excellent results in 21 of

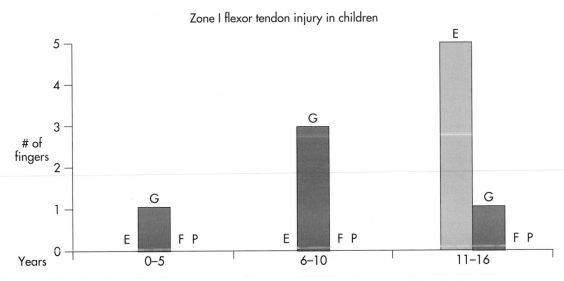

Fig. 64-2. Universally good results are seen in zone I repair using the Strickland criteria.

23 profundus lacerations. The good results were obtained regardless of location of laceration. Our experience with zone I repairs has also shown uniformly good or excellent results, with primary suture, carried out under 4 weeks, regardless of age (Fig. 64-2).

Some authors feel that the tendon can be advanced into the bone up to 1 cm.[9] In general we use advancement only for the flexor pollicus longus, because of concern about tethering of the adjacent finger profundus, that is *the quadrigia effect.* We prefer direct end-to-end repair using a buried core suture.[6] The surgeon should remember to attach the tendon into the metaphysis in the skeletally immature child. In cases where the proximal stump has retracted into the palm, the surgeon may elect to redirect the profundus tendon around the chiasm of the superficialis instead of passing through or sacrificing one limb of the superficialis.

Late. In chronic cases where the superficialis is intact, one option is to live with the lack of DIP joint flexion (Fig. 64-3). Another is to stabilize the DIP joint by soft tissue or bony fusion. The latter is not done until skeletal maturity is reached. A later consideration could be to graft through the intact superficialis with one- or two-stage reconstruction.[3] This is generally reserved for a child over 10 years old, because the rehabilitation protocol requires cooperation. When grafting, a tendon weave can be used proximally. The plantaris or palmaris longus are our first choice. Distally the growth plate must be avoided. The surgeon may attach the tendon into the epiphyseal bone via a pullout suture and avoid the growth plate.

Zone II

Previously called "no man's land," Arons[1] referred to it as "some man's land." Repair in this region has been and remains the source of most controversy, particularly in children. The main issues in this regard are as follows:
1. Primary repair versus grafting

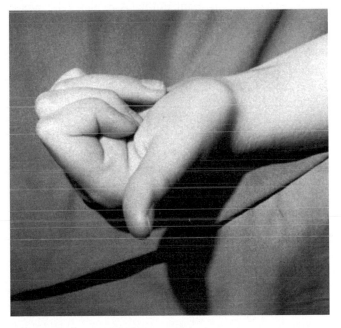

Fig. 64-3. A 10-year-old boy with flexor profundus avulsion of the right ring finger. Note the absence of DIP joint flexion on full fist making.

2. The timing of the repair
3. Repair of both tendons, versus repair of the profundus only
4. Associated digital nerve repair
5. Patient age and compliance with rehabilitation
6. Postoperative protocol

Entin, in 1965[6] stated that if the superficialis alone is cut, then no further treatment is necessary. If both superficilias and profundus were lacerated, he favored discarding the superficilias and primarily repairing the profundus. Vahvanen, in 1981[25] reported on 50 zone II repairs.

In his series the superficialis was excised and the profundus repaired primarily. He found that primary repair yielded superior results to tendon grafting at all levels, and in conclusion he recommended primary repair of both tendons in zone II by experienced hand surgeons. Wakefield, in 1964[26] advocated direct repair of the profundus only, with excision of the superficialis. He noted that direct repair was superior in children under 4 years and that tendon grafting was superior in children over 4 years old and stated that recurvatum at the PIP joint was not a clinically significant problem in digits with superficialis excision. In 1975 Strickland[21] advocated direct repair of the profundus alone, in cases when both tendons are lacerated. Tang, in 1994,[24] further subdivides zone II into four additional regions. Region 2A is the area from the distal margin of the superficilias insertion to the proximal margin of the insertion. Region 2B is from the proximal margin of the superficialis insertion to the distal border of the A_2 pulley. Region 2C is the area covered by the A_2 pulley, within the fibro-osseous sheath. Region 2D is the area from the proximal border of the A_2 pulley to the proximal margin of zone II. Results of region 2C repair of both tendons are compared with repair of the profundus only. In this study both tendon lacerations sustained in region 2C (that area covered by the A_2 pulley) fared better and had fewer reoperations if the superficialis was excised and the profundus alone was repaired.

If the superficialis is to be excised, we recommend leaving the distal stump to minimize weakening of the volar plate. Preservation of the superficialis becomes most important in the index and long fingers, for pinch and strength purposes.

Tendon grafting also has much support in the literature.[4] Bora, in 1970[3] reported on zone II injuries in which the profundus was cut, but the superficialis was functional. Using a plantaris graft on a delayed basis (6 weeks to 4 years), 17 of 20 cases were rated satisfactory. Hunter and Salisbury[10] reported on their results in 1970 using gliding artificial implants to produce acceptable functional results.

These findings were consistent regardless of the age, timing of repair (all under 4 weeks), the finger injured, multiple digit involvement, or if an associated digital nerve laceration was present and was primarily repaired.

TECHNIQUE

Meticulous handling of the small tissues, under magnification, by experienced hand surgeons must be observed when dealing with these delicate and complex structures. Midlateral or Bruner's incisions are used and incorporate the laceration. Accurate placement of the incisions will ensure less scar formation as the finger grows and the relationship of the structures change. Small mistakes can be amplified as the part grows! Careful and meticulous handling of these delicate structures using jeweler's forceps is essential. Preservation of the pulleys is critical, especially the A_2 and A_4 pulleys. We attempt to perform the repairs through the cruciate windows between the annular pulleys.

Many suture techniques have been described. In our experience a core stitch, using a modified Kessler technique with a 4-0 (or 5-0 for the younger child) synthetic, braided suture has given good results. When the tendon was of appropriate size, usually the index or long finger of a child over the age of 8, epitenon sutures of 6-0 or 7-0 nylon were also used to reinforce the repair. Each slip of the superficialis was repaired with a simple figure-of-eight suture. If the laceration was in the body of the superficialis, proximal to the chiasm, a mattress suture was used.

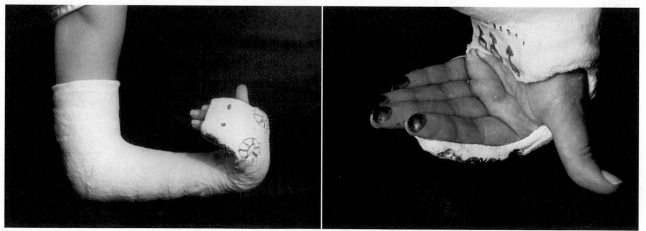

A   **B**

Fig. 64-4. A, Typical long arm cast with wrist flexed at 30° and metacarpophalangeal joints flexed at 70° and the interphalangeal joints extended. We trimmed this cast to allow the child to use finger motion without any constraints of the cast position. **B,** The child can elevate the digits. Games emphasizing active finger flexion can be played by bringing the fingers in to meet the palmar portion of the cast. Here we painted faces on the finger that then touch the face on the palm portion of the cast.

POSTOPERATIVE REHABILITATION

The postoperative care of these injuries is often the most challenging component. While some form of early postoperative mobilization is the norm in most adults,[12,23] this is not the same in children. Difficulties with comprehension and cooperation with the postoperative protocol are limiting factors.

The length of time of immobilization has been studied and most authors agree that the period of immobilization should not exceed 4 weeks.[6,9,24] O'Connell et al.,[18] in 1994 found that immobilization beyond 4 weeks dramatically increased the number of poor results. Vahvanen[25] recommended that in children under 6 years, the plaster should extend from the shoulder to the tip of the finger. The period of immobilization was under 4 weeks for the majority of his patients. Our postoperative protocol has consisted of immobilization for 4 weeks in children under 8 years. The child is placed in a long arm cast with the wrist at 60°, metacarpophalangeal (MP) joints at 70°, and the IP joints fully extended, leaving the palm and fingers free (Fig. 64-4, *A*). Active motion within these constraints is encouraged with the use of games involving faces drawn on the volar aspect of the cast, that the child plays under the supervision of the hand therapist (Fig. 64-4, *B*). During the active rehabilitation phase in young children, particularly when they have multiple tendon lacerations, we may often resort to immobilizing the uninjured hand to encourage use of the injured hand. Children over 8 years old are started immediately in the Duran passive protocol.

Following the initial 6 weeks of healing, age-appropriate rehabilitation activities are useful to maintain the child's interest and encourage finger motion and use. Nintendo games may have found their one true indication in that they help maintain a child's enthusiasm to use the injured finger in propelling Super Mario on his video journey (Fig. 64-5).

Seventy-four percent good or excellent results were obtained using the above protocol, regardless of the age, timing of repair (always under 4 weeks), or the presence of a concomitant digital nerve injury (Fig. 64-6).

When faced with the acute injury, several principles should be kept in mind.

1. Sharp lacerations can and should be repaired primarily at all levels and at all ages.

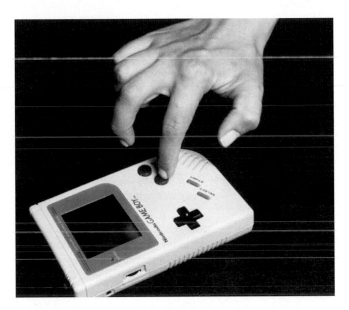

Fig. 64-5. The use of video games during rehabilitation encourages enthusiastic use of the injured index finger.

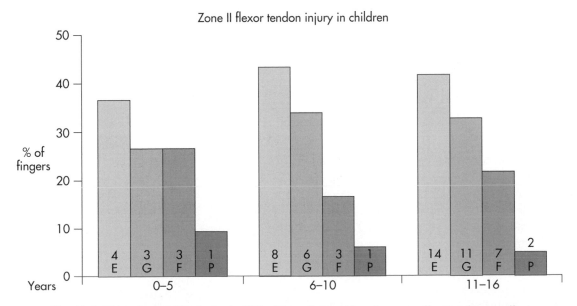

Fig. 64-6. Using the Strickland criteria, 74% of the patients achieved near excellent results regardless of age, timing of the repair when done under 4 weeks, or the presence of the concomitant digital nerve injury.

2. Exploration of digital nerves and the articular surface may be indicated.
3. The exploration and repair should be carried out in the operating room, under controlled conditions, using magnification and meticulous tissue-handling technique by an experienced hand surgeon.
4. Keeping in mind the regenerative capacity of the child, all available structures should be preserved.
5. A plan for definitive care should be made after the exploration.
6. Primary repair can usually be performed within 4 weeks of the injury.
7. In crush injuries with substance loss, primary repair is not recommended; definitive treatment must be carried out at a later date.

ZONES III, IV, AND V

We agree that these injuries should be treated with direct repair. Some special considerations include the following:

1. Injuries at or proximal to the myotendinous junction. Sutures are difficult to place in the muscle belly and overtensioning can cause necrosis; however, a few sutures placed in the fascia to reapproximate muscle ends are advisable. The entire arm should be protected by casting for 3 weeks.[9]
2. Injuries in the carpal tunnel. If the entire transverse carpal ligament has been incised, postoperative immobilization should be with the wrist in neutral to avoid bowstringing. Consideration should be given to reconstruction of the transverse carpal ligament as long as pressure within the canal will not be elevated.
3. Lacerations in the palm. If the lumbrical muscle has been injured, it must be allowed to heal in its resting position and not pulled distally or an imbalance of the intrinsic muscles can occur. The palmar fascia over the tendon junction should be excised to reduce scarring.

FLEXOR POLLICIS LONGUS

Primary repair, at any level, at any age has yielded good results in this simpler, one-pulley system. If tendon advancement becomes necessary, it should be limited to 1 cm.[9,22,26]

TENOLYSIS

Several factors must be observed when considering tenolysis. First, full passive motion should be present and active motion shown to be less than passive motion, and nonfunctional. Second, adequate time must be allowed to maximize conservative therapy, stretching, and exercise. Adhesions are more pliable and less extensive in children and can often be treated nonsurgically.[1] Third, the soft tissue envelope of the digit must be adequate; tenolysis should not be undertaken in the presence of inflammation.

There are two problems that are unique to children undergoing tenolysis. Ideally, tenolysis should be carried out under local anesthesia, so that the active excursion of the tendons can be documented. This also serves as a valuable psychologic tool for the patient, who can see the digit flex and work towards that goal in therapy. In children this poses an obvious difficulty because most young children cannot tolerate the operation under local anesthesia. When general anesthesia is used, a more proximal incision must be made to passively check the tendon excursion.

The other special problem in children is difficulty with the posttenolysis protocol. Birnie et al.[2] reported that all of the poor results following tenolysis in their series were in children under 11 years. They attributed the poor results to poor participation in the rehabilitation protocol and to the use of general anesthesia.

In our experience, vigilance in the postoperative period combined with aggressive therapy has proven effective in dealing with peritendinous scarring. In the cases that have required tenolysis, we prefer to wait until the child is old enough to participate in the rehabilitation.

REFERENCES

1. Arons MS: Purposeful delay of the primary repair of cut flexor tendons in "some man's land" in children, *Plast Reconstr Surg* 1974; 53(6):638-641.
2. Birnie RH, Idler RS: Flexor tenolysis in children. *J Hand Surg* 1995; 20A(2):254-257.
3. Bora FW: Profundus tendon grafting with unimpaired sublimis function in children, *Clin Orthop Rel Res* 1970; 71:118-123.
4. Boyes JH, Stark HH: Flexor tendon grafts in the fingers and thumb, *J Bone Joint Surg* 1971; 53A:1332-1342.
5. Cunningham MW, Yousif NJ, Matloub HS, et al: Retardation of tendon growth after injury to the flexor tendons, *J Hand Surg* 1985; 10A(1):115-117.
6. Entin MA: Flexor tendon repair and grafting in children, *Am J Surg* 1965; 109:287-292.
7. Gaisford JC, Fleegler EJ: Alterations in finger growth following flexor tendon injuries, *Plast Reconstr Surg* 1973; 51(2):164-168.
8. Grobbelaar AO, Hudson DA: Flexor tendon injuries in children, *J Hand Surg* 1994; 19B(6):696-698.
9. Herndon JH: Treatment of tendon injuries in children, *Orthop Clin North Am* 1976; 7(3):717-731.
10. Hunter JM, Salisbury RE: Use of gliding artificial implants to produce tendon sheaths, *Plast Reconstr Surg* 1970; 45(6):564-572.
11. Kleinert HE, Verdan C: Report of the committee on tendon injuries, *J Hand Surg* 1983; 8(5):part 2, 794-798.
12. Lister GD, Kleinert HE, Kutz JE, Atasoy E: Primary flexor tendon repair followed by immediate controlled mobilization, *J Hand Surg* 1977; 2(6):441-451.
13. Lundborg G, Rank F: Experimental intrinsic healing of flexor tendons based upon synovial nutrition, *J Hand Surg* 1978; 3:21.
14. Malek R: Embryology of the hand. In Tubiana R, ed: *The hand*, Philadelphia, 1981, Saunders.
15. Manske PR, Lesker PA, Bridwell K: Experimental studies in chickens on the initial nutrition of tendon grafts, *J Hand Surg* 1979; 4:545.
16. Nishijima N, Fujio K, Yamamuro T: Growth of severed flexor tendons in chickens, *J Orthop Res* 1995; 13(1):138-142.
17. Nishijima N, Yamamuro T, Ueba Y: Flexor tendon growth in chickens, *J Orthop Res* 1994; 12(4):576-581.
18. O'Connell SJ, Moore MM, Strickland JW, et al: Results of zone one and zone two flexor tendon repairs in children, *J Hand Surg* 1994; 19A(1):48-52.

19. Smith JW, Bellinger CG: The blood supply of tendons. In Tubiana R, ed: *The hand,* Philadelphia, 1981, Saunders.

20. Sasaki Y, Nomura S: An unusual role of the vinculum after complete laceration of the flexor tendons, *J Hand Surg* 1987; 12B(1):105-108.

21. Strickland JW: Bone, nerve, and tendon injuries of the hand in children, *Pediatr Clin North Am* 1975; 22(2):78-87.

22. Strickland JW: Flexor tendon surgery, part 1: primary flexor tendon repair, *J Hand Surg* 1989; 14B(3):261-272.

23. Strickland JW, Glogovac SV: Digital function following flexor tendon repair in zone two: a comparison of immobilization and controlled passive motion techniques, *J Hand Surg* 1980; 5(6):537-543.

24. Tang JB: Flexor tendon repair in zone 2C, *J Hand Surg* 1994; 19B(1):72-75.

25. Vahvanen V, Gripenberg L, Nuutinen P: Flexor tendon injury of the hand in children, a long term follow up study of 84 patient, *Scand J Plast Reconstr Surg* 1981; 15:43-48.

26. Wakefield AR: Hand injuries in children, *J Bone Joint Surg* 1964; 46A(6):1226-1234.

1) Kim Cúc, 17 ♀ — Hot water burn in childhood L. severe contracture of all fingers especially long and ring.

♀: a) "Z" plasty, index.
b) ◇ grafts (full thickness from L. inguinal region — long and Ring fingers. PIP Transarticular K.W. fixation (max. ext.)

DIP ___ axis
PIP ___ deficit
(normal diamond patterns of finger)
▦ = grafted area.

mid-axial line
incision from PIP axis·
bisects angle of contracture.
finger opens leaving ◇ deficit.
Some nerve shortening, etc.!

2) Chanh (see consult. p. 60)
Resection of mid. portion of central extensor tendon, leaving bi-lateral bands intact, released the check-rein effect on the PIP joint.

——— " ———

- Discussion of Ext. + Sup. fl. Tendon releases with AP crush injuries of prox. phalanx.
- P.O. check on earlier cases.

Part XVI

AESTHETIC CONSIDERATIONS

Sketch by J. William Littler, from his "A Surgical Diary: Viet Nam 1969."

Chapter 65

THE MUTILATED HAND AND ITS PATIENT

Jean Pillet

The indications for prosthetic treatment of an amputated hand depend more on patient behavior than on the actual amputation. This behavior varies considerably from one patient to another and changes over time. In general, we think of recent amputations, the surgical procedure involved, and rehabilitation. Yet patients with long-term amputations exist. Why are they forgotten? Generally, surgeons and therapists are familiar with the problems of recent amputees, who are often considered severely handicapped patients who need functional assistance. They tend to ignore the changes that occur with time, believing that long-term amputees no longer require their services. It is important to acquire an understanding of how the needs of recent amputees change over time and to get to know the situation of long-term amputees better. Analyzing all aspects of their behavior highlights two major attributes of the hand—function and aesthetics. When these two are not combined, they can cause an individual's hand to no longer seem human.

FUNCTION

First and foremost, the human hand is a functional organ, considered the universal functional tool. It can carry out not only complex prehensile but also extremely precise percussion activities. Given today's level of technology, the hand's connections via the brain with sight, nerves, muscles, tendons, and joints ensure that it remains irreplaceable. Only touch can provide us with genuine feelings of consistency, shape, and softness. The hand characterizes a human individual's own specific harmony, indispensable for the person as well as for those close to him or her.

AESTHETICS

The hand is also an aesthetic organ. How these aesthetic qualities evolve and are perceived varies from individual to individual as well as from one ethnic group to another. In general, Latin and Mediterranean peoples are more conscious of the beauty of the hand than are Anglo-Saxons or Scandinavians. In the United States, because ethnic groups intermix from one generation to another, characteristics regarding how the hand is viewed are not as sharply defined, but do not completely disappear.

Based on these functional and aesthetic concerns, we consider hand amputees, whether total or partial, not as disabled patients, but rather as victims of an abnormality or of a difference.

AMPUTEE BEHAVIOR

The behavior of accident victims must be distinguished from that of patients who have undergone disease-related amputation.

Accident victims

Two different stages are seen in accident victims: those of recent amputation, with which surgeons are familiar, and those of less recent amputation, usually less well known.

Recent amputees

The behavior of recent amputees changes over two well-defined stages. The first stage—during the hospital stay—is characterized by emotional shock followed by unreasonable expectations. Patients, often in a state of prostration and apparently indifferent, are told of the sacrifice needed because of the extent of their lesions. But explanations can never alleviate the emotional shock. These surgery patients often anticipate a dark professional and personal future. However, while they remain in a hospital environment, and at least as long as the bandages have not come off, these patients feel supported and, even more importantly, understood, because during the healing process they find it normal to be assisted in every movement of everyday life. These persons who have become handicapped try to envision the various solutions available to them, either through surgery or through the fitting of a prosthesis. They have faith in science and believe in miracles, whether transplants or the possibility of a real artificial hand.

The second stage—after leaving the hospital—is often a time of shame followed by hope and then disappointment. These patients have healed or almost healed physically after surgery and consult surgeons as a part of follow-up procedures. We can advise and reassure them, but these patients must return to family and friends, to their own environment. Usually such patients act disabled, hiding their stump and not using it, for psychologic and material reasons. Because the scar is still recent, they become dependent on the family environment, which often operates out of poor advice, feeling sorry for the patient, who finds this painful. At this time of shame, patients should not be pitied or helped unnecessarily. Indeed, however well-meant or loving the protection given recent amputees, these patients will always rapidly find themselves on their own. The amputees, without help from family or friends, must adapt to everyday life. Thus the role of physicians, physical therapists, psychologists, and, in the case of young amputees, the mother is crucial during this confusing stage. It is a time full of hope and disappointments but, because the future depends on it, it is nevertheless essential.

Long-term amputees

Whereas recent amputees are, at least temporarily, heavily disabled, long-term amputees may or may not be disabled, depending on how they have been guided, first by the family and medical environment and then by the different welfare bodies involved. Amputees will be skillful or clumsy and well adjusted or not. Motivation is entirely psychologic and essentially depends on how they view the consequences of amputation.

Poorly adjusted patients are a minority. Some amputees hide their stump and refuse to use it. Others may wear their functional prosthesis but do not use it, as if its very presence could justify their behavior. Yet others accept their condition too well, being pleased to be constantly helped by others either because they have a psychologic or emotional need to be treated like children, which reflects a psychologic disorder, or because they are receiving financial compensation, which turns them into beneficiaries within an economically strong and socially sophisticated environment.

Contrary to this minority, most amputees return to a normal life as *well-adjusted individuals.* They return to their family and friends, although a change may be needed in

professional occupation. Generally, they have managed to assess their situation realistically. Those fitted with a prosthesis have usually stopped wearing it; those who are not fitted have rapidly adapted their remaining capacities to cope with situations functionally. However, most also retain a well-defined feeling of frustration concerning aesthetic aspects.

Disease-related amputation patients

The behavior of patients who have undergone a disease-related amputation differs significantly from that of accident victims. Although they do not have to face the brutal psychologic trauma of amputation, they are confronted with the more emotional one of necessary mutilation. Sometimes this is perceived as a sound solution to a problem, and functional and aesthetic handicaps are seen as the price paid for success. In other cases the amputation is rejected or acceptance is deferred because the prospect is too traumatic. The patient must understand how necessary the sacrifice is, with stress placed on the fact that the anticipated disfigurement is likely to be of relative unimportance with the use of an aesthetic prosthesis.

Amputee children and their parents

To better understand the behavior of young amputees, it is necessary to distinguish between the behavior of these children and that of their parents. In addition, surgeons must understand the behavior of adult amputees because children will grow up to be adult amputees.

The parents of amputee children have the functional and aesthetic needs to make a normal child out of a child perceived as abnormal. When we inquire about a child's behavior, the parents will be the ones who answer. The difficulties encountered in dealing with amputee children are generally caused by the parents' projections. Such children are seen as disabled and therefore functionally incomplete, although they are not. Contrary to adults, children have marvelous adaptation capabilities, and it is adults' preconceived ideas that cause them difficulties.

As a first step, parents must come to accept their child as he or she is, that is, different. If this stage is overlooked, any decision is likely to be wrong. Therefore clinicians must be aware of the parents' unconscious wish to make a normal child out of one perceived as disabled. They expect a miracle, and the usual outcome will be disappointment. Parents must face the following truth: An aesthetic or functional prosthesis will never be able to fully replace the lost hand of their young amputee. However, prescribing the fitting of a prosthesis does not imply an irreparable case and irrevocable decision, as with a surgical procedure.

The young amputee's first prosthetic consultation

For parents, the first consultation is essential, so it is also crucial for the child. Parents must understand what their child's functional capabilities will be. Specifically, these children will be able to do everything other children the same age can do, but will do it by using different techniques. Parents and others around the child can offer help, unobtrusively, to find individualized replacement and substitution solutions.

In a world where everything is designed to be used with both hands, where the environment is based on normal possibilities, it seems inconceivable that it is possible to do everything with just a stump, or even two, but this is exactly what long-term amputees manage to do. When observing them, we feel convinced that we are confronted with an exceptionally gifted individual. Even amputees can be surprised when another, with a higher level of amputation, can carry out the same activities as rapidly and as well as they can.

Some authors recommend fitting functional prosthesis on very young children with unilateral distal amputation because this ensures excellent results. But are these good results helpful to the patient or do they only illustrate the soundness of a theory? Even without prostheses these young amputees achieve—just as those with agenesis can— amazing functional results. Without wearing a prosthesis they can develop personal techniques, so why should we insist that they use our techniques, making them dependent on a prosthesis?

Adolescence is the most crucial period for amputees. At this age, any kind of maladjustment tends to be overestimated and parents who are disconcerted by these difficulties often grant whatever their children request. We do not believe that unreasonable requests should be rejected outright, but we prefer to carefully evaluate the situation, including the adolescent's psychologic problems and problems related to amputation. This careful assessment enables us to see how we can help these adolescents to understand what is really going on and to express a genuine need based on the nature of the existing problems. A prosthesis will not solve all their problems, particularly their social problems or those accompanying the choice of profession. Adolescent patients will have to face the intervention of teachers and guidance counselors, who may be more or less well informed on the subject of functional possibilities related to unilateral distal amputation.

FITTING OF FUNCTIONAL PROSTHESES
Compensating for the functional deficits of a totally amputated hand

Active functional prostheses
The main quality of a hand is sensation, which no functional prosthesis can provide. This explains why, with unilateral distal amputees, prosthetic replacements are almost always failures even though everything is done to ensure that the prosthesis provides satisfactory functional results.

As soon as patients have healed, they are referred to a specialized rehabilitation center. The whole rehabilitation process centers on the prosthesis. Rehabilitation requires a long time, even in the best of cases where it is geared to eventual professional requalification.

Most patients who have undergone amputation of the hand do not use their functional prosthesis because they find it awkward, compared with their stump, which is much more efficient. A prosthesis can encourage the patient to remain physically and psychologically handicapped. By refusing the prosthesis, these patients liberate themselves and progressively adapt their abilities, finding solutions that are at least as efficient as with a prosthesis.

Level of amputation in fitting functional prosthesis. It was generally believed that correct adaptation of prostheses was only possible if the amputation was carried out at the level of, or above, the lower third of the forearm. However, this type of amputation, considered ideal for fitting a prosthesis, is obsolete. We do not believe that, in an emergency, a surgeon must deliberately sacrifice what could be preserved to conform to this preprosthetic amputation approach. With an accident victim, amputation should be as economical as possible, preserving as much as can be salvaged. Modern techniques make this possible, so the prosthesis must adapt to a stump that is not necessarily in conformity with previous standards. As Dautry recommends, "Keep everything you can in order to obtain as long a stump as possible, covered with healthy skin, well vascularized and having sensation, avoiding, as much as possible, distal scar tissue." Amputees who have long stumps are aware that a functional prosthesis, cumbersome and lacking in sensation, will not improve their situation. When an amputation at a higher level is proposed, under the pretext of fitting a prosthesis, they reject it because of the fear of no longer being able to do anything. In fact, the more distal the level of the amputation, the lesser the handicap. A long stump that preserves sensation, pronation, and supination is extremely functional.

Working prostheses
Aristotle described the hand of a manual worker as "the tool of tools," the holder of tools. Working prostheses, which we call *tool-holding prostheses,* are always well accepted because they are considered fully part of a worker's normal equipment. Both amputees and their workmates invest such devices with the dignity of a tool.

This tool-holding prosthesis should be limited to precisely this important role, designed around a specific instrument to obtain a specific result. Generally, it is put on at the factory door and removed when leaving, like an overall.

Usually a tool-holding prosthesis is very simple, light, and easy to fit onto the stump. The amputee participates in its design, either at the factory or at a prosthesis center. In fact, amputees often invent clever ways of improving these devices. An intelligent amputee often develops, on a do-it-yourself basis, small accessories to be attached either

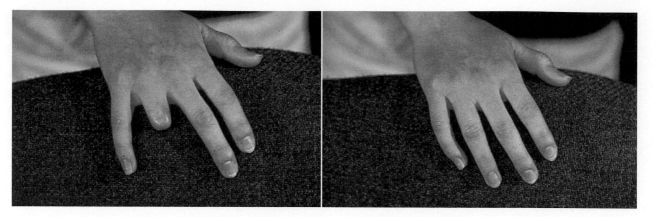

Figs. 65-1 and 65-2. The more the stump is pain free, well vascularized, without trophic disorders, fleshy, and, most importantly, has sensation, the better the prosthesis is accepted. It must be well-oriented, have a perimeter smaller than that of the opposite side, and be longer than 1 cm.

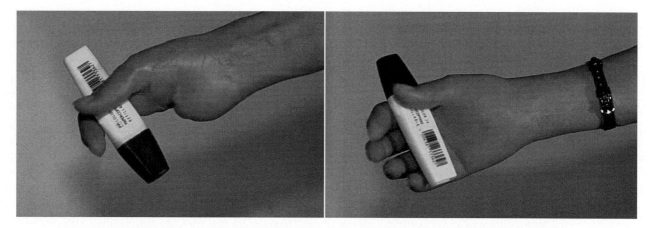

Figs. 65-3 and 65-4. Fitting prostheses on partial hands is still difficult. The range of physical problems encountered is huge, and potential solutions vary according to patient needs. Usually it is best to leave the remaining fingers outside the prosthesis, as long as the distal border is fine enough not to attract attention.

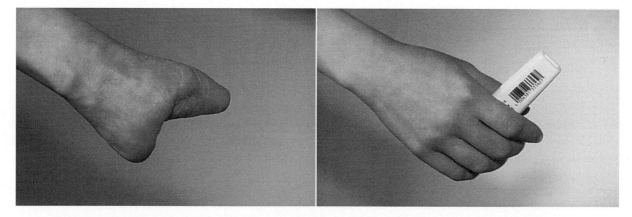

Figs. 65-5 and 65-6. The prosthesis that preserves the metacarpals and the carpal provides support for the palm and enables two-handed prehension of heavy objects. Also, because of the elastic memory of its components, it can hold lightweight objects.

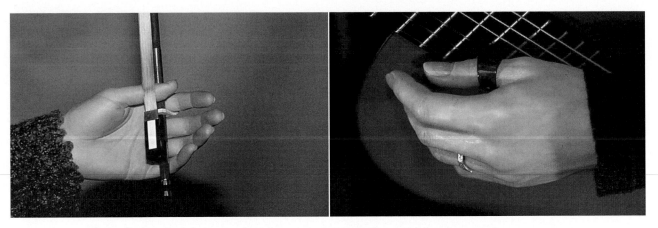

Figs. 65-7 and 65-8. Should a child or an adult, having undergone total amputation of a hand or a forearm, wish to play a musical instrument, aesthetic prostheses, usually with some adjustments, can be perfect. Obviously, these musicians will most likely not play professionally, but they have a good time, play music for their own pleasure and that of their family and friends, and enhance their own well-being.

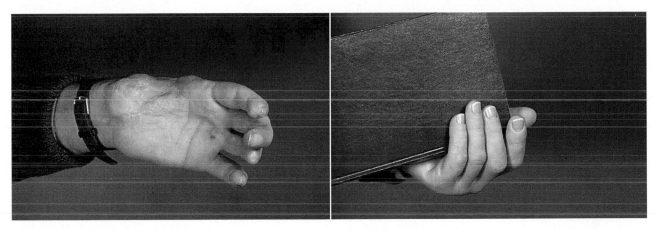

Figs. 65-9 and 65-10. This patient, highly motivated as to the appearance of his hand, has chosen to wear a prosthesis that covers all of the palm and fingers. For the last 12 years he has worn it from morning to evening at work (in a bank) and for social activities.

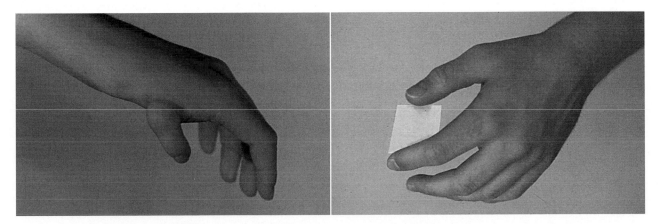

Figs. 65-11 and 65-12. On the basis of our latest experimental techniques for the fixation of prosthesis on short or floating stumps, we have achieved results such as this, but follow-up has been only a few months.

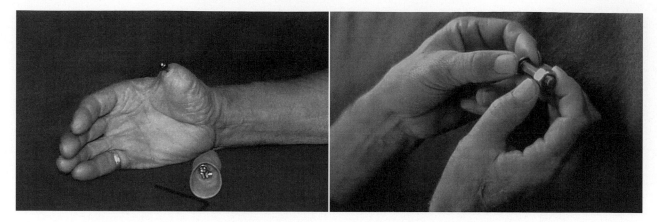

Figs. 65-13 and 65-14. Dental-type implants (Branemark and Lundborg) showed that the force of the pinch can be transmitted from the bone to the prosthesis. The patient can also feel feedback pressure. However, our follow-up has been only 2 years thus far.

to the stump or to the prosthesis using an ordinary leather strap; these accessories are mainly used at work.

Compensating for the functional deficits of a partially amputated hand

Passive functional prostheses

In general, a passive functional prosthesis is a palette that provides apposition to the remaining fingers. It is often used in response to specific professional requirements and is essential for manual workers. The passive functional prosthesis is supported by the metacarpals and allows the fingers and the wrist to move freely. It requires perfect adjustment to avoid pain at the level of the more sensitive areas, whether during use or during fixation. The shape must be adapted not only to the stump but also to the tool used and the mobility of the remaining fingers. Modifications should be possible as rehabilitation progresses. The material it is made from must be resistant and rigid, with antiskid contact points to ensure good functional stability.

Levels of amputation and related fitting problems

Digital amputation

Although patients are always anxious to obtain their prostheses, it is necessary to wait for the size of the stump to stabilize. Initial postsurgery care consists of controlling edema. At first, applying a Coban bandage can help reduce stump size. Coban must be applied in a distal to proximal manner, using a figure-of-eight pattern. The area is tightly bandaged but compression is avoided. Very importantly, the joints must be allowed to move freely. When the stump circumference stabilizes, it is time to start designing the prosthesis.

Long stumps. Frequently, long stumps are spatula shaped and voluminous. In some cases they cannot be fitted without surgical alterations.

The prosthesis, which is very thin, covers the whole distal phalanx, like a thimble. The drawbacks are obvious. If the consistency of the fingernail is natural, it can easily wound the sensitive skin of the stump underneath. If the fingernail is flexible and comfortable, it will be difficult to use nail polish on it.

The benefit of this type of prosthesis is that it can give the finger the added length necessary, for example, for a secretary to work at a computer or a flutist to return to his or her instrument.

Short stumps. By definition, short stumps are less than 1 cm long. Therefore the problem is attaching the prosthesis. Both surgical alteration and ring or glue fixation must be considered.

1. *Surgical alteration.* After healing, the shape of the stump must be cylindrical, not conical. There must be no lateral-palmar ligaments extending from the commisure to the opening of the fingers, and the minimum length is 1.5 cm.
2. *Ring fixation.* This implies making two or three rings, which are then linked together, an adaptation of the technique used for dental bridges. One ring is for the prosthetic finger, whereas the other (or others) is for the adjacent finger (or fingers). This technique is complex but remains a viable option for patients who refuse any form of surgical procedure but require an improvement in their condition.
3. *Glue fixation.* This technique almost always causes problems. If the glue sticks, the area is difficult to clean. This hardens and thickens the prosthesis, which should be extremely thin. Glue can prove irritating to the skin when the prosthesis is removed day after day. Irritation can also ensue if the prosthesis is not removed for several days, because of lack of exposure of the skin to air. If the glue does not stick, the prosthesis is not solidly attached and can fail.

Medium-size stumps. Medium-size stumps must be appropriately oriented, with the perimeter smaller than that of the opposite side, and they must be more than 1 cm long. Prostheses for these stumps must be flexible, but not exceedingly so, because a number of light tasks require stronger apposition, for example, in the case of a punch card operator.

For these stumps, a dorsal orthosis, such as specially designed silver rings, adjusted and placed on the prosthesis, provide resistance to counterforce pressures. Because of its stability, this system offers greatly improved function.

The attachment of these prostheses must be secure, comfortable, and simple. Removing the prosthesis creates negative pressure, which must be eliminated by pinching the side in order to create, voluntarily, an air tunnel. The stump must also be well filled with bone and be cylinder shaped.

Amputation of the thumb. Partial amputation of the thumb can be compared with that of the fingers. However, amputation of the first ray implies that the prosthesis, for secure attachment, must cover all of the palm and go over the wrist, which is a considerable drawback. Depending on patient motivation, this reduced sensitivity of the hand is perceived differently.

Multidigit amputation. Several fingers can be replaced with a prosthesis if the stumps are sufficiently long to ensure that each one is solidly attached. Should this not be the case, a hand glove will be needed, leaving the thumb free to ensure adequate sensation.

Problem cases. The following are difficult cases to address:

1. *Large stumps.* In general, without surgical removal of fatty tissues, large stumps cannot be fitted. In some cases surgery can be avoided by bandaging the stump with Coban for approximately 1 month.
2. *Hyperflexed stumps.* Hyperflexed stumps usually result from poorly done amputations and often result in prostheses that are overly voluminous and poorly oriented. Our experience in this area has proved the superiority, at both functional and aesthetic levels, of disarticulation over salvaging a small area of the distal phalanx. This latter approach provides a longer stump but one that rapidly becomes stiff and fixed in a hyperflexed position.
3. *Painful stumps.* A patient who has a painful stump will not be able to stand wearing a prosthesis. These patients should be referred for classic desensitizing techniques. If after 1 month, no progress has been achieved, surgical alteration may be necessary. However, with hypersensitive stumps, a prosthesis can offer a two-fold benefit: providing a comfortable constant pressure and giving a reassuring protection against impacts.
4. *Toe transfer.* When patients find toe transfers ugly, they can be covered with an aesthetic prosthesis, worn only for social activities. However, this prosthesis can, in certain cases, be worn permanently if the patient feels that this toe-finger attracts too much attention from

other individuals, becoming, as the patient says, a "focal point of morbid curiosity."

Amputation of the hand

Partial amputation of the hand. With the so-called metacarpal hand, where there is preservation of one or several fingers, the lack of any one ideal solution means that there are a large number of possibilities, which must be carefully evaluated. The range of physical problems involved with fitting prostheses on partial hands is huge, and potential solutions must be carefully reviewed, taking into account patient needs, which are just as varied. These prostheses must be perfectly adjusted. They must be fine enough to preserve skin sensation and enable free movement of the remaining fingers as well as the wrist. Partial metacarpal amputations can be oblique or central, with part or total preservation of one or several fingers, as follows:

1. *Partial preservation of one or several fingers.* Digital stumps are covered with hand prostheses, restoring their normal length and natural aspect.
2. *Total preservation of one or several fingers.* It is best for the preserved fingers to remain outside the prosthesis, as long as the outer limit of the prosthesis, at the basis of the fingers, is thin enough not to attract attention.

Total amputation of the hand. Preserving the metacarpals, or the carpal, naturally enables two-handed prehension of heavy objects, as well as the supporting function of the palm. Initially, the degree of handicap is greater for patients disarticulated at the radiocarpal level, but they are potentially just as capable as others of leading a normal life. In general, the patients do not find difficulty in making any movements they wish. Any difficulties that may occur do not interfere with everyday activities.

Amputation of the forearm

Long or short forearm stumps can be fitted with aesthetic prostheses. These simple prostheses, which are lengthening devices, improve two-handed prehension and provide better balance to the way children handle their body. Even a very short forearm stump is long enough to enable attachment of such a prosthesis. The cap slips over the stump, leaving the elbow free, and therefore, totally preserving its mobility. A thin suction sleeve holds the prosthesis in place, overlapping the cap by a few centimeters.

Bilateral amputees. Fortunately, bilateral amputations, except in the case of fingers, are fairly rare. The physical handicap is such that, normally, it overshadows the aesthetic issue. However, this problem sometimes does arise, acutely, and in such situations, it may prove beneficial to fit the amputee with a prosthesis on one side only.

Fitting children with a prosthesis

The age at which a child is fitted with an aesthetic prosthesis depends on the existence of a functional pinch, as follows:

1. *The stump with no pinch.* Theoretically it is possible to fit a baby amputee as young as 18 months, but not earlier because of the skin reactions caused by attaching a prosthesis to the stump. Generally, the prosthesis is a simple lengthening device, which allows the child to adapt to its balance and encourages two-handed activities.
2. *The stump with pinch.* If there is still a pinch, however rudimentary, a prosthesis is definitely not advisable because it would prove more of a nuisance than useful. Without the prosthesis the patient will be able to undertake all the movements required for everyday activities. Therefore it is preferable to wait for adolescence, and for a greater degree of motivation, before designing an aesthetic prosthesis. At that stage, it might become a psychologic necessity.

Regardless of whether pinch is or is not present, it is sometimes necessary to fit a prosthesis on a very young child, especially if the parents are suffering from severe psychologic trauma. This is therapy for the parents, unfortunately provided via the child.

The future of aesthetic prostheses for providing improved function

Secure prosthetic attachment on a short stump is important and we believe it will be achieved in the very near future. Specific advances to be seen are as follows:

1. *Active function aesthetic prostheses.* Thanks to dental implants (Branemark and Lundborg), the force of pinch can be transmitted from the bone to the prosthesis. The patient can also feel feedback pressure. Gosset notes that "Obviously an implant in the maxilla does not entail the same consequences as an implant—external attachment—in another bone." One year ago, we fitted a prosthesis on a patient who had this type of experimental implant in the right first metacarpal bone. Although our follow-up period has been short, the patient is having encouraging results.
2. *Passive function aesthetic prostheses.* Thanks to the latest techniques for attaching prostheses, we can place a simple thumb device on a floating thumb, without having to cover the palm. Follow-up in this area has been, so far, only a few months.

Iselin has said, "We must be cautious vis-a-vis our 'champion patients' because the quality of their results does not necessarily depend upon the quality of our technique."

FITTING WITH AESTHETIC PROSTHESES
Motivations and expectations

Amputees who desire aesthetic prostheses are often exigent, even perfectionists and therefore difficult to please. Thus it is necessary to take time and listen to them carefully to clearly define individual prosthetic needs. Many aspects must be taken into account, including the analysis of the patient's unspoken motivations and his or her real expectations.

Motivations

It is important to verify whether, as far as the appearance of the hand is concerned, patients are highly motivated or if they are coming to satisfy their family or simply because an insurance company has agreed to pay for the prosthesis.

Aesthetic prostheses satisfy a deeply felt need for those born with agenesis and for amputees, specifically, the desire to go unnoticed and to have two hands, just like everybody else. Therefore the more beautiful aesthetic prostheses are the ones that are not noticed. Wearing these prostheses has a genuine psychotherapeutic effect for those highly motivated individuals. Formerly handicapped patients are now able to go out; to go to the swimming pool; to wear short-sleeved shirts, a bracelet, or rings. Easy to put on and to take off, these prostheses are considered an accessory that covers up an undesirable feature and enables these individuals to escape unwelcome curiosity.

The psychologic role, which is of paramount importance for the patient, is not always clearly perceived, even by experienced professionals. Indeed, people who attach a great deal of importance to the aesthetic appearance of their hand wish to see it improved, even sometimes acting against the advice of their own physician or surgeon, who may claim that this prosthesis would delay rehabilitation. Nothing could be further from the truth. Amputees who have lost not only function but are also aesthetically impaired are mainly concerned, at least at first, with hiding their mutilation. This is, as stated earlier, the period of shame.

Case study. We fitted a farmer from Georgia, a simple man, approximately 60 years old, who had undergone a metacarpal amputation with preservation of the thumb. When we suggested leaving his thumb outside the prosthesis to preserve as much function as possible, he told us that he preferred to see it covered in order to achieve as high a level of aesthetic attractiveness as possible. He planned to wear his prosthesis only on Sundays, to go to church. He did not want to have to hide his hand anymore. He wanted to be "beautiful for God."

When patients are sufficiently motivated to improve the appearance of their hand, it is important to explain to them why they will not wear their prosthesis. Indeed, they will not be satisfied with the prognosis and will have to endure all of its drawbacks, a prospect that is quite unacceptable. To better understand this future refusal, they should bear in mind the proverb, "Love is blind."

Expectations

Patients' expectations must be realistic. If they expect too much, they will be disappointed and will never be satisfied simply by wearing a prosthesis, which, however sophisticated, can never replace a lost hand. Sometimes a patient will request a prosthesis knowing that it will cause discomfort and functional loss, and will only provide mediocre aesthetic results. For example, off-center digital stumps always lead to unattractive prostheses. Several digital prostheses, fitted on the same hand, reduce its sensation and prehensile strength. Disarticulation of several fingers, at the metacarpal phalanx level, means that the prosthesis will have to cover the whole hand and trophic changes will make it difficult to bear. These patients should be advised against prostheses, unless the psychologic aspects outweigh their drawbacks. The patient must be able to face the following truth: An aesthetic prosthesis is not a panacea for each and every amputee.

Is the aesthetic prosthesis functional?

Mechanically speaking, the answer to this question is no, yet patients tell us it is functional. Why? Because they use it. This may be easier to understand if one looks at the psychologic reasons why patients wear a prosthesis. An aesthetic prosthesis satisfies a genuine need and thus is psychologically acceptable and considered useful (functional).

Genuine function of aesthetic prostheses

Genuine function is mainly observed in social and professional activities. Here the prosthesis enables the use of remaining structures, as follows:

- Extends stumps that are too short, enabling them to be used in apposition to the other fingers
- Ensures preservation of joint mobility and skin sensation because of its extreme thinness
- Protects a sensitive stump with its thickness, thereby freeing the patient from the fear of using it
- Supports pushing, especially important for activities requiring two hands
- Holds lightweight objects because of the elastic memory nature of its components

Relative function of aesthetic prostheses

Frequently an amputee will feel that a functional pinch, surgically salvaged on a heavily damaged hand, is too repulsive to be used in public. With an aesthetic prosthesis, the patient will take the stump out of a pocket and use it. This illustrates the value of these prostheses, which, by restoring a normal appearance to the stump, makes it operational even while reducing function.

Relationship of prosthesis to professions and hobbies

Interruption of professional activities

In numerous contacts with the public, aesthetic prostheses are often the key that allows patients to return to occupations for which they are already qualified. For example, a railway conductor, the victim of an accident at work who had a right metacarpal hand with a salvaged thumb, was able to go back to work using an aesthetic prosthesis. In public, this restored a normal appearance to the hand and, more importantly, enabled him to punch tickets because of the index finger on the prosthesis, which could be apposed to the pressure of the thumb. This patient wore an aestetic prosthesis everyday at work for 25 years, until he retired.

Need for retraining

Prostheses broaden the scope of professional possibilities and allow the choice of certain occupations that require contacts with clients.

Case study. A 16-year-old boy had been involved in a workshop explosion, resulting in total amputation of the first ray and partial amputation of the last three fingers on the right side and radial carpal amputation on the left. He had wanted to become a dentist. The left side was fitted with an aesthetic prosthesis covering the whole hand. This helped him to become a high level civil servant. He has worn this prosthesis every day for the last 37 years, except when he was at home.

A special case: musicians. The amputee musician has lost function and become handicapped with regard to his or her instrument. Expectations are often unrealistic, including retrieving a lost hand or lost dexterity. If the amputee is already a professional musician, any amputation will be perceived as a disaster, but prostheses can prove helpful. Unfortunately, if the musician is a virtuoso performer, amputation can mean extreme psychologic distress, and no prosthesis will be able to restore lost physical and mental virtuosity. What prostheses can do for amputee musicians is, in general, not significant, except in the case of distal finger amputations. Hand or forearm prostheses for musicians are extremely rare. Usually these individuals must find another profession.

If, after complete amputation of the hand or even of the forearm, a child or adult wishes to play a musical instrument, aesthetic prostheses with some clever adjustments are perfect. For example, small elastic straps can easily attach a bow to the prosthetic fingers. A mediator, fixed on a ring set onto the thumb of the prosthesis, will make guitar playing possible. Thus an aesthetic prosthesis can provide many hours of pleasure by really helping the patient overcome technical difficulties and restoring a normal appearance. Obviously, a patient who must attach a bow to a prosthesis will never sound like a virtuoso, but he or she can play for personal pleasure or for family and friends, enhancing personal well-being.

RESULTS AND CONCLUSIONS

It is always difficult to analyze the results of 40 years of experience because results essentially depend on the personality of each individual patient. Patients are entitled to competence. Thus each patient, or parent in the case of young children, is entitled to expect the very best results. We must know how to channel the patient's expectations by providing, at length and patiently, information on what can be done professionally. This information must be understood and accepted before any prosthetic treatment is undertaken, because the level of expectation must not exceed professional capabilities. This principle is crucial because it will avoid conflict when evaluating short-term and long-term results.

Wearing an aesthetic prosthesis

The cause of amputation has very little influence on the actual use of the aesthetic prosthesis. There can be very significant differences between patients. They generally fall into two categories, as follows:

1. The broadest category comprises patients who consider the prosthesis a piece of clothing. They put it on each day when they leave home. Some wear it from morning to night—it is a part of themselves.

2. In the minority category are patients who keep their prosthesis on, night and day, as well as those who wear it only once or twice a year, on special occasions. Still others in this category never wear the prosthesis, but refuse to give it up because they feel they can wear it if they ever need to. These consider the prosthesis as medication.

Wearing a prosthesis is not necessarily permanent and final. Usually an aesthetic prosthesis is removed as soon as the socialization requirements no longer make it necessary. It is abandoned by those who have lost their inhibitions. Whether wearing an aesthetic prosthesis is temporary or long-term, the device does help patients get through a difficult period of life. If wearing the prosthesis is temporary, this does not reflect the failure of the therapeutic approach, but rather proves its psychologic efficacy. The prosthesis is worn when patients feel they need it and set aside when they feel well again.

As with any reconstructive method, aesthetic prostheses have pros and cons. Their major drawback is that they are a foreign body. Their significant advantage is that they do not impair the patient's surgical future.

BIBLIOGRAPHY

Dautry P, Pillet J, Apoil A, Biteau O: A La Recherche d'une main perdue, *Revue du Praticien* 1971; 21:603 .

Iselin M, Pillet J: Possibilites actuelles de la prothese plastique, Association a la Chirurgie dans les Mutilations de la Main, *La presse Medicales-6eme Annee* 1953; 82:1766-1767.

Pillet J: La Prothese plastique et restauratrice chez les amputes partiels du membre superieur, *Acta Chir Belg* 1958; 57:319-322.

Pillet J: Evolution psychologique des amputes, *Chirurgie (Memoires de l'Academie)* 1977; 8:708-713.

Pillet J: La Prothese dans les amputations des extremites digitales, 2eme ed, *G.E.M. Monographie* 1981; 9:123-127.

Pillet J: The aesthetic hand prosthesis, *Orthop Clin North Am* 1981; 12:961-969.

Pillet J: Aesthetic hand prosthesis, *J Hand Surg* 1983; 8(5):part 2.

Pillet J: Psychologic assessment of the patient with unilateral upper extremity (ch 27) and Cosmetic prosthesis (ch 28). In Boswick J Jr, ed: *Current concept in hand surgery,* Philadelphia, 1983, Lea and Febiger.

Pillet J: Digital and hand prosthetic fitting microsurgery for major limb reconstruction, In Urbanniak R, ed: *Microsurgery for major limb reconstruction,* St Louis, 1987, Mosby.

Pillet J: *La Chirurgie secondaire dans les mutilations de la main,* 1989, Souquet Mansat.

Pillet J: The aesthetic and functional replacement. "Reconstruction of the thumb." In Landi A, De Lucia S, Desantis G, eds: *Reconstruction of the thumb,* London, 1989, Chapman and Hall.

Pillet J, Biteau O: La Prothese plastique du membre superieur, *Gazette Medicale Fr* 1969; 87:3421-3425.

Pillet J, Dufourmentel C: La Substitution prothetique de l'ongle, *G.E.M. Monographie,* 1978; 9:118-122.

Pillet J, Guyaux MC, Le Gall CA: Prostheses ungueales, *Ann Dermatol Venereol* 1987; 114:425-428.

Pillet J, Mackin E: Aesthetic hand prosthesis—its psychological and functional potential. In Hunter JM, Schneider LH, Mackin EJ, eds: *Rehabilation of the hand,* ed 2, St Louis, 1984, Mosby.

Pillet J, Mackin E: Aesthetic restoration. In Bowker JH, Michael JW, eds: *AAOS atlas of limb prosthetics: surgical, prosthetic and rehabilitation principles,* ed 2, St Louis, 1992, Mosby.

Pillet J, Mackin E: Prosthetic contribution to distal amputations. In Foucher G, ed: *Fingertip and nailbed injuries,* New York, 1990, Churchill Livingstone.

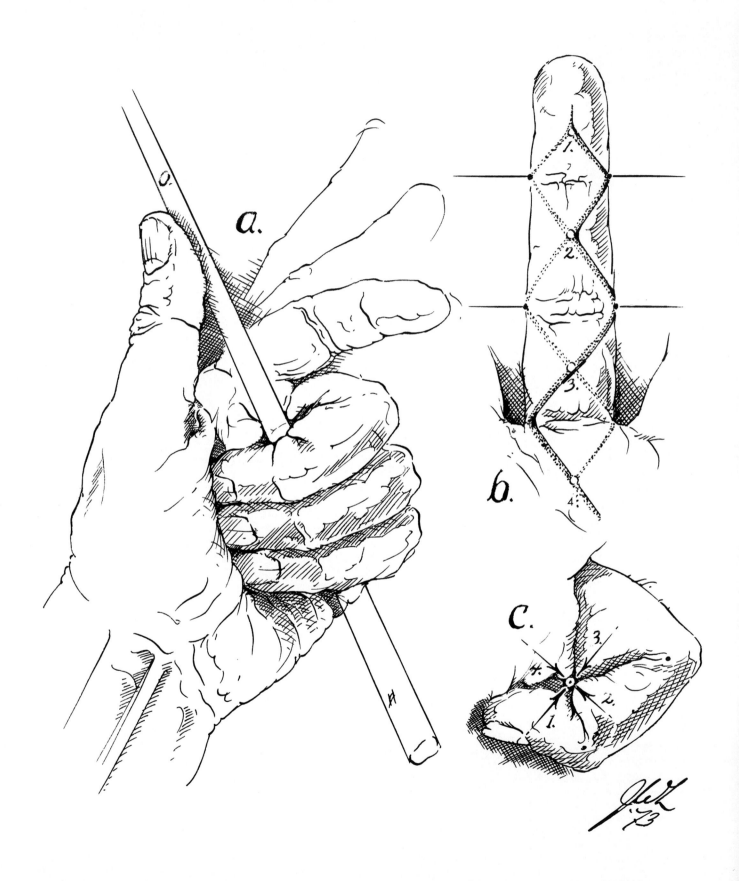

Part XVII

IMPAIRMENT EVALUATION

The areas of cutaneous contact in the flexed digits (Littler, 1974). These contact regions are diamond shaped when the digit is extended. The sides of the diamond undergo little variation in length during flexion-extension movements, and any incision made along their lines will not retract. When the digits are flexed against the palm, the radial digits whose palmar integument is innervated by the median nerve touch the skin of the thenar eminence, which is also innervated by the median nerve. The ulnar digits whose palmar integument is innervated by the ulnar nerve touch the skin of the palm innervated by the ulnar nerve. When a fist is formed, the palmar face of the thumb innervated by the median nerve comes into contact with the dorsal skin of the middle phalanges of the index and middle fingers, also innervated by the median nerve. (From Tubiana R, et al: Examination of the hand. In Littler JW, ed: *Architecture and function of the hand,* Philadelphia, 1984, Saunders.)

Chapter 66

EVALUATION OF IMPAIRMENT OF HAND FUNCTION*

Alfred B. Swanson
Geneviève de Groot Swanson
Carl Göran-Hagert

There are millions of people in the world who are suffering the residual effects of injury or destructive diseases to the hand and upper extremity. Physicians interested in treating disabilities of the hand should accept the responsibility for accurate evaluation of the patient's physical condition and be able to compute the permanent anatomic and functional impairment. This evaluation is usually limited to the analysis of the anatomic, functional, and cosmetic effect loss after optimal surgical and physical rehabilitation. The physician is responsible for a medical evaluation of impairment, not a rating of disability. The latter is an administrative function that relates to the patient's ability to engage in gainful activity as this affects his or her social and economic standards of living.

Determination of treatment programs and proper evaluation of the results depend on accurate and complete patient records. Records of examinations, operations, and treatment are increasingly under review by insurance companies, law courts, and other judicial bodies.

Techniques for recording the history and for measuring anatomic, functional, and cosmetic deficits should be standard and routine and are facilitated by an orderly and convenient method of examination. Evaluations should be made after consistent and thorough histories are taken and careful observations, examinations, and tests are performed.

The proper evaluation of impairment presumes knowledge of the normal functional anatomy of the part.

Evaluation is usually a determination of loss of structure, motion, strength, presence of pain, and/or loss of sensibility as compared with the opposite normal limb; if both are impaired, comparison with an average limb is made.

In 1966 Dr. A.B. Swanson was chairman of a special committee of the International Federation of Societies for Surgery of the Hand (IFSSH), whose charge was to develop a system for evaluation of physical impairment in the hand and upper extremity that would be reliable and easy to use. The authors have brought together systems of medical societies and classic works, and with the participation of many hand surgeons, they have refined and extended the evaluation methods of physical impairment of the hand and upper extremity. The system developed has been tested and used by many hand surgeons around the world and was approved for international application by the IFSSH at its first congress, held in Rotterdam, Holland, in 1980. The evaluation system recently has been endorsed by the American Society for Surgery of the Hand (ASSH), the American Academy of Orthopaedic Surgeons (AAOS), and the American Medical Association (AMA) for national usage and has been included in the *Guide to the Evaluation of Permanent Impairment of the Extremities and Back,* third and fourth editions.

Evaluation methods

Evaluation of the upper extremity can be arbitrarily divided into anatomic, cosmetic, and functional categories. A method that combines these categories is necessary to show an accurate profile of the patient's condition. The

*From Hunter JM, Mackin EJ, Callahan AD, eds: *Rehabilitation of the hand: surgery and therapy,* ed 4, St Louis, 1995, Mosby.

617

patient's psychologic, sociologic, environmental, and economic status also must be considered. The *physical evaluation* determines the anatomic impairment and is based on the history and a detailed examination of the upper extremity and patient. The *cosmetic evaluation* concerns the patient's and society's reaction to the patient's condition. The *functional evaluation* is more involved and measures the patient's motor performance of functional activities. Functional studies are increasingly sophisticated and can complement the evaluation process. However, the necessary level of precision and reproducibility has not yet been developed to derive a numerical impairment rating. Evaluation of the anatomic impairment is considered the most reliable system at present.

A complete and detailed examination of the upper extremity is facilitated by the use of a printed chart that lists in an orderly fashion the various tests and measurements. A sketch of the hand with dorsal and palmar views simplifies the description of loss of parts and the location of scars or other defects. An example of a chart used for evaluation of the rheumatoid hand is shown in Fig. 66-1. The evaluation record includes a checklist for the common information necessary to record the history, type of disease, onset, duration, distribution of disease process, laboratory tests, and treatment. Organized columns are provided to record the range of motion (ROM) and strength of each joint, prehensile patterns, ability to perform activities of daily living (ADL), and ambulatory status. Specific clinical abnormalities are recorded and classified as mild, moderate, or severe (see the box on p. 619).

We have devised specific charts to help record and calculate impairments of the hand and upper extremity according to the method presented in this chapter (Fig. 66-2).

PRINCIPLES AND METHODS OF HISTORY TAKING

History taking should record the necessary information: identification, vital statistics, diagnosis, history of the disease. Additionally, in the case of trauma, it should narrate the accident, how and where it happened, the mechanics and severity of the injury, and the time sequence of treatment relative to emergency care, definitive care, and postoperative therapy. The complaint of how the residual difficulty affects the patient's activities should be recorded in his or her own words. Any history of previous difficulty in the same extremity and general conditions that would influence the patient's recovery also are noted.

The patient's hand can be observed as the examiner is taking a history and measuring the upper portion of the limb. The general posture of the hand, the position of its various joints as active motion of the upper extremity is carried out, and the state of nutrition, color, moisture, swelling, or muscle weakness can be subtly checked without the patient's awareness.

Malingering or psychogenic overlay may make it difficult to obtain an accurate estimate of impairment. The patient whose complaints are not justified by objective findings or whose response to testing varies widely from time to time should put the examiner on guard. It may be impossible to identify the malingerer without the help of evidence gathered outside the examining room when the patient does not think he or she is being observed.

PHOTOGRAPHIC RECORD

A set of standard position photographs of the hand is essential for the record. Suggested sequences should include views of the hand from various positions, carrying out flexion-extension of the fingers, and the functions of grasp and pinch. Film sequences can help evaluate the patient's adaptation to needs of daily living. Manipulating buttons and safety pins, threading a needle, turning the screw-top lid of a jar, writing, picking up and releasing objects, and turning a nut on and off a bolt are but a few of the activities that are suitable for recording on film.

RADIOLOGIC EVALUATION

A standard series of roentgenograms including anterior, posterior, lateral, and oblique views of the hand and wrist should be part of the record. Films of the other joints of the upper extremity also may be included. The films should be taken without jewelry or other items about the extremity. The anatomic extended position is desired but must not be forced, so that the degree of deformity also can be evaluated on the roentgenogram. Cineradiography can help show the range of movement of the various joints.

ANATOMIC EVALUATION METHODS

The hand is primarily a grasping or prehensile organ. The action of the shoulder, elbow, and wrist joints enables the hand to be placed at almost any area of the body or to be pulled toward or pushed away from the body. It is obvious, therefore, that every examination should include an evaluation of the entire limb and the condition of all the structures, including skin, nails, neurovascular musculotendinous structures, bones, and joints. Digits are named rather than numbered. Circumferential measurements of both extremities are recorded. The evaluation includes measuremnt of the ROM of individual joints, strength of pinch and grasp, muscle testing, sensory evaluation, and pain assessment.

The cutaneous coverage of the limb should be evaluated for scars, abnormal pigmentation, redundancy, ulcerations, loss of subcutaneous tissues, and adhesions or contractures and their effect on function. Temperature, color, swelling, texture, and tenderness should be noted, as well as nail-bed deformities.

For each joint, the ROM or position of ankylosis, the presence and degree of synovitis, instability, subluxation, lateral deviation, and rotation are recorded. The circumference of individual joints is measured in centimeters, and angulation and rotation is measured in degrees. The musculotendinous system is evaluated for tendon ruptures, constrictive tenosynovitis, extensor tendon subluxations, and intrinsic tightness. The presence and severity of collapse deformities are described for each digit. Disturbances of the normal carpal and metacarpal transverse arches and digital longitudinal arches are noted. The description of the thumb includes length, mobility, stability, capacity for placement to the hand, flexibility, and depth of the first web space.

Important tools for a good examination include goniometer, dynamometer, pinch meter, ruler, sensory testing devices, a two-point compass, familiar objects for tactile identification and the pickup test, and cylinders of various sizes to measure the effective grasp (Fig. 66-3).

Range of motion measurement

The range of motion should be recorded on the principle that neutral position equals 0°, as accepted by the AAOS in

---

Severity index arbitrarily classifies common deformities and degree of involvement as mild, moderate, or severe

Thumb swan-neck—flexion limit of MP joint
a. Mild = MP ROM + 10° to 50°
b. Moderate = MP ROM + 20° to 30°
c. Severe = MP ROM + 30° to 10°
Thumb boutonnière—extension limit of MP joint
a. Mild = MP −5° to −20°
b. Moderate = MP −20° to −40°
c. Severe = MP more than −40°
Swan-neck fingers—flexion limit of PIP joint
a. Mild = PIP ROM +10° to 50°
b. Moderate = PIP ROM +20° to 30°
c. Severe = PIP ROM +30° to 10°
Boutonnière—extension limit of PIP joint
a. Mild = PIP extension limit −5° to −10°
b. Moderate = PIP extension limit −10° to −30°
c. Severe = PIP extension limit more than −30°
Instability—measure excess of passive mediolateral motion compared with a normal joint
a. Mild = less than 10°
b. Moderate = 10° to 20°
c. Severe = more than 20°
Subluxation to dislocation
a. Mild = capable of reduction manually
b. Moderate = incomplete reduction manually
c. Severe = irreducible dislocation
Ulnar or radial joint deviation—digits
a. Mild = less than 10°
b. Moderate = 10° to 30°
c. Severe = more than 30°
Rotational deformity—digits
a. Mild = less than 15°
b. Moderate = 15° to 30°
c. Severe = more than 30°
Lateral deviation—wrist or elbow
a. Mild = less than 20°
b. Moderate = 20° to 30°
c. Severe = more than 30°
Crepitation with motion
a. Mild = inconstant during active ROM
b. Moderate = constant during active ROM
c. Severe = constant during passive ROM

Synovial hypertrophy
a. Mild = visual increase in joint size
b. Moderate = palpable increase in joint size
c. Severe = more than 10% increase in joint size by measure
Contrictive tenosynovitis
a. Mild = inconstant triggering during active ROM
b. Moderate = constant triggering during active ROM
c. Severe = prevents active ROM
Intrinsic tightness—with MP joint extended
a. Mild = PIP flexion more than 60°
b. Moderate = PIP flexion 20° to 60°
c. Severe = PIP flexion less than 20°
Extensor tendon subluxation
a. Mild = subluxes on MP flexion
b. Moderate = reducible subluxation in intermetacarpal groove
c. Severe = nonreducible subluxation in intermetacarpal groove
Painful joint with motion
a. Mild = pain with active motion
b. Moderate = pain with active motion that interferes with activity
c. Severe = pain at rest that prevents activity
Subchondral sclerosis
a. Mild, when present
Erosions—x-ray examination
a. Mild = one erosion
b. Moderate = two erosions
c. Severe = three or more erosions
Joint narrowing—x-ray examination
a. Mild = ⅓ narrowing
b. Moderate = ⅔ narrowing
c. Severe = obliteration of joint space
Vasculitis
a. Mild = paronychial hemorrhages and/or subcutaneous nodules
b. Moderate = peripheral neuropathy
c. Severe = cutaneous gangrene
Nodules
a. Mild = one nodule, mobile and nontender
b. Moderate = two nodules, fixed and tender
c. Severe = more than three nodules, fixed, tender, with skin breakdown

RHEUMATOID ARTHRITIS EVALUATION RECORD

Name _____ ; Sex ☐ Male ☐ Female; Hand ☐ R ☐ L; Birth date _____

Address _____

Occupation _____ Dominant hand: ☐ R ☐ L; ☐ Hospital _____ Examiner _____

Diagnosis: ☐ Juvenile rheumatoid ☐ Adult rheumatoid ☐ Erosive arthritis ☐ Osteoarthritis ☐ Psoriatic arthritis   Date _____

☐ Ankylosing spondylitis ☐ Sjögren's syndrome ☐ Systemic lupus erythematosus ☐ Trauma

Onset date _____ Sedimentation rate: ☐ Wintrobe ☐ Westergren ☐ Rourke   Rheumatoid test ☐ (+) ☐ (−)

Onset distribution ☐ Peripheral ☐ Central ☐ Both; Remission ☐ Yes ☐ No; Anemia ☐ Yes ☐ No   Family Hx ☐ (+) ☐ (−)

Check if the following has been completed: ☐ X-rays ☐ Photographs ☐ Movies ☐ Cineradiography

Range of motion (ROM) use neutral = zero method of American Academy of Orthopedic Surgeons 1965.

Codes 1-25 represent observed and measured abnormalities. Use as indicated in appropriate sections.

Severity indices mild, moderate, and severe are represented by a, b, & c and further categorize codes 1-25.

The code 1-25 is below on this sheet. Severity indices are on separate detachable sheet.

This evaluation record has been designed for computer analysis. Responses must be complete.

	Thumb codes 1, 2, 3, 9-14, 19, & 22	Joints		ROM		
Thumb		MC	Abd			
			Add			
			Opp			
				Flex	Ext	Ank
		MP				
		IP				

	Finger codes 3-15, 19, 22-25	Joints	Flex	Ext	Ank
Index		MP			
		PIP			
		DIP			
	Flex DIP crease to palmar crease (cm)				
Middle		MP			
		PIP			
		DIP			
	Flex DIP crease to palmar crease (cm)				
Ring		MP			
		PIP			
		DIP			
	Flex DIP crease to palmar crease (cm)				
Little		MP			
		PIP			
		DIP			
	Flex DIP crease to palmar crease (cm)				
Wrist	Codes 3, 7-14, 19, 20, 22, 23	Flex			
		Ext			
		U. Dev.			
		R. Dev.			

Prehensile patterns: Check if able to perform.

Grasp:		
Cylinders	2.5 cm	
	5 cm	
	7.5 cm	
	10 cm	
Spheres	5 cm	
	7.5 cm	
	10 cm	
	12.5 cm	

Strength: ☐ Lb ☐ Kg ☐ mm Hg		
Pulp pinch	Index	
	Middle	
	Ring	
	Little	
Lateral or key pinch		
Grip		

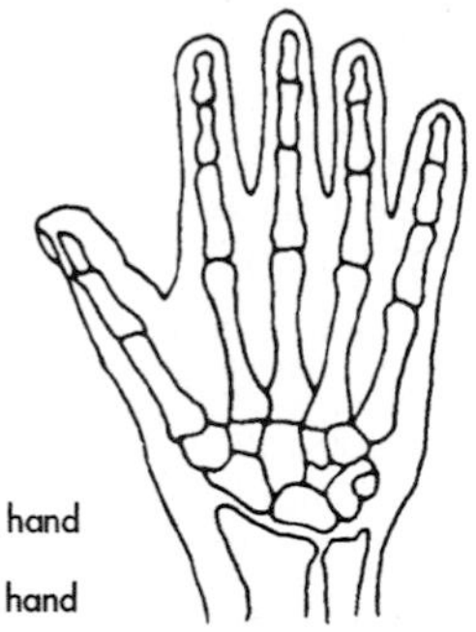

Dorsum L hand
or
Palmar R hand

Sketch implant into appropriate site

Code for clinical abnormality:

1—Thumb swan neck
2—Thumb boutonnière
3—Subluxation—dislocation
4—Swan neck, finger
5—Boutonnière, finger
6—Intrinsic tightness
7—Ulnar drift
8—Radial drift
9—Ankylosis
10—Instability
11—Tendon rupture
12—Constrictive tenosynovitis
13—Synovial hypertrophy
14—Crepitation with motion
15—Extensor tendon subluxation
16—Varus angle
17—Valgus angle
18—Rotational deformity
19—Erosions

20—Joint narrowing
21—Subchondral sclerosis
22—Painful joint with motion
23—Nerve compression: M, U, R
24—Vasculitis
25—Nodules

Severity index:
a—Mild
b—Moderate
c—Severe

ADL	I = Independent			A = Assisted				U = Unable							
Dressing	I	A	U	Hygiene	I	A	U		I	A	U		I	A	U
Upper ext.				Teeth				Eating				Doorknob			
Trunk				Hair				Toilet				Car door			
Lower ext.				Shave				Telephone				Screw top jar			
Bath				Pickup coin				Typewrite				Aerosol can			
Shower				Turn key				Write				Fasteners			

Ambulatory status:
☐ Independent   ☐ Wheelchair with partial walking
☐ Assisted walk   ☐ Bedfast

Fig. 66-1. Preoperative evaluation record. This form is designed for evaluation of rheumatoid and arthritic hands. (Modified from Swanson AB: *Flexible implant resection arthroplasty in the hand and extremities,* St Louis, 1973, Mosby.)

A. Upper Extremity Impairment Evaluation Record—Part I (Hand)　　　　　Side ☐ R　☐ L

Name _____ Age _____ Sex ☐ M ☐ F　Dominant hand ☐ R ☐ L　Date _____

Occupation _____ Diagnosis _____

Abnormal motion						Amputation	Sensory loss	Other disorders	Hand impairment %
Record motion, ankylosis, and impairment %						Mark level & impairment %	Mark type, level, & impairment %	List type & impairment %	• Combine digit IMP% ★ Convert to hand IMP%

Thumb

			Flexion	Extension	Ankylosis	IMP% 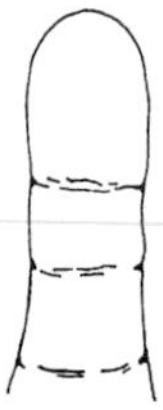 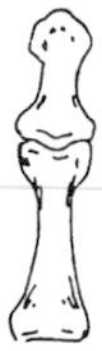				
	IP	Angle °								
		IMP%								
	MP	Angle °								
		IMP%								
			Motion	Ankylosis	IMP%					
	CMC	Radial abduction Angle °								Abnormal motion [1]
		IMP%								Amputation [2]
		Adduction Cms								Sensory loss [3]
		IMP%								Other disorders [4]
		Opposition Cms								Digit impairment % • Combine 1, 2, 3, 4
		IMP%								

Add impairment %　CMC + MP + IP = 　[1]　IMP % = [2]　IMP % = [3]　IMP % = [4]　**Hand impairment % ★ Convert above**

Index

		Flexion	Extension	Ankylosis	IMP%				
DIP	Angle °					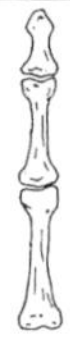	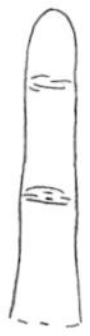		Abnormal motion [1]
	IMP%								Amputation [2]
PIP	Angle °								Sensory loss [3]
	IMP%								Other disorders [4]
MP	Angle °								Digit impairment % • Combine 1, 2, 3, 4
	IMP%								

• Combine impairment %　MP + PIP + DIP = 　[1]　IMP % = [2]　IMP % = [3]　IMP % = [4]　**Hand impairment % ★ Convert above**

Middle

DIP	Angle °								Abnormal motion [1]
	IMP%								Amputation [2]
PIP	Angle °								Sensory loss [3]
	IMP%								Other disorders [4]
MP	Angle °								Digit impairment % • Combine 1, 2, 3, 4
	IMP%								

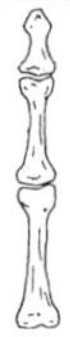

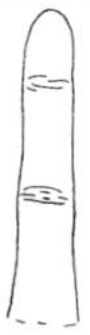

• Combine impairment %　MP + PIP + DIP = 　[1]　IMP % = [2]　IMP % = [3]　IMP % = [4]　**Hand impairment % ★ Convert above**

Ring

DIP	Angle °								Abnormal motion [1]
	IMP%								Amputation [2]
PIP	Angle °								Sensory loss [3]
	IMP%								Other disorders [4]
MP	Angle °								Digit impairment % • Combine 1, 2, 3, 4
	IMP%								

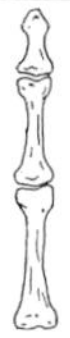

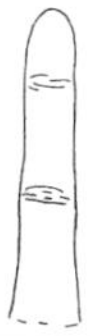

• Combine impairment %　MP + PIP + DIP = 　[1]　IMP % = [2]　IMP % = [3]　IMP % = [4]　**Hand impairment % ★ Convert above**

Little

DIP	Angle °								Abnormal motion [1]
	IMP%								Amputation [2]
PIP	Angle °								Sensory loss [3]
	IMP%								Other disorders [4]
MP	Angle °								Digit impairment % • Combine 1, 2, 3, 4
	IMP%								

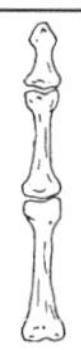

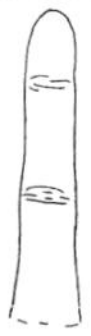

• Combine impairment %　MP + PIP + DIP = 　[1]　IMP % = [2]　IMP % = [3]　IMP % = [4]　**Hand impairment % ★ Convert above**

Total hand impairment (Add hand impairment % for thumb + index + middle + ring + little finger) =	%
Upper extremity impairment (†Convert total hand impairment % to upper extremity impairment %) =	%; enter on Part II, Line II
If hand region impairment is only impairment, convert upper extremity impairment to whole person impairment:‡ =	%

• Combined Values Chart: Table 66-5; ★ Use Table 66-2 (Digits to hand); † Use Table 66-3 (Hand to upper extremity); ‡ Use Table 66-4
　Courtesy of G. de Groot Swanson, MD

Fig. 66-2. A, Upper extremity impairment evaluation record—part 1 (hand).

B. Upper Extremity Impairment Evaluation Record—Part 2 (Wrist, elbow, and shoulder) Side ☐ R ☐ L

Name_____ Age _____ Sex ☐ M ☐ F Dominant hand ☐ R ☐ L Date _____

Occupation _____ Diagnosis_____

Abnormal motion					Other disorders	Regional impairment %	Amputation
Record motion, ankylosis, and impairment %					List type & impairment %	• Combine [1] + [2]	Mark level & impairment %
Wrist		Flexion	Extension	Ankylosis	IMP%			
	Angle°							
	IMP%							
		RD	UD	Ankylosis	IMP%			
	Angle°							
	IMP%							
Add IMP% FLEX/EXT + RD/UD =					[1]	IMP% =	[2]	
Elbow		Flexion	Extension	Ankylosis	IMP%			
	Angle°							
	IMP%							
		Pronation	Supination	Ankylosis	IMP%			
	Angle°							
	IMP%							
Add IMP% FLEX/EXT + PRO/SUP =					[1]	IMP% =	[2]	
Shoulder		Flexion	Extension	Ankylosis	IMP%			
	Angle°							
	IMP%							
		Adduction	Abduction	Ankylosis	IMP%			
	Angle°							
	IMP%							
		Int Rot	Ext Rot	Ankylosis	IMP%			
	Angle°							
	IMP%							
Add IMP% FLEX/EXT + ADD/ABD + INT ROT/EXT ROT =					[1]	IMP% =	[2]	IMP%

I. **Amputation impairment (other than digits)**		=	%
II. **Regional impairment of upper extremity** • (Combine hand _____% + wrist _____% + elbow _____% + shoulder _____%)		=	%
III. **Peripheral nerve system impairment**		=	%
IV. **Peripheral vascular system impairment**		=	%
V. **Other disorders (not included in regional impairment)**		=	%

Total upper extremity impairment (• Combine I + II + III + IV + V)		=	%
Impairment of the whole person (Use table 66-4, upper extremity to whole person)		=	%

If both limbs are involved, calculate the whole person impairment for each on a separate chart and combine the percents.
• Use Combined Values Chart, Table 66-5.

Fig. 66-2, cont'd. B, Upper extremity impairment evaluation record—part 2 (wrist, elbow, and shoulder).

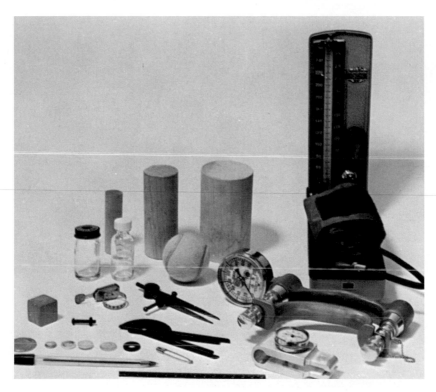

Fig. 66-3. Equipment suggested for evaluation of upper extremity. (From Swanson AB: *Flexible implant resection arthroplasty in the hand and extremities,* St Louis, 1973, Mosby.)

1965 (Fig. 66-4). In this method all motions of the joint are measured from defined zero as the starting position. The "extended anatomic position" of an extremity is therefore accepted as 0° rather than 180°. The degrees of motion of a joint are added in the direction the joint moves from the zero starting position. Active motion is obtained with full flexion or extension muscle force. Passive motion is measured after normal soft-tissue resistance to movement is overcome; in the finger joints this is approximately 0.5 kg of force.

The term *extension* describes motion opposite to flexion at the zero starting position. Extension exceeding the neutral position, as seen at the metacarpophalangeal (MP), elbow, or knee joints, is referred to as "hyperextension," and is recorded with a plus (+) symbol. Incomplete extension from a flexed position to the neutral position represents extension lag and is recorded with a minus (−) symbol. The plus and minus signs have no mathematical significance.

Example. The motion of a finger joint with a 15° flexion contracture and 90° of flexion is recorded as −15° to 90°. A finger joint with 15° of hyperextension and 45° of flexion has a recorded motion of +15° to 45°.

Digital joints are measured with the proximal joints in neutral or straight-line position (Fig. 66-5). Active motion or ankylosis is recorded. The spread of the fingers and its strength are measured. Measurement of thumb motions includes radial abduction, adduction, opposition, and flexion-extension of the metacarpophalangeal and interphalangeal (IP) joints. At the wrist, extension and flexion, and

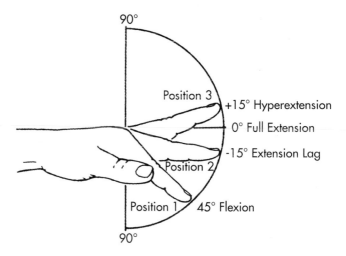

Fig. 66-4. Range of motion of index finger metacarpophalangeal joint. Measure hyperextension as plus (+) value, extension lag as minus (−) value, and neutral position as 0°, as suggested by the American Academy of Orthopaedic Surgeons.

radial and ulnar deviations are measured. Elbow flexion, extension, pronation, and supination are recorded. Shoulder motions include flexion/extension, abduction/adduction, and internal/external rotation.

Neurologic examination

The neurologic examination includes a complete motor and sensory evaluation of the hand and upper extremity to

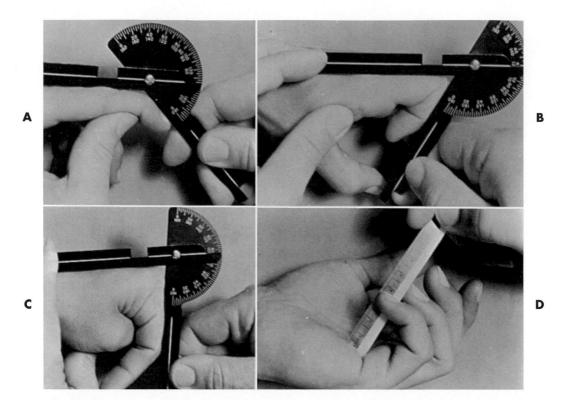

Fig. 66-5. Techniques of measurement of digital joints. **A,** Distal interphalangeal joint. **B,** Proximal interphalangeal joint. **C,** Metacarpophalangeal joint. **D,** Maximal flexion distance measured from pulp of the finger to the distal palmar crease (Boyes' method). (From swanson AB: *Flexible implant resection arthroplasty in the hand and extremities,* St Louis, 1973, Mosby.)

determine the presence and location of peripheral nerve disorders, including those of the nerve roots, brachial plexus, and major peripheral nerves. Digital nerve loss and the presence and location of neuromas are evaluated. Tenderness, sensitivity, and painful states such as causalgias and other sympathetic dystrophies are appraised.

Muscle power testing. Muscle power testing is important to evaluate the upper extremity disabled by paralysis or paresis resulting from nervous system disorders. It is based on the ability of the muscle to contract, move a joint through its ROM against gravity, and hold that motion against resistance. Muscle power loss can be classified as shown in Table 66-14, p. 655.

Sensory evaluation. Evaluation of sensory function in the hand should consider all sensory submodalities, including perception of pain, heat, cold, and touch. The grading system introduced by the Nerve Injuries Committee of the British Medical Research Council in 1954 (S0, S1, S2, S3, S3+, S4), grades the sensory recovery after nerve injury as follows: first, no sensation; then a spectrum of protective sensations including perception of pain, heat, cold, and some degree of light touch; and finally, recovery of fine discriminative touch functions. However, if the two-point discrimination test is normal, it is not necessary to test sensory submodalities, because they are assumed to be present.

The moving two-point discrimination test can help assess the regenerating nerve, because this function recovers before the static two-point discrimination. The classic Weber static two-point discrimination test is more practical.

Moberg originally described the use of a paper clip opened and bent into a caliper. However, more accurate instruments are also available.* With the patient's eyes closed, the device tips are lightly touched to the digit in the longitudinal axis, without blanching or indenting the skin. A series of one or two points is applied, and the subject indicates whether he or she feels one or two points. The distance of the tips is first set at 15 mm and is progressively decreased with accurate responses. Testing is started distally and proceeds proximally to determine the longitudinal level of involvement. The minimum distance at which the patient can discriminate between one-point and two-point applications in two out of three trials is recorded. Two-point discrimination values greater than 15 mm represent a total sensory loss; values between 15 and 7 mm represent a partial sensory loss; and values equal to or less than 6 mm are considered normal. The distribution of the sensory loss is

*Aesthesiometer, Fred Sammon, Inc., Box 32, Brookfield, IL 60513; Disk-Criminator, P.O. Box 16392, Baltimore, MD 21210; DeMayo 2-Point Discrimination Device, Padgett Instrument Co., 2838 Warwick Traffic Way, Kansas City, MO 64108.

noted according to the involvement of one or both digital nerves and to the length of the digit affected.

Objective tests for sensory impairment are limited and one must rely on the patient's honesty. When malingering is suspected, more objective methods include the ninhydrin test for sudomotor function and antegrade or orthograde electrodiagnostic testing. It also may be possible to prick the patient's fingertip to see whether the finger is withdrawn from this painful stimulus. Functional isolation of the finger, as noted in the blindfolded pickup test, will aid the examiner in determining the presence or absence of any useful sensation in the digit.

The ninhydrin test for sudomotor function can be a useful method for documenting the interruption of the digital nerves. However, it has limitations in evaluation of the "recovering" nerve, because there is not a direct relationship between return of sudomotor function and return of tactile gnosis.

Pain evaluation

Pain is difficult to evaluate because it is a subjective symptom. Pain can be defined as a disagreeable sensation that has as its basis a highly variable complex made up of afferent nerve stimuli interacting with the emotional state of the individual and modified by his or her experience, motivation, and state of mind. Pain may be verified and the intensity of pain may be evaluated in a thorough physical examination. Pretended pain may be detected by tests that confuse the patient into responding with signs that are contradictory to the usual clinical examination. Examination can further demonstrate whether the pain has an anatomic background or whether it is associated with other signs of nerve dysfunction. Impairment caused by pain associated with peripheral nerve disorders can be classified according to how the pain interferes with performance of activities.

Grip and pinch strength measurements

Strength is measured with properly gauged mechanical devices. The *strength of the grip* is measured with the adjustable handle of a Jamar dynamometer spaced at 4 cm (second position) or 6 cm (third position) according to the size of the hand. The mechanical dynamometer may be too gross to measure the grasp in the weak, arthritic hand. A sphygmomanometer may be used to record grips of lesser power. The blood pressure cuff is rolled to 5 cm diameter and inflated to 50 mm Hg; the cuff is then squeezed and the change in millimeters of mercury from 50 mm Hg is recorded as the power of grip. An electronic pinch meter based on the strain-gauge principle has been used by us for measuring the strength of pinch in pounds or kilograms of pressure. Other devices used for pinch or grasp measurement include a variety of mechanical pinch meters and the force-pressure measuring device of Mannerfelt (see Suggested Readings at the end of this chapter).

Many factors, including fatigue, handedness, time of day, age, stage of nutrition, pain, cooperation of the patient, and presence of amputations, restricted motion, pain, and sensory loss, can influence the strength of the grip. The tests are repeated three times with each hand at different times during the examination and are reliable if the readings have less than 20% variation.

Two techniques have been reported to help detect individuals who exert less than maximal effort on grip strength testing. Stokes pointed out that the plotting of grip strength measurements from each of the five handle settings of the Jamar dynamometer would produce a bell-shaped curve. Those individuals not exerting maximal effort will produce results yielding a straight line or a flat curve.

The rapid exchange grip technique may help identify malingerers. The grip strength is first determined by standard methods. The subject is then instructed to grip the dynamometer as hard as possible, first with one hand, and then quickly with the other hand for at least five exchanges. Patients who did not apply maximal effort with the standard technique will show significantly higher strength; if they become aware of this, the strength of both hands will drop significantly. Decreased strength can also be due to fatigue. When there is suspicion or evidence that the subject is exerting less than maximal effort, grip strength measurements become invalid for impairment determination.

A baseline of normal grip and pinch strength was studied in our clinic by testing a group of 100 healthy people (Table 66-1). The strength of the grip was measured with the adjustable handle of a Jamar dynamometer spaced at 6 cm. The minimal and maximal strength of the grip measurement ranged from 30.4 to 70.4 kg in the male group and 14 to 38.6 kg in the female group. The strength of chuck, pulp, and lateral pinch was tested with an electronic pinch meter based on the strain-gauge principle. However, similar findings were obtained with the standard pinch meter. The majority of patients preferred chuck pinch to any other type of pinch for applying the most force. The IP joint of the thumb was hyperextended in most cases when maximal force of chuck pinch was applied. A tendency to hyperextend either the proximal interphalangeal (PIP) or the distal interphalangeal (DIP) joints was evident when maximal pulp pinch with separate fingers was applied. For the PIP joint, this tendency increased from the radial to the ulnar sides of the hand. Lateral pinch is a strong type of pinch that may be an important adaptation in the disabled hand and may provide a very useful function when pulp pinch is lost.

The dominant hand was usually stronger in heavy manual workers; however, the nondominant hand may be stronger in a significant percentage of other individuals tested. Grip strength of the nondominant hand was weaker in 5.4% of males and 8.9% of females. The strength of pinch in the nondominant hand was weaker by only 4% in males and 6% in females. The data obtained in our study indicated that there is less difference in strength of the dominant and

Table 66-1. Average hand strength in 100 subjects

	Strength (kg)			
	Men		Women	
Category	Dominant hand	Non-dominant hand	Dominant hand	Non-dominant hand
Occupation	Unsupported grip			
Skilled labor	47.0	45.4	26.8	24.4
Sedentary	47.2	44.1	23.1	21.1
Manual labor	48.5	44.6	24.2	22.0
Average	47.6	45.0	24.6	22.4
Age (yr)	Unsupported grip			
20	45.2	42.6	23.8	22.8
21 to 30	48.5	46.2	24.6	22.7
31 to 40	49.2	44.5	30.8	28.0
41 to 50	49.0	47.3	23.4	21.5
51 to 60	45.9	43.5	22.3	18.2
Occupation	Lateral pinch			
Skilled labor	6.6	6.4	4.4	4.3
Sedentary	6.3	6.1	4.1	3.9
Manual labor	8.5	7.7	6.0	5.5
Average	7.5	7.1	4.9	4.7
Occupation	Chuck pinch			
Skilled labor	7.3	7.2	5.4	4.6
Sedentary	8.4	7.3	4.2	4.0
Manual labor	8.5	7.6	6.1	5.6
Average	7.9	7.5	5.2	4.9
Digit	Pulp pinch with separate digits			
Index	5.3	4.8	3.6	3.3
Middle	5.6	5.7	3.8	3.4
Ring	3.8	3.6	2.5	2.4
Little	2.3	2.2	1.7	1.6

Adapted from Swanson AB, Matev IB, de Groot Swanson G: The strength of the hand, *Bull Prosthet Res,* p 145, Fall, 1970.

nondominant hands than has generally been thought. It has been demonstrated that approximately 4 kg of force is needed for adequate grip to perform 90% of ADL. Patients usually can manipulate the objects of their environment, such as door handles, if they have this degree of strength. The majority of simple activities can be accomplished with approximately 1 kg of pinch strength.

Principles and methods of impairment evaluation

The most practical and useful approach to the evaluation of digit impairment is to compare the current loss of function with the loss resulting from an amputation. Total loss of motion of a digit and total loss of sensation, or ankylosis and severe malposition that would render the digit essentially useless, are considered about the same as amputation of the part.

Ankylosis in the optimum functional position of joints is given the least impairment on the charts. Impairment resulting from total sensory loss is considered to be 50% of that caused by amputation.

The upper limb is considered as a unit of the whole person and is divided into hand, wrist, elbow, and shoulder. The hand is further separated into digits and their parts. The regional evaluation rates impairments caused by amputation, sensory loss, and abnormal motion of the digits, wrist, elbow, and shoulder. Techniques to rate impairments of the upper extremity caused by lesions of the peripheral vascular system, peripheral nervous system, and other specific disorders are described. A method to combine two or more impairments of a specific unit or of the entire upper extremity will be defined.

PREVIOUS INJURY OR ILLNESS

Impairment evaluations should be based on the examiner's actual findings. A prior injury or illness should receive consideration only if evidence, such as x-ray film, indicates that it was present before the impairment being evaluated was incurred.

CUMULATIVE TRAUMA DISORDER

A patient with work-related symptoms may not show any sign of permanent impairment, and alteration of the patient's work tasks may reduce the symptoms. Such an individual should not be considered to be permanently impaired.

Example: A 50-year-old woman, an assembly line worker doing repetitive motion activities with her hands, complained of a 3-month history of pain and swelling in the hand and wrist with occasional radiation to the elbow and shoulder. Physical examination and laboratory studies, including electrodiagnostic studies, were negative.

The worker was treated symptomatically with splints, flexibility exercises, and antiinflammatory medications and was given 3 weeks' vacation with pay. On follow-up evaluation she had no symptoms. She returned to work and 2 weeks later complained of recurrence of the same symptoms. The physical examination and laboratory studies still were normal. The same conservative therapy was prescribed, and after 3 weeks the symptoms were relieved.

It was concluded that the woman should be assigned to a different job. Because the physical examination remained normal, she was given no permanent impairment rating.

AMPUTATION IMPAIRMENT EVALUATION

Amputation of the entire extremity or 100% loss of the limb is considered 60% impairment of the whole person. Amputations at levels below the elbow, distal to the biceps insertion and proximal to the MP level, are considered a 95% loss of the total limb (Fig. 66-6, *A*). Amputation of the fingers and thumb through the MP joint removes the most essential parts and is considered 100% impairment of the hand or 90% impairment of the total limb; because loss of the entire limb equals 60% impairment of the whole person, 90% impairment of the limb equals 54% impairment of the person.

The digits represent five coordinated units into which all hand function is unequally divided. When evaluating the impaired function of the entire hand, one evaluates each finger and thumb separately on a 100% scale in relation to the entire digit. Each digit is then given a relative value to the entire hand as follows: thumb, 40%; index and middle fingers, 20% each; and ring and little fingers, 10% each (Fig. 66-6, *B*). Amputation through each portion of a digit is given a relative value as follows: digit MP joint, 100%; finger PIP joint, 80%; finger DIP joint, 45%; and thumb IP, 50% (Figs. 66-6, *B,* 66-11, and 66-15). The value of each portion of a digit can be related to the entire hand by multiplying it by the digit's relative value to the hand.

Example: Amputation through the PIP joint of the index finger represents 80% impairment of the finger; the index finger's relative hand value is 20%; therefore this amputation represents 80% × 20%, or 16%, impairment of the hand (Fig. 66-6, *B,* and Table 66-2).

When amputations of multiple digits or parts of digits are present, the hand impairment values for each digit are *added* directly together to obtain the total hand impairment.

Hand impairment values are multipled by 90% to obtain upper extremity impairments, and then by 60% to obtain impairments of the whole person (Tables 66-3 and 66-4). Using this principle of progressive multiplication of percentage values, one can relate the impairment of each digit or portion thereof to the hand, the upper limb, and eventually to the whole person.

Example: Amputation of the entire thumb (40% hand impairment) with amputation through the DIP joint of the index finger (45% × 20% = 9% hand impairment) equals 49% impairment of the hand (Fig. 66-6, *B*);

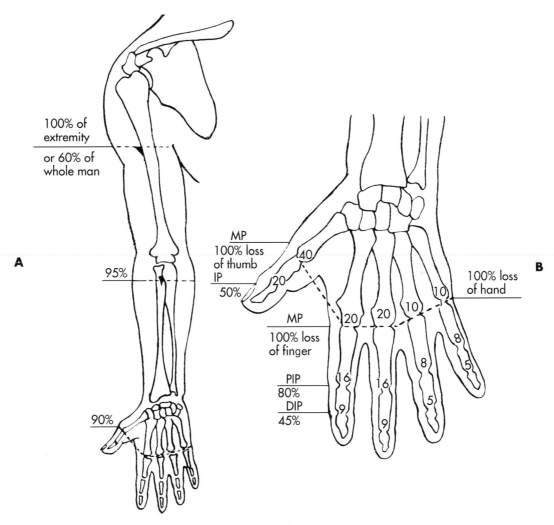

Fig. 66-6. Amputation impairments: percentage of impairments related to whole person, extremity, hand, or digit. **A,** Impairments of the upper extremity for amputation at various levels. **B,** Impairments of the digits (numbers, outside drawing) and hand (numbers, inside drawing) for amputation at various levels. (*MP,* metacarpophalangeal; *IP,* interphalangeal; *PIP,* proximal interphalangeal; *DIP,* distal interphalangeal.)

$49\% \times 90\% = 44\%$ impairment of the upper extremity (see Table 66-3); and $44\% \times 60\% = 26\%$ impairment of the whole person (see Table 66-4).

SENSORY IMPAIRMENT EVALUATION OF THE DIGITS

Any loss resulting from a sensory deficit that contributes to permanent impairment must be unequivocal and permanent. Sensibility of the palmar surface of the distal segment contributes to the function of the digit. Sensory loss on the least often opposed surfaces of the fingers and thumb should be given less value than the more important surfaces used in the usual pinch and grasp activities. Loss of sensibility on the dorsal surface of the digits is not considered disabling. Sensory deficits proximal to the level of the digits and symptomatic neuromas are rated according to the peripheral nervous system disorders section (p. 650). The two-point discrimination test, and other techniques for sensibility assessment are discussed on pp. 624 and 625.

Table 66-2. Relationship of impairment of the digits to impairment of the hand

% Impairment of		% Impairment of		% Impairment of	
Thumb	Hand	Index or middle finger	Hand	Ring or little finger	Hand
0-1 =	0	0-2 =	0	0-4 =	0
2-3 =	1	3-7 =	1	5-14 =	1
4-6 =	2	8-12 =	2	15-24 =	2
7-8 =	3	13-17 =	3	25-34 =	3
9-11 =	4	18-22 =	4	35-44 =	4
12-13 =	5	23-27 =	5	45-54 =	5
14-16 =	6	28-32 =	6	55-64 =	6
17-18 =	7	33-37 =	7	65-74 =	7
19-21 =	8	38-42 =	8	75-84 =	8
22-23 =	9	43-47 =	9	85-94 =	9
24-26 =	10	48-52 =	10	95-100 =	10
27-28 =	11	53-57 =	11		
29-31 =	12	58-62 =	12		
32-33 =	13	63-67 =	13		
34-36 =	14	68-72 =	14		
37-38 =	15	73-77 =	15		
39-41 =	16	78-82 =	16		
42-43 =	17	83-87 =	17		
44-46 =	18	88-92 =	18		
47-48 =	19	93-97 =	19		
49-51 =	20	98-100 =	20		
52-53 =	21				
54-56 =	22				
57-58 =	23				
59-61 =	24				
62-63 =	25				
64-66 =	26				
67-68 =	27				
69-71 =	28				
72-73 =	29				
74-76 =	30				
77-78 =	31				
79-81 =	32				
82-83 =	33				
84-86 =	34				
87-88 =	35				
89-91 =	36				
92-93 =	37				
94-96 =	38				
97-98 =	39				
99-100 =	40				

From *Guides to the evaluation of permanent impairment,* ed 4, Chicago, 1994, American Medical Association.

Table 66-3. Relationship of impairment of the hand to impairment of the upper extremity

% Impairment of		% Impairment of		% Impairment of	
Hand	Upper extremity	Hand	Upper extremity	Hand	Upper extremity
0 =	0	35 =	32	70 =	63
1 =	1	36 =	32	71 =	64
2 =	2	37 =	33	72 =	65
3 =	3	38 =	34	73 =	66
4 =	4	39 =	35	74 =	67
5 =	5	40 =	36	75 =	68
6 =	5	41 =	37	76 =	68
7 =	6	42 =	38	77 =	69
8 =	7	43 =	39	78 =	70
9 =	8	44 =	40	79 =	71
10 =	9	45 =	41	80 =	72
11 =	10	46 =	41	81 =	73
12 =	11	47 =	42	82 =	74
13 =	12	48 =	43	83 =	75
14 =	13	49 =	44	84 =	76
15 =	14	50 =	45	85 =	77
16 =	14	51 =	46	86 =	77
17 =	15	52 =	47	87 =	78
18 =	16	53 =	48	88 =	79
19 =	17	54 =	49	89 =	80
20 =	18	55 =	50	90 =	81
21 =	19	56 =	50	91 =	82
22 =	20	57 =	51	92 =	83
23 =	21	58 =	52	93 =	84
24 =	22	59 =	53	94 =	85
25 =	23	60 =	54	95 =	86
26 =	23	61 =	55	96 =	86
27 =	24	62 =	56	97 =	87
28 =	25	63 =	57	98 =	88
29 =	26	64 =	58	99 =	89
30 =	27	65 =	59	100 =	90
31 =	28	66 =	59		
32 =	29	67 =	60		
33 =	30	68 =	61		
34 =	31	69 =	62		

From Principles and methods of impairment evaluation in the hand and upper extremity. In: *Guides to the evaluation of permanent impairment,* ed 4, Chicago, 1994, American Medical Association.

The sensory impairment is based on the results of the two-point discrimination test over the distal palmar area of the digit, or over the most distal area of the digital stump in the presence of a partial amputation. The sensory impairment is rated according to the *sensory quality* and the *distribution of the sensory loss.*

The *sensory quality* is classified based on the results of the two-point discrimination test, and the impairment is rated as follows:

Sensory loss	Two-point discrimination	Sensory impairment
Total	>15 mm	100%
Partial	15 to 7 mm	50%
None	6 mm or less	0%

The *distribution of the sensory* loss is determined by the level of involvement of one or both digital nerves and is classified as follows:

1. *Transverse sensory loss:* both digital nerves involved.
2. *Longitudinal sensory loss:* one digital nerve involved on either the radial or ulnar side of the digit.

The *level of involvement* is determined by the area of sensory loss and is calculated as a percentage of the length of the digit.

Total transverse sensory loss (greater than 15 mm) represents a 100% sensory loss involving both digital nerves and receives 50% of the amputation impairment value for that level of involvement (Figs. 66-6, *B,* 66-7, 66-11, and 66-15). Complete loss of both digital nerves at the level of the MP joint therefore receives the following hand impairment values: thumb, 20%; index and middle fingers, 10%; ring and little fingers, 5% (see Fig. 66-7).

Partial transverse sensory loss (15 to 7 mm) represents a 50% sensory loss involving both digital nerves and receives 25% of the amputation impairment value for that level of involvement.

Longitudinal sensory loss impairments are calculated according to the relative importance of the side of the digit for sensory function as follows: thumb and little finger, radial side 40% and ulnar side 60%; index, middle, and ring fingers, radial side 60% and ulnar side 40%. The corresponding hand impairment values for total longitudinal sensory loss of the entire length of each side of each digit are shown in Fig. 66-7.

Impairment values for total and partial transverse and longitudinal sensory losses are calculated according to *the level of involvement,* taking into consideration the percentage of the length of the digit affected by the sensory loss. In the presence of amputation, the sensory impairment is similarly rated according to the length of the digital stump. For ease of determination, total and partial transverse and longitudinal sensory impairment values at various levels

have been computed for the index, middle, and ring fingers (see Table 66-6) and for the thumb and little finger (see Table 66-7).

Example: Total sensory loss (50% amputation impairment) along the distribution of the ulnar nerve of the thumb starting at the level of the IP joint represents a 60% sensory loss of 50% of the thumb length, or 50% × 60% × 50% = 15% thumb impairment and a 6% hand impairment (see Tables 66-2 and 66-7).

Sensibility on the ulnar aspect of the border finger is rated more highly. Therefore, if the little finger has been amputated, the relative value of the ulnar side of the ring finger becomes 60%, and that of the radial side 40%.

Table 66-4. Relationship of impairment of the upper extremity to impairment of the whole person

% Impairment of		% Impairment of		% Impairment of	
Upper extremity	Whole person	Upper extremity	Whole person	Upper extremity	Whole person
0 = 0		35 = 21		70 = 42	
1 = 1		36 = 22		71 = 43	
2 = 1		37 = 22		72 = 43	
3 = 2		38 = 23		73 = 44	
4 = 2		39 = 23		74 = 44	
5 = 3		40 = 24		75 = 45	
6 = 4		41 = 25		76 = 46	
7 = 4		42 = 25		77 = 46	
8 = 5		43 = 26		78 = 47	
9 = 5		44 = 26		79 = 47	
10 = 6		45 = 27		80 = 48	
11 = 7		46 = 28		81 = 49	
12 = 7		47 = 28		82 = 49	
13 = 8		48 = 29		83 = 50	
14 = 8		49 = 29		84 = 50	
15 = 9		50 = 30		85 = 51	
16 = 10		51 = 31		86 = 52	
17 = 10		52 = 31		87 = 52	
18 = 11		53 = 32		88 = 53	
19 = 11		54 = 32		89 = 53	
20 = 12		55 = 33		90 = 54	
21 = 13		56 = 34		91 = 55	
22 = 13		57 = 34		92 = 55	
23 = 14		58 = 35		93 = 56	
24 = 14		59 = 35		94 = 56	
25 = 15		60 = 36		95 = 57	
26 = 16		61 = 37		96 = 58	
27 = 16		62 = 37		97 = 58	
28 = 17		63 = 38		98 = 59	
29 = 17		64 = 38		99 = 59	
30 = 18		65 = 39		100 = 60	
31 = 19		66 = 40			
32 = 19		67 = 40			
33 = 20		68 = 41			
34 = 20		69 = 41			

From *Guides to the evaluation of permanent impairment,* ed 4, Chicago, 1994, American Medical Association.

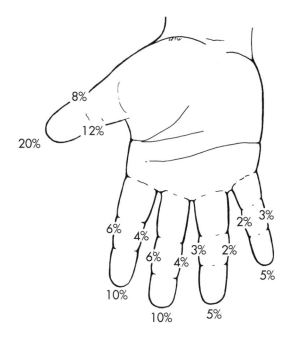

Fig. 66-7. Hand impairments for total transverse sensory loss of entire length of digit (number at tips of digits) and total longitudinal sensory loss of entire radial and ulnar sides (numbers at sides of digits). Total transverse sensory loss is calculated as 50% that of amputation.

Loss of palmar cutaneous nerve sensibility is considered to be a 5% impairment of the hand. Zero to 10% impairment of the upper extremity may be given for loss of sensibility of the palmar or dorsal ulnar cutaneous nerve, the palmar branch of the median nerve, or the superficial branch of the radial nerve (Fig. 66-31, p. 654).

FINGER MOTION IMPAIRMENT EVALUATION "A = E + F" METHOD

The arc of motion is the total number of degrees of excursion of a joint between the two extremes of motion, for example, from maximum extension to maximum flexion. When there is ankylosis the degrees of lost motion (A), equal the sum of lost extension degrees (E) and lost flexion degrees (F), or $A = E + F$. A always equals the number of degrees of normal arc of motion of the joint.

The measured angles of flexion and extension are represented by V_{flex} and F_{ext}. Assuming that a joint that would have ROM from 0° extension (theoretically smallest V_{ext}) to 90° flexion (theoretically largest V_{flex}), actually has a measured V_{flex} of 90° and measured V_{ext} of 0°, there is no loss of motion.

When joint extension is decreased, E (lost extension degrees) equals the measured V_{ext} minus the theoretically smallest V_{ext}.

Example: If a joint that would have a normal extension to 0° actually has a measured V_{ext} of 20°, $E = 20° - 0°$, or 20° (Fig. 66-8).

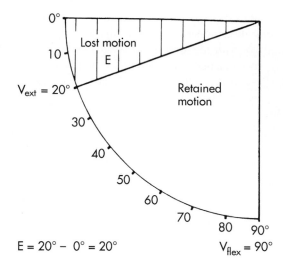

$$E = 20° - 0° = 20°$$

Fig. 66-8. Example of metacarpophalangeal joint presenting motion from 20° extension lag to 90° flexion; lost extension E, is equal to measured extension angle ($V_{ext} = 20°$) minus theoretically smallest possible extension angle (0°), or $E = 20°$.

When joint flexion is decreased, F (lost flexion degrees) equals the theoretically largest V_{flex} minus the measured V_{flex}.

Example: If a joint that would have a normal flexion to 90°, actually has a measured V_{flex} of 60°, $F = 90° - 60°$ or 30° (Fig. 66-9).

With decreasing flexion, V_{flex} decreases, and with impaired extension, V_{ext} increases. These values will finally meet at the same point on the arc of motion, or $V_{flex} = V_{ext}$. When this occurs, there is ankylosis or loss of the total arc of motion degrees (A).

Example: If a joint that would have a normal extension to 0° and a normal flexion to 90° is ankylosed in 40° of flexion (Fig. 66-10),

$V_{ext} = V_{flex}$
$E = 40° - 0°$, or 40°;
$F = 90° - 40°$, or 50°;
$A = E (40°) + F (50°)$, or 90°.

The preceding formula is of basic importance in the discussion and evaluation of impaired function. Impairment of finger function may be caused by lack of extension (E) with or without lack of flexion (F) or ankylosis (A). The restricted motion impairment percentages are called I_E, I_F, and I_A respectively, and are functions of the angle (V) measured at examination. $I_E\%$ is a function of V_{ext} and goes to 0% when V_{ext} reaches its theoretically smallest value; $I_F\%$ is a function of V_{flex} and goes to 0% when V_{flex} reaches its theoretically largest value; $I_A\%$ is a function of V when $V_{ext} = V_{flex}$ and similarly, $I_A\% = I_E\% + I_F\%$.

Note that $I_A\%$ varies according to the angle at which the ankylosis occurs on the potential arc of motion and that it reaches its lowest value when the angle of ankylosis corresponds to the functional position of the joint.

The formula, $A = E + F$, also can be written $E = A - F$; therefore impairment values for lack of extension ($I_E\%$)

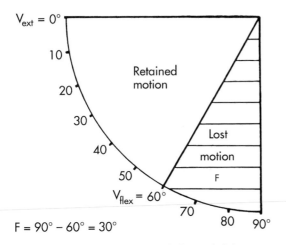

$$F = 90° - 60° = 30°$$

Fig. 66-9. Example of metacarpophalangeal joint presenting motion from 0° extension to 60° flexion; lost flexion, F, is equal to theoretically largest possible angle of flexion (90°) minus measured flexion angle ($V_{flex} = 60°$), or $F = 90° - 60° = 30°$.

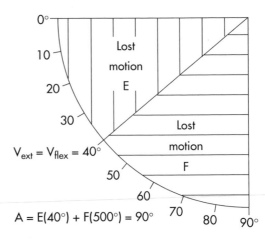

$$A = E(40°) + F(500°) = 90°$$

Fig. 66-10. When no motion is retained, ankylosis is present—in this example at 40°. As can be seen, total motion lost to ankylosis (A) is equal to 40° of lack of extension, E, plus 50° lack of flexion, F; sum of E (40°) and F (50°) equals A (90°).

can be calculated for any measured angle on the basis that $I_E\% = I_A\% - I_F\%$. The derivation of $I_E\%$ is of fundamental importance for adequate evaluation of impairment caused by restricted joint motion. The values of both $I_E\%$ and $I_F\%$ are available to estimate impairment percentages relating not only to the number of degrees of lost motion, but most important, to the location of the loss on the arc of motion.

Impairment curves based on the preceding formula were derived on a 100% scale for each motion of each joint of the upper extremity, assigning the position of function according to the literature recommendations for fusion. The values of $I_A\%$ vary according to the angle of ankylosis. $I_A\%$ reaches its maximum value or 100% at the two extreme positions of the arc of motion and drops to its lowest value when ankylosis occurs in the functional position of the joint. The impairment curves were then converted to pie graphs of motion impairment by applying the relative value of each unit of motion as a conversion factor.

IMPAIRMENT ESTIMATION FOR COMBINED VALUES

The method to *combine* various impairments is based on the principle that each impairment acts not on the whole part (for example, the whole finger) but on the portion that remains (for example, the PIP joint and proximally) after the preceding impairment has acted (for example, on the DIP joint). When there is more than one impairment to a given part, these impairments must be *combined* before the conversion to a larger part is made. The *combined* values determination is based on the formula:

$A\% + B\% (100\% - A\%) = $ the combined values of $A\% + B\%$

When this formula is used, all percentages combined must be expressed on a common denominator. For example, multiple impairments of a finger are *combined* as expressed on the 100% relative value of the finger. The combined value

is converted to the next larger part, for example, the hand. If three or more values are to be *combined*, two may be selected and their *combined* value found. This *combined* value and the third value are *combined* to give the total value. This procedure can be repeated indefinitely, with the value obtained in each case being a combination of all the previous values. Combined Value Tables for ease of determination are provided in Table 66-5.

Example: An index finger presents an amputation at the DIP joint and ankylosis of the PIP joint at 90°; the *combined* impairment to the index finger can be computed according to the formula as follows: amputation of the DIP joint represents a 45% impairment to the index finger (see Fig. 66-6, *B*) and ankylosis of the PIP joint at 90° represents a 75% impairment to the index finger (Fig. 66-13). These can be *combined* as follows:

45% + 75% (100% − 45%) = 45% + 75% (55%) =
45% + 41% = 86% impairment to the index finger.

The index finger represents 20% to the hand, and the above impairment would represent a 20% × 86% impairment to the hand, or 17% (see Table 66-2). The *combined* impairment value of the above example also can be found quickly in Table 66-5 at the intersection of the vertical and horizontal coordinates represented by 45% and 75% finger impairment.

When multiple impairments of a digit are present, such as abnormal motion, sensory loss, or amputation, these are expressed in terms of digit impairment and are *combined* using the combined values chart, Table 66-5. Similarly, multiple regional impairments such as those of the hand, wrist, elbow, and shoulder are expressed individually in terms of the upper extremity before being *combined* together. Note that when more than one digit is involved, the hand impairments contributed by each digit are *added* directly together before relating the hand impairment to upper extremity impairment.

Table 66-5. Combined values chart

	1	2	3	4	5	6	7	8	9	10	11	12	13	14	15	16	17	18	19	20	21	22	23	24	25	26	27	28	29	30	31	32	33	34	35	36	37	38	39	40	41	42	43	44	45	46	47	48	49
1	2
2	3	4
3	4	5	6
4	5	6	7	8
5	6	7	8	9	10
6	7	8	9	10	11	12
7	8	9	10	11	12	13	14
8	9	10	11	12	13	14	14	15
9	10	11	12	13	14	14	15	16	17
10	11	12	13	14	15	15	16	17	18	19
11	12	13	14	15	15	16	17	18	19	20	21
12	13	14	15	16	16	17	18	19	20	21	22	23
13	14	15	16	16	17	18	19	20	21	22	23	23	24
14	15	16	17	17	18	19	20	21	22	23	23	24	25	26
15	16	17	18	18	19	20	21	22	23	24	24	25	26	27	28
16	17	18	19	19	20	21	22	23	24	24	25	26	27	28	29	29
17	18	19	19	20	21	22	23	24	24	25	26	27	28	29	29	30	31
18	19	20	20	21	22	23	24	25	25	26	27	28	29	29	30	31	32	33
19	20	21	21	22	23	24	25	25	26	27	28	29	30	30	31	32	33	34	34
20	21	22	22	23	24	25	26	26	27	28	29	30	30	31	32	33	34	34	35	36
21	22	23	23	24	25	26	27	27	28	29	30	30	31	32	33	34	34	35	36	37	38
22	23	24	24	25	26	27	27	28	29	30	31	31	32	33	34	34	35	36	37	38	38	39
23	24	25	25	26	27	28	28	29	30	31	31	32	33	34	35	35	36	37	38	38	39	40	41
24	25	26	26	27	28	29	29	31	31	32	32	33	34	35	35	36	37	38	38	39	40	41	41	42
25	26	27	27	28	29	30	30	31	32	33	33	34	35	36	36	37	38	39	39	40	41	42	42	43	44
26	27	27	28	29	30	30	31	32	33	33	34	35	36	36	37	38	39	39	40	41	42	42	43	44	45	45
27	28	28	29	30	31	31	32	33	34	34	35	36	36	37	38	39	39	40	41	42	42	43	44	45	45	46	47
28	29	29	30	31	32	32	33	34	34	35	36	37	37	38	39	40	40	41	42	42	43	44	45	45	46	47	47	48
29	30	30	31	32	33	33	34	35	35	36	37	38	38	39	40	40	41	42	42	43	44	45	45	46	47	47	48	49	50
30	31	31	32	33	34	34	35	36	36	37	38	38	39	40	41	41	42	43	43	44	45	45	46	47	48	48	49	50	50	51
31	32	32	33	34	34	35	36	37	37	38	39	39	40	41	41	42	43	43	44	45	45	46	47	48	48	49	50	50	51	52	52
32	33	33	34	35	35	36	37	37	38	39	39	40	41	42	42	43	44	44	45	46	46	47	48	48	49	50	50	51	52	52	53	54
33	34	34	35	36	36	37	38	38	39	40	40	41	42	42	43	44	44	45	46	46	47	48	48	49	50	50	51	52	52	53	54	54	55
34	35	35	36	37	37	38	39	39	40	41	41	42	43	43	44	45	45	46	47	47	48	49	49	50	51	51	52	52	53	54	54	55	56	56
35	36	36	37	38	38	39	40	40	41	42	42	43	43	44	45	45	46	47	47	48	49	49	50	51	51	52	53	53	54	55	55	56	56	57	58
36	37	37	38	39	39	40	40	41	42	42	43	44	44	45	46	46	47	48	48	49	49	50	51	51	52	53	53	54	55	55	56	56	57	58	58	59
37	38	38	39	40	40	41	41	42	43	43	44	45	45	46	46	47	48	48	49	50	50	51	51	52	53	53	54	55	55	56	57	57	58	58	59	60	60
38	39	39	40	40	41	42	42	43	44	44	45	45	46	47	47	48	49	49	50	50	51	52	52	53	54	54	55	55	56	57	57	58	58	59	60	60	61	62
39	40	40	41	41	42	43	43	44	44	45	46	46	47	48	48	49	49	50	51	51	52	52	53	54	54	55	55	56	57	57	58	59	59	60	60	61	62	62	63
40	41	41	42	42	43	44	44	45	45	46	47	47	48	48	49	50	50	51	51	52	53	53	54	54	55	56	56	57	57	58	59	59	60	60	61	62	62	63	63	64
41	42	42	43	43	44	45	45	46	46	47	47	48	49	49	50	50	51	52	52	53	53	54	55	55	56	56	57	58	58	59	59	60	60	61	62	62	63	63	64	64	65
42	43	43	44	44	45	45	46	47	47	48	48	49	50	50	51	51	52	52	53	54	54	55	55	56	57	57	58	58	59	59	60	61	61	62	62	63	63	64	65	65	66	66
43	44	44	45	45	46	46	47	48	48	49	49	50	50	51	52	52	53	53	54	54	55	56	56	57	57	58	58	59	60	60	61	61	62	62	63	64	64	65	65	66	66	67	68
44	45	45	46	46	47	47	48	48	49	50	50	51	51	52	52	53	54	54	55	55	56	56	57	57	58	59	59	60	60	61	61	62	62	63	64	64	65	65	66	66	67	68	68	69
45	46	46	47	47	48	48	49	49	50	51	51	52	52	53	53	54	54	55	55	56	57	57	58	58	59	59	60	60	61	62	62	63	63	64	64	65	65	66	66	67	68	68	69	69	70
46	47	47	48	48	49	49	50	50	51	51	52	52	53	54	54	55	55	56	56	57	57	58	58	59	60	60	61	61	62	62	63	63	64	64	65	65	66	67	67	68	68	69	69	70	70	71
47	48	48	49	49	50	50	51	51	52	52	53	53	54	54	55	55	56	57	57	58	58	59	59	60	60	61	61	62	62	63	63	64	64	65	66	66	67	67	68	68	69	69	70	70	71	71	72
48	49	49	50	50	51	51	52	52	53	53	54	54	55	55	56	56	57	57	58	58	59	59	60	60	61	62	62	63	63	64	64	65	65	66	66	67	68	68	69	69	70	70	71	71	72	72	73
49	50	50	51	51	52	52	53	53	54	54	55	55	56	56	57	57	58	58	59	59	60	60	61	61	62	62	63	63	64	64	65	65	66	66	67	67	68	68	69	69	70	70	71	71	72	72	73	73	74

From *Guides to the evaluation of permanent impairment*, ed 4, Chicago, 1994, American Medical Association.

The values are derived from the formula: $A\% + B\% (100\% - A\%)$ = combined values of A and B. To combine any two impairment values, locate the larger of the values on the side of the chart and read along that row until reaching the column indicated by the smaller value at the bottom of the chart. At the intersection of the row and the column is the combined value.

Table 66-5. Combined values chart—cont'd

	1	2	3	4	5	6	7	8	9	10	11	12	13	14	15	16	17	18	19	20	21	22	23	24	25	26	27	28	29	30	31	32	33	34	35	36	37	38	39	40	41	42	43	44	45	46	47	48	49	50
50	51	51	52	52	53	53	54	54	55	55	56	56	57	57	58	58	59	59	60	60	61	61	62	62	63	63	64	64	65	65	66	66	67	67	68	68	69	69	70	70	71	71	72	72	73	73	74	74	75	75
51	51	52	52	53	53	54	54	55	55	56	56	57	57	58	58	59	59	60	60	61	61	62	62	63	63	64	64	65	65	66	66	67	67	68	68	69	69	70	70	71	71	72	72	73	73	74	74	75	75	76
52	52	53	53	54	54	55	55	56	56	57	57	58	58	59	59	60	60	61	61	62	62	63	63	64	64	64	65	65	66	66	67	67	68	68	69	69	70	70	71	71	72	72	73	73	74	74	75	75	76	76
53	53	54	54	55	55	56	56	57	57	58	58	59	59	60	60	61	61	61	62	62	63	63	64	64	65	65	66	66	67	67	68	68	69	69	69	70	70	71	71	72	72	73	73	74	74	75	75	76	76	77
54	54	55	55	56	56	57	57	58	58	59	59	59	60	60	61	61	62	62	63	63	64	64	65	65	66	66	66	67	67	68	68	69	69	70	70	71	71	71	72	72	73	73	74	74	75	75	76	76	77	77
55	55	56	56	57	57	58	58	59	59	60	60	60	61	61	62	62	63	63	64	64	64	65	65	66	66	67	67	68	68	69	69	69	70	70	71	71	72	72	73	73	73	74	74	75	75	76	76	77	77	78
56	56	57	57	58	58	59	59	60	60	60	61	61	62	62	63	63	63	64	64	65	65	66	66	67	67	67	68	68	69	69	70	70	71	71	71	72	72	73	73	74	74	74	75	75	76	76	77	77	78	78
57	57	58	58	59	59	60	60	60	61	61	62	62	63	63	63	64	64	65	65	66	66	66	67	67	68	68	69	69	69	70	70	71	71	72	72	72	73	73	74	74	75	75	75	76	76	77	77	78	78	79
58	58	59	59	60	60	61	61	61	62	62	63	63	63	64	64	65	65	66	66	66	67	67	68	68	68	69	69	70	70	71	71	71	72	72	73	73	74	74	74	75	75	76	76	76	77	77	78	78	79	79
59	59	60	60	61	61	61	62	62	63	63	64	64	64	65	65	66	66	66	67	67	68	68	68	69	69	70	70	70	71	71	72	72	73	73	73	74	74	75	75	75	76	76	77	77	77	78	78	79	79	80
60	60	61	61	62	62	62	63	63	64	64	64	65	65	66	66	66	67	67	68	68	68	69	69	70	70	70	71	71	72	72	72	73	73	74	74	74	75	75	76	76	76	77	77	78	78	78	79	79	80	80
61	61	62	62	63	63	63	64	64	65	65	65	66	66	66	67	67	68	68	68	69	69	70	70	70	71	71	72	72	72	73	73	73	74	74	75	75	75	76	76	77	77	77	78	78	79	79	79	80	80	81
62	62	63	63	64	64	64	65	65	65	66	66	67	67	67	68	68	68	69	69	70	70	70	71	71	72	72	72	73	73	73	74	74	75	75	75	76	76	76	77	77	78	78	78	79	79	79	80	80	81	81
63	63	64	64	64	65	65	66	66	66	67	67	67	68	68	69	69	69	70	70	70	71	71	72	72	72	73	73	73	74	74	74	75	75	76	76	76	77	77	77	78	78	79	79	79	80	80	80	81	81	82
64	64	65	65	65	66	66	67	67	67	68	68	68	69	69	69	70	70	70	71	71	72	72	72	73	73	73	74	74	74	75	75	76	76	76	77	77	77	78	78	78	79	79	79	80	80	81	81	81	82	82
65	65	66	66	66	67	67	67	68	68	69	69	69	70	70	70	71	71	71	72	72	72	73	73	73	74	74	74	75	75	76	76	76	77	77	77	78	78	78	79	79	79	80	80	80	81	81	81	82	82	83
66	66	67	67	67	68	68	68	69	69	69	70	70	70	71	71	71	72	72	72	73	73	73	74	74	75	75	75	76	76	76	77	77	77	78	78	78	79	79	79	80	80	80	81	81	81	82	82	82	83	83
67	67	68	68	68	69	69	69	70	70	70	71	71	71	72	72	72	73	73	73	74	74	74	75	75	75	76	76	76	77	77	77	78	78	78	79	79	79	80	80	80	81	81	81	82	82	82	83	83	83	84
68	68	69	69	69	70	70	70	71	71	71	72	72	72	72	73	73	73	74	74	74	75	75	75	76	76	76	77	77	77	78	78	78	79	79	79	80	80	80	80	81	81	81	82	82	82	83	83	83	84	84
69	69	70	70	70	71	71	71	71	72	72	72	73	73	73	74	74	74	75	75	75	76	76	76	76	77	77	77	78	78	78	79	79	79	80	80	80	80	81	81	81	82	82	82	83	83	83	84	84	84	85
70	70	71	71	71	72	72	72	72	73	73	73	74	74	74	75	75	75	75	76	76	76	77	77	77	78	78	78	78	79	79	79	80	80	80	81	81	81	81	82	82	82	83	83	83	84	84	84	84	85	85
71	71	72	72	72	72	73	73	73	74	74	74	74	75	75	75	76	76	76	77	77	77	77	78	78	78	79	79	79	79	80	80	80	81	81	81	81	82	82	82	83	83	83	83	84	84	84	85	85	85	86
72	72	73	73	73	73	74	74	74	75	75	75	75	76	76	76	76	77	77	77	78	78	78	78	79	79	79	80	80	80	80	81	81	81	82	82	82	82	83	83	83	84	84	84	84	85	85	85	85	86	86
73	73	74	74	74	74	75	75	75	75	76	76	76	77	77	77	77	78	78	78	78	79	79	79	79	80	80	80	81	81	81	81	82	82	82	82	83	83	83	84	84	84	84	85	85	85	85	86	86	86	87
74	74	75	75	75	75	76	76	76	76	77	77	77	77	78	78	78	78	79	79	79	79	80	80	80	81	81	81	81	82	82	82	82	83	83	83	83	84	84	84	84	85	85	85	85	86	86	86	86	87	87
75	75	76	76	76	76	77	77	77	77	78	78	78	78	79	79	79	79	80	80	80	80	81	81	81	81	82	82	82	82	83	83	83	83	84	84	84	84	85	85	85	85	86	86	86	86	87	87	87	87	88
76	76	76	77	77	77	77	78	78	78	78	79	79	79	79	80	80	80	80	81	81	81	81	82	82	82	82	82	83	83	83	83	84	84	84	84	85	85	85	85	86	86	86	86	87	87	87	87	88	88	88
77	77	77	78	78	78	78	79	79	79	79	80	80	80	80	80	81	81	81	81	82	82	82	82	83	83	83	83	83	84	84	84	84	85	85	85	85	86	86	86	86	86	87	87	87	87	88	88	88	88	89
78	78	78	79	79	79	79	80	80	80	80	80	81	81	81	81	82	82	82	82	82	83	83	83	83	84	84	84	84	84	85	85	85	85	85	86	86	86	86	87	87	87	87	87	88	88	88	88	89	89	89
79	79	79	80	80	80	80	80	81	81	81	81	82	82	82	82	82	83	83	83	83	83	84	84	84	84	84	85	85	85	85	86	86	86	86	86	87	87	87	87	87	88	88	88	88	88	89	89	89	89	90
80	80	80	81	81	81	81	81	82	82	82	82	82	83	83	83	83	83	84	84	84	84	84	85	85	85	85	85	86	86	86	86	86	87	87	87	87	87	88	88	88	88	88	89	89	89	89	89	90	90	90
81	81	81	82	82	82	82	82	83	83	83	83	83	83	84	84	84	84	84	85	85	85	85	85	86	86	86	86	86	87	87	87	87	87	87	88	88	88	88	88	89	89	89	89	89	90	90	90	90	90	91
82	82	82	83	83	83	83	83	83	84	84	84	84	84	85	85	85	85	85	85	86	86	86	86	86	87	87	87	87	87	87	88	88	88	88	88	88	89	89	89	89	89	90	90	90	90	90	90	91	91	91
83	83	83	84	84	84	84	84	84	85	85	85	85	85	85	86	86	86	86	86	86	87	87	87	87	87	87	88	88	88	88	88	88	89	89	89	89	89	89	90	90	90	90	90	90	91	91	91	91	91	92
84	84	84	84	85	85	85	85	85	85	86	86	86	86	86	86	87	87	87	87	87	87	88	88	88	88	88	88	88	89	89	89	89	89	89	90	90	90	90	90	90	91	91	91	91	91	91	92	92	92	92
85	85	85	85	86	86	86	86	86	86	87	87	87	87	87	87	87	88	88	88	88	88	88	88	89	89	89	89	89	89	90	90	90	90	90	90	90	91	91	91	91	91	91	91	92	92	92	92	92	92	93
86	86	86	86	87	87	87	87	87	87	87	88	88	88	88	88	88	88	89	89	89	89	89	89	89	90	90	90	90	90	90	90	90	91	91	91	91	91	91	91	92	92	92	92	92	92	92	93	93	93	93
87	87	87	87	88	88	88	88	88	88	88	88	89	89	89	89	89	89	89	89	90	90	90	90	90	90	90	91	91	91	91	91	91	91	91	92	92	92	92	92	92	92	92	93	93	93	93	93	93	93	94
88	88	88	88	88	89	89	89	89	89	89	89	89	90	90	90	90	90	90	90	90	91	91	91	91	91	91	91	91	91	92	92	92	92	92	92	92	92	93	93	93	93	93	93	93	93	94	94	94	94	94
89	89	89	89	89	90	90	90	90	90	90	90	90	90	91	91	91	91	91	91	91	91	91	92	92	92	92	92	92	92	92	92	93	93	93	93	93	93	93	93	93	94	94	94	94	94	94	94	94	94	95
90	90	90	90	90	91	91	91	91	91	91	91	91	91	91	92	92	92	92	92	92	92	92	92	92	93	93	93	93	93	93	93	93	93	93	94	94	94	94	94	94	94	94	94	94	95	95	95	95	95	95
91	91	91	91	91	91	92	92	92	92	92	92	92	92	92	92	92	93	93	93	93	93	93	93	93	93	93	93	94	94	94	94	94	94	94	94	94	94	94	95	95	95	95	95	95	95	95	95	95	95	96
92	92	92	92	92	92	92	93	93	93	93	93	93	93	93	93	93	93	93	94	94	94	94	94	94	94	94	94	94	94	94	94	95	95	95	95	95	95	95	95	95	95	95	95	96	96	96	96	96	96	96
93	93	93	93	93	93	93	93	94	94	94	94	94	94	94	94	94	94	94	94	94	94	95	95	95	95	95	95	95	95	95	95	95	95	95	95	96	96	96	96	96	96	96	96	96	96	96	96	96	96	97
94	94	94	94	94	94	94	94	94	95	95	95	95	95	95	95	95	95	95	95	95	95	95	95	95	96	96	96	96	96	96	96	96	96	96	96	96	96	96	96	96	96	97	97	97	97	97	97	97	97	97
95	95	95	95	95	95	95	95	95	95	96	96	96	96	96	96	96	96	96	96	96	96	96	96	96	96	96	96	96	96	96	97	97	97	97	97	97	97	97	97	97	97	97	97	97	97	97	97	97	97	98
96	96	96	96	96	96	96	96	96	96	96	96	96	97	97	97	97	97	97	97	97	97	97	97	97	97	97	97	97	97	97	97	97	97	97	97	97	97	98	98	98	98	98	98	98	98	98	98	98	98	98
97	97	97	97	97	97	97	97	97	97	97	97	97	97	97	97	97	98	98	98	98	98	98	98	98	98	98	98	98	98	98	98	98	98	98	98	98	98	98	98	98	98	98	98	98	98	98	98	98	98	99
98	98	98	98	98	98	98	98	98	98	98	98	98	98	98	98	98	98	98	98	98	98	98	98	98	99	99	99	99	99	99	99	99	99	99	99	99	99	99	99	99	99	99	99	99	99	99	99	99	99	99
99	99	99	99	99	99	99	99	99	99	99	99	99	99	99	99	99	99	99	99	99	99	99	99	99	99	99	99	99	99	99	99	99	99	99	99	99	99	99	99	99	99	99	99	99	99	99	99	99	99	100
	1	**2**	**3**	**4**	**5**	**6**	**7**	**8**	**9**	**10**	**11**	**12**	**13**	**14**	**15**	**16**	**17**	**18**	**19**	**20**	**21**	**22**	**23**	**24**	**25**	**26**	**27**	**28**	**29**	**30**	**31**	**32**	**33**	**34**	**35**	**36**	**37**	**38**	**39**	**40**	**41**	**42**	**43**	**44**	**45**	**46**	**47**	**48**	**49**	**50**

Continued.

Table 66-5. Combined values chart—cont'd

	51	52	53	54	55	56	57	58	59	60	61	62	63	64	65	66	67	68	69	70	71	72	73	74	75	76	77	78	79	80	81	82	83	84	85	86	87	88	89	90	91	92	93	94	95	96	97	98	99
51	76																																																
52	76	77																																															
53	77	77	78																																														
54	77	78	78	79																																													
55	78	78	79	79	80																																												
56	78	79	79	80	80	81																																											
57	79	79	80	80	81	81	82																																										
58	79	80	80	81	81	82	82	82																																									
59	80	80	81	81	82	82	82	83	83																																								
60	80	81	81	82	82	82	83	83	84	84																																							
61	81	81	82	82	82	83	83	84	84	84	85																																						
62	81	82	82	83	83	83	84	84	84	85	85	86																																					
63	82	82	83	83	83	84	84	84	85	85	86	86	86																																				
64	82	83	83	83	84	84	85	85	85	86	86	86	87	87																																			
65	83	83	84	84	84	85	85	85	86	86	86	87	87	87	88																																		
66	83	84	84	84	85	85	85	86	86	86	87	87	87	88	88	88																																	
67	84	84	84	85	85	85	86	86	86	87	87	87	88	88	88	89	89																																
68	84	85	85	85	86	86	86	87	87	87	88	88	88	88	89	89	89	90																															
69	85	85	85	86	86	86	87	87	87	88	88	88	89	89	89	89	90	90	90																														
70	85	86	86	86	87	87	87	87	88	88	88	89	89	89	90	90	90	90	91	91																													
71	86	86	86	87	87	87	88	88	88	88	89	89	89	90	90	90	90	91	91	91	92																												
72	86	87	87	87	87	88	88	88	89	89	89	89	90	90	90	90	91	91	91	92	92	92																												
73	87	87	87	88	88	88	88	89	89	89	89	90	90	90	91	91	91	91	92	92	92	92	93																											
74	87	88	88	88	88	89	89	89	89	90	90	90	90	91	91	91	91	92	92	92	92	93	93	93																										
75	88	88	88	89	89	89	89	90	90	90	90	91	91	91	91	92	92	92	92	93	93	93	93	94	94																									
76	88	88	89	89	89	89	90	90	90	90	91	91	91	91	92	92	92	92	93	93	93	93	94	94	94	94																								
77	89	89	89	89	90	90	90	90	91	91	91	91	91	92	92	92	92	93	93	93	93	94	94	94	94	94	95																							
78	89	89	90	90	90	90	91	91	91	91	91	92	92	92	92	93	93	93	93	93	94	94	94	94	95	95	95	95																						
79	90	90	90	90	91	91	91	91	91	92	92	92	92	92	93	93	93	93	93	94	94	94	94	95	95	95	95	95	96																				
80	90	90	91	91	91	91	91	92	92	92	92	92	93	93	93	93	93	94	94	94	94	94	95	95	95	95	95	96	96	96																			
81	91	91	91	91	91	92	92	92	92	92	93	93	93	93	93	94	94	94	94	94	94	95	95	95	95	95	96	96	96	96	96																		
82	91	91	92	92	92	92	92	92	93	93	93	93	93	94	94	94	94	94	94	95	95	95	95	95	96	96	96	96	96	96	97	97																	
83	92	92	92	92	92	93	93	93	93	93	93	94	94	94	94	94	94	95	95	95	95	95	95	96	96	96	96	96	96	97	97	97	97																
84	92	92	92	93	93	93	93	93	93	94	94	94	94	94	94	95	95	95	95	95	95	96	96	96	96	96	96	96	97	97	97	97	97	97															
85	93	93	93	93	93	93	94	94	94	94	94	94	94	95	95	95	95	95	95	96	96	96	96	96	96	96	97	97	97	97	97	97	97	98	98														
86	93	93	93	94	94	94	94	94	94	94	95	95	95	95	95	95	95	96	96	96	96	96	96	96	97	97	97	97	97	97	97	97	98	98	98	98													
87	94	94	94	94	94	94	94	95	95	95	95	95	95	95	95	96	96	96	96	96	96	96	96	97	97	97	97	97	97	97	98	98	98	98	98	98	98												
88	94	94	94	94	95	95	95	95	95	95	95	95	96	96	96	96	96	96	96	96	97	97	97	97	97	97	97	97	97	98	98	98	98	98	98	98	98	99											
89	95	95	95	95	95	95	95	95	95	96	96	96	96	96	96	96	96	96	97	97	97	97	97	97	97	97	97	98	98	98	98	98	98	98	98	98	99	99	99										
90	95	95	95	95	96	96	96	96	96	96	96	96	96	96	97	97	97	97	97	97	97	97	97	97	98	98	98	98	98	98	98	98	98	98	99	99	99	99	99	99									
91	96	96	96	96	96	96	96	96	96	96	96	97	97	97	97	97	97	97	97	97	97	97	98	98	98	98	98	98	98	98	98	98	98	99	99	99	99	99	99	99	99								
92	96	96	96	96	96	96	97	97	97	97	97	97	97	97	97	97	97	97	98	98	98	98	98	98	98	98	98	98	98	98	98	99	99	99	99	99	99	99	99	99	99	99							
93	97	97	97	97	97	97	97	97	97	97	97	97	97	97	98	98	98	98	98	98	98	98	98	98	98	98	98	98	99	99	99	99	99	99	99	99	99	99	99	99	99	99	100						
94	97	97	97	97	97	97	97	97	98	98	98	98	98	98	98	98	98	98	98	98	98	98	98	98	99	99	99	99	99	99	99	99	99	99	99	99	99	99	99	99	99	100	100	100					
95	98	98	98	98	98	98	98	98	98	98	98	98	98	98	98	98	98	98	98	99	99	99	99	99	99	99	99	99	99	99	99	99	99	99	99	99	99	99	99	100	100	100	100	100	100				
96	98	98	98	98	98	98	98	98	98	98	98	98	99	99	99	99	99	99	99	99	99	99	99	99	99	99	99	99	99	99	99	99	99	99	99	99	99	100	100	100	100	100	100	100	100	100			
97	99	99	99	99	99	99	99	99	99	99	99	99	99	99	99	99	99	99	99	99	99	99	99	99	99	99	99	99	99	99	99	99	99	100	100	100	100	100	100	100	100	100	100	100	100	100	100		
98	99	99	99	99	99	99	99	99	99	99	99	99	99	99	99	99	99	99	99	99	99	99	99	99	100	100	100	100	100	100	100	100	100	100	100	100	100	100	100	100	100	100	100	100	100	100	100	100	
99	100	100	100	100	100	100	100	100	100	100	100	100	100	100	100	100	100	100	100	100	100	100	100	100	100	100	100	100	100	100	100	100	100	100	100	100	100	100	100	100	100	100	100	100	100	100	100	100	100

Regional evaluation

FINGERS

Amputation impairment of fingers

1. Use Fig. 66-11, top scale, to determine the impairment of the finger caused by amputation at various lengths. Amputations through the metacarpal represent a 100% finger impairment and are not given extra values.
2. Use Tables 66-2, 66-3, and 66-4 to relate the finger impairment to the hand, upper extremity, and whole person.

Example: Amputation of the index finger through the DIP joint is equivalent to a 45% finger impairment, 9% hand impairment, 8% upper extremity impairment, and 5% whole person impairment.

Sensory impairment of fingers

See pp. 624 and 625 for a description of the sensory assessment methods and pp. 628 to 630 for the principles of sensory impairment evaluation.

1. Use the two-point discrimination test to identify the type of sensory loss as total (greater than 15 mm) or partial (7 to 15 mm).
2. Determine whether one (longitudinal sensory loss) or both (transverse sensory loss) digital nerves are involved.
3. Identify the level of involvement or percentage of finger length involved (Fig. 66-11, top scale).
4. Consult Table 66-6 for the index, middle, and ring fingers and Table 66-7 for the thumb and little finger to determine the digit impairment for total or partial, transverse, and longitudinal (ulnar or radial) sensory loss according to the percentage of digit length involved.
5. Convert the digit impairment to hand, upper extremity, and whole person impairment using Tables 66-2, 66-3, and 66-4.

Examples: A *total transverse* sensory loss (greater than 15 mm) over the index finger palmar surface starting at the level of the PIP joint (80% finger length) is equivalent to a 40% finger impairment (see Table 66-6) and an 8% hand impairment (see Table 66-2).

A *partial transverse* sensory loss (7 to 15 mm) involving the full length of the palmar surface of the little finger starting at the level of the MP joint gives a 25% impairment of the finger (see Table 66-7) and a 3% impairment of the hand (see Table 66-2).

A *total longitudinal* sensory loss (greater than 15 mm) over the distribution of the index radial digital nerve starting at the level of the MP joint (100% finger length) is equivalent to a 30% finger impairment (see Table 66-6) or a 6% hand impairment (see Table 66-2).

A *partial longitudinal* sensory loss (7 to 15 mm) over the distribution of the ulnar nerve of the little finger starting at the level of the PIP joint (80% finger length) is equivalent to

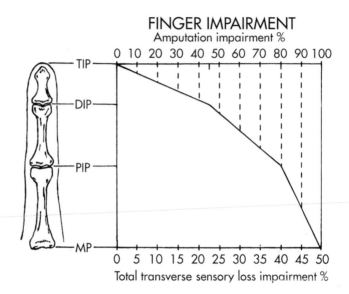

Fig. 66-11. Finger impairments for amputation at various lengths *(top scale)* and total transverse sensory loss *(bottom scale)*. Total transverse sensory loss impairments correspond to 50% of amputation values.

a 12% finger impairment (see Table 66-7) or a 1% hand impairment (see Table 66-2).

Motion impairment of fingers

See pp. 619 and 623 and Figs. 66-4 and 66-5 for a description of the motion measurement methods and pp. 630 and 631 for the principles of motion impairment evaluation. The goniometer readings are rounded to the nearest 10°. The motion impairment relative value given to each finger joint is the same as that found in amputation impairments: DIP, 45%; PIP, 80%; and MP, 100% (Figs. 66-6, *B,* and 66-11).

Impairment curves for lack of flexion, lack of extension, and ankylosis were derived on the 100% scale for each joint according to the formula $A = E + F$. Pie graphs of finger impairment were then derived by applying the relative value of each joint as a conversion factor (Figs. 66-12, 66-13, and 66-14).

In the normal hand, the MP joint can hyperextend usefully to 20°; a small percentage of extension impairment has been assigned to the loss of hyperextension, or $I_E\% = 5\%$ at 0° extension (see Fig. 66-14). The PIP and DIP joints normally extend to 0°, and $I_E\%$ equals 0% at this angle; between the angles of 0° of extension and +30° of hyperextension, impairment values are given for lack of flexion and not for hyperextension. Consideration for positions of hyperextension allows us to rate impairment of flexion when ankylosis occurs in a hyperextended position. For example, ankylosis of the PIP joint in 30° hyperextension equals 80% finger impairment (see Fig. 66-13). Note that for each joint, the ankylosis impairment value is at its lowest for the angle of functional position.

Table 66-6. Finger impairments for transverse and longitudinal sensory loss of index, middle, and ring fingers based on percentage of digit length involved

% Value of digit length	Transverse sensory loss %		Longitudinal sensory loss %			
			Ulnar digital nerve		Radial digital nerve	
	Total loss	Partial loss	Total loss	Partial loss	Total loss	Partial loss
100	50	25	20	10	30	15
90	45	23	18	9	27	14
80	40	20	16	8	24	12
70	35	18	14	7	21	11
60	30	15	12	6	18	9
50	25	13	10	5	15	8
40	20	10	8	4	12	6
30	15	8	6	3	9	5
20	10	5	4	2	6	3
10	5	3	2	1	3	2

Table 66-7. Digit impairments for transverse and longitudinal sensory loss of thumb and little finger based on percentage of digit length involved

% Value of digit length	Transverse sensory loss %		Longitudinal sensory loss %			
			Ulnar digital nerve		Radial digital nerve	
	Total loss	Partial loss	Total loss	Partial loss	Total loss	Partial loss
100	50	25	30	15	20	10
90	45	23	27	14	18	9
80	40	20	24	12	16	8
70	35	18	21	11	14	7
60	30	15	18	9	12	6
50	25	13	15	8	10	5
40	20	10	12	6	8	4
30	15	8	9	5	6	3
20	10	5	6	3	4	2
10	5	3	3	2	2	1

Distal interphalangeal joint flexion and extension. The finger DIP joint has a normal motion of 0° extension to 70° flexion. The position of function is 20° flexion.

1. In Fig. 66-12, locate the measured angles of flexion and extension (row labeled *V*) and match to the impairments of flexion (row labeled $I_F\%$) and extension (row labeled $I_E\%$). Impairment values for hyperextension are read above the 0° neutral position.
2. *Add* I_F and $I_E\%$ to obtain the finger motion impairment at the DIP joint.
3. In the presence of ankylosis, match the measured angle *(V)* to its corresponding ankylosis impairment under the row labeled $I_A\%$ (see Fig. 66-12).

Examples: The middle finger DIP joint has motion of −20° extension to 70° flexion: $I_E\% = 4\%$; $I_F\% = 0\%$ (see Fig. 66-12); 4% + 0% = 4% middle finger impairment, or 1% hand impairment (Table 66-2).

The index finger DIP joint has motion of +20° hyperextension to 30° flexion: $I_E\% = 0\%$; $I_F = 21\%$; 0% + 21% = 21% index finger impairment, or 4% hand impairment.

The ring finger DIP joint is ankylosed in 30° hyperextension: $I_A\% = 45\%$ ring finger impairment, or 5% hand impairment.

Proximal interphalangeal joint flexion and extension. The PIP joint has a normal motion from 0° extension to 100° flexion. The position of function is 40° flexion.

1. In Fig. 66-13, locate the measured angles of flexion and extension (row headed *V*) and match to the impairments of flexion (row labeled $I_F\%$) and extension (row labeled $I_E\%$). Impairment values for hyperextension are read above the 0° neutral position.
2. *Add* $I_F\%$ and $I_E\%$ to obtain the finger motion impairment at the PIP joint.

3. In the presence of ankylosis, match the measured angle *(V)* to its corresponding ankylosis impairment under the row labeled $I_A\%$ (see Fig. 66-13).

Examples: The index finger PIP joint has motion of +30° hyperextension to 30° flexion: $I_E\% = 0\%$; $I_F\% = 42\%$ (Fig. 66-13); 0% + 42% = 42% index finger impairment, or 8% hand impairment (see Table 66-2).

The index finger PIP joint has motion of −30° extension lag to 100° flexion: $I_E\% = 11\%$; $I_F\% = 0\%$; 11% + 0% = 11% index finger impairment, or 2% hand impairment.

The middle finger PIP joint is ankylosed in 30° hyperextension: $I_A\% = 80\%$ middle finger impairment, or 16% hand impairment.

Metacarpophalangeal joint flexion and extension. The finger MP joint motion ranges from +20° hyperextension to 90° flexion. The position of function is 30° flexion.

1. In Fig. 66-14, locate the measured angles of flexion and extension (row labeled *V*) and match to the corresponding impairment of flexion (row labeled $I_F\%$) and extension (row labeled $I_E\%$). Impairment values for hyperextension are read above the 0° neutral position.
2. *Add* $I_F\%$ and $I_E\%$ to obtain the finger motion impairment at the MP joint.
3. In the presence of ankylosis, match the measured angle *(V)* to its corresponding ankylosis impairment under the row labeled $I_A\%$ (see Fig. 66-14).

Examples: The index finger MP joint has a motion of −10° extension to 60° flexion: $I_E\% = 7\%$; $I_F\% = 17\%$ (Fig. 66-14); 7% + 17% = 24% index finger impairment, or 5% hand impairment (see Table 66-2).

The middle finger MP joint is ankylosed in 10° hyperextension: $I_A\% = 57\%$ middle finger impairment, or 11% hand impairment.

IA% = impairment due to ankylosis
IE% = impairment due to loss of extension
IF% = impairment due to loss of flexion
V = measured angles of motion
* = position of function

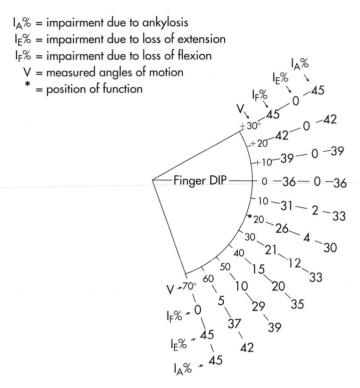

Fig. 66-12. Pie graph for finger impairments caused by abnormal motion at the DIP joint. Relative value of functional unit is 45% of finger. Ankylosis in functional position (20° flexion) receives the lowest $I_A\%$, or 30%.

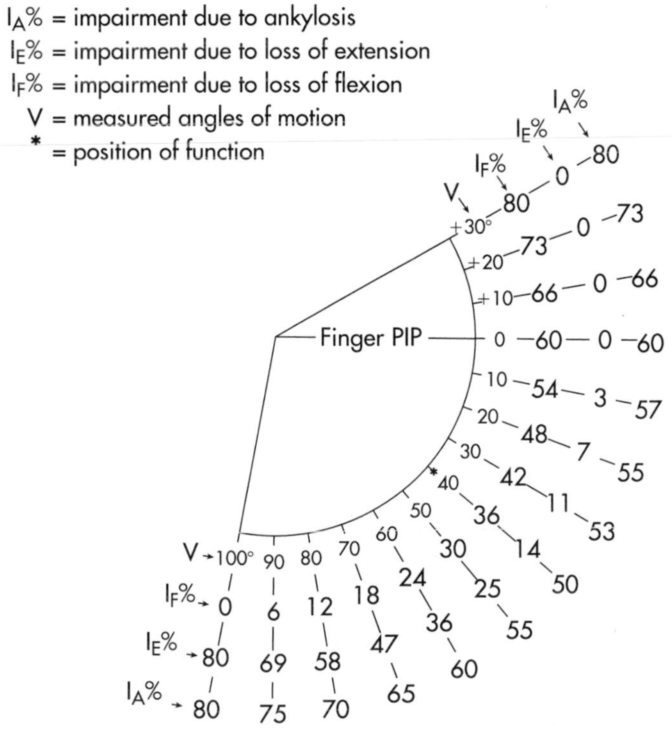

IA% = impairment due to ankylosis
IE% = impairment due to loss of extension
IF% = impairment due to loss of flexion
V = measured angles of motion
* = position of function

Fig. 66-13. Pie graph for finger impairments caused by abnormal motion at the PIP joint. Relative value of functional unit is 80% of finger. Ankylosis in functional position (40° flexion) receives the lowest $I_A\%$, or 50%.

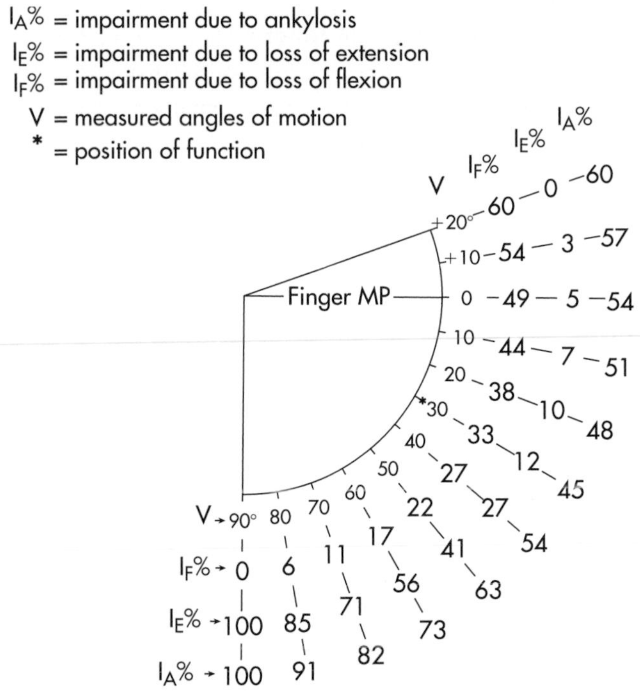

IA% = impairment due to ankylosis
IE% = impairment due to loss of extension
IF% = impairment due to loss of flexion
V = measured angles of motion
* = position of function

Fig. 66-14. Pie graph for finger impairments caused by abnormal motion at the MP joint. Relative value of functional unit is 100% of finger. Ankylosis in functional position (30° flexion) receives the lowest $I_A\%$, or 45%.

Combining abnormal motion impairments for more than one finger joint

The finger motion impairment values of the DIP, PIP, and MP joints are calculated separately and then *combined* to derive the entire finger motion impairment (see Table 66-5). The finger impairment is then expressed in terms of the hand, upper extremity, and whole person using Tables 66-2, 66-3, and 66-4.

Example: Index finger motion impairments are 40%, DIP joint; 30%, PIP joint; and 20%, MP joint: 40% *combined* with 30% = 58%; 58% *combined* with 20% = 66% index finger impairment, or 13% hand impairment, 12% upper extremity impairment, and 7% impairment of the whole person (see Tables 66-2, 66-3, and 66-4).

Combining finger impairments caused by amputation, sensory loss, and abnormal motion

Finger impairment values resulting from amputation, sensory loss, and abnormal motion are calculated separately and then *combined* to obtain the entire finger impairment (see Table 66-5). Use Tables 66-2, 66-3, and 66-4 to relate the finger impairment to the hand, upper extremity, and whole person.

Example: Ring finger amputation impairment is 45%; sensory impairment, 10%; and abnormal motion impairment, 50%: 45% *combined* with 10% = 51%; 51% *combined* with 10% = 56% ring finger impairment, or 6% hand impairment, 5% upper extremity impairment, and 3% impairment of the whole person (see Tables 66-2, 66-3, and 66-4).

THUMB
Amputation impairment of thumb

1. Use Fig. 66-15, top scale, to determine the impairment of the thumb resulting from amputation at various lengths. Amputations through the metacarpal represent a 100% thumb impairment and are not given extra values.
2. Use Tables 66-2, 66-3, and 66-4 to relate the thumb impairment to the hand, upper extremity, and whole person.

Example: Thumb amputation through the IP joint rates as 50% thumb impairment, 20% hand impairment, 18% impairment of the upper extremity, and 11% impairment of the whole person (see Tables 66-2, 66-3, and 66-4).

Sensory impairment of thumb

See pp. 624 and 625 for a description of the sensory assessment methods and pp. 628 to 630 for the principles of sensory impairment evaluation.

1. Use the two-point discrimination test to identify the type of sensory loss as total (greater than 15 mm) or partial (7 to 15 mm).
2. Determine whether one (longitudinal sensory loss) or both (transverse sensory loss) digital nerves are involved.
3. Identify the percentage of thumb length involved (see Fig. 66-15, top scale).
4. Consult Table 66-7 (p. 636) to determine the thumb impairment for total or partial transverse and longitudinal (ulnar or radial) sensory loss according to the percentage of thumb length involved.
5. Convert the thumb impairment to hand, upper extremity, and whole person impairment using Tables 66-2, 66-3, and 66-4.

Examples: A total transverse sensory loss (greater than 15 mm) over the thumb pulp starting at the level of the IP joint (50% thumb length) is equivalent to a 25% thumb impairment (see Table 66-7) or 10% hand impairment (see Table 66-2).

A partial transverse sensory loss (7 to 15 mm) involving the full length of the palmar surface of the thumb starting at the MP joint gives a 25% thumb impairment, or 10% hand impairment.

A total longitudinal sensory loss (greater than 15 mm) over the distribution of the thumb ulnar digital nerve starting at the level of the IP joint (50% thumb length) is equivalent to a 15% thumb impairment (see Table 66-7) or a 6% hand impairment (see Table 66-2).

A partial sensory loss (7 to 15 mm) over the distribution of the thumb radial nerve starting at the level of the MP joint is equivalent to a 10% thumb impairment (see Table 66-7) or 4% hand impairment.

Motion impairment of thumb

See pp. 619 and 623 for a description of the motion measurement method and pp. 630 and 631 for the principles

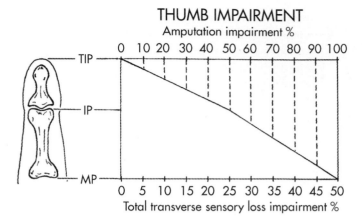

Fig. 66-15. Thumb impairments for amputation at various lengths *(top scale)* and total transverse sensory loss *(bottom scale).* Total transverse sensory loss impairment corresponds to 50% of amputation values.

of motion impairment evaluation. The goniometer readings are rounded to the nearest 10°.

The thumb has five functional units of motion, each contributing a relative value to the total thumb ray motion as follows:

1. Flexion and extension of the IP joint: 15%
2. Flexion and extension of the MP joint: 10%
3. Adduction: 20%
4. Radial abduction: 10%
5. Opposition: 45%

Impairment curves were derived on a 100% scale for each unit of motion based on the formula $A = E + F$. Pie graphs and Tables of thumb motion impairment were derived from these graphs by applying the relative value of each unit of motion as a conversion factor (Figs. 66-16 through 66-20, 66-22, and Tables 66-8 through 66-10).

Interphalangeal joint flexion and extension. The thumb IP joint motion ranges from 30° hyperextension to 80° flexion. The position of function is 20° flexion.

1. In Fig. 66-17, locate the measured angles of flexion and extension (row labeled *V*) and match to the impairments of flexion (row labeled $I_F\%$) and extension (row labeled $I_E\%$). Impairment values for hyperextension are read above the 0° neutral position.
2. *Add* $I_F\%$ and $I_E\%$ to obtain the thumb motion impairment at the IP joint.
3. In the presence of ankylosis, match the measured angle *(V)* to its corresponding ankylosis impairment under the row labeled $I_A\%$ (see Fig. 66-17).

Examples: Thumb IP joint motion is +30° hyperextension to 10° flexion: $I_E\% = 0\%$; $I_F\% = 6\%$ (see Fig. 66-17); $0\% + 6\% = 6\%$ thumb impairment or 2% hand impairment (see Table 66-2).

Thumb IP joint motion is −30° extension to 50° flexion: $I_E\% = 5\%$; $I_F\% = 2\%$; $5\% + 2\% = 7\%$ thumb impairment or 3% hand impairment.

Thumb IP joint ankylosis in 60° flexion: $I_A\% = 12\%$ thumb impairment or 5% hand impairment.

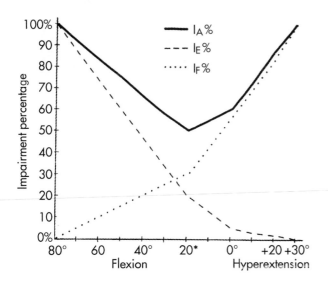

Fig. 66-16. Impairment curves for ankylosis ($I_A\%$) and for loss of flexion ($I_F\%$) and extension ($I_E\%$) of interphalangeal joint of the thumb. Ankylosis in functional position (20° flexion receives the lowest $I_A\%$, or 50%.

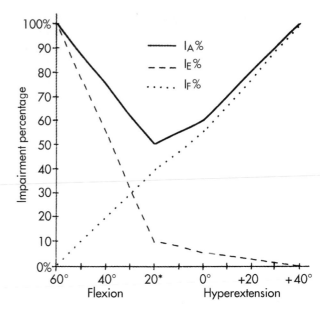

Fig. 66-18. Impairment curves for ankylosis ($I_A\%$) and for loss of flexion ($I_F\%$) and extension ($I_E\%$) of the metacarpophalangeal joint of the thumb. Ankylosis in functional position (20° flexion) receives the lowest $I_A\%$, or 50%.

$I_A\%$ = impairment due to ankylosis
$I_E\%$ = impairment due to loss of extension
$I_F\%$ = impairment due to loss of flexion
V = measured angles of motion
* = position of function

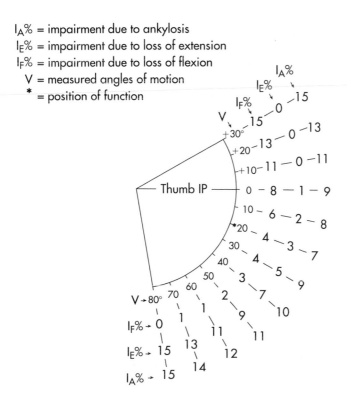

Fig. 66-17. Pie graph for thumb impairments caused by abnormal motion at the interphalangeal joint. Relative value of functional unit is 15% of thumb ray motion.

$I_A\%$ = impairment due to ankylosis
$I_E\%$ = impairment due to loss of extension
$I_F\%$ = impairment due to loss of flexion
V = measured angles of motion
* = position of function

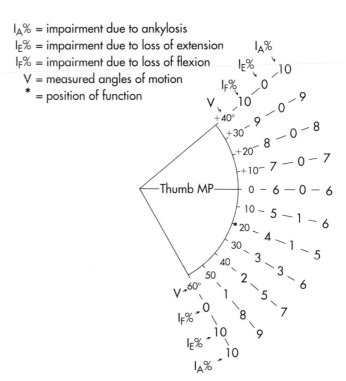

Fig. 66-19. Pie graph for thumb impairments caused by abnormal motion at the metacarpophalangeal (MP) joint. Relative value of functional unit is 10% of thumb ray motion.

Thumb metacarpophalangeal joint flexion and extension. The thumb MP joint motion ranges from +40° hyperextension to 60° flexion. The position of function is considered to be 20° flexion.

1. In Fig. 66-19, match the measured angles *(V)* of flexion and extension degrees to their corresponding impairments of flexion (row labeled $I_F\%$) and extension (row labeled $I_E\%$). Impairment values for positions of hyperextension are read above the 0° neutral position.

2. The values of $I_F\%$ and $I_E\%$ are *added* to obtain the thumb impairment resulting from loss of motion at the MP joint.

3. If the MP joint is ankylosed, the measured angle *(V)* is matched to its corresponding ankylosis impairment under the row headed $I_A\%$ (see Fig. 66-19). Note that ankylosis in the position of function (20°) is given the lowest $I_A\%$ value, 5%.

Examples: Thumb MP joint has +20° hyperextension to 20° flexion: $I_E\% = 0\%$; $I_F\% = 4\%$ (see Fig. 66-19); 0% + 4% = 4% thumb impairment or 2% hand impairment (see Table 66-2).

Thumb MP joint has −20° extension to 50° flexion: $I_E = 1\%$; $I_F\% = 1\%$; 1% + 1% = 2% thumb impairment or 1% hand impairment.

Thumb adduction. Adduction is measured as the smallest possible distance in centimeters from the flexion crease of the thumb IP joint to the distal palmar crease over the level of the fifth MP joint. The normal ROM is from 8 to 0 cm of adduction (see Fig. 66-20).

In Table 66-8, match the measured adduction angle to the thumb impairment value for lost motion or ankylosis.

Examples: Measured thumb adduction at 6 cm gives an 8% thumb impairment (see Table 66-8) or 3% hand impairment (see Table 66-2).

Thumb ankylosis in either 8 or 0 cm adduction corresponds to a 20% thumb impairment.

Thumb radial abduction. Radial abduction is measured as the largest achievable angle between the first and second metacarpals. The normal range of radial abduction is from 0° to 50° (Fig. 66-21).

In Table 66-9, match the measured angle of radial abduction to the thumb impairment value for lost motion or ankylosis. Ankylosis in any position of radial abduction corresponds to a full impairment of this function or 10% thumb impairment.

Example: Thumb radial abduction to 10° is equivalent to 9% thumb impairment (see Table 66-9) or 4% hand impairment (see Table 66-2).

Thumb opposition. Thumb opposition is measured as the largest achievable distance between the flexor crease of the thumb IP joint and the distal palmar crease over the third MP joint. The normal range of opposition is from 0 to 8 cm (see Fig. 66-22).

In Table 66-10, match the measured angle of opposition to the thumb impairment for lost motion of ankylosis.

Examples: Thumb opposition measured at 5 cm corresponds to a 5% thumb impairment (see Table 66-10) or a 2% hand impairment (see Table 66-2).

Thumb ankylosis in 8 cm of opposition gives a 29% thumb impairment (see Table 66-10) or a 12% hand impairment.

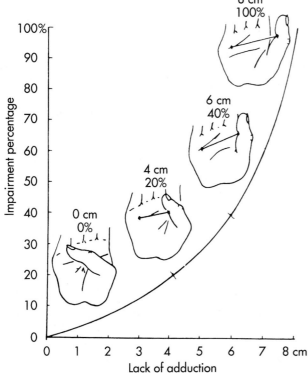

Fig. 66-20. Linear measure of thumb adduction in centimeters at various positions and impairment curve for lack of adduction. Adduction to 0 cm gives 0% impairment; 8 cm lack of adduction gives 100% impairment.

Table 66-8. Thumb impairment values for lack of adduction and ankylosis. Relative value of functional unit is 20% of thumb motion

Lack of adduction (cm)	Thumb impairment %	
	Lost motion	Ankylosis
0	0	20
1	0	19
2	1	17
3	3	15
4	4	10
5	6	15
6	8	17
7	13	19
8	20	20

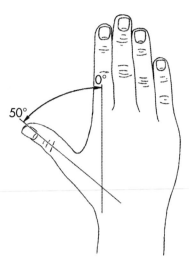

Fig. 66-21. Radial abduction of the thumb measured in degrees.

Table 66-9. Thumb impairment values for lack of radial abduction and ankylosis. Relative value of functional unit is 10% of thumb motion

Measured radial abduction (degrees)	Thumb impairment %	
	Lost motion	Ankylosis
50	0	10
40	1	10
30	3	10
20	7	10
10	9	10
0	10	10

THUMB OPPOSITION IMPAIRMENT %

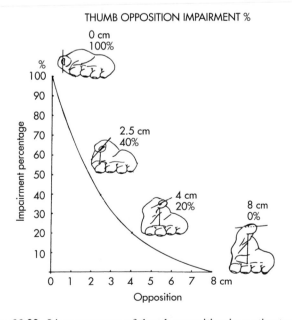

Fig. 66-22. Linear measure of thumb opposition in centimeters at various postions and impairment curve for loss of motion.

Adding impairments for two or more abnormal thumb motions

Because the relative value of each thumb unit of motion was assigned in the impairment charts, the thumb impairment values for each abnormal motion (see Figs. 66-17 and 66-19 and Tables 66-8 through 66-10) are *added* directly together to determine the thumb impairment. If each unit of motion was fully impaired, the thumb motion impairments would add to 100%. Note that motion impairments of the finger DIP, PIP, and MP joints are *combined* rather than added.

Example: IP joint $I_F\%$ (12%) + $I_E\%$ (3%) = 15%; MP joint $I_A\% = 10\%$; adduction impairment = 20%; radial abduction impairment = 10%; opposition impairment = 45%: 15% + 10% + 20% + 10% + 45% = 100% thumb impairment, or 40% hand impairment.

Combining thumb impairments resulting from amputation, sensory loss, and abnormal motion

Thumb impairment values resulting from amputation, sensory loss, and abnormal motion are calculated separately and then combined using the *combined* values chart (see Table 66-5) to obtain the entire thumb impairment. Use Tables 66-2, 66-3, and 66-4 to relate the thumb impairment to the hand, upper extremity, and whole person.

Note that if motion measurements are affected by the presence of an amputation, only the amputation impairment is given. For example, amputation proximal to the MP joint affects measurements of adduction and opposition, and only amputation impairment is considered.

Example: Thumb amputation impairment = 10%; sensory impairment = 20%; and abnormal motion impairment = 30%: 10% *combined* with 20% = 28%; 28% *combined* with 30% = 50% thumb impairment or 20% hand impairment, 18% upper extremity impairment, and 11% impairment of the whole person (see Tables 66-2, 66-3, and 66-4).

Table 66-10. Thumb impairment values for lack of opposition and ankylosis. Relative value of functional unit is 45% of thumb motion

Measured opposition (cm)	Thumb impairment %	
	Lost motion	Ankylosis
0	45	45
1	31	40
2	22	36
3	13	31
4	9	27
5	5	22
6	3	24
7	1	27
8	0	29

DETERMINING IMPAIRMENTS OF TWO OR MORE DIGITS

1. Impairment values are calculated separately for each digit involved.
2. Digit impairment values are converted to hand impairment values (see Table 66-2).
3. Hand impairment values contributed by each digit involved are *added* to obtain the total hand impairment.
4. The hand impairment is then converted to impairments of the upper extremity and the whole person (see Tables 66-3 and 66-4).

Example: A hand presents impairments of several digits as follows:

	% Digit impairment	% Hand impairment
Middle finger	10	2
Index finger	30	6
Thumb	50	20
Total hand impairment		28

A 28% hand impairment represents 25% impairment of the upper extremity and 15% impairment of the whole person.

WRIST
Amputation impairment

Amputations at levels below the elbow, distal to the biceps tendon insertion, and proximal to the MP joints are rated as a 90% to 95% impairment of the upper extremity according to the level of occurrence (see Fig. 66-6, *A*). This corresponds to a 54% to 57% impairment of the whole person (see Table 66-4).

Example: An amputation through the radiocarpal joint is considered a 92% impairment of the upper extremity and a 55% impairment of the whole person.

Motion impairment of wrist

The wrist functional unit represents 60% of the upper extremity function. Two units of motion contribute a relative value to wrist function as follows:

1. Flexion and extension: 70% of wrist function, or $70\% \times 60\% = 42\%$ of upper extremity.
2. Radial and ulnar deviation: 30% of wrist function, or $30\% \times 60\% = 18\%$ of upper extremity.

For each functional unit, impairment curves for abnormal motion and ankylosis were derived based on the formula $A = E + F$ and were expressed on a 100% scale (Figs. 66-23, *A*, and 66-24, *A*). These were converted to pie graphs of upper extremity impairment values by applying the value of

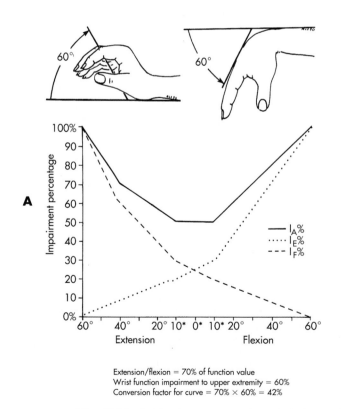

Extension/flexion = 70% of function value
Wrist function impairment to upper extremity = 60%
Conversion factor for curve = 70% × 60% = 42%

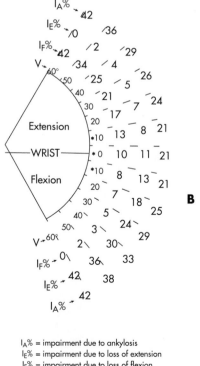

$I_A\%$ = impairment due to ankylosis
$I_E\%$ = impairment due to loss of extension
$I_F\%$ = impairment due to loss of flexion
V = measured angles of motion
* = positions of function

Fig. 66-23. A, Impairment curves for ankylosis ($I_A\%$) and for loss of flexion ($I_F\%$) and extension ($I_E\%$) of the wrist joint. Ankylosis in functional psoitions (10° extension to 10° flexion) receives the lowest $I_A\%$, 50%. **B,** Pie graph for upper extremity impairments caused by abnormal wrist flexion and extension. Relative value of functional unit is 42%.

each unit as a conversion factor (Figs. 66-23, *B,* and 66-24, *B*). Note that the goniometer readings are rounded to the nearest 10°.

Wrist flexion and extension. The usual range of wrist motion is from 60° extension to 60° flexion. The position of function is from 10° extension to 10° flexion.

1. In Fig. 66-23, *B,* locate the measured angles of flexion and extension (row labeled *V*) and match to the impairment of flexion (row labeled $I_F\%$) and extension (row labeled $I_E\%$).
2. *Add* $I_F\%$ and $I_E\%$ to obtain the upper extremity impairment resulting from this abnormal motion.
3. In the presence of ankylosis, match the measured angle *(V)* to its corresponding ankylosis impairment under the row labeled $I_A\%$ (see Fig. 66-23, *B*).

Examples: Wrist extension 20° and wrist flexion 40°: $I_E\% = 7\%$; $I_F\% = 3\%$ (see Fig. 66-23, *B*); 7% + 3% = 10% impairment of the upper extremity.

Wrist ankylosis in 60° flexion: $I_A\% = 42\%$ impairment of the upper extremity.

Wrist ankylosis in 30° ulnar deviation: $I_A\% = 18\%$ upper extremity impairment.

Wrist radial and ulnar deviation. Lateral wrist motion ranges from 20° radial deviation to 30° ulnar deviation. The position of function is from 0° to 10° ulnar deviation.

1. In Fig. 66-24, *B,* locate the measured angles of radial and ulnar deviation (row labeled *V*) and match to the impairments of radial deviation (row labeled $I_{RD}\%$) and ulnar deviation (row labeled $I_{UD}\%$).
2. *Add* $I_{RD}\%$ and $I_{UD}\%$ to obtain the impairment of the upper extremity resulting from this abnormal motion.
3. In the presence of ankylosis in lateral deviation, match the measured angle *(V)* to its corresponding ankylosis impairment under the row labeled $I_A\%$ (see Fig. 66-24, *B*).

Examples: Wrist radial deviation 20° and ulnar deviation 10°: $I_{RD}\% = 0\%$; $I_{UD}\% = 4\%$ (see Fig. 66-24, *B*); 0%+ 4% = 4% upper extremity impairment.

Determining abnormal motion impairments at the wrist joint

Upper extremity impairment values resulting from abnormal motion of ankylosis are calculated separately for each wrist unit of motion. Because the relative value of each unit of motion was assigned in the impairment graphs, the impairment values for each abnormal wrist motion (see Figs. 66-23, *B,* and 66-24, *B*) are *added* directly together to obtain the upper extremity impairment.

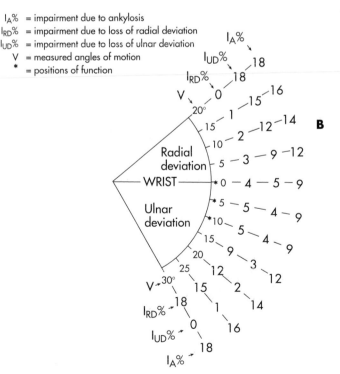

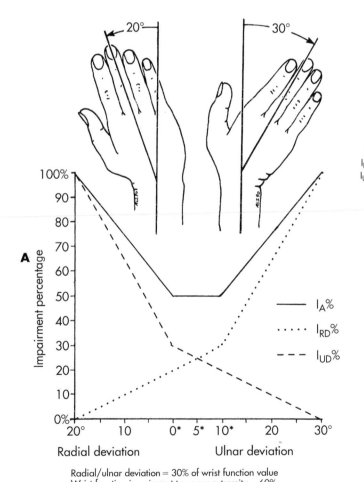

A

Radial/ulnar deviation = 30% of wrist function value
Wrist function impairment to upper extremity = 60%
Conversion factor for curve = 30% × 60% = 18%

Fig. 66-24. A, Impairment curves for ankylosis ($I_A\%$) and for loss of radial deviation ($I_{RD}\%$) and ulnar deviation ($I_{UD}\%$) of the wrist joint. Ankylosis in functional positions (0° to 10° ulnar deviation) receive the lowest $I_A\%$, or 50%. **B,** Pie graph for upper extremity impairments caused by abnormal wrist ulnar and radial deviation. Relative value of functional unit is 18%.

Using Table 66-4, relate the upper extremity impairment to impairment of the whole person.

Example: Upper extremity impairment of 20% caused by loss of wrist flexion and extension, and of 10% caused by loss of ulnar and radial deviation: 20% + 10% = 30% impairment of the upper extremity, or 18% impairment of the whole person.

ELBOW
Amputation impairment

Amputations below the axilla and proximal to the biceps tendon insertion are rated as a 95% to 100% impairment of the upper extremity according to the level of occurrence (see Fig. 66-6, *A*). This corresponds to a 57% to 60% impairment of the whole person (see Table 66-4).

Motion impairment of elbow

The elbow functional unit respresents 70% of the upper extremity function. Two units of motion contribute the relative value to elbow function as follows:

1. Flexion and extension: 60% of elbow function, or 60% × 70% = 42% of upper extremity.
2. Pronation and supination: 40% of elbow function, or 40% × 70% = 28% of upper extremity.

Note that impairments of forearm pronation and supination are ascribed to the elbow because the major motors for this function are inserted about the elbow. For each functional unit, impairment curves for abnormal motion and ankylosis were derived based on the formula $A = E + F$ and expressed on a 100% scale (Figs. 66-25, *A*, and 66-26, *A*). These were converted to pie graphs of upper extremity impairment values by applying the value of each unit as a conversion factor (Figs. 66-25, *B*, and 66-26, *B*). The goniometer readings are rounded to the nearest 10°.

Elbow flexion and extension. The usual range of elbow motion is from 0° extension to 140° flexion. The position of function is 80° flexion. The most useful ROM from a functional point of view is considered to be from 45° to 110° of flexion. Therefore lack of extension less than 45° and lack of flexion beyond 110° are given relatively small impairment values.

1. In Fig. 66-25, *B*, locate the measured angles of flexion and extension (row labeled *V*) and match the impairments of flexion (row labeled $I_F\%$) and extension (row labeled $I_E\%$).
2. *Add* $I_F\%$ and $I_E\%$ to obtain the upper extremity impairment resulting from this abnormal motion.
3. In the presence of ankylosis, match the measured angle *(V)* to its corresponding ankylosis impairment under the row labeled $I_A\%$ (see Fig. 66-25, *B*).

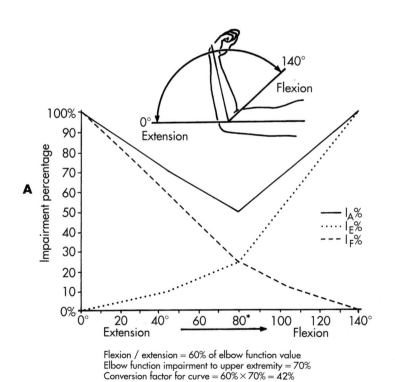

Flexion / extension = 60% of elbow function value
Elbow function impairment to upper extremity = 70%
Conversion factor for curve = 60% × 70% = 42%

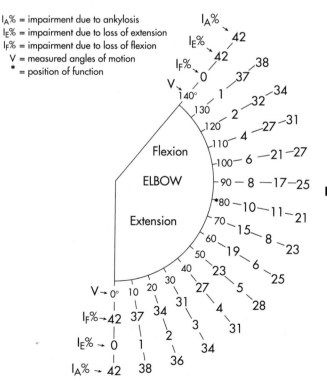

Fig. 66-25. A, Impairment curves for ankylosis ($I_A\%$) and for loss of flexion ($I_F\%$) and extension ($I_E\%$) of the elbow joint. Ankylosis in functional position (80° flexion) is given the lowest $I_A\%$, or 50%. **B,** Pie graph for upper extremity impairments caused by abnormal flexion and extension of elbow. Relative value of functional unit is 42%.

Examples: Elbow extension 30° and flexion 100°: $I_E\% = 3\%$; $I_F\% = 6\%$; $3\% + 6\% = 9\%$ impairment of the upper extremity.

Elbow ankylosis in 120° flexion: $I_A\% = 34\%$ impairment of the upper extremity.

Elbow pronation and supination. The usual range of forearm rotation is from 80° supination to 80° pronation. The position of function is 20° pronation.

1. In Fig. 66-26, *B*, locate the measured angles of pronation and supination (row labeled *V*) and match to the impairments of pronation (row labeled $I_P\%$) and supination (row labeled $I_S\%$).
2. *Add* $I_P\%$ and $I_S\%$ to obtain the upper extremity impairment resulting from this abnormal elbow motion.
3. In the presence of ankylosis, match the measured angle *(V)* to its corresponding ankylosis impairment under the row labeled $I_A\%$ (see Fig. 66-26, *B*).

Examples: Elbow pronation 60° and supination 40°: $I_P\% = 1\%$; $I_S\% = 2\%$; $1\% + 2\% = 3\%$ upper extremity impairment.

Elbow ankylosis in 20° pronation: $I_A\% = 8\%$ upper extremity impairment.

Determining abnormal motion impairments at the elbow joint

Upper extremity impairment values resulting from abnormal motion or ankylosis are calculated separately for each elbow unit of motion. Because the relative value of each unit of motion was assigned in the impairment graphs, the impairment values for each abnormal elbow motion (see Figs. 66-25, *B*, and 66-26, *B*) are *added* directly together to obtain the upper extremity impairment.

Using Table 66-4, relate the upper extremity impairment to impairment of the whole person.

Examples: Upper extremity impairment of 42% resulting from loss of elbow flexion and extension, and of 28% resulting from loss of pronation and supination: $42\% + 28\% = 70\%$ impairment of the upper extremity, or 42% impairment of the whole person.

Elbow ankylosis in 80° flexion and 20° pronation: Flexion $I_A\% = 21\%$; pronation $I_A\% = 8\%$: $21\% + 8\% = 29\%$ upper extremity impairment.

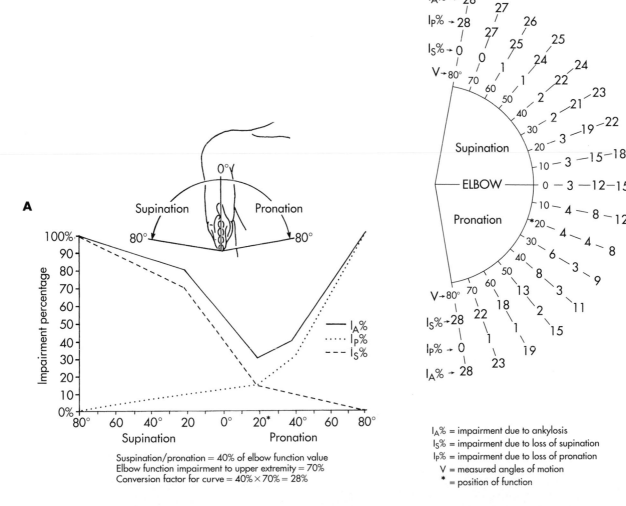

Suspination/pronation = 40% of elbow function value
Elbow function impairment to upper extremity = 70%
Conversion factor for curve = 40% × 70% = 28%

$I_A\%$ = impairment due to ankylosis
$I_S\%$ = impairment due to loss of supination
$I_P\%$ = impairment due to loss of pronation
V = measured angles of motion
* = position of function

Fig. 66-26. A, Impairment curves for ankylosis ($I_A\%$) and for loss of supination ($I_S\%$) and pronation ($I_P\%$) of the forearm. Ankylosis in functional position (20° pronation) is given the lowest $I_A\%$, or 30%. **B,** Pie graph for upper extremity impairments caused by abnormal supination and pronation of forearm. Relative value of functional unit is 28%.

SHOULDER

Amputation impairment

Amputation of the arm at the shoulder level represents a 100% impairment of the upper extremity (Fig. 66-6, *A*, p. 627) and a 60% impairment of the whole person.

Motion impairment of shoulder

The shoulder functional unit represents 60% of the upper extremity function. Three units of motion contribute a relative value to shoulder function as follows:

1. Flexion: 40% of shoulder function; extension: 10% of shoulder function; flexion and extension: 50% of shoulder function, or 50% × 60% = 30% of upper extremity.
2. Abduction: 20% of shoulder function; adduction: 10% of shoulder function; abduction and adduction: 30% of shoulder function, or 30% × 60% = 18% of upper extremity.

3. Internal rotation: 10% of shoulder function; external rotation: 10% of shoulder function; internal and external rotation: 20% of shoulder function, or 20% × 60% = 12% of upper extremity.

For each functional unit, impairment curves for abnormal motion and ankylosis were derived based on the formula $A = E + F$ and expressed on a 100% scale (Figs. 66-27, *A*, 66-28, *A*, and 66-29, *A*). These graphs are converted to pie graphs of upper extremity impairment values by applying the value of each unit as a conversion factor (Figs. 66-27, *B*, 66-28, *B*, and 66-29, *B*).

For each unit of motion, the position(s) of function were chosen according to the recommendations in the literature concerning arthrodesis of the glenohumeral joint even though motions of different joints are involved in each, including the glenohumeral joint, acromioclavicular joint, sternoclavicular joint, and the movement between the scapula and the chest wall. The goniometer readings are rounded to the nearest 10°.

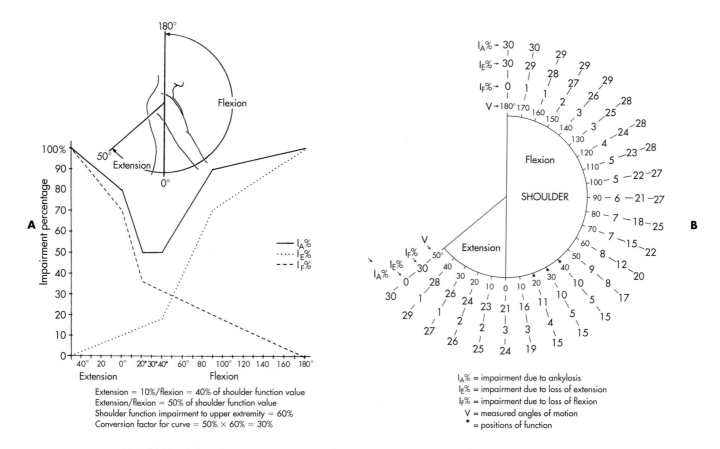

Extension = 10%/flexion = 40% of shoulder function value
Extension/flexion = 50% of shoulder function value
Shoulder function impairment to upper extremity = 60%
Conversion factor for curve = 50% × 60% = 30%

I_A% = impairment due to ankylosis
I_E% = impairment due to loss of extension
I_F% = impairment due to loss of flexion
V = measured angles of motion
* = positions of function

Fig. 66-27. A, Impairment curves for ankylosis (I_A%) and for loss of flexion (I_F%) and extension (I_E%) of the shoulder. Ankylosis in functional positions (20° to 40° flexion) are given the lowest I_A%, or 50%. **B,** Pie graph for upper extremity impairments caused by abnormal shoulder flexion and extension. Relative value of functional unit is 30%.

Shoulder flexion and extension. The usual range of shoulder motion is from 50° extension to 180° flexion. The position of function is from 20° to 40° flexion, and $I_A\%$ receives its lowest value (50%) at these angles (see Fig. 66-27, A). The most important range of flexion is from 0° to the position of function with a decrease of impairment from 70% at 0° to 35% at 20° flexion. From there on, the flexion impairment curve decreases to 0% at 180° flexion. The most important function of extension is to bring the arm from 90° flexion to the position of function; therefore the extension impairment decreases from 70% at 90° flexion to 20% at 40° flexion. From there on the extension impairment curve decreases to 0% at 50° extension.

1. In Figure 66-27, B, locate the measured angles of flexion and extension (row labeled V) and match to the impairments of flexion (row labeled $I_F\%$) and extension (row labeled $I_E\%$).
2. *Add* $I_F\%$ and $I_E\%$ to obtain the upper extremity impairment resulting from this abnormal motion.

3. In the presence of ankylosis, match the measured angle *(V)* to its corresponding ankylosis impairment under the row labeled $I_A\%$ (Fig. 66-27, B).

Examples: Shoulder extension 0° and flexion 40°: $I_E\% = 3\%$; $I_F\% = 10\%$; 3% + 13% upper extremity impairment.

Shoulder ankylosis in 30° flexion: $I_A\% = 15\%$ upper extremity impairment.

Shoulder abduction and adduction. The usual range of shoulder motion is from 180° abduction to 50° adduction. The position of function is from 20° to 50° abduction, and $I_A\%$ receives its lowest value (50%) at these angles (Fig. 66-28, A). The most important range of abduction is from 0° to the position of function with a decrease of impairment from 70% at 0° to 35% in the functional position range. From there on, the abduction impairment curve decreases to 0% at 180° abduction. The most important function of adduction is to bring the arm from 90° abduction to the position of function; therefore the adduction impairment curve decreases from 65% at 90° abduction to 15% at 50° adduction.

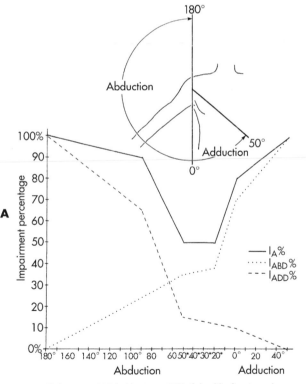

Abduction = 20%/adduction = 10% of shoulder function value
Abduction/adduction = 30% of shoulder function value
Shoulder function impairment to upper extremity = 60%
Conversion factor for curve = 30% × 60% = 18%

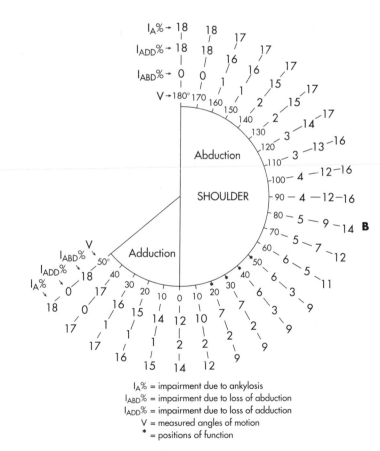

$I_A\%$ = impairment due to ankylosis
$I_{ABD}\%$ = impairment due to loss of abduction
$I_{ADD}\%$ = impairment due to loss of adduction
V = measured angles of motion
* = positions of function

Fig. 66-28. A, Impairment curves for ankylosis ($I_A\%$) and for loss of abduction ($I_{ABD}\%$) and adduction ($I_{ADD}\%$) of the shoulder. Ankylosis in functional positions (20° to 50° abduction) are given the lowest $I_A\%$, or 50%. **B,** Pie graph for upper extremity impairments caused by abnormal shoulder abduction and adduction. Relative value of functional unit is 18%.

From there on, the adduction impairment curve decreases to 0% at 50° adduction.

1. In Fig. 66-28, *B,* locate the measured angles of abduction and adduction (row labeled *V*) and match to the impairments of abduction (row labeled $I_{ABD}\%$) and adduction (row labeled $I_{ADD}\%$).
2. *Add* $I_{ABD}\%$ and $I_{ADD}\%$ to obtain the impairment of the upper extremity resulting from abnormal motion.
3. In the presence of ankylosis of the shoulder, the measured angle *(V)* is matched to its corresponding ankylosis impairment under the row labeled $I_A\%$ (Fig. 66-28, *B*).

Note that ankyloses in functional positions (20° to 50° abduction) receive the lowest $I_A\%$ value, or 9%.

Examples: Shoulder adduction of 0° and abduction of 50°: $I_{ADD}\% = 2\%$; $I_{ABD}\% = 6\%$; $2\% + 6\% = 8\%$ upper extremity impairment.

Shoulder ankylosis in 20° abduction: $I_A\% = 9\%$ upper extremity impairment.

Shoulder internal and external rotation. The usual range of shoulder motion is from 90° internal rotation to 90° external rotation. The position of function is from 30° to 50° internal rotation, and $I_A\%$ receives its lowest value (50%) at these angles (Fig. 66-29, *A*). The most important range of internal rotation is from 50° external rotation to the position of function, with a decrease of impairment from 80% at 50° external rotation to 25% at 40° internal rotation. From there on, the internal rotation impairment curve decreases to 0% at 90° internal rotation. The most important function of

external rotation is to bring the arm to the position of function with a decrease of impairment from 100% at 90° internal rotation to 30% at 50° internal rotation. From there on, the external rotation impairment curve decreases to 0% at 90° external rotation.

1. In Fig. 66-29, *B,* locate the measured angles *(V)* of internal and external rotation and match to the corresponding impairments of internal rotation (row labeled $I_{IR}\%$) and external rotation (row labeled $I_{ER}\%$).
2. *Add* $I_{IR}\%$ and $I_{ER}\%$ to obtain the impairment of the upper extremity resulting from this abnormal motion.
3. In the presence of ankylosis, match the measured angle *(V)* to its corresponding ankylosis impairment under the row labeled $I_A\%$ (Fig. 6-29, *B*).

Note that ankyloses in the functional positions (30° to 50° internal rotation) receive the lowest $I_A\%$ value, or 6%.

Examples: Shoulder internal rotation of 0° and external rotation of 50°: $I_{IR} = 5\%$; $I_{ER} = 1\%$; $5\% + 1\% = 6\%$ upper extremity impairment.

Shoulder ankylosis in 10° internal rotation: $I_A\% = 7\%$ upper extremity impairment.

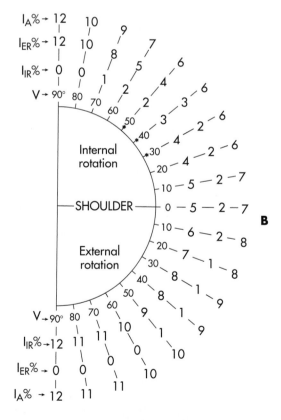

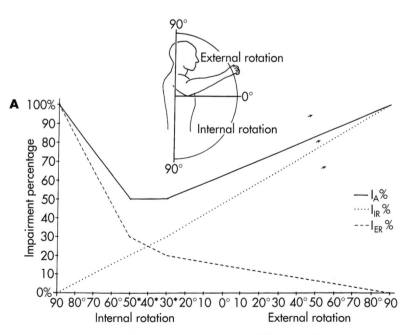

External/internal rotation = 20% of shoulder function value
Shoulder function impairment to upper extremity = 60%
Conversion factor for curve = 20% × 60% = 12%

$I_A\%$ = impairment due to ankylosis
$I_{IR}\%$ = impairment due to loss of internal rotation
$I_{ER}\%$ = impairment due to loss of external rotation
V = measured angles of motion
* = positions of function

Fig. 66-29. **A,** Impairment curve for ankylosis ($I_A\%$) and for loss of internal rotation ($I_{IR}\%$) and external rotation ($I_{ER}\%$) of the shoulder. Ankylosis in functional positions (30° to 50° internal rotation) are given the lowest $I_A\%$, or 50%. **B,** Pie graph for upper extremity impairments caused by abnormal shoulder internal and external rotation. Relative value of functional unit is 12%.

Determining abnormal motion impairments at the shoulder joint

Upper extremity impairment values resulting from abnormal motion or ankylosis are calculated separately for each shoulder unit of motion. Because the relative value of each unit of motion was assigned in the impairment graphs, the impairment values for each abnormal shoulder motion (see Figs. 66-27, *B,* 66-28, *B,* and 66-29, *B*) are *added* directly together to obtain the upper extremity impairment.

Using Table 66-4, relate the upper extremity impairment to impairment of the whole person.

Example: Upper extremity impairment of 20% resulting from loss of shoulder flexion/extension, of 10% resulting from loss of abduction/adduction, and of 6% resulting from loss of internal/external rotation: 20% + 10% + 6% = 36% upper extremity impairment, or 22% impairment of the whole person.

Impairment resulting from peripheral vascular disorders

Impairment of the upper extremity can result from peripheral vascular disorders involving the arteries, veins, or lymphatics. The estimated amount of impairment is based on the severity and extent of the signs and symptoms, rather than on a specific diagnosis.

A classification system for impairment of the upper extremity based on the severity of peripheral vascular disease is provided in Table 66-11. If amputations are present, the resultant impairment is determined separately according to the criteria discussed in the appropriate regional impairment sections. The upper extremity impairment value resulting from amputation is then *combined* with the value resulting from peripheral vascular disease through the combined values chart (see Table 66-6, p. 636). Impairment resulting from pain is not rated separately because this factor already has been considered in Table 66-11.

Impairment resulting from peripheral nerve system disorders

This section presents criteria for the evaluation of permanent impairments of the upper extremity resulting from disorders of the spinal nerves, C5 to C8 and T1, of the brachial plexus, and of major peripheral nerves.

Permanent impairment of the upper extremity resulting from peripheral nerve system disorders results from abnormalities of the motor and/or sensory function that remain after appropriate treatment and a sufficient length of time to allow optimal regeneration and the appearance of signs of physiologic recovery.

Table 66-11. Impairment of upper extremity resulting from peripheral vascular disease

Symptoms	Severity, classification and upper extremity impairment %				
	Class 1 (0–9%)	Class 2 (10–39%)	Class 3 (40–69%)	Class 4 (70–89%)	Class 5 (90–100%)
Claudication and	None	Intermittent on severe usage	Intermittent on moderate usage	Intermittent on mild usage	Persistent
Pain at rest	None	None	None	Intermittent	Severe and constant
Edema and	Transient	Persistent and moderate	Marked	Marked	Marked
Elastic support control		Incomplete	Partial	None	None
Signs of vascular damage	Loss of pulses; minimal loss of subcutaneous tissue of fingertips; arterial calcifications on x-ray film; asymptomatic dilation of veins or arteries not requiring surgery; no decreased activity	Healed painless amputation stump of one digit with persistent vascular disease or healed ulcer	Healed amputation stump of two or more digits with persistent vascular disease or superficial ulceration	Amputation of two or more digits of both extremities or amputation at or above the wrist of one extremity with persistent widespread or deep ulceration of one extremity	Amputation of all digits, or amputation at or above the wrist of both extremities with persistent vascular disease or widespread or deep ulcerations of both extremities
Raynaud's phenomenon and	At < 0° C (32° F)	At < 4° C (39° F)	At < 10° C (50° F)	At < 15° C (59° F)	At < 20° C (58° F)
Medication control	Good	Good	Partial	Partial	Poor

Adapted from *Guides to the evaluation of permanent impairment,* ed 4, Chicago, 1994, American Medical Association.

The impairment determination is based on the extent of loss of function resulting from (1) sensory deficits or pain and (2) motor deficits. It is not necessary to rate separately certain characteristic deformities and manifestations of peripheral nerve lesions such as restricted motion, atrophy, and vasomotor, trophic, and reflex changes, because these deficits have been reflected in the sensory and/or motor impairment values presented. If restricted motion cannot be attributed to a major peripheral nerve lesion, the motion impairment values are rated separately and then *combined* with the peripheral nerve system impairment values.

Accurate diagnosis is based on a complete medical history, a thorough medical and neurologic examination, and appropriate laboratory testing. The anatomic distribution and severity of the motor and/or sensory loss must be verified and related to dysfunction of specific peripheral nerves, spinal nerves, or the brachial plexus.

The origins and functions of the peripheral nerves of the upper extremity are summarized in Table 66-14. The motor and sensory innervation and cutaneous dermatomes of the upper extremity are illustrated in Figs. 66-30 through 66-32. A schematic diagram of the brachial plexus is shown in Fig. 66-33.

IMPAIRMENT EVALUATION METHODS

The impairment evaluation is based on the anatomic distribution of the motor and/or sensory loss and its severity. The severity of loss of function caused by sensory deficits or pain (Table 66-12) and/or motor deficits (Table 66-13) is appropriately graded and related to the anatomic structure(s) involved. Maximum percentages of impairment caused by sensory and motor deficits have been derived for the spinal nerves (Table 66-15), brachial plexus (Table 66-16), and major peripheral nerves (Table 66-17). For each structure involved, impairment percentages are calculated by *multiplying* the maximum impairment value of the nerve structure caused by motor or sensory deficit (see Tables 66-15 through 66-17) by the grade of severity of sensory or motor loss (see Tables 66-12 and 66-13). When both functions are involved, the impairment percentages derived for each are *combined.*

Sensory deficits and pain

A wide range of abnormal sensations can be associated with peripheral nerve lesions and can include: anesthesia, dysesthesia, paresthesia, hyperesthesia, cold intolerance, and an intense burning pain. Pain and sensory deficits associated with peripheral nerve disorders must be evaluated according to the following criteria: (1) degree of interference with performance of activities; (2) distribution along defined anatomic pathways; (3) description consistent with characteristics of peripheral nerve involvement; and (4) consistent correspondence with other disturbances of the involved nerve structure. Permanent loss of function because of pain or discomfort is described as a condition that exists after

Table 66-12. Classification of severity of sensory deficits or pain caused by peripheral nerve disorders

Grade	Description of sensory deficit or pain	% Sensory deficit
1	No loss of sensibility, abnormal sensations, or pain	0
2	Decreased sensibility with or without abnormal sensations or pain that is forgotten during activity	1–25
3	Decreased to absent sensibility, with or without abnormal sensations or pain, that interferes with activity	26–60
4	Decreased to absent sensibility, with or without abnormal sensations or pain, that may prevent activity, and/or minor causalgia	61–80
5	Decreased to absent sensibility with abnormal sensations and severe pain that prevents activity, and/or major causalgia	81–100

From Swanson AB, de Groot Swanson G: Principles and methods of impairment evaluation in the hand and upper extremity. In: *Guides to the evaluation of permanent impairment,* ed 4, Chicago, 1994, American Medical Association.

optimum physiologic adjustment and maximum medical rehabilitation have been administered. Subjective complaints of pain that cannot be substantiated along these lines should not be considered for impairment.

The upper extremity impairment caused by sensory deficits or pain is calculated as follows:

1. Localize the distribution of cutaneous sensory deficits using Figs. 66-31 and 66-32.
2. Determine the severity of sensory deficit or pain according to the classification shown in Table 66-12.
3. Identify the nerve structure(s) involved (see Table 66-14 and Figs. 66-31 through 66-33).
4. Find the maximum impairment of the upper extremity caused by sensory deficit for each structure involved: spinal nerves (see Table 66-15), brachial plexus (see Table 66-16), and major peripheral nerves (see Table 66-17).
5. Multiply the severity of sensory deficit by the maximum impairment value to obtain the upper extremity impairment for each structure involved.

Sensibility losses caused by digital nerve lesions are rated according to the method described in the regional evaluation of the hand. Symptomatic neuromas are evaluated with the criteria presented in this section (see Tables 66-12 and 66-17). Both methods should not be used in the same patient.

Motor deficits

Muscle testing can help evaluate the motor function of specific nerves. Muscle testing rates the ability of a muscle unit to contract, move a joint through its full ROM against gravity, and hold the part against resistance. Both upper

Table 66-13. Classification of severity of motor deficits caused by peripheral nerve disorders based on individual muscle rating

Grade	Description of muscle function	% Motor deficit
5	Active movement against gravity with full resistance	0
4	Active movement against gravity with some resistance	1–25
3	Active movement against gravity only, without resistance	26–50
2	Active movement with gravity eliminated	51–75
1	Slight contraction and no movement	76–99
0	No contraction	100

Adapted from the Medical Research Council: *Aids to the examination of the peripheral nerve system,* Memorandum No. 45, London, 1976, Her Majesty's Stationery Office.

extremities should be tested and the results compared. The upper extremity impairment caused by motor deficits is calculated as follows:

1. Identify the motion and muscles involved.
2. Determine the severity of motor deficiency according to the classification shown in Table 66-13.
3. Identify the nerve structure(s) involved (see Table 66-14, and Figs. 66-30 and 66-33). Find the maximum impairment of the upper extremity caused by motor deficit for each structure involved: spinal nerves (see Table 66-15), brachial plexus (see Table 66-16), and major peripheral nerves (see Table 66-17).
4. Multiply the severity of motor deficit by the maximum impairment value to obtain the upper extremity impairment for each structure involved.

Loss of grip and pinch strength relating to other conditions is discussed on p. 664. The evaluator should not apply impairment values from both sections to the same condition.

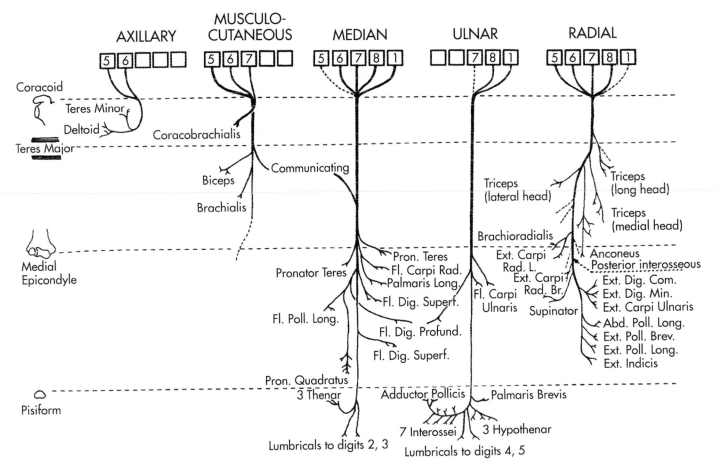

Fig. 66-30. Motor innervation of the upper extremity. (Reproduced from Swanson AB, deGroot Swanson G: Principles and methods of impairment evaluation in the hand and upper extremity. In: *Guides to the evaluation of permanent impairment,* ed 4, Chicago, 1994, American Medical Association.)

Table 66-14. Origins and functions of the peripheral nerves of the upper extremity emanating from the brachial plexus

Nerves of plexus	Primary branches	Secondary branches	Function
Muscular branches Dorsal scapular (C5) Long thoracic (C5, 6, 7) Suprascapular (C5, 6) Lateral pectoral (C5, 6, 7) Medial pectoral (C8, T1) Upper subscapular (C5, 6) Lower subscapular (C5, 6) Thoracodorsal (±C6, C7, 8)	Unnamed		Motor to Longus colli, Scalenes, and Subclavius Motor to Rhomboideus major and minor, Levator scapulae Motor to Serratus anterior Motor to Supraspinatus and Infraspinatus Motor to Pectoralis major Motor to Pectoralis major and minor Motor to Subscapularis Motor to Teres major and Subscapularis Motor to Latissimus dorsi
Medial brachial cutaneous (T1)			Sensory to anteromedial surface of arm (with intercostobrachial)
Medial antebrachial cutaneous (C8, T1)			Sensory to anteromedial surface of arm and ulnar surface of forearm
Musculocutaneous (C5, 6, 7)	Unnamed Lateral antebrachial cutaneous		Motor to Coracobrachialis, Biceps brachii, Brachialis Sensory to radial surface of forearm
Axillary (C5, C6)	Posterior Anterior	Teres minor branch Superior lateral brachial cutaneous	Motor to Teres minor Motor to posterior part of Deltoid Sensory to skin over lower two thirds of Deltoid Motor to central and anterior parts of Deltoid
Radial (C5, 6, 7, 8, ±T1)	Unnamed Ulnar collateral Posterior brachial cutaneous Inferior lateral brachial cutaneous Posterior antebrachial cutaneous Superficial and dorsal digitalis Posterior interosseous	 Unnamed branch Superficial branch Deep branch Terminal branch	Motor to Triceps Brachii, Anconeus, Brachioradialis, Extensor carpi radialis longus, Brachialis (lateral part only) Motor to medial head of Triceps brachii Sensory to posteromedial surface of arm (with intercostobrachial) as far as olecranon Sensory to distal posterolateral surface of arm Sensory to dorsal surface of arm and forearm and distal posterolateral one third of arm Sensory to dorsum of radial one half of wrist and hand; thumb, index, middle, and radial one half of ring finger to middle phalanx Motor to Extensor carpi radialis brevis, Supinator Motor to Extensor digitorum communis, Extensor digiti quinti proprius, Extensor carpi ulnaris Motor to Extensor pollicis longus, Extensor pollicis brevis, Abductor pollicis longus, Extensor indicis proprius Sensory to wrist joint capsule
Median (±C5, C6, 7, 8, T1)	Unnamed Anterior interosseus Palmar cutaneous Common palmar radial digital Common palmar central digital Common palmar ulnar digital	Cubital fossa and forearm branches Thenar muscular branch Proper palmar digitals (1st, 2nd, 3rd) Proper palmar digital (4th) Proper palmar digital (5th)	Motor to Pronator teres, Flexor carpi radialis, Palmaris longus, Flexor digitorum superficialis Motor to radial half of Flexor digitorum profundus of the index and middle fingers, Flexor pollicis longus, Pronator quadratus Sensory to radial surface of palm Motor to Abductor pollicis brevis, Flexor pollicis brevis, and Opponens pollicis Motor to first Lumbrical; sensory to 1st web space, to palmar and distal dorsal surfaces of thumb, and to index palmar surface and distal dorsal surface on radial side Motor to second Lumbrical; sensory to 2nd web space and to palmar surfaces and distal dorsal surfaces of contiguous sides of index and middle fingers Sensory to 3rd web space and to palmar surfaces and distal dorsal surfaces of contiguous sides of middle and ring fingers
Ulnar (±C7, C8, T1)	Unnamed Palmar and dorsal cutaneous Superficial palmar Deep palmar		Motor to Flexor carpi ulnaris, ulnar half of Flexor digitorum profundus of ring and little fingers Sensory to ulnar half of hand, little finger and ulnar half of ring finger Motor to Palmaris brevis Motor to Abductor pollicis, deep head of Flexor pollicis brevis, Abductor digiti quinti, Flexor digiti quinti brevis, Opponens digiti quinti, third and fourth Lumbricals, all Interossei

Modified from Swanson AB, de Groot Swanson G: Principles and methods of impairment evaluation in the hand and upper extremity. In: *Guides to the evaluation of permanent impairment,* ed 4, Chicago, 1994, American Medical Association.

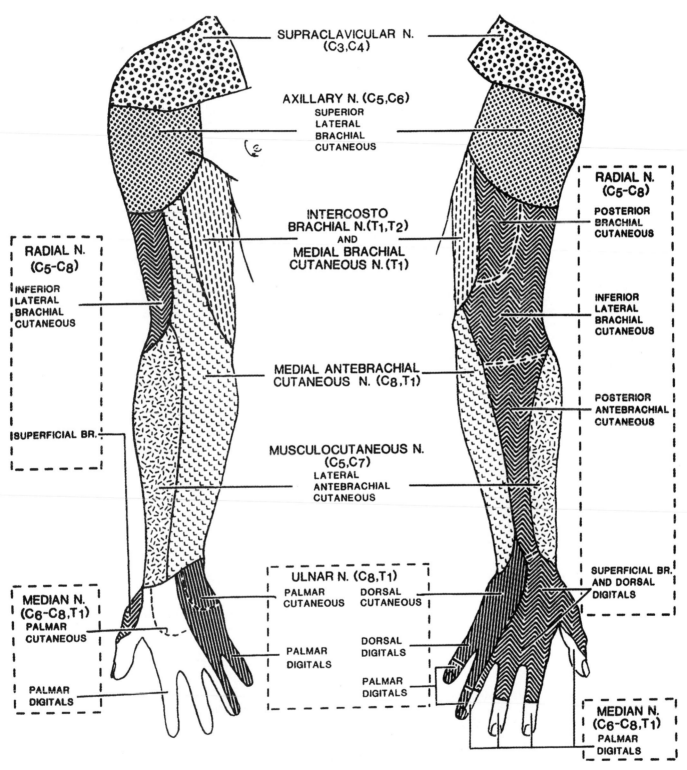

Fig. 66-31. Cutaneous nerves of the upper limb. (Adapted from Netter FH: *The atlas of human anatomy,* Summit, NJ, 1989, CIBA-GEIGY Corp.)

PERIPHERAL NERVE SYSTEM IMPAIRMENT DETERMINATION

The determination of impairment of the peripheral nerve system includes the following:

1. Spinal nerves, C5 to C8 and T1
2. Brachial plexus
3. Major peripheral nerves
4. Entrapment neuropathies
5. Causalgia and reflex sympathetic dystrophy (RSD)

Spinal nerves

The impairment due to injuries or diseases of spinal nerves is based on the severity of loss of function of the peripheral nerves receiving fibers from a specific spinal nerve. Because peripheral nerves receive fibers from more than one spinal root, involvement of two or more spinal nerves giving fibers to the same peripheral nerve produces a greater loss of function of a specific nerve, and the impairment is then rated according to the brachial plexus values (see Table 66-16) rather than combining the individual spinal nerve values (see Table 66-15). For example, the maximum upper extremity impairment caused by *combined* motor and sensory deficits resulting from a lesion of the lower trunk (C8 and T1) is 76% (see Table 66-16); the combination of the impairment values for C8 (48%) and T1 (24%), as shown on Table 66-15, gives a 60% upper extremity impairment and does not reflect the severity of loss of function.

The spinal nerve related impairment is derived as follows:

1. Localize the distribution of the cutaneous sensory deficit according to the dermatome involved (see Figs. 66-31 and 66-32). Evaluate the motor deficit and identify the muscles involved (see Table 66-14 and Fig. 66-30).
2. Identify the spinal nerve involved.

Table 66-15. Maximum upper extremity impairments caused by unilateral sensory and/or motor deficits of individual spinal nerves

| Spinal nerve | Maximum % upper extremity impairment* | | |
	Caused by sensory deficit or pain†	Caused by motor deficit‡	Caused by *combined* motor and sensory deficits
C5	5	30	34
C6	8	35	40
C7	5	35	38
C8	5	45	48
T1	5	20	24

*See Table 66-4 for converting upper extremity impairments to whole person impairments.

†See Table 66-12 for grading loss of function caused by sensory deficit or pain.

‡See Table 66-13 for grading loss of function caused by motor deficit.

Reproduced from Swanson AB, de Groot Swanson G: Principles and methods of impairment evaluation in the hand and upper extremity. In: *Guides to the evaluation of permanent impairment,* ed 4, Chicago, 1994, American Medical Association.

3. Rate the severity of sensory (see Table 66-12) and motor (see Table 66-13) deficit.
4. Find the values for maximum impairment of the upper extremity caused by motor and/or sensory deficits of individual spinal nerves (see Table 66-15).
5. Multiply the severity of sensory (see Table 66-12) and/or motor (see Table 66-13) deficits by the appropriate values from Table 66-15 to obtain upper extremity impairment values for each function.
6. Combine the impairment values for motor and sensory deficits to obtain the total upper extremity impairment value.
7. Convert the impairment value of the upper extremity to the whole person impairment (see Table 66-4).

Example: After a neck injury, a 50-year-old man presents with neck pain radiating down the right arm. The examination shows a 25% sensory deficit of the C5 dermatome and a 25% motor deficit of the muscles innervated by C5. The loss of function is determined as a permanent impairment.

1. Sensory impairment: $25\% \times 5\%$ (see Table 66-15) = 1% upper extremity.
2. Motor impairment: $25\% \times 30\%$ (see Table 66-15) = 8% upper extremity.
3. 1% *combined* with 8% equals 9% impairment of the upper extremity (combined values chart) (see Table 66-5) or 5% of the whole person (see Table 66-4).

Brachial plexus

The brachial plexus innervates the shoulder girdle and upper extremity and is formed by the anterior primary divisions of the fifth through eighth cervical roots and the first thoracic root. These roots anastomose to form three primary trunks: upper trunk (C5 and C6), middle trunk (C7), and lower trunk (C8 and T1) (see Fig. 66-33). Specific findings result from the involvement of these structures.

Total brachial plexus paralysis is seen as: flail arm, paralysis of all muscles of the hand, and no sensibility. Sudorific function is intact when lesion is preganglionic.

Upper-trunk paralysis (C5, C6), Erb-Duchenne type, is seen as: paralysis of biceps, deltoid, brachialis, supraspinatus, infraspinatus, and rhomboids; weakness of triceps, pectoralis major, and extensor carpi radialis brevis and longus; most finger movements are intact; biceps reflex is absent; and sensory deficit of C5 and C6 dermatomes (see Fig. 66-33).

Lower trunk paralysis (C8, T1), Déjerine-Klumpke type, is seen as: paralysis of all intrinsic muscles of the hand; weakness of the flexor carpi ulnaris (FCU) and flexor digitorum profundus (FDP) of the little finger; Horner syndrome (ptosis, mitosis, enophthalmos) if T1 root is avulsed from spinal cord; and sensory deficit of C8 and T1 dermatomes (see Fig. 66-33).

The brachial-plexus-related impairment is derived as follows:

1. Localize the distribution of the sensory deficit according to the dermatomes involved (see Figs. 66-32 and

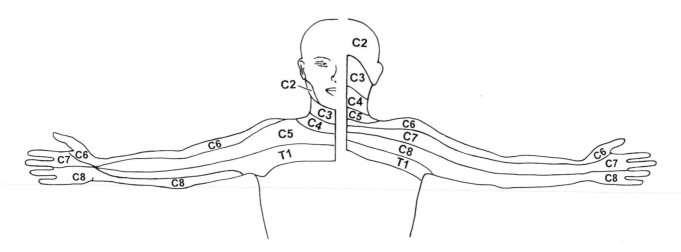

Fig. 66-32. Dermatomes of the upper limb.

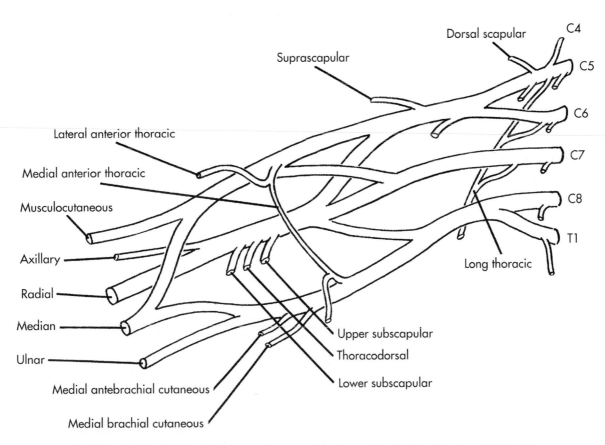

Fig. 66-33. The brachial plexus. (Reproduced from Swanson AB, de Groot Swanson G: Principles and methods of impairment evaluation in the hand and upper extremity. In: *Guides to the evaluation of permanent impairment,* ed 4, Chicago, 1994, American Medical Association.)

Table 66-16. Maximum upper extremity impairments caused by unilateral sensory and/or motor deficits of brachial plexus

Brachial plexus trunk	Maximum % upper extremity impairment*		
	Caused by sensory deficit or pain†	Caused by motor deficit‡	Caused by *combined* motor and sensory deficits
Brachial plexus (C5–C8, T-1)	100	100	100
Upper trunk (C5, C6) (Erb-Duchenne)	25	75	81
Middle Trunk (C7)	5	35	38
Lower trunk (C8, T1) (Dejerine-Klumpke)	20	70	76

*See Table 66-4 for converting upper extremity impairments to whole person impairments.

†See Table 66-12 for grading loss of function caused by sensory deficit or pain.

‡See Table 66-13 for grading loss of function caused by motor deficit.

Reproduced from Swanson AB, de Groot Swanson G: Principles and methods of impairment evaluation in the hand and upper extremity. In: *Guides to the evaluation of permanent impairment,* ed 4, Chicago, 1994, American Medical Association.

66-33). Evaluate the motor deficit and identify the muscles involved (see Table 66-14 and Fig. 66-30).
2. Identify the brachial plexus trunk involved.
3. Rate the severity of sensory (see Table 66-12) and motor (see Table 66-13) deficits.
4. Find the values for maximum impairment of the upper extremity caused by motor and sensory deficits of the brachial plexus and its trunks for the level of involvement (see Table 66-16).
5. Multiply the severity of sensory (see Table 66-12) and motor (see Table 66-13) deficits by the appropriate values from Table 66-16 to obtain upper extremity impairment values for each function.
6. *Combine* the impairment values for motor and sensory deficits to obtain the total upper extremity impairment value.
7. Convert the impairment value of the upper extremity to the whole person value (see Table 66-4).

Major peripheral nerves

The sensory and motor innervation of the upper extremity is summarized in Figs. 66-30 and 66-31 and Table 66-14. Impairment of major peripheral nerves is derived as follows:

1. Identify the nerve(s) involved and determine the level of the lesion.
2. Rate the severity of loss of sensory (see Table 66-12) and motor (see Table 66-13) function.
3. Find the value(s) for maximum impairment of the upper extremity caused by motor and/or sensory deficits of each major peripheral nerve involved (see Table 66-17).
4. Multiply the degree of sensory (see Table 66-12) and/or motor (see Table 66-13) deficit by the appropriate values from Table 66-17 to obtain upper extremity impairment values for each function of each nerve involved.
5. For mixed nerves, *combine* the impairment values for motor and sensory deficits to obtain the total upper extremity impairment value (see Table 66-5).
6. If more than one nerve is involved, *combine* the upper extremity impairment derived for each nerve (see Table 66-5).
7. Convert the impairment value of the upper extremity to a whole person impairment value (see Table 66-4).

Example: A patient had a subluxation of the right shoulder that was reduced anatomically. After an appropriate course of treatment, the patient, while standing, had full shoulder abduction against gravity and some resistance, starting with the arm alongside the body. There was some hypesthesia of the skin over the lower two thirds of the deltoid, which did not interfere with activity. The impairment was classified as permanent.

The impairment evaluation is based on the sensory and motor deficits. The sensory deficit is determined as follows:

1. Cutaneous sensory defect distribution involved: axillary nerve (see Fig. 66-31).
2. Maximum upper extremity impairment caused by sensory deficit of axillary nerve: 5% (see Table 66-17).
3. Gradation of severity of sensory deficit: 25% (see Table 66-12).
4. Impairment of the upper extremity caused by sensory deficit of the axillary nerve: $25\% \times 5\% = 1\%$.

The motor deficit is determined as follows:
1. Muscle involved: deltoid
2. Nerve involved: axillary (see Table 66-14 and Fig. 66-30).
3. Maximum upper extremity impairment caused by motor deficit of the axillary nerve: 35% (see Table 66-17).
4. Gradation of loss of muscle strength: 25% (see Table 66-13).
5. Impairment of the upper extremity caused by motor deficit of the axillary nerve: $25\% \times 35\% = 9\%$.

Combined motor and sensory deficit caused by involvement of the axillary nerve: 9% combined with 1% = 10% upper extremity impairment, or 6% whole person impairment (see Table 66-4).

Table 66-17. Maximum upper extremity impairments caused by unilateral sensory or motor deficits of the major peripheral nerves

Nerves	Maximum % upper extremity impairment*		
	Caused by sensory deficit or pain†	Caused by motor deficit‡	Caused by *combined* motor and sensory deficits
Pectorals (medial and lateral)	0	5	5
Axillary	5	35	38
Dorsal scapular	0	5	5
Long thoracic	0	15	15
Medial antebrachial cutaneous	5	0	5
Medial brachial cutaneous	5	0	5
Median (above midforearm)	39	44	66
Median (anterior interosseous branch)	0	15	15
Median (below midforearm)	39	10	45
Radial palmar digital of thumb	7	0	7
Ulnar palmar digital of thumb	11	0	11
Radial palmar digital of index finger	5	0	5
Ulnar palmar digital of index finger	4	0	4
Radial palmar digital of middle finger	5	0	5
Ulnar palmar digital of middle finger	4	0	4
Radial palmar digital of ring finger	3	0	3
Musculocutaneous	5	25	29
Radial (upper arm with loss of triceps)	5	42	45
Radial (elbow with sparing of triceps)	5	35	38
Subscapulars (upper and lower)	0	5	5
Suprascapular	5	16	20
Thoracodorsal	0	10	10
Ulnar (above midforearm)	7	46	50
Ulnar (below midforearm)	7	35	40
Ulnar palmar digital of ring finger	2	0	2
Radial palmar digital of little finger	2	0	2
Ulnar palmar digital of little finger	3	0	3

*See Table 66-4 for converting upper extremity impairments to whole person impairments.
†See Table 66-12 for grading loss of function caused by sensory deficit or pain.
‡See Table 66-13 for grading loss of function caused by motor deficit.
Reproduced from Swanson AB, de Groot Swanson G: Principles and methods of impairment evaluation in the hand and upper extremity. In: *Guides to the evaluation of permanent impairment,* ed 4, Chicago, 1994, American Medical Asociation.

Entrapment neuropathy

Only cases of permanent damage not responding to treatment qualify for impairment ratings. Impairment values caused by entrapment neuropathy can be calculated from the motor and/or sensory deficits of each nerve involved as described earlier. For ease of determination, Table 66-18 provides upper extremity impairment values for each major nerve and site of entrapment according to its degree of severity. Do not use both methods.

Example: A 40-year-old landscaper presented with a 1-year history of median nerve compression in the right dominant hand with abnormal median nerve conduc-

tion studies and an abnormal electromyogram. Six months after surgical decompression of the median nerve in the right carpal tunnel, followed by a change of occupation to salesman, his only symptoms were infrequent transient episodes of numbness in the thumb and index finger after 40 minutes of driving. Examination showed a full range of movement of all joints and a normal two-point discrimination sensory testing. Compared with the left hand, he had a 40% strength loss index (see p. 664).

The upper extremity impairment caused by a mild residual carpal tunnel syndrome was rated at 10% (Table

Table 66-18. Upper extremity impairment caused by entrapment neuropathy

| Entrapped nerve | Entrapment site | Degree of severity and % upper extremity impairment | | |
		Mild	Moderate	Severe
Suprascapular		5	10	20
Axillary		10	20	38
Radial	Upper Arm	15	25	45
Posterior interosseous	Forearm	10	20	35
Median	Elbow	15	35	55
Anterior interosseous	Proximal forearm	5	10	15
Median	Wrist	10	20	40
Ulnar	Elbow	10	30	50
Ulnar	Wrist	10	30	40

Reproduced from Swanson AB, de Groot Swanson G: Principles and methods of impairment evaluation in the hand and upper extremity. In: *Guides to the evaluation of permanent impairment,* ed 4, Chicago, 1994, American Medical Association.

66-18) or 6% of the whole person (see Table 66-4). No additional rating was given for loss of grip strength.

Causalgia and reflex sympathetic dystrophy

Causalgia is a term that describes the constant and intense burning pain usually seen with RSD when the causative painful lesion involves injury to a nerve.

The term *major causalgia* designates an extremely serious form of RSD produced by a partial injury to a major mixed nerve in the proximal portion of the extremity. The term *minor causalgia* designates a more common form of RSD produced by an injury to the distal part of the extremity involving a purely sensory nerve.

Other clinical forms of RSD not associated with injury of a peripheral nerve include: minor traumatic dystrophy, shoulder-hand syndrome, and major traumatic dystrophy.

The four cardinal symptoms of RSD are pain, swelling, stiffness, and discoloration. The diagnosis of RSD can be supported with a three-phase nucleotide flow study, cold-stress testing, recurrence of pain after previously successful stellate ganglion (Horner's syndrome must be present) or Bier blocks.

The impairment secondary to RSD is usually calculated by first separately rating: (1) the upper extremity impairment caused by loss of motion of each joint involved; (2) the sensory deficit or pain impairment according to the guidelines of this section (see Table 66-12); and (3) the motor deficit impairment of the injured peripheral nerve, if it applies (see Table 66-13). The appropriate impairment values for loss of motion, pain and sensory deficits, and motor deficits (if applicable) are then *combined* to obtain the impairment of the upper extremity. Major causalgia that persists despite appropriate treatment can result in a complete loss of function of the upper extremity or an impairment as great as 100%.

COMBINING IMPAIRMENTS CAUSED BY MULTIPLE DEFICITS OF THE PERIPHERAL NERVE SYSTEM

When a structure with mixed sensory and motor fibers is involved, the sensory impairment is *combined* with the motor impairment through the combined values chart (see Table 66-5).

When more than one peripheral nerve system structure is involved, their respective upper extremity impairments are *combined*.

When multiple impairments of the extremity are present (e.g., amputation, loss of motion, vascular disorders, or other conditions), the peripheral nerve system impairment is *combined* with the other impairments to obtain the total upper extremity impairment.

When both upper extremities are involved, the respective upper extremity impairments are converted to whole person impairments and then *combined* through the combined values chart.

Impairments caused by other disorders of the upper extremity

Disorders of the upper extremity that have not been previously rated by other methods and that can contribute to additional impairment should be considered in the final impairment determination. These include the following:

1. Bone and joint disorders
2. Arthroplasty procedures (resection or implant)
3. Musculotendinous disorders
4. Loss of strength

The impairment values derived from these disorders are rated separately and *combined* with appropriate values through the combined values chart (see Table 66-5).

Table 66-19. Impairment values for digits, hand, upper extremity, and whole person for disorders of specific joints

Units and joints	Unit	Hand	Upper extremity	Whole person
Shoulder				
Glenohumeral	—	—	60	36
Acromioclavicular	—	—	25	15
Elbow				
Entire elbow	—	—	70	42
Ulnohumeral	—	—	50	30
Proximal radioulnar	—	—	20	12
Wrist				
Entire wrist	—	—	60	36
Radiocarpal	—	—	40	24
Distal radioulnar	—	—	20	12
Proximal carpal row	—	—	30	18
Entire hand	—	100	90	54
Thumb				
Entire thumb	100	40	36	22
CMC	75	30	27	16
MP	10	4	4	2
IP	15	6	5	3
Index and middle fingers				
Entire finger	100	20	18	11
MP	100	20	18	11
PIP	80	16	14	8
DIP	45	9	8	5
Ring and little fingers				
Entire finger	100	10	9	5
MP	100	10	9	5
PIP	80	8	7	4
DIP	45	4	4	2

Adapted from Swanson AB, de Groot Swanson G: Principles and methods of impairment evaluation in the hand and upper extremity. In: *Guides to the evaluation of permanent impairment,* ed 4, Chicago, 1994, American Medical Association.

These disorders are included in the impairment determination only when they contribute additional impairment not previously rated by other parameters. The evaluator must use appropriate judgment to avoid duplication of impairment when other findings are present.

Relative impairment values for loss of function of the digits, hand, wrist, elbow, and shoulder are shown in Table 66-19. Note that these values differ from amputation impairment values shown in Fig. 66-8, except at the finger levels. The severity of bone, joint, and musculotendinous disorders has been classified into mild, moderate, and severe degrees. Appropriate impairment percentages were given to each grade of severity as shown in pp. 659 to 665. The appropriate impairment percentages shown are multiplied by the relative impairment value of each unit or joint from Table 66-19 to obtain the digit, hand, and upper extremity impairments. The impairment values for resection and implant arthroplasty of various joints are expressed in terms of upper extremity impairment in Table 66-20. Loss of strength is discussed on p. 664.

BONE AND JOINT DEFORMITIES
Joint crepitation with motion

Joint crepitation with motion can indicate synovitis or cartilage degeneration. The impairment of a specific joint is found by multiplying its relative value (see Table 66-19) by the percentage of joint impairment caused by crepitation.

SEVERITY OF JOINT CREPITATION WITH MOTION	% JOINT IMPAIRMENT*
Mild: Inconstant during active ROM	10
Moderate: Constant during active ROM	20
Severe: Constant during passive ROM	30

*Multiply by relative value of joint (Table 66-19) to find joint impairment caused by crepitation.
ROM, Range of motion.
Adapted from Swanson AB, Mays JD, Yamauci Y: A rheumatoid evaluation record for the upper extremity, *Surg Clin North Am* 1968; 48:1003-1013.

Other findings, such as synovial hypertrophy, carpal collapse with arthritic changes, or restricted motion, can indicate a greater severity of the same pathologic process and take precedence over joint crepitation, which should not be rated in these cases.

Example: Mild crepitation of proximal radiolunar joint without other symptoms would result in a 10% × 20% = 2% impairment of the upper extremity (see Tables 66-19 and above).

Joint swelling from synovial hypertrophy

This condition is usually rated by decreased joint motion and is considered for impairment rating only when there is full ROM of the joint. The impairment value of a specific joint is found by multiplying its relative value (see Table 66-19) by the percentage of joint impairment caused by synovial hypertrophy.

JOINT SWELLING FROM SYNOVIAL HYPERTROPHY	% JOINT IMPAIRMENT*
Mild: Visually apparent	10
Moderate: Palpably apparent	20
Severe: >10% increase in size	30

*Multiply by relative value of joint (Table 66-19) to find joint impairment caused by synovial hypertrophy.
Adapted from Swanson AB, Mays JD, Yamauci Y: A rheumatoid evaluation record for the upper extremity, *Surg Clin North Am* 1968; 48:1003-1013.

Digital lateral deviation

The longitudinal alignment of the DIP, PIP, or MP joint is measured in degrees during full active extension. Because the longitudinal arch of the digits is affected by lateral deviation at any level, the *entire digit is considered impaired.*

The impairment value of a specific digit is found by multiplying its relative value (see Table 66-19) by the percentage of digit impairment caused by lateral deviation.

DIGIT ULNAR OR RADIAL DEVIATION	% DIGIT IMPAIRMENT*
Mild: < 10°	10
Moderate: 10° to 30°	20
Severe: > 30°	30

*Multiply by relative value of digit (Table 66-19) to find digit impairment caused by lateral deviation.
Adapted from Swanson AB, Mays JD, Yamauci Y: A rheumatoid evaluation record for the upper extremity, *Surg Clin North Am* 1968; 48:1003-1013.

If other impairments of the same digit are present, they are *combined* using the combined values chart (see Table 66-5).

Example: Ligamentous injury of middle finger DIP joint results in 9° ulnar deviation and a ROM of −10° extension to 30° flexion:

1. Ulnar deviation (mild) impairment: $10\% \times 100\% =$ 10% finger impairment (see Tables 66-19 and above).
2. Motion impairment: $I_E\% = 2\%$; $I_F = 21\%$ (Fig. 66-12); $2\% + 21\% = 23\%$ finger motion impairment.
3. Middle finger impairment: 10% *combined* with $23\% = 31\%$ finger impairment (combined values chart), or 6% impairment of the hand, 5% of the upper extremity, and 3% of the whole person (see Tables 66-2, 66-3, and 66-4).

Digit rotational deformity

The rotational alignment of the DIP, PIP, or MP joint is measured in degrees during full active flexion of the digit. Because rotational deformity at any level affects the function of the entire digit, the *impairment percentage is applied to the entire digit.*

The impairment percentage of a specific digit is found by multiplying its relative value (see Table 66-19) by the percentage of digit impairment caused by rotational deformity. If other impairments of the same digit are present, they are *combined* using the combined values chart.

DIGIT ROTATIONAL DEFORMITY	% DIGIT IMPAIRMENT*
Mild: < 15°	20
Moderate: 15° to 30°	40
Severe: > 30°	60

*Multiply by relative value of digit (Table 66-19) to find digit impairment caused by rotational deformity.
Adapted from Swanson AB, Mays JD, Yamauci Y: A rheumatoid evaluation record for the upper extremity, *Surg Clin North Am* 1968; 48:1003-1013.

Example: Healed fracture of fifth metacarpal results in 20° pronation deformity of little finger with MP joint motion from +20° extension to 60° flexion.

1. Rotational impairment (moderate): $40\% \times 100\% =$ 40% finger impairment (see Table 66-19).
2. Motion impairment of MP joint: $I_E\% = 0\%$; $I_F\% = 17\%$ (see Fig. 66-14); $0\% + 17\% = 17\%$ finger impairment caused by decreased motion.
3. Little finger impairment: 40% *combined* with $17\% = 50\%$ finger impairment, or 5% hand impairment (Table 66-2).

Persistent joint subluxation or dislocation

When persistent joint subluxation or dislocation results in decreased motion of the joint, impairment percentages are given only for lack of motion (see regional evaluation, pp. 635 to 649). When motion is not restricted, the percentage of joint impairment is found by mulitplying its relative value (see Table 66-19) by the percentage of joint impairment caused by joint subluxation or dislocation.

JOINT SUBLUXATION OR DISLOCATION	% JOINT IMPAIRMENT*
Mild: Complete reduction manually	20
Moderate: Incomplete reduction manually	40
Severe: Cannot be reduced	60

*Multiply by relative value of joint (Table 66-19) to find joint impairment caused by subluxation or dislocation.
Adapted from Swanson AB, Mays JD, Yamauci Y: A rheumatoid evaluation record for the upper extremity, *Surg Clin North Am* 1968; 48:1003-1013.

Joint mediolateral instability

The excessive passive mediolateral motion of a joint is appraised by comparison with a normal joint and graded according to the degree of severity.

EXCESSIVE PASSIVE MEDIOLATERAL JOINT MOTION	% JOINT IMPAIRMENT*
Mild: < 10°	20
Moderate: 10° to 20°	40
Severe: > 20°	60

*Multiply by relative value of joint (Table 66-19) to find joint impairment caused by mediolateral instability.
Adapted from Swanson AB, Mays JD, Yamauci Y: A rheumatoid evaluation record for the upper extremity, *Surg Clin North Am* 1968; 48:1003-1013.

The percentage of joint impairment resulting from instability is then multiplied by the relative value of the joint involved (see Table 66-19). Other impairments of the same joint, if present, are *combined* with the combined values chart, Table 66-5.

Example: A patient who is not a candidate for surgery has a 20° passive radial deviation of the thumb MP joint after a ligamentous injury:

1. Radial instability impairment (moderate): 40% joint impairment.
2. Relative value of thumb MP joint function: 10% (Table 66-19).
3. Thumb impairment: 40% × 10% = 4% thumb impairment, or 2% hand impairment and 2% upper extremity impairment (see Tables 66-2 and 66-3).

Radial and ulnar deviation of wrist and elbow joints

Lateral deviation of the wrist and elbow is measured during maximum active joint extension. Note that the normal carrying angle at the elbow should be taken into consideration. The percentage of joint impairment caused by lateral deviation is multiplied by the relative value of the joint (see Table 66-19) to derive the upper exremity impairment.

WRIST AND ELBOW JOINT LATERAL DEVIATION	% JOINT IMPAIRMENT*
Mild: < 20°	10
Moderate: 20° to 30°	20
Severe: > 30°	30

*Multiply by relative value of joint (Table 66-19) to find the upper extremity impairment caused by wrist and elbow lateral deviation.
Adapted from Swanson AB, Mays JD, Yamauci Y: A rheumatoid evaluation record for the upper extremity, *Surg Clin North Am* 1968; 48:1003-1013.

Other impairment of the same joint, if present, are *combined* using the combined values chart (see Table 66-5).

Example: One year after simple radial head resection for fracture, the patient presents with a 15° lateral deviation of the elbow:

1. Lateral deviation impairment (mild): 10% joint impairment. Relative value of elbow function: 70% of upper extremity (see Table 66-19). Impairment caused by elbow lateral deviation: 10% × 70% = 7% upper extremity impairment.
2. Simple resection of the radial head: 8% upper extremity impairment (see Table 66-20).
3. The elbow lateral deviation impairment (7%) is *combined* with the radial head resection impairment (8%) to obtain the total upper extremity impairment derived from the elbow joint, 14%.

Carpal instability

Based on the severity of the radiographic findings, carpal instability patterns can be classified as mild, moderate, or severe. The proximal carpal row represents half of the wrist value, or 30%. Therefore the carpal instability severity grades of mild (20%), moderate (40%), or severe (60%) corresponding to the upper extremity are 6%, 12%, and 18%, respectively.

RADIOGRAPHIC FINDINGS	% UPPER EXTREMITY IMPAIRMENT		
	MILD (6%)	MODERATE (12%)	SEVERE (18%)
Radioscaphoid angle	45-59°	60-70°	> 70°
Radiolunate angle	< 10°	10-30°	> 30°
Carpal height collapse	< 5%	5%-10%	> 10%
Carpal translation	Mild	Moderate	Severe
Arthritic changes	Mild	Moderate	Severe

Modified from Swanson AB, de Groot Swanson G: Principles and methods of impairment evaluation in the hand and upper extremity. In: *Guides to the evaluation of permanent impairment,* ed 4, Chicago, 1994, American Medical Association.

Only one category of impairment (mild, moderate, or severe) is selected based on the greatest severity of the radiographic findings listed under each column; values shown cannot be added or combined between grades of severity.

The evaluator must use judgment to avoid duplicating impairment ratings. These radiographic parameters are used only when all other wrist factors are normal, except after carpal bone resection or implant arthroplasty. In the latter situation, the carpal instability impairment (see above) is *combined* with the arthroplasty impairment (see Table 66-20) through the combined values chart, Table 66-5.

Certain cases may present wrist pain and loss of strength related to a dynamic or nondissociative carpal instability that cannot be measured by changes of angles on the radiograms. The examiner must use appropriate clinical sense to determine the severity of this type of instability and rate the resulting upper extremity impairment as mild (6%), moderate (12%), or severe (18%). Pain and loss of strength are not rated separately.

Example: The patient has radioscaphoid angle of 65°, radiolunate angle of 5°, and moderate arthritic changes. The upper extremity impairment caused by carpal instability patterns is moderate, or 12%.

Arthroplasty

Simple resection arthroplasty is given 40% impairment of the joint value, and implant arthroplasty is given 50% impairment of the joint value. Impairments of the upper extremity after arthroplasty of specific joints or bones are listed in Table 66-20.

In the presence of decreased motion or ankylosis, motion impairments are derived separately (see pp. 635 to 649) and combined with arthroplasty in using the combined values chart (see Table 66-5).

After arthrodesis procedures, the impairment determination is based on the measured angle of fusion according to the ankylois impairment ($I_A\%$) guidelines presented for each joint in the regional evaluation section.

Example: An osteoarthritic patient has an implant arthroplasty of the PIP joint of the middle and ring fingers with a ROM of $-10°$ extension to $60°$ flexion and fusion of the DIP joint of the middle finger in $20°$ flexion:

1. Middle finger impairment:

PIP joint implant arthroplasty: 50% impairment of the joint or $50\% \times 80\% = 40\%$ finger impairment (see Table 66-19). PIP joint, $-10°$ extension to $60°$ flexion: $I_E\% = 3\%$ and $I_F\% = 24\%$ finger impairment (see Fig. 66-13).

Restricted motion impairment: $3\% + 24\% = 27\%$ finger impairment.

The middle finger PIP joint impairment is found by *combining* the arthroplasty impairment with the restricted motion impairment using the combined values chart, or 40% *combined* with $27\% = 56\%$ finger impairment at the PIP joint.

DIP joint fusion in $20°$ flexion: $I_A\% = 30\%$ finger impairment at the DIP joint (see Fig. 66-12).

Table 66-20. Impairment of the upper extremity after arthroplasty of specific bones or joints

Level of arthroplasty*	% Impairment of upper extremity	
	Resection arthroplasty (40%)	Implant arthroplasty (50%)
Shoulder	24	30
Distal clavicle (isolated)	10	—
Total elbow	28	35
Radial head (isolated)	8	10
Total wrist	24	30
Ulnar head (isolated)	8	10
Proximal carpal row	12	15
Carpal bones	12	15
Thumb†		
CMC	11	13
MP	1	2
IP	2	3
Index or middle finger‡		
MP	7	9
PIP	6	7
DIP	3	4
Ring or little finger‡		
MP	3	4
PIP	3	3
DIP	2	2

*If more than one level is involved, *combine* from distal to proximal.
†If more than one thumb joint is involved, *add* impairments.
‡If more than one joint is involved in the same finger, *combine* impairments. If multiple digits are involved, *add* impairments for each.
Adapted from Swanson AB, de Groot Swanson G: Principles and methods of impairment evaluation in the hand and upper extremity. In: *Guides to the evaluation of permanent impairment,* ed 4, Chicago, 1994, American Medical Association.

The impairment for the middle finger is found by *combining* the impairment at the level of the DIP and PIP joints, or 30% *combined* with $56\% = 69\%$ middle finger impairment. The middle finger represents 20% of the hand (see Table 66-19). Therefore the middle finger contributes $69\% \times 20\% = 14\%$ hand impairment. The finger to hand impairment conversion is also found in Table 66-2.

2. Ring finger impairment:

The calculation for PIP joint impairments caused by implant arthroplasty and restricted motion are the same as those for the PIP joint of the middle finger, or 56% finger impairment. This corresponds to a $56\% \times 10\% = 6\%$ hand impairment (see Table 66-2).

3. Total hand and upper extremity impairment:

The total hand impairment is obtained by *adding* the hand impairments derived from the middle and ring fingers, or $14\% + 6\% = 20\%$ hand impairment. This corresponds to a $20\% \times 90\% = 18\%$ upper extremity impairment (see Table 66-3) and 11% whole person impairment (see Table 66-4).

MUSCULOTENDINOUS IMPAIRMENTS
Constrictive tenosynovitis

Impairment caused by constrictive tenosynovitis may be *combined* with other digit impairments. However, when the active ROM is restricted, no additional rating is given for constrictive tenosynovitis. The impairment caused by constrictive tenosynovitis is multiplied by the relative value of the digit (see Table 66-19).

CONSTRICTIVE TENOSYNOVITIS	% DIGIT IMPAIRMENT*
Mild: Inconstant triggering on active ROM	20
Moderate: Constant triggering on active ROM	40
Severe: Constant triggering on passive ROM	60

*Multiply by relative value of each digit (Table 66-19) to find digit impairment.
ROM, Range of motion.
Adapted from Swanson AB, Mays JD, Yamauci Y: A rheumatoid evaluation record for the upper extremity, *Surg Clin North Am* 1968; 48:1003-1013.

Intrinsic tightness

The Bunnell test is used to demonstrate intrinsic tightness in the hand. In a normal hand, passive flexion of the PIP joint still can be obtained when the MP joint is hyperextended. When the intrinsic muscles are tight, their available stretch is taken up by the MP joint hyperextension, and passive flexion of the PIP joint becomes restricted.

Impairment caused by intrinsic tightness can be *combined* with other digit impairments. However, when active motion at the MP and/or PIP joints is already restricted, no additional rating is given for intrinsic tightness. The impairment caused by intrinsic tightness is multiplied by the relative value of the digit (see Table 66-19) to obtain the digit impairment.

INTRINSIC TIGHTNESS (PASSIVE PIP JOINT FLEXION WITH MP JOINT HYPEREXTENDED)	% DIGIT IMPAIRMENT*
Mild: PIP flexion > 60°	20
Moderate: PIP flexion 60° to 20°	40
Severe: PIP flexion < 20°	60

*Multiply by relative value of each digit (Table 66-19) to find digit impairment.
Adapted from Swanson AB, Mays JD, Yamauci Y: A rheumatoid evaluation record for the upper extremity, *Surg Clin North Am* 1968; 48:1003-1013.

Extensor tendon subluxation at MP joint

Impairment caused by extensor subluxation at the MP joint can be *combined* with other joint or digit impairments. However, when persistent tendon subluxation results in restrictive motion, only impairment values for lost motion are given (see regional evaluation, p. 638).

Multiply the extensor tendon subluxation impairment at the MP joint by the relative value of the digit (see Table 66-19) to obtain the digit impairment.

EXTENSOR TENDON SUBLUXATION AT MP JOINT	% DIGIT IMPAIRMENT
Mild: Subluxation on MP joint flexion only	10
Moderate: Reducible subluxation in IMC groove	20
Severe: Nonreducible subluxation in IMC groove	30

*Multiply by relative value of each digit (Table 66-19) to find relative digit impairment.
IMC, Intermetacarpal; MP, metacarpophalangeal.
Adapted from Swanson AB, Mays JD, Yamauci Y: A rheumatoid evaluation record for the upper extremity, *Surg Clin North Am* 1968; 48:1003-1013.

Other musculoskeletal system defects

If the measured anatomic impairment (e.g., loss of shoulder motion) does not adequately reflect the extent of a musculoskeletal defect as demonstrated on MRI or at surgery, in rare cases additional impairment can be given at discretion.

LOSS OF STRENGTH

Because strength measurements are functional tests that are influenced by incentives and other subjective factors that are difficult to control, we decided not to assign a large role to these values in an evaluation system based on anatomic impairment. This view is not universally held by physicians doing impairment evaluations. Further research is needed

before grip and pinch strength loss can assume a larger place in impairment evaluations. However, in rare cases, if the examiner believes that loss of strength represents an additional impairing factor not already taken into consideration, it may be rated separately. This impairment is then *combined* with other hand impairments. As in any impairment evaluation, the examiner must be sure that the patient has reached maximal improvement and that the condition is permanent.

Hand strength and its measurements can be affected by the presence of amputations, pain, sensory loss, restricted motion of the digits, and disorders of the bones, joints, and musculotendinous and nervous systems. In these cases, no separate loss of strength impairment is given, and the anatomic impairments are evaluted according to the guidelines described for each.

Impairments caused by motor deficits secondary to disorders of the peripheral nerve system and various degenerative neuromuscular conditions are rated only according to the peripheral nerve system evaluation criteria. Note that weakness of strength can occur without muscle atrophy.

Grip or pinch strength are measured according to the techniques described on p. 625. For each hand, three readings of grip, lateral, and key pinch are taken and averaged. The strength of the affected extremity is compared with that of the normal opposite side to derive an index of strength loss as follows:

$$\frac{\text{Normal strength} - \text{Abnormal strength}}{\text{Normal strength}} = \% \text{ Strength Loss Index}$$

The upper extremity impairment is based on the strength loss index range as shown below.

% STRENGTH LOSS INDEX	% UPPER EXTREMITY IMPAIRMENT
10–30	10
31–60	20
61–100	30

Reproduced from Swanson AB, de Groot Swanson G: Principles and methods of impairment evaluation in the hand and upper extremity. In: *Guides to the evaluation of permanent impairment,* ed 4, Chicago, 1994, American Medical Association.

If both grip and pinch strength are decreased, the function with the highest loss (greatest Strength Loss Index) is used to determine the upper extremity impairment. Both values are not used at the same time. If both extremities are abnormal, comparison is made with average normal strengths listed in Table 66-1 (p. 626) and originally described by Swanson, Matev, and de Groot.

Example: Grip strength of right hand is 10 kg and of left (normal) hand is 45 kg:

$$\frac{45 \text{ kg} - 10 \text{ kg}}{45 \text{ kg}} = 78\% \text{ Strength Loss Index}$$

A 78% Strength Loss Index corresponds to a 30% impairment of the upper extremity.

Combining regional impairments to obtain upper extremity and whole person impairment

1. Determine regional impairments for the hand, wrist, elbow, and shoulder.
2. *Combine* regional impairments with combined values chart, Table 66-5 (pp. 632 to 634). Note that digit and hand impairments must be converted to upper extremity impairments (Tables 66-2 and 66-3, p. 628) before combining with other upper extremity impairments.
3. Use Table 66-4 (p. 629) to convert upper extremity to whole person impairments.

Example: A patient with multiple injuries to the upper extremity presents with the following impairments: thumb 100%; index, 80%; upper extremity impairment due to wrist, 10%; and upper extermity impairment due to elbow, 40%.

1. Digit impairments are converted to hand and upper extremity impairments: 100% thumb impairment = 40% hand impairment; 80% index impairment = 16% hand impairment (see Table 66-2, p. 628). Hand impairments are *added* to obtain a 56% hand impairment or 50% upper extremity impairment (see Table 66-3, p. 628).
2. Regional upper extremity impairments are then combined as follows: 50% (hand) *combined* with 10% (wrist) is 55%; 55% *combined* with 40% (elbow) is 73% impairment of the upper extremity or 44% impairment of the whole person (see Table 66-4, p. 629).

Summary of steps to evaluate impairments of the upper extremity

1. **Hand region.** Use upper extremity evaluation record part 1 (Fig. 66-2, *A*, p. 621).
   a. Determine level of *amputation(s)* if present and record digit impairment (thumb, p. 638; fingers, p. 635).
   b. Measure two-point discrimination and record *sensory* impairment for each digit (thumb, p. 638; fingers, p. 635).
   c. Measure ROM and record motion impairment for each digital joint (thumb IP, p. 638; MP, p. 640; CMC, p. 640; fingers DIP, PIP, MP, p. 636).
   For the thumb, *add* individual joint impairments. For each finger, *combine* impairments of individual joints using combined values chart (see Table 66-5, pp. 632 to 634).
   d. Determine digit impairments caused by *other disorders* (pp. 658 to 663) for each joint or digit.
   e. For each digit, *combine* impairments caused by *amputation, sensory loss, loss of motion,* and

other disorders (when appropriate) to obtain individual digit impairments.
   f. *Convert* digit impairments to hand impairments (see Table 66-2, p. 628).
   g. *Add* hand impairment value for each digit involved to obtain total hand impairment.
   h. *Convert* the hand impairment to upper extremity impairment (see Table 66-3, p. 628).
   i. If additional upper extremity impairment is present because of *loss of strength* (p. 663), *combine* with other upper extremity impairment values (see Table 66-5, pp. 632 to 634).
   j. If no other upper extremity impairment is present, convert the upper extremity impairment related to the hand region to whole person impairment (see Table 66-4, p. 629).

For steps 2 to 11 use the upper extremity impairment evaluation chart, part 2 (see Fig. 66-2, *B*, p. 622).

2. **Wrist region.** Determine the upper extremity impairment caused by *loss of motion* and *other disorders* (p. 658). *Combine* values to obtain upper extremity impairment of the wrist region.
3. **Elbow region.** Determine the upper extremity impairment caused by *loss of motion* and *other disorders* (p. 658). *Combine* the values to obtain upper extremity impairment of the elbow region.
4. **Shoulder region.** Determine the upper extremity impairment caused by *loss of motion* and *other disorders. Combine* the values to obtain upper extremity impairment of the shoulder region.
5. **Amputation proximal to digit level.** Determine level of *amputation* of upper extremity if present (see Fig. 66-6, *A*, p. 621), and record upper extremity impairment caused by amputation (see Fig. 66-2, *B*, p. 622).
6. **Peripheral nerve disorders.** Rate impairments caused by peripheral nerve disorders, including entrapment neuropathy, causalgia, and RSD (pp. 657 to 658).
7. **Peripheral vascular disorders.** Consult p. 649 to rate impairment caused by *peripheral vascular disorders.*
8. **Other disorders** not included in regioal impairment. Consult pp. 658 to 662 to rate upper extremity impairment caused by other disorders.
9. **Total upper extremity impairment.** Use the combined values chart (see Table 66-5, pp. 632 to 634) to combine upper extremity impairments caused by *amputation* (other than hand), *regional disorders* (hand, wrist, elbow, shoulder), *peripheral vascular system involvement, peripheral nerve system involvement,* and *other disorders.*
10. **Whole person impairment.** *Convert* upper extremity impairment to whole person impairment (see Table 66-4, p. 629).

A. Upper Extremity Impairment Evaluation Record—Part I (Hand) Side ☒ R ☐ L

Name _J.D._ Age _45_ Sex ☒ M ☐ F Dominant hand ☒ R ☐ L Date _____
Occupation _Carpenter_ Diagnosis _multiple amputations + neuroma_

Abnormal motion						Amputation	Sensory loss	Other disorders	Hand impairment %
Record motion, ankylosis, and impairment %						Mark level & impairment %	Mark type, level, & impairment %	List type & impairment %	• Combine digit IMP% ★ Convert to hand IMP%

Thumb

			Flexion	Extension	Ankylosis	IMP%				
IP	Angle °									
	IMP%									
MP	Angle °									
	IMP%									
			Motion	Ankylosis	IMP%					
CMC	Radial abduction	Angle °								Abnormal motion [1]
		IMP%								Amputation [2]
	Adduction	Cms								Sensory loss [3]
		IMP%								Other disorders [4]
	Opposition	Cms								Digit impairment % • Combine 1, 2, 3, 4
		IMP%								

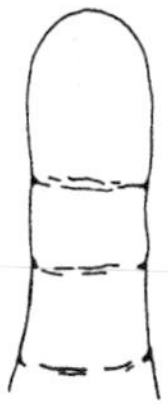

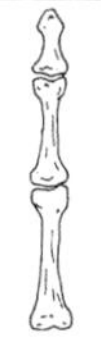

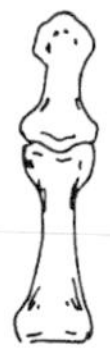

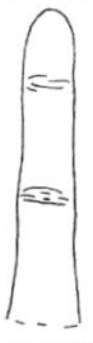

Add impairment % CMC + MP + IP = [1] IMP % = [2] IMP % = [3] IMP % = [4] **Hand impairment % ★ Convert above**

Index

		Flexion	Extension	Ankylosis	IMP%	Amputation	Sensory loss		Hand impairment %	
DIP	Angle °					U R	Abnormal motion [1]	17
	IMP%						Amputation [2]	80
PIP	Angle °						Sensory loss [3]	
	IMP%					neuroma grade 4 (see part 2)	Other disorders [4]	
MP	Angle °	60	+20		17		Digit impairment % • Combine 1, 2, 3, 4	83
	IMP%	17	0					

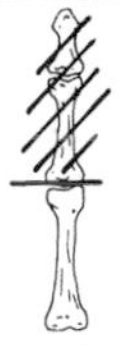

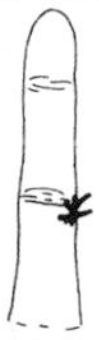

• Combine impairment % MP + PIP + DIP = 17 [1] IMP % = 80 [2] IMP % = [3] IMP % = [4] **Hand impairment % ★ Convert above** 17

Middle

		Flexion	Extension	Ankylosis	IMP%	Amputation		Hand impairment %	
DIP	Angle °						Abnormal motion [1]	48
	IMP%						Amputation [2]	60
PIP	Angle °	30	0		42		Sensory loss [3]	
	IMP%	42	0				Other disorders [4]	
MP	Angle °	70	+20		11		Digit impairment % • Combine 1, 2, 3, 4	79
	IMP%	11	0					

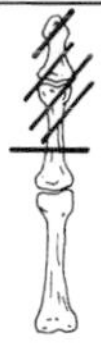

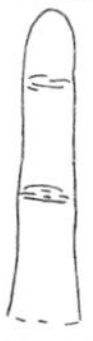

• Combine impairment % MP + PIP + DIP = 48 [1] IMP % = 60 [2] IMP % = [3] IMP % = [4] **Hand impairment % ★ Convert above** 16

Ring

		Flexion	Extension	Ankylosis	IMP%	Amputation		Hand impairment %	
DIP	Angle °	30	-10		23		Abnormal motion [1]	41
	IMP%	21	2				Amputation [2]	25
PIP	Angle °	70	0		18		Sensory loss [3]	
	IMP%	18	0				Other disorders [4]	
MP	Angle °	80	+20		6		Digit impairment % • Combine 1, 2, 3, 4	56
	IMP%	6	0					

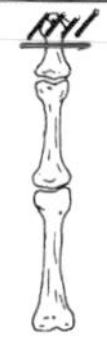

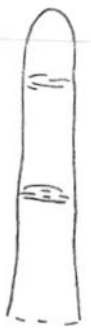

• Combine impairment % MP + PIP + DIP = 41 [1] IMP % = 25 [2] IMP % = [3] IMP % = [4] **Hand impairment % ★ Convert above** 6

Little

		Flexion	Extension	Ankylosis	IMP%		Hand impairment %	
DIP	Angle °						Abnormal motion [1]	
	IMP%						Amputation [2]	
PIP	Angle °						Sensory loss [3]	
	IMP%						Other disorders [4]	
MP	Angle °						Digit impairment % • Combine 1, 2, 3, 4	
	IMP%							

• Combine impairment % MP + PIP + DIP = [1] IMP % = [2] IMP % = [3] IMP % = [4] **Hand impairment % ★ Convert above**

Total hand impairment (Add hand impairment % for thumb + index + middle + ring + little finger) =	% 17 + 16 + 6 = 39%
Upper extremity impairment (†Convert total hand impairment % to upper extremity impairment %) = 35 %; enter on Part II, Line II	
If hand region impairment is only impairment, convert upper extremity impairment to whole person impairment:‡ = %	

• Combined Values Chart: Table 66-5; ★ Use Table 66-2 (Digits to hand); † Use Table 66-3 (Hand to upper extremity); ‡ Use Table 66-4
Courtesy of G. de Groot Swanson, MD

Fig. 66-34. *Example 1.* Upper extremity impairment evaluation record. **A,** Part 1 (hand). *Continued on the next page.*

B. Upper Extremity Impairment Evaluation Record—Part 2 (Wrist, elbow, and shoulder)　　　　　Side ☒ R ☐ L

Name _J. D._　　　　　　　Age _45_　Sex ☒ M ☐ F　Dominant hand ☒ R ☐ L　Date _____
Occupation _Carpenter_　　　　　　　　　Diagnosis _Multiple amputations + neuroma_

		Abnormal motion				Other disorders	Regional impairment %	Amputation
		Record motion, ankylosis, and impairment %				List type & impairment %	• Combine [1] + [2]	Mark level & impairment %
Wrist		Flexion	Extension	Ankylosis	IMP%			
	Angle°							
	IMP%							
		RD	UD	Ankylosis	IMP%			
	Angle°							
	IMP%							
					[1]	[2]		
	Add IMP% FLEX/EXT + RD/UD =					IMP% =		
Elbow		Flexion	Extension	Ankylosis	IMP%			
	Angle°							
	IMP%							
		Pronation	Supination	Ankylosis	IMP%			
	Angle°							
	IMP%							
					[1]	[2]		
	Add IMP% FLEX/EXT + PRO/SUP =					IMP% =		
Shoulder		Flexion	Extension	Ankylosis	IMP%			
	Angle°							
	IMP%							
		Adduction	Abduction	Ankylosis	IMP%			
	Angle°							
	IMP%							
		Int Rot	Ext Rot	Ankylosis	IMP%			
	Angle°							
	IMP							
					[1]	[2]		
	Add IMP% FLEX/EXT + ADD/ABD + INT ROT/EXT ROT =					IMP% =		IMP%

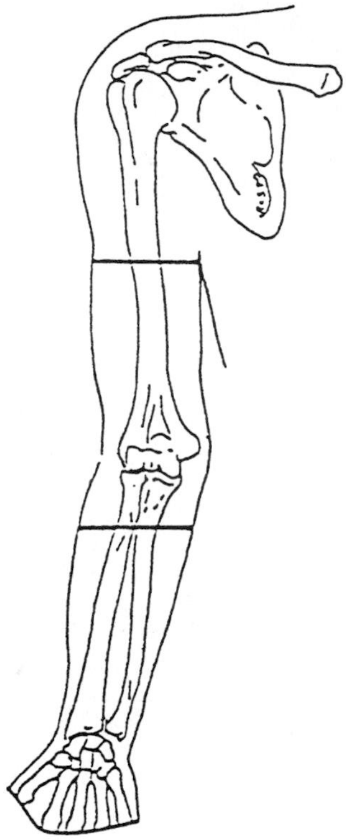

I. Amputation impairment (other than digits)　　　　　　　　　　　　=

II. Regional impairment of upper extremity
　• (Combine hand _35_ % + wrist _____ % + elbow _____ % + shoulder _____ %)　= _35 %_

III. Peripheral nerve system impairment _Neuroma Grade 4 of index Radial Digital_
Nerve 80% (table 13) × 5 % (table 17) = 4 %　= _4 %_

IV. Peripheral vascular system impairment　　　　　　　　　　　　=

V. Other disorders (not included in regional impairment)　　　　　　　=

Total upper extremity impairment (• Combine I + II + III + IV + V)
　　　　　　_35 % + 4 %_　　　= _38 %_

Impairment of the whole person (Use table 66-4, upper extremity to whole person)　= _23 %_

If both limbs are involved, calculate the whole person impairment for each on a separate chart and *combine* the percents (Combined Values Chart).
• Use Combined Values Chart, Table 66-5

Fig. 66-34 cont'd. B, Part 2 (wrist, elbow, and shoulder).

A. Upper Extremity Impairment Evaluation Record—Part I (Hand)   Side ☑ R ☐ L

Name _A.B. Example 2_ Age _50_ Sex ☐ M ☑ F Dominant hand ☑ R ☐ L Date _____
Occupation _Factory worker_ Diagnosis _Flexor tendons and Digital nerve Lacerations; Colle's Fracture_

			Abnormal motion			Amputation	Sensory loss	Other disorders	Hand impairment %
		Record motion, ankylosis, and impairment %				Mark level & impairment %	Mark type, level, & impairment %	List type & impairment %	• Combine digit IMP% ★ Convert to hand IMP%

Thumb

			Flexion	Extension	Ankylosis	IMP%				
IP	Angle °									
	IMP%									
MP	Angle °									
	IMP%									
			Motion	Ankylosis	IMP%					
CMC	Radial abduction	Angle °								Abnormal motion [1]
		IMP%								Amputation [2]
	Adduction	CMS								Sensory loss [3]
		IMP%								Other disorders [4]
	Opposition	CMS								Digit impairment % • Combine 1, 2, 3, 4
		IMP%								

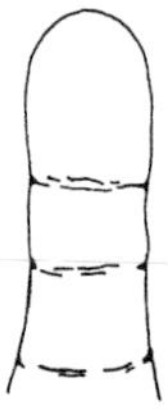

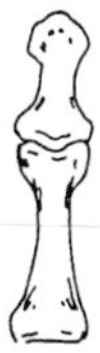

Add impairment % CMC + MP + IP = ___ [1] IMP % = ___ [2] IMP % = ___ [3] IMP % = ___ [4] **Hand impairment % ★ Convert above**

Index

		Flexion	Extension	Ankylosis	IMP%				
DIP	Angle °								Abnormal motion [1]
	IMP%								Amputation [2]
PIP	Angle °								Sensory loss [3]
	IMP%								Other disorders [4]
MP	Angle °								Digit impairment % • Combine 1, 2, 3, 4
	IMP%								

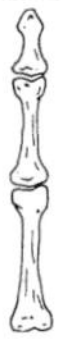

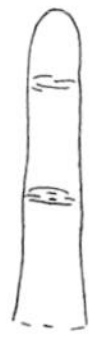

• Combine impairment % MP + PIP + DIP = ___ [1] IMP % = ___ [2] IMP % = ___ [3] IMP % = ___ [4] **Hand impairment % ★ Convert above**

Middle

		Flexion	Extension	Ankylosis	IMP%				
DIP	Angle °	30	−10						Abnormal motion [1] 57
	IMP%	21	2		23				Amputation [2]
PIP	Angle °	70	−10						Sensory loss [3] 12
	IMP%	18	3		21				Other disorders [4]
MP	Angle °	50	−10						Digit impairment % • Combine 1, 2, 3, 4 62
	IMP%	22	7		29				

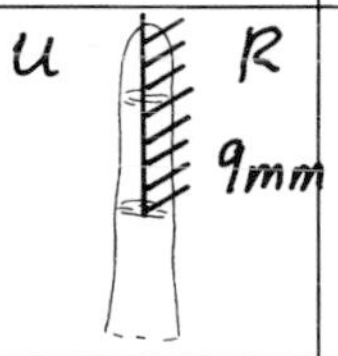

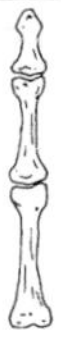

(Amputation sketch: U / R 9mm)

• Combine impairment % MP + PIP + DIP = 57 [1] IMP % = ___ [2] IMP % = 12 % [3] IMP % = ___ [4] **Hand impairment % ★ Convert above 12**

Ring

		Flexion	Extension	Ankylosis	IMP%				
DIP	Angle °								Abnormal motion [1]
	IMP%								Amputation [2]
PIP	Angle °								Sensory loss [3]
	IMP%								Other disorders [4]
MP	Angle °								Digit impairment % • Combine 1, 2, 3, 4
	IMP%								

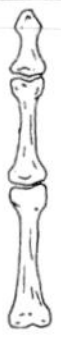

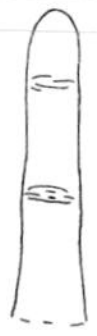

• Combine impairment % MP + PIP + DIP = ___ [1] IMP % = ___ [2] IMP % = ___ [3] IMP % = ___ [4] **Hand impairment % ★ Convert above**

Little

		Flexion	Extension	Ankylosis	IMP%				
DIP	Angle °								Abnormal motion [1]
	IMP%								Amputation [2]
PIP	Angle °								Sensory loss [3]
	IMP%								Other disorders [4]
MP	Angle °								Digit impairment % • Combine 1, 2, 3, 4
	IMP%								

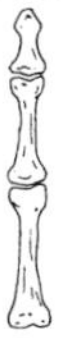

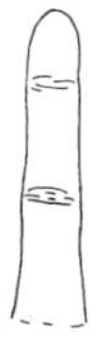

• Combine impairment % MP + PIP + DIP = ___ [1] IMP % = ___ [2] IMP % = ___ [3] IMP % = ___ [4] **Hand impairment % ★ Convert above**

Total hand impairment (Add hand impairment % for thumb + index + middle + ring + little finger) = **12** %

Upper extremity impairment (†Convert total hand impairment % to upper extremity impairment %) = **11** %; enter on Part II, Line II

If hand region impairment is only impairment, convert upper extremity impairment to whole person impairment:‡ = ___ %

• Combined Values Chart: Table 66-5; ★ Use Table 66-2 (Digits to hand); † Use Table 66-3 (Hand to upper extremity); ‡ Use Table 66-4
Courtesy of G. de Groot Swanson, MD

Fig. 66-35. *Example 2.* Upper extremity evaluation record. **A,** Part 1 (hand). *Continued on the next page.*

B. Upper Extremity Impairment Evaluation Record—Part 2 (Wrist, elbow, and shoulder) Side ☒ R ☐ L

Name *A.B. Example 2*   Age *50*   Sex ☐ M ☒ F   Dominant hand ☒ R ☐ L   Date _____
Occupation *Factory worker*   Diagnosis *Flexor tendons and Digital nerve Lacerations: Colle's Fracture*

	Abnormal motion				Other disorders	Regional impairment %	Amputation
	Record motion, ankylosis, and impairment %				List type & impairment %	• Combine [1] + [2]	Mark level & impairment %

Wrist

	Flexion	Extension	Ankylosis	IMP%
Angle°	40°	30°		8
IMP%	3	5		
	RD	UD	Ankylosis	IMP%
Angle°	20°	10°		4
IMP%	0	4		

Add IMP% FLEX/EXT + RD/UD = *12*   [1]   IMP% =   [2]

Elbow

	Flexion	Extension	Ankylosis	IMP%
Angle°	140°	0°		0
IMP%	0	0		
	Pronation	Supination	Ankylosis	IMP%
Angle°	40°	30°		5
IMP%	3	2		

Add IMP% FLEX/EXT + PRO/SUP = *5*   [1]   IMP% =   [2]

Shoulder

	Flexion	Extension	Ankylosis	IMP%
Angle°				
IMP%				
	Adduction	Abduction	Ankylosis	IMP%
Angle°				
IMP%				
	Int Rot	Ext Rot	Ankylosis	IMP%
Angle°				
IMP				

Add IMP% FLEX/EXT + ADD/ABD + INT ROT/EXT ROT =   [1]   IMP% =   [2]   IMP%

I. Amputation impairment (other than digits)   =

II. Regional impairment of upper extremity
• (Combine hand *11* % + wrist *12* % + elbow *5* % + shoulder _____ %)   = *26%*

III. Peripheral nerve system impairment   =

IV. Peripheral vascular system impairment   =

V. Other disorders (not included in regional impairment)   =

Total upper extremity impairment (• Combine I + II + III + IV + V)   = *26%*

Impairment of the whole person (Use table 66-4, upper extremity to whole person)   = *16%*

If both limbs are involved, calculate the whole person impairment for each on a separate chart and *combine* the percents (Combined Values Chart).
• Use Combined Values Chart, Table 66-5

Fig. 66-35 cont'd. B, Part 2 (wrist, elbow, and shoulder).

11. **Bilateral upper extremity impairment.** If both upper extremities are involved, the whole person impairment value for each upper extremity is derived as above and then *combined* using the combined values chart (see Table 66-5, pp. 632 to 634).

Example 1: Multiple finger amputations and neuroma. While working with a band saw, a carpenter sustained amputations through the index, middle, and ring fingers. After 6 months he had good skin coverage and no pain in the middle and ring fingers. He presented with a painful neuroma on the radial side of the index finger stump that made him bypass the finger. He refused surgery because there was no guarantee for full sensory recovery. His complaints included finger amputations, painful neuroma (see Tables 66-13 and 66-17), decreased finger motion (see Figs. 66-12 through 66-14), and weakness of grip. The examination results and impairment calculations are shown on the upper extremity evaluation form (Fig. 66-34). The weakness of grip was satisfactorily considered in the anatomic impairment percentages given, and no extra values were given.

Example 2: Deep palmar laceration of the right middle finger and Colles' fracture of right wrist. Complete lacerations of the FDP and FDS, sustained by a 50-year-old woman when she fell in a glass factory, were repaired with primary flexor tenorrhaphies. The radial digital nerve was repaired with a microneurorrhaphy. There was no involvement of the PIP joint. The right distal radius fracture was appropriately reduced and immobilzied. After 16 months and an adequate course of rehabilitation, the patient was evaluated for impairment. The patient's complaints included numbness of the radial side of the middle finger, decreased motion of the middle finger, decreased wrist motion and forearm rotation, moderate wrist pain with heavy activity and some deformity, and a 40% Strength Loss Index.

The factors considered for impairment rating were sensory loss of the middle finger, decreased motion of the finger and wrist, and limited forearm rotation (see Table 66-5 and Figs. 66-12 through 66-14, 66-23, *B,* 66-24, *B,* and 66-26, *B*). Strength loss was not rated because it was not thought to be an additional impairing factor. No additional impairment was given for deformity or pain. The impairment evaluation is shown in Fig. 66-35.

SUGGESTED READINGS

American Academy of Orthopaedic Surgeons: *Joint motion, method of measuring and recording,* Chicago, 1965.

Bateman JE: Disability evaluation about the shoulder, *Surg Clin North Am* 1963; 43:1721.

Beasley WC: Quantitative muscle testing: principles and applications to research and clinical service, *Arch Physiol Med* 1961; 42:398.

Bechtol CO: Grip test, the use of a dynamometer with adjustable handle spacings, *J Bone Joint Surg* 1954; 36A:820.

Bertelsen A, Capener N: Fingers, compensations and King Canute, *J Bone Joint Surg* 1960; 42B:390.

Boyes JH: Flexor tendon grafts in the fingers and thumb, *J Bone Joint Surg* 1950; 32A:489.

Boyes JH: *Bunnell's surgery of the hand,* ed 5, Philadelphia, 1970, JB Lippincott.

Bunnell S: The management of the non-functional hand—reconstruction vs. prosthesis, *Artif Limbs* 1957; 4:76.

Carroll D: A quantitative test of upper extremity function, *J Chron Dis* 1965; 18:479.

Crenshaw AH, ed: *Campbell's operative orthopaedics,* ed 8, St Louis, 1992, Mosby.

Culver J: Personal written and oral communication, The Cleveland Clinic, Cleveland, 1990-1992.

Dellon AL, Kallman CH: Evaluation of functional sensation in the hand, *J Hand Surg* 1983; 8:865-870.

De Palma A: *Surgery of the shoulder,* ed 2, Philadelphia, 1973, JB Lippincott.

Garrett JW: The adult human hand: some anthropometric and biomechanic considerations, *Hum Factors* 1971; 13:117.

Goldner JL: Pain: extremities and spine: evaluation and differential diagnosis. In Omer GE Jr, Spinner M, eds: *Management of peripheral nerve problems,* Philadelphia, 1980, Saunders.

Guide to the evaluation of permanent impairment of the extremities and back, *JAMA* 1958; 166:February 16 (special edition).

Guide to the evaluation of permanent impairment of the peripheral spinal nerves, American Medical Association Committee on Medical Rating of Physical Impairment, 1962.

Hamasaki K: The study of the hand, lost digit, *Acta Med* Kyushu University, 1961; 31:53.

Hollander JL: *Arthritis and allied conditions, a textbook of rheumatology,* ed 8, Philadelphia, 1972, Lea & Febiger.

Hunter JM, Salisbury RF: Flexor tendon reconstruction in severely damaged hands, *J Bone Joint Surg* 1971; 53A:829.

Karger DW, Bayha FH: *Engineered work measurement,* ed 2, New York, 1965, Industrial Press.

Kirkpatrick EJ: Evaluation of grip loss, *Calif Med* 1956; 85:314.

Kline DG: Caution in the evaluation of results of peripheral nerve surgery. In Smit M, ed: *Peripheral nerve lesions,* Berlin, 1990, Springer-Verlag.

Kroemer KHE, Howard JM: Towards standardization of muscle strength testing, *Med Sci Sports* 1970; 2:224.

Lankford LL: Reflex sympathetic dystrophy. In Omer GE Jr, Spinner M, eds: *Management of peripheral nerve problems,* Philadelphia, 1980, Saunders.

Lewey FH, Kuhn WG, Juditski JT: A standardized method for assessing the strength of hand and foot muscles, *Surg Gynecol Obstet* 1947; 85:785.

Litcman HM, Paslay PR: Determination of finger-motion impairment by linear measurement, *J Bone Joint Surg* 1974; 56A:85.

Littler JW: The physiology and dynamic function of the hand, *Surg Clin North Am* 1960; 40:259.

Luck JV Jr, Florence DW: A brief history and comparative analysis of disability systems and impairment rating guides, *Orthop Clin North Am* 1988; 19:839-844.

Mannerfelt L: Studies on the hand in ulnar nerve paralysis, *Acta Orthop Scand* (Suppl) 1966; 87:63.

Mannerfelt L: Motor function testing. In Omer GE, Spinner M, eds: *Management of peripheral nerve problems,* Philadelphia, 1980, Saunders.

McBride ED: *Disability evaluation,* ed 6, Philadelphia, 1963, JB Lippincott.

Medical Research Council: *Aids to the examination of the peripheral nervous system,* Memorandum No 45, London, 1976, Her Majesty's Stationery Office.

Moberg E: Objective methods for determining the functional value of sensibility in the hand, *J Bone Joint Surg* 1958; 40B:454.

Omer GE Jr: Nerve compression syndromes, *Hand Clin* 1992; 8:317-324.

Omer GE Jr: Management techniques for the painful upper extremity. In Murray JA, ed: *Instructional course lectures,* American Academy of Orthopaedic Surgeons, St Louis, 1984, Mosby.

Omer GE Jr: Report of the committee for evaluation of the clinical result in peripheral nerve injury, *J Hand Surg* 1983; 8(part 2):754-758.

Omer GE Jr: Physical diagnosis of peripheral nerve injuries, *Orthop Clin North Am* 1981; 12:207-228.

Omer GE Jr: Methods of assessment of injury and recovery of peripheral nerves, *Surg Clin North Am* 1981; 61:303-319.

Omer GE Jr: Sensibility testing. In Omer GE, Spinner M, eds: *Management of peripheral nerve problems,* Philadelphia, 1980, Saunders.

Patterson HMcL: Grip mreasurements as a part of the pre-placement evaluation, *Ind Med Surg* 1965; 34:555.

Rattner IN: *Injury ratings,* New York, 1970, Crescent Publishing.

Slocum DB, Pratt DR: The principles of amputation of the fingers and hand, *J Bone Joint Surg* 1944; 26:535.

Slocum DB, Pratt DR: Disability evaluation for the hand, *J Bone Joint Surg* 1946; 28:491.

Smith HB: Smith hand function evaluation, *Am J Occup Ther* 1973; 27:244.

Smith WC: *Principles of disability evaluation,* Philadelphia, 1959, JB Lippincott.

Stack G, ed: Internal publication, International Federation of Societies for Surgery of the Hand, 1970.

Stokes HM: The seriously injured hand: weakness of grip, *J Occup Med* 1983; 25:683-684.

Swanson AB: Evaluation of impairment of function in the hand, *Surg Clin North Am* 1964; 44:925.

Swanson AB: Multiple finger amputations: concepts of treatment, *J Mich Med Soc* 1962; 61:316.

Swanson AB: Restoration of hand function by the use of partial or total prosthetic replacement, *J Bone Joint Surg* 1963; 45A:276.

Swanson AB: Levels of amputation of fingers and hand: considerations for treatment, *Surg Clin North Am* 1964; 44:1115.

Swanson AB: Evaluation of disabilities and recordkeeping. In Swanson AB, ed: *Flexible implant resection arthroplasty in the hand and extremities,* St Louis, 1973, Mosby.

Swanson AB: Evaluation of impairment of hand and upper extremity function. In: *Japanese journal of traumatology and occupational medicine,* vol 40, no 6, 1992, pp 355-358.

Swanson AB, de Grooot Swanson G: Principles and methods of impairment evaluation in the hand and upper extremity. In Engelberg AL, ed: *Guides to the evaluation of permanent impairment,* ed 3, Chicago, 1988, the American Medical Association.

Swnason AB, de Groot Swanson G: Evaluation and treatment of the upper extremity in the stroke patient, *Hand Clin* 1989; 5:75-96.

Swanson AB, de Groot Swanson G: Principles and methods of impairment evaluation in the hand and upper extremity. In: *Guides to the evaluation of permanent impairment,* ed 3 revised, Chicago, 1990, the American Medical Association.

Swanson AB, de Groot Swanson G: Evaluation and treatment of the upper extremity in the stroke patient. In Tubiana R, ed: *The hand,* vol 4, Philadelphia, 1991, Saunders.

Swanson AB, de Groot Swanson G: Principles and methods of impairment evaluation in the hand and upper extremity. In: *Guides to the evaluation of permanent impairment,* ed 4, Chicago, 1993, the American Medical Association.

Swanson AB, de Groot Swanson G: Principles and methods of impairment evaluation in the hand and upper extremity. In: *Guides to the evaluation of permanent impairment,* ed 4 revised, Chicago, 1994, American Medical Association.

Swanson AB, de Groot Swanson G, Blair SJ: Evaluation of impairment of hand and upper extremity function. In Barr JS Jr, ed: *Instructional course lectures,* American Academy of Orthopaedic Surgeons, St Louis, 1989, Mosby.

Swanson AB, de Groot Swanson G, Göran-Hagert C: Evaluations of impairment of hand function. In Hunter JM, Schneider LH, Mackin EJ, Callahan AD, eds: *Rehabilitation of the hand: surgery and therapy,* ed 3, St Louis, 1990, Mosby.

Swanson AB, de Groot Swanson G, Kaplan E: Amputations in the hand, concepts and treatment. In Spinner M, ed: *Kaplan's functional and surgical anatomy of the hand,* ed 3, Philadelphia, 1984, JP Lippincott.

Swanson AB, Göran-Hagert C, de Groot Swanson G: Evaluation of impairment of hand function. In Hunter JM, Schneider LH, Mackin E, Callahan AD, eds: *Rehabilitation of the hand,* St Louis, 1978, Mosby.

Swanson AB, Göran-Hagert C, de Groot Swanson G: Evaluation of impairment of hand function. In Hunter JM, Schneider LH, Mackin E, Callahan AD, eds: *Rehabilitation of the hand,* ed 2, St Louis, 1984, Mosby.

Swanson AB, Hagert CG, de Groot Swanson G: Evaluation of impairment of hand function, *J Hand Surg* 1983; 8(part 2):709-722.

Swanson AB, Matev IB, de Groot G: The strength of the hand, *Bull Prosthet Res* p 145, Fall, 1970.

Swanson AB, Mays JD, Yamauchi Y: A rheumatoid arthritis evaluation record for the upper extremity, *Surg Clin North Am* 1968; 48:1003.

Taylor CL: Biomechanics of the normal and the amputated upper extremity. In Klopsteg PE, Wilson PD, eds: *Human limbs and their substitutes,* New York, 1954, McGraw-Hill.

Taylor CL, Schwartz RJ: The anatomy and mechanics of the human hand, *Artif Limbs* 1955; 2:22.

Tubiana R, Michon J, Thomine J: Scheme for assessment of deformities of Dupuytren's disease, *Surg Clin North Am* 1968; 48:979.

Van't Hof A, Heiple KG: Flexor tendon injuries of the fingers and thumb: a comparative study, *J Bone Joint Surg* 1958; 40A:256.

Wechesser EC: Reconstruction of a grasping mechanism following loss of digitus, *Clin Orthop* 1959; 15:69.

INDEX

A

AA; *see* Amino acid content
AAEM; *see* American Board of Electrodiagnostic Medicine
AAOS; *see* American Academy of Orthopaedic Surgeons
Abductor digiti minimi (ADM), 551
Abductor digiti quinti (ADQ), 562
Abductor pollicis brevis (APB), 214
Abductor pollicis longus (APL), 214
Abilities Test, 231
ABPN; *see* American Board of Psychiatry and Neurology
Accident, amputee victims, 603-604
Active motion, early
  estimating internal tendon forces, 371-376
  postoperative tendon programs, 362
  repair design, 371
Active range of motion (AROM), 195
Active tendon reconstruction, types, 530-531
Activities, bilateral, *200*
Activities of daily living (ADL), 149, 231
  checklist, *151*
  independence rating, 231
Adhesion
  bone, *387*
  formation, growth factor stimulation, *292*
  molecules, 287
Adhesions, flexor tendons, 450
ADL; *see* Activities of daily living
ADM; *see* Abductor digiti minimi
ADQ; *see* Abductor digiti quinti
Adventitectomy, 112
AGA therovision system, 78
Age, force threshold, 73-74
AHC; *see* Anterior horncells
Albinus, Bernard Siegfried, 252
Aldo Leopold Rule, 159
Allodynia, 101
Allografts, 398
AMA; *see* American Medical Association
American Academy of Orthopaedic Surgeons (AAOS), 617
American Board of Electrodiagnostic Medicine (AAEM), 32
American Board of Psychiatry and Neurology (ABPN), 32
American Medical Association (AMA), 617
American Society for Surgery of the Hand (ASSH), 54, 94, 314, 617
American Society of Hand Therapists Splint Classification System, 96
  Annual Meeting of (1970), 70
American Spinal Injury Association (ASIA), 226
Amino acid (AA) content, *302*
Amputations
  bilateral, 609
  digital, 100, 608
  disease-related, 604
  elbow, determining impairment of, 644
  fingers, determining impairment of, 635, *635*
  fitting functional prosthesis, 605
  fitting problems, 608-609
  functional deficits, 608

Amputations—cont'd
  hand, 609, 664
  impairment evaluation, 626-628
  impairments, percentage relations, *627*
  multidigit, 609
  multiple finger, 669
  patient adjustment, 603-605
  shoulder, determining impairment of, 646
  reimplantation, *479-480, 481*
  thumb
    determining impairment of, 638, *638*
    combining impairments, 641
  total hand, *607*
  wrist, determining impairment of, 642
Amputees
  behavior, 603-605
  children and parents, 604-605
  long-term, 604
  recent, 603-604
Anatomic pulley, dorsal convex, 558, *559*
Anatomy
  axillary, 15
  brachial plexus, 14-15
  functional flexor tendon, 237-252
  median, 16-17
  musculocutaneous, 16
  neural gross, 14
  surgical, 20
Anesthesia, 355
  dolorosa, 101
  reconstruction of flexor tendon function, 529-530
Ankylosis
  impairment curves, *639*
  loss of total motion, *631*
Anterior horncells (AHC), 32
Anterior transpositions, 185-187
APB; *see* Abductor policis brevis
APL; *see* Abductor policis longus
Arcade of Struthers, 17
ARC motion
  active short, 362
  bilateral, *204*
  following tendon repair, 362-391
Arm awareness, 203
AROM; *see* Active range of motion
Art, 4
Arthritis, rheumatoid; *see* Rheumatoid arthritis
Arthroplastics, 429
Arthroplasty, 661-662
ASIA; *see* American Spinal Injury Association
ASSH; *see* American Society for Surgery of the Hand
ATT; *see* Automated tactile tester
Automated tactile tester (ATT), 52, 63, 66, 73
Available excursion, 259
Axon(al)
  loss, 33
  regeneration, 85-88
  transport, 137-138
Axonotomesis, *34*, 140-141
  affects, 34

Page numbers in italics indicate illustrations; *t* indicates tables.